£40 -

D1808599

Treatment of Cancer

Treatment of Cancer

EDITED BY

Keith E. Halnan

MD, FRCP, FRCR, FRSE, Hon. MD(Gdansk)

Director, Department of Radiotherapy and Oncology,
Royal Postgraduate Medical School,
Hammersmith Hospital, London

LONDON

Chapman and Hall

First published 1982
by Chapman and Hall Ltd.
11 New Fetter Lane, London EC4P 4EE

© Chapman and Hall Ltd.

Printed in Great Britain at the University Press,
Cambridge

ISBN 0 412 21850 X

All rights reserved. No part of this book may be
reprinted, or reproduced or utilized in any form or by
any electronic, mechanical or other means, now known
or hereafter invented, including photocopying and
recording, or in any information storage or retrieval
system, without permission in writing from the
publisher.

British Library Cataloguing in Publication Data

Treatment of cancer.
 1. Cancer
 I. Halnan, Keith Edward
 616.9′94′06   RC262

 ISBN 0-412-21850-X

Contents

vi *Contents*

ASSOCIATE EDITORS

J.L. Boak, MD, MChir, FRCS
*Formerly Senior Lecturer in Surgery, Royal
Postgraduate Medical School, Hammersmith
Hospital, London*

Derek Crowther, PhD, MA, MB, BChir, FRCP
*Professor of Medical Oncology, Cancer Research
Campaign, Department of Medical Oncology,
Christie Hospital and Holt Radium Institute,
Manchester, England*

Carl F. von Essen, MD
*Pion Therapy Project,
Schweizerisches Institute für Nuklear Forschung,
Villigen, Switzerland, formerly Professor of Radiology
and Oncology, University of California, San Diego,
USA*

J. Stewart Orr, DSc, F Inst P, FRSE
*Professor of Medical Physics,
Royal Postgraduate Medical School, Hammersmith
Hospital, London*

M.J. Peckham, MD, FRCP, FRCR
*Professor of Radiotherapy, Institute of Cancer
Research and The Royal Marsden Hospital, London
and Surrey*

Contributors

K.D. Bagshawe, MD, FRCP, FRCOG
  Professor of Medical Oncology, Department of
  Medical Oncology, Charing Cross Hospital,
  Fulham Palace Road, London

Joan W. Baker, MB, BS, FRCR
  Consultant Radiotherapist and Oncologist,
  Radiotherapy Department, The Royal Marsden
  Hospital, London and Surrey

Ann Barrett, MB, BS, MRCS, LRCP, FFR, DMRT
  Senior Lecturer in Radiotherapy, The Royal
  Marsden Hospital, London and Surrey

J.L. Boak, MD, MChir, FRCS
  Former Senior Lecturer in Surgery, Royal
  Postgraduate Medical School, Hammersmith
  Hospital, London

Vivien H. C. Bramwell, MB, BS, BSc, MRCP
  Senior Registrar in Medical Oncology Cancer
  Research Campaign Department of Medical
  Oncology, Christie Hospital and Holt Radium
  Institute, Manchester

Jill A. Bullimore, MB, BS, DMRT, FRCR
  Consultant Radiotherapist and Oncologist,
  Radiotherapy Centre, Bristol Royal Infirmary

Haydn Bush, PhD, MB, MRCP, DMRT
  Former Senior Lecturer and Consultant in
  Medical Oncology, Christie Hospital and
  University Hospitals of South Manchester,
  Manchester. Director, Ontario Cancer Research
  and Teaching Foundation, London Clinic,
  London, Ontario, Canada

Kenneth C. Calman, MD, PhD, FRCS, FRSE
  Cancer Research Campaign, Professor of
  Oncology, 1 Horselethill Road, Glasgow

Alistair J. Cochran, MD, MRCPath
  Professor of Pathology and Surgery, University
  of California, Los Angeles, 924 Westwood
  Blvd., Suite 400, Los Angeles

R. C. Coombes, PhD, MB, MRCP
  Honorary Senior Registrar, Department of
  Medicine, The Royal Marsden Hospital, and
  Clinical Scientist, Ludwig Institute for Cancer
  Research, Clifton Avenue, Sutton, Surrey

Derek Crowther, PhD, MA, MB, BChir, FRCP
  Professor of Medical Oncology, Cancer
  Research Campaign Department of Medical
  Oncology, Manchester University and Christie
  Hospital and Holt Radium Institute,
  Manchester

John Currie, MA, MChir Camb, FRCS
  Consultant Neurological Surgeon, St.
  Bartholomew's Hospital, London, and Regional
  Neurosurgical Centre, Oldchurch Hospital,
  Romford

Thomas J. Deeley, FRCR
  Director, South Wales Radiotherapy and
  Oncology Service, Velindre Hospital,
  Whitchurch, Cardiff

Peter Diggory, MB, BS, BSc, FRCS, FRCOG
  Senior Consultant Gynaecologist to Kingston
  and Richmond Group of Hospitals, Honorary
  Consultant to The Royal Marsden Hospital,
  London and Surrey

William Duncan, FRCS, FRCP, FRCR
  Professor of Radiotherapy, University of
  Edinburgh, Chairman of Department of
  Radiation Oncology, Western General Hospital
  and Royal Infirmary, Edinburgh

The late Roy E. Ellis, BSc, PhD
  Formerly Head of Department of Medical
  Physics, University of Leeds, General Infirmary,
  Leeds

Carl F. von Essen, MD
  Pion Therapy Project, Swiss Institute for
  Nuclear Research, Villigen 5234, Switzerland.
  Former Professor of Radiology and Oncology,
  University of California, San Diego, USA.

J. M. Ford, MB, BS, MRCP
Clinical Scientific Officer for the Imperial Cancer Research Fund, Lincolns Inn Fields. Honorary Senior Registrar, Department of Medical Oncology, St. Bartholomew's Hospital, London

C. S. B. Galasko, ChM, FRCS, FRCSE
Professor of Orthopaedic Surgery, University of Manchester

Neville Gleave, FRCS
Senior Lecturer and Honorary Consultant Surgeon, Christie Hospital and Holt Radium Institute, Manchester

Keith E. Halnan, MD, FRCP, FRCR, FRSE
Director, Department of Radiotherapy and Oncology, Royal Postgraduate Medical School, Hammersmith Hospital, London

John L. Haybittle, MA, PhD
Chief Physicist, Physics Department, Addenbrooke's Hospital, Hills Road, Cambridge

W.F. Hendry, ChM, FRCS
Consultant Genito-urinary surgeon, Royal Marsden and St. Bartholomew's Hospitals, and Chelsea Hospital for Women, London

J. M. Henk, MA, FRCR
Consultant and Honorary Senior Lecturer in Radiotherapy and Oncology, Royal Marsden Hospital and Institute of Cancer Research, London. Honorary Consultant, St. George's Hospital, and Moorfields Eye Hospital, London

John H.C. Ho, MD, DSc(Hon), FRCP, FRCR, FRACR(Hon), FACR(Hon)
Consultant in Charge of Medical and Health Department, Institute of Radiology and Oncology, Hong Kong, Honorary Lecturer in Radiology, University of Hong Kong. Institute of Radiology and Oncology, Queen Elizabeth Hospital, Kowloon, Hong Kong

John Hermon-Taylor, MChir, FRCS
Professor of Surgery, St. George's Hospital Medical School, London

A. M. Jelliffe, MD, FRCP, FRCR
Chairman, Meyerstein Institute of Radiotherapy and Oncology, Middlesex Hospital, London.

Stephen N. Joffe, BSc, MD, FRCS
Professor of Surgery, College of Medicine, Department of Surgery, University of Cincinnati

Arthur Jones, MD, FRCP, FRCS, FRCR, Hon. FACR
Professor of Radiotherapy in the University of London. Director, Department of Radiotherapy, St. Bartholomew's Hospital, London

Charles A. F. Joslin, MB, BS, FRCR, DMRT
Professor of Radiotherapy, University of Leeds and Honorary Consultant Radiotherapist, Leeds Area Health Authority (Teaching)

C. J. Karzmark, PhD
Associate Professor of Radiology. Chief, Radiological Physics Section, Department of Radiology, Stanford University School of Medicine, 300 Pasteur Drive, Stanford, California

T. J. McElwain, MB, BS, FRCP
Head, Academic Division of Medicine, Institute of Cancer Research. Consultant Physician, The Royal Marsden Hospital, Sutton, Surrey

David Machin, MS
Community Medicine, University of Southampton, Southampton General Hospital, Southampton

Christopher Mallinson, FRCP
Consultant Physician, Lewisham Hospital, London. Honorary Lecturer in Medicine, Guy's Hospital Medical School, London

Walter M. Melia, MB, BCh, MRCP
Clinical Research Fellow, King's College Hospital Medical School, London

Martin G. Mott, MB, ChB, MRCP, DCH
Consultant Senior Lecturer in Paediatric Oncology, University of Bristol Department of Child Health, Royal Hospital for Sick Children, Bristol

A. H. W. Nias, DM, FRCR
The Richard Dimbleby Professor of Cancer Research, St. Thomas's Hospital Medical School, London

J. Stewart Orr, DSc, FInstP, FRSE
Professor of Medical Physics, Royal Postgraduate Medical School, Hammersmith Hospital, London

M.J. Peckham, MD, FRCP, FRCR
    Professor of Radiotherapy, Institute of Cancer
    Research and The Royal Marsden Hospital,
    London and Surrey

K. R. Peel, MB, ChB, FRCS, FRCOG
    Senior Clinical Lecturer in Obstetrics and
    Gynaecology, University of Leeds,
    Gynaecological Surgeon, Hospital for Women
    at Leeds, Honorary Consultant Gynaecologist,
    Regional Radiotherapy Centre, Cookridge
    Hospital, Leeds

Richard Peto, PhD
    Reader in Cancer Studies, Department of
    Medicine, University of Oxford

R.C.S. Pointon, MA, MRCP, FRCR
    Director of Radiotherapy, Christie Hospital and
    Holt Radium Institute, Manchester

Trevor J. Powles, PhD, MRCP
    Senior Lecturer in Medicine at the Institute of
    Cancer Research and Honorary Consultant
    Physician at The Royal Marsden Hospital,
    London and Surrey

Karl H. Proppe, MD
    Assistant Pathologist, Massachusetts General
    Hospital, Assistant Professor of Pathology,
    Harvard Medical School, Boston

S. Rafla, MD, PhD, FFR, FRCR
    Director, Radiation Therapy Department,
    Methodist Hospital, Lutheran Medical Centre
    and Maimonides Medical Centre, Brooklyn,
    New York

R.C.G. Russell, FRCS
    Consultant Surgeon, The Middlesex Hospital
    and St. John's Hospital for Diseases of the Skin,
    London

M. Ruth Sandland, FRCS, FRCR
    Consultant Radiotherapist, St. Bartholomew's
    Hospital, and Hospital for Sick Children,
    London

Ralph N. Sapsford, ChM, FRCS
    Consultant Cardiothoracic Surgeon and Senior
    Lecturer in Cardiothoracic Surgery, Royal
    Postgraduate Medical School, Hammersmith
    Hospital, London

J. Howard Scarffe, MB, MRCP
    Lecturer and Honorary Senior Registrar, Cancer

Research Department of Medical Oncology,
Christie Hospital and Holt Radium Institute,
and Manchester University, Manchester

Fritz H. Schroeder, MD
    Professor of Urology, Head, Institute and
    Department of Urology, Erasmus University
    Rotterdam, Rotterdam

Ian E. Smith, MD, MRCP
    Consultant Medical Oncologist, The Royal
    Marsden Hospital, Honorary Senior Lecturer,
    Institute of Cancer Research, London and
    Surrey

Margaret F. Spittle, FRCR, MSc, DMRT
    Consultant in Radiotherapy and Oncology, The
    Meyerstein Institute of Radiotherapy and
    Oncology, The Middlesex Hospital, London

Maurice J. Staquet, MD, MS
    Director, EORTC Data Center, Institut Jules
    Bordet, Université Libre de Bruxelles, Brussels

Herman D. Suit, MD, DPhil
    Chief, Department of Radiation Medicine,
    Massachusetts General Hospital, Professor of
    Radiation Therapy, Harvard Medical School,
    Boston

Malcolm L. Sutton, MA, BM, BCh, MRCP, FRCR
    Consultant in Radiotherapy and Oncology,
    Christie Hospital and Holt Radium Institute,
    Manchester

Richard J. Sylvester, MS
    Assistant Director, EORTC Data Center,
    Institut Jules Bordet, Université Libre de
    Bruxelles, Brussels

Nicholas Thatcher, PhD, MB, BChir, MRCP, DMRT
    Senior Lecturer and Honorary Consultant,
    Cancer Research Campaign, Department of
    Medical Oncology, University of Manchester
    and Christie Hospital and Holt Radium
    Institute, Manchester

Brigit van der Werf-Messing, MD
    Professor and Chairman, Department of
    Radiation Therapy of the Rotterdam
    Radiotherapy Institute and of the Erasmus
    University, Rotterdam

J. M. A. Whitehouse, MA, MD, FRCP
    Professor of Medical Oncology, Southampton
    General Hospital, Southampton

David E. Whittam, FRCS
    Consultant Otolaryngologist, St. George's
    Hospital, London

Roger S. Williams, MD, FRCP
    Director, The Liver Unit, King's College
    Hospital, London

J. E. Wright, MD, FRCS, DO
    Consultant Ophthalmic Surgeon, Moorfields
    Eye Hospital, London

Preface

Attainment of the best treatment of cancer will continue to be of paramount importance for the foreseeable future. One of the current dogmas, almost a cliché, is the importance of integration and of team work, of the main methods – surgery, radiotherapy, and chemotherapy. Yet this is still often much more precept than practice. This book is an attempt towards achieving this important goal. It describes *cancer treatment of all kinds*, everyday and esoteric, so that anyone interested in the optimum management of cancer can read sufficiently to know something sensible and up to date about the particular tumour or particular treatment method that concerns him, whatever his specialty. This is meant to be an international textbook, considerably based on distinguished British authors but with contributors also from North America, Asia and the continent of Europe.

Like Gaul, the book is divided into three parts – principles, practice and techniques. The first part – Principles of Treatment – reviews the roles and rationales of Surgery, Radiotherapy (with a section on the newest radiations – nuclear particles), Chemotherapy, Endocrine treatment, and Immunotherapy. The second main part – Clinical Practice – is an extensive series of chapters in every individual class of tumour. Some of these chapters are purposely more expansive then others, to allow world authorities, such as John Ho on nasopharyngeal cancer, to let us all have the benefit of much wider experience than most of us can hope to achieve, and others to give space for the very interesting newly described tumours such as the apudomas. Some are comprehensive summaries mainly based on the outstanding experience of one particular centre, such as the unique experience of the Christie Hospital in cancer of the mouth. Others are on tumours only now beginning to be attacked by the modern combined approach, such as tumours of the liver and pancreas. All should give a guide sufficient to point the way to the best contemporary treatment protocols. The final part – Methods and Techniques – gives more essential detail which will be of value in deciding on technique including medical management; the extremely important practical and psychological handling of patients (sometimes terminal) and of their relatives; and radiation equipment and treatment planning. Lastly, there are two essential chapters on statistics and trial protocols.

I have been greatly helped, not only by the authors, usually working in teams of two or three, but especially by five associate editors who have given advice on their areas of expertise: James Boak on surgery, Carl von Essen on particle radiotherapy and the American viewpoint, Derek Crowther on chemotherapy, Stewart Orr on physics and science, and Michael Peckham on radiotherapy. Barry Shurlock and the publishing staff of Chapman and Hall have been most helpful and tolerant. Finally, I wish to urge all doctors (surgical, medical and radiation) to read about all that can be done by their colleagues with even more attention than they give to their own roles.

London   Keith E. Halnan

A note on radiation units

In this book the current units the rad, curie and rem are used. New SI (Systeme Internationale) units are about to come in; in Britain they will be legally authorized from 1981 and will be in sole use by 1986. Their introduction in the European Economic Community (EEC) had been authorized since 1978. In many other parts of the world there are no plans yet for change. Tables of the new units are given below.

Quantity	New named unit and symbol	In other SI units	Old special unit and symbol	Relationship old to new units
Exposure	–	C/kg	röntgen (R)	1 R = 2.58 × 10^{-4} C/kg
Absorbed dose	gray (Gy)	J/kg	rad (rad)	1 rad = 0.01 Gy
Dose equivalent	sievert (Sv)	J/kg	rem (rem)	1 rem = 0.01 Sv
Activity	becquerel (Bq)	s^{-1}	curie (Ci)	1 Ci = 3.7 × 10^{10} Bq

The table below gives the prefixes to be used with SI units

Multiples			Sub-multiples		
Factor	Prefix	Symbol	Factor	Prefix	Symbol
10^{18}	exa	E	10^{-1}	deci	d
10^{15}	peta	P	10^{-2}	centi	c
10^{12}	tera	T	10^{-3}	milli	m
10^{9}	giga	G	10^{-6}	micro	μ
10^{6}	mega	M	10^{-9}	nano	n
10^{3}	kilo	k	10^{-12}	pico	p
10^{2}	hecto	h	10^{-15}	femto	f
10^{1}	deca	da	10^{-18}	atto	a

Part One: Principles of Treatment

1 Introduction
An approach to the treatment of cancer: past, present and future

Keith E. Halnan

This book is written by many authors with one common theme – the optimal treatment of cancer. Sir George Pickering has discussed the aims of treatment, and his views on hypertension can equally well be applied to cancer. Doctors have different attitudes to treatment. Some treat their patients as human individuals; some treat the labels which they have fixed to their patients, perhaps as cases in a scientific randomly controlled trial protocol; some treat the patient's relatives and a few treat the doctor himself. *The main object of treatment should be that expressed by the American Declaration of Independence in 1776, namely: 'Life, liberty and the pursuit of happiness'.* Many oncologists may too easily concentrate on the first, at the expense of the second and third – the quality of life must not be disregarded.

Basic concepts: the nature, growth and spread of cancer

Cancers can arise in any organ of the body, but some sites are more frequent than others. Each cancer is descended from a single cell that at some stage became free from its normal territorial restraints and so was able to form a family of cells that could multiply without limit. (Cairns, 1978)

There are about 10^{13} cells in the human body and from start to finish, from the fertilized egg to death in old age, a human being is the product of about 10^{16} cell divisions.

The layman often thinks that cancer is a single incurable disease that can begin anywhere in the body, and that it spreads throughout the body, causing much pain and other unpleasant symptoms before inevitable death. Similarly, it may be thought that surgery is unpleasant and mutilating, that radiotherapy burns the patient and makes him sick, and that chemotherapy not only makes him sick but does this repeatedly and interminably, usually removing all his hair also. This is the main cause of unnecessary fear and of the highly undesirable delay before diagnosis.

In fact the definition of cancer or 'malignancy' is extremely difficult. Firstly, perhaps one should state that cancer is a disease in which a family of cells will grow progressively, with permanent impairment of normal growth control, resulting in spread of the primary group of tumour cells – the primary tumour – which penetrates the capsule of the parent organ. Secondly, the cancer cells will penetrate the walls of either lymphatic or blood vessels, and will be capable of implantation and growth in secondary or metastatic sites, especially in lymph nodes from lymphatic spread, and in any organ from blood-borne spread, especially lungs, bones, liver and brain.

Either of these criteria can be sufficient. For example a basal cell carcinoma of skin or a glioma of the brain will be capable of killing the patient without any distant metastasis, lymphatic or blood-borne. Similarly, there may be widespread distant metastases from a tiny thyroid carcinoma or a small cell bronchial carcinoma while the primary carcinoma is still small and well confined to the primary organ. The histologist or cytologist will then recognize criteria for malignancy in individual cells: abnormal nuclei, frequent abnormal mitoses and changes in the ultrastructure. There may also be changes in the structure and arrangement of the tumour compared with normal parent tissue.

It is this last kind of diagnosis that is more debatable, when the transition occurs between a papilloma and carcinoma of the bladder, or a malignant or benign ovarian cyst. Pre-malignancy or carcinoma-in-situ is one very arguable field; good examples are carcinoma *in situ* of the uterine cervix which may not become invasive at all, or tiny latent carcinomas of the prostate, apparently present in a majority of very elderly men and often never causing any symptoms at all.

The cancer may sometimes be multicentric but will more often be considered to arise from mutations of one cell into a new permanently malignant cell. The tumour may grow exponentially or more likely at decreasing rate as a 'Gompertz' growth curve. A just perceptible tumour of 1 g contains 10^9 cells, and 10^{12} cells or 1 kg will often be more than enough to kill the patient (dependent upon patterns of spread). It becomes clear that many cancers must have originated for a substantial period, certainly months and often years before becoming clinically detectable or before causing symptoms and becoming apparent to the patient last of all. It also becomes obvious that latent microscopic metastases may well be present in very many patients and that treatment must be far more vigorous or must continue for much longer than needed to induce a 'complete remission', i.e. result in no clinical evidence of disease (Fig. 1.1).

Epidemiology: present and future

The total incidence of cancer seems from past ex-

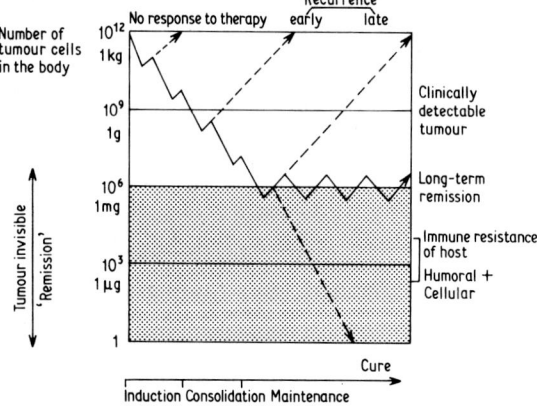

Fig. 1.1 This diagram shows the successive response of a tumour to cycles of chemotherapy but the reduction in numbers from 'induction' therapy might well have been caused by surgery, the 'consolidation' by post-operative radiotherapy, with final reduction for long-term cure being caused by chemotherapy.

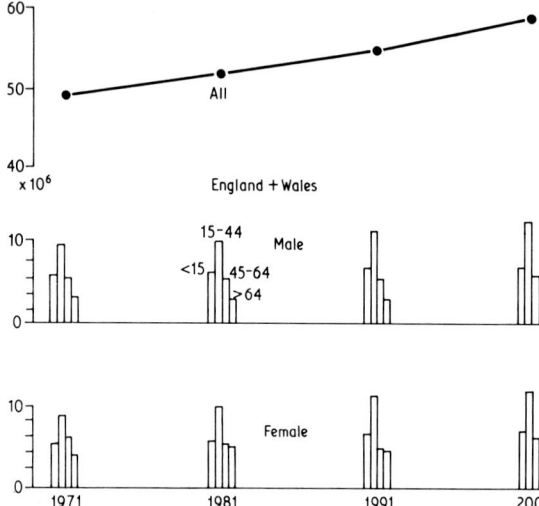

Fig. 1.2 Population projection for England and Wales, with histograms showing age distribution.

perience unlikely to change very much over the next ten years, particularly if one is considering incidence on an age-corrected basis. Most cancers have a steep increase in incidence with age; in most parts of the world the proportion of elderly people is itself increasing, as population control methods become so widely available and because of increasing success in treatment of disease, infectious especially, other than cancer and cardiovascular disease.

Population changes will vary considerably but most 'developed' or Western countries are now only expanding relatively slowly as shown in Fig. 1.2 for England and Wales. The population group aged 75 and over is likely to increase by over 25%, and will have a considerable incidence of cancer.

Past experience (in Scotland as an example) will show us how these changes will alter the incidence of cancer. Over the last 50 years cancer has been increasing, this has mainly been occuring in the elderly (Fig. 1.3) as well as in the numerically very small group of children.

Major differences are occurring in different sites, the most important being the lung, responsible for most of the last 30 years' increase in cancer in men and likely to do the same for women if present trends continue and smoking continues unabated.

Detailed very interesting analyses for world trends are given in the recent report *Cancer Services in Scotland* from the Scottish Health Service Planning Council (1980). In Scotland itself the size of change expected in registration by 1991 is given in Table 1.1 based both on

Table 1.1. Projected change in cancer registration to 1991 in Scotland.

All sites: + 4–5%
Specific sites:

– 8–10%	Little change	+ 1–3%	+ 3–5%	+ 5–7%
Cervix uteri	Ovary Lymphatic system	Stomach	Breast Leukaemia	Lung Colon and rectum Pancreas Bladder Prostate

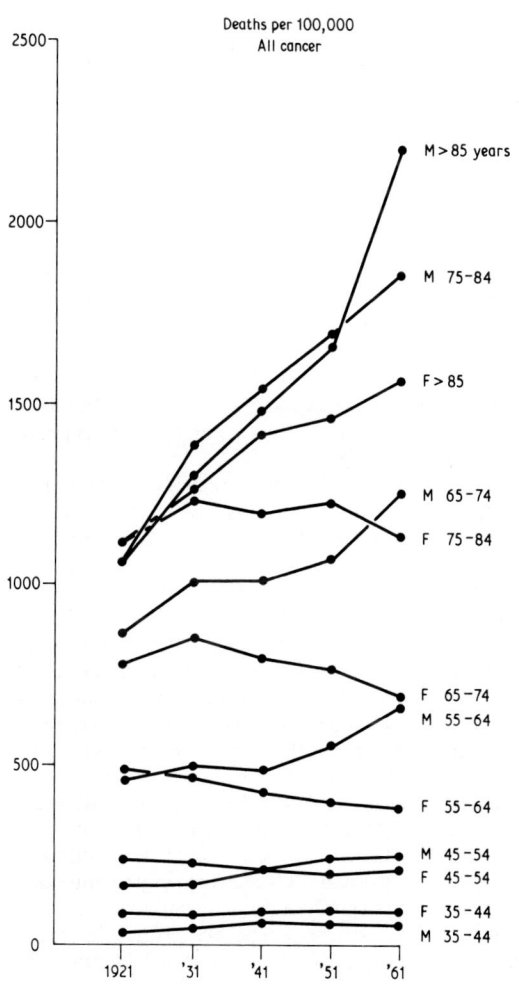

Deaths per 100,000
All cancer

M > 85 years

M 75-84

F > 85

M 65-74

F 75-84

F 65-74
M 55-64

F 55-64

M 45-54
F 45-54

F 35-44
M 35-44

Fig. 1.3 Cancer death rates in age groups in Scotland for men (M) and women (F).

recent trends and on population change.

Changing death rates in England and Wales make an interesting comparison with those from the USA given below. They show that the overall age-standardized death rate for all cancers is apparently not changing significantly, though there are very steep increases in death rates in both sexes for lung cancer, and reduction in cancer of the stomach, and cervix uteri. There has been a reduction in deaths from cancers of the colon and rectum also, possibly now levelling off, with similar increase in the pancreas, prostate and ovary. It should be stressed that these are age-corrected and that population changes, especially increase in the elderly, can still cause considerable overall increase (Fig. 1.4a, b, (Kemp and Toms, 1979)).

Changes in the USA are well summarized in the American Cancer Society's *Cancer Facts and Figures* (1978), they are similar to those seen in Britain, and likely in Europe (Figs. 1.4, 1.5a, b).

Estimates in 1978 of both incidence and death rates also make the position very clear (Figs 1.6, 1.7).

Estimates for other countries can similarly be made. In general, populations will often be increasing much more rapidly, such as in Egypt or Sri Lanka. Cancer incidence may at present be much lower but is likely to increase similarly. There are of course major site differences such as the increased prevalence of nasopharyngeal cancer in parts of China, the liver in parts of Africa, the stomach in Japan, the skin in Australia and New Zealand, and so on (see Table 1.7 below). Treatment itself may not need to be different.

Diagnosis and referral

Many patients will come to the clinical oncologist with a ready-made diagnosis and more or less complete investigation or 'staging'. It is wise to be sceptical and iconoclastic; *no diagnosis should be taken for granted and this is more true the more eminent the physician or surgeon from whom the patient has come.*

The histology should be reviewed in all cases if pos-

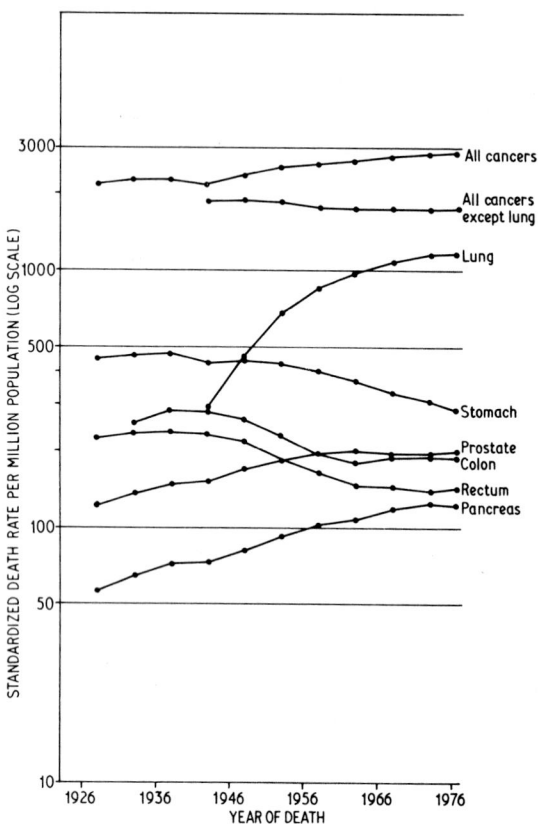

Fig. 1.4a Age standardized death rates for selected cancers in males 1926–1977 (Kemp and Toms, 1979).

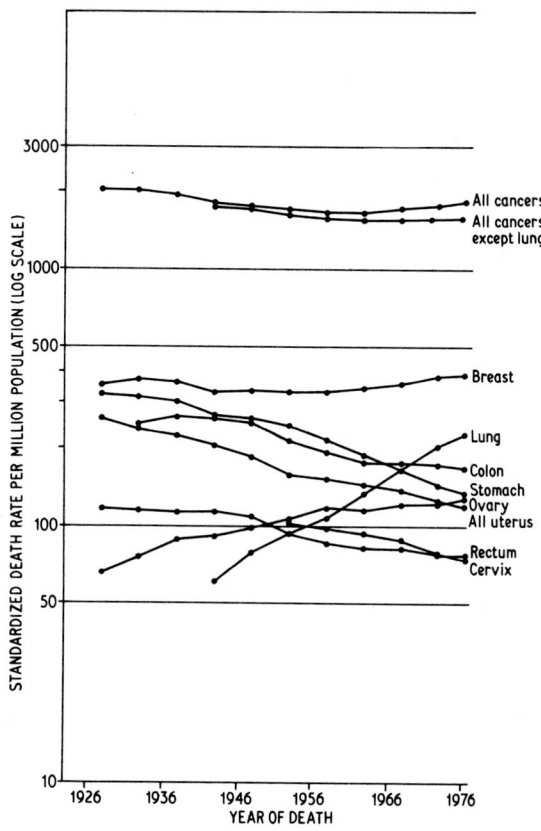

Fig. 1.4b Age standardized death rates for selected cancers in females 1926–1977 (Kemp and Toms, 1979).

sible and for tumours with notoriously difficult histology such as leukaemia, lymphoma, thyroid and salivary tumours this is particularly important. Even for the common bronchial carcinoma it is essential to know whether the tumour is small cell or large for example, rather than only 'undoubtedly malignant' or even 'anaplastic carcinoma'. A full detailed report is essential, with knowledge of tumour size, numbers and proportion of involved lymph nodes, evidence of capsular, lymphatic and blood vessel spread, and so on. It is obviously of great help to discuss cases both with the pathologist involved and also with any surgeon or physician who has investigated the patient, performed any biopsy or explorative operation.

It is naturally helpful to see the patient before any definitive operation if possible, though some tumours may have clinically appeared benign and the diagnosis of malignancy made for the first time by the pathologist on the operation specimen.

Investigations and staging

Full investigation is especially important in cancer, firstly because it can spread to almost any site in the body, secondly because of the effect of spread upon prognosis and most importantly because of the need for treatment planning to be altered appropriately according to *stage*. Every method of treatment carries its own hazards and we need to give the optimum first treatment, optimum for each individual patient, with likely benefits outweighing potential hazards. At one extreme the small early skin cancer can be almost universally cured by local treatment – surgical or radiation; at the other extreme, the moribund patient with widespread metastasis from a highly malignant insensitive tumour such as a fibrosarcoma, will not benefit from any anti-cancer treatment, he will need very good and careful general medical care. Many patients in the intermediate groups will benefit from combinations of

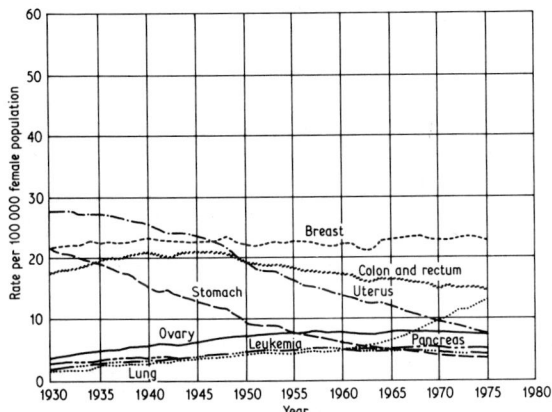

Fig. 1.5a Female cancer death rates (age-standardized) in the United States 1930–75 (National Vital Statistics Division and Bureau of the Census, 1940).

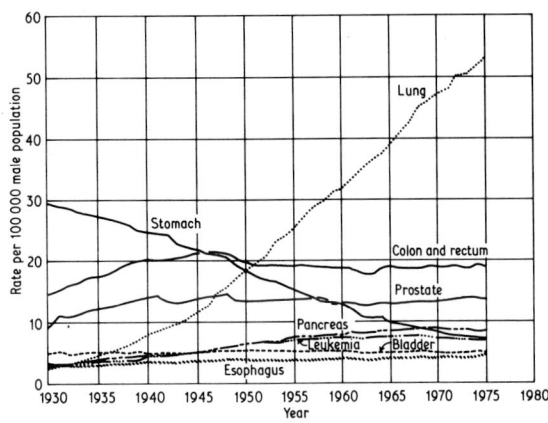

Fig. 1.5b Male cancer death rates (age-standardized) in the United States 1930–75 (National Vital Statistics Division and Bureau of the Census, 1940).

treatment, which need to be carefully planned in full knowledge of the histological classification and anatomical spread of the tumour.

Clinical history

The traditional or classical history-taking is of great importance and should not be regarded as tedious and time-wasting in comparison with the scientific investigation and evaluation, let alone the treatment itself. Nearly every patient will be frightened or nervous, and establishment of a sympathetic rapport at this first meeting may be of considerable value later when it may be necessary to persuade the patient of the value of apparently unpleasant treatment, or even more of the need to continue treatment for a long period extending into years.

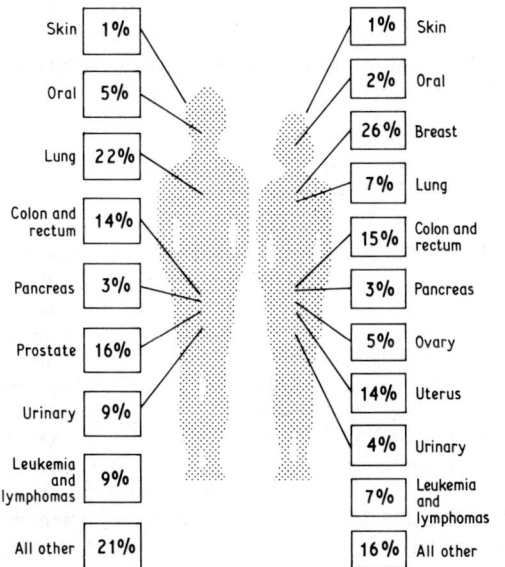

Fig. 1.6 Estimates of cancer incidence in USA by site and sex, 1978 (excluding non-melanoma skin cancer and carcinoma in situ of uterine cervix).

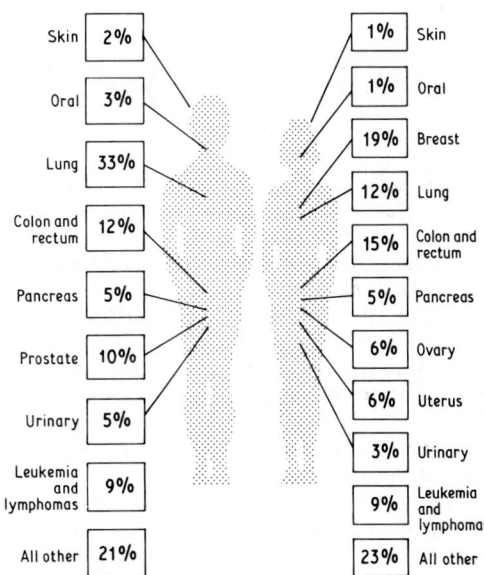

Fig. 1.7 Estimates of cancer deaths in USA by site and sex, 1978.

Length of history, speed of growth of the tumour, both primary and any metastases, are obvious fruitful subjects of enquiry. General or paraneoplastic symptoms, pain, tenderness, nausea, appetite and weight change will need to be known. Occupations, family history and previous medical history are of obvious value. Even religion can be interesting relevant knowledge related to habits of different kinds, Mormons and nuns being outstanding examples. Exposure to carcinogens of all kinds should be known, cigarettes and alcohol being only the two most clear examples. Finally it will be helpful for follow-up in future to know not only the names and addresses of the nearest relatives, but also of a close reliable relative or friend at a second address.

Clinical examination

This also must be complete and reminds one, as in all scientific work, *that measurement in numbers is necessary* – all measurable tumour deposits should be entered on an anatomical diagram with measurements in at least two dimensions. Photography is of value in addition to, rather than instead of, careful measurement and description.

All organ systems will need clinical assessment for tumour involvement or functional impairment. A good physician never neglects to do a rectal examination, the good oncologist will do no less and will also benefit from doing all the old fashioned inspections of facies, skin, tongue, eyelids and so on; the supraclavicular fossae are one particularly worthwhile region for examination.

Diagnostic imaging

X-ray diagnostic investigations are similarly essential. The normal series of examinations are now reinforced by a new method – computerized axial tomography (EMI, CT, or CAT scanning). CT-scanning can often detect smaller tumour deposits than was possible hitherto, for example in the lungs, brain and liver, and can also detect very small density differences; tumours that are difficult to outline by contrast medium can still be seen, such as retroperitoneal, para-aortic, and pelvic tumours – even lymph node masses, whether or not they take up contrast medium in a lymphangiogram. A further method of perhaps even more future and dynamic value is nuclear magnetic resonance (NMR), which has no radiation hazard. Nuclear medicine, bone scans and ultrasonic investigations, and also contributing to tumour evaluation.

Laboratory investigations

The whole range of laboratory examinations can be, but should not be, automatically requested, dependent on the tumour and its stage. Initial full blood and biochemical screening will almost always be required. The haematological examination is of major importance. Bone marrow examination, better by trephine than by aspiration, can show the presence of tumour cells as well as more direct causes of anaemia or cytopenia. Renal and hepatic function equally well need to be known because of possible impairment by tumour and by treatment.

Bacteriology, urology and immunology are all three of relevance. Tuberculosis and syphilis are no longer the major diagnostic competitors but they and their modern successors can still mimic tumours and tumour effects. Immunological defences are of clear relevance, as detailed later.

Tumour markers or index substances is rightly a field of great current interest, shown to be of most value probably in trophoblastic tumours. There are at least six of major value, almost all in rare tumours. The exception is one of the oldest – acid phosphatase for prostatic carcinoma – the others being α-foetoprotein for hepatomas and teratomas, chorionic gonadotrophin for chorion-carcinoma, thyroglobulin for thyroid adenocarcinoma, calcitonin for medullary thyroid carcinoma, and the immunoglobulins for myeloma and some other lymphomas. Ideally the tumour marker can be used to monitor progress of the tumour as it is destroyed by treatment, particularly after clinical, radiological and other anatomical measures can no longer give evidence of tumour, and may be the key to successful but minimal treatment.

The physician's ability to use his eyes has been aided dramatically by the use of fibre-optics, so that there can be both more flexible and efficient transmission of images. 'Was Man kennt, Man sicht!' – *endoscopy* is now an invaluable diagnostic aid.

Clinical classification and staging

Improvement in the results of treatment is such a gradual and multifactorial exercise that valid assessment and evaluation of treatment is essential. Equally well, progress is highly dependent upon the extent and spread of each individual tumour. It is therefore now, as stated by the International Union Against Cancer, a 'hallowed tradition' to *stage* cancer, and this is essential for adequate analysis. The stated objectives of classification are:

1. To aid the clinician in planning treatment.
2. To give some indication of prognosis.
3. To assist in evaluation of treatment results.

4. To facilitate exchange of information between treatment centres, without ambiguity.
5. To contribute to the continuing investigation of human cancer.

To achieve these objectives we need a system whose basic principles can be applied to all sites, irrespective of treatment, and which may be supplemented by information which becomes available later from histopathology and from surgery. *The 'TNM System' meets these requirements*. It provides an essential communication and information exchange device and a useful guide for prognosis and for therapy.

The convenient, inexpensive, pocket-book edition published by the UICC (1978) should be used by all oncologists, it describes the whole system clearly and in detail. The system is based on the assessment of the primary tumour T, the regional lymph nodes N, and on the absence or presence of distant metastases M. Numbers are then added to these three components (e.g. T1, T2, NO, N1, MO, M1 etc.) to indicate the extent of the disease. Additional pathological information can be added by P categories, and grading by G categories. Twenty-eight different sites have now been classified. *Staging* is then also done. The TNM classification can lead to thirty or more groups, easy to record individually but impracticable to subdivide into the tables of results unless numbers are very large indeed.

Broad grouping or staging is older than the TNM system and goes back, for example, to the Heymans 'League of Nations' staging for carcinoma of the cervix uteri. Four stages are commonly used, with Roman numbers, and for many sites can fit into the following kind of definitions, as shown in Table 1.2.

In recent years, the term 'staging' has been applied to the increasingly complex investigation of patients, such as those with leukaemia, Hodgkin's lymphoma, or testicular tumours, including not only full radiology with lymphangiography and CT-scanning, but also needle or other biopsies of organs such as the kidneys and testes, and even 'staging laparotomy' with splenectomy and lymph node biopsy. The information gained becomes useful not only in planning initial treatment but also when repeated later, in deciding on continuation or change in treatment.

Treatment

Introduction

The treatment of cancer used to be simple. Many cases would be advanced and their diagnosis obvious but most would come first to the surgeon who would attempt radical excision of the earlier cases and would biopsy the remainder. Radiotherapy would be used for cure of a few tumours, skin cancer, cancer of cervix and larynx being obvious examples, 'palliative' treatment being given to many others. It was early recognized that a few very radiosensitive tumours such as lymphomas would be preferentially treated by biopsy only and radiotherapy. Hormone treatment was poorly understood and effective for an unselected proportion of cancers, breast especially. Chemotherapy, nitrogen mustard in particular, had a dramatic effect on Hodgkin's disease but was of little value otherwise. Widespread pessimism among the medical profession as much as the general public, had some foundation.

Today the position is transformed; surgery remains the main initial approach but is increasingly frequently followed, preceded or accompanied by other treatment. Radiotherapy is much more exact and better localized; sensitizers and high LET radiation are promising even better results. Effective systemic treatment of microscopic as well as macroscopic metastases is being developed using chemotherapy, and sometimes endocrine and immune treatments. Interaction between different treatment methods is very important. Team work and integration becomes essential with mutual consultation from the beginning. One of the old dogmas of oncology is that '*the first treatment should be the best; it will certainly give the best chance of success*' and this is even more true today. Good cancer treatment therefore requires knowledge from the beginning of the possibilities, achievements and hazards, of *all* methods of treatment.

The treatment of the tumour is described, usually in some detail, in the chapters that follow, and only a few preliminary comments will be appropriate here.

The constant re-iteration of the need for *combined* team planning is necessary. This is firstly required before *any* treatment is given. This is required in fair-

Table 1.2 Typical clinical staging.

Stage	Primary tumour		Regional lymph nodes	Distant metastases
I	mobile ('operable')		none	none
II	mobile ('operable')		mobile ('operable')	none
III	fixed ('inoperable')	or	fixed ('inoperable')	none
IV	any of above		any of above	present

ness to both the patient and the other colleagues concerned. It is not only that there is interaction, in side-effects especially, between different methods of treatment, but also it is obvious that any treatment of any kind cannot be revised or altered once it has been given. This does not mean that every patient has to be seen by two, three or more consultants. For the more common tumour there will be a mutually approved protocol or policy, and even more importantly there will be regular contact and collaboration between the consultants concerned, they will know and respect each other's point of view. A few simple points can be outlined here.

Surgery

Surgical removal has obvious advantages and disadvantages (see Chapter 2). Once a block of tissues has been removed it can do no harm in a specimen container, but equally well there can be no direct effect of surgery except on the tissue that has been excised. Even nowadays there remain limits to the extent of reasonable excision without undue multilation or hazard. Surgery will retain an important place in oncology for a long time to come, but ultraradical surgery may lead to no better results because of the obvious spread of the tumour, so much that if ultraradical surgery is necessary it may also imply that there are microscopic distant metastases outside the reach of the surgeon's knife.

Radiotherapy

This is the second main method of treatment (see Chapters 3, 4, 40, 41). It should first be made clear that this implies the use of ionizing rather than all electromagnetic radiation, and that this class of radiation has a selective unique effect on tumour cells. Radiotherapy should not be classed with the non-specific destruction of tumour and normal cells alike that can be accomplished by many methods, from the primitive use of caustics to the sophisticated use of laser beams or of cryosurgery – all these should be considered as methods of surgery. The sensitivity of individual tumours will vary considerably; some, such as seminomas, will be very sensitive and all cells will be sterilized, but in general there will not be the 'all or none' effect of surgery but only a chance, perhaps 60%, perhaps 99%, that there will be a permanent complete response. To counterbalance this there will be no need to remove any normal tissue and, if dosage and conditions are correct, normal tissue damage will be repairable. Thus if, for example, either a tongue or laryngeal tumour can be destroyed or removed by either radiotherapy or by surgery and the chances of survival are the same, the advantages of retaining normal speech will be well

worth considering. The acute and long term hazards of radiotherapy are very well documented (see Chapter 38) and must be taken into account, but only in comparison with those of the alternatives, often less well known.

Chemotherapy

This is correctly the most promising of current methods of treatment (see Chapter 5). The 'magic bullet' or 'wonder drug' will continue to be searched for and may indeed arrive. Cancer chemotherapy is, however, still a relatively young discipline though being applied with wisdom and discretion. Its practitioners are beginning to learn the lessons that come to all doctors who treat cancer. Long-term complete and careful follow up is necessary. Hazards as well as benefits must be assessed and cure may not be certain in many tumours for many years. Carcinogenesis and genetic hazards are becoming apparent as they have done from ionizing radiation. The great advantage of chemotherapy is that it is almost, but not quite completely, systemic, reaching to nearly all body organs. It will in suitable circumstances be of great value in an 'adjuvant' prophylactic role, and this needs continued very careful assessment.

Endocrine or hormone treatment

This can be used for certain tumours, usually well differentiated, very similar to their parent organs which are under endocrine control (see Chapter 6). This kind of treatment is often very attractive in that it may be very free from side-effects and hazards and may seem to offer considerable advantages over the more obviously 'toxic' alternatives such as radiotherapy or chemotherapy. It must be realized, however, that hormonal dependence or control cannot always be accurately predicted, even with receptor analysis, and that any effect may even then only be temporary. There may be side-effects, as for example, the cardiovascular complications and indeed deaths from oestrogens given for prostatic cancer. It would be regrettable if potentially curative treatment was delayed until its chances of success were lessened, and it will often be appropriate to give hormone treatment as an *addition* rather than an alternative to whatever other treatment is suitable.

Immunotherapy

This is at present in favour, though perhaps the pendulum is beginning to swing against it, as has happened before. As with hormone treatment there is much attraction in the concept of harnessing natural immune defences – 'mother nature' in fact – to control a tumour.

Table 1.3 Performance status.

Swiss	Karnofsky
0 Able to carry on normal activity	100 Normal, no complaints
	90 Normal activity, minimal signs or symptoms
1 Able to live at home, with tolerable symptoms	80 Normal activity with effort, some symptoms
	70 Caring for self, unable to work
2 Disabling symptoms but < 50% of time in bed	60 Needs occasional assistance, but able to care for most needs
	50 Needs considerable assistance and frequent medical care
3 Severely disabled, > 50% of time in bed but able to stand	40 Disabled, needs special care
	30 Severely disabled, needs hospital care
4 Very ill, confined to bed	20 Very ill, in hospital, needs supportive care
	10 Moribund
5 Dead	0 Dead

There are of course obvious hazards too, as are pointed out very clearly by Cochran (see Chapter 7), and the consensus of opinion seems to be that if immunotherapy can be of value it will usually be to control no more than a relatively small number of potentially active tumour cells remaining after the majority has been destroyed by other methods.

Combined treatment is the essence of many advances. It is increasingly important to study not only addition, potentiation and perhaps synergistic good effects but also the combined hazards and toxicities.

Evaluation and assessment: results

Most improvements in treatment are relatively modest, and their quality and validity need time and adequate numbers of patients, with good protocols and statistics as outlined in Chapters 43 and 44. Adequate evaluation and assessment is increasingly important. As always it is essential for this to be *exact, objective, and numerical* rather than subjective and qualitative. There are three main parameters:

1. *Tumour size* which should be measured as the mean of two perpendicular diameters.
2. *Remission duration*, measured from the beginning of treatment until two consecutive measurements show increase of tumour size of 25%.
3. *Survival* since start of therapy.

Five definitions of *response* in solid tumours are used:

1. *Complete remission* (CR) – disappearance of all tumour, usually for a defined remission duration.

2. *Partial remission* (PR) – tumour shrinkage of more than 50% of initial size.
3. *Improvement* – significant shrinkage of less than 50%.
4. *No change.*
5. *Progression* of tumour size during treatment.

It is often found helpful to evaluate the *general condition* of the patient before or after treatment, the pre-treatment evaluation often correlates well with the response to treatment. The *Karnofsky Performance Status* (Table 1.3) is one good method of doing this and there are many simpler indices.

Symptoms, signs and toxic effects can be similarly 'scored', usually on a 5-digit scale, this can include pain, weight change, renal, hepatic and other functions, blood counts, upper gastrointestinal effects, bowel movement changes, and other specific effects. All can usefully be scored in a similar way (Table 1.4).

Table 1.4 Symptoms or toxic effect score.

0 –	none
1 –	mild, tolerable
2 –	moderate
3 –	severe
4 –	life-threatening
5 –	death caused

It is essentially helpful to use standard forms, reports or flow sheets and good examples are given in Figs. 1.8, 1.9, 1.10 and 1.11.

Date of Observation								
Day of Study								
Observer's Initials								

GIVE COORDINATES FOR ALL MEASUREMENTS (include Liver and Spleen)

Lesions Measured								
Liver (cm)								
Spleen (cm)								

Did new lesions appear during treatment?   YES_____ NO_____

Give coordinates for new lesions: _____

INDICATE ON DIAGRAM ALL MEASURABLE AND PALPABLE LESIONS AT START OF THERAPY
(include Liver and Spleen)

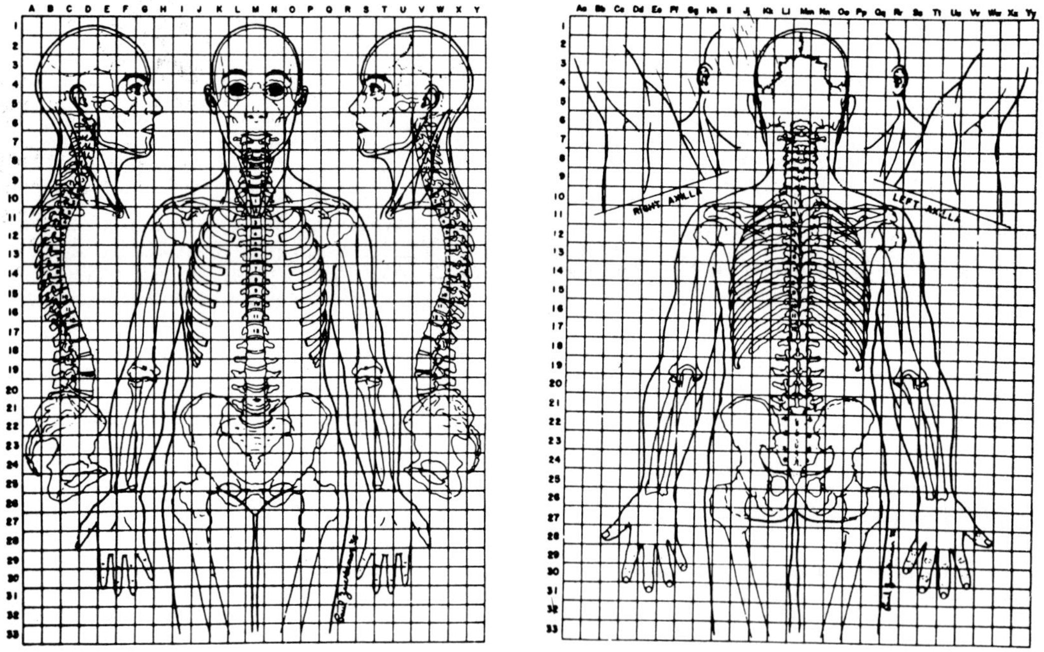

Patient Name _____ Institution _____

Protocol # EST _____ Page _____ of _____ pages

ECOG FORM C
3/69

Fig. 1.8 Patient measurement form used by Eastern Cooperative Oncology Group (USA).

SUMMARY AND EVALUATION FORM - ECOG FORM D

INSTRUCTIONS: This form is to be completed and submitted, together with the appropriate flow sheets and measurement forms, whenever a patient completes or is removed from a treatment program of a study. Unless otherwise specified, use "N/A", "N/D", or "UNKN" to indicate "not applicable", "not done", or "unknown" respectively. Do not write in shaded boxes.

Patient's Name ______ Protocol No. ______ Protocol Case No. ______

Institution ______

COMPLICATIONS AND TOXICITY

0=none 4=life-threatening
1=mild 5=lethal
2=moderate 9=unknown
3=severe

	MOST SEVERE DUE TO PROTOCOL TREATMENT ONLY	MOST SEVERE DUE TO ALL CAUSES
G.I. (other than the specific toxicities in this list)	☐	☐
Vomiting	☐	☐
Diarrhea	☐	☐
Infection	☐	☐
Bleeding	☐	☐
Skin and mucosa	☐	☐
Neurologic	☐	☐
Respiratory	☐	☐
GU	☐	☐
Hematologic	☐	☐
Liver	☐	☐
Other	☐	☐

☐ "Other" toxicity specified:
0-not applicable 7-other(single),specify: ______
1-fever
2-chills
3-alopecia 8-other(multiple),specify: ______
4-edema
5-ascites
6-cardiac 9-unknown

DISEASE RESPONSE

☐ Objective response (consult protocol for definitions; enter first applicable code)
1-complete response
2-partial response
4-progression(or recurrence for surgical adj. studies only)
3-no change
8-unevaluable
9-unknown

if complete response, partial response, or progression:
☐☐ ☐☐ ☐☐ Date of onset (m,d,y)

if complete or partial response:
☐ Continuation of response
1-response continuing
2-relapse occurred after a response was achieved; give date of relapse: ☐☐ ☐☐ ☐☐
3-no relapse occurred, but no further information obtainable or patient lost to follow-up
4-no relapse observed, but patient died

☐ Subjective response
1-marked improvement 4-worsening
2-moderate improvement 8-unevaluable
3-no improvement 9-unknown

☐ Did new metastases, lesions, or other areas of new disease appear? (1-no 2-yes 9-unknown)

Organ involvement at end of treatment (circle appropriate items)

BONE	CNS	REGIONAL LYMPH NODES
SKIN	LUNG(S)	DISTANT METASTASES
LIVER	SOFT TISSUE	OTHER, SPECIFY ______

TREATMENT

☐☐ ☐☐ ☐☐ Day of first dose of treatment (m,d,y) ☐☐ ☐☐ ☐☐ Day of last dose of treatment (m,d,y)

AGENT NAME	TOTAL AMOUNT GIVEN DURING TREATMENT PROGRAM	TREATMENT MODIFICATIONS (CIRCLE APPROPRIATE ITEMS)			
		DOSAGE INCREASED	DOSAGE DECREASED	RX INTERRUPTED	RX TERMINATED EARLY
		DOSAGE INCREASED	DOSAGE DECREASED	RX INTERRUPTED	RX TERMINATED EARLY
		DOSAGE INCREASED	DOSAGE DECREASED	RX INTERRUPTED	RX TERMINATED EARLY
		DOSAGE INCREASED	DOSAGE DECREASED	RX INTERRUPTED	RX TERMINATED EARLY
		DOSAGE INCREASED	DOSAGE DECREASED	RX INTERRUPTED	RX TERMINATED EARLY

Reasons for treatment modifications: ______

☐☐ ☐☐ ☐☐ Date removed from study/program
M D Y

☐ Survival status
1-alive
2-dead
9-lost to follow-up

☐☐ ☐☐ ☐☐ Date last known alive or date of death
M D Y

☐ Was patient eligible for this treatment program? (1-no, 2-yes, 9-unknown)

☐ If patient is unevaluable, enter first applicable reason:
8-wrong therapy 6-inadequate data
4-patient refused therapy 9-other, specify ______
7-patient lost to follow-up
2-inadequate therapy 5-early death
3-protocol violation 1-non-randomized

☐ Performance status at start of treatment program

______
Investigator (please print) Date (m,d,y)

Investigator: Keep last copy and send remaining top copies to Operations Office.

ECOG - 9/77

Fig. 1.9 Patient evaluation form used by Eastern Cooperative Oncology Group (USA).

Patient's Name_____ Hosp. or Soc. Sec. No._____

Institution_____ Protocol Number_____

									REMARKS (R_1, R_2, R_3, etc.)
PROTOCOL TREATMENT	1. Date 197____(mo./day)								
	2. Initials								
	RECORD ACTUAL DOSE; IF MODIFIED OR NOT GIVEN, EXPLAIN								
	3. Rx 1 (dose/day)								
	4. Rx 2 (dose/day)								
	5. Rx 3 (dose/day)								
	6. Rx 4 (dose/day)								
	7. Rx 5 (dose/day)								
OTHER THERAPY	SPECIFY AMOUNT; GIVE DETAILS								
	8. Antibiotics/Analgesics								
	9. Radiation (rads/day)								
	10. Transfusions (units)								
	11.								
PATIENT STATUS	12. PERFORMANCE STATUS*								
	13. Weight (kg)								
	14. Temperature								
ABNORMALITIES (Grade 0-5)**	CIRCLE REACTIONS DUE TO PROTOCOL THERAPY								
	15. Anemia								
	16. Hemorrhage								
	17. Infection								
	18. GU								
	19. Hepatic								
	20. Nausea & Vomiting								
	21. Other GI								
	22. Pulmonary								
	23. Cardiac								
	24. Neurologic—PN								
	25. Neurologic—CNS								
	26. Skin								
	27. Allergy								
	28. Fever								
	29. Pain								
	30. Other (specify)								
LABORATORY VALUES	REFER TO PROTOCOL FOR TEST SCHEDULES								
	31. HGB (gm %)]								
	32. HCT (%)								
	33 WBC (x 1000)								
	34. Neutrophyls (%)								
	35. Lymphs (%)								
	36. Platelets (x 1000)								
	37. Retic (%)								
	38. BUN (mg %)								
	39. Serum Creatinine (mg %)								
	40. Alk. Ptase (units)								
	41. Bilirubin (mg %)								
	42. SGOT (units)								
	43. SGPT (units)								
	44. LDH (units)								
	45. Uric Acid (mg %)								
	46. Total Protein (gm %)								
	47. Albumin (gm %)								
	48. Abnormal Protein (gm %)								
	49. Calcium (mg %)								
	50. Phosphorus (mg %)								
	51.								
SKIN TESTS†	52. PPD Int (mm)								
	53. Mumps (mm)								
	54. Varidase (dose & mm)								
	55. Dermatophytin 0 (1:100) (mm)								
	56. Other:								

† Measure at 48 hours induration as the mean of two diameters measured at right angles in mm.

*PERFORMANCE STATUS KEY	**PATIENT STATUS KEY
0—Normal activity	0—None or Normal
1—Symptoms but ambulatory	1—Mild
2—In bed < 50% of time	2—Moderate
3—In bed > 50% of time	3—Severe
4—100% bedridden	4—Life-Threatening
	5—Lethal

Fig. 1.10 Patient flow sheet form used by Eastern Cooperative Oncology Group (USA).

		0	1	2	3	4
Leuko-penia	WBC × 10³	≥4.5	3.0−<4.5	2.0−<3.0	1.0−<2.0	<1.0
	Neut × 10³	≥1.9	1.5−<1.9	1.0−<1.5	0.5−<1.0	<0.5
Thrombo-cytopenia	Plt × 10³	≥130	90−<130	50−<90	25−<50	<25
Anemia	Hgb gm%	≥11	9.5−10.9	<9.5		
	Hct %	≥32	28−31.9	<28		
	Clinical			Sx of anemia	Req transfusions	
Hemorrhage		None	Minimal	Mod—Not debilitating	Debilitating	Life threatening
Infection		None	No active Rx	Requires active Rx	Debilitating	Life threatening
GU	BUN mg%	≤20	21−40	41−60	>60	Symptomatic uremia
	Creatinine	≤1.2	1.3−2.0	2.1−4.0	>4.0	
	Proteinuria	Neg	1+	2+−3+	4+	
	Hematuria	Neg	Micro-Cult−positive	Gross-Cult−positive	Gross+Clots	c̄ obst uropathy

Urinary tract infection should be graded under infection, not GU.
Hematuria resulting from thrombocytopenia is graded under hemorrhage.

		0	1	2	3	4
Hepatic	SGOT	<1.5 × nl	1.5−2 × normal	2.1−5 × normal	>5 × normal	
	Alk Phos	<1.5 × nl	1.5−2 × normal	2.1−5 × normal	>5 × normal	
	Bilirubin	<1.5 × nl	1.5−2 × normal	2.1−5 × normal	>5 × normal	
	Clinical				Precoma	Hepatic coma

Viral hepatitis should be recorded as infection rather than liver toxicity.

		0	1	2	3	4
N & V		None	Nausea	N & V controllable	Vomiting intractable	
Diarrhea		None	No dehydration	Dehydration	Grossly bloody	
Pulm	PFT	Nl	25−50% decrease in Dco or VC	>50% decrease in Dco or VC		
	Clinical		Mild Sx	Moderate Sx	Severe Sx-Intermittent O_2	Assisted vent or continuous O_2

Pneumonia is considered infection and not graded as pulmonary toxicity unless felt to be resultant from pulmonary changes directly induced by treatment.

		0	1	2	3	4
Cardiac		Nl	ST—T changes	Atrial arrhythmias	Mild CHF	Severe or refract CHF
		Nl	Sinus tachy >110 at rest	Unifocal PVC's	Multifocal PVC's	Ventric tachy
					Pericarditis	Tamponade
Neuro	PN	None	Decr DTR's	Absent DTR's*	Disabling sens loss	Resp dysfunction 2° to weakness
			Mild paresthesias	Severe paresthesias	Severe PN pain	Obstipation req surg
			Mild constipation	Severe constipation	Obstipation	Paralysis—confining pt to bed/wheelchair
				Mild weakness	Severe weakness	
					Bladder dysfunct	
	CNS	None	Mild anxiety	Severe anxiety	Confused or manic	Seizures
			Mild depression	Mod depression	Severe depression	Suicidal
			Mild headache	Mod headache	Severe headache	Coma
			Lethargy	Somnolence	Cord dysfunction	
				Tremor	Confined to bed due to CNS dysfunct	
				Mild hyperactivity		
Skin & Mucosa		Nl	Transient erythema Pigmentation, atrophy	Vesticulation Subepidermal fibrosis	Ulceration Necrosis	
	Stomatitis	None	Soreness	Ulcers—can eat	Ulcers—cannot eat	
Alopecia		None	Alopecia—mild	Alopecia—severe		
Allergy		None	Transient rash Drug fever ≤38°C (≤100.4°F)	Urticaria Drug fever >38°C (>100.4°F) Mild bronchospasm	Serum sickness Bronchospasm—req parenteral meds	Anaphylaxis
Fever		≤37.5°C	≤38°C (≤100.4°F)	>38°C (>100.4°F)	Severe c̄ chills (>40°C)	Fever c̄ hypotension

Fever felt to be caused by drug allergy should be graded as allergy.
Fever due to infection is graded under infection only.

		0	1	2	3	4
Local Tox		None	Pain	Pain + Phlebitis	Ulceration	

1. The toxicity grade should reflect the most severe degree occurring during the evaluated period, not an average.
2. When two criteria are available for similar toxicities, e.g., leukopenia, neutropenia, the one resulting in the more severe toxicity grade should be used.
3. Toxicity grade = 5 if that toxicity caused the death of the patient.
4. Refer to detailed toxicity guidelines or to study chairman for toxicity not covered on this table.

Fig. 1.11 Toxicity criteria form used by Eastern Cooperative Oncology Group (USA).

Key for Fig 1.11

Sx = Symptoms
Rx = Therapy
N&V = Nausea & vomiting
PFT = Pulmonary function test
DCO = Diffusing capacity for CO
VC = Vital capacity
Nl = Normal
PVC = Premature ventricular contractions (extra-systoles)
CHF = Congestive heart failure
PN = Peripheral neuropathy
DTR = Deep tendon reflexes

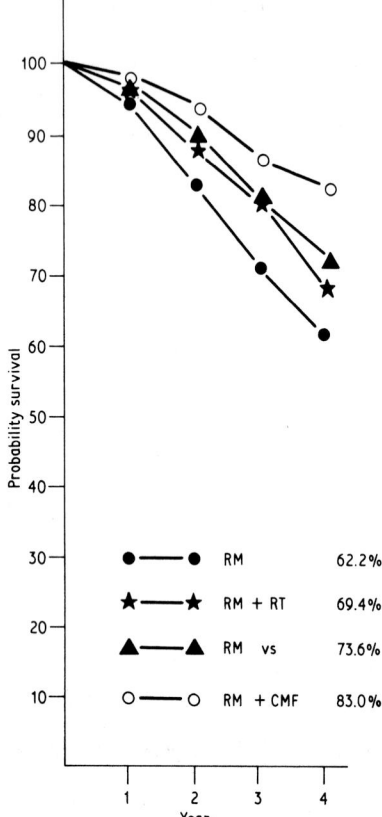

Fig. 1.12 Overall survival for breast cancer (Stages 1 and 2) at the National Cancer Institute, Milan. RM – radical mastectomy only, 1964–67; RM + RT – radical mastectomy and radiotherapy, 1968–72; RM – radical mastectomy only, 1973–75; RM +CMF – radical mastectomy and chemotherapy, 1973–75 (Bonadonna, Valagussa and Veronesi, 1978).

Statistical analysis

Correct and good statistical analysis of results, very often from random controlled trials, is essential. It is unfortunately unlikely that many, perhaps any, new method of treatment will be more than partially effective in inducing complete remission, let alone long-term cure. Comparison with alternative treatment is very difficult, and historical controls are usually not a valid comparison. The results of treatment seem to be improving in most tumours from various causes, from general improvements in medical care. A good recent example of this comes from the National Cancer Institute in Milan, regarding breast cancer. Good results were being obtained from radical mastectomy only in

1964–67 but they were improved even further, apparently, by adding radiotherapy during 1968 to 1972. The current trial of adjuvant chemotherapy was then begun with encouraging results so far. The interesting point however is that the survival curves for 1973–1975 were better than the previous ones, even for the control arm alone, and thus in this context at least, use of historical controls, even very recent ones, is obviously misleading (Fig. 1.12; see also Chapter 16).

This is perhaps true indeed in some less obvious areas, such as in the use of the historical control survival curves, leading to a plateau of only about 20%, for osteosarcoma, to assess the apparently considerable success of adjuvant treatment. Examination of survival through the years at the Mayo Clinic shows that even this may not be as valid and certain as most of us thought (Fig. 1.13; see also Chapter 29).

Historical controls are perhaps sometimes adequate and unavoidable as in the assessment of acute leukaemia but in most trials it will be more than helpful to undertake random controlled trials with adequate statistical evaluation, such as by the log-rank method comparing actuarial survival or recurrence-free curves.

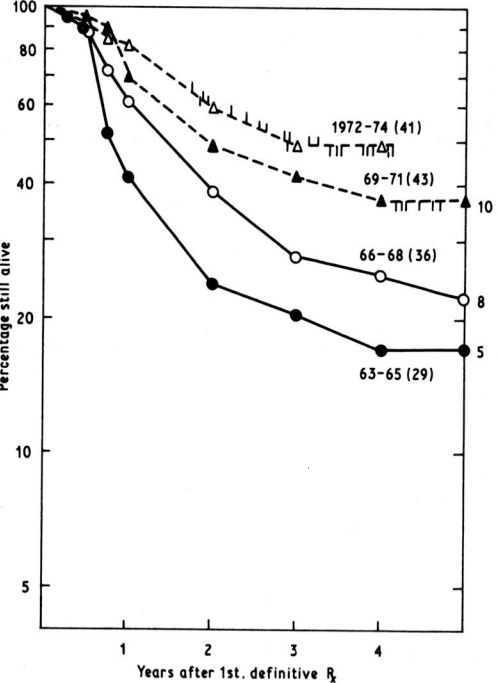

Fig. 1.13 Overall survival for osteosarcoma at the Mayo Clinic for time periods 1963–65, 1966–68, 1969–71 and 1972–74, showing successive improvement *not* related to adjuvant chemotherapy which was given most commonly in 1963–65 and 1969–71.

Table 1.5   Total numbers of patients needed for 80% probability of detection of difference at 5% significance in a random controlled trial comparing two treatment regimes.

		Probability of survival in one arm					
		0.20	0.25	0.30	0.35	0.40	0.45
Probability of survival in other arm	0.25	2180	–	–	–	–	–
	0.30	580	2500	–	–	–	–
	0.35	270	600	2700	–	–	–
	0.40	160	300	720	2940	–	–
	0.45	106	176	320	760	3066	–
	0.50	76	114	186	340	780	3120

Numbers are of the greatest importance (see Table 1.5 and Chapters 43 and 44).

Organization of cancer services

The most advanced methods of diagnosis and treatment are of no value to the individual patient if he cannot arrive at a hospital where they are in use. At the same time it is clearly uneconomic and impracticable to consider having in, say, every town or community of 50–100 000 people a cancer unit complete with adequate staff experienced in diagnosis, surgical, radiation and medical treatment, in all the specialities, and with equipment including, say, a whole-body computerized tomography X-ray scanner, a linear accelerator and simulator let alone neutron or pion units, full laboratory facilities, and medical treatment facilities for acute leukaemia, and surgical facilities for major surgery up to those for organ transplants! Yet these should

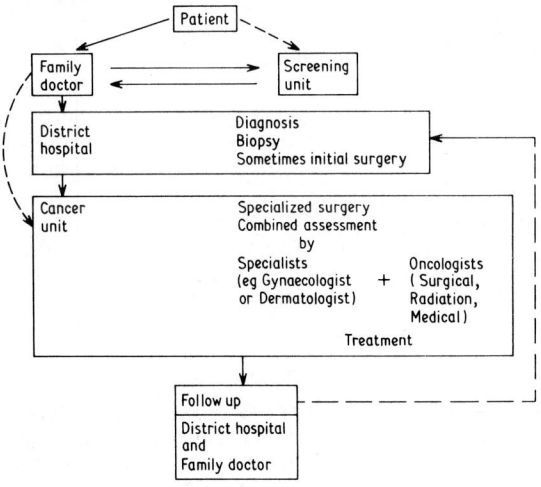

Fig. 1.14 Patient flow chart.

be available to all those who can benefit from them.

The need therefore is for comprehensive cancer centres distributed as widely as possible, and for adequate professional education and referral or linkage arrangements so that all patients can come, wherever they live.

The cancer unit or centre

The objective of this organization should be the availability of the highest standards of care for all. It must be accepted and taken for granted that no single doctor will now have all the skill, training and experience necessary. Cancer is a group of diseases that must be treated by multidisciplinary groups of doctors. On the other hand it would equally be wrong and indeed impracticable for all cancer to be treated in a specialist cancer hospital, not only for geographical reasons, but also because so many (perhaps half) of all cases present with non-specific symptoms such as cough or haematuria. The patient will begin as always by seeing his family doctor or general practitioner. He will then be referred usually to the neighbouring district general hospital, to a general physician or surgeon or to an appropriate specialist such as a gynaecologist or dermatologist. A minority of patients will have obvious cancer and be sent directly to the cancer centre. An additional minority may have come directly or indirectly through a screening service for breast, uterine cervix or other cancer.

At the general hospital there must be linkage with a cancer centre and the best way for this to develop is by the establishment of a weekly clinic by a visiting oncologist (radiation, medical, or both) from the centre. Secondarily there should be professional education – meetings, seminars, study groups – at the general hospital and the cancer centre, with full knowledge of treatment policies and possibilities, and agreement to treatment protocols and trials. This should be a development of the present British system of peripheral clinics from the larger radiotherapy and oncology centres (Fig. 1.14). Every consultant should be able to feel himself to be part of the cancer services.

The cancer centre or unit should not be an isolated specialist hospital. Consultation, discussion and collaboration with the main streams of medicine and surgery is vital. The well-known few cancer hospitals have accomplished much and will continue to do so but they could surely do even more as part of one of the best general hospitals, preferably university or teaching when appropriate. The new cancer centres then should be part of, or as a minimum on the same site or campus, as one of the best general hospitals.

The main core component of the cancer unit will be an integrated clinical oncology unit, including medical and radiation oncology. Staff from other disciplines would have part-time or even full-time appointments. Most of the diagnostic and supporting facilities such as radiology and laboratory medicine would be part of the main general hospital departments. It is difficult to envisage a wide role for many full-time surgical oncologists, with the possible exception of 'head and neck' surgeons. Details of the framework for a centre are outlined in Table 1.6.

This will then also allow the development of specialist groups or units with not only medical, radiation and surgical oncology expertise but also with gynaecologists for female genital cancer, urologists, paediatricians, dermatologists and haematologists as appropriate, indeed units in virtually every specialty. A few very uncommon highly specialized tumours such as retinoblastoma or chorion carcinoma may well be treated at only a few or even one national centre.

It is not appropriate to discuss further here all the associated features of a centre but social, nursing, other ancillary workers, community and general practice links are essential. Cancer education of all kinds and the best communications should be features of any centre.

Study or cooperative oncology groups

A recent important development is the organization of several groups of workers interested in one particular tumour, or a particular kind of treatment. In North America these are usually called 'cooperative oncology groups' and good examples are ECOG (the Eastern Cooperative Oncology Group) and SWOG (the South Western Oncology Group). In Europe they have developed as 'study groups', commonly under the aegis of the EORTC (European Organization for Research in Treatment of Cancer). National groups have also been effective, often under research foundations, in Britain the Medical Research Council and Cancer Research Campaign. Most will collect data and organize clinical

Table 1.6   Framework for a cancer centre.

CANCER UNIT – minimum population served 500 000; ideal probably $1-2 \times 10^6$

Facilities

Out-patient Department – facilities for combined clinics, day-care for investigation and treatment, especially chemotherapy

In-patient beds – about 100 per million population (75 radiotherapy, 25 chemotherapy mainly)

Hostels – patients from long distances needing only limited care

Diagnostic facilities – Radiology: comprehensive to include CT-scanning
Ultrasonics
Nuclear medicine
– Laboratory medicine: Histopathology and cytology
Haematology
Clinical chemistry
Microbiology
Immunology

Linked general hospital – integrated or on same site, neighbouring special units if not on site, e.g. neurology and neurosurgery, plastic surgery

Cancer intelligence unit – library, teaching and meeting facilities, cancer registration, follow up and statistics

Staff

Clinical oncologists with much common training, with main interest in radiation and medical treatment, usually with part-time (once-weekly) appointment at peripheral district hospitals. Limited number of surgical oncologists with main appointment in cancer unit. Most will work also in general or special hospitals.

trials. Membership can be of very considerable benefit, giving access to the most up to date methods of treatment and requiring detailed evaluation and investigation of patients, and indeed 'quality control'. Most groups will give at least limited financial support dependent upon entry of patients into trials with a published 'track record'. Further development of groups of these kinds is strongly advocated.

Research and the future

It is commonplace to state that most cancers (60 to 90%) are caused by environmental factors and to assume that this implies that most cancers are therefore preventable. This often leads to consequent assumption that most cancers are caused by 'pollution' – a

Table 1.7 Variation in incidence of common cancers (Doll, 1977).

Type of cancer	Region of highest incidence	Risk up to age 75 (%)	Range of variation*	Region of lowest incidence
		Men		
Skin	Queensland	Over 20	Over 200	Bombay
Esophagus	North-east Iran	20	300	Nigeria
Lung	Great Britain	11	35	Nigeria
Stomach	Japan	11	25	Uganda
Liver	Mozambique	8	70	Norway
Prostate	USA blacks	7	30	Japan
Colon	Connecticut	3	10	Nigeria
Mouth	India	Over 2	Over 25	Denmark
Rectum	Denmark	2	20	Nigeria
Bladder	Connecticut	2	4	Japan
		Women		
Cervix	Columbia	10	15	Israel (Jews)
Breast	Connecticut	7	15	Uganda

* The highest incidence observed in any country divided by the lowest observed incidence.

currently fashionable target to blame for many of the maladies of our civilization – or even more specifically industrial chemicals in air, water, or food. This is, however, too simple; it is better to state no more than that most cancers are caused by extrinsic or exogenous factors, many of which may originate in our 'life style', not only cigarettes but also diet in general. The best evidence for this comes from the interesting geographical variation in incidence of common cancers (Table 1.7).

Genetic influence seems relatively slight in comparison, one important piece of evidence being the conclusion that identical twins are not much more alike in the cancers they suffer from than are non-identical twins. Improvement in life-style is difficult to achieve but the Mormons have provided recent evidence that it can be of considerable value (Enstrom, 1978).

However, since we know that most cancers take so many years to develop it seems sensible to conclude that the incidence is unlikely to change much over the next ten, twenty-five or perhaps fifty years. Screening and early detection will have no more than slight impact. Improvement in treatment thus will continue to be needed.

Transplants and better reconstruction may come from surgery. Radiotherapy will remain an important method of localized treatment to main tumour bulk or masses. Fast neutrons, perhaps even pions may become a major method. Systemic regional or whole body radiotherapy may be regarded as almost 'one drug' of combined chemotherapy. New drugs will continue to be discovered but better treatment will more likely come from better combinations and timing of existing drugs. Early, or 'adjuvant' treatment, may have an increasing role for the more malignant tumours. Endocrine treatment will be improved by new analogues, such as the anti-hormones, but more by better selection of tumours by knowledge of hormone receptors. Wide use of immunotherapy seems doubtful at present, but by no means impossible. One contemporary new field of study is the 'interferons' (see Chapter 7).

The literature: continuing education and keeping up to date

Every good oncologist will wish to keep up to date; text books can do no more than help with the basic groundwork and can point towards more detailed sources. Nevertheless reading the literature remains essential and one should begin with a few general journals such as *Nature*, the *Lancet*, the *New England Journal of Medicine*, and the *British Medical Journal*, or one's national equivalents. General cancer journals follow, both the monthlies, with *Cancer* remaining perhaps most important, together with another such as the *British Journal of Cancer*; the recent review periodicals such as *Cancer Treatment Reviews*, and *Seminars in Oncology* being useful. The more specialist journals come next: *Cancer Treatment Reports*, the surgical, radiation and medical oncology journals and two newer very valuable ones being *Clinical Oncology* (from the British Association of Surgical Oncologists) and the *International Journal of Radiation Oncology*, as well as the regional specialist journals devoted to the blood, gut, chest, skin and so on. The *Year Books*,

Surgical Clinics and similar reviews are useful in addition to abstract journals such as *Excerpta Medica*.

Attendance at meetings can be a serious problem since most of us will try to keep up both with cancer treatment in general and with one's parent specialty. In general, of course, a symposium for under a hundred active participants will be of great value than the continental or international conferences with thousands of members. The small 'visiting clubs' are particularly valuable, meeting twice a year in different members' centres, giving one an opportunity of getting to know what really goes on in a friend's department. The 'cooperative oncology groups' already referred to can serve the same purpose.

It is hoped that this text book can be an initial source of guidance, that will then need taking further into current work both listened to, and seen, as well as being read from the printed word.

Conclusions

Wider use of existing methods of treatment and better professional organization of cancer management seem as likely to improve overall results in the community as improvements in methods, agents and techniques; at least both are equally important. One should paraphrase Calman and Paul (1978):

> Cancer is almost always treatable and often curable.
> The diagnosis must always be confirmed and its extent re-investigated.
> Evaluation of treatment is continually necessary.
> Full communication is vital at all levels.
> Every symptom is not sinister.

and finally: Guerir quelquefois, soulager souvent, consoler toujours (Cure sometimes, help often, comfort always).

Further reading

General

Ackerman, L.V. and Regato, J.A. Del (1977), *Cancer: Diagnosis, Treatment and Prognosis*. 5th edn, Mosby, St. Louis.

Advances in Cancer Research. (1953 onwards), Academic Press, New York.

Becker, F.F. (ed.) (1975 onwards), *Cancer: a Comprehensive Treatise.* (several volumes), Plenum Press, New York and London.

Cairns, J. (1978), *Cancer: Science and Society*. W.H. Freeman, San Francisco.

Calman, K.C. and Paul, J. (1978), *An Introduction to Cancer Medicine*. MacMillan, London.

Rubin, P. (ed.) (1978), *Clinical Oncology for Medical Students and Physicians*. American Cancer Society, University of Rochester, New York.

Smithers, D.W. (1964), *On Nature of Neoplasia in Man*. Livingstone, London.

Symington, T. and Carter, R.L. (eds) (1976), (Supplement, 1980), *Scientific Foundations of Oncology*. Heinemann, London.

Year Book of Cancer (annually), Academic Press, New York.

Epidemiology

Schottenfeld, D. (ed.) (1975), *Cancer Epidemiology and Prevention: Current Concepts*. C.C. Thomas, Springfield, Illinois.

Genetics

Schimke, R.N. (1979), *Genetics and Cancer in Man*. Churchill, London.

Immunity

Cochran, A.J. (1978), *Man, Cancer and Immunity*. Academic Press, New York.

Pathology

Evans, R.W. (1978), *Histological Appearances of Tumours*. 3rd edn, Churchill, London.

Willis, R.A. (1979), *Pathology of Tumours*. 5th edn, Butterworths, London.

Atlas of Tumour Pathology (1969 onwards), Second series (Various fascicles), Armed Forces Institute of Pathology, Washington DC, USA.

Surgery

Nealon, T.F. (ed.) (1976), *Management of the Patient with Cancer*. 2nd edn, W.B. Saunders, Philadelphia.

Raven, R.W. (ed.) (1977), *Principles of Surgical Oncology*. Baillière-Tindal, London.

Radiotherapy

Fletcher, G.H. (ed.) (1980), *Textbook of Radiotherapy*. 3rd edn. Lea and Febiger, Philadelphia.

Hall, E.J. (1978), *Radiobiology for the Radiologist*. 2nd edn, Harper and Row, New York.

Moss, W.T., Brand, W.N. and Battifora, H. (1979) *Radiation Oncology*. 5th edn, C.V. Mosby, St. Louis.

Paterson, R. (ed.) (1963), *Textbook of Radiotherapy*. 2nd edn, Arnold, London.

Medical Treatment

Clarysse, A., Kenis, Y. and Mathé, G. (1976), *Cancer Chemotherapy*. Springer-Verlag, Berlin.

Holland, J.F. and Frei, E. (eds) (1980), *Cancer Medicine*. 2edn, Lea and Febiger, Philadelphia.

Horton, J. and Hill, G.J. (1977), *Clinical Oncology*. W.B. Saunders, Philadelphia.

Salmon, S.E. and Jones, S.E. (eds) (1981), *Adjuvant Therapy of Cancer* **III**. Grune and Stratton, New York.

Dermatology

Helm, T. (ed.) (1979), *Cancer Dermatology*. Lea and Febiger; Henry Kimpton, London and New York.

Gynaecology

Bush, R.S. (1979), *Malignancies of the ovary, uterus, and cervix,* Edward Arnold, London.

McGowan, L. (1978), *Gynecologic Oncology*. Appleton-Century-Crofts; Prentice-Hall, London and New York.

Rutledge, F. (ed.) (1976), *Gynecologic Oncology*. Wiley, New York.

Pediatrics

Sutow, W.W., Vietti, T.J. and Fernback, D.J. (eds) (1977), *Clinical Pediatric Oncology*. C.V. Mosby, St. Louis.

References

American Cancer Society (1978), *Cancer Facts and Figures*.

Bonadonna, G., Valagussa, P. and Veronesi, U. (1978), Is adjuvant Therapy altering the cause of breast cancer? *Sem. Oncol.*, **5**, 450–64.

Calman, K.C. and Paul, J. (1978), *An Introduction to Cancer Medicine*. MacMillan, London.

Carter, S.K. (1978), The analysis of adjuvant trials. *Cancer Treat. Rev.*, **5**, 1–5.

Doll, R. (1977), Strategy for detection of cancer hazards to man. *Nature*, **265**, 589–96.

Enstrom, J.E. (1978), Cancer in Mormons. *Cancer*, **42**, 1943–51.

Halnan, K.E. (1973), Cancer – the future. *Br. J. Radiol.*, **46**, 793–8.

Kemp, N.H. and Toms, J. (1979), Cancer statistics 1977, In: *Cancer Research Campaign 56th Annual Report 1978*, 54–65.

Monfardini, S., Brunner, K. and Crowther, D. (1977), *Cancer Chemotherapy Course Manual*, UICC, Geneva.

National Vital Statistics Division and Bureau of the Census (1940), USA.

Scottish Health Service Planning Council, Cancer Programme Planning Group (1980), *Cancer Services in Scotland*, Scottish Home and Health Department, Edinburgh.

Taylor, W.F., Ivins, J.C., Danlin, D.C. and Pritchard, D.J. (1978), Osteogenic sarcoma experience at the Mayo Clinic 1963–1974, In: *Immunotherapy of Cancer: Present Status of Trials in Man* (eds W.D. Terry and D. Windhost), Raven Press, New York, pp. 257–69.

2 The place and scope of surgery

J.L. Boak

A majority of cancers will be seen first by the surgeon and their diagnosis will not always even be suspected until microscopic histological information is available. Surgery will often therefore be the first available, and often the most obvious, form of treatment. The surgeon must be grateful for this valuable opportunity but should certainly accept it with great caution and great care, since his actions may well prove the key to success or failure and could, sometimes unwittingly, prejudice the efforts of his colleagues. Preliminary consultation and discussion with colleagues of all kinds will always be of value, even at the time when there is no more than suspicion of cancer. The military maxim 'Time spent on reconnaissance is seldom wasted' will very much apply. Choice of surgical technique is of great importance for each individual tumour and will be discussed further in the chapters in Part two on clinical practice. This chapter will discuss the very important general principles, to help set the scene.

The surgery of cancer is sometimes represented as a specialist field but the majority of cancer patients are treated by general surgeons or surgeons specializing in special anatomical areas. The presenting symptoms of cancer patients are similar to those of patients with non-malignant conditions but the discovery of a neoplastic lesion tends to invoke a sense of urgency to carry out definitive treatment. While early definitive therapy is obviously desirable it is essential that adequate time be given to careful assessment and investigation of the patient. Histological confirmation of the lesion and evidence of metastatic spread provides some concept of the possible prognosis and suggests the surgical and ancillary therapeutic regimes which might be considered. The definitive treatment to be advised, however, must take into account the patient's age, sex, occupation, social and cultural background together with the prognosis of coexisting disease and the possible physical and psychological morbidity associated with the proposed therapy.

Most cancer patients are referred to surgical clinics and the surgeon plays a key role in ensuring each patient receives correct and efficient primary management. The surgeon's role in the management of cancer might be considered under six headings:

1. Screening and early detection.
2. Relief of acute symptoms.
3. Establishing the diagnosis.
4. Defining the extent of disease.
5. Defining coexisting disease.
6. Definitive treatment.

Screening and early detection

It is reasonable to believe that detection of a malignant lesion at a time when it is small, with minimal local infiltration and no regional or systemic spread, will facilitate efficient treatment and improve the patient's prognosis. To this end screening programmes have investigated normal populations for the commoner cancers.

In general terms the number of cancers detected in screening programmes is low; the process tends to be expensive and may subject patients to unnecessary surgical procedures. The possible value of screening normal populations has yet to be established and a sounder case may be made for periodic screening of high risk populations. Identification of high risk factors in individual patients should suggest they be advised to attend for routine screening procedures and in certain instances prophylactic surgery might be considered advisable.

In this context, the surgeon's main role is to identify those patients who are at increased risk of developing a neoplastic lesion and to arrange the appropriate follow-up programme or prophylactic surgery. It is generally accepted that such conditions as multiple polyposis coli, or long-duration ulcerative colitis, require prophylactic colectomy and other conditions, such as severe atypical epithelial changes in breasts of patients with close family histories of breast cancer, are being considered as indications for offering bilateral subcutaneous mastectomy and prosthesis implantation. As our knowledge of risk factors increases, the scope of this important preventative surgical role may well widen.

Relief of acute symptoms

Varying degrees of anxiety and fear are associated with the cancer patient's symptoms and it is important that comforting reassurance should be given, willingly inviting and answering questions relating to the diagnosis and proposed therapy.

It is unfortunate that many cancers are asymptomatic until haemorrhage, perforation, obstruction, compression, pain or pathological fracture precipitates their presentation as acute surgical emergencies. Under such circumstances, emergency surgical intervention is often indicated and is frequently undertaken without the advantage of full pre-operative investigations by surgeons in training. The general principles of cancer surgery should, however, be strictly observed and while the relief of acute symptoms is the primary aim, every effort should be made to obtain tissue from the primary lesion, associated lymph nodes or organs suspected of possible involvement by metastatic tumour. The site, size and attachments of the primary lesion, state of associated lymph nodes and related organs should be noted and a careful search made for evidence of co-existing disease. It is good discipline to specify in one's operation notes the international TNM classification of the lesion based on the operative findings (see page 9).

Definitive complete excision of primary lesion at the time of the emergency procedure may be justified if such excision is judged to be the correct treatment for the emergency condition and would be indicated whether the lesion proves to be benign or malignant. Before embarking on other extensive or mutilating procedures, however, histological confirmation of the lesion by frozen section is advisable.

If at emergency exploration the neoplastic lesion is thought to be inoperable, consideration should be given to marking the lesion's margins with metal clips possibly facilitating subsequent radiotherapy.

Establishing the diagnosis

Before initiating intensive special investigations or treatment it is essential that every effort be made to establish the definitive diagnosis of cancer by histological examination of a biopsy specimen. Failure to obtain histological confirmation of the diagnosis will inevitably lead to extensive mutilating surgical procedures being performed for inflammatory or benign lesions. It is admitted that certain tumours do not readily lend themselves to biopsy, e.g. proximal colonic cancer, and it is not unusual for the surgeon to proceed on the basis of operative and radiological findings. In experienced hands mistakes in diagnosis are rare, but they do occur, and it is therefore mandatory that histological confirmation of a malignant lesion is obtained when a less extensive surgical procedure would be indicated for a benign lesion at the same site.

Preliminary biopsy of some common tumours has been held to be dangerous on the grounds of increasing dissemination of cancer cells, producing haemorrhage or damaging associated anatomical structures. The evidence for biopsy increasing the dissemination or worsening the prognosis of cancer is mainly anecdotal and cannot constitute a contraindication to preliminary biopsy. Possible haemorrhage or damage to associated anatomical structures must be anticipated and due care exercised in obtaining the biopsy specimen.

Fibreoptic endoscopy has greatly increased the range of neoplasms amenable to pre-operative biopsy and the acceptance of drill, aspiration, needle and punch biopsies has greatly facilitated the efficient investigation and preparation of the patient for definitive surgical procedures.

Defining the extent of disease

The size of the primary lesion and degree of local infiltration constitutes the first step in the definition of the extent of neoplastic disease. On the basis of clinical findings the tumour is designated its international T classification and some judgement as to its operability made.

Clinical assessment of possible regional lymph node involvement is notoriously difficult and particularly inaccurate in patients with early lymph node involvement. In the absence of widespread metastases the degree of regional lymph node involvement is particularly important in assessing the patient's prognosis and deciding definitive therapy. Lymphography and lymphoscintigraphy may prove helpful in assessing regional lymph node involvement but accurate definition of secondary spread to regional lymph nodes at present demands histological verification of lymph node biopsy specimens. Preliminary biopsy of regional lymph nodes is seldom practical and is not widely practised save in routine staging laparotomy for Hodgkin's disease. Random biopsy of axillary (Forest, 1969) or internal mammary nodes (Haagensen and Obeid, 1959) has been advocated in deciding the definitive management of breast cancer, and preliminary lymph node biopsy should perhaps be considered in any situation where the patient's management might be altered if definitive evidence of regional lymph node involvement is available.

The primary surgical management is most frequently changed when evidence of distant metastatic spread is present and such evidence must be carefully sought. A knowledge of the organs or tissues most frequently secondarily involved by particular tumours focuses attention to those areas worthy of intensive investigation. Conventional radiology has been joined by computerized axial tomography, radioisotope scanning and ultrasound as diagnostic methods used in the search for overt and occult metastatic spread but, like conventional radiology, these new methods have limitations and the clinician must remain constantly aware of possible fallacies in their interpretation. The present inaccuracy of defining early occult disease is a great weakness in the management of patients with cancer and it is hoped that continuing research and refinement of the previously mentioned methods together with biochemical estimations of tumour marker substances, e.g. oncofoetal proteins, hydroxyproline and γ-glutamyl transpeptidase, will greatly facilitate the selection of those patients requiring systemic ancillary treatment.

At laparotomy prior to oophorectomy for advanced pre-menopausal breast cancer, performed on the basis of positive bone scans or X-rays, it is not unusual to discover evidence of unsuspected intra-abdominal disease further emphasizing the limitations of existing diagnostic methods. Diagnostic laparotomy is accepted in Hodgkin's disease as a necessary step in a patient's management and is also advocated as a 'second look' procedure in certain centres to detect recurrent disease following gastrointestinal resections. Such procedures frequently permit resection of early recurrent tumour either locally in the gastrointestinal tract or in the liver.

Laparotomy or laparoscopy are acceptable diagnostic procedures and may be considered in any situation where intra-abdominal metastatic deposits would contraindicate extensive local surgery or indicate adjuvant therapy to be necessary. It should be performed routinely for all abdominal malignancies but is also advocated for excluding occult intraperitoneal, lumboaortic or hepatic metastasis before considering hemipelvectomy for sarcoma, pneumonectomy for bronchial carcinoma and oesophagectomy for oesophageal carcinoma. Demonstration of such occult intra-abdominal spread would equally contraindicate radical surgery for breast, melanoma and other malignancies but laparotomy is not frequently performed simply as a staging procedure.

Careful and enthusiastic attempts to define the extent of neoplastic disease are essential to correct patient management but it should be recognized that clinical assessment and special investigations are fraught with pitfalls of fallacy and inaccuracy. It is frequently only after full histological examination of a resected specimen that the true extent of local tumour and lymph node involvement may be realized. Our present diagnostic methods allow identification of those patients with grossly advanced disease but do not allow confident staging of those patients with purely local disease curable by conservative local surgery or with minimal spread of tumour curable by extended surgery or energetic ancillary therapy.

Defining coexisting disease

Cancer increases in frequency with age reaching a peak between the sixth and seventh decade, and therefore occurs in a population most frequently afflicted with other maladies – particularly ischaemic heart, cerebral and peripheral vascular disease. Old age and debility do not usually constitute contraindications to surgery for emergency conditions but when considered in association with the natural history of the patient's neoplastic lesion may suggest a conservative approach is worthy of consideration.

The possibility of multiple or multicentric tumours should be considered and appropriate investigations carried out. A thorough assessment of coexisting conditions is essential before final decisions are made on definitive treatment, and it is at this stage that consultation with colleagues is very helpful.

Definitive treatment

When the diagnosis has been established and, as far as possible, the extent of disease defined, a final decision may be reached on possible definitive therapy. Curative surgical therapy aims to completely extirpate all existing tumour but, when the degree of spread precludes such surgery, palliative procedures attempt to allay symptoms and improve the quality of remaining life.

Curative surgery

Complete excision of all tumour requires careful assessment and planning. The aim is to excise the neoplastic lesion with a wide margin of normal surrounding tissue and all involved regional lymph nodes. In the absence of pre-existing occult metastatic deposits such a procedure carefully performed, avoiding local implantation or dissemination of tumour cells should provide the patient with a guaranteed cure.

How wide the area of normal tissue excised around a tumour should be is debatable. Arbitrary margins tend to be defined for individual tumours and are generally decided on the basis of anatomical and surgical convenience with consideration for the tumour's anticipated pattern of spread and probability of it to recur locally. While adequate local treatment is essential, a too radical approach excising excessive uninvolved normal tissue will do little to improve the prognosis and much to increase the morbidity of the procedure.

Excision of uninvolved lymph nodes cannot be expected to benefit the patient. Extension of a surgical procedure to include all regional lymph nodes can only be justified if such extended excision is likely to remove all residual tumour or where the histological verification of the degree of lymph node involvement will alter the patient's subsequent management. Experience with breast cancer and malignant melanoma has demonstrated no improvement in mortality by extending surgical procedures to include apparently uninvolved regional lymph nodes and much morbidity is avoided by adopting a watch policy treating regional nodes only when their progressive enlargement indicates metastatic involvement.

Failure of current pre-operative diagnostic methods to confidently identify all those patients who might be curable by conservative local surgery undoubtedly leads to more extensive procedures being performed than might be strictly necessary. Adequate wide local excision of a primary tumour frequently offers the best hope of cure for many solid tumours but the dividing line between being adequate and being excessively radical is often difficult to define.

Palliative surgery

Palliative surgery aims to relieve troublesome symptoms, prevent complications and prolong a life of improved quality. The majority of clinical cancers present late in their biological life with overt or occult metastatic foci already established and it should be conceded that most surgical procedures are probably palliative. The multidisciplinary approach to cancer therapy recognizes this fact and the combination of palliative surgery with radiotherapy and chemotherapy attempts to improve and prolong palliation or, in a few instances, achieve a cure.

There is much less justification for a radical approach to palliative surgery. Sound judgement and experience are necessary in the selection of the best palliative procedure but are probably most essential in deciding when not to interfere at all, thus avoiding unnecessary morbidity, inflicting and prolonging suffering in the name of palliation.

Palliative resection

Total resection of the primary tumour is frequently the best palliative procedure in certain cancers, e.g. colorectal and other gastrointestinal tumours. Successful removal of a locally advanced primary tumour occasionally including parts of other adherent or involved structures will frequently relieve or avoid particularly unpleasant complications. The difficulty of distinguishing macroscopically between inflammatory and neoplastic infiltratory changes, however, cannot be over emphasized. Histological confirmation of the extent of the neoplastic disease is important and it should be recognized that the attempted complete eradication of the disease by surgery is not feasible and is certainly not a matter of immediate urgency. Much morbidity and, in some cases, even mutilation can be avoided when a two-stage procedure is judged possible. The temporary colostomy or other bypass procedure performed after full laparotomy and biopsy, or conservative local excision of the main primary lesion, provides useful information regarding the tumour grade, probable extent of spread and above all, provides time for the resolution of associated inflammatory changes rendering any subsequent planned procedure technically simpler.

Failure to recognize and act on these principles may provide the personal satisfaction of having achieved the surgical goal in one operation but will inevitably lead to unnecessary complications and excision of non-cancerous lesions and organs. Total cystectomy and abdominoperineal resection of rectum have, and will probably continue to be occasionally performed for inflammatory or benign disease because a cavalier urgent approach rather than a patient, considered attitude of judgement is maintained during surgery.

It is important that the surgeon having gathered all possible relevant information has a clear concept of what might be achieved by a palliative procedure and consults with his colleagues in other disciplines regarding their views on proposed surgical procedures which may facilitate subsequent radio- or chemotherapeutic regimes. Palliative resection reducing tumour bulk, ligation of the hepatic artery, cannulation of the umbilical artery or local injection of 50% alcohol as a coeliac plexus block may be indicated in certain instances.

Regression of distant metastasis has been recorded following resection of primary choriocarcinoma (Baird, 1957), neuroblastoma (Koop *et al.*, 1955) and renal carcinoma (Everson and Cole, 1966) but metastases more usually only show some response to hormonal or other systemic therapy.

Palliative resection of localized metastatic deposits may occasionally be considered when the primary disease site is controlled and there is no evidence of metastasis to other organs. The results of surgical resection for pulmonary metastasis are variable and unpredictable. It would seem prudent only to consider pulmonary resection in patients with a solitary metastasis confined to one lung after a long disease-free interval (Alexander and Haight, 1947). Other reports, however, indicate that surgical resection for multiple and even bilateral lesions give favourable results (Thomford *et al.*, 1965; Holmes *et al.*, 1977).

Hepatic metastases carry a gloomy prognosis: 34% of patients with colorectal cancer, 13% with gastric and pancreatic cancer and 10% with gall bladder cancer, survive 6 months following detection of hepatic secondaries. At 12 months the survival changes to 18%, 9%, 3% and 0% (Bengmark *et al.*, 1970). Five year survivals are only obtained following surgical excision (Forster, 1970; McKenzie and Wilson, 1970), and as for pulmonary lesions, a more favourable prognosis is associated with small, solitary lesions occurring after a long disease-free interval.

Metastases to the central nervous system produce devastating neurological symptoms and the surgical excision of solitary intracranial metastatic lesions may afford many months of meaningful prolongation of life in carefully selected patients (Ranohoff, 1975). In general, the results of surgical extirpation of intracerebral metastasis are similar to radiotherapy and the latter is associated with lower morbidity.

Palliative bypass surgery
When palliative resection of tumours obstructing the gastrointestinal, biliary or renal tract is not feasible or advisable then useful palliation is frequently obtained by a simple bypass procedure. Bypass of biliary and gastrointestinal obstructions by assessory anastomotic techniques or occasionally by intubation, relieve troublesome symptoms and are greatly appreciated by many patients.

Small bowel obstruction is a common entity with only 10–20% of cases being related to malignancy (Daris and Sperling, 1969; Maver, 1977). Primary tumours of the small intestine are rare representing 1–3% of gastrointestinal tumours and the majority of obstructing lesions are secondary to primary lesions in colorectum (44.8%), ovary (16.8%), cervix (14.6%) or other sites (23.8%) (Glass and LeDuc, 1973).

Operative mortality in patients with abdominal carcinomatosis approaches 25% and a reasonable period of conservative gastrointestinal suction and electrolyte replacement therapy is indicated before embarking on emergency surgery. The palliative procedure of choice depends on the operative findings but there is general agreement that in coexisting large and small bowel disease, colostomy should be avoided for as long as possible; enteroanastomosis is preferable to dissecting free individual small bowel loops; the maximal length of small bowel should be preserved and if possible the

ileocaecal valve should not be sacrificed (Barnett, 1976).

Intestinal obstruction developing in a patient known to have carcinoma must not be assumed to be due to incurable recurrence; 25% of such patients (Ketcham, 1970) were found to have no residual tumour or a new primary as the cause for obstruction and 40% achieved long term palliation following surgery. Involvement of the small bowel by secondary tumour, however, is associated with an average survival of only 11 months (Barnett, 1976).

Colorectal obstruction occurs about half as frequently as small bowel obstruction but is caused by malignant lesions four times as frequently as by other causes. Treatment is surgical, delayed only to allow fluid and electrolyte resuscitation since perforation is associated with delay and increases operative mortality. 50% of obstructing colonic carcinomas are judged to be curable at the time of resection but in all major reported series the 5-year survival rate is approximately 20%.

The treatment of biliary obstruction is surgical but when due to a malignant lesion the possibility of performing a curative procedure is slight. Primary intrahepatic tumours account for less than 3% of biliary duct obstruction due to malignancy and the most common is intrahepatic biliary duct carcinoma. 75% of extrahepatic neoplastic biliary tract obstruction occurs in the periampullary region. More than 80% of these are carcinoma of the pancreas and 15% arise in the bile ducts (Williams *et al.*, 1960). Gall bladder carcinoma is commoner than primary biliary duct carcinoma but accounts for only 8% of cases presenting with neoplastic biliary obstruction. Resection of intrahepatic primary lesions is seldom technically feasible. Intrahepatic cholangiojejunostomy or permanent indwelling shunt may provide an average survival of some 8–12 months.

The prognosis for non-periampullary extrahepatic lesions is equally poor. Resectable primary bile duct carcinomas are associated with only a 4% 3-year survival and the average survival after choledochojejunostomy is less than 12 months (Yarborough, 1973). Periampullary lesions are more likely to be substantially benefited by surgery. Radical pancreaticoduodenectomy is particularly favoured in common bile duct (25% 5-year survival), ampulla of vater (32% 5-year survival) and duodenal (41% 5-year survival) lesions but in carcinoma of the pancreas affords only a 12.5% 5-year survival. Resection rates, however, vary greatly depending on the experience and judgement of the surgeon.

Oesophageal carcinoma has its peak incidence in the eighth decade and while operability may reach 67% only 45% prove resectable. In experienced hands operative mortality ranges from 6.2% for gastro-oesophageal growth to 30.8% for middle third growths (McKeown, 1974). Death during the first post-operative year however accounts for more than 50% of patients having lower third and 35.2% middle third neoplasms resected. Five-year survival ranges from 11 to 23.5% (Gunnlaugsson *et al.*, 1970; Nakayama, 1959; McKeown, 1974).

Recurrent and unresectable oesophageal carcinomas pose the distressing problems associated with oesophageal obstruction and in such cases dilatation and intubation of the strictured oesophagus offers the best palliation (Mousseau *et al.*, 1956; Celestin, 1959). Gastrostomy and jejunostomy do not prevent aspiration of secretions and are in themselves a poor choice of palliative procedure. Palliative intubation is associated with an operative mortality of less than 10% and a 73% successful alleviation of symptoms has been reported (Duvoisin *et al.*, 1967).

Gastroduodenal obstruction due to gastric carcinoma is a late feature of this disease but palliative sub-total resection is the preferred palliative procedure. Gastroenterostomy is a less desirable alternative and gastrostomy should not be considered.

Ureteric obstruction may be relieved by a choice of ureter transplantation procedures but it is important to consider that bilateral ureteric obstruction leads to a fairly rapid and painless demise. In performing a ureteric bypass procedure it must be ensured one is not simply substituting a more unpleasant prolonged terminal phase to the illness. Extension of pelvic or retroperitoneal malignancy to involve the ureter is usually a very late event. Brin *et al.* (1975) report a series of 47 patients undergoing ileal loop diversion for bilateral ureteric obstruction for pelvic tumour: 59% left hospital with only 50% survival at 3 months and only 22.7% being alive at 6 months. Patients with prostatic carcinoma made up the majority of patients surviving for 6 months.

Endocrine ablation

Certain tumours may be hormone-dependent and alteration of the host's hormonal levels may influence the tumour's growth. Endocrine ablation is most frequently practised in the palliative treatment of recurrent or advanced pre-menopausal breast cancer and those patients most likely to benefit from bilateral oophorectomy, adrenalectomy or hypophysectomy may be selected by estimating hormone receptor levels in the primary or secondary tumour (Chapter 6).

Bilateral orchiectomy frequently produces long remissions in patients with prostatic cancer and is frequently advocated as the palliative procedure of choice in this disease (Chapter 24).

Surgical relief of pain

Some care must be taken in establishing that pain is due to malignancy and not to some readily remediable condition such as local abscess or other complication of previous therapy. Cancer pain tends to be localized, gradually increasing in severity and by virtue of its duration frequently creates difficulty in management. The majority of patients are usually managed with analgesic drugs but many would benefit from palliative pain relieving procedures. Local injection of 50% alcohol into the coeliac plexus (Bridenbaugh *et al.*, 1964; Moore, 1965) relieves the pain of recurrent or inoperable carcinoma of stomach, pancreas, liver and biliary tree. Sub-arachnoid block with solutions of phenol (Gerbershagen *et al.*, 1972), chlorocresol (Maher, 1963) or alcohol (Hay, 1962) have all been reported to provide useful relief of prolonged pain. Similarly peripheral nerve block by local injection of phenol or alcohol may be employed in the localized pain of head and neck cancers not readily amenable to other blocking procedures (Mousel, 1967; DeKrey *et al.*, 1967) or rib metastasis (Riding and Lipton, 1973).

Spinothalamic cordotomy provides the most efficient method of relieving intractable pain and was first performed by Martin in 1911 (Spiller and Martin, 1912). Section of the anterolateral quadrant of the spinal cord interrupts pain and temperature appreciation for the contralateral side of the body inferior to the lesion and is particularly useful for intractable pain in the thoracoabdominal and pelvic areas.

Adequate relief of pain is reported in 70–80% of cases but the 20% incidence of urinary retention and other complications require careful selection of patients. The necessity for a major surgical procedure to perform cordotomy is largely being circumvented by the introduction of percutaneous procedures for interrupting the spinothalamic tracts (Mullan *et al.*, 1963; Rosomoff *et al.*, 1965; Lipton, 1968) and thus pain relief may be offered to patients who might otherwise be unsuitable for general anaesthesia and further surgery.

Extensive intracranial surgery in the debilitated cancer patient is associated with high morbidity and mortality, but spinothalamic interruption in the brain stem or mid-brain may control upper extremity and head and neck pain.

Sensory rhizotomy – the division of posterior spinal nerve roots – may be performed as an alternative to local blocking procedures and is particularly applicable to chest, abdominal and certain selected cases of pain in extremities (White, 1966).

Relief of spinal cord compression

Some patients with slow growing lesions may survive for prolonged periods following metastatic invasion of the spinal cord (Jameson, 1974) and it is essential that the diagnosis, evaluation and emergency treatment be completed expeditiously if permanent neurological sequelae are to be prevented.

The level of cord compression, nature of primary tumour, speed of onset, degree and duration of symptomatology determine the appropriate treatment. Following clinical and radiological confirmation of the diagnosis, high dose corticosteroid therapy should be instituted and local radiotherapy may be administered reserving surgery for those patients failing to show a rapid response. Rapidly progressing symptoms, severe neurological symptoms or myelographically demonstrated complete block are indications for early surgical treatment. Short duration paralysis warrants laminectomy as an emergency procedure. Operative mortality from laminectomy ranges from 6 to 13% depending on patient selection (Törmä, 1957; White *et al.*, 1971; Brice and McKissock, 1965) and the best prognostic indicator for functional neurological recovery is the pre-treatment status. 60% of patients ambulatory before therapy remain so. 35% of pre-operatively paretic patients achieve subsequent mobility and only 7% of paraplegic patients recover sufficiently to get about (Bruckman and Bloomer, 1978).

Plastic and reconstructive surgery

Following mutilating surgical procedures of the head and neck skilled plastic surgical management can do much to improve the appearance and general well-being of the patient. For many skin cancers careful planning of the pattern of skin excision and subsequent reconstruction of the defect is required. Diligence and meticulous technique are obligatory to avoid possible implantation of neoplastic cells into donor sites and when technically feasible free skin grafts are usually preferred to flaps and tube reconstruction.

In routine excision biopsy procedures of head, neck and breast, it is of particular importance to plan incisions and close the wound meticulously, producing the best possible scar and avoiding disfigurement. The majority of lesions biopsied in these sites are benign and will require no further surgery. The subsequent management of neoplastic lesions usually allows excision of the biopsy scar and ugly scars facilitating wide excision biopsy should be avoided whenever possible. An increasing number of patients are requesting breast reconstruction following mastectomy for carcinoma. Approximately 80% of patients developing local skin recurrence following mastectomy do so within two years (Karabali-Dalamaga *et al.*, 1978) and delayed prosthesis implantation is practised in some centres. Cosmetic results are only acceptable when the patient wears a bra or swimming costume.

Sub-cutaneous mastectomy and immediate reconstruction has been advocated in selected cases of established breast carcinoma, but the inaccuracy of existing methods to pre-operatively assess the extent of the disease perhaps renders this a hazardous procedure. A stronger case might be made for such conservative reconstructive surgery being offered prophylactically to high risk patients with severe histologically confined epithelial changes or carcinoma *in situ*.

Thermal knives in cancer surgery

The traditional surgical scalpel continues to be the instrument of choice in cancer surgery but the use of thermal knives or probes are under continuing investigation. Electrosurgery or diathermy was introduced into surgical procedures towards the end of the nineteenth century and prominent advantages claimed included speedier operations, less blood loss, fewer ligatures acting as foreign bodies and less oozing of serum and lymph from wounds. By the 1930s electrosurgery had gained wide acceptance in many fields. Improved technology now enables endoscopic excision biopsy and fulguration to be used routinely in the management of many tumours with a great deal of safety. More recently, investigators have been studying the use of other thermal knives, *viz.* cryosurgical probes, CO_2 lasers and plasma scalpels.

Cryosurgical techniques destroying tissue by local freezing are being increasingly advocated as a worthwhile palliative procedure in head and neck, prostatic, skin, breast and rectal cancers. As with diathermy fulguration it is claimed that useful palliation of local pain, reduction of tumour bulk, offensive discharges and capillary bleeding can be achieved (Cahan 1972).

The use of the CO_2 laser in cancer surgery has been enthusiastically acclaimed by Kaplan (1976) but others are more guarded in their appraisals. The newer plasma scalpel utilizing a jet of highly ionized argon to cut and coagulate tissues is presently being perfected and should shortly be available for wider clinical trials (Glover *et al.*, 1978).

It is difficult to see that these newer modalities will offer much more to cancer surgery than has already been achieved by electrosurgery, but final judgement must await wider experience in their use and with further technological improvements it is possible that each type of thermal knife may come to have a proper but particular role in cancer surgery.

Transplantation surgery in cancer

The risk of transplanting occult neoplastic foci disqualifies the cancer patient from acting as a live or cadaveric donor of tissues and organs. This risk does not, however, apply to potential donors with intracerebral tumours which do not metastasize outside the skull nor to transplanting the corneas of cancer patients. Renal homotransplant recipients have developed donor type cancer after receiving kidneys from donors suffering from carcinoma of bronchus (Martin *et al.*, 1965), larynx (McPhaul and McIntosh, 1965), kidney (Hume, 1966), and thyroid (Muiznieks *et al.*, 1968). The growth of transplanted neoplastic cells is facilitated by the immunosuppressive regime necessary to permit homograft survival but is likely to regress completely following removal of the kidney and cessation of immunotherapy (Wilson *et al.*, 1968).

The replacement of cancerous organs by homotransplantation is an attractive concept and would be particularly applicable to cancers effecting a solitary kidney or liver. Poor results obtained in treating primary hepatic and intrahepatic biliary cancers has determined that this vital, unpaired organ's complete excision and replacement by transplantation should receive most investigation. Results are, however, extremely disappointing since all patients develop recurrent cancer and survival does not exceed 18 months (Starzl *et al.*, 1969). Lung cancer has been treated by pulmonary homotransplantation but again no long-term survivors have been obtained (Hardy *et al.*, 1963).

As in conventional curative surgery success depends on the complete removal of all neoplastic cells with the primary excision procedure. The growth of residual neoplastic foci will probably always be facilitated by non-specific immunotherapeutic regimes and the results of cancerous organ replacement by transplantation will remain disappointing.

When a solitary kidney is excised for renal or pelviureteric cancer the patient may subsequently be maintained on haemodialysis for a prolonged period confirming whether or not the primary surgery has been curative. In such rare cases renal transplantation might be considered. Successful renal homotransplantation has been reported in a patient following resection of renal tumour (Woodruff *et al.*, 1969) but without the development of successful artificial live machines capable of maintaining patients for long periods, more specific immunosuppressive regimes and accurate methods defining the extent of neoplastic disease, it is difficult to foresee a major role for organ transplantation in cancer therapy (*Lancet*, 1969). This view must however be considered in association with the argument that homotransplantation offers the only possible hope of cure in certain young patients with primary hepatomas (Calne, 1969).

Conclusion

Surgery occupies a key role in the prophylaxis, diagnosis and treatment of cancer but the nature of the disease and uncertainty of its extent and aggressiveness requires a multidisciplinary approach. Constant appraisal of personal diagnostic accuracy, operative decision-making and performance, with ability and willingness to modify techniques is essential if advances are to be made in the successful management of the cancer patient. Dogma and anecdotal evidence frequently influence surgical decisions. Enthusiasm frequently accompanies the application of new methods or ideas. If cancer therapy is to achieve more cures and prolonged life of acceptable quality for more patients, it is essential that critical appraisal of all possible treatment modalities are fairly considered and, if used, fairly assessed on a sound scientifically controlled basis.

References

Alexander, J. and Haight, C. (1947), Pulmonary resection for solitary metastatic sarcomas and carcinomas. *Surgery Gynec. Obstet.*, **85**, 129.

Baird, D. (1957), *Combined Textbook of Obstetrics and Gynaecology*. E. and S. Livingstone, Edinburgh, p. 779.

Barnett, W.O. (1976), Problems in abdominal surgery. VI Intestinal obstruction from peritoneal carcinomatosis. *J. Mississippi State Med. Ass.*, **17**, 325.

Bengmark, S. *et al.* (1970), Treatment of hepatic tumours. *Digestion*, **3**, 309.

Brice, J. and McKissock, W. (1965), Surgical treatment of malignant extradural spinal tumours. *Br. Med. J.*, **2**, 1341.

Bridenbaugh, L.D., Moore, D.C. and Campbell, D.D. (1964), Management of upper abdominal cancer pain. *J. Am. Med. Ass.*, **190**, 877.

Brin, E.N., Schiff, M. and Weiss, R.M. (1975), Palliative urinary diversion for pelvic malignancy. *J. Urol.*, **113**, 619.

Bruckman, J.E. and Bloomer, W.D. (1978), Management of spinal cord compression. *Semin. Oncol.*, **5**, 135.

Cahan, W.G. (1972), The cryosurgical management of massive recurrent cancer. *Proc. Int. Cong. Cryosurg.* (Vienna), p. 295.

Calne, R.Y. (1969), Immunosuppression and cancer. *Lancet*, **i**, 625.

Celestin, L.R. (1959), Permanent intubation in

inoperable cancer of the oesophagus and cardia. *Ann. R. Coll. Surg.*, **25**, 165.

Daris, S.E. and Sperling, L. (1969), Obstruction of the small intestine. *Arch. Surg.*, **99**, 424.

DeKrey, J.A., Spragne, A.Y., Curanah, H. and Knox, P.R. (1967), Therapeutic blocks for intractable pain. *Anaesth. Analg. Curr. Res.*, **46**, 636.

Duvoisin, G.E., Ellis, F.H. and Payne, W.S. (1967), The value of palliative prosthesis in malignant lesions of the oesophagus. *Surg. Clinics N. Amer.*, **47**, 827.

Everson, T.C. and Cole, N.H. (1966), *Spontaneous regression of cancer.* W.B. Saunders, Philadelphia.

Forest, A.P. (1969), Points in the practical management of breast cancer. *Br. J. Surg.*, **56**, 782.

Forster, J.H. (1970), Survival after liver resection for cancer. *Cancer*, **26**, 493.

Gerbershagen, J.U., Baar, H.A. and Kreuscher, H. (1972), Langzeit nerv blockaden zur behandlung schwerer schnerzzurstande. *Anaesthesist*, **21**, 112.

Glass, R.L. and LeDuc, R.J. (1973), Small intestine obstruction from peritoneal metastasis. *Am. J. Surg.*, **125**, 316.

Glover, J.L., Bendick, P.J. and Link, W.J. (1978), The use of thermal knives in surgery. *Curr. Prob. Surg.*, **1**, 1.

Gunnlaugsson, G.H., Wychalis, A.R., Roland, C. and Ellis, F.H. (1970), Analysis of the records of 1,657 patients with carcinoma of the oesophagus and cardia of the stomach. *Surg., Gynec. Obstet.*, **130**, 997.

Haagensen, C.D. and Obeid, S.T. (1959), Biopsy of the apex of the axilla in carcinoma of the breast. *Ann. Surg.*, **149**, 149.

Hardy, J.D., Webb, W.R., Dalton, M.L. and Walker, G. (1963), Lung homotransplantation in man. *J. Am. Med. Ass.*, **186**, 1065.

Hay, R.C. (1962), Subarachnoid block in the control of intractable pain. *Anaesth. Analg. Curr. Res.*, **41**, 12.

Holmes, E.C., Ramming, K.P., Eilber, F.R. and Norton, D.L. (1977), The surgical management of pulmonary metastasis. *Sem. Oncol.*, **1**, 65.

Hume, D.M. (1966), Progress in clinical renal homotransplantation. *Adv. Surg.*, **2**, (ed. C.E. Wilch) Chicago Year Book. Med. Pub., p. 419.

Jameson, R.M. (1974), Prolonged survival in paraplegia due to metastatic spinal tumours. *Lancet*, **1**, 1209.

Kaplan, I. (ed.) (1976), *Laser Surgery.* Jerusalem Academic Press, Jerusalem.

Karabali-Dalamaga, S. *et al.* (1978), Natural history and prognosis of recurrent breast cancer. *Br. Med. J.*, **2**, 730.

Ketcham, A.S. (1970), Modern trends in the prevention of cancer recurrence. In: *Cancer Problems in*

Surgery: Surgical Oncology, Ben. H. Huber Pub.

Koop, C.E., Kiesewetter, W.B. and Horn, R.C. (1955), Neuroblastoma in childhood survival after major surgical treatment to the tumour. *Surgery*, **38**, 272.

Leading article (1969), Immunosuppression and cancer. *Lancet*, **1**, 505.

Lipton, S. (1968), Percutaneous electrical cardotomy in relief of intractable pain. *Br. Med. J.*, **2**, 210.

Maher, R.M. (1963), Intratheral chlorocresol in the treatment of pain in cancer. *Lancet*, **1**, 965.

Martin, D.C., Rubini, M. and Rosen, V.J. (1965), Cadaveric renal homotransplantation with inadvertent transplantation of carcinoma. *J. Am. Med. Ass.*, **192**, 752.

Maver, H.G. (1977), Small bowel obstruction in a community hospital. *Minnesota Med.*, **60**, 273.

McKenzie, A.D. and Wilson, J.W. (1970), Hepatic resection for blood bone metastasis from large bowel cancer. *Can. J. Surg.*, **13**, 159.

McKeown, K.C. (1974), Surgical treatment of carcinoma of the oesophagus. *Proc. Roy. Soc. Med.*, **67**, 389.

McPhaul, J.J. and McIntosh, D.A. (1965), Tissue transplantation still vexes. *New Engl. J. Med.*, **272**, 105.

Moore, D.C. (1965), *Regional Block,* 4th edn, Thomas, Springfield, Illinois.

Mousel, L.H. (1967), Treatment of intractable pain of the head and neck. *Anaesth. Analg. Curr. Res.*, **46**, 705.

Mousseau, M., Le Forestier, J., Barbin, J. and Hardy, M. (1956), Place de l'intubation a demeure dans le traitment palliatif du cancer de l'oesophage. *Arch. Malad. appar. Malad. Nutrit.*, **45**, 208.

Muiznieks, H.W., Berg, J.W., Lawrence, W. and Randall, H.T. (1968), Suitability of donor kidneys from patients with cancer. *Surgery*, **64**, 871.

Mullan, S. (1971), Percutaneous cordotomy. *J. Neurosurg.*, **35**, 360.

Mullan, S. *et al.* (1963), Percutaneous interruption of spinal pain tracts by means of a strontium-90 needle. *J. Neurosurg.*, **20**, 931.

Nakayama, K. (1959), Statistical review of five-year survivals after surgery for carcinoma of the oesophagus and cardiac portions of the stomach. *Surgery*, **45**, 883.

Ranohoff, J. (1975), Surgical management of metastatic tumours. *Sem. Oncol.*, **1**, 21.

Riding, J.E. and Lipton, S. (1973), Relief of pain. *Recent Adv. Surg.*, **8**, (ed. S. Taylor), Churchill Livingstone, p. 1.

Rosomoff, H.L., Carrol, F., Brown, J. and Sheptak, P. (1965), Percutaneous radiofrequency cervical cordotomy technique. *J. Neurosurg.*, **23**, 639.

Spiller, W.G. and Martin, E. (1912), The treatment of

persistent pain of organic origin in the lower part of the body by division of the anterolateral column of the spinal cord. *J. Am. Med. Ass.*, **58**, 1489.

Starzl, T.E. *et al.* (1969), Orthotopic liver transplantation in man. *Transplant. Proc.*, **1**, 216.

Thomford, N.R., Wollner, L.B. and Clugett, O.T. (1965), The surgical treatment of metastatic tumours in the lungs. *J. Thorac. Cardiovasc. Surg.*, **49**, 357.

Törmä, T. (1957), Malignant tumours of the spine and extradural space. A study based on 250 histologically verified cases. *Acta chir. Scand.* (Suppl), **225**, 1.

White, J.C. (1966), Posterior rhizotomy, a possible substitute for cordotomy in otherwise intractable neuralgias of the trunk and extremities of non-malignant origin, *Clin. Neurosurg.*, **13**, 20.

White, W.A., Patterson, R.H. and Bergland, R.M. (1971), Role of surgery in the treatment of spinal cord compression by metastatic neoplasms. *Cancer*, **27**, 558.

Williams, R.D., Elliot, D.W. and Zollinger, R.N. (1960), Surgery for malignant jaundice. *Arch. Surg.*, **80**, 992.

Wilson, R.E. *et al.* (1968), Immunological investigation of human cancer transplanted with renal homograft. *New Engl. J. Med.*, **278**, 479.

Woodruff, M.F.A., Rolan, B., Robson, J.S. and MacDonald, M.K. (1969), Renal transplantation in man. *Lancet*, **1**, 6.

Yarborough, D.R. (1973), Primary carcinoma of the extrahepatic bile ducts. *Am. J. Surg.*, **125**, 723.

3 Radiation biology – the basis of radiotherapy

A.H.W. Nias

Soon after the discovery of X-rays by Roentgen in 1895, their biological effects began to be apparent. Within four months there came a report of hair loss in a radiation worker and this led to the logical step of using X-rays in the treatment of a benign hairy naevus in 1897. Thus, within two years of their discovery, X-rays had been shown not only to be useful in the treatment of abnormal tissue but also to produce unacceptable changes in normal tissue. The problem of devising a clinically acceptable therapeutic ratio between normal and tumour tissue damage soon began to be solved by experience; namely, to deliver the radiation dosage in a number of exposures rather than one single treatment. Fractionated radiotherapy, as we know it today, was described in 1922 by Regaud and his colleagues in France where, of course, Becquerel and Curie had earlier discovered the radioactive properties of uranium and radium in 1896.

During the 85 and more years since those discoveries, radiotherapy has evolved into one of the most scientific branches of medicine and has established its role as the second line of attack, after surgery, in the treatment of primary cancers.

In this chapter the biological effects of ionizing radiation will be described to provide the scientific basis of radiotherapy. In order to devise a treatment schedule which delivers the maximum damage to the tumour, the clinician needs to know precisely how such a radiation schedule will damage the normal tissues. As in all branches of medicine there is a degree of risk which must be accepted but the radiotherapist has the advantage of knowing this risk from many years of experience with orthodox schedules. The science of radiobiology has helped to explain these empirical findings. Use of the various radiobiological principles enables new schedules to be devised which may improve the therapeutic ratio.

Two words need to be defined, to assist this understanding. From the clinician's point of view the effect of a radiation dose schedule will first be seen as some form of response in the treated area. Hopefully, this will show itself as a shrinkage of the tumour volume without too much reaction of the normal tissue. If palliation is all that can be achieved then such shrinkage is eventually followed by recurrent growth. The time scale of the shrinkage and possible recurrence depends upon the kinetics of the particular cell population (e.g. rapid with a lymphoma; slow with a basal cell carcinoma). This is *radioresponsiveness;* but it does not give a direct indication of the *radiosensitivity* of the tumour. The sensitivity of a cell population can only be measured by the number of cells which do not survive a radiation dosage. The extent of this cell killing will determine if the tumour can be cured.

The section on cell survival curves will show how radiosensitivity is determined. Other sections will show the variety of patterns of radioresponsiveness of normal tissues and tumours. Before that, the mode of action of radiation will be described in terms of the biophysical and biological mechanisms.

Biophysical events

The reason why X-rays are so damaging to tissues is quite simply because of their very short wavelength. Other electromagnetic radiations ranging from radio waves at the longest wavelength through visible light to ultraviolet light at the shortest extreme have varied biological effects, but none produce ionization. This is the removal of an electron from its atom or molecule as illustrated in Fig. 3.1, which shows the neutrons (n) and protons (p^+) that form the nucleus of an atom, together with the planetary electrons (e^-), one of which is shown to have been ejected by an incident photon (or packet of radiation energy).

This process of ionization should not be confused with the ionized state in which many molecules in aqueous solution exist under normal chemical conditions. This state is due to simple dissociation into positively and negatively charged ions which coexist in stable equilibrium (e.g. water dissociates into H^+ and OH^- ions). By contrast, the consequence of X-irradiation is the formation of pairs of free radical ions which are *not* in equilibrium. Instead of simple dissociation, water is ionized into H_2O^+ ions and free electrons, e^-. Such a free electron is shown in Fig. 3.1. These free radical ions are extremely unstable and quickly form neutral free radicals which are uncharged atoms or molecules with an unpaired electron in the outer orbit. So the very unstable H_2O^+ forms H^+ and $OH^.$ (where the dot signifies an unpaired electron). Although such free radicals are more stable, they are still very reactive. Both free radical ions and the resultant free radicals disrupt normal molecular structures and damage the biological target. This, then, is the primary mode of action of ionizing radiation. The most important free radicals have been mentioned in this paragraph, namely $OH^.$ and e^- aq. In the presence of water (omnipresent in biological systems) the free electrons (e^-) become hydrated and are called aqueous electrons, or e^-aq. They are reducing free radicals while $OH^.$ radicals are oxidative. The effect of oxygen will be shown to be very important in this radiobiology chapter and this is why it is necessary to appreciate at this stage that $OH^.$ radicals tend to produce more damage at the molecular level. Anything like oxygen that swings the

radiation chemical competition in favour of the oxidative pathway will therefore be more damaging to the biological target. Likewise, any agent that depletes the concentration of reducing radicals (like the nitro-imidazole compound, misonidazole, which is electron-affinic) will also increase the biological effect of radiation. On the other hand agents which are reducing, like -SH compounds, will tend to have a radio-protective effect. This is presumed to be the mode of action of WR–2721 (Yuhas, 1980) which is believed to protect normal tissues but not tumours. Most agents which are radioprotective (like cysteamine) or radio-sensitizing (like misonidazole) are toxic at the dose level required to be effective in man. The only non-toxic sensitizing agent is oxygen. It is also important to understand that such agents must be present at the time the radiation dose is delivered. The drugs may still be effective if given some time beforehand but there will be no action at all if they are given even a few microseconds after the end of the radiation dose.

Timing is also known to be important when certain cancer chemotherapy agents are used in conjunction with radiotherapy. This sort of combination relies upon secondary biochemical interactions rather than the primary radiation chemical effects described above for drugs which are true protectors or sensitizers. The complex mechanisms involved in a combination of chemotherapy with radiotherapy are discussed later in this chapter.

The biological target

However varied are the tissues of the body, the basic biological units of importance are the individual cells from which they are formed. At the level of dosage used in cancer treatment, the mode of action of radiotherapy is a sequence of molecular processes which bring about the cessation of cell division. A simplified diagram of a mammalian cell (Fig. 3.2) shows the number of different organelles which go to make up a single such unit of animal life. Each organelle has its own function but the whole cell is more than the sum of its parts. Interaction between the organelles is essential if the cell is to continue to do its work. In the context of the cancer cell, however, it is the property of proliferation that is of prime importance. Cancer represents the uncontrolled growth of a cell population. Radiotherapy seeks to inhibit such proliferation.

A beam of X-rays ionizes whatever lies in its path, in a random manner. An ionizing event may thus occur just as often in the cell nucleus or in the cytoplasm or outside the cell altogether, in the intercellular matrix. Only damage which affects the nucleus will have any significant effect, however. This is because, despite the

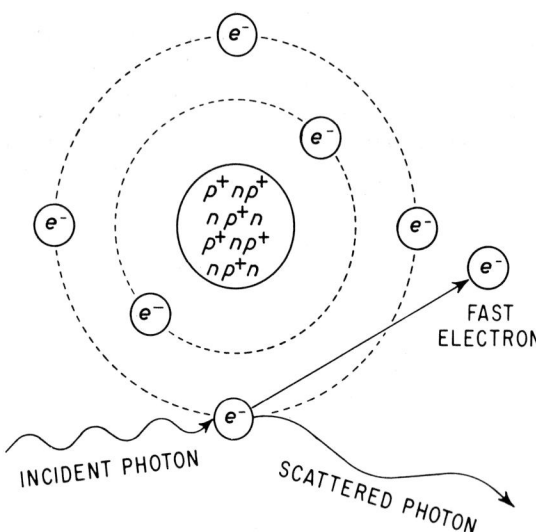

Fig. 3.1 Ionization of an atom by an X-ray photon (from Hall, 1978).

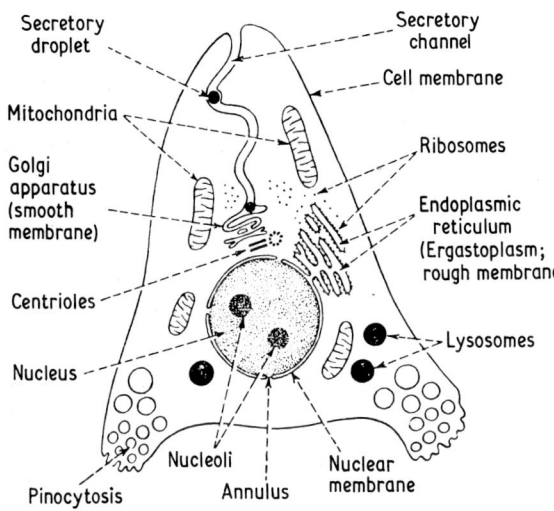

Fig. 3.2 Organelles of a typical cell.

interaction between those organelles shown in Fig. 3.2, it is the DNA which is the most sensitive target. If one considers the 'central dogma' of molecular biology:

$$\text{DNA} \xrightarrow{\text{Transcription}} \text{RNA} \xrightarrow{\text{Translation}} \text{PROTEIN}$$

it can easily be appreciated that damaged protein can be replaced so long as the RNA message remains available. Similarly, damaged RNA can also be replaced so long as normal DNA is available to transcribe it. If the DNA itself has been damaged, however, then the code may be irreparably destroyed. Such damage will not immediately kill a cell. Indeed it may continue to function for the whole of its normal life span as a single cellular entity. Only when the time comes for cell division to take place will the damage be revealed; mitosis will fail and the cell then dies a mitotic death. As far as cancer treatment is concerned, this failure to proliferate is a satisfactory conclusion, since the tumour will cease to grow if all the tumour cells with the capacity to proliferate are prevented from further cell division. For many normal tissues a failure of further proliferation may also be tolerated by the patient (neurones do not proliferate anyway, for example); but some normal cell populations, like gut epithelium, bone marrow and vascular endothelium *are* required to proliferate and radiation damage to such tissues may prove unacceptable if repopulation cannot keep pace with damage to a sufficient degree to preserve normal function.

The term 'radioresponsiveness' was defined in the introduction to this chapter, with reference to clinical observations of the rate of tumour shrinkage and pos-

sible recurrence. The time scale of this radiation response depends upon the growth kinetics of the cell populations in question. The next section is primarily devoted to tumour cell kinetics but the same principles can be applied to normal cell populations whose patterns of radioresponsiveness are just as important to the radiotherapist when he seeks guidance on the extent to which a treatment schedule can be tolerated by an individual patient.

Tumour cell kinetics

One of the most useful ways of explaining the growth and structure of tumours is the growth fraction model shown in Fig. 3.3. In this diagram the cell population is divided into four compartments (where 'compartment' describes function, not structure). The proliferating compartment represents the growth fraction (sometimes called P, for proliferating cells) from which cells may pass one way into compartments of either sterile or dead cells (cell loss). A reversible pathway exists between the growth fraction and a compartment containing cells in G_0; i.e. resting (or 'Q', for quiescent) cells. These can be recruited into the growth fraction by a suitable stimulus, such as depletion of proliferating cells by radiotherapy. This process of recruitment may apply to normal stem cell populations as well as to resting tumour cells. In a simpler form (i.e. without cell death), the model would divide the tumour cells into a proliferating and non-proliferating pool. The growth fraction is defined as the ratio of the proportion of proliferating cells to the total cell population. The growth fraction can be estimated from the disparity between the doubling time of the tumour and the generation time of the proliferating cells. In the presence of cell death, the growth fraction model becomes more complex and, after irradiation, changes in growth fraction, cell loss and intermitotic time are all likely to play some part in determining changes in

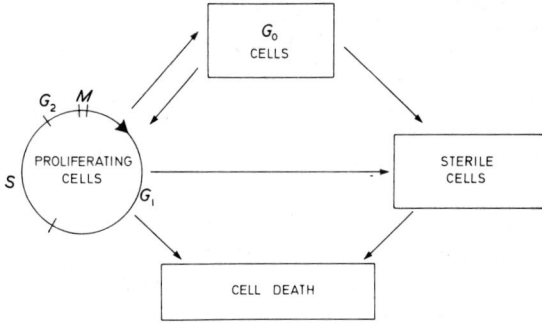

Fig. 3.3 Kinetic compartments of a cell population (from Mendelsohn and Dethlefsen, 1967).

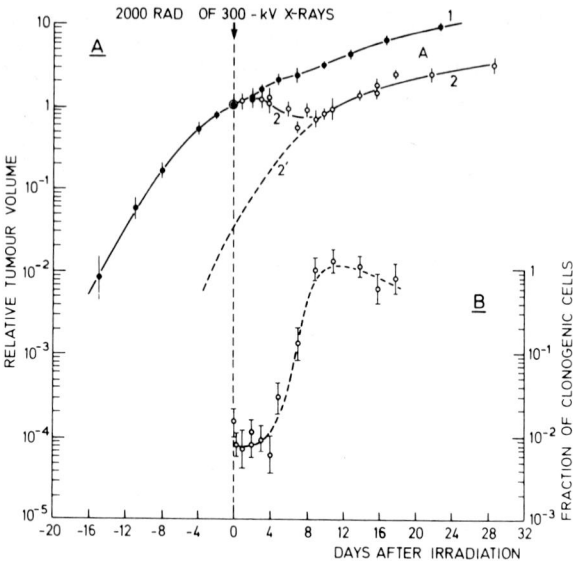

Fig. 3.4 Growth curves of a rat rhabdomyosarcoma (from Hermens and Barendsen, 1969).

growth rate during the repopulation process. Of these, it is considered that variation in growth fraction and rate of cell loss are the major factors and these in turn are likely to depend on changes in vascular architecture and function after irradiation.

The clinical use of measurements of tumour diameter may suggest that tumours grow logarithmically. By contrast Fig. 3.4 illustrates the non-exponential growth of a transplanted rhabdomyosarcoma where tumour volume is the parameter of repopulation. It is seen that with such serial measurements the growth curve does not remain exponential but bends towards the time axis. However, growth curves obtained from serial measurements of tumour diameter frequently do remain exponential during a relatively short period of observation. This paradox has been explained on the basis of central necrosis of a tumour with continued proliferation of the outer cell layers. These two processes acting together will often result in a linear increase of tumour diameter with time when a thin proliferating shell surrounds a necrotic core – the so-called 'orange skin' effect.

Central necrosis is not the only factor confusing the evidence from serial measurements of tumour diameter. Every tumour contains a stroma of normal tissue and the relative proportions of stromal cells to tumour cells vary in different tumours and at different times during the growth of the same tumour. For this reason serial estimates of tumour volume, whether obtained from total weight or merely from diameter,

provide only an indirect measure of the kinetics of the total tumour cell population.

The reason for the decrease in the rate of growth of a tumour with increasing size is probably because the supporting stroma cannot maintain a rate of growth equal to that of the parenchymal cells. The nutritional environment of the tumour cells becomes poorer as the distance between blood vessels increases, and this leads to a decreased rate of cell proliferation and cell death. The rate of proliferation of endothelial cells may also limit, indirectly, the rate of tumour growth but there have been few attempts to study the population kinetics of vascular endothelial cells and supporting connective tissue, possibly because endothelial cells of blood vessels are difficult to recognize in thin tumour sections. Values have been estimated for kinetic parameters for endothelial cells of capillary walls and for carcinoma cells of a transplanted C_3H mouse mammary tumour. The turnover time was about 50 hours for the endothelial cells compared with 22 hours for the carcinoma cells.

It should be noted that the turnover time is not the same as the cell cycle time. Nor can values for the kinetics of mouse cells be used to guide radiotherapists in the timing of the response of human cells. If the 2-year life-span of a laboratory mouse is compared with the 70 years expected of man then a considerable difference might be expected in kinetic values. This is not borne out in practice and the two mammalian species show relatively small differences when precise measurements have been possible. The values for colonic epithelial cells provide a typical example: S phase in mouse is 6·5 hours, in man 20 hours; G_2 phase in mouse is 1·5 hours, in man 8 hours; cell cycle in mouse is 16 hours, in man 45 hours. The human values are included in Table 3.1 where seven cell types are listed. Some values for Growth Fraction and Cell Loss Factor are included and those for Basal Cell Carcinoma provide a numerical explanation for the very slow clinical progress of rodent ulcers, both in their usually long history of growth before diagnosis and in their sometimes slow disappearance after radiotherapy. This is because of the very high cell loss factor (95%) and the low growth fraction (30%) of this cell population, apart from its relatively long cell cycle.

Table 3.1   Kinetics of some human cell populations (from Duncan and Nias, 1977).

Cell type	Length of S phase (h)	Cell cycle time (h)	Growth fraction (%)	Cell loss factor (%)
Basal cell carcinoma	19	72	30	95
Squamous cell carcinoma	12	38	24	90
Melanoma	25	80	25	70
Carcinoma cervix	10	15	50	
Acute leukaemia	10	20		
Bone marrow	13	24		
Normal colon	20	45		

Cell survival curves

Cell survival curves are used to show the response of single cells to increasing single doses of radiation of various qualities, delivered under various environmental conditions and at various rates of dose. The response of single cells is tested by their ability to grow into colonies (i.e. to proliferate) after the treatment. If a cell demonstrates this reproductive capacity during a minimum period after the treatment then that cell can be considered to have survived. In this context, survival requires not merely the continued existence of the cell as a living entity (i.e. functionally intact) but also the property of proliferation. When considering the radiotherapy of cancer cell populations, it is that property which is of greatest interest since the aim of treatment is to destroy the proliferative capacity of the cancer cells while leaving sufficient normal cells to maintain the function of the normal tissues in the treated volume. Some of the cancer cells may still 'survive', in the sense that they respire, synthesize macromolecules and exhibit other biochemical properties. In one sense these cells are still living but since they will play no further part in the growth of the tumour they can usually be ignored. This is why the information obtainable from cell survival curves is confined to the response of proliferating cells.

Compared to the number of colonies in an unirradiated aliquot of cells (defined as 100% or unity) the number of colonies formed in an irradiated aliquot will represent the fraction of the initial cell number which survived that dose of irradiation. If values for surviving fraction are plotted against values for radiation, dose–response curves such as those in Fig. 3.5. will be obtainable. The shape of these curves is characteristic for low LET radiation, i.e. it is the sort of dose response that is found with conventional radiotherapy. After an initial shoulder region the larger the dose – on a linear scale – the smaller the surviving fraction – on a logarithmic scale. This exponential relationship has been found for all mammalian tissues where it has been possible to test the radiation response of the constituent cells by some quantitative method. What this means is that the larger the tumour volume the larger the radiation dose will be needed to eradicate it, assuming that every single tumour cell must be 'sterilized'. The fact that the normal tissue tolerance dose is smaller for larger volumes is an unfortunate limitation in view of this theoretical requirement for a larger tumour dose. Be that as it may, the essential feature of mammalian cell survival curves is their exponential shape following the initial shoulder region.

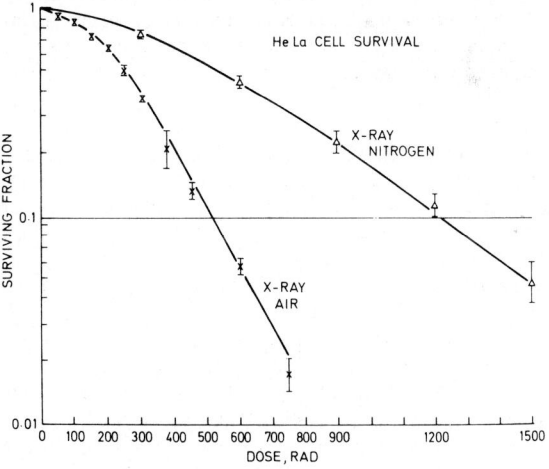

Fig. 3.5 X-ray survival curves of HeLa cells (from Duncan and Nias, 1977).

The curves in Fig. 3.5 illustrate the response of cells to single doses of radiation. The response of cells in a tissue to a dose fractionated over several weeks will depend upon a number of factors, including the size of the individual fraction doses. The biological effect of these doses can be predicted from the cell survival curves obtained with those cell populations which are relevant to the clinical problem. The usual method of comparison between such curves is by describing their shape using the two parameters D_0 and n. D_0 describes the slope of the exponential portion of the curve after the initial shoulder and it is the dose, in rads, required to reduce the surviving fraction to a value of $^1/e$ (where e is the exponential function and $^1/e$ equals 0.37). Thus D_0 is the mean lethal dose for that cell population and the value can be read off the graph as the extra dose required to reduce survival from 10% to 3.7% or 1% to 0.37%. The dose required to reduce survival from 100% to 37% might be called D_{37} but this is a misleading parameter since it includes the shoulder portion of the curve.

The size of the shoulder of a cell survival curve is described by extrapolating the exponential portion upwards to the vertical axis of the graph. This point on that logarithmic scale is then called, quite simply, the extrapolation number, n. The point where this extrapolated line crosses the horizontal axis (at 100% survival) may be described as the quasi-threshold dose D_q (in rads). This may loosely be considered as an amount of 'wasted' radiation attributable to sub-lethal damage, for that cell population, after a large dose has been given. The shapes of cell survival curves can thus be compared using the parameter D_0 to describe the exponential slope and either of the parameters n or D_q to describe the extent of the shoulder. The size of the shoulder itself determines the response to the multiple small doses of about 150–300 rad each, which are commonly used in radiotherapy.

Oxygen enhancement ratio

The difference between the exponential slopes of the two curves in Fig. 3.5 illustrates a well-known radiobiological phenomenon; namely, enhancement of the effect of radiation by oxygen. If the two curves can be fitted to the same shape, i.e. their exponential slopes can be shown to extrapolate to the same point on the vertical axis (the same extrapolation number, n), then this indicates that oxygen is a purely dose-modifying factor in the environment of the cells at the time of irradiation. In such a case, the ratio of the two values for D_0 provides a single value for the parameter called the oxygen enhancement ratio (OER). This is the ratio of doses given hypoxically or in air to produce a given level of cell killing. Thus, oxygen was purely a dose-

modifying factor, under the experimental conditions described and the OER obtainable from the ratio of the D_0 values of 150 rad for aerated cells and 360 rad for hypoxic cells was 2.39. Calculations of this sort can be applied to data obtained with any cell population which can be assayed for survival of the colony forming ability of single cells. The data in Fig. 3.5 were obtained using HeLa cells which were originally derived from a human carcinoma of cervix.

In many tumour tissues, however, the cell population will be some mixture of those two extremes and the actual dose–response curve will be biphasic. Fig. 3.6 illustrates this for a mouse tumour studied by the dilution assay technique of Hewitt and Wilson (1959). Leukaemic cells infiltrate the liver of the donor mouse and a cell suspension is then made. After increasing doses of radiation to the donor mice, increasing numbers of cells must be inoculated into the groups of recipient mice if tumours are to develop. By suitably varying the cell dilution, an average of one viable cell is inoculated into each mouse and the usual exponential dose–response is established. If the donor animal is alive at the time of irradiation then its tumour cells are oxygenated and the lowest curve is obtained. If the animal is killed long enough beforehand, all the cells will be anoxic and the uppermost curve is found. With intermediate time intervals, the other curves will be

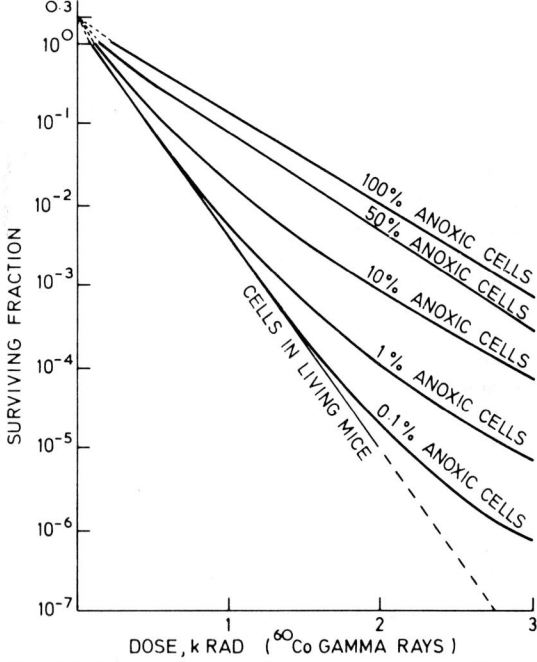

Fig. 3.6 Survival curves of cell populations with various proportions of anoxic cells (from Hewitt and Wilson, 1959).

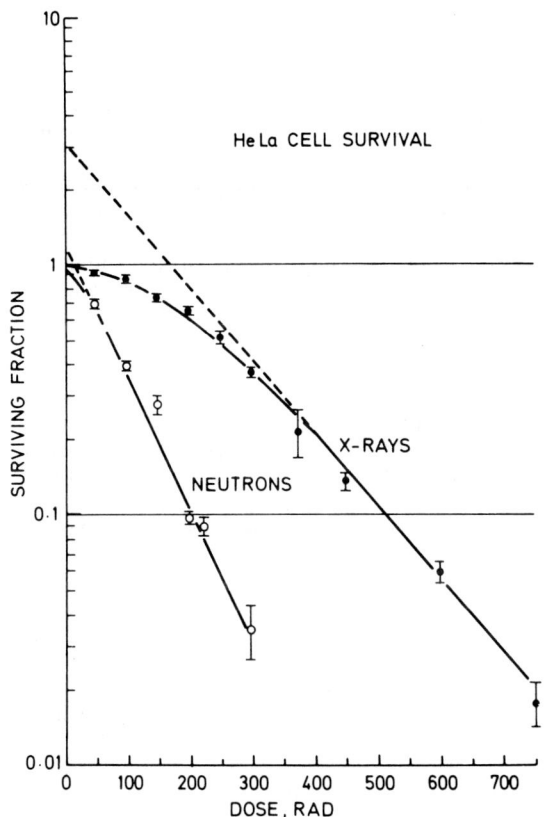

Fig. 3.7 Survival curves of HeLa cells irradiated with X-rays or fast neutrons (from Nias *et al.*, 1967).

compared after irradiation of cells with X-rays and fast neutrons. Fig. 3.7 shows a pair of survival curves of HeLa cells irradiated in air with 300 kV X-rays and 14.7 MeV monoenergetic neutrons from a D-T generator. The curves are obviously different; the extrapolation numbers are 3.2 for X-rays and 1.6 for neutrons. This provides an example of variation in biological response over the range of doses used for fractionated radiotherapy. This is the Relative Biological Efficiency (RBE) of fast neutrons compared with medium voltage X-rays. The data in Table 3.2 were obtained from the curves in Fig. 3.7.

Table 3.2 Variation of RBE with survival level (from Nias *et al.*, 1967).

Survival level (%)	Neutron dose (rad)	X-ray dose (rad)	RBE
90	15	65	4.3
80	30	115	3.8
70	45	160	3.6
60	60	200	3.3
50	80	240	3.0
40	100	280	2.8
30	125	335	2.7
20	160	400	2.4
10	210	515	2.4
3	305	695	2.3

obtained which are biphasic; starting with an aerated slope and changing to an anoxic slope when all the aerated cells have been sterilized. The relevant curve for radiotherapy is probably the 10% anoxic cell example, although information on the degree of hypoxia of human tumours is very inadequate and a broad range of values can be presumed to apply. The main conclusion from this is that hypoxia may not represent a clinical problem when small fraction doses are used over the range where the biphasic curve approaches the aerated slope. It follows from this, that any benefit from the use of hyperbaric oxygen is more likely to be found with larger fraction doses over the range where the biphasic curve deviates from the aerated slope. Here again a single value for OER cannot be applied over the range of fraction doses used in radiotherapy.

Relative biological efficiency

An analogous situation exists when survival curves are

The important conclusion to be drawn from these survival curves is that, because of the relatively small shoulder on the neutron curve compared with that on the X-ray curve, the value of RBE changes considerably over just that range of dosage most commonly employed in fractionated radiotherapy.

Cell survival through the cell cycle

Under the special conditions of a cell culture laboratory, it is possible to manipulate a cell population so that all the cells are passing through the phases of the cycle in synchrony. It is then found that, with the exception of mitosis, cells are most radiosensitive just towards the end of the G_1 phase. They then become progressively more resistant as they progress through the S phase but become more sensitive when they pass into the G_2 phase before the next mitosis. With certain drug combinations, cell populations may become synchronized to some extent and then this variation in radiosensitivity may occur under clinical conditions.

It is important to stress that it is not the whole of this

or that phase of the cell cycle that is radiosensitive or radioresistant, but rather that sensitivity varies throughout the phases of the whole cycle. Except for mitosis, it is the particular point in the cycle when cells are completing G_1 and beginning S (the $G_1 - S$ transition) that is the most radiosensitive. There are some cells with a long G_1 phase which are as radioresistant near the beginning of G_1 as they are near the end of S. This radioresistant portion of the cell cycle is absent, however, from cells with only a short G_1 phase, which progress quickly from mitosis to the $G_1 - S$ transition point, both of which are radiosensitive. Any such variation in radiosensitivity is likely to affect normal as well as tumour cells, however.

Recovery from radiation damage

Except for the treatment of small skin lesions, radiotherapy is almost always given as a series of fractionated doses. Fraction doses of a few hundred rad are delivered to the volume, often at daily intervals for five days per week over a period of three to six weeks. For this reason the single dose survival curves just described have only a limited application to the clinical situation, except as a basis for comparison of the radiosensitivity of different cell populations exposed to different forms of radiation under different environmental conditions. During fractionated radiotherapy, both recovery and repopulation will tend to reduce the effectiveness of the total radiation dosage. Repopulation was discussed in the context of tumour cell kinetics, but repopulation is a less important factor in fractionation than recovery. Some experimental animal studies certainly suggest that recovery is more important.

Pigs were irradiated either with one single dose or with 5 fractions in 4 days, or 5 fractions in 28 days. The doses required to produce the same skin reaction are shown in Table 3.3.

These observations lead to the conclusion that even fractionation over the shortest period necessitates 1600 rad extra to produce the same effect. This is mainly attributable to recovery since repopulation would be minimal over that 4-day period; and even over the 28-day period the dose increment for the same

Table 3.3.   Doses required to produce the same skin reaction (from Fowler *et al.*, 1963).

Fractionation	Total dose	Dose increment
1 Fraction	2000 rad	–
5 Fractions in 4 days	3600 rad	1600 rad
5 Fractions in 28 days	4200 rad	600 rad

number of fractions amounts to only another 600 rad. The recovery phenomenon was obviously more important than repopulation in that situation. Nevertheless, when large numbers of small fraction doses are given, so that recovery is quite small after each dose, then repopulation may be comparable to, or even greater than, recovery. This would apply to comparison of say, 25 with 35 fractions given, say over 5 or 7 weeks; not to small numbers of large doses as in the above comparison of 5 fractions with a single dose.

A sparing effect of radiation when fractionated or given at reduced dose-rate has been known for many years and Fig. 3.8 shows this in a schematic diagram which compares the surviving fractions of cells after either a single dose of 2000 rad (4.8×10^{-7} cells) or 5 fractions of 400 rad (10^{-5} cells) or 10 fractions of 200 rad (9×10^{-4} cells). The cell survival curve is drawn in full for the single dose regime; only the 'shoulders' are drawn for the two fractionated regimes. These shoulders have exactly the same shape as that for the single dose curve. The point is that they must be 'reconstructed' after each fraction dose and this is the reason why larger numbers of fractions are less effective. Fig. 3.8 shows that 10×200 rad is 90 times less effective than 5×400 rad; and 6×200 rad is 15 times less effective than 3×400 rad. In each case, the same total dose is most effective if given in one single treatment.

Recovery from sub-lethal damage is probably a metabolic process since although it is relatively insen-

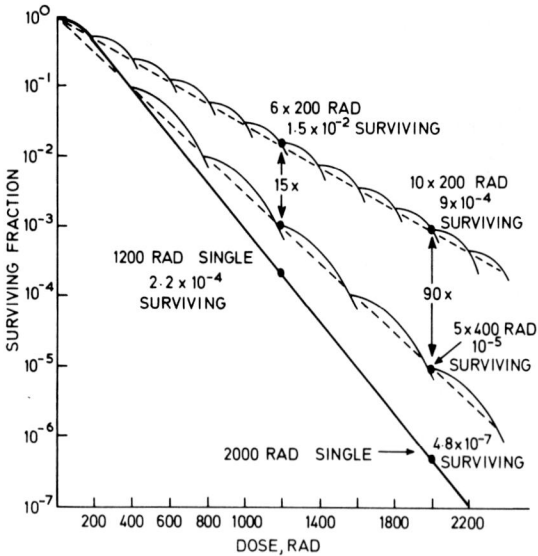

Fig. 3.8 Cell survival from single doses and from fractions of 400 rad or 200 rad each.

sitive to small reductions in temperature and to low oxygen tension (e.g. hypoxic cells at 340 ppm O_2 appear to be able to recover), it can be suppressed by some metabolic inhibitors, in particular those which are incorporated into DNA (IUdR, BUdR) or bind to the DNA (actinomycin D). It occurs fairly rapidly with a time constant of about one hour and it involves reconstruction of the shoulder of the survival curve. A two-dose (or 'split-dose') experiment is required to demonstrate it but the amount of recovery is not dose-dependent. Less recovery is seen in hypoxic cells, provided they remain hypoxic during the interval between the two doses; the recovery then appears to occur more slowly. Less recovery is also found after high LET radiation.

Recovery from potentially lethal damage (PLD) has begun to attract attention because it may be more evident in cell populations which are not actively proliferating. These would be tissues with a negligible growth fraction which will include many tumours but also some normal tissues. In this case, the amount of recovery is dose-dependent, the higher the dose the more recovery (in contrast to recovery from sub-lethal damage, SLD).

Whereas recovery from SLD is a fractionation phenomenon which occurs generally whenever two or more doses of radiation are delivered more than an hour apart, recovery from PLD is more difficult to demonstrate. If over-crowded cell cultures reflect a clinical situation this would be more likely to occur in the early stages of a course of radiotherapy when the tumour cell population has a lower growth fraction. Radio-therapeutic (and adjunctive) regimes which result in the majority of the cell population moving into proliferative activity will then be associated with a reduction in this form of recovery, although recovery from SLD remains (as depicted in Fig. 3.8). Finally, both forms of recovery occur during the first hours after a 'first' dose. The amount of SLD is measured by the response to a 'second' dose delivered at varying times after that first dose, whereas to measure the amount of PLD the important interval is that between the first dose and some stimulus which triggers more cell division. Both SLD and PLD are less evident after high LET radiation.

Although the size of the shoulder on a cell survival curve does not necessarily indicate the amount of sublethal damage from which such cells may recover, anything that increases the shoulder size (D_q value) will reduce the effectiveness of smaller fraction doses of radiotherapy compared wtih larger doses. There is evidence that the survival curves of cells irradiated in contact with each other (as in most tissues) have much larger shoulders. Thus the D_q value of Chinese hamster cell survival curves rises from 200 to 900 rad when the single cells are allowed to grow into multicellular spheroids. A possible therapeutic advantage would accrue if limiting normal tissues tended to have larger values for D_q than tumours but there is no evidence for this. Indeed, all the data reported so far from survival curves seem to show that there is no systematic difference between the radiosensitivity of normal and tumour cells from the same histological type of tissue.

Limiting normal tissues

Radiotherapists need to understand the response of those normal tissues which are likely to limit the dosage which is primarily intended for the tumour. The term 'radical' radiotherapy implies an attempt to cure a tumour by delivering the maximum dosage which the irradiated normal tissue can tolerate. The maximum dose which may safely be given to a particular type or volume of tissue is known as the tolerance dose. The normal tissues to be discussed in this chapter are therefore those which commonly limit radiotherapy in this respect. These 'limiting' normal tissues' include skin, gastrointestinal tract, bone marrow and blood vessels. Blood vessels may well be the most important of all, since damage to the vascular supply will eventually lead to damage to other tissues, discussed later on as late effects.

Vascular tissue

The larger vessels are apparently radioresistant, in contrast to the capillaries and small arteries which become occluded after moderate doses of irradiation. It will be damage to these smaller vessels which will delay wound healing and cause late damage to the skin and other tissues such as the kidney and the central nervous system (CNS). At the cellular level the endothelial lining of large vessels is probably as sensitive as that in capillaries but, because of the large diameter of those vessels, even if endothelial proliferation and swelling or blood clotting does occur, the vessels will not be occluded. The radiosensitivity of capillary endothelial cells from mouse kidney has been studied, in a comparison using *in vitro* tissue culture techniques. 'Typical' cell survival curves were found, having values for D_0 of 200 rad in air, 530 rad under hypoxic conditions, the same extrapolation number 2.3 and thus an oxygen enhancement ratio of 2.65. If these results are relevant to human blood vessels they show that vascular endothelial cells are just as radiosensitive as other cells.

Vascular endothelium is known to have rather slow tissue turnover times. Damage develops more slowly. The turnover time for endothelial cells in the capillaries of a mouse tumour is 50 hours (as compared with 22 hours for the tumour cells). Eventually, however, tissues and organs with the same order of kinetic parameters (liver, thyroid, connective tissue) and in the lower order of kinetics (e.g. CNS) will show radiation damage as an indirect result of vascular damage and this will be discussed later.

Intestine

In the whole digestive tract, the small intestine is the most important site of radiation injury. All three regions, the duodenum, jejunum and ileum are lined by a columnar epithelium consisting of mucus and columnar or 'chief' cells. The crypts which contain the generative cells for epithelial replacement are found in the mucosa at the bases of the villi. The cells of the crypts and of the related villi can be considered parts of a cell renewal system, which is in a state of kinetic equilibrium. Cell renewal occurs in the mitotic areas in the crypts. From these, newly formed cells migrate out and move from the base of the villi to the top. A survival curve for mouse jejunum has a D_0 value of 130 rad and is based upon the number of regenerating crypts of Lieberkuhn which can be counted around the circumference of a section of gut. Since the D_0 values for skin and intestinal cell populations are very similar, 130 rad and 150 rad, respectively, the more acute radiation response of intestine must be attributed to differences in the kinetics of the cell populations (the cycle time for intestinal stem cells is 12 hours; for skin it is 5 days).

Bone marrow

It is known that the haematopoietic bone marrow is composed principally of three renewal systems: erythropoietic, myelopoietic, and thrombopoietic, but the

morphological identity of the stem cell (or cells) of bone marrow and even the anatomical boundaries of its normal site of origin and its location are not known. The stem cell (or cells) is known to exist however, and its proliferative capacity can be characterized by indirect physiological means. The mature granulocyte and lymphocyte may spend a sizeable fraction of their life span outside of the blood vessels. There is good evidence to consider the division of this proliferative system into 'pools' and 'compartments' to characterize the normal and abnormal states and to allow systematic kinetic studies for the establishment of the key parameters of the system. Such division, however, into compartments can only be arbitrary and will depend to some extent on the technique and the judgement of the observer. Survival of bone marrow stem cells can be measured by the spleen colony method. D_0 varies between 60 and 105 rad, while n lies between 1.2 and 2.7. These values of D_0 overlap the range for cells cultured *in vitro*, although they fall at the lower end of the range.

The consequence of radiation depletion of the bone marrow stem-cell population is eventually seen in the form of a depression in the peripheral blood count. Fig. 3.9 shows the peripheral blood counts of rats after 500 rad of whole body irradiation. Time elapses after the bone marrow is irradiated before the maximum depression occurs followed by recovery to a normal level. This time interval depends upon the kinetics of the various types of stem cell population. Each of the marrow populations has its own kinetics and the time scale of the perturbation in the peripheral blood count varies accordingly.

The earlier 'compartments' of these blood cell populations will involve proliferation in the bone marrow and the peripheral blood counts show only the 'output' compartment. The total period of time from input to output starts the moment a stem cell is stimulated to begin proliferation along one of the three possible pathways of differentiation; erythroid, myeloid and platelet (e.g. the myeloid pathway ending up in a mature polymorphonuclear leucocyte). The stem cells initiate a variable number of cell divisions during which differentiation and maturation gradually supervene before the cells appear in the peripheral blood in their recognizable form. It is noteworthy that red cells have a relatively very long life span in the peripheral blood for all species; 110 days for man. The other two cell types have both a shorter total life span (from start to finish) and a shorter period in the peripheral blood. It is the total time, however, from start to finish, which determines the responses shown in Fig. 3.9. The peripheral blood count which shows the earliest depression of all is that for lymphocytes. This cell population is receiving increasing attention because recent advances in im-

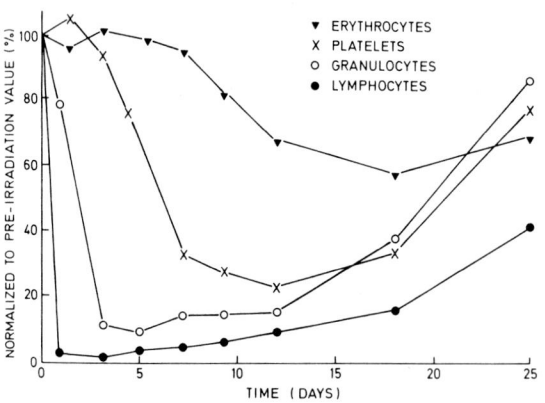

Fig. 3.9 Peripheral blood counts of irradiated rats.

munology are centred upon the phenomenon of cell-mediated immunity and the immune system must now be included in the category of limiting normal populations.

The response of the immune system to radiation can be considered both in terms of a reduction in the populations of lymphoid cells which perform the function of cell-mediated immunity, and also in terms of a depression of the humoral immunity from antibody production by such cells. Following whole-body irradiation the B-lymphocytes are much more radioresponsive than the T-cells. The evidence for this is both morphological and functional; primary nodules of lymphoid cells will reappear within 7 days, but restoration of the depleted thymus-dependent compartment may still take 4–5 weeks. Both active antibody synthesis and circulating antibody are radio-resistant, however.

Late effects on normal tissues

There is an indirect relationship between the degree of early reaction in a tissue and the probability of developing a late reaction, but the pathogenesis of early and late reactions is different. The immediate radiation reaction depends predominantly on the number of parenchymal cells killed by radiation, whereas the development of late reactions is also influenced by two other processes associated with progressive secondary damage. These changes are associated with ischaemia and fibrosis produced in the tissue. The ischaemia results from damage to the endothelial cells and walls of the blood vessels. Fibrosis may well also be directly related to the degree of cell killing in the vascular endothelium, resulting in protein fractions extravasating into the interstitial tissues. It must be noted, however, that the pathogenesis of radiation fibrosis is not properly understood. The actual late radiation effect will depend on the relative damage to the parenchymal cells and to the vascular endothelium. This will differ from tissue to tissue and may also be influenced by the quality of radiation and the method of dose fractionation. The interpretation of the differences seen in late reactions in normal tissues will depend on the relative extent of damage to the specific tissue cells and to their supporting vasculoconnective tissue.

Central nervous system

The central nervous system was considered at one time to consist of tissues of high radioresistance. It is now recognized that this false interpretation resulted from the commonly late manifestation of radiation injury which is related to the slow turnover of cells in nervous tissue. Depending upon the dose level there are two modes of radiation injury. One mode is vascular which predominates with single explosure of between 2000 and 3000 rad. The other affects white matter through damage to the supporting glia and is most clearly seen with single exposures of 3000–4000 rad. The two modes of damage can be explained in cellular terms and a cell-survival model may be assumed to explain the incidence of radiation myelitis as a function of dose. A survival curve for neuronal cells has been derived that is consistent with a D_0 value of 130 rad and an extrapolation number of 2, although it cannot be regarded as conclusive.

When the brain is irradiated to the high levels of dosage used in cancer therapy there is the risk of late brain necrosis. Chronic radiation encephalopathy usually presents three to 24 months after high-dose irradiation; the higher the dose the shorter the latent period. The injury is strikingly selective of the white matter indicated by wide-spread demyelinization. The cerebral cortex is least affected while the brain stem is particularly vulnerable. The blood vessels are also normally seen to be damaged with all degrees of degenerative change previously described and may include complete thrombosis, which will have grave clinical consequences in the brain. Similar changes may be found in the spinal cord. Sub-acute radiation myelopathy is usually a transient condition which occurs two to four months after irradiation, and may persist for several months. It is considered to be caused by the inhibition of myelinization due to loss of oligodendroglia and restitution occurs with time.

Chronic radiation myelopathy denotes severe and irreversible damage to the spinal cord (Fig. 3.10). The symptoms and signs are of partial and eventually complete transection of the cord. The white fibre tracts are greatly reduced, the grey columns standing out as pale areas, but often containing petechiae. The loss of tissue may be so great that the spinal cord almost disappears.

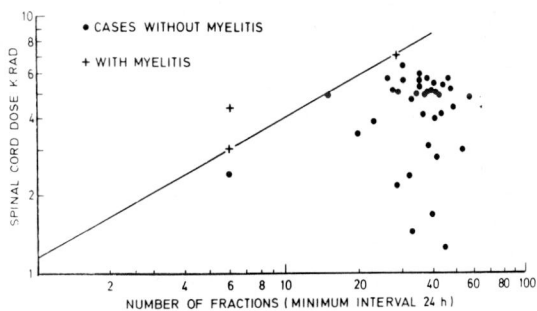

Fig. 3.10 Incidence of radiation myelitis of the spinal cord in the thoracic region (from Phillips and Buschke, 1969).

At the cellular level, these changes can be attributed to a greater sensitivity of oligodendrocytes in white matter than those in grey matter, with consequent demyelination. Vascular damage may lead eventually to ischaemic changes, but the acute response produces oedema due to increased vascular permeability.

The volume of brain or spinal cord irradiated is an important factor in the tolerance dose of radiation. It is suggested that, for orthovoltage radiation, the threshold dose is 4500 rad in 17 days for fields less than 50 cm² and should be reduced to 3500 rad when the fields are more than 100 cm². The tolerance doses in respect of thoracic spine are illustrated in Fig. 3.10.

Lung

The adult lung is a stable tissue with a very slow cellular proliferation in its differentiated cells and in the endothelial cells. This contrasts with the oesophagus which has a very rapid cell renewal system. Consequently the effects of radiation appear early in the oesophagus whereas the effects on the lung are seen much later. Radiation pneumonitis follows damage to either or both the cell populations found in the alveolar septa of the lungs: these are endothelial and alveolar cells. The response of capillary endothelial cells has already been mentioned and their damage may be the major factor in the development of pneumonitis. This may not be the only interpretation, however. The alveolar cells include a type which are vacuolated and secrete lung surfactant, a liquid material which, by reducing the surface tension of the fluid layer lining the alveoli, maintains their stability. Hydrostatic and osmotic pressures are balanced so as to prevent collapse of the alveoli upon expiration. Thus radiation pneumonitis may be just as much the consequence of dose-dependent loss of these alveolar cells as the result of capillary endothelial cell loss. In either or both cases there will be damage to the lung stroma characterized by oedema followed by hyalinization and fibrosis of the alveolar walls. Resulting impairment of ventilatory and diffusion capacities of the lung may be significant in the long-term effects of radiation (see Table 3.4). Haemorrhage into the lung may occur, also, as a result of radiation changes in the blood vessels.

Kidney

Late radiation injury to the kidney is commonly referred to as radiation 'nephritis' but it may be manifest in several different ways, and is really better described as radiation nephropathy. Hypertension is often a feature and radiation injury to the kidney is particularly likely to produce hypertension (Luxton and Kunkler, 1964). The kidney is an organ with many highly specialized functions and its cell systems all have very slow turnover rates. As a result radiation injury is usually not seen until some months after exposure. It depends both on the dose of irradiation and the volume of kidney irradiated.

Gonads

In the male gonad there is a stem cell population and progeny which are customarily categorized into spermatogonial stages, $A_0 - A_4$ and B, spermatocytes, spermatids and finally the mature spermatozoa. Spermatogonia are the most sensitive cells and are killed after exposure of the testes to relatively low doses of radiation and die in early prophase or later metaphase. As the supply of germ cells derived from spermatogonia becomes exhausted, the testes are progressively depleted of these cells until at two to four weeks after exposure mature sperm cells have disappeared. If the dose has not been excessive, regeneration from type A spermatogonia spared from radiation death begins. The time course of this phenomenon over a five-year period has been described for a man who had received an accidental dose of total body irradiation (Fig. 3.11). The sperm count reached its lowest level six months after irradiation and then recovered a normal level at two to three years. In contrast, the Leydig and Sertoli cells of the interstitial tissues are relatively radioresistant; testes atrophied because of radiation damage appear to contain more interstitial cells than germ cells.

Early in this century it was recognized that the ovaries atrophy after irradiation and that temporary or permanent sterility may result. In order to evaluate studies of irradiated ovaries, stress must be laid upon

Table 3.4 Development of radiation pneumonitis (from van den Brenk, 1971).

Phase	Sequence of events	Time span
Exudative	Cell damage, inflammatory exudates	0–40 days
Pneumonitis	Desquamation, consolidation, organization	20–60 days
Fibrosis	Fibrosis, devascularization	60–200 days
Secondary changes	Calcification, metaplasia, neoplasia	200 days

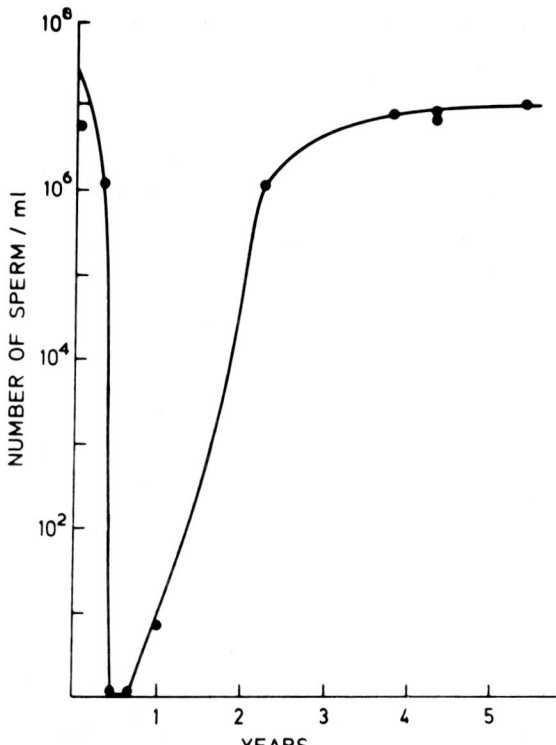

Fig. 3.11 Changes in sperm count after irradiation (from Oakes and Lushbaugh, 1952).

Effects on the embryo and foetus

Many physical, chemical and infective agents are known to carry high risks of producing damaging effects on the embryo and foetus and great care is taken to minimize such hazards. Severe effects will commonly follow the irradiation of the developing offspring. The important stages of growth in this respect are pre-implantation, organogenesis and foetal development. During the period of pre-implantation (0–9 days in man) the organism is particularly sensitive to radiation, the LD 50/30 in mice being one-third that of the mature animal. Irradiation at this stage usually results in death and those organisms that survive may show little abnormality, except those having sex chromosome aberrations. It is during the period of active organogenesis (9–42 days) that irradiation will produce severe anatomical malformation. During this phase of development in which major changes occur quickly in the organization of the embryo, the time of irradiation very much determines the nature and severity of the malformation. Although irradiation at this stage will normally result in severe structural abnormalities, high doses will prove lethal to most of the embryos. It is also extremely important to note that irradiation of the embryo and foetus increases the risk of the child developing some forms of cancer and leukaemia and this is discussed in the section on leukaemogenesis and carcinogenesis.

Radiation carcinogenesis and leukaemogenesis

Much concern is often expressed about the possible carcinogenic effects of ionizing radiations and yet, compared to many chemical agents, these radiations are not highly dangerous in this respect. It is clear that the leukaemias are the most important neoplastic diseases induced by ionizing radiations and their incidence in man may be accounted for in part by exposure to radiation. It has been estimated that perhaps over half the other forms of cancer in man are caused by chemicals, but the overall increase in incidence due to radiation is very small indeed.

The incidence of malignant change following irradiation is so small that large populations at risk have to be studied to allow reliable interpretation to be made of the observations. Since the latent period for the induction of cancer is so long, five to eight years for leukaemia and perhaps 15 or more years for most other forms of cancer, these observations have also to be made for very many years in most circumstances. Uncertainty of the spontaneous incidence rates of cancer and leukaemia in particular populations and the incidence of deaths from intercurrent diseases also makes comparative analysis of data from exposed

the fact that no other organ presents such large differences in response after irradiation between species or between individuals within a species. In the developing foetus, oogonia are relatively radioresistant, but oocytes in primordial follicles are extremely radio-sensitive ($D_0 = 90$ rad). Sensitivity diminishes as the follicles mature, and is low before ovulation. Thus, female (as well as male) germ cells are most sensitive during the last premeiotic prophase and the development into mature gametes. The crucial difference between male and female germ cells is that male germ cells represent a renewing cell population whereas female germ cells do not. The 'fertile-sterile-fertile' pattern often found in the ovaries after irradiation is not a result of regeneration from a stem-cell pool, as it is in males, but of the higher sensitivity of the intermediate follicular stages compared with that of the primitive and mature stages. Granulosa cells in the developing follicles are damaged even earlier than the oocytes, but in the mature follicles and the corpus luteum they appear more resistant.

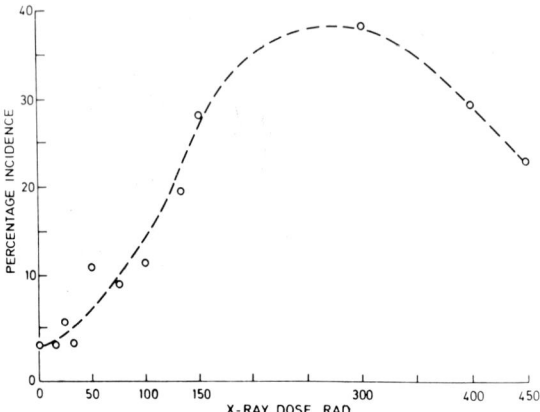

Fig. 3.12 Incidence of myeloid leukaemia in irradiated mice (from Upton, 1961).

populations a difficult exercise. The incidence of both cancer and leukaemia naturally increases with age and this factor must be carefully controlled in assessing the risks of radiation exposure. The International Commission for Radiological Protection has estimated that whole-body exposure to the adult population of 1 rad per year would result in two cases of leukaemia and two cases of other forms of cancer per 100 000 population per year. The total level of background radiation including natural and other sources in the United Kingdom is about 0.1 rad per year and the number of cancers produced by this order of dose is very small indeed (approximately 0.07%) compared to the number of cases from other causes. In respect of leukamia, however, it has been estimated that 10% of all cases may be due to radiation exposure.

It has been thought that the incidence of cancer was a linear function of radiation dose, but this implies a single event transformation with dose. It must be remembered that radiation also kills cells and that as the dose of radiation increases, the probability of cell death becomes much greater than neoplastic transformation. Therefore the incidence of malignant disease will decrease again at high doses. The most reasonable dose-response relationship for the induction of cancer and leukaemia is illustrated by the curve of Fig. 3.12. In this curve there is an initial ascending part rising to a summit before a final descending part. It is the accurate measurement of the initial part of the curve that has proved to be impossible to determine with animal experiments, as in this very low dose range (under 100 rad), unacceptably large numbers of animals would be required. Despite this uncertainty the International Commission on Radiation Protection assumes the hypothesis of a linear dose-response

relationship and this assumption may over-estimate the hazard of doses below 100 rad.

Response of tumours

It has already been described how the inevitable result of exposure to ionizing radiation is the destruction of biological material in the treated area. Earlier parts of the chapter have dealt with the immediate response of normal tissues which limit the tumour dose, either because of an upper limit of early damage to particular tissues (like skin, blood vessels, gut or bone marrow) or because the dose delivered to a tumour will also be limited by the risk of producing late damage which becomes manifest in certain organs (like CNS, lung and kidney). The control of malignant disease remains the prime object of radiotherapy, however, and this present section is devoted to the radiation response of tumours. The emphasis will be upon scientific laboratory observations of the response of experimental animal tumours to radiation, as distinct from those clinical observations (e.g. from controlled clinical trials) which are usually less well defined and relatively imprecise.

The rat rhabdomyosarcoma is a good example of an animal tumour model system. The growth curve was illustrated earlier, in the section on tumour cell kinetics, in Fig. 3.4. This shows (*A*) observations on the tumour measured as it grows in the animal and (*B*) its cells assayed *in vitro*. The shape of the upper growth curve (1) of the untreated tumour was discussed earlier. The lower growth curve (2) shows the response of the tumour to a single dose of 2000 rad. The tumour first stops growing and then shrinks, but by day 12 after treatment growth resumes at a rate similar to that of the untreated tumour. During this period the viability of cells taken from the treated tumour was assayed by a clonogenic test *in vitro*. The results of this are shown in the lowest curve in Fig. 3.4. The fraction of clonogenic cells falls to 10^{-2} (or 1%) immediately after irradiation and remains at this level during the 4-day period when the tumour has stopped growing in the animal. Then the clonogenic fraction begins to rise but the tumour shrinks because of death and removal of that 99% of the cells whose viability was destroyed by the irradiation dose. By day 12, however, the clonogenic fraction has returned to unity, all the cells in the tumour are now viable and the tumour resumes that growth rate which would be expected from the other measurements. This *in vitro* assay provides a clear explanation of the radiation response of the tumour *in vivo*. The *in vitro* assay can also be used to test cellular radiosensitivity in terms of survival curves. The survival curves obtained in air and under hypoxic conditions have D_0 values of 120 rad and 295 rad, respectively, so that the OER is 2.46, a typical value.

Oxygen effect

That is an over-simplification of the oxygen effect in a tumour cell population which almost always contains a proportion of hypoxic and aerated cells. In the case of the rhabdomyosarcoma, 15% of the tumour cells are estimated to be hypoxic. It follows that the survival curve for such tumour cells will be biphasic in shape, with the change from a steeper aerated slope to a flatter hypoxic slope occurring at a dose level which depends upon the proportion of hypoxic cells in the tumour at the time of irradiation and also on the slope of the curve for aerated cells. Single dose survival curves with such a shape were discussed earlier (Fig. 3.6) but such curves only measure the response of a tumour cell population to a 'first' dose.

It is worth noting the influence of anaemia on the proportion of hypoxic cells in a tumour. Radiotherapists usually maintain the haemoglobin level of their patients above the 70% level for this reason. Even then, the majority of tumours are believed to have regions where the vascular supply is inadequate so that even a patient with a normal haemoglobin level will be unable to maintain a physiological oxygen tension throughout the cells of the tumour. Fig. 3.13 is the classical diagram which shows the relatively small fall in radiosensitivity of tissues nourished by a normal blood supply, i.e. the usual gradient from arterial to venous blood. Diffusion studies suggest that oxygen cannot diffuse more than 150μm from capillaries so that any tissue with an intercapillary distance of more than 300 μm will contain anoxic cells. Other chemicals have different diffusion rates and the value of the new type of electron-affinic compounds is that they can diffuse further than oxygen and are not metabolized in the hypoxic human tumours which they are intended to sensitize.

Fig. 3.13 shows how the radiosensitivity of biological

material falls rapidly when the partial pressure of oxygen is decreased below 20 mm Hg; well outside the physiological range. It is assumed that such a phenomenon does not occur in most normal tissues but will be found in tumours. This assumption needs to be modified to take into account those tissues, like brain, where capillaries are known to undergo cycles of constriction and dilation. The time scale of those cycles is usually measured in minutes, whereas the undoubtedly dynamic state of a tumour blood supply is more likely to be measured in cycles of hours. For the purposes of fractionated radiotherapy, delivered at a normal dose-rate, the simplified assumption that normal tissue is well oxygenated whilst a proportion of tumour cells is not, would seem to be valid.

Cure

Since the aim of radiotherapy is to cure the primary human tumour it is useful to study an animal tumour where this end can be achieved. In clinical parlance the word 'cure' is usually replaced by a statistical parameter like 5-year survival. For the mouse an equivalent period of time is 120 or 150 days and this is used in the studies shown in Fig. 3.14. This is also part of a study of reoxygenation but this time the figure shows the results of an experiment using C$_3$H mice into whose chest wall the mammary tumour (which occurs spontaneously in this strain of mouse) has been transplanted. When the tumour measures 6 mm in diameter the experiment is begun with a 'priming' dose of 1500 rad. At time intervals thereafter the dose which cures 50% of a group of animals is determined (TCD$_{50}$). In this case that second dose was given when the tumour was hypoxic (using a clamp around the tumour), or aerated or hyperbaric (with the mouse in a hyperbaric chamber). 'Cure' meant that there was not palpable evidence of tumour in the irradiated volume at 150 days after treatment.

The statistical significance of results like those is superior to that from a clinical trial because the biological material is less variable. Thus hyperbaric oxygen is shown to sensitize the tumour to radiation and hypoxia to protect. In addition, patterns of reoxygenation for the C$_3$H tumour are shown for air and hyperbaric oxygen in that the tumour is most sensitive to a second dose delivered two to three days after a priming dose. This best interval for fractionation has also been shown to be an optimum interval for multifraction X-ray treatments of the same C$_3$H mouse tumour. Thus 5 fraction doses given over a 9-day period (5F/9d) gives much better tumour control than 5 daily fractions (5F/4d), at total doses which cause similar skin reactions in both schedules. Such multifraction studies can provide even more 'relevant' information for the better understanding of fraction-

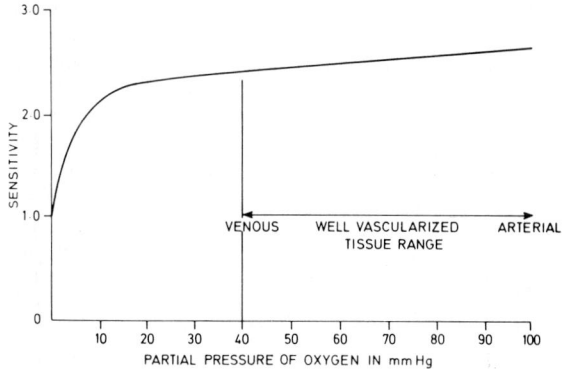

Fig. 3.13 Relationship of radiosensitivity to oxygen concentration (from Deschner and Gray, 1959).

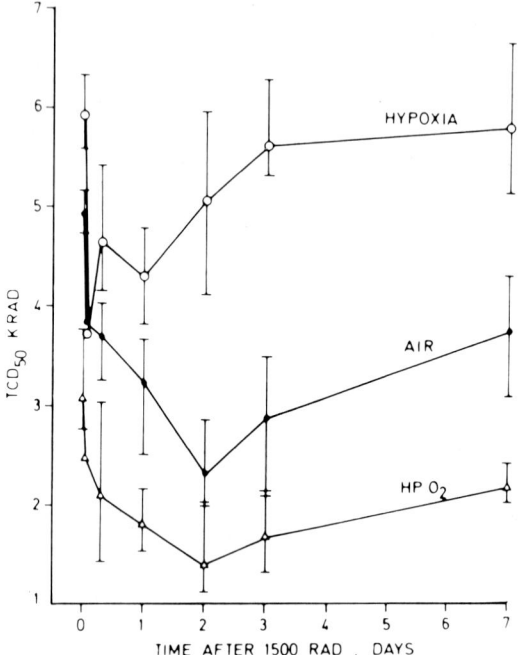

Fig. 3.14 Variation of TCD_{50} for C_3H mouse mammary carcinoma (from Howes, 1969).

ated radiotherapy, so long as the difference between mice and men is not forgotten.

Metastases

Until there is strong evidence to disprove it, the assumption can be made that metastatic deposits have a similar radiosensitivity to the primary tumour from which they originated. In terms of radioresponsiveness this would mean that a given volume of metastatic tumour should respond to the same extent as the same volume of primary tumour. The clinical situation very rarely allows such a comparison to be made – primary and secondaries are not often the same size at the same time. Patients with multiple metastases which require treatment provide a commoner opportunity for objective comparison and some of the fractionation problems to be discussed later can be answered just as well, or better, by using such clinical material, as by the use of animal tumours.

The best animal model for the study of distant metastases is the R1B5 fibrosarcoma since after transplantation the primary tumour grows subcutaneously, with a capsule and stroma like a clinical tumour. It is therefore possible to perform an apparently radical excision; local recurrence is uncommon after this procedure.

Such operations are quite commonly followed by pulmonary and other distant metastases, but the incidence of these metastases is significantly reduced if the animals are irradiated pre-operatively (Table 3.5). The use of pre-operative radiotherapy before radical surgery is often intended to reduce the incidence of local recurrence since this can more certainly be attributed to malignant cells newly 'spilt' at the time of operation. In most patients it is not easy to tell whether distant metastasis was not already present at the time of surgery, but the results shown in Table 3.5 show an obvious reduction in metastasis following pre-operative radiotherapy.

Table 3.5 Death from distant metastases after excision of R1B5 sarcoma (from Thomlinson, 1966).

Pre-operative dose	No. of animals	No. of deaths	% deaths
Nil	43	39	91
2000 rad	14	7	50
4000 rad	17	4	24

It must be said, however, that the best information on the direct response of human metastases remains that obtained from the irradiation of lung metastases clinically. This has shown that the kinetics of the human tumours remain unchanged, after the period of growth restraint, from that which existed before radiotherapy.

Fractionation

The practice of giving multiple small daily fractions of radiation was first introduced in an attempt to irradiate as many tumour cells as possible during mitosis since this was recognized as the most sensitive phase of the cell cycle. The use of multiple fractions had also been shown to spare overlying normal tissues while causing severe damage to relatively deep-seated structures. The early demonstration of this fact by Regaud et al. (1922) following experiments on the rat testes was confirmed by pioneer radiotherapists who found that fractionation of the total dose of radiation had a relatively favourable effect on normal tissues while still having a lethal effect on tumours. The object of fractionation in radiotherapy is to kill all tumour cells without producing serious damage to the surrounding normal tissues which necessarily must be included in the volume of high-dose irradiation. It is now clear that the clinical benefits of giving multiple dose fractions result from the complex interactions of many biological and physical factors. The cumulative effects of these factors will depend on the site, size and histological type of tumour, in addition to the radiotherapy technique employed.

The clinical effects of fractionated radiation are influenced primarily by the three 'Rs' of radiobiology already described. These are:

1. The capacity of mammalian cells to *Recover* from sublethal damage.
2. *Repopulation* of the tumour and normal tissues between fractions.
3. *Re-oxygenation* of the tumour during the course of treatment.

The third process is presumed to apply only to irradiated tumour tissue. The first two processes apply to normal tissues as well. Earlier in this chapter the recovery process was shown to be more important than repopulation (Table 3.3) and this is reflected in the fractionation formula proposed by Ellis (1965) for normal tissue tolerance which considers the number of fractions and the overall treatment time. Ellis related the physical dose given in a prescribed overall time in a specific number of fractions to what he called the nominal standard dose or NSD. The NSD of 'iso-effective' dose has been called the RET (rad equivalent therapy).

$$D_N = \text{NSD} \cdot T^{0.11} N^{0.24}$$

The use of the Ellis formula has provided a means for radiotherapists to compare the tolerance levels of doses delivered by different treatment regimes in respect of this effect on normal connective tissues. It should be remembered that it does not represent the iso-biological effect on all tissues or at all dose levels and does not, in itself, indicate the relative effectiveness of treatment techniques. Ellis has pointed out that it is meant to apply to connective tissue injury and so may be relevant to tissues other than skin, and he did include data on other organs such as the kidney. The Ellis formulation should not be used for less than 5 or for more than 30 fractions and the term ($T^{0.11}$) does not not apply beyond 100 days.

The concept of NSD may readily be misused in other ways. Commonly, for example, the calculated NSD for incomplete treatments (i.e. sub-tolerance levels) are added together although it is inherent in the NSD concept that it is applicable only to regimes of treatment delivering full tolerance doses of radiation. In order to simplify the system and make it more generally applicable, Orton and Ellis (1973) introduced factors which relate time, dose and fractionation and which are proportional to partial tolerance. These TDF factors provide a simple and more reliable way of comparing and equating all regimes of radiotherapy.

It has been recognized that the Ellis formulation does not represent all the physical factors which may influence the biological response. One of the most highly developed mathematical descriptions of the effects of radiotherapy is that reported by Kirk, Gray and Watson (1977). They believe that Ellis' formula is relevant to all degrees of biological effect on normal tissues and not just meaningful in relation to tolerance levels of radiation damage. If this is accepted the NSD notation may be replaced by a parameter which is a constant of proportionality (R), i.e.

$$D_N = R \cdot T^{0.11} \cdot N^{0.24}$$

Since R for fractionated treatments is simply a measure of the accumulated biological response, they have suggested that R becomes known as the cumulative radiation effect (or CRE), a scale of biological effect. The NSD is therefore the value of CRE at the tolerance level of normal tissue radiation reactions. The difference of this approach to that of Ellis is illustrated by developing the equation given above to describe R or the CRE.

$$R = D_N \cdot T^{-0.11} \cdot N^{-0.24}$$

Clearly the CRE is proportional to the total dose, whereas the NSD was chosen to be dependent on the number of fractions. The scale of radiation effect is, therefore, different in the CRE formulation although the effects are the same at tolerance levels of damage.

The concept of CRE has been applied to treatments by moulds and implants and extended to incorporate the influence of the volume factor. It is also possible for the analysis to deal with gaps which may be introduced into a radiotherapy fractionation scheme either inadvertently, or by design, to complete a comprehensive system which may allow the assessment and comparison of the effect of different treatments on normal tissues, allowing for a delay in CRE in intervals between treatments.

An important question which has yet to be answered is whether there is a direct correlation between the acute and late effects of radiation, particularly for limiting normal tissues. The various iso-effect formulae have either not been applied to enough different fractionation regimes or the end-points for early and late damage are not sufficiently comparable to provide a valid answer. Clearly this latter problem may be insoluble when, for example, an acute moist desquamation is to be compared with late fibrosis of deeper tissues. There is also the phenomenon of 'slow repair' which has recently been reported for slowly proliferating tissues like lung where the late effect is the primary problem.

New methods in radiotherapy

Accelerated 'heavy' particles

The improvements that can be expected in radio-therapy must increase the therapeutic ratio between tumour response and normal tissue damange. This can be achieved by the use of methods designed to reduce the radioresistance of hypoxic tumour cells (OER) or by improving the physical localization of radiation dose distribution. A new form of radiation which combines both a reduced OER and an improved dose-dis-tribution is the negative π-meson (or pion). Pions are sub-atomic particles with a mass 276 times that of an electron, but with the same negative charge. They are produced by accelerating extremely high energy protons (500 to 750 MeV) in a synchrocyclotron onto a graphite or lead target. Negative π-mesons are interesting because the deposition of energy occurs mainly in the Bragg ionization peak where the pions slow down and are captured by nuclei present in tissues. Pions produce densely ionizing particles when they are attentuated in tissues as a result of nuclear disintegrations releasing α-particles, neutrons and protons following their capture in the nuclei of carbon, oxygen and nitrogen. The entrance, or plateau, region of the depth-dose curve is produced by the much less densely ionizing fast particles and so in this region the

RBE of the pion beam is much lower (Fig. 3.15).

Under conditions of clinical pion radiotherapy, how-ever, a broader peak is required in order to encompass the volume of a typical tumour. As a result, many of the idealized values shown in Fig. 3.15 are reduced. While the plateau RBE remains at approximately 1.0, the peak RBE is 1.4 and the OER at the peak is about 2.2 (representing an 'oxygen gain factor' of only 1.3). Nevertheless, the biological and physical differences between the plateau and the peak still indicate a sig-nificant therapeutic advantage in the clinical appli-cation of pion beams. Use of pions, as well as of other particle beams, is discussed further in Chapter 4.

Other charged particles that have only been studied under experimental conditions include helium, carbon, neon and argon ions. Various RBE values have been reported at both plateau and peak positions but what is important is the peak to plateau ratio in each case. These ratios range from 1.9 for carbon down to 1.0 for argon. OER values range from 1.7 to 1.2. There are no more than very limited plans for the clinical use of those particles, unlike protons which have been used clini-cally for many years because of the depth-dose characteristics of beams in the range 150 to 200 MeV. Their biological qualities do not differ from those of low LET radiation, however.

The high LET radiation which has received the most clinical study is the fast neutron with a mean energy of at least 6 MeV. Fig. 3.16 shows four cell survival curves (three of which were shown in Figs. 3.5 and 3.7). The two X-ray curves were shown in Fig. 3.5 to illustrate the OER of 2.4 for low LET radiation. By comparison, the two neutron curves illustrate the smaller OER value of 1.5. The ratio of these two OER values represents a gain factor of 1.6 and this therapeutic advantage is the

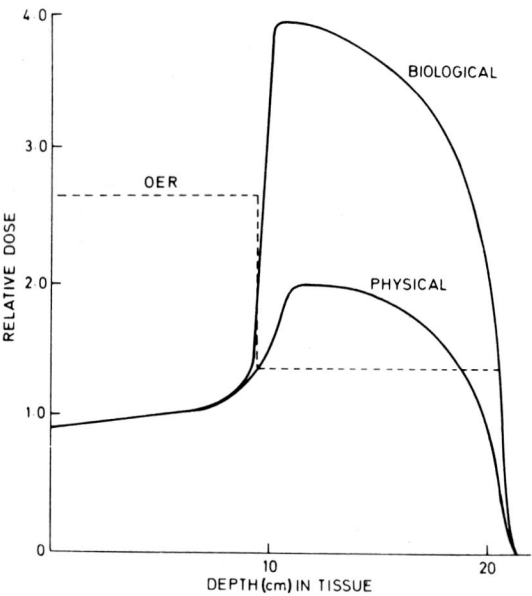

Fig. 3.15 Relative physical and biological dose distri-bution of negative π-mesons in tissues (from Duncan and Nias, 1977).

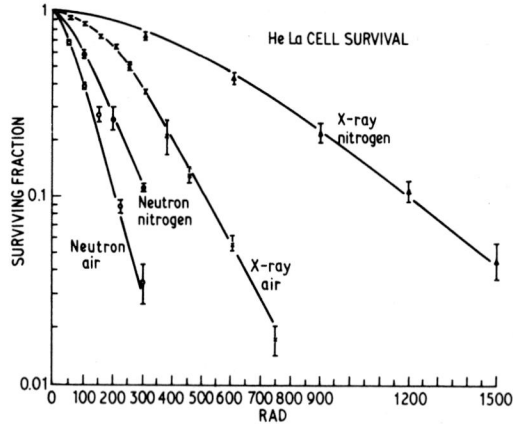

Fig. 3.16 Survival curves of HeLa cells irradiated with X-rays or fast neutrons in air or in nitrogen (from Nias *et al*., 1967).

main rationale for the use of fast neutrons in clinical radiotherapy. The other advantage would accrue from any difference in RBE values between tumour and limiting normal tissues and there are some examples which encourage this hope. Thus, tumour RBEs tend to be higher than those for haematological tissues. (The inverse relationship between RBE value and fraction-dose size was described earlier: see Fig. 3.7 and Table 3.2.) While fast neutron generators tend to be less expensive than charged particle generators and neutrons provide a reduction in OER, there is none of the advantage in dose distribution shown with pions.

Hyperthermia

There has recently been a rebirth of interest in the effects of hyperthermia on cancer and the demonstration that it is a powerful synergist of radiation effects. The mechanism of the action of hyperthermia on normal and cancer cells is still poorly understood, but it has been shown that some cancer cells are more sensitive to heat treatment than normal cells. This selective effect is much more marked above about 42°C. The mode of action is certainly different from that of irradiation and the effects of these differences may have important implications for radiotherapy. Cells in the late S-phase which are the most resistant to X-rays are found to be the most sensitive to the effects of heating. The combination of heating and X-radiation therefore produces a reduction in the differential radiosensitivity of cells, throughout the cell cycle potentiating the effects of radiation on asynchronous populations.

The quantitative cellular effects of heating depend critically on the temperature to which they are elevated and the period for which they are kept at that temperature. In general terms there is a complementary relationship between temperature and time so that the proportion of cells sterilized may be correlated with the total energy absorbed. If irradiated with simultaneous hyperthermia the radiation cell-survival curve shows a greatly reduced shoulder region and the slope of the exponential portion of the curve is much steeper. Cells show a phenomenon called thermal tolerance, i.e. they are less sensitive to a second heating. On the other hand, cells are more sensitive to heat at lower pH, as is found in hypoxic regions, where thermal tolerance is reduced.

At the tissue level, a combination of hyperthermia and radiation will also lead to increased damage. The amount of this increase can be expressed as a thermal enhancement ratio (TER) defined as the dose of irradiation without heat divided by the dose with heat required for a given biological effect. Fig. 3.17 shows how the TER varies with the time sequence of irradi-

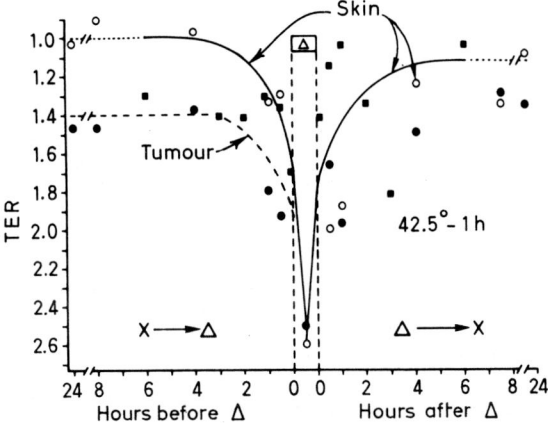

Fig. 3.17 Composite graph of thermal enhancement ratios (TER) for mouse skin and tumours after the application of radiation (×) before, during and after heating (Δ). The solid line and open circles (o) apply to skin reactions. The dotted line and closed symbols (■, •) are for tumour response (from Dewey *et al.*, 1980).

ation (×) and heating (Δ) at 42.5°C for one hour. Simultaneous treatment gives the largest effect. Irradiation before heating has the advantage that the TER for tumour is larger than for normal skin. This advantage is lost with the reverse sequence.

The techniques of inducing either systemic hyperthermia or localized heating (for example by microwave radiation) are currently being evaluated in a few cancer centres.

Basic radiobiological research continues to investigate the subject further as there is the possibility that the combination of hyperthemia and radiotherapy may prove to be of clinical benefit. It may well be that this benefit is the happy consequence of two opposing factors: (1) microscopic foci in tumours are less radiosensitive because inadequate blood supply leads to reduced oxygen tension and (2) the same foci will tend to be raised to a relatively high temperature during local heating because the inadequate blood supply results in less dissipation of heat. Thus the more radioresistant cells will be more affected by heat damage.

Unorthodox fractionation and hyperbaric oxygen

If reduction in OER is all that is being attempted then a number of options are open to the radiotherapist, including optimization of fractionated X-ray dosage from standard treatment machines. The practice of treating patients five days each week for three to six weeks has no scientific basis except for the original observation that some form of fractionation improves normal tissue tolerance compared with the effect of a single dose. That apart, the precise dose-time relationship has still to be established for each clinical situation. The fractionation formulae described above have emboldened some clinicians to try unorthodox regimes varying from three acute treatments per day over a short period (Svoboda, 1978) to multiple fractions of protracted irradiation over much longer periods than usual (Pierquin *et al.*, 1974). Information on the contribution of reoxygenation has been obtained indirectly from clinical trials with hyperbaric oxygen which show that fewer larger radiation doses delivered at longer intervals are then more effective than the standard number of smaller daily doses in air. With such optimization the use of hyperbaric oxygen has shown significant advantage in the treatment of malignancies in certain sites like head and neck, cervix and bronchus (squamous cell tumours) (Dische, 1978).

Adjuvant drugs

Hypoxic cell sensitizers

Another method of overcoming the oxygen problem is to use an adjuvant drug which selectively sensitizes hypoxic cells. The nitroimidazole drugs have this property by virtue of their electron-affinity. The radiosensitizing property of Misonidazole was described at the beginning of this chapter (i.e. affinity for the

hydrated electron e^-_{aq}). Unlike oxygen, this drug is not metabolized by hypoxic cells so that a sufficient concentration can effect the sort of enhanced radiation response shown in Fig. 3.18. An enhancement ratio of 2 is obtained with a dose level of the drug which is non-toxic in C_3H mice. The figure shows that only half the radiation dose is needed to produce the same delay in regrowth of tumours in mice treated with Misonidazole. Unfortunately the pharmacokinetics of Misonidazole are quite different between mice and men – a much longer half-life in man reduces the dosage level that can safely be given and the resultant enhancement ratio is not much higher than 1.2 for fractionated regimes of radiotherapy.

Perhaps the best results will be obtained by using a single large dose of Misonidazole with the first fraction of radiotherapy (when hyperbaric oxygen is less likely to be effective) and then using hyperbaric oxygen for subsequent X-ray treatments. If a fast neutron generator is available then this might also be used with hyperbaric oxygen to reduce the OER still further! The problem with all such regimes is lack of a direct clinical assay of the extent and localization of hypoxic cells in tumours. There is evidence that Misonidazole could be used for such a diagnostic assay if labelled with a gamma-emitting radionuclide (Chapman *et al.*, 1981).

Other drug – radiation combinations

Hypoxic cell sensitizers have been subjected to detailed laboratory and clinical research and their mode of action and efficacy are relatively well understood (see Adams *et al.*, 1978). It is regrettable that the same degree of detailed study has not been made of all the other chemotherapeutic agents in current use for cancer treatment in combination with radiotherapy. The extent of the problem is illustrated in Fig. 3.19 which illustrates the terminology used in the description of drug–radiation interactions. If an agent is completely inactive when used by itself, then evidence from sensitization or protection can be obtained without more detailed study (left-hand column of Fig. 3.19). Regrettably this requirement is not even satisfied for radiosensitization by oxygen since even this substance is toxic in certain circumstances.

In nearly every combination of drug and radiation both agents show some effect which is dose-dependent. The right-hand column of Fig. 3.19 illustrates the only sure way of determining the combination of dosage (timing will be discussed later) of the two agents which will produce the desired response: namely, positive interaction which provides the possibility of an improvement in tumour response without any increase in effect on normal tissues. Dose-effect curves are needed for *both* agents if this information is to be

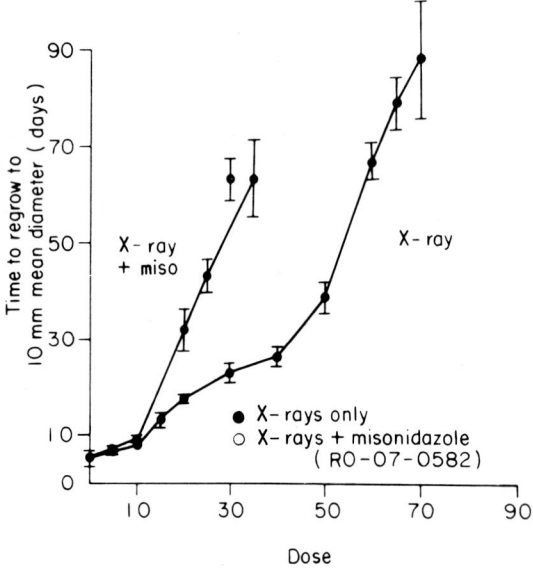

Fig. 3.18 Effect of Misonidazole on the radiation response of mouse tumours (from Abdelaal and Nias, 1979).

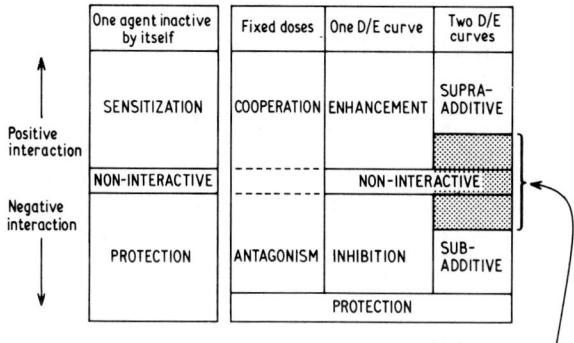

	One agent inactive by itself	Fixed doses	One D/E curve	Two D/E curves
Positive interaction ↑	SENSITIZATION	COOPERATION	ENHANCEMENT	SUPRA-ADDITIVE
	NON-INTERACTIVE	---	NON-INTERACTIVE	
Negative interaction ↓	PROTECTION	ANTAGONISM	INHIBITION	SUB-ADDITIVE
		PROTECTION		

CONCEIVABLY ADDITIVE RESPONSE

Fig. 3.19 Terminology of drug–radiation interaction (from Steele, 1979).

obtained. In nearly every example in both the clinical and experimental literature this requirement is not satisfied and conclusions are reached on the basis of insufficient data (e.g. the middle columns of Fig. 3.19).

The combination of radiation and drug may be more effective because of one or more of the following mechanisms: (a) interaction may occur due to presence of the drug during irradiation, (b) the drug may interfere with repair of radiation damage, (c) there may be some differential effect upon the proliferation kinetics of tumour and/or normal cells.

The presence of the drug during radiation should ideally be demonstrated by standard biochemical and pharmacological techniques. If the active moiety of the drug molecule can be labelled with radioactive isotope, this demonstration is relatively simple (although invasive methods of sampling such as biopsies are not always possible or ethically desirable with human subjects). If the active moiety cannot be labelled or tissue samples cannot be studied then indirect evidence of drug binding will have to suffice, but doubt must then remain if or how the drug interacted with the radiation. It will also be important to know whether the drug binds to the target molecules in the cell following passive diffusion or some mechanism of active transport.

Before studying repair of radiation damage in cells exposed to drug–radiation combination it is necessary to know the pattern of repair in that cell following damage by radiation alone and drug alone. Following radiation, it is known that the timing of events within a cell which is attempting to recover from damage to its DNA will depend upon four factors: (a) the nature and number of lesions produced in its DNA, (b) the ability of the cell to perform those different types of repair required by such lesions, (c) the growth conditions at the time which may help or hinder the cell's repair mechanism, (d) the efficiency of each repair event in

restoring the full competence of the original DNA in both its transcriptional and replicative roles.

The same sort of information should be sought for each drug before the repair mechanism can be expected to be understood in drug–radiation combinations. At the present time there is a relative dearth of information but such data as are available show that many drugs may reduce repair capacity following radiation. It is not clear if and how the molecular biological evidence for the repair of DNA strand breakage can be correlated with the biological phenomenon usually termed 'recovery from sub-lethal damage', but it is known that the drug actinomycin D which inhibits RNA synthesis also inhibits 'Elkind recovery'. Other drugs which are known to reduce the amount of Elkind recovery include 5-fluorouracil, BUdR and IUdR, vinblastine and platinum coordination complexes. A difference in the cellular environment at the time of radiation may influence the degree of recovery from potentially lethal damage independently from such effects on sub-lethal damage (Utsumi and Elkind, 1979).

Turning to the third mechanism, this is related to the proliferation kinetics of the cell populations affected by the drug–radiation combination treatment. This is the point to state what has so far only been inferred – namely, that DNA is considered to be the prime target of both radiation and drug therapy. This may be a misleading generalization as far as some cancer chemotherapeutic agents are concerned – some will undoubtedly bind to and damage organelles and molecules in the cell other than the nucleus and its DNA. The main objective of cytotoxic action in the context of cancer therapy must be loss of the proliferative capacity of malignant cells, however, and it can be stated that radiation in the therapeutic dose range damages DNA and its function more than any other cellular constituent.

The large amount of literature describing the mechanism of radiation is not matched by equivalent knowledge of the various drugs in common use. Dosimetry, for example, is a relatively very precise physical technique with radiation where the distribution in treated tissues can be precisely measured and the clinician can repeat a treatment in the confident knowledge that his prescribed dose will be faithfully delivered. For most drugs it is almost impossible to emulate this precision. Certain minimal information should nevertheless be available before a drug is used. What is the mode of action at the cellular level? Does the drug reach the intracellular target molecules by passive diffusion or active transport? Is the drug active in its original form or by some degradative product (e.g. after cyclization in the case of nitrogen mustard and by liver metabolism in the case of cyclophosphamide)?

What is the rate of degradation and loss of activity of the drug (e.g. the half-time of hydrolysis in water or preferably in some medium relevant to the *in vivo* milieu at 37°C)? Does the drug degrade to a final product which is non-toxic? What are the pharmacokinetics? Solubility of the drug is another consideration. Is the drug soluble in aqueous medium and (apart from temperature effects) is its activity influenced by pH? Does any other change in the substrate influence drug activity?

It is up to the clinician to design combination regimes based upon well established drug and radiation mechanisms. The designer should remember that single doses are the exception and that repeated treatments with combination regimes are the rule. The phenomenon of 'recruitment' will therefore apply; this is a term used to designate the induction of a resting cell into the mitotic cycle or the induction of a slowly proliferating cell population to increase its rate of cell replication.

The result of such recruitment (and other inevitable consequences of repeated treatments with both drug and radiation) will be a tendency for both normal and tumour cell populations to cycle randomly. The search for cycle phase-specific drugs has produced some important fundamental observations but unless a tumour cell population can be synchronized, this sort of information cannot be utilized.

It is difficult enough to synchronize a mammalian cell population under laboratory conditions and then only for one cycle, using physical methods *in vitro*. When it comes to drugs, the use of hydroxyurea *in vivo* has led to only partial synchrony. Perhaps more attention should be paid to normal circadian rhythms which may turn out to be sufficiently different from those of a particular tumour to provide some rationale for the optimal timing of drug–radiation therapy.

Selection of the optimum combinations of drug and radiation requires a wide spectrum of skills. Just as radiotherapy can only be practised with a knowledge of physics and radiobiology, so chemotherapy requires the equivalent knowledge of pharmacology and chemobiology. Few individuals can expect to acquire all these skills and the best solution is for a number of clinicians to design the treatment protocols in consultation with the appropriate basic scientists.

Further reading

Alper, T. (1979), *Cellular Radiobiology*. Cambridge University Press.

Duncan, W. and Nias, A.H.W. (1977), *Clinical Radiobiology*. Churchill Livingstone, Edinburgh.

Hall, E.J. (1978), *Radiobiology for the Radiologist*. 2nd ed, Harper and Row, New York.

References

Abdelaal, A.S. and Nias, A.H.W. (1979), Regression, recurrence and cure in an irradiated mouse tumour. *J. R. Soc. Med.*, **72**, 100–5.

Adams, G.E., Fowler, J.F. and Wardman, P. (eds) (1978), Hypoxic cell sensitisers in radiobiology and radiotherapy. *Br. J. Cancer*, **37**, Supplement III.

Chapman, J.D., Franko, A.J. and Sharplin, J. (1981), A marker for hypoxic cells in tumours with potential clinical applicability. *Br. J. Cancer*, **43**, 546–50.

Deschner, E.E. and Gray, L.H. (1959), Influence of oxygen tension on X-ray induced chromosomal damage in Ehrlich ascites tumour cells irradiated in vitro and in vivo. *Radiat. Research*, **11**, 115–46.

Dewey, W.C., Freeman, M.L., Raaphorst, G.P., Clark, E.P., Wong, R.S.L., Highfield, D.P., Spiro, I.J., Tomosovic, S.P., Denman, D.L. and Cross, R.A. (1980), Cell biology of hyperthermia and radiation. In *Radiation Biology in Cancer Research*. (eds R.E. Meyn and H.R. Withers), Raven Press, New York, pp. 589–621.

Dische, S. (1978), Hyperbaric oxygen: the Medical Research Council trials and their clinical significance. *Br. J. Radiol.*, **51**, 888–94.

Duncan, W. and Nias, A.H.W. (1977), *Clinical Radiobiology*. Churchill-Livingstone, Edinburgh, p.208.

Ellis, F. (1965), The relationship of biological effect to dose-time fractionation factors in radiotherapy. *Curr. Topics Radiat. Res.*, **4**, 357–97.

Fowler, J.F., Morgan, R.L., Silvester, J.A., Bewley, D.K. and Turner, B.A. (1963), Experiments with fractionated X-ray treatment of the skins of pigs. *Br. J. Radiol.*, **36**, 188–196.

Hall, E.J. (1978), *Radiobiology for the Radiologist*. 2nd edn, Harper and Row, London, p. 7.

Hermens, A.F. and Barendsen, G.W. (1969), Changes of cell proliferation characteristics in a rat rhabdomyosarcoma before and after X-irradiation. *Europ. J. Cancer*, **5**, 173–89.

Hewitt, H.B. and Wilson, C.W. (1959), The effect of tissue oxygen tension on the radiosensitivity of leukaemia cells irradiated in situ in the livers of leukaemic mice. *Br. J. Cancer*, **13**, 675–84.

Howes, A.E. (1969), An estimation of changes in the proportions and absolute numbers of hypoxic cells after irradiation of transplanted C₃H mouse mammary tumours. *Br. J. Radiol.*, **42**, 441–7.

Kirk, J., Gray, W.M. and Watson, E.R. (1977), Cumulative radiation effect. *Clin. Radiol.*, **28**, 29–92.

Luxton, R.W. and Kunkler, P.B. (1964), Radiation nephritis. *Acta Radiol.*, **2**, 169–78.

Mendelsohn, M.L. and Dethlefsen, L.A. (1967), Tumour growth and cellular kinetics, In: *The Proliferation and Spread of Neoplastic Cells*. M.D.

Anderson Hospital, Houston, p. 200.

Nias, A.H.W., Greene, D., Fox, M. and Thomas, R.L. (1967), Effect of 14 MeV monoenergetic neutrons on HeLa and P388F cells in vitro. *Int. J. Radiat. Biol.*, **13**, 449–56.

Oakes, W.R. and Lushbaugh, C.C. (1952), Course of testicular injury following accidental exposure to nuclear radiations. *Radiology*, **59**, 737–43.

Orton, C.G. and Ellis, F. (1973), A simplification of the use of the NSD concept in practical radiotherapy. *Br. J. Radiol.*, **46**, 529–37.

Phillips, T.L. and Buschke, F. (1969), Radiation tolerance of the thoracic spinal cord. *Am. J. Roentg.*, **105**, 659–64.

Pierquin, B., Baillet, F. and Brown, C. (1974), La téléradiotherapique continue et de faible débit. *J. Radiol. Electrol.*, **55**, 757–63.

Regaud, C., Coutard, H. and Hautant, A. (1922), Contribution en traitement des cancers endolarynges par les rayons. *Xth International Congress d'Otology*, 19–22.

Roentgen, W.C. (1895), Uber eine neue Art von Strahlen Erste Mitteilung. *Sber. Physik. Medizin. Ges. Wurzburg*, 132–41.

Steele, G.G. (1979), Terminology in the description of drug-radiation interactions. *In. J. Radiat. Oncol.*, **5**, 1145–50.

Svoboda, V.H.J. (1978), Further experience with radiotherapy by multiple daily sessions. *Br. J. Radiol.*, **51**, 363–9.

Thomlinson, R.H. (1966), Personal communication.

Upton, A.C. (1961), The dose response relation in radiation induced cancer. *Cancer Res.*, **21**, 717–29.

Utsumi, H. and Elkind, M.M. (1979), Potentially lethal damage versus sublethal damage: independent repair processes in actively growing Chinese hamster cells. *Radiat. Res.*, **77**, 346–60.

van den Brenk, H.A.S. (1971), Radiation effects on the pulmonary system, In: *Pathology of Radiation*, (ed. C.C. Berdjis), Williams and Wilkins, Baltimore.

Yuhas, J.M. (1980), A more general role for WR-2721 in cancer therapy. *Br. J. Cancer*, **41**, 832–34.

4 Heavy particle radiotherapy

Carl F. von Essen

In the survey of radiation therapy results by Suit (1969) it was calculated that at least one third of the failures related primarily to the persistence of local tumour. A significant percentage therefore of failure by radiation therapy is caused by the inability to ablate cancer at the site of origin. This limitation surely relates to the tumour lethal dose that can be delivered, to its distribution in the target volume and in the body, and to the relative specificity of damage upon tumour cells and malignant cells. How newer forms of radiation, heavy particles, charged or neutral, might interact in order to overcome these limitations in cancer therapy will herein be discussed.

The tumour lethal dose

As shown in Chapter 3, the survival of tumour (and other) cells has an exponential function following an initial insensitivity, D_q, a measure of the ability to repair sub-lethal damage. With the most extreme conditions of radioresistance such as anoxia of the tumour, the lethality curves, although less steep, still preserve an exponential form. Thus it is apparent, in contrast to most chemotherapeutic agents, that a sufficiently large dose of ionizing radiations can sterilize any known tumour. The critical difficulty in carrying out successfully the ablation of tumours is the tolerance of normal tissues within, and outside, the tumour. It is unacceptable to produce a degree of morbidity that results in years of suffering despite the ablation of a potentially malignant cancer. Two approaches can be made, however, to reach a more optimum level of tumour lethality; first, the reduction of the volume of unnecessary normal tissue exposure; second, the overcoming of radioresistant factors in the tumour.

Dose distribution

The principal cause of failure for all treatment modalities is the escape of tumour cells through vascu-lar pathways. Solutions for this problem are currently involving a major effort in cancer treatment research. However, as discussed by Suit, a significant fraction of failure relates to the localized, not yet metastasized, primary cancer.

Often within the volume of gross tumour (the tumour volume) are critical normal structures, i.e. oesophagus, bladder and bowel which can scarcely be spared from the dose required to ablate the cancer. Immediately surrounding this volume is a second zone termed the target volume. This incorporates the tumour volume plus a margin of normal tissue which includes both normal tissues and sub-clinical (i.e. invisible), actual or potential tumour cells. This total volume is one which, for any locoregional treatment modality, must be excised or treated sufficiently to sterilize every tumour cell therein. Finally, for most existing forms of radiation therapy the actual volume of tissue and tumour that is treated may be significantly larger than the target volume. The reason for this is due to limitations of a technical nature such as the exponential absorption characteristic of photon beams, the complexity of shaping such beams to the actual target volume, the uncertainty of accurate daily reproducibility of treatment, patient movements, and inherent errors in the beam geometry and dose delivery.

It has been well established that the tolerance of the body to withstand ionizing radiation in any significant dosage is strongly volume-dependent. This relates to the importance of repopulation of cells from unirradiated sites into the radiated zone in order to maintain tissue integrity. It is extremely likely that a significant advance can be made if the radiation volume is closely tailored to the target volume (Kramer and Suntharalingam, 1977). The tumour dose can then be raised to more effective levels, such as those achieved by radioactive implants, and radiation morbidity to surrounding normal tissues can simultaneously be reduced.

Heavy charged particles, including negative π-mesons (pions), protons, helium, carbon, neon and argon ions (Table 4.1) all share the characteristics of depositing the greatest dose at the *end* of their path through matter. This phenomenon is termed the Bragg peak (Fig. 4.1) and differs significantly from the more or less exponential absorption occurring with photon and neutron beams. Since the ideal goal of radiation therapy is to deliver the entire dose within the target volume and to completely spare non-target tissues it is apparent that these charged particles more closely approach that ideal.

Biological selectivity

As has been discussed in Chapter 3, heavy particles such as neutrons, carbon, neon and argon ions and also pions produce dense ionization patterns (high LET) which tend to reduce or eliminate radioresistant factors such as hypoxia and cell cycle insensitivity. Evidence that hypoxia is an important factor in clinical tumour radioresistance is now being established from recently published results of clinical utilization of hyperbaric oxygen therapy as an adjunct to conventional radiotherapy (Dische, 1978). This hypoxic radioresistance factor is termed the oxygen enhancement ratio (OER) and is extensively discussed in Chapter 3. Particles

heavier than protons but also including negative pions exhibit various degrees of OER reduction compared to low LET irradiations. Heavy charged particles have, generally, a higher LET in the Bragg peak than in the plateau, thus exhibiting both distribution and potential biological advantages. The LET in the peak, however, is generally lower than that for neutrons. Thus, if the biological advantages were considered of principal importance, then only neutrons would be worthwhile investigating, because of the high LET and reasonably comparable dose distribution to low LET radiations. However, at present, the degree to which dose distribution and biological selectivity separately contribute to improvement of results in radiotherapy is not known, and a variety of particles must be clinically investigated.

Neutrons

Fast neutrons

The development of the cyclotron in the 1930s permitted the acceleration of heavy charged particles such as deuterons which were able to generate useful beams of neutrons following collision with beryllium and other low atomic weight elements. Radiobiological studies showed that the RBE for neutrons appeared

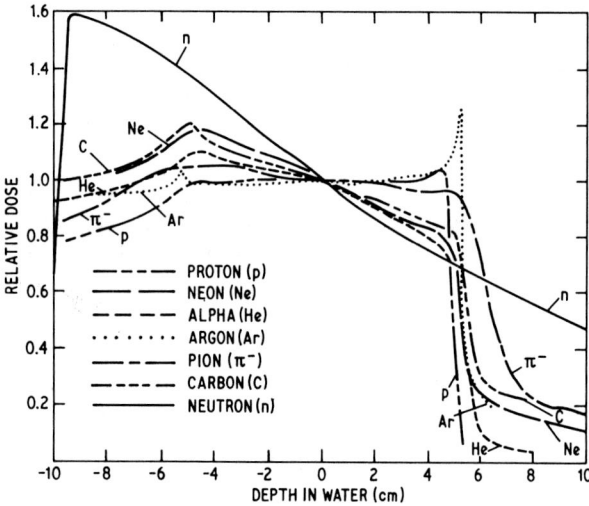

Fig. 4.1 Measured central axis depth-dose distributions for heavy particles. The Bragg peaks for charged particle beams are spread to 10 cm in width and the distributions are normalized at the peak centre. The depth-dose curve for a typical neutron beam is also shown. (Reproduced by courtesy of Raju *et al.*, 1978*a*.)

Table 4.1 Comparative theoretical advantages of heavy particle beams (adapted and modified from Castro *et al.*, 1979, and Raju, 1979).

	Improved dose distribution	Improved biological selectivity
Fast neutrons		***
Slow neutron capture	*	****
Protons	****	
Helium ions	****	*
Negative pions	***	**
Carbon ions	***	**
Neon ions	**	***
Argon ions	*	****

greater for the effects on animal tumours than upon normal tissues. Clinical trials were carried out between 1938 and 1943 and results were presented by Stone in 1948. He concluded that neutron therapy was not useful because of the marginal therapeutic ratio between tumour curve and normal tissue damage. The conclusions were reviewed by Fowler and his colleagues (1963) and a different view was reached that overdosage occurred in many cases because of a previously unsuspected increase of RBE with multiple fractionated treatments by neutrons. Subsequently an intensive radiobiological and clinical programme was initiated by the MRC Cyclotron Unit of the Hammersmith Hospital in London and continued by facilities throughout the world (Table 4.2).

Radiobiological characteristics of neutrons

A more detailed review of neutrons and other heavy particle radiotherapy is given in Chapter 3. In summary the RBE of neutrons varies inversely with neutron energy, is greater for smaller doses, for biological systems with large repair capacities (D_q), and for actively growing cell systems. Thus it is not possible to assign a single RBE value. However, in the clinical range of dosage, fractionation, and target tissues, RBE values of between 3 and 4 are commonly reported. The OER value is inversely related to the RBE value and has been shown to vary from as low as 1.1 to 1.8. In the clinical range the OER appears to lie between 1.5 and 1.8.

Dose distribution characteristics of neutrons

Neutron beams have depth dose curves similar to those of medium to high energy photons (Fig. 4.1). There is a small degree of skin sparing that increases with neutron energy. Because a D–T generator produces 14 MeV monoenergetic neutrons, it has a depth dose distribution similar to a neutron beam generated by 30 MeV peak deuterons in a cyclotron (Brennan, 1969). As with photons, the source skin distance is important but must be selected with regard to the available neutron flux. As is seen in Table 4.2 the 50% depth dose in tissue varies from 8 to 15 cm as compared to 11 cm for cobalt 60, 16 cm for 6 MeV X-rays, and 20 cm for 15 MeV X-rays. The modal number, 9 cm, refers to the majority of current beams in clinical use and constitutes a distinct drawback to the range of potential usefulness of these neutron beams in comparison with depth doses available with higher energy photons. Higher energy neutrons, which gain in penetration but lose little in OER advantages, such as at the facilities in Louvain and Batavia, can overcome these difficulties.

Results from recent clinical trials of fast neutron beams

Data were presented at the 3rd International Meeting of Fast Neutrons and other Fast Particles held at the Haague in late 1978 from the principal centres studying the experimental aspects of fast neutron therapy (see Table 4.2). Masterful reviews by Dutreix and Tubiana (1979) and Halnan (1979) and concluding discussions can be summarized as follows:

1. Certain tumour types in accessible sites appear to be more favourably affected by neutrons than by photons: these include relatively advanced epidermoid carcinomas of the head and neck, salivary gland adenocarcinomas, and some soft tissue sarcomas.
2. Certain other sites had promising results but evaluation remained problematic because of short follow-up experience, insufficient number of cases, or lack of controls. These include advanced cancer of the cervix, osteosarcoma, and carcinomas of the rectum.
3. At least one site showed clearly poorer results with neutron therapy: malignant glioma of the brain.
4. Results with 'mixed schedules' appeared in many hands to be better than results by pure neutron therapy. These schedules included alternating photons and neutron radiation or neutron 'boosts' to high dose photon therapy.
5. The high incidence of complications had to be compared to the therapeutic benefits. It was important to distinguish, if possible, 'tumour related' against 'treatment related' complications. It was apparent that many very advanced cancers, when eradicated, left significant anatomic and functional defects

Table 4.2 Fast neutron clinical facilities.

Site	Source type	Particle	Energy (MeV)	Reaction	Mean energy (MeV)	SSD (cm)	Tissue D_{50} (cm)	Dose rate (rad/min)
Univ. Calif., Berkeley	Cyclotron	d^+	16	$d^+ \rightarrow Be$	8	115	9	25
MRC Cyclotron Unit, London	Cyclotron	d^+	16	$d^+ \rightarrow Be$	8	120	9	40
Texas A & M (TAMVEC)	Cyclotron	d^+	50	$d^+ \rightarrow Be$	21	140	14	80
Univ. Washington, Seattle	Cyclotron	d^+	21	$d^+ \rightarrow Be$	8	150	9	50
MANTA Washington, D.C.	Cyclotron	d^+	35	$d^+ \rightarrow Be$	15	125	11	55
NIRS Chiba, Japan	Cyclotron	d^+	30	$d^+ \rightarrow Be$	12	200	10	60
University Hospital, Hamburg	D-T gener. (isocentric)	d^+	0.4	$d^+ \rightarrow T$	15 [1]	80	9	20
A.v.Leeuwenhoek Hospital, Amsterdam	D-T gener. (isocentric)	d^+	0.4	$d^+ \rightarrow T$	15 [1]	80	9	8
Fermilab. Batavia, Illinois	Linac	p^+	66	$p^+ \rightarrow Be$	25	153	15	45
W. General Hospital, Edinburgh	Cyclotron (isocentric)	d^+	15	$d^+ \rightarrow Be$	7	125	10	30
W. German Tumour Centre, Essen	Cyclotron	d^+	14	$d^+ \rightarrow Be$	7	125	10	40
Heidelberg, Deutsch. Krebsforschungs- zentrum	D-T gener. (isocentric)	d^+	0.4	$d^+ \rightarrow Be$	15 [1]	100	10	8
Louvain	Cyclotron	d^+	55	$d^+ \rightarrow Be$	21	155	14	150
Berlin DDR	Cyclotron	d^+	14	$d^+ \rightarrow Be$	6	100	8	20

References to Table 4.2
1. Stone (1948); 2. Catterall (1979); 3. Peters *et al.* (1978, 1979); 4. Griffin *et al.* (1979); 5. Ornitz *et al.* (1979); 6. Tsunemoto *et al.* (1979); 7. Tsunemoto *et al.* (1979); 8. Franke *et al.* (1978, 1979); 9. Batterman and Breur (1979); 10. Lawrence and Cohen (1979); 11. Duncan and Arnott (1979); 12. Maier and Hüdepohl (1979); 13. Schnabel (1979); 14. Wambersie *et al.* (1979); 15. Eichhorn *et al.* (1974, 1977, 1979).

Ref. (see below)	Clinical onset year	Representative dose schedules (rad/treatment/days)	Remarks
1	1939	Various	Trials completed 1943 Stone reported severe late effects RBE subsequently found higher due to fractionation.
2	1967	1560/12/26 [3]	Largest clinical results. Randomized trials of head and neck demonstrate neutron advantages. Long-term follow up provides assessment of late effect RBE.
3	1972	Various mixed schedules [2]	Neutron therapy alone abandoned 1974. Mixed schedule yielded improved results in advanced cervix cancer. Breast treatment gave high degree of fibrosis.
4	1973	1800/12/40 [2] 1800/18/40 1800/24/40	Mixed schedule also studied. No improvement in treatment of gliomas. Neutrons and mixed schedules of neutrons and photons appear to show advantages in intermediate and advanced head and neck tumours.
5	1973	2160/28/47 [2]	Head and neck sarcomas had high rate of local control. Poor results with gliomas. Late fibrosis considered higher than acceptable in certain cases.
6	1975	1560/12/28 [2] 1650/15/33 1620/18/40	Local control of radioresistant tumours appeared higher with concomitant increased late reaction in normal tissues.
7	1975	1560/12/28 1650/15/33 1620/ 8/40	Glioma data encouraging for mixed schedule with shrinking fields and maximum photon equivalent dose of 6000 rad.
8	1976	1560/12/26 [3] and mixed schedules	Abdominal treatments with mixed schedules. Neutron boost used for gliomas with promising results. Prostate and rectum treatments provided good palliation.
9	1976	1750/25/32 [4] 1600/20/26	No advantages with gliomas. Promising results with salivary gland and head and neck. Complicated rate higher with large fields and dose above 1700 rad.
10	1976	2000–2400 rad [2] 12–24 treatment 40 days	Mixed schedules also investigated. Glioma results poor. Head and neck sarcomas, adenocarcinoma results appear superior with neutrons.
11	1978	1600/20/26 [4]	Poor survival in glioma patients treated with neutrons. No major differences in control rate or morbidity in head and neck patients treated with neutrons or photons.
12	1978	1600/16/26 [4]	23/30 Patients with advanced tumours and full dose showed complete regression. Serious complications in 11/54 cases, all with advanced tumours.
13	1978	1800/20/33 [2]	Bronchus carcinoma trial: early improved survival with neutrons but increased lung fibrosis.
14	1978	Mixed schedule [2]	Pilot studies initiated.
15	1978	Mixed schedule [2]	Bronchus carcinoma treated by mixed schedule (40% neutron dose) with improved local control rate but poorer survival rate.

[1] Monoenergetic (14.5 MeV)
[2] Total dose (includes γ contribution)
[3] Neutron dose only

[4] Total effective dose = $(N + \frac{1}{3}\gamma)$
[5] Facilities in Glasgow, Manchester, Dresden, Zürich, Cleveland in preliminary phases

which could be directly attributed to normal tissue destruction by the pre-existing tumour.

6. It was concluded, during general discussions, that, although there exist conflicting data, a definite advantage existed in certain cases with neutron therapy, that the ratio of normal tissue damage to tumour control was favourable in these cases, but that the majority of existing beams had an inferior dose distribution which made it nearly impossible fairly to compare photons with neutrons.

7. It was considered that the advantages of neutrons over the best available photon modalities were still 'not proved', but warranted further study.

8. It was recommended that neutron beams with better dose distribution advantages, necessarily generated from higher energy cyclotrons or linacs, must be developed in order to provide a better basis for comparison with photons.

Slow neutron capture therapy

The potential benefit of nuclear interactions by slow neutrons with nuclides incorporated into malignant tissues was first proposed by Locher in 1936. In 1953–1961 clinical studies were carried out at the Brookhaven National Laboratory and the Massachusetts Institute of Technology on boron capture by slow neutrons generated in nuclear reactors. The patients treated had malignant brain tumours, generally glioblastoma multiforme (Farr *et al.*, 1961; Sweet *et al.*, 1962). The principles of therapy were the following: many compounds may enter brain tumours in preference to normal brain tissues because of the breakdown of the normal blood-brain barrier by cancer invasion; compounds containing boron-10 have a large capture cross-section for thermal (slow) neutrons. The ensuing reactor at the molecular level

$$^{10}_{5}B + ^{1}_{0}n \rightarrow (^{11}_{5}B) \rightarrow ^{7}_{3}Li + ^{4}_{2}He + 2.4 \text{ MeV}$$

produces a densely ionizing highly localized radiation of heavy nuclear fragments of lithium and α-particles. Assuming that normal brain tissue had no boron uptake and that adequate boron is taken up uniformly by the tumour and that a sufficient flux of thermal neutrons is available, then doses of the order of thousands of rad can be deposited in the tumour cells with relatively little radiation to normal brain. Because of the markedly localized effective range of the heavy fragments, the normal methods of dosimetric verification in rad was not possible. However, severe radiation effects were found in the tumours, but also, unfortunately, in the normal brain tissues presumably because of infracapillary alpha radiation from retained boron-10 in the blood.

Because of failure to demonstrate clinical advantages the trials were abandoned in 1961.

Japanese investigators continued studies and began treating patients in 1968 on the basis of new rationale and techniques as follows (Hatanaka and Sweet, 1978):

1. Intra-arterial infusion of boron-10 compounds.
2. Synthesis of compounds that rapidly clear from the blood.
3. Corticosteroid therapy to mitigate capillary damage.
4. Small fractionated doses.
5. Improved shielding of normal brain and insertion of ping-pong balls in the tumor bed to improve the radiation exposure.

A limited number of patients with malignant glioma were treated from 1968 to 1974 with a suggestive increase in average survival (Hatanaka, 1975).

Problems remaining are the poor depth dose characteristics of thermal neutrons and the uniformity and amount of uptake by the boron compounds in the tumour. This study continues following the installation of a new reactor facility in 1977 (Hatanaka *et al.*, 1975):

Protons

Introduction

Proton beams possess characteristics of great usefulness for radiation therapy of cancer (Wilson, 1946, Larsson, 1967). The dose at the Bragg peak is much greater than in the entry and plateau region (Fig. 4.1), and there is relatively little side-scatter, thus sharp-edged beams with favourable peak-plateau ratios can be used for very small treatment volumes such as the pituitary and for creating radiolesions in small areas of the brain. Spreading out the Bragg peak permits large volumes to be treated with very favourable dose distributions, even shaping in three dimensions. Protons were first used clinically in Berkeley in 1954 for pituitary irradiation (Lawrence, 1957); thereafter in Uppsala, also for cancer therapy, Harvard, and in the Soviet Union. Since it is not yet established in which direction the greatest improvement in the effectiveness of radiation therapy lies, dose distribution versus biological selectivity, a complete evaluation of a beam that comes closest to the optimum dose distribution is important. Clinical trials are now underway in Cambridge (Massachusetts), in the Soviet Union, and will begin again, after 1982, in Uppsala (Table 4.3).

Biological characteristics of protons

Proton beams with a clinically useful energy (150 to 200 MeV) demonstrate no biological qualities that differ from other low LET radiations. Numerous biological studies have repeated RBE values ranging from 0.7 to 1.2 and depending mainly on the energy of the reference photon radiation. Thus the dose response experience of megavoltage can be used without modification in developing proton radiotherapy (Raju *et al.*, 1978 *a, b, c*).

Dose distribution characteristics of protons

The proton beam exhibits the characteristic Bragg-Gray dose distribution in matter in common with other charged particles (Raju *et al.*, 1978*a*). Because range straggling is small the protons stop within 1% of the mean range. Multiple scattering gives a negligible penumbra for large beams and only becomes significant for beams of less than a few millimetres in cross-section (Koehler and Preston, 1972). The proton range is related to the energy and the clinically useful range of up to 26 cm can be developed by a beam of 200 MeV. Since the Bragg peak is quite narrow for monoenergetic proton beams it is necessary to spread the peak to the dimensions of the target volume. This is done by means of a ridge filter or a dynamic range shifter (Koehler *et al.*, 1975) (Fig. 4.2). It is obvious that the peak to plateau ratio decreases as the Bragg peak is spread. The penumbra that is seen with photon and, particularly, electron beams is strikingly diminished with proton beams. By utilizing opposing beams, and overlapping the spread-out Bragg peaks, the dose distribution is superior to that obtained with even high energy photon beams, i.e. the ratio of the

Table 4.3 Proton clinical facilities.

Site	Source type	Energy range (MeV)	Max. range in tissues (cm)	Clinical onset year	Remarks	References
University of California, Berkeley	Cyclotron	200	26	1954	Plateau protons used to ablate normal pituitary for metastatic breast cancer and diabetic retinopathy. Beam converted into helium ions, 1958	Lawrence (1957) Linfoot *et al.* (1963)
Gustaf Werner Institute, University of Uppsala	Synchro-cyclotron	187	23	1957	Variety of doses up to 3000 in one fraction to advanced cancers at various sites. Boost therapy also used. Several striking long-term regressions. Programme stopped in 1976 for up-grading of cyclotron.	Larsson (1967) Graffman and Jung (1970) Stenson (1971) Fors (1964)
Harvard University	Cyclotron	160	18	1960	Bragg peak irradiation for normal pituitary ablation, pituitary tumours. 15000 rad maximum single dose. Large field studies begun in 1973. Density corrections implemented. Promising high dose therapy of prostate and other sites.	Kjellberg *et al.* (1968) Suit *et al.* (1977) Gragordas *et al.* (1978)
Lab. for Nuclear Research, Dubna, USSR	Synchro-cyclotron	200	26	1967	Wide range of dose schedules for advanced cancers in many sites. Single doses up to 10 000 rad. Treatments completed c. 1973 and await development of new, dedicated facilities.	Abazov *et al.* (1971)
Inst. Theoretical and Experimental Physics, Moscow	Synchro-cyclotron	200	26	1967		Abazov *et al.* (1971)
Physiotechnical Institute, Gatchina, USSR	Synchro-cyclotron	1 GeV	extended range-plateau protons	1975	Used for small field therapy only.	Abazov *et al.* (1971)

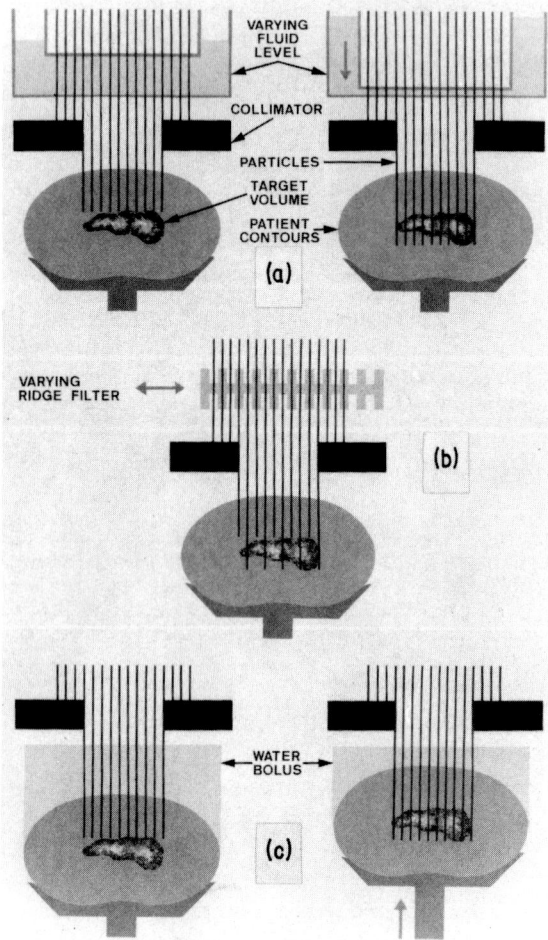

Fig. 4.2 Three methods for distributing Bragg peak ('stopping') particles within the target volume: (*a*) Dynamic range shifter – an oscillating piston displaces the level of an oil or other liquid so that the charged particles are uniformly dispersed in a given range of depth. (*b*) Ridge filter method – a variable thickness metal absorber oscillates in a lateral direction to displace the range of particles uniformly. (*c*) Water bolus method – the patient is translated in a water bolus so that the range of particles is uniformly dispersed. Not shown are methods to shape the particle distribution to complex contours of the target volume. These methods include the introduction of fixed bolus, moving collimators, and patient movement within a small focus of Bragg peak particles.

dose in the target volume to the integral dose in surrounding normal tissues is greater with protons (Suit *et al.*, 1975).

Results of clinical trials of proton therapy

As seen in Table 4.3, much of the early work involved the high dose, small volume, treatment on the pituitary in order to induce hormonal ablation for the management of advanced breast and prostate cancer and for diabetic retinopathy. It was demonstrated that ablative doses as high as 30 000 rad (fractionated) or 15 000 rad (single dose) were effective and relatively without morbidity because of the precision of the beam edges and the careful localization and treatment planning employed (Kjellberg, 1975). Results competitive with those of surgery were obtained, and although hypophysectomy for normal ablation is nowadays less common, proton therapy continues to be used for this purpose.

However, because of the excellent dose localization possibilities, the treatment of pituitary adenomas and eventually malignant tumours in various sites was initiated by the various centres. Reports of the earliest experiences came from Uppsala (Falkmer *et al.*, 1962; Sténson, 1971) and were particularly interesting because of the unusual dose-time schedule: single doses of as high as 3000 rad. Total regression of several advanced carcinomas was reported. Fractionated radiotherapy at 500 rad per fraction to total doses of 6000 rad in 6 weeks also gives excellent regression with low morbidity. These early data seem to indicate that the better dose localization possible with protons permits more intensive therapy to be delivered.

The experience in the Soviet Union is similar: single doses as high as 10 000 rad have been given without apparent difficulty. The general experience reported indicates the relative low incidences of normal tissue complications considering the intensive dosage delivered. There is now a major particle therapy project dedicated to medical use under development.

The cancer therapy programme at Harvard began in 1973 and concentrated on planning large field therapy with corrections for inhomogeneities in the beam path. The simultaneous development of computerized axial tomography (CT) was fortunate in view of the complex problems of calculating and correcting for heterodense structures. In contrast to Uppsala and Moscow, the dosage was in the conventional range using five fractions a week. Treatment of cancer of the prostate using proton 'boosts' was particularly extensive and the ability to give doses at least 10% higher than considered tolerable with conventional radiotherapy was found feasible. Other sites treated included head and neck carcinomas, salivary gland, para-aortic nodes, and retinal tumours (Suit *et al.*, 1977). At Berkeley the use of protons for large field therapy was not pursued; the development of heavy ion therapy will be discussed in the section on heavy ions.

In summary: The dose localization potential of proton beams approaches more closely to the ideal goal of radiotherapy than that of any other reasonably available particle: this goal is the uniform deposition of 100% of the dose within the target volume. No significant additional selectivity due to increased RBE or decreased OER is expected or has been experienced in the clinical studies.

Proton therapy has not yet been evaluated by randomized clinical trials. Pilot studies to date at the centres in Berkeley, Cambridge (Massachusetts), Uppsala and the USSR all indicate the expected advantages of superior dose localization. The unique properties of protons for small beam radiotherapy make them also useful as a form of 'radiosurgery' (Larsson *et al.*, 1963).

Negative pions

Introduction

The negative pion (π-meson) was originally observed in nuclear emulsions exposed to cosmic rays (Occhialini and Powell, 1947) and first generated by the Berkeley cyclotron (Gardner and Lattes, 1948). It has qualities that make it uniquely interesting for the radiation therapy of cancer; it has a charge equal to an electron but 273 times its mass. When a proton beam disintegrates atoms of a target material, negative pions of various kinetic energies fly in all directions. They respond to magnetic fields and may be collected into beams that can be directed as desired by additional magnetic systems. Their range in matter, for example human tissue, is a function of their initial kinetic energy and the stopping power of the material. When a negative pion comes to rest it is attached to a nucleus of nearby O, N or C atoms and cascades down the atomic orbit layers towards the attracting nucleus with the emission of mesic X-rays. When it reaches the nucleus its entire mass is converted into energy as the capturing nucleus literally explodes, throwing out nuclear fragments in all directions. The total energy thus produced is almost 140 MeV; 40 MeV is used to overcome the binding energy of the capturing nucleus, about 70 MeV is kinetic energy of emerging neutrons and about 30 MeV becomes kinetic energy of protons, α particles, and heavier nuclear fragments. Neutrons, α particles, and heavier nuclei produce dense, short-ranged ionization and are responsible for the greatest amount of local damage. The patterns of tracks formed are known

Table 4.4 Negative pion clinical facilities. [1]

Institution and location	Pion source	Available proton current	Type of applicator	Type of medical beam	Initiation of climical testing	Results of clinical trials
Los Alamos Scientific Laboratory and University of New Mexico, Los Alamos	600 MeV proton Linac	300 μa	11 quadrupole focusing and bending magnets	single-vertical	1974	Phase II trials under way; marked regression with low or absent morbidity in many cases [2]
TRIUMF Vancouver	[3] 500 MeV proton isochronous cyclotron	100 μa	9 quadrupole and 2 sextrupole focusing and bending magnets	single-horizontal	1979	Phase I trials completed
SIN Villigen Switzerland	[4] 590 MeV proton isochronous cyclotron	100 μa	0.9 Steradian solid-angle acceptance spectrometer	60 radially concentric	1980	Phase I trials completed

[1] Facilities at Stanford, USA and Dubna, USSR at various stages of development. No clinical trials foreseen for several years.

[2] Kligerman *et al.* (1979)
[3] Henkelmann *et al.* (1977)
[4] von Essen *et al.* (1979)

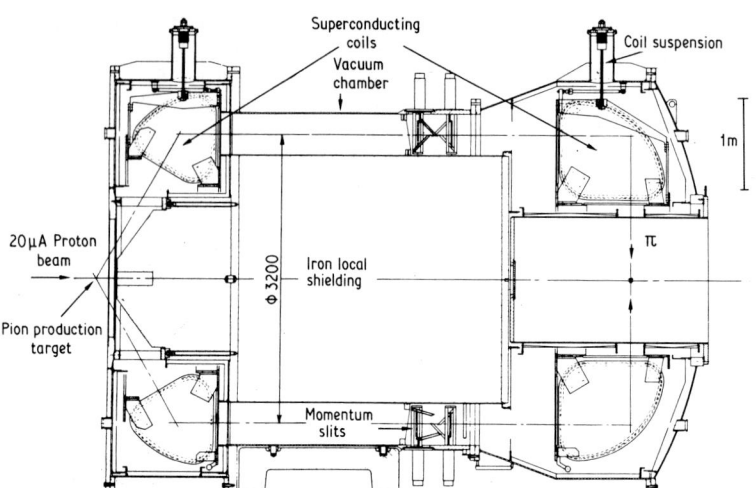

Superconducting coils
Vacuum chamber
Coil suspension
1m
20μA Proton beam
Iron local shielding
π
Φ 3200
Pion production target
Momentum slits

Fig. 4.3 View of the SIN Pion therapy applicator. The proton beam generates pions from a target which are captured by a large superconducting torus consisting of 60 electromagnetic coils. The pions are directed along 60 radially parallel channels, each controlled by a separate momentum slit to a second torus and there focused to an isocentre in the treatment chamber. The principle and prototype were developed at Stanford University (Boyd and Schwettman).

as pion 'stars'. All these important events occur in the stopping region of the π-, while the area of plateau during the entrance of the π- at high velocity is irradiated to a relatively small extent. There the particle is sparsely ionizing with an RBE less than one or approaching one for damaging normal tissues on the way into the tumor. Negative pions were considered potentially useful for radiation therapy (Fowler, 1965, Bond, 1971) and programmes for their utilization were developed with the building of the large medium energy accelerators in Los Alamos, New Mexico, Vancouver, British Columbia, and Villigen, Switzerland (Table 4.4). Clinical programmes have developed or are in progress at these sites. A potentially unique design for the medical use of pions was proposed and constructed at Stanford University, Calfornia (Kaplan *et al.*, 1973) (Fig. 4.3). This is a double-toroidal spectrometer that collects pions emerging from the bombarded target material over a large solid angle (0.9 Steradian), divides them into 60 separate, individually controlled beams that are focused by the second torus to an isocentre. The Stanford concept involved the generation of pions by an electron beam from a small linac in order to develop a facility that could potentially be based in a hospital. The dose rate available has been marginal and the project has not progressed. However, the facility at SIN (Swiss Institute for Nuclear Research) has taken up the design concept but utilizes a proton beam that will provide a generous dose rate (von Essen *et al.*, 1979).

Biological characteristics of negative pions

A large number of biological studies from various pion beams has yielded a wide range of RBE values for the peak region and plateau regions. These values range from 1.0 to 5.4 and 1.0 to 1.8 respectively (Raju *et al.*, 1977). The data covers a variety of biological systems and physical parameters including dose-rate, peak locus and peak spread.

The reference radiation parameters have also varied greatly. With experiments on normal tissues with fractionated pion radiation at dose rates approximating the clinical situation, the RBE values ranged from about 1.4 to 1.7 (Raju *et al.*, 1980). Because the pion star component predominates in the distal region of the Bragg peak it was expected and found that the RBE was greatest at that location. The OER was reduced to levels of about 2.4 in the plateau and to 2.2 in the peak (Hall and Astor, 1979; Raju *et al.*, 1979). These values alter with the peak, but OER appears to vary less than the RBE. The effect of pions on the shape of the cell survival function appears to be predominantly to reduce the shoulder (D_q) in some *in vitro* systems (Yuhas *et al.*, 1979). The development of an *in vitro* cell culture gel system by Skarsgard and Palcic (1974) and developed further by others (Raju *et al.*, 1975; Tremp and Rao, 1979) has permitted the calculation of cell killing to be directly correlated to the geographic position of the cells in the pion beam. In this way RBE differences for various doses at various positions of the plateau and the peak could be experimentally confirmed. The RBE of single and fractionated dose RBE for mouse skin reaction ranged from 1.1 to 1.4 for 1 to 5 fractions (Raju *et al.*, 1980). In clinical studies on the reaction of human skin to fractionated pion radiation an RBE value of 1.4 was calculated (Kligerman *et al.*, 1977).

In summary, for conditions of clinical pion radiotherapy, experimental data suggest that the plateau RBE is approximately 1.0 and the peak RBE is approximately 1.4. The OER in the peak is about 2.2.

This compares with the neutron values of 3 to 4 for RBE and 1.5 to 1.8 for OER. These data confirm the expected intermediate positions of pions in the LET spectrum. However, the biological and physical differences between the plateau and the peak suggest a significant therapeutic gain factor in the clinical application of pion beams.

Dose distribution characteristics of negative pions

As with other charged particle beams, the depth of the Bragg peak is dependent upon the initial particle momentum. In the clinical range of about 12 to 20 cm penetration the momentum ranges from 140 to 176 MeV/c (Salzmann, 1979). The peak-plateau ratio diminishes with increasing momentum, as it does when the peak is broadened by a dynamic range shifter or a ridge filter. Three-dimensional beam shaping becomes possible if the beam is swept through the target volume in the form of a small spot or cylinder of 'stopping' pions. This possibility of dynamic treatment is being planned by the facilities at Los Alamos and Villigen. As mentioned in the previous section the distribution of LET in the stopping region (Bragg peak) varies with position of the peak. Therefore, in order to achieve a uniform biological effective dose it is necessary to modulate the shape of the Bragg peak to compensate for RBE or to use opposing beams. The SIN facility will use up to 60 radially opposing beams to form a small focal spot that will be swept through the tumour by either positional change (raster scan) or momentum change (ring scan) (Pedroni, 1979).

Results of clinical trials with negative pions

The major experience with treatment of human cancer to date comes from Los Alamos. The study began in 1974 with evaluations of metastatic lesions and surrounding tissues. A clinical RBE factor of 1.4 was calculated (Kligerman *et al.*, 1977). Only in 1977 was it possible to begin the treatment of a series of patients with a phase II protocol (the treatment of advanced but localized malignant disease). In this trial 28 phase II patients received pion therapy only between 1977 and 1978. Evaluation of results at least two years after treatment of the last patient and three years after treatment of the first patient indicate the following:

1. For doses of 24–28 fractions (5 treatments weekly) and for target volumes from 700 cc to 4.6 l the RBE for normal mucosa appears to be between 1.6 and 1.7.
2. The percentage of local control is dose-dependent. For doses of 3100 ±200 rad the control rate is about 75%.
3. Late morbidity was not encountered in patients with at least two years follow-up.

The initial experience with pion radiotherapy appears promising. Phase III trials at Los Alamos will compare the effects of pions with conventional supervoltage radiation modalities in a variety of sites at stages of disease where local control can be expected in a reasonable but minimal percentage with conventional techniques. The clinical programme at Vancouver will utilize a single horizontal beam while the Swiss Institute for Nuclear Research programme will embark directly into a unique dynamic scanning method of three-dimensional beam shaping.

Heavy ions

Introduction

Alpha particles (helium ions) were observed to have a dense ionization pattern in experiments carried out as early as 1935 by Zirkle. It was predicted that not only they, but also heavier ions such as carbon, neon, and argon would be useful in the treatment of cancer, not only because of their high LET (linear energy transfer) but also because of the characteristic Bragg peak shared by all charged particles heavier than electrons. The clinical development of these various particle beams has come from the University of California at Berkeley, which was also the site of the first artificially produced negative pions, and the first clinical proton and neutron programmes.

Radiobiological characteristics of heavy ion beams

Helium ions
Experimental studies in cell culture by several investigators (Raju *et al.*, 1978c; Todd *et al.*, 1974; Ward *et al.*, 1976) have confirmed that the spread-out helium peak tended to reduce the RBE towards unity. For single doses of helium ions the RBE values have ranged from 1.1 to 1.4 while the plateau generally has a value close to 1.0. However, the OER was found to be significantly reduced, e.g. values of 1.8 to 2.3 in various experiments compared to 2.9 for low LET X- or γ-rays.

Carbon ions
The experimentally observed RBE values for a variety of *in vitro* cell culture systems ranges from 1.3 to 2.3 in the peak and 1.0 to 1.3 in the plateau. The OER values range from 1.7 to 2.2 and 1.7 to 3.3 respectively (Raju *et al.*, 1980; Chapman *et al.*, 1978; Goldstein *et al.*, 1979). The peak-plateau RBE ratio (for 4-cm spread peak) then is from 1.3 to 2.3, which is greater than for helium and neon.

Neon
Similar studies (Fu *et al*., 1979) indicate peak-plateau RBE ratios (for 4-cm spread peak) of about 1.2 with RBEs of 1.9 to 2.5 in the peak. OER values as low as 1.6 in the peak were found.

Argon
Peak-plateau RBE ratios of 1 to less than 1 by the same investigators indicate the limited clinical usefulness of argon beams from a dose-distribution standpoint although OER values as low as 1.2 were found in the peak region.

Dose-distribution characteristics of heavy ions

Helium
The depth-dose characteristics of α-particles are quite similar to those of protons (Fig. 4.1). Because of the doubling of mass to charge ratio the scattering of the helium beam is even less, however, than that of the proton beam. Using the 910 MeV Synchro-cyclotron the position of the Bragg peak is 32 cm in water.

Carbon, neon, argon
As the charge of a heavy ion increases, the energy needed to give a clinically useful beam also increases, therefore only very large accelerators such as the Berkeley BEVELAC (6.2 GeV protons) are capable of generating clinical beams of carbon, neon or argon. With heavier ions such as argon the peak to plateau

ratio diminishes, because of nuclear interaction, thus the geographic advantage of charged particle beams begins to diminish as the total mass increases (Fig. 4.1).

Results of clinical trials with heavy ion beams
(Table 4.5)

Helium
During the improvement of the Berkeley 184-in Synchro-cyclotron it was found advantageous to change from proton to helium in order to exploit the Bragg peak and the favourable low multiple scatter characteristics of helium ions. Thus, from 1958 to the present day a large number of patients have been treated for a variety of pituitary conditions including chromophobe pituitary adenomas, Nelson syndrome, acromegaly, and Cushing's disease. As with the experience with proton beams, both in Berkeley and Harvard, it was shown that, with proper planning and beam localization, high dosage helium therapy could effectively ablate normal function for both normal and abnormal pituitary glands (Lawrence and Tobias, 1965). For normal pituitary ablation, which was useful in some cases of metastatic breast cancer and diabetic retinopathy, doses from 13 000 to 30 000 rad were possible with only occasional morbidity produced as symptomatic cranial nerve paresis. Lower doses were highly effective for acromegaly, Cushing's disease, and Nelson's syndrome (post-adrenalectomy pituitary adenoma). Following pilot studies in the treatment of

Table 4.5   Heavy ion clinical facilities.

Site [1]	Ion source	Type	Range (cm)	Year of onset	Clinical experiences
	910 MeV Synchro-cyclotron	Helium	32	1958	*Pituitary ablation*: Produced by 13 000 to [2] 31 000 rad, fractionated.
				1958	*Pituitary adenomas*: Controlled by 3500 to [3] 10 000 rad in 6 fractions.
				1975	*Large field therapy*: Promising results in [4] carcinoma of pancreas, esophogus, and cervix. Randomized trials started.
Berkeley					
	BEVELAC (heavy ion linac plus 6.2 GeV proton Synchrotron (Bevatron)	Carbon Neon Argon	24 14 12	1978 1978 1979	Early phase I experience indicates expected [5] RBE of 2.7 for carbon and 3.4 for neon.

[1] Synchrotron at Saclay is being prepared for heavy ion radiotherapy
[2] Lawrence *et al*. (1965)
[3] Linfoot *et al*. (1963)
[4] Castro and Quivey (1977)
[5] Castro *et al*. (1979)

metastatic lesions the Berkeley programme embarked in 1975 on a large field programme for the treatment of cancer at various sites. The largest experience to date has been the treatment of unresectable carcinoma of the pancreas. Castro and coworkers (1979) reported disease-free survival of 7/24 evaluable patients who received a total dose equivalent to at least 5000 rad of cobalt γ-irradiation. These patients have survived for periods of 6–39 months after treatment. Early promising results have also been obtained on the treatment of cancer of the oesophagus. Randomized clinical trials are being established in a cooperative regional group to compare helium with the best available conventional radiation modalities.

Carbon and neon
Pilot studies are in progress with these particles. The expected skin and mucosal reactions for the predicted RBEs of 2.7 for carbon and 3.4 for neon have developed. An analysis of potentially favourable tumour types and sites will map out the future for this programme.

Discussion

It must be emphasized that, with the advent of these new beams, a particular incentive exists to determine very accurately the target volume in three dimensions and to assess radiation tolerance of normal tissues within this target volume more carefully (Suit and Goitein, 1974). This is because particle beams, specifically charged particle beams, have a finite range in tissue and thus can be exploited to improve dose distribution but also can be a handicap if the target volume is not well known and tissue density inhomogeneities in the beam path are not compensated (Goitein, 1977). With the advent of computerized tomography (CT) not only can the radiotherapist map out the target volume and identify normal structures much better but the physicist can also develop techniques for compensation of heterodensities and evolve three-dimensional optimization treatment planning programmes. Naturally, all these considerations apply to photon beams as well. A true comparison of photons and heavy particles must be based on similar efforts in treatment planning and accuracy of treatment. However, often it will be found that small errors can produce greater dose inhomogeneities with charged particle beams than with photon beams. The technical developments in improving treatment accuracy should provide a general benefit in radiotherapy. Dedicated CT-facilities for all the charged particle projects are being planned.

The development of randomized clinical trials is necessary to evaluate the various beams accurately (Breur, 1974) as well as cooperation between groups on a regional or particle-type basis (Parker *et al.*, 1977, Hussey *et al.*, 1977). It is likely that intercomparison with various types of particles will be important in order to reach conclusions eventually about relative benefits.

Eventually attention should be given to the financial cost-benefit of these very expensive projects. If they show any advantages over the best techniques of conventional radiation then it should be determined in which way they can be best utilized. One frequently discussed approach is the method of 'boost' therapy in which the patient would be treated primarily by conventional radiation to generous fields that include areas of micrometastases, and secondarily by particle therapy to the actual tumour volume in a small number of fractions or even a single treatment. In this way one particle facility could serve a large geographic area and the expense of such treatment could be diluted through a large cancer patient population.

Conclusions

The theoretical attributes of heavy particles vary between dose distribution and high LET advantages, both of which have been found to be important considerations in seeking improvement in radiation therapy (Table 4.1). Initial clinical experiences are favourable in many sites. Ultimately, randomized clinical trials must compare the effects of these particle beams, not only with the best conventional radiotherapy but also with each other. Improvements in beam volume delineation, heterodensity compensation, and three-dimensional treatment planning with computerized tomography (CT) should benefit radiation therapy as a whole. If heavy particles are shown to have advantages in achieving better local control on cancer it will still be important to plan comprehensive programmes involving chemotherapy and immunotherapy in order to deal with metastatic disease, the principal cause of failure.

Further reading

American College of Radiology (1977), *Particles and Radiation Therapy, Second International Conference,* Pergamon Press, New York.
Barendsen, G.W., Broerse, J.J. and Breur, K. (eds) (1979), *High-LET Radiations in Clinical Radiotherapy,* Proceedings of the 3rd meeting on Fundamental and Practical Aspects of the Application of Fast Neutons and other High-LET Particles in Clinical Radiotherapy, *Eur. J. Cancer,* Supplement, Pergamon, Oxford.*

*Appreviated in this listing to *Eur. J. Cancer* Supplement.

Catterall, M., Bewley, D.K. (1979), *Fast neutrons in the treatment of cancer.* Academic Press, London. Grune and Stratton, New York.

Raju, M.R. (1980), *Heavy Particle Radiotherapy.* Academic Press.

Tobias, C.A., Lyman, J.T. and Lawrence, J.H. (1971), Some considerations of physical and biological factors in radiotherapy with high-LET radiation including heavy particles, pi-mesons, and fast neutrons. *Prog. Atomic Med.: Recent Adv. Nucl. Med.,* **3,** 167–218.

Von Essen, C.F. (1980), The pi-meson therapy program at SIN. *J. Can. Assoc. Radiologists,* **31,** 19–25.

References

Abazov, V.I. *et al.* (1971), Use of proton beams in the USSR for medical and biological purposes. *JINR,* E – 5854, 1–21.

Batterman, J.J. and Breur K. (1979), Results of Fast Neutron Radiotherapy at Amsterdam. In *Eur J. Cancer* Supplement, pp. 17–22.

Bond, V.P. (1971), Negative pions: their possible use in radiotherapy. *Am. J. Roentg. Radiat. Ther. Nucl. Med.,* **111,** 9–26.

Brennan, J.T. (1969), Fast neutrons for radiation therapy. *Radiol. Clinics N. Am.,* **7,** 365–74.

Breur, K. (1974), International cooperation with regard to clinical trials of fast neutron radiotherapy. *Eur. J. Cancer,* **10,** 385–6.

Castro, J.R. and Quivey, J.M. (1977), Clinical experience and expectations with helium and heavy ion irradiation. *Int. J. Radiat. Oncol. Biol. Phys.,* **3,** 127–31.

Castro, J.R. *et al.* (1979), Results of tumor treatment with alpha particles and heavy ions at the Lawrence Berkeley laboratory, *Eur. J. Cancer,* Supplement pp.67–74.

Catterall, M. (1977), The results of randomized and other clinical trials of fast neutrons from the Medical Research Council Cyclotron, London. *Int. J. Radiat. Oncol. Biol. Phys.,* **3,** 247–53.

Catterall, M. (1979), Observations on the reactions of normal and malignant tissues to a standard dose of neutrons. In *Eur. J. Cancer* Supplement, pp. 11–16.

Chapman, J.D. *et al.* (1978), Radiation biophysical studies with mammalian cells and a modulated carbon ion beam. *Radiat. Res.,* **74,** 101–11.

Dische, S. (1978), Medical Research Council trials and their clinical significance. *Br. J. Radiol.,* **51,** 888–95.

Duncan, W. and Arnott, S.J. (1979), Results of clinical applications with fast neutrons in Edinburgh. In: *Eur. J. Cancer* Supplement, pp. 31–36.

Dutreix, J. and Tubiana, M. (1979), Evaluation of clinical experience concerning evaluation of tumour response to hig-LET radiation. In *Eur. J. Cancer* Supplement, pp. 243–250.

Eichhorn, H.J., Lersel, A. and Matschke, S. (1974), Comparison between neutron therapy and ^{60}Co gamma ray therapy of bronchial, gastric and oesophagus carcinomata. *Eur. J. Cancer,* **10,** 361–4.

Eichhorn, H.J. (1977), Four years' experience with combined neutron-telecobalt therapy (investigations on tumour-reaction of lung cancer). *Int. J. Radiat. Oncol. Biol. Phys.,* **3,** 277–80.

Eichhorn, H.J., Lersel, A. and Dalliige, K. (1979), Five years of clinical experience with a combination of neutrons and photons. In *Eur. J. Cancer* Supplement, pp. 79–82.

Falkmer, S. *et al.* (1962), Pilot study on proton irradiation of human carcinoma. *Acta Radiol.,* **58,** 33–51.

Farr, L.E. *et al.* (1961), Effect of thermal neutrons on central nervous system structures in man. *Arch. Neurol.,* **4,** 246.

Fors, B. *et al.* (1964), Effect of high energy protons on human genital carcinoma. *Acta Radiol. Ther. Biol. Phys.,* **2,** 384–98.

Fowler, J.F., Morgan, R.L. and Wood, C.A.P. (1963), Pre-therapeutic experiments with fast neutron beam from the Medical Research Council Cyclotron. I. The biological and physical advantages and problems of neutron therapy. *Br. J. Radiol.,* **36,** 77–80.

Fowler, P.H. (1965), 1964 Rutherford Memorial Lecture. Pi-mesons versus cancer? *Proc. Phys. Soc.,* **85,** 1051–66.

Franke, H.D. *et al.* (1978), The neutron therapy facility (DT, 14 MeV) at the radiotherapy department of the University Hospital Hamburg-Eppendorf. *Strahlentherapie,* **154,** 225–32.

Franke, H.D. (1979), Results of clinical applications of fast neutrons at Hamburg-Eppendorf. In *Eur. J. Cancer* Supplement, pp. 51–60.

Fu, K.K. *et al.* (1979), Biological effects of single doses of accelerated heavy ions: III. Neons. *Radiat. Res.* (in press).

Gardner, E. and Lattes, C.M.G. (1948), Production of mesons by the 184-inch Berkeley Cyclotron. *Science,* **107,** 270–1.

Goitein, M. (1977), The measurement of tissue heterodensity to guide charged particle radiotherapy. *Int. J. Radiat. Oncol. Biol. Phys.,* **3,** 27–33.

Goldstein, L.S. *et al.* (1979), Biological effects of single doses: II Carbon. *Radiat. Res.* (in press).

Graffman, S. and Jung, B. (1970), Clinical trials in radiotherapy and the merits of high energy protons. *Acta Radiol. Ther. Phys. Biol.,* **9,** 1–23.

Gragodas, E.S. *et al.* (1978), Proton irradiation of choroidal melanomas. Preliminary results. *Arch. Ophthal.,* **96,** 1583–91.

Griffin, T.W., Blasko, J.C. and Laramore, G.E. (1979), Results of fast neutron beam radiotherapy pilot studies at the University of Washington. In *Eur. J. Cancer* Supplement, pp. 23–30.

Hall, E.I. and Astor, M. (1979), The oxygen enhancement ratio for negative pi-mesons. *Int. J. Radiat. Oncol. Biol. Phys.*, **5**, 55–60.

Halnan, K.E. (1979), Evaluation of normal tissue responses of high LET radiations. In *Eur. J. Cancer* Supplement, pp. 251–6.

Hatanaka, H. (1975), A revised boron-neutron capture therapy for malignant brain tumors. *J. Neurol.*, **209**, 81–94.

Hatanaka, H. and Sweet, H.W. (1975), Slow-neutron capture therapy for malignant tumors. Its history and recent development, In *Biomedical Dosimetry*, IAEA, Vienna.

Hatanaka, H. and Sweet, H.W. (1975), In *Biomedical Dosimetry*, IAEA-SM-193/79, International Atomic Energy Agency, Vienna, pp. 147–78.

Hatanaka, H. Amano *et al.* (1978), Boron-neutron capture therapy in relation to immunotherapy. *Acta Neurochirurg.*, **42**, 57–72.

Henkelmann, R.M. *et al.* (1977), Recent developments at the pi-meson radiotherapy facility at TRIUMF. *Int. J. Radiat. Oncol. Biol. Phys.*, **2**, 123–7.

Hussey, D.H., Fletcher, G.H. and Caderao, J.B. (1974), Experience with fast neutron therapy using the Texas A & M Variable Energy Cyclotron. *Cancer*, **34**, 65–77.

Hussey, D.H., Parker, R.G. and Rogers, R.C. (1977), Evolution of dosage schedules at the fast neutron therapy facilities in the United States. *Int. J. Radiat. Oncol. Biol. Phys.*, **3**, 255–60.

Kaplan, H.S. *et al.* (1973), A hospital-based superconducting accelerator for negative pi-meson beam radiotherapy. *Radiology*, **108**, 159–72.

Kjellberg, R.N. *et al.* (1968), Proton-beam therapy in acromegaly. *New Engl. J. Med.*, **278**, 689–95.

Kjellberg, R.N. (1975), A system of therapy of pituitary tumors – Bragg peak proton hypophysectomy, In *Tumors of the Nervous System*, (ed. H.G. Seydel), John Wiley and Sons Inc., NY, pp. 144–74.

Kligerman, M.M. *et al.* (1977), The relative biological effectiveness of pions in the acute response of human skin. *Int. J. Radiat. Oncol. Biol. Phys.*, **3**, 335–9.

Kligerman, M.M. *et al.* (1979), Results of clinical applications of negative pions at Los Alamos, In *Eur J. Cancer* Supplement, pp. 61–6.

Koehler, A.M. and Preston, W.M. (1972), Protons in radiation therapy. *Radiology*, **104**, 191–5.

Koehler, A.M., Schneider, R.J. and Sisterson, J.M. (1975), Range modulators for protons and heavy ions. *Nucl. Instrum. Meth.*, **131**, 437–40.

Kramer, S. and Suntharalingam, N. (1977), Low-LET alternatives to particle irradiation. *Int. J. Radiat. Oncol. Biol. Phys.*, **3**, 343–9.

Larsson, B., Leksell, L. and Rexed, B. (1963), The use of high energy protons for cerebral surgery in man. *Acta Chir. Scand.*, **125**, 1–7.

Larsson, B. (1967), Radiological properties of beams of high-energy protons. *Radiat. Res.*, Suppl. 7, 304–11.

Lawrence, G.A. (1979), Fast neutron project at Fermilab. In *Eur. J. Cancer* Supplement, pp. 37–42.

Lawrence, J.H. (1957), Proton irradiation of the pituitary. *Cancer*, **10**, 795–8.

Lawrence, J.H. and Tobias, C.A. (1965), Heavy particles in medicine, In *Progress in Atomic Medicine*, (ed. J.H. Lawrence), Grune and Stratton Inc., NY, pp. 127–46.

Linfoot, J.A. *et al.* (1963), The alpha particle or proton beam in radiosurgery of the pituitary gland for Cushing's disease. *New Engl. J. Med.*, **269**, 597–601.

Locher, G.L. (1936), Biological effects and therapeutic possibilities of neutrons. *Am. J. Roentg.*, **36**, 1.

Maier, E. and Hüdepohl, C. (1979), Dosimetric results for d(14)+Be neutrons of cyclotron isocentric neutron facility CIRCE in Essen. In *Eur. J. Cancer* Supplement, pp. 143–4.

Occhialini, G.P.S. and Powell, C.F. (1947), Nuclear disintegrations by slow charged particles of small mass. *Nature*, **159**, 186–90.

Ornitz, R.D. *et al.* (1979), Clinical observations of early and late normal tissue injury and tumor control in patients receiving fast neutron irradiation. *Eur. J. Cancer* Supplement pp. 43–50.

Parker, R.G. *et al.* (1977), Preliminary clinical results from US fast neutron teletherapy studies. *Cancer*, **40**, 1434–8.

Pedroni, E. (1979), Development of the therapy planning programs for the 60 beams SIN pion applicator. *Radiat. Environ. Biophys.*, **16**, 211–18.

Peters, L.J. *et al.* (1978), A preliminary report of the MDAH-TAMVEC fast neutron therapy pilot study. *Am. J. Roentg.*, **130**, 374–86.

Peters, L.J., Hussey, D.H. and Wharton, J.T. (1979), Second preliminary report of the M.D. Anderson Study of neutron therapy for locally advanced gynecological tumors. In *Eur. J. Cancer* Supplement, pp. 3–10.

Raju, M.R. (1979), A heavy-particle comparative study: p, He, C, Ne, Ar, $\pi-$, n. In *Eur. J. Cancer* Supplement, pp. 230–2.

Raju, M.R. and Richman, C. (1972), Negative pion radiotherapy: physical and biological aspects. *Curr. Top. Radiat. Res. Quart.*, **8**, 159–233.

Raju, M.R. *et al.* (1975), Biological effects of the Los Alamos meson beam on cells in culture. *Radiology*, **116**, 191–3.

Raju, R.R. *et al.* (1977), Biological effects of negative pions. *Int. Radiat. Oncol. Biol. Phys.*, **3**, 327–34.

Raju, M.R. *et al.* (1978*a*), A heavy particle comparative study Part I: depth-dose distributions. *Br. J. Radiol.*, **51**, 699–703.

Raju, M.R. *et al.* (1978*b*), A comparative study of heavy particles in radiation therapy (n, $\pi-$, p, He, C, Ne, Ar). Part II. Cell survival as a function of depth of penetration. *Br. J. Radiol.*, **51**, 704–11.

Raju, M.R. *et al.* (1978*c*), A heavy particle comparative study. Part III. OER and RBE. *Br. J. Radiol.*, **51**, 712–19.

Raju, M.R. *et al.* (1979), OER and RBE for negative pion beams of different peak widths. *Br. J. Radiol.* **52**, 494–98.

Raju, M.R. *et al.* (1980), Effect of fractionated doses of pions on normal tissues: Part I Mouse skin. *Int. J. Radiation Oncology Biol. Phys.*, **6**, 1663–66.

Salzmann, M. (1979), Measurement at the πE3 single beam correlated to dosimetry and therapy planning for the pion applicator at SIN. *Radiat. Environ. Biophys.*, **16**, 219–24.

Schnabel, K. (1979), (personal communication).

Skarsgard, L.D. and Palcic, B. (1974), Pretherapeutic research programmes at π-meson facilities. In *Proceedings of the XIIIth International Congress of Radiology*, International Congress Series No. 339, Radiology, Excerpta Medica, Amsterdam.

Sténson, S. (1971), Clinical experience with proton-beams. In *Proceedings of the Symposium of Pion and Proton Radiotherapy*, National Accelerator Laboratory, Batavia, Illinois, pp. 89–106.

Stewart, J.G. and Jackson, A.W. (1975), The steepness of the dose response curve both for tumor cure and normal tissue injury. *Laryngoscope*, **85**, 1107–11.

Stone, R.S. (1948), Neutron therapy and specific ionization. *Am. J. Roentg.*, **59**, 771–85.

Suit, H.D. (1969), Statement of the problem pertaining to the effect of dose fractionation and total treatment time in response of tissue to X-irradiation. In: *Time and Dose Relationships in Radiation Biology as Applied to Radiotherapy, Carmel Conference*, Brookhaven National Laboratory Report BNL-50203 (C-57), pp. vii–x.

Suit, H.D. and Goitein, M. (1974), Dose-limiting tissues in relation to types and location of tumors: implications for effects to improve radiation dose distribution. *Eur. J. Cancer*, **10**, 217–24.

Suit, H.D. *et al.* (1975), Exploratory study of proton radiation therapy using large field techniques and fractionated dose schedules. *Cancer*, **35**, 1646–57.

Suit, H.D. *et al.* (1977), Clinical experience with protons and heavy ions. *Int. J. Radiat. Oncol. Biol. Phys.*, **3**, 115–25.

Sweet, W.H., Soloway, A.H. and Wright, R.L. (1962), Evaluation of boron compounds for use in neutron capture therapy of brain tumors. II. Studies in Man. *J. Pharmac. Exp. Ther.*, **137**, 263.

Todd, P. *et al.* (1974), Spatial distribution of human cell survival and oxygen effect in a therapeutic helium ion beam, *Cancer*, **34**, 1–5.

Tremp, J. and Rao, K.R. (1979), Survival of normal and malignant cells after irradiation with the SIN negative pion beam over the depth profile. In *Eur J. Cancer* Supplement, pp. 234–5.

Tsunemoto, H. *et al.* (1979), Results of clinical application of fast neutrons in Japan. In *Eur. J. Cancer* Supplement, pp. 75–8.

von Essen, C.F. *et al.* (1979), The medical pi-meson project at SIN. In *Eur. J. Cancer* Supplement, pp. 222–3.

Wambersie, A., Meulders, J.P. and Winant, M. (1979), The fast neutron therapy facility at Cyclone, Louvain-la-Neuve. In *Eur. J. Cancer* Supplement, pp. 145–6.

Ward, W.F. *et al.* (1976), RBE and OER of extended Bragg peak helium ions; survival and development of rat embryos. *Int. J. Radiat. Biol.*, **30**, 317–26.

Wilson, R.R. (1946), Radiological use of fast protons. *Radiology*, **47**, 487–91.

Yuhas, J.M., Li, A.P. and Kligerman, M.M. (1979), Present status of the proposed use of negative pi-mesons in radiotherapy. *Adv. Radiat. Biol.*, **8** (in press).

Zirkle, R.E. (1935), Biological effectiveness of alpha particles as a function of ion concentration produced in their path. *Am. J. Cancer*, **23**, 558–67.

5 Cancer chemotherapy

Derek Crowther

History

The concept of a chemotherapeutic agent arose in ancient medicine but the use of the elements arsenic, mercury, bismuth and antimony which were in vogue in Europe during the Renaissance were toxic and of little value. World War I led to the experimental use of the sulphur mustards after the observation that exposure to sulphur mustard gas was followed by bone marrow hypoplasia and severe damage to lymphoid organs. Following these studies, many alkylating agents were developed during or shortly after World War II, such as mechlorethamine, myeleran, chlorambucil and melphalan. The folic acid antagonists were developed and Farber *et al.* (1974) showed aminopterin to be the first chemotherapeutic agent capable of regularly producing remissions in lymphoblastic leukaemia of childhood. These initial successes led to a large profusion of chemotherapeutic agents until today, over 30 agents are in constant use in most departments of chemotherapy and more than 20 others are being actively studied in man.

The development of effective intermittent combination chemotherapy and its integration with other modalities of treatment such as surgery and radiotherapy has greatly increased the complexity of our approach to the management of the cancer patient but, undoubtedly, has already led to a revolution in the way that many patients with cancer are successfully managed.

Questions which must be asked and answered before prescribing an anti-tumour agent

The decisions and considerations to be made in connection with prescribing an anti-tumour agent for a patient with cancer are the following:

1. *Name.* What is the approved or generic name of the drug to be used?
2. *Class.* To which class does the drug belong (e.g. hormone, anti-metabolite, alkylating agent)?
3. *Aim.* What aim is to be achieved? (cure or palliation, tumour regression or maintenance of remission).
4. *Alternatives.* What other form of therapy might have been chosen instead? Is chemotherapy a good choice? Consider efficacy, safety and cost.
5. *Route and dosage.* By what route, in what dose and at what intervals is each drug to be given and why? In what form(s) does the drug come?
6. *Evaluation.* What observations should be made to determine whether the aim has been achieved? When should they be made?
7. *Duration.* How long should the treatment continue?
8. *Elimination.* How is the drug eliminated? Will the patient's illness change the usual pattern of distribution and effects of the drug?
9. *Side-effects.* What undesirable effects accompany the use of the drug and what is the approximate frequency? Are there any absolute contra-indications such as pregnancy?
10. *Interactions.* Are there any drugs which should be avoided while the patient is receiving his treatment?
11. *Patient's information.* Does the patient understand enough about the nature of his illness and the drugs used to be able to fully participate in the treatment? What has he been told, what has he remembered and what additional information does he need?

There are inevitably many factors which influence the choice of drug and the way in which it is used in a particular patient. These factors are listed in Table 5.1.

Screening and evaluation of anti-tumour agents

Following the early clinical observations that folic acid

Table 5.1   Factors to be considered when using an anti-tumour agent.

(A) Drug-dependent

1. Type of drug – mode of action, selectivity, phase dependency, metabolism, distribution and excretion
2. Dose
3. Route
4. Schedule of drug administration
5. Combination chemotherapy – synchronous or sequential, effects of other non-cytotoxic drugs
6. Relationship with other treatment modalities radiotherapeutic, surgical or hormonal

(B) Patient-dependent

1. Individual response – dependent upon age, sex, body weight and nutritional status, socioeconomic, psychological and genetic considerations, performance status, renal and hepatic function, bone marrow reserve and gastrointestinal abnormalities
2. Type of disease – tumour type, histology and proliferative characteristics, primary or metastatic disease, site of metastases and prognosis
3. Drug resistance – dependent upon both host and tumour

---

antagonists could induce remissions in childhood leukaemia and that nitrogen mustard could cause regression of certain forms of lymphoma, it became apparent that a method for screening and evaluating anti-tumour agents was required. This experimental approach now provides the basis for drug selection for use against human cancer.

The choice of drug for initial screening depends on both logical design and random selection. The agents are tested in both *in vitro* and *in vivo* systems against a range of experimental tumours (both slow and fast growing) and any activity documented. The optimal mode of administration is then determined and subsequently a detailed toxicologic and pharmacologic evaluation is carried out in experimental animals. Of the many thousands of agents tested each year, only a minority are selected for clinical evaluation. Such stringent testing is essential but it undoubtedly means that some potentially useful anti-tumour agents are excluded from human evaluation and a great deal of work is currently being carried out to ensure that the screening methods are optimum. Vincristine, a leading agent in the curative treatment of acute lymphoblastic leukaemia, is notoriously ineffective in leukaemia L1210 but fortunately, proved to be effective in other animal model systems and was submitted for clinical study. Clearly, pre-clinical efficacy screening cannot rest on one or two animal tumour systems. *In vitro* testing and xenografts may also be of value. The development of new agents has often rested with random

selection and empirical methods but an increasing number of drugs have been developed by biochemical reasoning (e.g. 6-mercaptopurine, 5-fluorouracil, cytosine arabinoside, 6-azauridine, 3-deazauridine, deoxycoformycin).

The clinical evaluation of a new agent may be divided into three phases:

Phase I   – determine clinical pharmacology (toxicity and maximum tolerated dose).
Phase II   – determine clinical activity against different but measurable malignant diseases.
Phase III – studies to establish role in cancer therapy; this will involve comparative randomized trials and studies of combined therapy.

The cancer chemotherapist should be familiar with this approach to evaluation since new drug development has an essential role in improving the results of a systemic approach to cancer treatment and the field is rapidly changing.

Classification of anti-tumour agents

Most anti-cancer drugs can be grouped into chemical classifications indicating the major property associated with their mechanism of action, e.g. alkylating agents, folate antagonists etc. (see Table 5.2). Hormones have been excluded from this table and will be considered in Chapter 6. An understanding of the biochemical locus of drug action may provide important guidelines for their use in combination and for suggesting the most appropriate schedule. It is salutary to remember, however, that we do not completely understand the mechanisms by which any one anti-cancer agent destroys a tumour cell *in vivo* and selection of agents on a rational basis is difficult. Inhibitory and cytotoxic effects may act as different points in the growth cycle and we can rarely point to a single phase of the growth cycle and say that is where a particular agent has its main effect. The alkylating agents, for example, alkylate nucleic acids and this appears to be the most important effect of these agents *in vitro* and *in vivo*. Nevertheless, their clinical effects are varied and there is a spectrum of anti-neoplastic activity against human as well as animal tumours. This perhaps reflects differences in membrane transport requirements, sites of alkylation and secondary mechanisms of action. In support of this concept, recent animal studies have indicated a lack of cross-resistance in some situations and in man the use of intermittent high dose cyclophosphamide has proved to be of help in myeloma patients resistant to melphalan.

Nearly all anti-tumour agents act by interfering with the cell replication. The cell cycle is represented in diagrammatic form in Fig. 5.1. There are several well

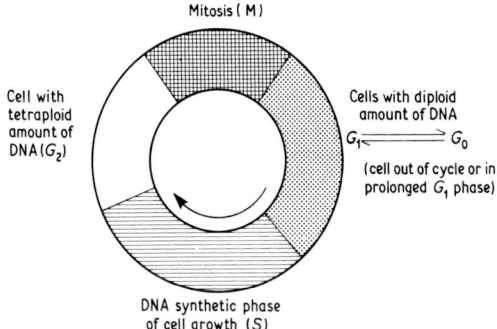

Fig. 5.1 Diagrammatic representation of the cell cycle.

defined phases before cell division takes place, G_1, a phase in which the cell prepares itself for the S or DNA-synthetic phase of cell growth and a premitotic phase (G_2) in which the cell prepares for mitosis (M). The term G_0 is applied to cells considered to be out of cycle and not preparing for DNA synthesis. In the case of tumour cells, an appreciable proportion may be out of cycle but at least some are known to have the capacity of entering the growth cycle again under the appropriate conditions.

The anti-tumour agents can be broadly classified into predominantly phase-dependent drugs which kill exponentially at lower doses but reach a plateau at higher doses and predominantly non-phase dependent drugs which kill cells exponentially with increasing dose (Fig. 5.2). The phase dependency of different anti-tumour agents is listed in Table 5.3. The alkylating agents and anthracyclines are predominantly non-phase dependent and the anti-metabolites and vinca alkaloids are examples of phase-dependent agents. Knowledge of the phase specificity/dependency of anti-cancer drugs is useful in clinical practice since some generalizations can be made concerning the ways

these groups of drugs can be used to optimize tumour response and minimize toxicity.

Table 5.2 Classification of anti-tumour agents.

Alkylating agents	Anti-metabolites
Busulfan	Cytosine arabinoside
Chlorambucil	5-Fluorouracil
Cyclophosphamide	5-FUdr
Nitrogen mustard (mechlorethamine)	6-Mercaptopurine
Phenylalanine mustard (melphalan)	Methotrexate
Pipobroman	6-Thioguanine
Dibromomannitol	6-Azauridine
Thio-TEPA	3-Deazauridine
Tri-ethylenemelamine	
Mitotic Inhibitors	*Enzymes*
Vincristine	L-Asparaginase
Vinblastine	
Antibiotics	*Unclassified*
Anthracyclines – Adriamycin	Nitrosoureas – BCNU
Daunorubicin	CCNU
Bleomycin	Methyl CCNU
Mitomycin C	Streptozotocin
Actinomycin D	Procarbazine
Mithramycin	Imidazole carboxamide (DTIC)

Table 5.3 Classification of anti-tumour agents according to their effects on cell cycle.

Predominantly non-phase dependent	Predominantly phase-dependent
Alkylating agents	Vinca alkaloids
Nitrosoureas	Hydroxyurea
Anthracyclines	Cytosine arabinoside
Imidazole carboxamide (DTIC)	Methotrexate
Mitomycin C	6-Mercaptopurine
Actinomycin D	6-Thioguanine
	Procarbazine
	Podophyllotoxins VM26
	VP 16–213

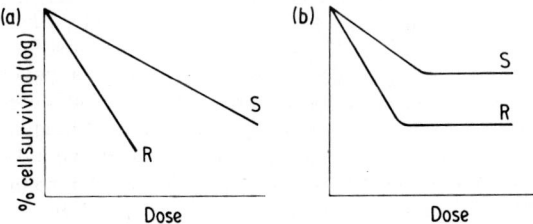

Fig. 5.2 The relationships between tumour cell kill and the dose of two main classes of antitumour agent. (a) Pre-dominantly non-phase-dependent agents which kill cells exponentially with increasing dosage. (b) Predominantly phase-dependent agents which kill cells exponentially at lower doses but reach a plateau at higher doses. (S = slowly proliferating cells; R = rapidly proliferating cells.)

Phase-dependent agents exert an increasingly toxic effect the longer an effective concentration is maintained for the cells in the sensitive phase, since more cells have time to enter the phase (provided the drug does not prevent entry). Given over a short period, even at high dose level, these agents are not very toxic. Cells not in the sensitive phase, at the time of the brief exposure, will not be affected. Phase-specific agents should be administered in fractionated schedules or infusions unless they have a long half-life. The toxicity of predominantly non-phase dependent agents which can affect cells at all phases of the cell cycle in both malignant and normal cells depends on the drug concentration. To achieve maximum effect, it is therefore logical to administer the drugs intermittently at the highest dose, allowing recovery of normal tissues in the intervening two- to three-week period. Some drugs interfere with progression from one phase to another in the cell cycle. Cytosine arabinoside and hydroxyurea, for example, inhibit the progression of G_1 cells into S and therefore cells in S are protected. This protective effect can be overcome by giving the drug intermittently at intervals that permit the non-S phase cells to enter S during the drug-free period. Most chemotherapeutic agents with any given dose kill the same percentage not the same number of cells. This concept of 'first order cell kill' is illustrated in Table 5.4. It follows that therapy will be more effective if started when the tumour mass is small.

Table 5.4 First order cell kill induced by chemotherapy.

Injection No.	Surviving cells	% killed	No. killed each time
Start	1 000 000		
1	100 000	90	900 000
2	10 000	90	90 000
3	1000	90	9000
4	100	90	900
5	10	90	90
6	1	90	9

Drug absorption, distribution, metabolism and excretion

Drugs have characteristic physicochemical and pharmacokinetic properties and a knowledge of these helps to predict the behaviour of the drug in the body and is an important guide in the selection of dose and schedule of administration. Only a small proportion of the drug administered actually reaches and reacts with its receptor in the tumour cell, the absolute amount depends to a great extent on factors influencing the concentration of free drug in the plasma. This is diagrammatically represented in Fig. 5.3. The rate at which these processes (absorption, distribution, biotransformation and excretion) are carried out will influence the concentration of active drug available to the tumour and is itself influenced by many factors such as the individual characteristics of the drug, pathological and physiological variations within the indi-

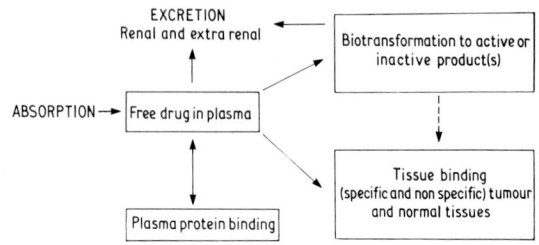

Fig. 5.3 Drug absorption, distribution and excretion patterns.

vidual patient and the effects of other drugs taken concurrently.

Individual patients show a wide variation in response to the same dose of drug. Much of this variability in drug response between patients can be explained by individual kinetic factors, particularly genetically determined differences in drug metabolism and by the effects of intercurrent illness or disease states on pharmacokinetics or tissue response.

The plasma half-time is the time during which the concentration of a drug is decreased by 50%. This is a reflection of an initial distribution into body compartments followed by metabolism and excretion. All other factors being equal, plasma half-time indicates the time available for drug–target cell interaction and is one factor to be considered in designing a drug schedule. If there is a large reservoir or 'third' compartment for drug sequestration such as ascites or pleural effusion, the plasma half-time may be prolonged and the area under the concentration/time curve may be larger with consequent increased drug toxicity. A good example of this is the increased toxicity of methotrexate in patients with ascites or a large pleural effusion. Drug dosage must be individualized if the desired therapeutic response with minimum side effects is to be obtained. The response to some drugs is better correlated with steady-state plasma concentrations than to dosage.

Tissue perfusion

The uptake of an active agent by tumour cells depends upon the rate of blood flow through the tumour, the tumour mass and the relative partitioning of drug between the plasma and the tumour tissue. With highly lipid-soluble drugs, penetration into highly vascular tissues may be sufficiently rapid for equilibration between plasma and tissue to become established after only a single passage of blood through the tissue. Clearly, the possibility of using agents to alter the blood flow through a tumour and improve drug access is an exciting one.

The aim of chemotherapy is to obtain an effective drug concentration at the tumour site for a long enough period to kill the tumour cells. Drug diffusion into the tumour will be helped by maintaining a high plasma/tumour concentration gradient but using conventional methods, this usually means intolerable toxicity in view of the low therapeutic indices of the anti-tumour agents. The use of drug analogues which competitively reverse the effect of a chemotherapeutic agent is important in this context and one of the best known examples is the use of high dose methotrexate followed by rescue with folinic acid. A few hours at high plasma concentration will be accompanied by high tumour levels of methotrexate; folinic acid then given at moderate dosage will effectively 'reverse' the effect of methotrexate on normal tissues and the slow diffusion of the rescue agent into the tumour works in favour of the host but against the tumour. Other agents have been found to reduce the toxicity of methotrexate and have a capacity for 'rescue' such as thymidine and L-asparaginase but in their clinical role is not yet established. Indeed, it is salutary to remember that there have been no good studies comparing high dose methotrexate with optimal low dose treatment which indicate that high dose methotrexate is superior in human cancer and any role for high dose methotrexate is still highly controversial. Nevertheless, the principle of high dose treatments with 'rescue' is an important one and 'rescue' methods are being devised for other drugs.

Lipid solubility and degree of ionization

Drugs in solution can pass through cell layers by three general mechanisms: passive diffusion through the lipid bilayer, filtration through pores in the membrane and transport by specialized 'carrier' systems which move water soluble compounds through lipid membranes. Drugs will diffuse through the lipid bilayer of the cell membrane at rates proportional to their lipid/water partition coefficient and to their concentration gradient. The majority of common drugs are weak electrolytes which ionize in aqueous solution. Only the non-ionized form may dissolve in lipid. This proportion can be calculated from the Henderson-Hasselbach equation:

$$\text{For weak acids} \quad pH - pK_a = \log \frac{\text{ionized}}{\text{non-ionized}}$$

$$\text{For weak bases} \quad pH - pK_a = \log \frac{\text{ionized}}{\text{non-ionized}}$$

The Ka is a function for the ionization constant of the drug. If a drug is a strong acid or base it tends to be more highly ionized at physiological pH and will cross membranes more slowly.

It follows that analogues of existing anti-tumour agents with different lipid/water solubility characteristics could have quite different distribution and effects. Platinum compounds are proving to be of great interest since, cis-dichlorodiammine platinum II is a drug of value in the treatment of advanced testicular teratoma, ovarian and bladder cancer. New platinum analogues with varying lipid/water solubility have been developed in the hope that improved antitumour effect with reduced renal toxicity can be obtained and these analogues should be available for clinical studies in the near future.

Access to the central nervous system (CNS)

Infiltration of the meninges is a common feature of acute lymphoblastic leukaemia and some forms of lymphoma. Primary or secondary brain tumours are important causes of death in both adults and children and it is important to consider the possibility of drug activity reaching the CNS. The blood-cerebrospinal fluid (CSF) barrier represents a tight membrane with lipid characteristics; the CSF-brain barrier, on the other hand, is relatively loose and can be traversed by lipid insoluble substances. It is important to recognize that the diffusion can occur in both directions and systemic toxicity may occur following cytotoxic drug administration intrathecally. Methotrexate is indeed more toxic on the bone marrow when given using the intrathecal route than when the same dose is given intravenously.

Drugs such as cytosine arabinoside, 6-mercaptopurine, procarbazine and dianhydro-galactitol all enter the CSF readily when given systemically. The amount diffusing into the CSF depends on the quantity of drug is given and effective CSF methotrexate levels are only obtained when high dose regimes with rescue are used since the agent is not lipid-soluble. This realization has enabled high dose methotrexate to be used as treatment for leukaemia and lymphoma involving the CNS but its role in treatment and prophylaxis needs to be further evaluated. The use of high dose methotrexate would be more likely to give a more homogenous distribution in the CNS and this could be an important advantage over intrathecal therapy. Other drugs such as the vinca alkaloids, anthracyclines (daunorubicin and adriamycin), alkylating agents and enzymes (L-asparaginase) do not enter the CSF readily following systemic administration.

Consideration of drug access to the CSF will undoubtedly be of great importance in the future development of therapeutic procedures designed to improve the treatment of malignant disease involving the CNS. Rescue agents are being developed which do not cross the blood-brain barrier in appreciable amounts and can be used to reverse the systemic effects of an anti-cancer agent allowing a prolonged period of CNS treatment. One example of this is carboxy-peptidase G_1, an enzyme which does not penetrate the CSF but can allow larger doses of methotrexate to be tolerated in experimental systems. Carboxypeptidase G_1 is a high molecular weight (92000) enzyme synthesized by a micro-organism (*Ps. stutzeri*) and is capable of rapidly hydrolysing methotrexate.

Cytosine arabinoside, methotrexate and hydro-cortisone may all be given intrathecally and the first two are of particular value in the treatment of leu-kaemic infiltration of the CNS provided careful attention is given to dose, dilution, diluent and schedule.

Considerations of lipid solubility and molecular weight do not give absolute indications of whether a particular drug is likely to be effective against tumours of the CNS. Compounds of intermediate lipid/water partition coefficients seem to have the best activity, although the balance is in favour of drugs which are more lipid-soluble. Compounds with very high lipid solubility have not proved to be of great value in prac-tice and this merely emphasizes the diversity of factors influencing the response of a tumour to an anti-tumour agent and the need for adequate *in vivo* testing.

Receptors for dopamine, serotonin, opiates, gluco-corticoids, nerve growth factor and adrenergic drugs are present in the CNS and the future use of these as carriers for an active agent can be considered.

Protein binding

Reversible binding to plasma protein is important in determining the distribution of a drug and its com-bination with receptors. Only unbound drug is dif-fusible and pharmacologically active. The degree of binding will depend upon the amount of drug, the affinity of the drug for protein and the amount of binding protein. In plasma the protein most frequently involved in drug binding is albumin and levels of this are known to be markedly reduced in some patients with malignant disease. Displacement is an important mechanism in drug interaction, particularly in the case of cytotoxic drugs which usually have a low therapeutic ratio.

Drugs vary quite markedly in the extent of albumin binding, pyrimidine analogues for example, (e.g. 5-fluorouracil, cytosine arabinoside) do not seem to bind significantly, whereas about 50% of methotrexate is bound in the serum concentration range 0.1 to 1000 μg/ml. Displacement of methotrexate from albumin binding occurs with sodium salicylate, phenylbutazone and sulphonamides.

The albumin displacement phenomenon is known to

be of particular importance during control of anti-coagulation with coumarin derivatives and the control of diabetes with the sulphonylureas. The chemo-therapist should be aware that these considerations are likely to become of increasing importance in the development of optimum programmes of chemo-therapy.

Active transport across membranes

Most drugs pass across cell membranes by diffusion but special 'pump' mechanisms can exist which transport drugs *against* a concentration gradient. Such mechanisms are important, for example, between urine and the renal tubule and between bile and hepatocyte. Some drugs are actively transported because they are structurally similar to important endogenous com-pounds, e.g. the pyrimidine analogue 5-fluorouracil. Others such as Melphalan and Chloranbucil use amino acid transport mechanisms.

Drug metabolism

Most anti-cancer agents are metabolized in the body, usually to products which are inactive with lower lipid solubility and are excreted. In some instances, active metabolites are produced. In the case of cyclo-phosphamide, the parent drug is inactive but several alkylating agents are produced during catabolism. The rationale for the development of this drug was that it would be cleaved to form nor-HN_2 by phosphora-midase enzymes reported to be present in high con-centrations in malignant human tumours. However, it was soon found that the drug was inactive against tumour cells *in vitro* and required activation by liver microsomes. Cyclophosphamide is converted in the liver into 4-hydroxycyclophosphamide which may exist in equilibrium with aldophosphamide. These inter-mediates can be further enzymatically oxidized to 4-ketocyclophosphamide and carboxyphosphamide, both urinary excretion products of low cytotoxicity. A competing β-elimination reaction releases acrolein and phosphoramide mustard. The latter is the most cyto-toxic metabolite discovered and this product is pro-posed as being responsible in large part for the activity of cyclophosphamide (Fig. 5.4).

Anabolic activation is particularly important in the case of anti-metabolites. The role of anabolic and cata-bolic activation and deactivation is of great importance since it may form the basis of selective activity in dif-ferent cell types (normal and malignant).

Usually, drug metabolism occurs in two phases:
1. Biotransformation – involving hydroxylation, oxi-dation, reduction or hydrolysis.
2. Conjugation – e.g. with sulphate, acetyl or a glucuronyl group.

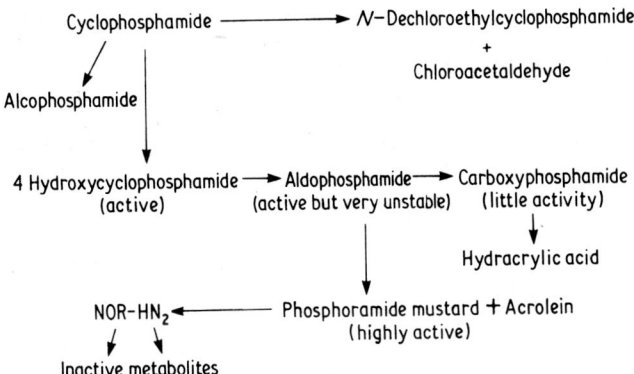

Fig. 5.4 The major metabolites of cyclophosphamide.

Drug metabolism chiefly occurs in the liver but can also occur in the plasma, gastrointestinal tract, kidneys and lungs. For this reason, hepatic function is an important consideration in the choice of dose of some anti-tumour agents. The anthracyclines (e.g. adriamycin and daunorubicin) are excreted mainly in the bile and the agents have enhanced toxicity in patients with hepatic failure or biliary obstruction.

The activity of the enzymes which metabolize drugs may themselves be altered by other drugs and this forms the basis of one type of drug interaction. Pretreatment with barbiturates, for example, will increase hepatic microsomal enzyme activity leading to alterations in the metabolism of cyclophosphamide but this has not yet been shown to be clinically important.

Another more important example of drug interaction is the three-fold increase in toxicity for 6-mercaptopurine in patients receiving the xanthine oxidase inhibitor allopurinol for hyperuricaemia. Under normal circumstances, xanthine oxidase plays an important role in detoxifying 6-mercaptopurine and about one third of intravenously administered 6-mercaptopurine is metabolized by xanthine oxidase to 6-thiouric acid and excreted in the urine.

This type of drug interaction can be used to enhance the effect of an anti-tumour agent. Cytosine arabinoside is inactivated by a pyrimidine nucleoside deaminase which can be inhibited by tetrahydrouridine. The latter, although it has no antileukaemic action by itself, can potentiate the activity of cytosine arabinoside in experimental leukaemia.

Excretion

Most anti-tumour agents are excreted in the bile and urine. Drugs not bound to albumin are filtered by the glomerulus. The proximal tubule possesses two pump systems which transport drugs from plasma to urine,

one for the acidic and the other for the basic drugs. Acidic drugs compete with one another for the secretory mechanism and probenecid can be used to reduce the elimination of acidic drugs (e.g. penicillins and possibly anti-cancer agents such as methotrexate). Passive reabsorption of lipid-soluble drugs and the non-ionized fraction of drugs which are weak electrolytes takes place in the renal tubule. Elimination of weak acids by the kidney is increased by alkalinizing the urine. The reverse is true for weak bases. Active tubular resorption of ions and various solutes can also take place in the proximal tubule (Fig. 5.5).

Excretion in tears, sweat, saliva and in the breath is relatively unimportant but may be the cause of unusual toxicity such as the conjunctivitis seen following the use of high dose methotrexate.

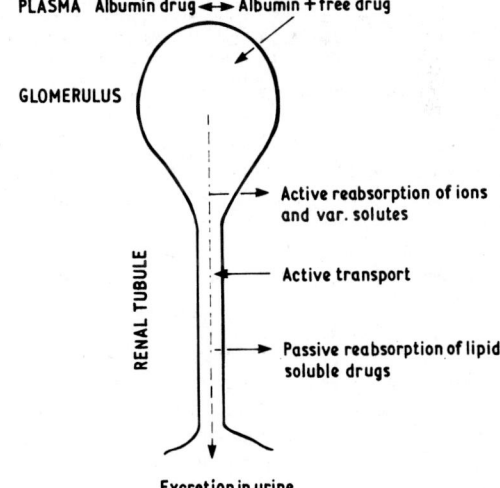

Fig. 5.5 The mechanism of renal excretion for anti-tumour agents.

Factors affecting pharmacokinetics

Several host-dependent factors have important influences on drug absorption, distribution, metabolism and excretion and these have been listed in Table 5.1. Illness which affects renal and hepatic function, bone marrow reserve or gastrointestinal function may well have a marked influence on the efficacy and toxicity of a drug. Individual characteristics such as age, the ability of the patient to attend for treatment, socioeconomic and psychological factors will all have an important influence on therapy.

Age

Elderly patients are particularly susceptible to adverse drug reactions and bear the brunt of unwanted drug effects. Absorption and elimination rates are both frequently reduced in the elderly. Responsiveness to drug is altered in infants and young children because of progressive changes with growth and development in the processes of drug handling in the body. On occasions, children may tolerate a relatively high dose of a drug compared with an adult. For example, 1–2 mg weekly doses of vincristine are well tolerated by children for several weeks but in adults the same dose can cause considerable neurotoxicity, particularly in the elderly.

Genetic factors

Hereditary differences in the amount or structure of a key enzyme can lead to major differences in drug metabolism and effect. Clinically important examples of this are abnormal plasma pseudocholinesterase (leading to increased toxicity of suxamethonium), rapid or slow acetylation of drugs such as isoniazid, sulphonamides etc. and glucose-6-phosphate dehydrogenase differences (leading to increased toxicity of a number of oxidizing drugs resulting in haemolysis). The role of genetic differences in the metabolism of anti-tumour agents is currently being investigated and it seems likely that these differences could prove to be important in the control of dose using these agents which have a low therapeutic index.

Dose

The dose of an anti-tumour agent is clearly of great importance in maximizing the anti-tumoural effect and minimizing toxicity. The relationship between the desired and undesired effects of a drug is termed its 'therapeutic index'. In an experimental situation this can be defined more clearly:

$$\text{Therapeutic index} = \frac{\text{Dose required to produce tumour responses/cure in 50\% animals}}{\text{Dose required to kill 50\% animals (LD}_{50})}$$

Therapeutic indices for most anti-cancer drugs are low, hence dose considerations are most important. It must not be inferred, however, that higher and higher doses are always associated with better response, albeit with increased toxicity. In clinical practice, the optimum dose for tumour response may well be below the dose producing life-threatening toxicity. This phenomenon is likely to be more common when agents with a higher therapeutic index are considered such as L-asparaginase. Such considerations are important before embarking on studies of high dose chemotherapy necessitating bone marrow transplantation. Dose-response curves should first be plotted in the lower dose range before moving to life-threatening doses which may not be more effective.

Route of administration

The route by which a drug is given is an important consideration because some drugs are poorly absorbed or badly tolerated when given by mouth, others are highly caustic substances which can cause extensive tissue necrosis if given subcutaneously and intramuscularly or if inadvertently any drug should leak out of a vein during intravenous administration. Particularly caustic agents are mechlorethamine, cyclophosphamide, imidazole carboxamide, the vinca alkaloids and the anthracycline antibiotics. These agents should be injected slowly into the rubber tubing of a fast flowing saline or dextrose infusion.

Consideration of the route of administration is also of importance in determining drug efficacy. The route by which a drug is administered may be extremely important in experimental systems and may make the difference between cure of a tumour and complete failure (Table 5.5). Thus intraperitoneal or intraportal injection of nitrogen mustard was found to have less than one quarter of the effect on the Walker tumour than the same amount of drug given intravenously. In man, cytotoxic drugs are frequently given by mouth and most of the absorbed material passes through the liver before reaching the tumour and this is important for agents metabolized in the liver and may reduce the effective concentration of drug reaching the tumour considerably. Patients are notoriously unreliable in taking medication by mouth and in addition, intestinal absorption normally varies a great deal and as little as 20% of the dose may be absorbed. Nausea and vomiting with many of the drugs may lead to little being absorbed.

Agents may be given by intra-arterial infusion in order to improve access to the tumour and reduce remote effects. Agents are available with extremely short half-lives in the plasma (a few seconds) and this means that systemic toxicity can be minimal. Unfortunately, tumour blood flow can be erratic and the normal surrounding tissues may be better perfused, leading to necrotic effects at these sites (e.g. pinnae in the case of head and neck tumours). The difficulty of the methods and the lack of a clear advantage have made this approach unpopular.

Table 5.5   Influence of route administration on the anti-tumour activity of nitrogen mustard on the Walker tumour (Cobb, 1966).

Intravenous		Intraportal	
Tumour curative dose	LD$_{50}$	Tumour curative dose	LD$_{50}$
0.1 mg	1.5 mg	None	1.8 mg

Tumour cell proliferation characteristics

Chemotherapy is largely based empirically on observed differences between normal and tumour cells in response to anti-tumour agents. Part of this difference can be explained by consideration of proliferative characteristics but it must be emphasized that cell kinetics cannot explain all the interactions seen between drugs and cells and such considerations are also dependent upon pharmacokinetics, biochemistry and tumour biology.

The proliferation of tumour cells is not entirely autonomous, neither is it constant for it varies with the size of the tumour and is related to its blood supply. Animal studies show that the characteristics of tumour cell proliferation have an important influence on the response to chemotherapy. Skipper (1971) has reviewed some of the principles concerned and the following generalizations can be made for experimental tumours:

1. The doubling time of a tumour increases with the tumour mass and the thymidine labelling index decreases (Table 5.6). The growth of most experimental tumours can be described as Gompertzian rather than linear after the statistician who first described the mathematics (Fig. 5.6).
2. The response to chemotherapy is proportional to the thymidine labelling index (the number of cells synthesizing DNA).
3. The shorter the doubling time at the onset of treatment, the better the response to chemotherapy.
4. As the tumour grows, the disease becomes less easy to cure.
5. Non-phase-dependent agents are generally more effective than phase-dependent agents against

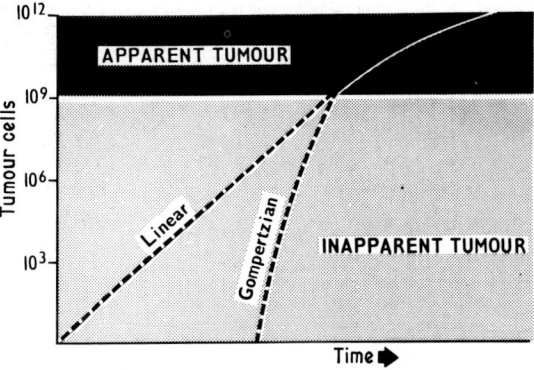

Fig. 5.6 Hypothetical growth curves for subclinical tumour, the Gompertzian growth showing prolongation of the tumour-doubling time as the tumour mass increases and linear growth.

tumours with longer doubling times and lower thymidine labelling indices.

Though the data are more sparse for human tumours, there are suggestions that these generalizations also apply to human cancer and proliferation studies are proving useful in the choice of chemotherapy and in predicting duration of remission and survival.

Table 5.6   Mass of tumour and doubling time (Carcinoma 755 System) (Skipper, 1971).

Days post-implant	Average mass (mg)	Doubling time (days)
8	220	1.2
16	3400	7.4
20	5200	>10

Tumours induced by fragments taken from small, rapidly growing tumours and from large slowly growing tumours grow at the same rates

Timing of drug administration

The time at which drugs are given has an important influence on toxicity and may make a difference between success and failure of a therapeutic regimen. Table 5.7 gives an example illustrating the importance of this from Skipper's work. Fig. 5.7 illustrates the importance of scheduling when a combination of two agents is used. Should they be given together or sequentially? Using one schedule, the effect may be

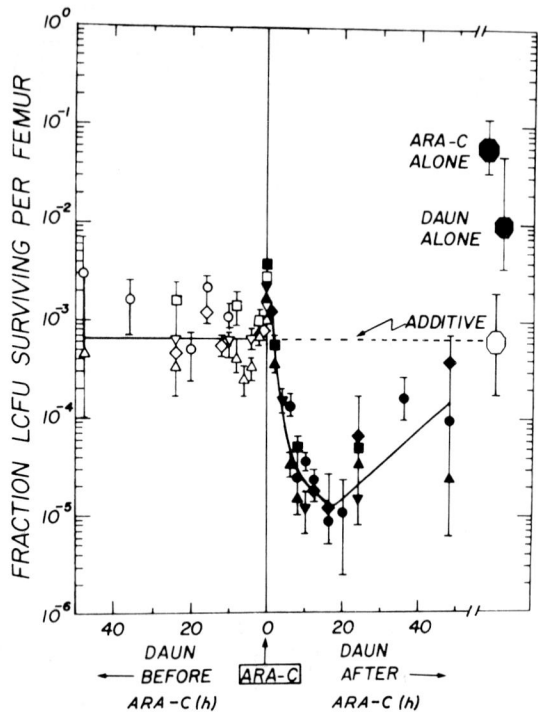

Table 5.7 Timing of cytosine arabinoside and response of L1210 leukaemia (Skipper *et al.*, 1967).

mg/kg/dose	No. of doses	Interval between doses	% cures with 10^6 cells
15	8	10 min – 1 h	0
15	8	3 h	60
15	8	8 h	30
15	8	9 h	0

Fig. 5.7 The importance of schedule of drug administration in combination chemotherapy. LCFU = leukaemia colony forming units; Daun = daunorubicin; AraC = cytosine arabinoside. (Reproduced by courtesy from Edelstein *et al.*, 1974.)

synergistic and using another, antagonistic.

The effects of dose and scheduling may be quite different for normal and tumour cells and this can be exploited to minimize toxicity and improve efficacy. Significant schedule dependency has been shown to exist between methotrexate and cytosine arabinoside and between L-asparaginase and methotrexate. Attempts are being made in man to alter the timing of cytotoxic drugs in such a way as to increase the effect on tumour cells and reduce the effect on normal cells. The effect may be increased by attempting to synchronize division of the tumour cells. The synchronization process entails the selective killing of a certain fraction of the proliferating tumour cell population, leaving the remaining cells in the non-sensitive phases of the cell cycle. The latter may then continue the growth cycle or be 'recruited' into it, thus allowing a second drug to be administered when the remaining cells are most sensitive to its action. A drug may be used to 'recruit' cells from the non-proliferating compartment to the proliferating compartment allowing subsequent chemotherapy to be of greater effect. A good example of this

approach is provided by treating an experimental plasmacytoma with cyclophosphamide. The recruited cells were then effectively destroyed by administration of the phase-specific agent cytosine arabinoside which initially was ineffective against the tumour (Griswold *et al.*, 1968). Synchrony can be achieved in man but appropriate studies have not yet been undertaken to determine whether the procedure has an advantage over empirical measures.

Knowledge that the proliferation characteristics of normal and tumour cells can vary with the time of day has suggested that timing of drug administration within the 24-hour period could be important and has lead to a new term being applied to this work: 'chronotherapy'.

Anti-tumour agents are usually used intermittently to allow regrowth of normal marrow and gut epithelium. In this way, the toxicity of a drug may be reduced and its efficacy improved. A clear example of this is the use of intermittent methotrexate during remission in childhood acute lymphoblastic leukaemia (ALL). Twice weekly methotrexate is much more effective in maintaining remission than a daily dose schedule for the same toxicity (Selawry, 1965).

It should be remembered that it may be misleading to directly apply schedule and sequence data derived from animal or cell culture studies to clinical practice or for that matter, from one human neoplastic disease, to another. Appropriate clinicopharmacological studies in man provide the best guide for therapeutic design.

Combination chemotherapy

Combination chemotherapy has been shown to be of great value in improving the results of treating cancer patients when compared with single agent therapy. Combinations of drugs are not always better than the same agents used singly but there are good examples in clinical practice where this is the case. This is true for example, in improving the response rates and survival in patients with Hodgkin's disease and some other lymphomas, acute leukaemia in both adults and children, testicular teratocarcinoma, breast cancer and a

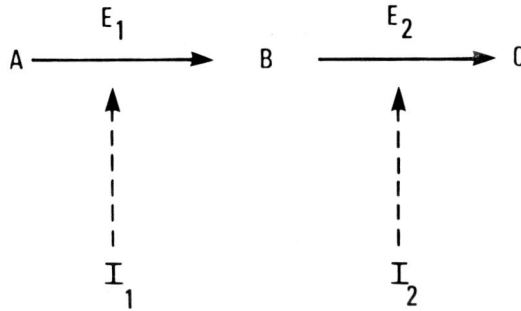

Sequential blockage of pathway synthesizing end product C. E_1 and E_2
are intermediary enzymes and I_1 and I_2 chemotherapeutic inhibitions
of these reactions.

Fig. 5.8 The mechanism of sequential blockade by anti-tumour agents of a pathway synthesizing snd product C. E_1 and E_2 are intermediary enzymes and I_1 and I_2 are chemotherapeutic inhibitions of these reactions.

variety of other cancers of adults and children. Examples may be found elsewhere in this textbook.

A word of caution is required about the use of drug combinations in human cancer since not all combinations in animal systems are advantageous: some are antagonistic. For example, a combination of methotrexate and cytosine arabinoside has proved disadvantageous in some experimental tumours. Possibly this is because methotrexate kills cells by inhibiting thymidylate synthesis but, in addition, has some inhibitory activity of purine synthesis which protects some cells by preventing DNA synthesis. A combination of methotrexate and a pure DNA inhibitor such as cytosine arabinoside would not be curative since some cells would be held in G_1.

If three or four drugs are active as single agents against a particular tumour, the number of possible drug combinations which could be tested is very large and is enormous if dose/schedule differences are considered. For this reason, it is important that a rational guess be made in selecting combinations most likely to be of value. Most combinations in the past have been chosen on the basis of minimal overlapping toxicity. By selecting active agents with minimal or non-overlapping toxicities, full doses of each component can be used with tolerable host toxicity. A good example of this is the combined use of vinblastine and bleomycin for testicular teratocarcinoma (see Chapter 26), nevertheless, toxicity to one agent may be enhanced by the addition of another and this is becoming increasingly important in clinical practice. Pulmonary toxicity with bleomycin may be made worse by the addition of adriamycin, cyclophosphamide and vin-

cristine as in the BACOP regime for non-Hodgkin lymphomas. This necessitated a marked reduction in bleomycin dose when this combination was used. Lethal toxicity with the rapid development of pulmonary fibrosis has followed the use of bleomycin and cyclophosphamide in combination.

It is possible to devise a combination of drugs which have a different mechanism of action and provide greater benefit than the single agents do individually. If

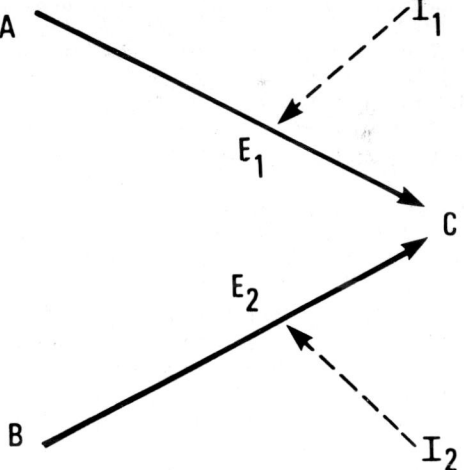

Fig. 5.9 The mechanism of concurrent inhibition by anti-tumour agents. End product C has two alternative pathways which are concurrently inhibited by chemotherapeutic inhibitions I_1 and I_2.

the side-effects are different these should not be additive and the combination need be no more toxic than the agents used singly. In some experimental systems it can be shown that the benefit produced by a combination of two drugs can be greater than the additive effect of the agents used singly. This effect is known as 'synergism', and is accompanied by an improvement in the therapeutic index.

The terms sequential, concurrent and complementary inhibition have been coined to describe certain biochemical approaches to combination chemotherapy and are explained in diagrammatic form in Figs. 5.8, 9 and 10. The rationale for using sequential blockade is that a single inhibition of one enzyme would allow accumulation of the substrate which might protect the enzyme from further attack; the second inhibitor would prevent this. The combined use of hydroxyurea and cytosine arabinoside results in synergistic tumour cell destruction in the L1210 system and is an example of this type of combined approach. The rationale for concurrent inhibition lies in blocking more than one alternative pathway leading to the production of an essential end product, and in this way preventing the utilization of an alternative pathway which could lead to resistance. An example of this would be the combined use of cytosine arabinoside and 3-deazauridine. Cytosine arabinoside is an antimetabolite that must be activated by conversion into the triphosphate nucleotide Ara-CTP which produces inhibition of DNA synthesis primarily through the inhibition of DNA polymerase. It also blocks the conversion of cytidine into deoxycytidine (inhibiting the salvage pathway). *De novo* synthesis of pyrimidine can continue and in patients with leukaemia, resistant to cytosine arabinoside with high cytosine deaminase levels, the resistant cells mainly use the *de novo* pathway. Any agent blocking this would be expected to increase the effect of cytosine arabinoside. 3-Deazauridine inhibits *de novo* pyrimidine synthesis. 3-Deazauridine is converted into the triphosphate 3-Deaza-UTP which inhibits the conversion of uridine

triphosphate into cytidine triphosphate by CTP synthetase. The drug is also a competitive inhibitor of cytidine deaminase (the enzyme degrading cytosine arabinoside). The phenomenon where treatment with one agent results in the development of resistance to this agent but the tumour becomes sensitive to a new agent, is known as 'collateral' sensitivity. In the example given above, 3-deazauridine would be expected to have a greatly enhanced effect in cells resistant to cytosine arabinoside.

An example of complementary inhibition is provided by the treatment of adults with acute myelogenous leukaemia (AML) using a combination of cytosine arabinoside to inhibit DNA synthesis and an anthracycline (daunorubicin or adriamycin) which intercalates with DNA. The use of these two agents in combination is the basis for most remission induction programmes for AML and results in remissions of up to 70% in some series. The agents used singly produce remissions in only about 25% of patients.

Drug resistance

Resistance to a chemotherapeutic agent may be considered under two main headings: primary and acquired, which together constitute the major problem in cancer chemotherapy. The experimental approach in man has largely been directed against the problem of acquired resistance, and the systems involved have been found to be highly complex. Several mechanisms may be operative, such as selective killing of a sensitive population leaving resistant cells, or an adaptive change by the tumour cell. Some of these adaptive changes are listed in Table 5.8. A scientific study of drug resistance in man is inevitably complex for these reasons and the problem is compounded by the lack of a clear definition of drug resistance in clinical practice. A tumour may be unresponsive to an agent used at one dose or schedule but responsive at another. In view of this, it is difficult in human cancer to pinpoint a particular defect being responsible for drug resistance, although this can be done in the more well defined animal and *in vitro* model systems.

Preparation of new agents with different lipid solubility characteristics is important in the development of improved chemotherapy and could overcome problems of resistance due to altered drug transport by the cancer cell. Analogues of currently useful anti-tumour agents are being developed which use different cell membrane transport mechanisms in the hope that drug resistance due to altered transport of one drug may be overcome by giving the analogue. For example, antifolates are known with different transport mechanisms from methotrexate.

Changes in tumour cell proliferation characteristics

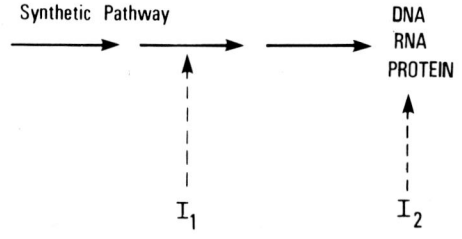

Fig. 5.10 The mechanism of complementary inhibition by antitumour agents. Inhibition of synthetic pathway, I_1, and of activity against the product, I_2.

may be an important feature in clinical resistance to therapy. In patients with chronic granulocytic leukaemia (CGL) or myeloma, for example, the disease frequently terminates in a more aggressive form with increased proliferation and resistance to chemotherapy. In CGL this involves a transition to an acute blast cell crisis of myeloblastic or lymphoblastic nature. Drugs such as busulphan which are so useful at controlling the chronic phase of the disease are almost completely ineffective at this time and drugs used for the treatment of acute leukaemia are more appropriate.

Several important questions must be answered concerning primary drug resistance. The part played by defective drug membrane transport, metabolic alterations, poor tumour blood supply and proliferative characteristics in naturally resistant solid human tumours should be studied. Measurement of drug sensitivity in young rapidly growing tumours compared with older, larger tumours would provide useful information and comparisons between the responsiveness of primary tumours and metastatic disease at different sites would also be of great value.

Evaluation

Proper evaluation of the cancer patient and his response to treatment is of fundamental importance. This has already been outlined in Chapter 1 but is sufficiently important to be re-emphasized with special relevance to chemotherapy.

Essential investigations before treatment

Before starting treatment it is essential to obtain information on the patient's past and present history, carry out a complete clinical examination with appropriate radiological and laboratory investigations, obtain a histological diagnosis and determine the extent of disease.

Clinical history
1. Onset of first symptoms of primary and/or metastatic disease.
2. Description of symptoms and direct questioning for other organ involvement.
3. Weight and weight changes during last year.
4. Past, family and social history.

Clinical examination
1. Size and extent of primary or metastatic disease; measurement of all measurable tumours in two perpendicular diameters for follow up measurements during therapy; photography may be of value.

Table 5.8. Types of drug resistance.

1. Primary		
2. Secondary	–	selective killing, leaving a resistant population of cells
		adaptive change by the tumour cell
		(a) inhibition of membrane transport
		(b) a change in the conformation of an enzyme rendering it insensitive to the drug
		(c) deletion of any enzyme necessary to activate the drug
		(d) detoxification of the drug to an inactive compound (the normal tissues may also contribute to this)
		(e) an increase in concentration of a metabolite which can overcome the biochemical lesion produced by the drug
		(f) an increase in concentration of target enzyme
		(g) a reduced requirement for the metabolite which is the product of the inhibited reaction
		(h) development of an alternative pathway which is not inhibited by the drug
		(i) change in proliferative characteristics of the tumour population

2. Examination of all organ systems for possible metastatic involvement or functional disturbances: all clinically palpable lymph nodes, liver, spleen, physical examination of respiratory and cardiovascular symptoms, oral cavity, skeletal and nervous system, abdominal palpation, rectal and gynaecological examination.
3. Performance status.
4. Weight, body surface area in m².

Routine laboratory investigations
1. Hb, WBC, differential film, platelet count and ESR.
2. Bone marrow aspiration, usually with trephine is indicated for all haematologic neoplastic disorders including leukaemias, myeloproliferative diseases, myeloma, malignant lymphomas; in solid tumours, it is indicated if there are peripheral blood abnormalities such as anaemia, immature white or red cells or thrombocytopenia which may indicate bone marrow infiltration.
3. Biochemical profile to assess organ function: blood urea and electrolytes, serum creatinine, total protein, albumin, calcium and liver function tests; further tests may be required depending on suspected abnormalities and biochemical markers are available for some tumours.

Radiology
1. A chest X-ray is always necessary and a limited skeletal survey is necessary in all diseases with a high incidence of bone metastases (e.g. breast, lung, thyroid, renal and prostatic cancer and melanoma).
2. Other radiodiagnostic procedures should be performed according to the individual problem.
3. Abdominal lymphography is useful for detecting enlarged nodes in malignant lymphoma, testicular cancer or whenever lower retroperitoneal lymph node enlargement is suspected; computerized axial tomography of the abdomen is proving to be of great value in this context and can replace abdominal lymphography in the investigation of enlarged intra-abdominal nodes in some centres where this facility is available; the technique is also proving of great value in the detection and evaluation of disease at other sites.

Scintigraphic or sonographic examinations
1. Bone scan may be performed instead of a skeletal survey in asymptomatic patients with tumours with a high incidence of osseous metastases but these scans are of little value for follow up evaluation of treatment results in metastatic bone disease.
2. Liver scan is not of great value since there is a high false positive and false negative rate.
3. Sonography can be used to evaluate the size and extent of abdominal disease.
4. Thyroid scan may be of value in suspected or manifest thyroid cancer.

All normal and pathological findings should be documented on special flow and tumour measurement sheets.

With few exceptions, the chemotherapy of solid malignant tumours is not a curative treatment. When confronted with a cancer patient, the first question must be: Is the cancer amenable to other perhaps more appropriate forms of therapy, namely surgery, radiotherapy or hormone therapy?

Absolute contraindications to chemotherapy include pregnancy, terminal disease (patients with a very short life expectancy), severe infection (e.g. first 24 hours of treatment for septicaemia) and coma. Other relative contraindications include old age (particularly in elderly patients with unresponsive tumours), very poor performance status, severe organ failure (kidney, heart, liver, bone marrow), brain metastases (if not treatable by radiotherapy), infection (until under control), dementia, inability of patient to attend clinic regularly, lack of patient cooperation and unsuccessful prior chemotherapy.

An example of the relationship between response to chemotherapy and performance status is provided by the treatment of gastrointestinal cancer and illustrated in Table 5.9. Performance status is therefore an important measure in evaluating a patient for chemotherapy.

Evaluation of response to treatment

In order to evaluate response to treatment, measurement of tumour must be undertaken at each consultation and any decrease in size in the primary or metastases carefully noted using two perpendicular measurements. Non-measurable improvement in tumour manifestations should also be assessed such as recalcification of osteolytic bone lesions and an estimate made of any decrease in size of poorly measurable lesions such as abdominal masses, liver and spleen size. Any change in weight should be noted together with an assessment of pain, appetite etc. Performance status may be graded as in Table 1.3. Any changes in laboratory parameters should be looked for.

Findings from many investigators suggest that many genes acquired at early stages of evolution may appear during ontogeny and are repressed after birth but can be reactivated and expressed in neoplasia. These gene products, although not entirely specific for the cancer concerned, may be used as a diagnostic tool and may provide a measure of the amount of tumour present. Biochemical markers such as this can help evaluation of response and hormone markers already have an important role in evaluating patients with placental choriocarcinoma.

It is convenient to have definitions for evaluating solid tumour response. Definitions for haematological malignant disease such as leukaemia will be found in Chapter 33.

Table 5.9   Relationship between performance status and response to 5-fluorouracil.

Performance status	Number of patients	Response %
0–1	66	39
2	47	26
3	21	4

Gastric carcinoma $p = < 0.01$

0	97	31
1	145	17
2	163	9
3	15	7

Colorectal carcinoma $p = < 0.05$

A 'response' is defined as a greater than 50% reduction in the product of two perpendicular diameters which is not accompanied by the appearance of tumour at any new site nor an increase in size of any known tumour deposit. The decrease must last for at least one to two months.

A 'complete response' or remission is defined as disappearance of all evidence of tumour (clinical, radiological, haematological and biochemical).

'Remission duration' is the duration of response since the start of treatment until renewed increase of tumour size to more than 25% of the product of two perpendicular diameters measured on two consultations during therapy.

Flow sheets indicating haematological, radiological and biochemical changes, in addition to clinical response, are essential for the proper management of patients on chemotherapy. There is little doubt that therapy will be suboptimal if this is not carried out and subsequent analysis frequently impossible.

Toxicity

All forms of anti-cancer therapy have their side-effects or complications. These must be carefully weighed against useful effects of the treatment. The complications of chemotherapy may be classified as immediate, early, intermediate and delayed and this classification is shown in Table 5.10.

Patterns of bone marrow toxicity may be rapid or delayed and not all chemotherapeutic agents which cause bone marrow depression do so in the same way. This is an important consideration in determining the appropriate schedule of administration. Drugs such as mechlorethamine, cyclophosphamide, vinca alkaloids and most anti-metabolites produce a nadir in the blood count at eight to ten days followed by a rapid recovery which is complete by two to three weeks. Other drugs such as the nitrosoureas have a greatly delayed recovery with a nadir at four to five weeks and should not be given more frequently than every six weeks. Other alkylating agents such as melphalan, chlorambucil and busulphan can have cumulative effects leading to prolonged bone marrow depression when a long course of treatment is completed. This is particularly important for busulphan where the count may continue to fall for several weeks after therapy has stopped and may take several months to recover. Melphalan produces the first nadir at eight to ten days followed by recovery and a further nadir at about four weeks. Mitomycin C also has a delayed bone marrow recovery pattern and tends to be cumulative. It is not wise to give this drug in combination with the nitrosoureas.

Some important organ effects are shown in Table 5.11.

Table 5.10   Complications of chemotherapy.

A. *Immediate* (within seconds)	anaphylactic shock cardiac arrhythmia pain at site of injection (this may later lead to tissue necrosis)
B. *Early* (within hours)	nausea, vomiting fever hypersensitivity reactions flu-like syndrome cystitis (this may also be delayed)
C. *Intermediate* (within days)	bone marrow depression stomatitis diarrhoea alopecia peripheral neuropathy (including paralytic ileus) renal failure immunosuppression
D. *Late* (within months)	injury to vital organs (e.g. heart – adriamycin; lung – bleomycin; liver – methotrexate; kidney – platinum compounds) skin hyperpigmentation effects on reproductive capacity (amenorrhea, subfertility) endocrinological changes (feminization, virilization etc.) teratogenic effects psychological effects of prolonged toxic therapy

The current vogue of combined therapies has resulted in important potentiation of some toxic side-effects. The pulmonary fibrosis of bleomycin may develop rapidly when this drug is combined with radiotherapy to the lung. The cardiotoxicity of the anthracyclines is increased by cyclophosphamide or radiotherapy and combined chemotherapy with radiotherapy to the mediastinum for Hodgkin's disease has been shown to be accompanied by increased cardiotoxicity and mediastinal effects. Mucositis and skin reactions caused by irradiation may be made worse by agents such as bleomycin and methotrexate. Indeed, several agents may cause 'recall' of the epithelial reaction due to radiotherapy given several weeks or even months previously. Exposure to sunlight in a patient treated with radiotherapy or chemotherapy (e.g. with methotrexate) may cause extensive skin ulceration. These combined toxicities are becoming increasingly important and schedules for minimizing the complications are currently under investigation.

Bone marrow toxicity is one of the most important

Table 5.11   Drug related side-effects related to target organ.

Target organ	Toxicity	Major implicated drugs
Bone marrow	Leucopenia	Nearly all drugs with the exception of bleomycin and L-asparaginase
Gastrointestinal tract	Stomatitis	Adriamycin, bleomycin, methotrexate, 5-fluorouracil, actinomycin D
	Gastritis	Many drugs, e.g. procarbazine
	Diarrhoea	Methotrexate, 5-fluorouracil
	Constipation or ileus	Vincristine
Skin	Hyperpigmentation	Bleomycin, busulphan
	Alopecia	Adriamycin, cyclophosphamide, vinca alkaloids, bleomycin
	Ulceration	Bleomycin, methotrexate
Nervous system	Peripheral neuropathy	Vinca alkaloids
	Cerebral dysfunction	Methotrexate, L-asparaginase
	Deafness	Platinum compounds
Heart	Arrhythmia and Cardiac failure (long term)	Adriamycin, daunorubicin Cyclophosphamide
Lungs	Fibrosis	Bleomycin, busulphan, methotrexate, cyclophosphamide
Pancreas	Pancreatitis	L-Asparaginase
Bladder	Cystitis	Cyclophosphamide
Liver	Abnormal liver function	Methotrexate, cytosine arabinoside, 6-mercaptopurine, L-asparaginase, DTIC
Kidney	Renal failure	Methotrexate, platinum compounds, mithramycin

side-effects of chemotherapy and it must be stressed that the development of granulocytopenia is much more important than other side-effects such as nausea or alopecia. Granulocytopenia is life-threatening whereas other side-effects which the patient might notice more readily may not be. Non-life-threatening side-effects are, however, usually the ones the patients worry about the most and psychological disturbances in the patient and his family are recognized to be of great importance. Dose modifications must be made in the presence of leucopenia or thrombocytopenia and a suggested modification is given in Table 5.12. In general, it is better to wait for recovery where possible and give full doses rather than modify the dose. The procedure in my own clinics is to wait for recovery for one week, if the blood count is low the dose modification is then accepted. It should be remembered, however, that a trend is much more important than a single count and flow charts are necessary to anticipate

haematologic toxicity. Obviously, these dose modifications do not necessarily apply in situations where there is bone marrow involvement or in haematologic malignant disease where evaluation of the bone marrow is essential.

Toxicity should be graded during follow up to allow full analysis and typical criteria adopted by the Eastern Cooperative Group in the USA have already been shown in Fig. 1.11.

Present status of chemotherapy in the treatment of the cancer patient

The introduction of intermittent combined chemotherapy has resulted in a marked improvement in survival for some malignant diseases such as acute lymphoblastic leukaemia of childhood, lymphomas, testicular tumours, placental choriocarcinoma, Wilm's tumour and various forms of sarcoma including osteo-

Table 5.12 Suggested dose reduction in chemotherapy of solid tumours.

Toxity grade	WBC/μl	Platelets/μl	Next dose
0	> 3500	> 100 000	100%
1	2500–3500	50 000–100 000	50%
2	< 2500	< 50 000	0% (wait until marrow recovers)

genic sarcoma. At least some of the patients in these groups can be considered to be cured by chemotherapy. In other malignant disease, the response rates may be relatively good but any improvement in survival, though useful, is modest. Examples in this category include breast cancer, ovarian cancer, myeloma and small cell carcinoma of lung. In many other malignant diseases, the response rates are low or of short duration and any improvement in survival is too small to be of real value, although tumour responses may provide useful palliation. Examples in this group include gastrintestinal, bronchial, bladder, cervix and uterine cancer, melanoma and hypernephroma. We must learn how to devise new approaches to deal with these problems. Undoubtedly, systemic therapy will play a major part in the future curative treatment of these forms of cancer and a knowledge of the principles of chemotherapy will help in considering the types of approach which can be used.

An integrated treatment approach to the cancer patient is necessary. We must not only optimize the individual types of therapy (systemic, radiotherapeutic and surgical) but we must also ensure their integration is carried out in the best possible manner. Chemotherapy may be very effective in reducing tumour volume for subsequent surgery or radiotherapy. 'Adjuvant' chemotherapy may be useful in eliminating residual disease following surgery or radiotherapy. There are good theoretical reasons for believing that adjuvant chemotherapy is more effective than chemotherapy given when obvious disease is present (Table 5.13). This prediction has been confirmed in clinical practice and exciting developments have taken place using this approach during the last few years. Adjuvant chemotherapy now is of documented value in improving survival in children with Wilm's tumour, Ewing's sarcoma and rhabdomyosarcoma, in adults with lymphoma and in some groups of women with breast cancer.

Organizational requirements

The aim of good patient management should be to provide effective treatment in the most convenient manner for the patient. For effective chemotherapy to be given safely there are many requirements. Both medical and nursing staff must be experienced in administering anti-tumour drugs. Nurses specially trained in this aspect of cancer treatment are of great value and proper facilities must be available for drug preparation for parenteral administration in order to avoid mistakes. Both ward and outpatient clinic facilities are required and in addition, a 'Day Ward' for patients staying for up to a few hours for minor investigations and treatment is important if more than a few patients are to be dealt with. Some facility for overnight stay following chemotherapy must be available. Multiple short admissions cause excessive problems for an acute medical or surgical ward and these are best dealt with on a Day Ward or short stay ward.

Table 5.13 Theoretical advantages of chemotherapy for patients with small tumour mass (minimal residual disease).

1. Experimental animals with tumours are more easily cured by chemotherapy when the tumour mass is small
2. Small tumour foci are associated with better drug access to the tumour cells
3. Low tumour mass is associated with reduced cell cycle times and greater susceptibility to most chemotherapeutic agents
4. Host has minimal immunosuppression
5. Better tolerance to drug toxicity
6. Reduced likelihood of competitive inhibitors for the chemotherapeutic agent
7. Potentially reduced number of drug resistant mutants

There must be appropriate collaboration with the Haematology Service and since blood counts and bone marrow results will usually be required within a two hour period, this will have staffing implications. Good contacts with the Pharmacy are essential and a Pharmacology service for appropriate drug assays may be required. A supportive care service must be closely associated with the chemotherapy team in order to manage haemorrhage and infection in the best possible manner. Appropriate group meetings or clinics should be held where patients' problems and treatment policies can be discussed on an interdisciplinary basis.

A coordinated approach to the treatment of most forms of cancer is now essential for it is only in this way that an integration of new developments in radiotherapy, surgery, chemotherapy and other potentially useful forms of systemic therapy can lead to improvements in patient management.

New approaches

A new approach in the development of more effective combined drug treatment has followed the recognition that agents which may have little anti-tumour effect when given alone may potentiate the effect of known anti-cancer agents. I have already alluded to drugs which alter the protein binding, metabolism or excretion of cytotoxic drugs. Agents such as amphotericin may increase membrane transport of drugs such as the nitrosoureas. Other agents such as thymidine may shunt a pyrimidine analogue such as 5-fluorouracil into a more toxic pathway. The inclusion of an anti-tumour agent within liposomes may improve tumour localization if the tumour cells can engulf these reagents

more readily than normal cells and marked changes in tissue distribution and toxicity of actinomycin D have been demonstrated using this technique. Several other 'carriers' may be developed to 'target' drugs (Gregoriadis, 1981).

Some tumour cells contain receptors for endogenous hormones (breast, prostate, uterus etc.) and this information has led to the development of steroid esters of alkylating agents in the hope that the hormone may act as a selective carrier. Unfortunately, information that these agents are taken up selectively with an improvement in therapeutic efficacy over the same drugs used separately is not available and in general the results of this approach have been disappointing.

In reviewing the achievements of the last ten years, it is easy to be impressed but a sobering feature is the realization of progress still to be made, particularly in the therapy for solid tumours. We must learn how to use existing chemotherapeutic agents in the best possible way and be ready to accept new agents for study. The study of tumour biology is already indicating mechanisms of invasion and the role and control of the blood supply in developing tumours. Agents which affect these processes could prove useful. Clearly the future outlook is an exciting one and the path to success will surely be one that links, even more closely, clinical observation with the basic sciences.

Appendix. Chemotherapeutic drugs and their characteristics

Alkylating agents

1. *Generic name*   MECHLORETHAMINE (Mustine, nitrogen mustard: HN_2)

Trade name   Mustargen

Presentation   10 mg/vials

Storage   Room temperature

Mode of administration   Intravenously over 30 s to 1 min into the tubing of a running intravenous infusion. Dilute ampoule in 10 ml water and use immediately
Other routes: intracavitary to control recurrent effusions

Dose and usual schedules
  – as single agent   0.4 mg/kg every 3–4 weeks or 0.1 mg/kg/week
  – in combinations   6 mg/m² day 1 and 8 (MOPP, MVPP)

Toxicity   Nausea and vomiting, moderate leukopenia, thrombocytopenia, possible chemical phlebitis at the site of injection

Comments and special precautions   Administer anti-emetics before injection. Local vesicant. If soft tissue infiltration occurs, application of ice compresses and/or infiltration with 1% procaine may relieve pain

2. *Generic name*   CYCLOPHOSPHAMIDE

Trade name   Cytoxan, Endoxana

Presentation   100 mg, 200 mg and 500 mg/vials
50 mg/tablets

Storage   Room temperature

Mode of administration   Intravenous sterile water 20 mg/ml (dissolve all crystals)
Oral

Dose and usual schedules
  – as single agent   Intravenous: 25–40 mg/kg in single dose, repeated every 3 weeks
Oral: 2–4 mg/kg/day for 10 days; adjust for maintenance
  – in combinations   100 mg/m²/day × 14 every month (CMF)
200 mg/m²/day × 4 every 3 weeks (+ adriamycin)
400 mg/m²/day × 5 every 3 weeks (CVP)

Toxicity   Leukopenia, thrombocytopenia, alopecia, cystitis, nausea and vomiting, not usually severe
Occasional pulmonary fibrosis and cardiotoxicity

Comments and special precautions   Warn patients about possibility of alopecia. Liberal fluid intake will minimize the risk of cystitis and the use of Mesna to prevent cystitis may be indicated

3. *Generic name*   CHLORAMBUCIL
   Trade name   Leukeran

Presentation   2 mg/tablets

Storage   Room temperature, stable for 1 year

Mode of administration	Oral
Dose and usual schedule	0.1–0.2 mg/kg/day
Toxicity	Leukopenia, thrombocytopenia
Comments and special precautions	Little toxicity when used for maintenance chemotherapy. Easy to administer to ambulatory patients
4. *Generic name*	MELPHALAN
Trade name	Alkeran, L.PAM
Presentation	2 mg/tablets, 5 mg/tablets; 100 mg/vial
Storage	Room temperature
Mode of administration	Oral, intravenous
Dose and usual schedule	0.25 mg/kg/day × 4 every 5–6 weeks
	50–100 mg/m² intravenously every 3 weeks Use diluent provided in 100–150 ml infusion NS
Toxicity	Leukopenia, thrombocytopenia. NB: toxicity more severe with intravenous regime
Comments and special precautions	Haemopoietic toxicity is cumulative and may sometimes be delayed.
5. *Generic name*	TRIETHYLENEPHOSPHORAMIDE
Trade name	Thio-Tepa
Presentation	15 mg/vials
Storage	Room temperature
Mode of administration	Intravenous, intramuscular (deep) Other routes: intracavitary to control local effusions
Dose and usual schedule – as single agent	0.8 mg/kg as a single dose or as 2–4 divided doses on successive days
– in combinations	12 mg/m² on days 1 and 8 (instead of HN₂ in MOPP)
Toxicity	Leukopenia, thrombocytopenia
Comments and special precautions	Rarely induces nausea and vomiting. Local reactions are minimal, and it can be administered by deep intramuscular injection in patients with inaccessible veins
6. *Generic name*	BUSULFAN
Trade name	Myleran
Presentation	2 mg/tablets
Storage	Room temperature, stable 1 year
Mode of administration	Oral

Dose and usual schedule in chronic granulocytic leukaemia	Initially 6–8 mg/day until WBC is halved; then half of initial dose until WBC falls below 20 000μl; then wait until WBC rises above 10 000. Try to keep WBC between 10 000 and 20 000 (usual dose 1–4 mg/day)
Toxicity	Leukopenia, thrombocytopenia, interstitial pulmonary fibrosis after prolonged treatment, amenorrhea, skin hyperpigmentation Gynaecomastia rare
Comments and special precautions	Convenient for administration to ambulatory patients but the drug is potentially highly dangerous in view of the very slow recovery of marrow reserve

Plant alkaloids

1. *Generic name*	VINBLASTINE
Trade name	Velban, Velbe
Presentation	10 mg/vials
Storage	Refrigerator
Mode of administration	Intravenous, 1 mg/ml
Dose and usual schedule – as single agent – in combinations	0.1–0.15 mg/kg/week 6 mg/m² on days 1 and 8 every 6 weeks (MVPP)
Toxicity	Nausea and vomiting, leukopenia, thrombocytopenia, alopecia, loss of reflexes, muscular weakness, paralytic ileus, stomatitis; beware of extravasation; neurological side effects not as severe as with vincristine
Comments and special precautions	Prolonged inflammatory reactions occur on extravasation. If paralytic ileus occurs, prostigmine can be used to stimulate intestinal peristalsis

2. *Generic name*	VINCRISTINE
Trade name	Oncovin
Presentation	1 mg/vials
Storage	Refrigerator
Mode of administration	Intravenous, 0.1 mg/ml
Dose and usual schedule – as single agent – in combinations	1.4 mg/m² weekly (6 weeks) maximum single 1.4 mg/m² every 3 weeks (CVP) dose is 2 mg
Toxicity	Peripheral neuropathy, paraesthesia, loss of deep tendon reflexes, constipation, paralytic ileus, mild leukopenia, thrombocytopenia; avoid extravasation
Comments and special precautions	This agent produces less bone marrow depression than vinblastine and can be given to leukopenic patients. If paralytic ileus occurs, prostigmine can be used to stimulate intestinal peristalsis

Anti-metabolites

1. *Generic name*	METHOTREXATE
Trade name	Methotrexate
Presentation	5, 50, 500 mg and 1 g/vials for parenteral use 2.5 mg/tablets for oral use
Mode of administration	Intravenous, intramuscular, oral, intrathecal
Dose and usual schedule – as single agent	2.5–5 mg/day or 15–50 mg/m² every 1–2 weeks. Intrathecal 8 mg/m² twice weekly (max. dose 12.5 mg) until symptoms of meningeal leukaemia have cleared
– in combinations	40 mg/m² on days 1 and 8, monthly (CMF)
Toxicity	Nausea and vomiting, leukopenia, thrombocytopenia, stomatitis, diarrhoea, occasional alopecia, hepatic and lung fibrosis (rare)
Comments and special precautions	If renal function is impaired, systemic toxicity is greatly enhanced. Elevation of BUN is a contra-indication for methotrexate. Leucovorin is a competitive inhibitor of methotrexate, and rescue using this agent will allow administration of much higher doses This agent may also be used in the treatment of methotrexate toxicity when given up to 72 h after the last methotrexate administration. Dosage 6–9 mg/m² every 6 h up to 72 h.
2. *Generic name*	6-MERCAPTOPURINE
Trade name	Purinethol
Presentation	50 mg/tablets, 500mg/vial
Storage	Room temperature
Mode of administration	Oral, intravenous (50 mg/ml)
Dose and usual schedule	2.5 mg/kg/day oral
Toxicity	Leukopenia, thrombocytopenia, occasional gastric intolerance, occasional liver damage (jaundice)
Comments and special precautions	If allopurinol is used concomitantly, the 6-mercaptopurine dose should be reduced to 25% of usual level
3. *Generic name*	CYTOSINE ARABINOSIDE
Trade name	Cytosar, Alexan Cytarabine
Presentation	100 mg/vials
Storage	Refrigerator, room temperature for 1 year
Mode of administration	Intravenous, intrathecal, subcutaneous
Dose and usual schedule in acute leukaemia – as single agent	2–3 mg/kg until response or toxicity or 1–3 mg/kg in 24 h infusion for up to 7 days

– in combinations	Intrathecal 50 mg twice weekly 100–150 mg/m² day × 5, every 10–14 days
Toxicity	Nausea and vomiting, leukopenia, thrombocytopenia, stomatitis, liver toxicity (rare)
Comments and special precautions	Blood count and marrow control of therapy essential in acute leukaemia. Support facilities should be available
4. *Generic name*	6-THIOGUANINE
Trade name	Thioguanine
Presentation	40 mg/tablets
Storage	Room temperature
Mode of administration	Oral
Dose and usual schedule	2'mg/kg/day
Toxicity	Leukopenia, thrombocytopenia, gastric intolerance (rare), jaundice (very rare)
Comments and special precautions	When 6-thioguanine is used together with allopurinol the dose remains unchanged.
5. *Generic name*	5-FLUOROURACIL
Trade name	Flourouracil
Presentation	250 and 500 mg/ampoules
Storage	Room temperature
Mode of administration	Intravenous, oral
Dose and usual schedule – as single agent	(a) 15 mg/kg/day × 3, followed after a 1 day rest, by 7.5 mg/kg every other day until toxicity occurs (b) 15 mg/kg weekly
– in combinations	(a) 10 mg/kg/day × 3–5 days every 6 weeks (b) 12 mg/kg/weekly on days 1 and 8 (CMF)
Toxicity	Nausea, stomatitis, diarrhoea, leukopenia, thrombocytopenia
Comments and special precautions	Individual patients tolerate a wide range in the total dose. Contra-indicated in patients in a poor nutritional state, with azotaemia or impaired liver function
Antibiotics 1. *Generic name*	ACTINOMYCIN D
Trade name	Cosmegen
Presentation	0.5 mg/vials
Storage	Room temperature

Mode of administration	Intravenous, $500 \mu g/ml$. Infuse in NS drip
Dose and usual schedule – as single agent	0.5 mg/day for 5 days (1.5 mg/m^2 intravenous may be given every 3 weeks)
Toxicity	Nausea, vomiting, stomatitis, leukopenia, thrombocytopenia, alopecia, liver toxicity
Comments and special precautions	Pain and severe local reaction on extravasation Skin reaction in previously or simultaneously irradiated areas of the skin may be severely exacerbated
2. *Generic name*	DOXORUBICIN; ADRIBLASTIN
Trade name	Adriamycin
Presentation	10 mg/vials
Storage	Refrigerator
Mode of administration	Intravenous, 2 mg/ml. Infuse in NS drip
Dose and usual schedule – as single agent	75 mg/m^2 every 3 weeks up to a total of 550 mg/m^2
– in combinations	$30–60 \text{ mg/m}^2$ every 3 weeks
Toxicity	Nausea, leukopenia, thrombocytopenia, alopecia, stomatitis, cardiotoxicity (usually only after 550 mg/m^2 total dose)
Comments and special precautions	Avoid extravasation: produces severe necrosis A total dose of 550 mg/m^2 should not be exceeded because of the risk of cardiac toxicity Potentiates toxicity of radiotherapy (e.g. irradiation mediastinum or liver)
3. *Generic name*	DAUNORUBICIN
Trade name	Daunomycin, Cerubidine
Presentation	20 mg/vials
Storage	Refrigerator
Mode of administration	Intravenous, 2 mg/ml. Infuse in NS drip
Dose and usual schedule – as single agent	$40–60 \text{ mg/m}^2$ once every 10 days
– in combinations	40 mg/m^2 on 2–3 successive days (combined with cytosine arabinoside)
Toxicity	as for adriamycin
Comments and special precautions	as for adriamycin
4. *Generic name*	BLEOMYCIN
Trade name	Blenoxane

Presentation	15 unit/vials
Storage	Room temperature
Mode of administration	Intravenous, intramuscular
Dose and usual schedule — as single agent	(a) 10–15 mg/m² every week or every 2 weeks (b) 7.5–15 mg/m²/day for 5 days by continuous intravenous infusion
– in combinations	the same as for use as single agent
Toxicity	Stomatitis, alopecia, oedema of fingers, skin hyperpigmentation, lung fibrosis, painful scarring extensor surfaces, rash
Comments and special precautions	Auscultate lung carefully during treatment to detect the appearance of lung toxicity. A total dose of 200–250 mg/m² should not be exceeded owing to the risk of pulmonary toxicity which is potentiated by drug combinations (e.g. cyclophosphamide)
5. *Generic name*	MITHRAMICIN
Trade name	Mithracin
Presentation	2.5 mg/vials
Storage	Refrigerator
Mode of administration	25–50 μg/kg/day × 7–10 days
Toxicity	Thrombocytopenia, bleeding, hypocalcaemia, hepatic toxicity, renal toxicity
Comments and special precautions	Avoid extravasation. This drug may produce very severe secondary effects (haemorrhages) and is used mainly for hospitalized patients May be used for hypercalcaemia
6. *Generic name*	MITOMYCIN C
Trade name	Mutamycin
Presentation	5 mg/vials
Storage	Refrigerator
Mode of administration	Intravenous. Infuse in NS drip
Dose and usual schedule — as single agent	10 mg/m² intravenously every 3–4 weeks
– in combinations	5–10 mg/m² (+5-fluorouracil + adriamycin)
Toxicity	Nausea and vomiting, thrombocytopenia, leukopenia, stomatitis, alopecia
Comments and special precautions	Avoid extravasation

Miscellaneous drugs

1. *Generic name*	L-ASPARAGINASE
Trade name	Elspar, Crasnitine, Porton brand (prepared from Erwinia sp.)
Presentation	10 000 international unit vials
Storage	Refrigerator
Mode of administration	Intravenous, dilute in sterile water or saline
Dose and usual schedule	10 000–20 000 U/m² intravenous, daily (for 2 weeks) or twice weekly for 4–6 weeks.
Toxicity	Possible hypersensitivity reactions and even anaphylactic shock, anorexia, nausea and vomiting, somnolence, confusion, hypoproteinaemia (lowering of fibrinogen), hypocholesterolaemia, abnormal liver function tests, very mild leukipenia and thrombocytopenia, pancreatis (rare), hyperglycaemia
Comments and special precautions	Bone marrow toxicity is practically absent; however, a strict check must be kept on liver toxicity Porton brand may be used if hypersensitivity occurs

2. *Generic name*	NITROSOUREAS (BCNU, CCNU, methyl-CCNU)
Trade name	BCNU: Carmustine CCNU: Lomustine Methyl-CCNU: Semustine
Presentation	BCNU: 100 mg/vials CCNU: 10, 40, 100 mg/capsules Methyl-CCNU: 50, 100mg/capsules
Storage	Refrigerator, stable 1 year
Mode of administration	BCNU: intravenous, dilute 3 ml alcohol and 17 ml water. Infuse in NS drip CCNU and methyl-CCNU: oral
Dose and usual schedule	BCNU: 150–200 mg/m² intravenous, single dose every 5–6 weeks CCNU: 100/130 mg/m² single dose every 5–6 weeks Methyl-CCNU: 150 mg/m² single dose every 5–6 weeks
Toxicity	Nausea, vomiting, thrombocytopenia, leukopenia (after 3–4 weeks)
Comments and special precautions	BCNU should be administered into the tubing of a running infusion to avoid pain due to venous cramps. Treatment with nitrosoureas cannot usually be resumed within 1 month of the initial administration owing to the occurrence of late bone marrow depression. Nitrosoureas should not be combined with mitomycin C owing to cumulative toxicity

3. *Generic name*	PROCARBAZINE
Trade name	Natulane
Presentation	50 mg/capsules
Storage	Room temperature, stable 1 year
Mode of administration	Oral
Dose and usual schedule – in combinations	100 mg/m²/day (MVPP and MOPP)
Toxicity	Nausea, vomiting, leukopenia, thrombocytopenia, CNS depression, skin eruption and flush syndrome produced by alcohol intake
Comments and special precautions	This agent potentiates psychotropic drugs. (Avoid monoamine oxidase inhibitors). Administer anti-emetics as from the first day of the course, gradually increase dose of procarbazine up to optimal daily level and also administer immediately prior to sleep to reduce nausea and vomiting Patients should not consume alcoholic beverages during the course of treatment.
4. *Generic name*	HYDROXYUREA
Trade name	Hydrea
Presentation	500 mg/capsules, 2 g/vials
Storage	Room temperature
Mode of administration	Oral, intravenous
Dose and usual schedule	1–2 g/m² orally daily for 2–4 weeks
Toxicity	Mild nausea and vomiting, leukopenia, thrombocytopenia
Comments and special precautions	The drug's major side effect is haematologic toxicity. Severe megaloblastic change is seen on bone marrow aspiration
5. *Generic name*	DIMETHYL-TRIAZENO-IMIDAZOLE CARBOXAMIDE (DTIC)
Trade name	Dome, Dacarbazine
Presentation	100 and 200 mg/ampoules
Storage	Refrigerator: Avoid exposure to light
Mode of administration	Intravenous. Use solution immediately
Dose and usual schedule	200–250 mg/m²/day × 5 every three weeks
Toxicity	Nausea and vomiting, flu-like syndrome (fever, muscular pain), leukopenia, thrombocytopenia uncommon
Comments and special precautions	The drug has a slight myelodepressive action. Symptomatic treatment of nausea and vomiting is required

6. *Generic name*	4'-DEMETHYLEPIPODOPHYLLOTOXIN 9-(4,6–0–2–THENYLDENE-β-D-GLUCOPYRANOSIDE (VM26)
Presentation	50 mg/vials
Storage	Room temperature
Mode of administriation	Intravenous by slow infusion (30–40 min) in 150 ml 5% normal saline (use dilution immediately)
Dose and usual schedule	50–150 mg/m² intravenous, repeated weekly
Toxicity	Nausea, vomiting, leukopenia, thrombocytopenia, hypotension and flushing, alopecia
Comments and special precautions	Avoid extravasation or fast injection
7. *Generic name*	4'-DEMETHYLEPIPODOPHYLLOTOXIN 9-(4,6–0–ETHYLIDENE-β-D-GLUCOPYRANOSIDE) (VP 16.213) (etoposide)
Trade name	Vepesid
Presentation	100 mg/vials 100 mg/capsules
Storage	Room temperature
Mode of administration	Oral or intravenous by slow infusion in 150 ml NS (use dilution immediately) There is some evidence that the drug is unstable in dextrose
Dose and usual schedule	Oral, 100–150 mg/m² daily × 5 every 3 weeks Intravenous, same as VM26
Toxicity	Same as VM26
Comments and special precautions	Same as VM26
8. *Generic name*	CIS DIAMMINEDICHLOROPLATINUM (II) (Cis-platinum)
Trade name	Neoplatin
Presentation	10 mg, 50 mg/vials
Storage	Refrigeration 2–8°C stable 2 years
Mode of administration	100 mg/m² usually intravenous infusion over 12 hours
	Alternative schedule: 20 mg/m² intravenously daily for 5 days
Toxicity	Nb. Prehydration is essential and at least 4 litres of fluid should be given over the first 24 hours. Mannitol or Frusemide should be given during this time if an adequate diuresis does not occur. An accurate assessment of renal function is important before treatment since renal impairment increases toxicity
Comments and special precautions	Side affects are severe. Severe nausea and vomiting electrolyte imbalance including hypomagnesaemia, renal failure, peripheral neuropathy, ototoxicity
	Potentially dangerous agent which should only be given by experienced chemotherapists

Further Reading

Textbooks

Avery, G.S. (ed.) (1976), *Drug Treatment: Principles and Practice of Clinical Pharmacology and Therapeutics.* Churchill Livingstone, Edinburgh and London.

Clarysse, A., Kenis, Y. and Mathe, G. (eds) (1976), *Cancer Chemotherapy: Its role in the treatment strategy of haematologic malignancies and solid tumours.* Springer Verlag, Berlin, Heidelberg and New York.

Goodman, L.S. and Gilman, A. (eds) (1970), *The Pharmacological Basis of Therapeutics.* 4th edn, Macmillan Ltd., London.

Holland, J.F. and Frei III, E. (eds) (1980), *Cancer Medicine* 2nd edn. Lea and Febiger, Philadelphia. (Sections on principles of chemotherapy and the chemotherapeutic agents).

Sartorelli, A.C. and Johns, D.G. (1974), *Antineoplastic and Immunosuppressive Agents*, I and II. Springer Verlag, Berlin, Heidelberg and New York.

Useful reviews

Gregoriadis, G. (1981), Targeting of drugs. *Lancet,* **ii**, 241–46.

Lant, A. (1978), Drugs: their action and therapeutic use. *Medicine,* **2**, 99.

Schabel, F.M. (1969), The use of tumour growth kinetics in planning 'curative' chemotherapy of advanced solid tumours. *Canc. Res.,* **29**, 2384.

Schabel, F.M. Jr. (1976), Concepts for treatment of micrometastases developed in murine systems. *Am. J. Roentg.,* **126**, 500.

Skipper, H.E. (1978), Adjuvant chemotherapy. *Cancer,* **41**, 936.

The pharmacologic basis of cancer chemotherapy, (1977). *Sem. Oncol.,* **4**, 131.

References

Cobb, L.M. (1966), *Int. J. Cancer,* **1**, 329.

Edelstein, M., Vietti, T. and Valeriote, F. (1974), Schedule-dependent synergism for the combination of 1-β-D-arabinofuranosylcytosine and daunorubicin. *Canc. Res.,* **34**, 293–97.

Farber, S. *et al.* (1948), Temporary remissions in acute leukaemia in children produced by folic acid antagonist, 4-aminopteroyl-glutamic acid. *New Engl. J. Med.,* **238**, 787.

Griswold, D.P. *et al.* (1968), Success and failure in the treatment of solid tumours. *Cancer Chemother. Rep.,* **52**, 345.

Selawry, O.S. (1965), New treatment schedule with improved survival in childhood leukaemia: Intermittent parenteral versus daily oral administration of methotrexate for maintenance of induced remission. *J. Am. Med. Ass.,* **194**, 75.

Skipper, H.E. (1971), *Natl. Cancer Inst. Mono.,* **34**, 2.

Skipper, H.E., Schabel, F.M. and Wilcox, W.S. (1967), Experimental evaluation of potential anticancer agents XXI Scheduling of arabinosyl cystone to take advantage of its S-phase specificity against leukaemia cells. *Cancer Chemother. Rep.,* **51**, 125.

6 Endocrine therapy

Trevor J. Powles, I.E Smith
and R.C. Coombes

Oncologists, trained in chemotherapy, clinical phar-macology and cell kinetics tend to approach endocrine therapy in a spirit restricted to their disciplines. Unfortunately, the principles involved are different and depend on a biological balance between host and tumour.

Many tissues in the body are influenced or controlled by hormones. They possess specific receptors to the relevant hormones which, when circulating, can stimu-late growth and function. It is hardly surprising that tumours which arise in endocrine-sensitive tissues may sometimes retain some endocrine control of growth. Changes in the endocrine environment in which the tumours develop may, therefore, inhibit further tumour development or even cause tumour regression. Unlike cytotoxic chemotherapy, changes in the endoc-rine status of the host which give rise to tumour regression do not cause inhibitory effects on essential host tissues such as bone marrow or gut. The endocrine effects on the host can often be minimized by selective hormone treatment or replacement which results in excellent symptomatic remissions. The tumours which are associated with hormone-stimulated changes in growth are particularly carcinoma of the prostate, breast, thyroid and uterus. The most important hormones to influence these tumours are the steroid hormones, thyroxine and the pituitary hormones. If hormone-sensitive tumours arise in an established endocrine environment, then presumably the tumour cells are able to divide in the presence of these hor-mones. Changes in the endocrine status may, therefore, be associated with inhibition of tumour growth and regression of the tumour. To effect these changes it is necessary to understand the basic relevant endocrin-ology.

Although only a few tumour types are potentially endocrine-sensitive, they are common and involve a large number of patients. The aim of this chapter is to describe the theoretical principles for endocrine therapy, outline the tumours and manoeuvres involved

and thereby establish the basic methods of treatment.

Endocrine basis of tumour response

Relevant endocrine physiology

Generally the hypothalamus produces polypeptide hormones which control the release of various anterior pituitary hormones which, in turn, control the function of various glands, including the breasts, prostate, thy-roid, ovaries, testes and adrenals.

Release of adrenocorticotrophic hormone (ACTH) controls steroid synthesis by the adrenals, particularly synthesis of cortisol and sex hormones from cholesterol (Fig. 6.1). Cortisol acts as a feed-back on the hypo-thalamus to inhibit corticotrophin-releasing factor and thereby release of further ACTH. The ovary is able to synthesize progesterone from cholesterol. It can also irreversibly synthesize oestradiol and oestrone from circulating Δ-4-androstenedione by aromatization of the A-ring (Fig. 6.2). Oestriole, another oestrogen associated with pregnancy is produced in variable amounts and it has been claimed that the balance of these oestrogens may be important in breast cancer (MacMahon et al., 1971).

Circulating oestrogens have several functions on the hypothalamus which may be relevant to cancer. Firstly, they inhibit luteinizing hormone (LH) and follicle-stimulating hormone (FSH) release from the pituitary which controls progesterone and oestrogen synthesis by the pre-menopausal functioning ovary. Increasing levels of oestrogen inhibit further release of LH/FSH by the pituitary. Secondly, low doses of oestrogen stimulate prolactin secretion as does thyrotropin-releasing hormone (TRH) whereas high levels of oestrogen inhibit prolactin release. At the menopause the ovaries gradually lose the ability to synthesize oestrogens with levels approximately half the peak values which occur in cycling pre-menopausal women.

Cholesterol

|(20,22-Desmolase)

(17-Hydroxylase)
Pregnenolone ⟶ 17-Hydroxypregnenolone ⟶ Dehydroepiandrosterone

|(3-β-Dehydrogenase)

(17-Hydroxylase)
Progesterone ⟶ 17-Hydroxyprogesterone ⟶ Δ-4-Androstenedione

|(11-Hydroxylase)- - - - - - - - - -|(11-Hydroxylase)

Desoxycorticosterone   Desoxycortisol (S)   Testosterone

|(21-Hydroxylase) - - - - - - - - - -|(21-Hydroxylase) |(Aromatization)

Corticosterone   Cortisol   Oestradiol ⇌ Oestrone

|(3-β-Hydroxylase)

Aldosterone

Fig. 6.1 Steroid hormone synthesis.

These reduced levels are associated with increased pituitary release of LH/FSH.

Testosterone is synthesized from Δ-4-androstenedione by the testes of the male and to a lesser extent by the ovary of the female and adrenal gland of both sexes. Before becoming active, testosterone must be converted into dihydrotestosterone.

From this outline it is quite obvious that apparently simple hormone manoeuvres such as administration of oestrogen or removal of the adrenal glands may have quite complex effects on many other hormones. For example, administration of a synthetic oestrogen like stilboestrol will act on the hypothalamus to inhibit or stimulate prolactin synthesis as well as inhibit release of LH and FSH with associated reduction in natural synthesis of various sex steroids. Stilboestrol will also compete for and induce enzymes and binding proteins involved in degradation and carriage of these hormones. By these means the body will attempt to correct and adapt to the induced endocrine changes. Administered steroid hormones such as androgens may be converted into other steroid hormones particularly oestrogens, a metabolic pathway which may be gradually induced by medication (Fig. 6.1). These factors may account for the relapse after response and subsequent withdrawal response which sometimes occurs with successful endocrine therapy.

Two types of endocrine manoeuvre may be attempted. Firstly, administration of hormones such as oestrogens, androgens, progestins, thyroxine etc., normally referred to as 'hormone therapy'. Alternatively, ablative therapy may be attempted by removal of endocrine glands (for example, adrenalectomy) or inhibition of enzymes by medical means (for example, aminoglutethimide which inhibits steroid synthesis).

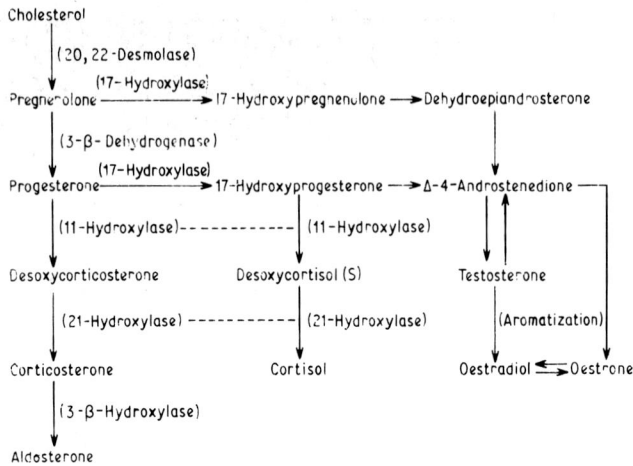

Experimental tumours

Many of the features of human endocrine therapy are mimicked by the rat 7, 12-dimethylbenz (a) anthracene

(DMBA)-induced and nitrosomethylurea (NMU)-induced mammary tumours (Table 6.1). Both these tumours possess oestrogen receptors and manipulation of the oestrogen status of the host will influence the induction rate of new tumours and growth rate of established tumours. An example is the regression of the DMBA-induced mammary tumour which occurs after removal of the ovaries or pituitary of the host (De Sombre *et al.*, 1976). Unfortunately, like human breast cancer, after a period of a few days or weeks the tumours start to grow again. Sometimes administration of oestrogens will now give rise to a further remission analogous to the withdrawal response seen with some patients after successful hormone therapy. This is not usually as good or as long as the primary remission.

Whether relapse after endocrine remission results from cloning of endocrine insensitive cells, or induced changes in hormone synthesis or metabolism is not clear, and further research is indicated in this area in order to attempt prolongation of endocrine remission.

How changes in endocrine status induce remissions remains a complete mystery. It seems probable that successful endocrine therapy is not cytotoxic as such, but rather induces differentiation and inhibition of cell division in tumours. Further research is needed in this area particularly in relation to development of combined endocrine and cytotoxic chemotherapeutic treatment.

Mechanisms of actions of hormones on tumours

Beatson first observed tumour regression of breast cancer in some patients following oophorectomy in 1896 (Beatson, 1896). Since this time various endocrine manoeuvres have been shown to influence the growth of many other clinical and experimental tumours (Table 6.1).

How hormones influence growth and behaviour of malignant tissues is not known. It is probable that endocrine changes are associated, in some tumours, with inhibition of cell division and stimulation of the cells into a more differentiated form. If sufficient, this will result, by natural wastage, in apparent tumour regression. Most hormones will stimulate changes in cyclic nucleotide and prostaglandin synthesis and these agents are known to modify cell division and differentiation. They may, therefore, be mediators or modulators of endocrine-induced regression of tumours. In total contrast to other forms of anti-cancer therapy, there is no evidence that hormones are cytotoxic, apart from perhaps the effects of corticosteroids on haematolymphoid neoplasms.

At an early stage in the development of endocrine therapy for breast cancer, three features become apparent: firstly, only a small proportion of patients

Table 6.1 Endocrine therapy in experimental and human tumours.

Experimental tumours	Endocrine response
DMBA	oophorectomy
	anti-oestrogens
NMU	oophorectomy
Human tumours	
Prostatic carcinoma	orchidectomy
	oestrogens
	hypophysectomy
Breast carcinoma	oophorectomy
	oestrogens
	androgens
	progestins
	adrenalectomy
	hypophysectomy
Thyroid carcinoma	thyroxine
Endometrial carcinoma	progestins
Renal carcinoma	progestins

respond (approximately 30%); secondly, most if not all who respond eventually relapse; and thirdly, those who respond to one form of endocrine manipulation have a high probability of responding to further manipulation. No real advance was made into understanding these problems until the discovery in tumour cells of hormone receptors similar to those identified in normal tissues under endocrine control.

Hormones generally act inside the nucleus of cells. Protein hormones, which are unable to cross the cell membranes, attach to specific membrane receptors to stimulate required processes within the cell. Each hormone has its own special receptor and therefore only cells possessing this receptor can be affected by the hormone and this allows hormones to have a selective effect on certain tissues.

Steroid hormones are able to pass through the cell membrane, but need to combine with specific cytoplasmic receptors in order to pass into the nucleus and become effective.

Simple reproducible and specific methods for measurement of hormone receptors in tissue specimens have now been developed.

Understandably, most studies have been carried out on mammary tumours, but several groups are beginning to apply these research techniques to other tumours. Studies of mammary carcinoma have shown that some tumour cells contain specific cytoplasmic receptors for some of the steroid hormones and cell-membrane receptors for some of the peptide hormones (for review see McGuire *et al*., 1977).

It is not unreasonable to suppose that it is necessary for tumour cells to possess hormone receptors in order to react to changes in the host endocrine status. This is confirmed by the correlation between the levels of oestrogen receptors present in tumours and the subsequent response to oophorectomy in pre-menopausal patients and oestrogen therapy or tamoxifen in post-menopausal patients (Table 6.2). What is rather curious is that this test also predicts likely response to other endocrine manoeuvres such as adrenalectomy, corticosteroid or androgen therapy. This implies coincidental presence of other receptors such as those for cortisol or androgens and therefore indirectly suggests that hormone reactive tumour cells arise from a multisensitive breast cell. This is not unreasonable in view of the variety of hormones to which the normal breast reacts.

The mechanism for translocation of the hormone/receptor complex into the nucleus is unknown, but once in the nucleus, the hormone remains bound to the receptor and associated with the centrioles during subsequent cell division (Nenci, 1978).

Following entry into the nucleus, oestrogen has mitogenic effects on some cells stimulating DNA replication and messenger RNA production associated with synthesis of further oestrogen and progesterone receptor. In this respect it is also of interest that prolactin and insulin will stimulate oestrogen receptor synthesis whereas dibutyryl cyclic AMP and oophorectomy will reduce receptor content.

Although these observations indicate a possible mechanism for response to oestrogens and oophorectomy, responses to progesterone are more difficult to explain. Progesterone receptors are present in 30–65% of human breast cancer, but their estimation has proved difficult due to the affinity of progesterone with corticosteroid binding sites. The biological effect of such bound progesterone is unclear since, unlike corticosteroids, progesterone does not inhibit thymidine incorporation in human breast cancer cells *in vitro*. It is possible that progesterone acts by modifying corticosteroid action (Lippman *et al.,* 1976).

Glucocorticoid receptors are found in 40–70% of human breast cancers and as in the case of lymphoma and leukaemia, binding of corticosteroid has an inhibitory effect resulting in cell death. Glucocorticoid-resistant leukaemia cells have been found to have lost their correct receptor action, some losing the ability to translocate the complex to the nucleus, and others having a non-functional receptor. The proper evaluation of the mechanisms of corticosteroid and receptors in human breast cancer has been hampered by the binding of progesterone to steroid receptor sites and the binding of steroid to contaminating plasma corticosteroid-binding protein, transcortin.

Androgen action in cancer has been studied *in vitro* using a human breast cell line. It seems that high dose testosterone is metabolized, in part to dihydrotestosterone, which binds to oestrogen receptor, therby mimicking the effects of oestrogen. Low dose testosterone, i.e. physiological levels, will also translocate the receptor through to the nucleus, but has no mitogenic effect. In support of this concept, it is known that high doses of androgen can stimulate tumour growth *in vivo*. It is possible that, *in vivo*, androgens have a similar action to oestrogens in post-menopausal women by sharing a common receptor site (McGuire *et al.*, 1977).

The relationship of peptide hormones to human tumour growth is complex. Although prolactin has been shown to have multiple effects in rat mammary tumour models, the relevance of this information to humans is dubious. Hypophysectomy may well effect its action via suppression of ovarian and adrenal function.

Receptor assay techniques

Application of oestrogen and progesterone receptors will mainly be considered here since they have been most extensively studied in human breast cancer. Receptor assays for corticosteroids and androgens have only recently been developed.

There are several methods used for measurement of oestrogen receptors in target tissues, but the simplest involves incubating aliquots of the tumour cytosol with tritiated oestradiol, and then removing free tritiated oestradiol with dextran-coated charcoal. If knowledge of the number or affinity of the binding sites is required, different dilutions of hormone are incubated with the receptor and the method of Scatchard is used to calculate these parameters. Sometimes a significant quantity of receptor sites is occupied by endogenous oestradiol and these sites can be displaced by incubation at body temperature. If the nuclear receptor content is required, a homogenate of the nuclei is made and incubated with tritiated oestradiol (for details of method see McGuire *et al.*, 1975).

The importance of progesterone receptors has recently been highlighted since the presence of these receptors has been shown to reflect activity of bound cytoplasmic oestradiol, and thus could be expected to predict the outcome of hormone therapy with a greater degree of certainty. The assay is carried out in a similar way to oestrogen receptors but a more stable analogue of progesterone (R2050) is utilized which does not bind to other hormone binding sites or to plasma.

Several problems exist with both assays. First of all, falsely positive results will occur if an unrepresentative section of tumour is examined, since distribution of hormone-responsive cells has been shown to be uneven by immunochemical staining techniques. Further, distribution of oestrogen receptor in metastatic tissue is inconsistent, so that some metastases may contain receptor and others may not. The major cause of false positivity, however, is that the receptor, although occurring in the cytoplasm, may not be biologically active. The cause of the biological inactivity is not known, but the explanation could be analogous to ectopic hormone production where high molecular weight forms of hormone exist with little biological activity.

False negatives are most often caused by collection and storage problems since even when stored at $-50°C$ the receptor deteriorates at a significant rate. At room temperature oestrogen receptor has a half-life of about twenty minutes. This rapid deterioration can be prevented by transportation at $0-4°C$ and storage at $-196°C$ (i.e. in liquid nitrogen). A high circulating level of oestradiol could occupy all available receptor sites and thus, without an assay of nucleus receptor or without an attempt at dislodging the bound receptor, false negative results will be obtained.

Clinical significance of receptor assay techniques

Prostate and uterine carcinomas contain significant oestrogen receptor content in 75% and 25% of cases respectively. Breast tumours are positive in 50–60% of cases (Table 6.2) and about two thirds of these demonstrate the presence of progesterone receptor (Table 6.3). Only very rarely do progesterone receptors exist in the absence of cytoplasmic oestrogen receptors; 25–

Table 6.2 Relationship of oestrogen receptor status to response to various endocrine treatments.

Treatment	Oestrogen Receptor positive	Oestrogen Receptor negative
Tamoxifen	32/67	1/15
Nafoxidene	7/10	0/8
Stilboestrol	12/9	1/17
Oophorectomy	28/43	2/74
Adrenalectomy	15/22	1/9
Androgens	10/28	2/22
Glucocorticoids	15/32	0/19
Hypophysectomy	9/14	0/12
Total response rate	128/235	7/176
Percentages	54.5%	4%

Table 6.3 Consideration of progesterone receptor (PGR) and oestrogen receptor (ER) status and relationship to response to hormone therapy (from McGuire *et al.*, 1977).

Status	ER^-PGR^-	ER^-PGR^+	ER^+PGR^-	ER^+PGR^+
Response	9/64 (14%)	3/6 (50%)	20/71 (28%)	67/91 (74%)

30% of benign breast tumours contain oestrogen receptor and normal breast contains very little receptor.

Receptor content in breast carcinomas is influenced by menopausal status, so that pre-menopausal women are less likely to have detectable cytoplasmic receptor (30% vs 50–60%). Oestrogen receptor is sometimes positive in metastases whilst negative in the primary and *vice versa*, but discordance is estimated to occur in only 20% of cases.

Although there is no clear correlation of oestrogen receptor content and the degree of cellularity, some workers have found that poorly differentiated tumours are more likely to be oestrogen-receptor negative, as are those with a prominent local lymphocytic reaction. On the other hand, invasive lobular carcinomas are more likely to be positive, as are those tumours that contain significant quantities of carcinoembryonic antigen.

It seems that patients whose tumours contain oestrogen receptors may have a better prognosis than those who do not (Knight *et al.*, 1977) even though there appears to be no relationship between receptor content and stage at presentation (Maynard *et al.*, 1978). This perhaps indicates that receptors are more likely to occur in well differentiated slowly growing tumours. Oestrogen-receptor positive tumours appear more likely to spread to bone, which is interesting in relation to the relatively high response rate of bone versus other metastases to endocrine ablative procedures.

The presence of oestrogen receptor in tumours indicates an approximately 50% chance of response to any of several types of endocrine therapy (Table 6.2). The presence of both progesterone and oestrogen receptor increases the chance of response (Table 6.3). On the other hand, absence of oestrogen receptor indicates little chance (4%) of response to any type of hormone or ablative therapy. It seems probable that measurement of receptors indicates the likelihood of response to endocrine therapy more accurately than clinical criteria, although this has never been confirmed in a clinical trial. These clinical criteria include: (a) menopausal status, since post-menopausal women are more

Table 6.4   Commonly used oestrogens in carcinoma of the breast and prostate.

Route and oestrogen	'Low' dose*	'High' dose*	Breast	Prostate
Oral				
Ethinyl oestradiol	0.3	1.0–3.0	+	–
Premarin	15	–	+	–
Stilboestrol	5–15	50–100	–	+
Intramuscular				
Estradurin	100 mg/	–	–	+
(polyoestradiol	month			
phosphate)				
Intravenous				
Honvan	250–500	–	–	+
(stilboestral	mg/day			
diphosphate)				

*mg/day unless otherwise stated

likely to have hormone-sensitive tumours than pre-menopausal; (b) disease-free interval since, as mentioned above, tumours containing receptor protein appear to grow more slowly than those lacking receptor and hence a long disease-free interval suggests that the tumour is hormone-sensitive; (c) response to previous hormone manipulation, and (d) site of dominant lesion, since hepatic metastases respond poorly to any form of endocrine therapy.

Endocrine manoeuvres

Oestrogens

The use of oestrogens in clinical cancer medicine was first described by Huggins and Hodges in 1941 with the report of regression of prostatic carcinoma in patients treated with stilboestrol. Three years later, Alexander Haddow reported similar regressions in some patients with breast cancer (Haddow *et al.*, 1944). Since then, oestrogen therapy has been widely used as an alternative to orchidectomy for prostatic cancer and standard

first-line treatment for post-menopausal patients with advanced breast cancer (Table 6.4).

Breast cancer (see Chapter 16)
Clinical response. Approximately 30% of post-menopausal women with breast carcinoma respond to oestrogen therapy; occasional regressions have also been claimed in pre-menopausal patients with very high dosage, but such treatment is rarely effective and may even have a tumour-stimulating effect. It is now, therefore, generally agreed that oestrogen therapy should be reserved for the post-menopausal patient.

The likelihood of response increases with age after the menopause; responses are seen in only 10% of patients within the first five years of the menopause compared with almost 50% in patients over 70 years. Prior radiotherapy has been reported to reduce the response to oestrogens of soft tissue metastases by 50% and it is our opinion that endocrine treatment should be tried before radiotherapy in such patients.

Site of metastatic disease is another factor in determining response to oestrogens. Soft tissue disease has the highest chance of regression with reported response rates of up to 50% and lung metastases respond in 25–30% of patients although responses for lymphangitis carcinomatosis are uncommon and of short duration. On the other hand, unlike other forms of endocrine therapy, responses in bone are seen in less than 10% of patients and oestrogen therapy for osseous metastases carries with it the added risk of precipitating life-threatening hypercalcaemia. Responses for liver and CNS metastases are extremely rare. These factors should be considered when planning appropriate therapy for individual patients, and oestrogens should not be used as first line treatment of disease principally involving bone, liver or pulmonary lymphatics (Table 6.5).

As mentioned above, another factor of value in predicting the chance of response to oestrogen treatment, and indeed to other forms of endocrine therapy, is the interval between the discovery of the primary tumour and the first clinical evidence of metastases. The longer this tumour-free interval, the greater the likelihood of tumour regression.

Table 6.5   Overall response and response by site for premarin compared with synthetic oestrogens in post menopausal patients with metastatic breast carcinoma.

	Overall response	Soft tissue	Lung	Bone	Liver	Marrow
Premarin	14/31 (45%)	13/23 (57%)	6/16 (38%)	2/11 (18%)	0/3	0/3
Synthetic oestrogens	12/30 (40%)	12/21 (57%)	2/11 (18%)	0/9 (0%)	0/1	0/3

The histological features of the primary tumour do not appear to correlate with response to oestrogen therapy. Recently, however, the development of techniques for measuring oestrogen receptors in breast cancer tissue (see above) has provided another important predictive indicator of response.

Response duration and survival. The average duration of response to oestrogen therapy is about sixteen months with individual patients occasionally maintaining a response for up to five years. Likewise, responding patients have been reported as surviving almost three times as long as non-responders. Despite this evidence for effective short-term improvement, cures after established metastatic disease are almost never described and oestrogen treatment, like all other forms of endocrine therapy for breast cancer remains purely palliative.

Withdrawal response. Once a patient has relapsed on oestrogen therapy, stopping treatment may result in a further period of tumour regression in up to 30% of patients. This so-called 'withdrawal response' is seen more frequently in patients whose original response has been of long duration, and is only very rarely seen in those who have not responded to the initial treatment. The duration of withdrawal response is usually shorter than that of the original response, and is on average nine to ten months' duration.

It is therefore important to wait at least six weeks after stopping oestrogen therapy before starting secondary treatment, to see whether a withdrawal response will occur.

Prostatic cancer (see Chapter 24)
Oestrogen therapy is effective in achieving pain relief in approximately 85% of patients with metastatic prostatic carcinoma, although the incidence of documented objective remissions is considerably lower. The mechanism of action is unknown but probably involves androgen suppression.

Although oral administration is satisfactory for most patients, intravenous therapy is sometimes indicated for urgent palliation, particularly in patients with impending urinary obstruction. Usually stilboestrol diphosphate (Honvan) is used for this purpose, and may bring about dramatic improvement, removing the need for later surgery (for review see Fergusson, 1972) (Table 6.4).

The dosage usually employed for each oestrogen compound is the same as for breast carcinoma with no convincing advantage demonstrated for very high dosage.

The median duration of response to oestrogen

therapy in prostatic carcinoma is around eighteen to twenty-four months. Responses of many years' duration have been reported, but as with breast cancer, cures are exceedingly rare, and treatment is again merely palliative. In view of the risks involved with this type of treatment, oestrogen therapy should be reserved for palliative treatment of symptomatic disease and only after orchidectomy has been considered.

Side-effects and toxicity
In women, oestrogens, although usually better tolerated than chemotherapy, do cause symptomatic side-effects in approximately 30% of patients, particularly in the early part of treatment. These include anorexia, nausea and even vomiting. Sodium retention with ankle swelling may occur with the associated risk of precipitating or exacerbating cardiac failure. For reasons which are not clear, thrombophlebitis is not usually a problem. Uterine bleeding usually occurs when treatment is discontinued and may occur during therapy, particularly if the patient is unreliable about taking the hormone. It can be stopped sometimes by increasing the dosage, but usually it is necessary to stop medication, wait for bleeding to stop, then restart with a higher dose. Hypercalcaemia which can be lethal (Cornbleet *et al.*, 1976) occurs in approximately 20% of patients. In men, oestrogen therapy has the disadvantage of causing feminization including gynaecomastia which may require surgical attention, but most patients will accept these problems in preference to orchidectomy. The cardiovascular complications are very much more serious with significant increase in cardiovascular death, so much so that in one large series, stilboestrol caused more deaths than the disease. This is particularly important in the elderly and, unfortunately, most patients with prostatic cancer are old.

Although oestrogen therapy is easy to administer, these unpleasant and often dangerous side-effects indicate the need for special caution before recommencing treatment.

Types of oestrogen and dosage
Details of the more commonly used oestrogens in the treatment of breast cancer are given in Table 6.4. The most commonly used synthetic oestrogens are diethylstilboestrol and ethinyl oestradiol. Premarin, a preparation of natural conjugate oestrogens is as effective as its synthetic counterparts and although more expensive, has the advantage of better tolerance (Table 6.5).

Parenteral preparations including stilboestrol diphosphate (Honvan), oestradiol undecylate, and hexoestrol are rarely required, and the latter two have the disadvantage of prolonged activity, which cannot be readily reversed if tumour stimulation or hyper-calcaemia occurs.

The dose of oestrogens necessary to achieve an anti-tumour effect has been a matter of some controversy. Usual dosages are also given in Table 6.4 and it is important to notice that these doses are higher than would be required for the treatment of most non-malignant endocrine conditions. On the other hand, there is little evidence that increasing standard dosage increases remission rate.

Oophorectomy

The beneficial effect of bilateral oophorectomy was first recorded by Beatson in 1896, when he recorded that two of six patients with breast cancer improved following this procedure. In the ten years that followed approximately one hundred patients were reported and 24% had attained a remission, with 15% attaining a remission of more than one year. Bilateral oophor-ectomy is now considered to be the primary treatment of choice for some pre-menopausal patients with disseminated breast cancer.

Clinical response

Overall responses vary between 24.5 and 37.0% depending largely on criteria of response. A fairly representative response rate of 29.5% was reported by Veronesi *et al.* (1975), and the mean duration of response in these patients was 16 months. The mean survival of responders was 31 months, whereas that of the non-responders was only 9 months. The 5-year survival of the former was 19% and that of the latter group 0%.

Over the years, as with other forms of endocrine response, certain clinical criteria have been identified which indicate likelihood of response to oophor-ectomy.

For example, several larger series have confirmed that a long recurrence-free interval following mastectomy is associated with a greater chance of response to oophorectomy. Thus in one series, 28% of those who relapsed within one year of mastectomy showed some response; 34% of those who relapsed between two and four years showed a response, and those patients who relapsed after five years demonstrated a 55% response. As already implied, these differences may well be related to the presence of less oestrogen receptor in faster growing anaplastic tumours.

Post-menopausal patients are most unlikely to respond to oophorectomy. Thus, in one series, 85 post-menopausal patients were castrated and none of those who were more than one year post-menopausal responded. The response rate in patients who were within one year of their last period was 7.1%.

Of the pre-menopausal patients, approximately 16% of patients under the age of 35 years respond compared with 32% of those over the age of 35. Patients with regular periods appear more likely to respond than those with irregular menses. The influence of metastatic disease in the ovaries on menstruation is not clear, but response is not influenced by the presence of metastases in this site.

However, the sites of other metastases do seem to influence the likelihood of response. Certain sites such as brain, seem unaffected by this procedure. The response rate for liver metastases are reportedly 9–16% and pulmonary lymphangitis 15–19%. The sites that respond most often include bone (25–35%) in which a dramatic resolution of bone pain often occurs within a few days or even hours of operation, 'soft tissue' including lymph nodes (35–40%) and often pleural effusions respond fairly rapidly, in contrast to lymphangitis.

It has been suggested that the response rates to oophorectomy can be increased from 30 to 50% by the administration of corticosteroids, but the mechanism of this is not clear since that the likelihood of clinical benefit is not related to the degree of adrenal suppression as shown by the ketosteroid or oestrogen excretion levels. Neither the addition of androgens nor progesterones appears to increase the response rate to oophorectomy. As has already been shown (Table 6.2) patients are more likely to respond to oophorectomy if their tumours contain significant quantities of oestrogen receptor.

Methods of castration

The ovaries can be ablated by surgical, radiotherapeutic and medical means. In this discussion, medical means will not be considered since these methods, utilizing anti-oestrogens, gonadotrophin inhibitors and agents inhibiting the synthesis of steroids, are still in the experimental stages, and none, as yet, have been shown to be of definite benefit.

Various large series have been reported in which response rate for radiotherapeutic castration is similar to that for surgical oophorectomy. However, time to remission takes longer because hormone levels take 3–5 months to fall following radiation at a dose of 1200 to 1600 rad in 4 days, compared with 2–3 days after surgical castration. If rapid relief of symptoms is required, then surgical oophorectomy is indicated. Should surgery be contra-indicated, radiation castration may be preferred (Stoll, 1972).

Bilateral oophorectomy, carried out surgically, provides a simple, quick and effective means for palliating breast cancer in a proportion of pre-menopausal patients whose tumours contain oestrogen receptors. The quality of life and duration of remission in these patients is excellent and thus oophorectomy should always be considered as first-line treatment in patients with symptomatic metastases.

In summary, responses are most likely to occur in patients whose tumours contain oestrogen receptor, who have a long 'tumour-free' interval, who have soft tissue and osteolytic lesions and who are pre-menopausal, but older than 35 years of age.

Adjuvant oophorectomy carried out following mastectomy has been shown to be of little value in either prolonging life or preventing the development of symptomatic metastases.

Androgen therapy for human breast cancer

It has been recognized for some time that androgen therapy can arrest and even reverse the progress of disseminated breast cancer although the mechanism still remains obscure (see earlier section). Although androgen receptor is present in about 20% of human breast tumours it has not been established whether androgens act directly on the tumour or indirectly as an oestrogen-like agent on the tumour hypothalamus. Nonetheless, there is now considerable clinical experience in their use for treatment of metastatic breast cancer.

Clinical response

For the most part, androgens are now only used for treatment of metastatic carcinoma of the breast and not other tumours. Approximately 10–20% of such patients will show 'objective' response (Table 6.6) with as many again having good symptomatic relief.

Pre-menopausal patients and those within five years of the menopause, are less likely to respond (14%) than those who are more than five years post-menopausal (25%). Some physicians have advocated androgen therapy immediately after oophorectomy in pre- and peri-menopausal patients, but there is little evidence for improved response in these patients.

Although there remains some controversy about the importance of site of metastases, most clinicians now agree that bone metastases are more likely to respond

Table 6.6

Treatment	No. responses/ no. patients	Response rate (%)
Fluoxymesterone or testosterone	17/106	16
Testosterone propionate	24/253	10
Testolactone	5/103	5
Testolactone	21/115	18
Calusterone	30/109	28
7-α-methyl-19-nortestosterone	73/335	22

(20–25%) than soft tissue or visceral disease. It has been claimed that up to 80% of patients with bone metastases have significant pain relief (Stoll, 1967).

Bone marrow failure, with leukoerythroblastic anaemia often responds to androgen therapy, attributed in part, to the anabolic properties of these hormones. For this reason androgens have been used in combination with marrow-depressant cytotoxic chemotherapy often with good results. Unfortunately, although this may be beneficial for bone marrow, little is known about the interactions of endocrine and chemotherapy on the tumour cells. For this reason, combination therapy is not indicated at present.

There is a close correlation of prediction of response and the presence of oestrogen receptor in the cytoplasm of the tumour cells and in view of the relatively low response rate and rather distressing side-effects it is unjustifiable to treat patients whose tumours are 'receptor-negative'.

Concerning the likelihood of response following temporary remission due to other forms of endocrine treatment in the pre-menopausal group who have responded to oophorectomy, some 10% will subsequently respond to androgens. Following oestrogens in the post-menopausal patients, about 30% will respond. Following relapse after a trial of androgen therapy, 10% will obtain a 'withdrawal' response lasting 6–10 months.

Types of androgen and side-effects

Table 6.7 lists the dose and method of administration of some commonly used androgens. The major disadvantage with the earlier testosterone preparations was virilization. This is generally an insidious process not initially noticed by the patient. The face becomes plethoric and often hirsute, the features become coarse and the voice deepens so that the patient is often unrecognizable. This is compensated by a feeling of euphoria, energy and well being. In view of the low probability of response, most clinicians feel that these side-effects are not acceptable if alternative therapy is available. Fortunately, some of the more modern preparations (e.g. fluoxymesterone) do not have such marked virilizing activity and, since the remission rates are similar, are therefore preferable for clinical use.

Nausea and vomiting are not as common as with oestrogens and neither is hypercalcaemia, reportedly occurring in only 5–10% of patients with skeletal metastases in the first week of treatment. Hepatotoxicity, in the form of cholestatic jaundice, occurs extremely rarely in patients taking modern testosterone preparations but used to be fairly common in those taking the oral androgens which are substituted in the 17a position. Calusterone has been incriminated in several cases of hepatic damage following its use

Table 6.7 Androgens in common use.

Generic name	Trade name	Route of administration	Dose
1. Fluoxymesterone	Halotensin	oral	30 mg/day
2. Nandrolone phenpropionate	Durabolin	intramuscular	50–100 mg/week
3. Calusterone	Calusterone	oral	200 mg/day
4. Testololactone	Teslac	intramuscular	100 mg 3 × weekly
5. Testosterone propionate	Oreton Propionate	intramuscular	25–50 mg 3 × weekly

(Goldenburg *et al.*, 1973).

Of all the agents used, probably fluoxymesterone is best tolerated and is the most suitable oral preparation (Stoll, 1972). Alternatively Durabolin, an anabolic androgen with relatively low virilization, may be conveniently given as a weekly intramuscular injection.

Anti-oestrogens

One of the more important advances in endocrine therapy in recent years has been the development of a group of non-steroidal oestrogen antagonists or anti-oestrogens for clinical use in the treatment of breast cancer. At present, the most widely used of these is tamoxifen (Nolvadex) (Ward, 1973); two others, nafoxidine and clomiphene are also in clinical use.

These agents compete with oestradiol for cytoplasmic oestrogen receptors but fail to have an oestrogenic effect on the cell. How this causes tumour regression in some patients is not known, but may be related to gradual depletion of receptor observed with continued medication.

Clinical response
The overall clinical response rate to tamoxifen is similar to other forms of endocrine therapy (approximately 30%). For example, out of 1269 patients with metastatic breast cancer, reviewed by Mourisden *et al.* (1978), 32% showed objective response to tamoxifen. The average duration of response to anti-oestrogens appears to be in excess of ten months, although individual responses in excess of four years have been reported. Responses are more common in patients who have previously responded to other forms of endocrine therapy (67% vs 15%) and in patients whose tumours contain oestrogen receptors (49% vs 7%). Soft tissue (35%) and visceral metastases (29%) frequently respond whereas response in bone appears at present controversial, with reported rates of between 9 and 50%.

There is probably an increase in the likelihood of response to anti-oestrogens with age past the menopause, but in contrast to oestrogen therapy, responses also occur in pre-menopausal women (27%).

Dosage
Tamoxifen is usually administered in an oral dose of 10–20 mg twice daily. Several studies have failed to show an increase in response rate by increasing this dosage, and individual patients resistant to conventional dosage do not appear to respond to a two-fold or three-fold increase.

Toxicity
The clinical value of tamoxifen is greatly enhanced by its remarkable freedom from toxicity, and the majority of patients tolerate the drug without any side-effects. About 15% of patients experience 'hot flushes' and about 10% initial nausea; vaginal bleeding is reported in less than 5% of patients. In 5 to 10% of patients a transient mild thrombocytopenia or leukopenia has been noted, for which the mechanism is at present unknown. Occasionally, a characteristic 'flare' has been described with increased tumour pain, and sometimes associated with hypercalcaemia. No life-threatening reaction appears to have been reported in any patient so far treated with this drug.

Clomiphene is likewise usually well tolerated with nausea the commonest side-effect; visual blurring is also occasionally reported. Nafoxidine is often associated with skin dryness, photosensitivity and ichthyosis, which frequently requires interruption of therapy. For this reason its clinical role appears to have been superseded by tamoxifen.

Conclusions
Anti-oestrogens have unquestionably made a major impact on the endocrine therapy of advanced breast cancer, and their very low instance of side-effects suggests that they may replace oestrogens as first line additive hormone therapy in the post-menopausal patient. Clinical studies on the role of these agents in the treatment of premenopausal patients, and in com-

bination therapy with cytotoxic drugs, are currently in progress, and the outcome of these may represent a significant advance in the management of metastatic breast carcinoma.

Major endocrine ablation

In 1952 adrenalectomy with cortisone replacement was first described by Huggins and Bergenstal for patients with advanced breast carcinoma, and in France transcranial hypophysectomy for this disease was reported by Perrault the same year (Perrault *et al.*, 1952). Since that time, both these major ablative endocrine operations have been widely used in the treatment of breast cancer and to a lesser extent in advanced carcinoma of the prostate.

Adrenalectomy

Bilateral adrenalectomy has been reported as achieving a response of 23–58% of patients with advanced breast cancer, usually as a 'second line' endocrine procedure. Short-lived subjective responses, particularly in association with relief of bone pain, occur in the majority of patients, but the overall objective response rate of 35% reported in a large series of 560 patients probably represents a fair average (Fraccia *et al.*, 1971). The mean duration of response for patients with objective remission varies from 1–2 years. Occasionally very long remissions have been reported. The operation is most effective for bone metastases, especially relief of pain which can be dramatic, occurring in some patients almost immediately. Responses in soft tissue are also common, but regressions in viscera, and in particular liver and brain, are rare. A differential response, with for example, resclerosis of lytic bone deposits but progressive liver metastases is not uncommon.

Patients who have responded to a previous endocrine procedure and then relapsed have a very much higher chance of achieving a further regression with adrenalectomy than previous non-responders. Likewise, the presence of oestrogen receptor in the tumour and a long tumour-free interval are favourable prognostic factors, as with other forms of endocrine treatment.

Although there are reports that the pain from bone metastases in patients with prostatic cancer may be relieved by adrenalectomy, objective responses only rarely occur. This treatment is, therefore, not usually used.

The main problem with this otherwise excellent palliative procedure is its operative morbidity and even mortality. Two approaches to surgery can be used, transabdominal or posterior, the latter being slightly safer but more time-consuming. Peri-operative mortalities of up to 25% with a post-operative morbidity of approximately 40% has been reported. As one might anticipate, these are related to the age and poor condition of the patient prior to surgery.

Cortisone replacement therapy is required permanently after operation. Although the physiological replacement dose is said to be 37.5 mg daily, most patients with advanced breast carcinoma require larger doses of around 50 mg daily. Mineralocorticoid replacement with fluorocortisone 0.05 mg daily is also usually required. It is important to stress that steroid replacement will need to be increased in association with infection, gastrointestinal upset or other medical problems however mild, and acute hypoadrenalism must always be considered for unexplained malaise.

Hypophysectomy

The rationale for pituitary ablation is the removal of the pituitary gonadotrophic and ACTH stimulus to sex hormone secretion by the gonads and adrenals respectively. Pituitary hormones, including prolactin, have themselves been implicated in the control of experimental mammary carcinoma, although at present there is no definitive evidence for this in humans.

Surgical ablation of the pituitary achieves a response rate at least as good as that for adrenalectomy in patients with advanced breast cancer and like the latter, can provide excellent palliation for an average of two years or more (Hayward *et al.*, 1970). As with adrenalectomy the procedure is particularly useful for painful metastases but is rarely effective for disease in the liver or brain. Other prognostic factors favouring a response are the same as for adrenalectomy.

Originally, pituitary ablation was carried out by transfrontal hypophysectomy. This procedure, though effective, is a major one involving frontal craniotomy, and has a mortality of between 1 and 17%. In recent years, the trans-sphenoidal approach has been developed with less trauma to the patient and reduced mortality and morbidity. The disadvantage of this technique is that of post-operative rhinorrhoea with risk of meningitis and incomplete removal of the pituitary which usually renders the operation ineffective.

Pituitary ablation has also been carried out by implantation of radioactive yttrium through the nose into the pituitary fossa (Forrest *et al.*, 1958). This is effective and carries a low mortality, but is also associated with rhinorrhea. Other techniques including cryosurgery, ultrasonic destruction and external beam radiation have their advocates but have not gained wide general acceptance.

Cortisone replacement therapy is of course required after pituitary ablation as is thyroxine. Transient diabetes insipidus usually occurs in the immediate post-operative period and is usually controlled with either pitressin snuff or AVP nasal drops. Patients who respond to adrenalectomy do not subsequently respond to hypophysectomy and *vice versa*. Therefore, the choice of hypophysectomy versus adrenalectomy for treatment of metastatic breast cancer has to be made.

The overall response rate and duration of response for hypophysectomy is probably slightly better than for adrenalectomy, and mortality/morbidity probably less. Nevertheless, mortality and morbidity for both procedures diminish with the experience of the surgeon involved and the facilities available and, therefore, the choice of operation for the individual patient should probably depend on these criteria.

Pituitary ablation is sometimes used as secondary endocrine therapy for advanced prostatic carcinoma, although the age and general debility of most patients limit its scope in this disease. It is often associated with rapid and marked relief of bone pain but objective parameters of tumour regression are less commonly seen. Subjective responses, in most patients, are short with an average duration of only a few months (Fergusson, 1972).

Aminoglutethimide

Previous attempts to inhibit adrenal steroid synthesis with high dose glucocorticoids or with $o-p$ DDD in the treatment of advanced breast carcinoma have been largely unsuccessful because of high toxicity and low response rates.

Aminoglutethimide, originally developed as an anticonvulsant agent, is a drug which inhibits the enzyme conversion of cholesterol into pregnenolone, the initial step in all adrenal steroid synthesis (Fig. 6.1). It is also believed to inhibit the conversion of androgens into oestrogens in peripheral tissues and, therefore, might be used as an alternative to major ablative endocrine surgery in breast carcinoma (Santen *et al.*, 1977; Smith *et al.*, 1978).

Table 6.8   Progestins in common use in the treatment of breast and uterine carcinomas.

Progestins	Dose (mg/day)
19-Nortestosterone derivatives	
Norethisterone acetate	60
17-α-hydroxyprogesterone derivatives	
Medroxyprogesterone	200–400
Megestrol	30–120
Testosterone derivatives	
Dimethisterone	300

Clinical response

Objective remission of metastases occurs in approximately 30% of patients treated with aminoglutethimide. The factors which predict response are very similar to those for major ablative surgery. Responses are commonest in soft tissues and bone, and the relief of bone pain is often dramatic, occurring within 24–48 hours after starting therapy. Patients who have previously responded to other endocrine therapy are more likely to respond than those who have failed to respond. Responses are more likely in other patients particularly those with a long tumour-free interval (Smith *et al.*, 1978).

Dosage

The usual dosage is 250 mg three or four times daily. Patients require replacement with cortisone acetate 25 mg twice daily or hydrocortisone 20 mg twice daily.

Toxicity

The drug is well tolerated without side-effects in the majority of patients. Some patients experience an initial dose-related lethargy, somnolence and unsteadiness. A transient maculopapular rash occurs in about 30% of patients approximately one week after the start of treatment. The rash, although dramatic, lasts for only a few days and is sometimes associated with fever. Although increased steroid replacement is necessary, a reduction in dosage of aminoglutethimide is not usually necessary.

Adrenal steroid synthesis rapidly returns to normal when the drugs is discontinued. Ease of administration, low toxicity and reversibility if ineffective, are important advantages for this drug over ablative surgery, but further studies are required to evaluate its place in the management of breast cancer. Its activity in prostatic carcinoma is not known but preliminary data suggest that responses in some patients do occur.

Progestins (Progestogens)

Progestins are derivatives of 17α-hydroxyprogesterone, testosterone or 19-nortestosterone. They possess varying degrees of oestrogenic, anti-oestrogenic and androgenic properties (Table 6.8). The most important role for progestin therapy in malignant disease is in the treatment of endometrial carcinoma of the uterus: progestins are also sometimes effective in the treatment of metastatic breast carcinoma, prostatic carcinoma and occasionally renal carcinoma.

Clinical response

The importance of progesterone in the maturation of normal endometrium and the fact that endometrial carcinoma is often a well differentiated tumour retaining considerable similarity to normal endometrium suggested that progestins might have a role in the treatment of advanced endometrial carcinoma no longer amenable to surgical control.

Various progestins have been shown to be active against endometrial carcinoma, with reported response rates of around 30% (Kennedy, 1963). Responses are commonest in bone and lung: somewhat surprising, responses are less likely for pelvic recurrence. In contrast to breast carcinoma, impressive regressions of extensive liver metastases with relief of jaundice have also been well described.

Factors favouring the likelihood of response include a long tumour-free interval between original diagnosis and recurrence, histologically well differentiated tumours, a slow rate of growth clinically and the presence of pulmonary metastases.

Regressions often occur slowly, becoming apparent after two months or more of treatment, but eventually complete remissions are sometimes achieved. Responses once achieved are often of long duration and survival is markedly prolonged. The average survival of responders is reported as being between 2.5 and 4.5 years after the start of treatment and up to 8 years in individual patients, compared with 5–6 months for non-responders.

In contrast to other forms of additive endocrine therapy, there is some evidence of a dose-response effect for progestins in endometrial carcinoma. It has also been suggested that increasing the initial loading dose is associated with a more rapid response.

In the treatment of breast carcinoma, progestins have been used largely as second-line therapy. The overall objective response rate is approximately 20% and is best for soft tissue metastases, including local recurrence. Response usually only occurs in post-menopausal patients and in contrast to oestrogens, is unrelated to age. In fact, responses are as likely during the first five post-menopausal years as later (Stoll, 1967).

An important aspect of therapy is the length of time between start of treatment and first signs of response: this is an average 6–8 weeks but may not occur for up to 4 months and, therefore, a long therapeutic trial is indicated before concluding that treatment is ineffective. The duration of response is usually only 6–9 months shorter than for other forms of endocrine therapy in breast cancer, but responses of up to 2 years' duration are occasionally reported.

Occasional subjective and objective responses have been reported in patients with prostatic carcinoma treated with progestins as second-line therapy (Brendler and Prout, 1962). In some non-castrated patients, plasma testosterone levels have been shown to fall during progestin therapy, without any change in plasma LH levels. Progestin therapy with Provera has been reported by Bloom to achieve objective tumour regressions in about 10% of patients with advanced metastatic renal carcinoma and testosterone in about another 5% (Bloom, 1967). Significant subjective improvement was claimed in up to 50% of patients. Evidence of tumour regression was seen between 2 and 8 weeks of starting therapy and response duration ranged from 2 to 35 months. Survival was significantly prolonged in responding patients compared with non-responders. Responses were much commoner in males than females and appeared to be associated with increasing age.

In a few patients, progestins and testosterone appeared to accelerate tumour growth and in some of these regressions were subsequently achieved by switching hormones.

Subsequent studies have failed to confirm these initial encouraging results, and most clinicians consider that useful remissions are probably rare. Nonetheless, in view of the poor response to chemotherapy with the relatively low toxicity of progestins, a therapeutic trial in metastatic disease is usually indicated.

Drugs and dosage
The most commonly used progestins in breast carcinoma are listed in Table 6.8. No overall difference in response rate has been found between them, but patients failing to respond to one agent have been reported as subsequently responding to another. Generally, norethisterone has been used mostly for breast cancer, progesterone and its derivatives for prostatic and uterine cancer and provera for renal carcinoma. There seems no rational basis for this.

Toxicity
In general, these agents are well tolerated. Occasionally nausea, vomiting, headaches, breast tension and leg cramps have been reported; a few patients complain of depression and irritability, but a larger number report therapeutically useful euphoria, increase in appetite and weight gain. The 19-nortestosterone group of agents are occasionally associated with biochemical and histological evidence of liver damage and this appears to be dose related. As with oestrogens, hypercalcaemia can occur following progestin administration.

Miscellaneous tumours

Malignant melanoma (see Chapter 30)

An endocrine influence in malignant melanoma is suggested by its extremely low incidence before puberty, by its exacerbation or in some patients, regression during pregnancy, and by a significantly increased survival in females compared with males.

Nevertheless, despite isolated case reports of responses to hypophysectomy, androgens or oestrogens, no convincing evidence of a significant role for endocrine therapy in the treatment of this malignancy has so far been established.

Thyroid carcinoma (see Chapter 15)

The majority of thyroid carcinomas are not clinically sensitive to endocrine therapy. However, dramatic responses to thyroxine or thyroid extract are often seen in young patients with papillary cancer, including a small sub-group of patients who have developed papillary carcinoma of the thyroid secondary to irradiation for benign disease. Most of these patients are women under 40 years of age (corresponding to a period when radiotherapy for benign disease in the neck and chest was in vogue) and remissions once achieved nearly always last indefinitely as long as treatment is continued. Tumour control is believed to be mediated through TSH suppression (see Chapter 15).

Further reading

Stoll, B.A. (1977), Palliation by castration and by hormone administration. In: *Breast Cancer Management – Early and Late* (ed. B.A. Stoll), Heinemann.

References

Beatson, G.T. (1896), On the treatment of inoperable cases of carcinoma of the mamma: suggestions for a new method of treatment with illustrative cases. *Lancet*, 2, 104–7.

Bloom, H.J.G. (1967), Treatment of renal cell carcinoma with steroid hormones: observations with transplanted tumours in the hamster and incurable cancer in man. In: *Renal Neoplasia* (ed. J.S. King), Little and Brown, Boston, p. 605.

Brendler, H. and Prout, G. (1962), A co-operative group study of prostatic cancer: stilboestrol versus placebo in advanced progressive disease. *Cancer Chemother. Rep.*, 16, 323–8.

Cornbleet, M., Bondy, P.K. and Powles, T.J. (1976), Acute fatal irreversible hypercalcaemia in breast cancer following oestrogen therapy. *Br. Med. J.*, i, 145.

De Sombre, E.R. *et al.* (1976), Estrogen and prolactin receptor concentrations in rat mammary tumours and response to endocrine ablation. *Cancer Res.*, 36, 354–8.

Fergusson, J.D. (1972), Prostatic cancer – endocrine therapy. In: *Endocrine Therapy in Malignant Disease* (ed. B.A. Stoll), W.B. Saunders, London, pp. 237–99.

Forrest, A.P.M., Blair, D.W. and Valentine, J.M. (1958), Screen implantation of the pituitary with yttrium-90. *Lancet*, ii, 192.

Fraccia, A.A. *et al.* (1971), Hypophysectomy as compared to adrenalectomy for advanced breast cancer. *Surgery, Gynec. Obstet.*, 133, 241.

Goldenburg, I.S. *et al.* (1973), Androgenic therapy for advanced breast cancer in women. *J. Am. Med. Ass.*, 223, 1267–8.

Haddow, A., Watkinson, J.M. and Patterson, E. (1944), Influence of synthetic oestrogens upon advanced malignant disease. *Br. Med. J.*, ii, 393–8.

Hayward, J.L. *et al.* (1970), Clinical trials comparing transfrontal hypophysectomy with adrenalectomy and with transethmoidal hypophysectomy. In: *Second Tenovus Workshop on Breast Cancer* (eds C.A.F. Joslin and E.N. Gleave), Tenovus Workshop, Cardiff.

Huggins, C. and Bergenstal, D.M. (1952), Inhibition of human mammary and prostatic cancers by adrenalectomy. *Cancer Res.*, 12, 134–41.

Huggins, C. and Hodges, C.V. (1941), Studies on prostatic cancer. *Cancer Res.*, 1, 293–7.

Kennedy, B.J. (1963), Progestogen for the treatment of advanced endometrial cancer. *J. Am. Med. Ass.*, 184, 758.

Knight, W.A. *et al.* (1977), Estrogen receptor as an independent prognostic factor for early recurrence in breast cancer. *Cancer Res.*, 37, 4669–71.

Lippman, M., Bolan, G. and Huff, K. (1976), The effects of glucocorticoids and progesterone on hormone-responsive human breast cancer in long-term tissue culture. *Cancer Res.*, 36, 4602–9.

McGuire, W.L. *et al.* (1975), Estrogen receptors in human breast cancer: an overview. In: *Estrogen Receptors in Human Breast Cancer.* (eds W.L. McGuire, P.P. Carbone and E.P. Vollner), Raven Press, New York, pp. 1–7.

McGuire, W.L. *et al.* (1977), Steroid receptors in breast tumours – current status. *Curr. Top. Exp. Endocr.*, 3, 93–129.

MacMahon, B. *et al.* (1971), Oestrogen profiles of Asian and North American women. *Lancet*, i, 900–2.

Maynard, P.V. et al. (1978), Estrogen receptor assay in primary breast cancer and early recurrence of the disease. *Cancer Res.*, 38, 4292.

Mourisden, H. *et al.* (1978), Tamoxifen in advanced breast cancer. *Cancer Treat. Rev.*, 5, 131–41.

Nenci, I. (1978), Receptor and centriole pathways of steroid activity in normal and neoplastic cells. *Cancer Res.*, 38, 4204–11.

Perrault, M. *et al*. (1952), L'hypophysectomie totale change le traitment de cancer du sein. Premier cas français, avein de la methode. *Therapie*, **7**, 290.

Santen, R.J. *et al*. (1977), Aminoglutethimide therapy of breast cancer. *Cancer*, **39**, 2948.

Smith, I.E. *et al*. (1978), Aminoglutethimide in the treatment of metastatic breast carcinoma. *Lancet*, **ii**, 646.

Stoll, B.A. (1967), Progestin therapy of breast cancer – comparison of agents. *Br. Med. J.*, **2**, 338.

Stoll, B.A. (1972), Castration and oestrogen therapy, In: *Endocrine Therapy in Malignant Disease*. (ed. B.A. Stoll), W.B. Saunders, London. pp. 139–64.

Veronesi, U., Pizzocaro, G. and Rossi, A. (1975), Oophorectomy for advanced carcinoma of the breast. *Surgery, Gynec. Obstet.*, **141**, 569.

Ward, H.W.C. (1973), Antioestrogen therapy for breast cancer: a trial of tamoxifen at two dose levels. *Br. Med. J.*, **1**, 13–14.

7 Immunity and cancer

Alistair J. Cochran

There is only limited satisfaction for the cancer therapist when reviewing the survival of his cancer patients. A sizeable proportion of patients with accessible primary cancers diagnosed early do survive for significantly long periods and may die of causes other than their cancer, but the outlook for those with established metastatic disease is gloomy, especially if the metastases have been blood-borne to viscera.

Two main tactical approaches are available to those attempting to remedy this situation. The first is to improve available forms of therapy, by attention to the techniques and timing of surgery and the techniques, timing and dose of radiotherapy and chemotherapy. This approach, which is an implicit part of good medical practice, has been associated over the years with a small but real and progressive increase in absolute survival and in the length of tumour-free intervals. The rate of advance is slow and it is difficult to see how these techniques alone will ever achieve acceptable control of metastatic malignancy. The alternative is to devise new forms of cancer therapy and considerable ingenuity has been shown, in devising and applying novel therapies. The failure of such approaches to attain an established place in cancer therapy indicates that, ingenious as they may be, none have represented a really significant advance. This rather depressing observation should not, however, inhibit cancer researchers and developmental therapists from continuing the search.

Since cancer is a disease in which there is a failure of cellular control, an important area of investigation is into the mechanisms whereby cells are maintained in their proper place and at a relatively defined number in absolute terms and relative to other cells. Once a sufficient understanding of these mechanisms has been achieved, the capacity to augment diminished control of division, proliferation and movement of tumour cells or perhaps inhibit relatively excessive control of the activities of non-tumour cell populations with natural activities which contain tumour cells, may provide a very powerful means of controlling the cancer cell.

Systems involved in the control of cell division, positioning and movement include the endocrine system, locally active humoral factors, such as chalones, cell-to-cell contacts and, to some extent, the immunological system. It remains an open question as to which systems are defective in cancer and the enthusiasm for studying individual systems has depended largely on the availability of techniques for their examination. There has been an enormous explosion of interest and knowledge of the immune system and its involvement in a variety of disease states, such as the autoimmune diseases during the past twenty years. This has led to the development of many new techniques for studying immune function *in vivo* and *in vitro* and added impetus has come from recently developed enthusiasm for and expertise in organ transplantation. The availability of techniques and personnel trained to think about medical problems from an immunological standpoint, has led to a renewal of enthusiasm for studies of immunity in cancer patients. This does not imply that those involved believe that the immune response is the sole, or most important mechanism in cancer control. Tumour immunology is regarded as an area of investigation which might yield significant insights into tumour cell biology.

The study of immunology in relation to cancer divides readily into two areas: firstly there are studies attempting to assess whether tumour-bearing individuals have depressed immunological functions and if so whether such depression is significantly involved in the development of tumours or is a result of the presence of a growing tumour mass; secondly there are attempts to demonstrate whether the membrane of the tumour cell contains molecules which differ from those in comparable adult cells and which are autoimmunogenic, evoking antibodies and specifically sensitized lymphoid cells. If such antibodies and lymphocytes do exist it is clearly crucial to know whether they are capable of killing or inhibiting tumour cells bearing the appropriate molecules.

Can we apply the findings and techniques of experimental tumour immunology in the management of the patients with cancer? Potential applications include tumour diagnosis, the monitoring of patients with proven cancer for the development of metastatic disease and the treatment of cancer by immunological methods. Immunological diagnosis and monitoring seem reasonably attainable if modest contributions to the management of cancer patients. The development of effective immunotherapy is likely to be a markedly more difficult task but would certainly represent a major advance in cancer treatment. Despite the daunting problems associated with immunotherapy numerous studies have been undertaken in animals and in man, in which attempts have been made to modify the immune system to produce tumour inhibition or regression.

The whole edifice of immunotherapy is based upon a foundation of theoretical and experimental tumour immunology. An understanding of the aims and strategies of immunotherapists therefore depends upon some knowledge of the current findings and beliefs of tumour immunology and I have therefore devoted the first part of this chapter to a summary of the available information on immunological aspects of cancer.

Animal studies

Animal studies of tumour immunology commenced in the latter years of the 19th century but were frustrated by the non-availability of inbred strains of animals and ignorance of the existence and role of transplantation antigens. Transplantation of tumour from one animal to another was usually followed by regression of that tumour. The frequency of this observation and the ease of its demonstration, led to undue optimism that some form of immunotherapy would soon be available. When it was realized that the effects being demonstrated were certainly not tumour-related, a period of extreme pessimism followed, epitomized by a paper by Woglom in 1929. The study of tumour immunology in animals continued at a low level, but advanced very little until inbred strains of mice became available: this permitted studies in which the effect of transplantation antigen disparity could be discounted and attempts to study tumour-associated antigens became more practicable. Further advances were the realization that one could titrate tumour resistance by challenging syngeneic animals with graded doses of tumour cells and that the maximum number of tumour cells which could be rejected was relatively small.

The classic experiment which suggests most strongly that tumour cells bear tumour-associated antigens is that in which a group of animals is immunized by exposure to tumour cells, or tumour cell membranes or extracts of tumour cells. Animals prepared in this way and comparable animals which have not been exposed to tumour materials are then challenged with varying numbers of viable tumour cells and the frequency of tumour development in the protected and unmodified animals is compared. Within a genetically identical (syngeneic) system if immunized mice reject a larger number of tumour cells than do non-immunized mice, it can be concluded that the tumour cells bear molecules which can function as tumour-associated antigens and which can induce an immune response in syngeneic animals. The most important fact is that this immune response has some capacity to bring about the rejection of tumour cells.

Studies with tumours induced by different types of carcinogens revealed that tumours induced by an oncogenic virus possessed at their membranes, antigens which were shared between tumours arising in different members of the same species and even in animals of different species exposed to the appropriate virus. This observation is fundamental as cross-protection within and between species is thus possible in the case of virus-induced tumours. By contrast, tumours arising as a result of chemical or physical carcinogenesis possess tumour-associated antigens which are primarily linked to the individual, so-called private antigens; shared-antigens may also exist on these tumours but are likely to be relatively weak. Thus, an animal which has methylcholanthrene painted on a number of areas of its skin will develop several tumours, each of which will have separate tumour-associated antigens. Cross-protection in this situation is not feasible.

It was early realized that this excellent system for studying tumour immunity was not generally available in man, and much effort has been expended in attempting to investigate tumour immunity using *in vitro* test systems which are potentially applicable to man. Anti-tumour humoral and cell-mediated immunity have been demonstrated in animal models by *in vitro* techniques, but mainly in animals with early or regressing tumours.

In animals, regimes of tumour exposure, not very dissimilar from those which can produce immunization and protection against subsequent tumour challenge, may in fact render the animal more susceptible to tumour challenge or augment the growth of an already existing tumour, a process known as *enhancement*. Subsequent *in vitro* studies have led to the suggestion that immunological factors such as free tumour-associated antigen, free antibody or antigen–antibody complexes may prevent the interaction of effector cells and cytotoxic antibodies with tumour cells and thus *block* the effect of the anti-tumour immune response, leading to the enhancement of tumour growth.

The main criticism of the very large volume of animal

work is that much of it bears little relevance to the human tumour situation. We know that tumour-associated antigens vary very widely in their ability to induce an immune response and thus may be spoken of as weak or strong antigens. We know too, that animals have a genetically inherited ability to respond to a particular antigen or antigens (immune responsiveness or IR genes). In order to obtain the most readily interpretable results, much research on animal tumour immunology has employed tumours in which the tumour-associated antigens (TAA) were strong and the IR genes inductive of strong immune responses. This understandable bias may prove in the long run to have been strongly counter-productive. It seems likely that most human tumours are at best possessed of weakly immunogenic TAA and that the immune responses against these TAA may be comparatively weak. Another problem is that the major killing malignant diseases in man, lung cancer, breast cancer in women and colon cancer, metastasize early and extensively, whereas this behaviour is exceptional with animal tumours. The realization of the inappropriateness of many animal models has grown recently and strenuous efforts are being expended to produce more realistic studies.

Studies in man

Clinical background

Before considering the experimental approach to human tumour immunology it is appropriate to look for clinical observations which suggest that whether or nor a tumour grows or metastasizes depends on host factors as well as features of the tumour itself. It must be emphasized that the evidence that such responses are substantially immunologically based is not strong, but there are some indications that the immune system may have a role in certain situations.

Immunological integrity and cancer

It has been postulated that one of the functions of the immune system is to identify antigenically abnormal cells including tumour cells, which may arise within the body by mutation and destroy these (Thomas, 1959; Burnet, 1967). If this is the case any situation or circumstances which would lead to a lowering of the efficiency of this 'immunological surveillance' mechanism would be associated with an increase in cancer incidence. There is some evidence that this is so, but the situation is complicated. In man, immune deficiency may occur as an inherited abnormality, may be imposed as a result of therapeutic manipulation

(mainly in relation to organ grafts, but also in individuals with perverted immune responses) or may be associated with non-malignant conditions including the ageing process. In the first two situations there is an increase in the frequency of tumours in immunologically depressed individuals but the surprising finding is that this increase is overwhelmingly in tumours of the lymphoreticular system. If 'immunological surveillance' as originally conceived were active, one would expect that removal of surveillance would lead to an increase in tumours of all kinds at a frequency similar to that seen with 'spontaneous' tumours. Other evidence regarded as being against the original concept of immune surveillance includes the monoclonality of many tumours, the relative rarity of multiple spontaneous tumours, the low incidence of spontaneous tumours in 'nude' (athymic) mice and immune-suppressed mice and the low frequency of tumours in 'immunologically privileged sites', such as the anterior chamber of the eye and the hamster cheek pouch.

The age-related increase in tumour incidence seems more likely to be due to cumulative carcinogen exposure than to any age-related decline in immune reactivity.

The concept of immunological surveillance has been a useful one in acting as a stimulus to research but clearly has to be modified and the present consensus is that while immunological surveillance may in fact be active in certain limited model systems and perhaps occasionally in man, it is not the universally active agency originally conceived. It is now believed that natural killer (NK) cells may provide a degree of surveillance, at least against some types of tumours.

Tumour regression

Most malignant tumours grow progressively and transient size reductions are usually due to necrosis. There are records of apparently spontaneous regression of histologically proved tumours which have totally (seldom) or partially (more common, but still infrequent) disappeared (Everson and Cole, 1966). The immunological basis of such regressions is by no means certain although tumours which most frequently regress include melanoma, renal carcinoma and choriocarcinoma in which recent studies suggest a host immune reaction. The fact that tumours can undergo retrogressive changes, encourages the search for methods of inducing this desirable event.

Variations in the rate of tumour progression

Histologically similar tumours progress at varying rates in different individuals which reflects tumour cell characteristics but could also indicate that antitumour immunity varies between individuals, possibly as a result of immune response (IR) gene activity. Metabolic or infective intercurrent disease must also be taken into account.

Tumour latency and dormancy
It is a relatively common observation that some ostensibly cured patients may, after many years, develop metastases which are identical to the original tumour. It is possible that the tumour cells may be held in symbiosis until an environment develops which is favourable to tumour growth.

Histological observations
A proportion of tumours are associated with cells of the reticuloendothelial and immunological systems, particularly during the early part of their evolution. Thus, many cells in a tumour mass are macrophages, lymphocytes or plasma cells rather than tumour cells. Patients with infiltrated tumours have generally a better than average prognosis, e.g. gastric carcinoma, neuroblastoma and choriocarcinoma. In animal studies tumours heavily infiltrated with macrophages are less likely to metastasize than those with infrequent macrophages. However, limited studies of peritumoural lymphoreticular cells have not shown them to have a strong antitumour effect on tumour cells *in vitro*. This may merely reflect the difficulty of obtaining this population in a condition suitable for investigation.

It has been claimed that certain patterns in tumour-free reactive lymph nodes such as sinus histiocytosis and sarcoid-like patterns, may have a favourable prognostic significance. Other histological features such as lymphocytic and macrophage infiltration, scar tissue formation in tumours and the extracellular deposition of normally intracellular materials (e.g. melanin) may indicate partial regression. The desmoplastic reaction and capsule formation possibly indicate a host response. If desmoplasia indicates a host response, it is ineffective, as patients with scirrhous breast carcinomas have no survival advantage.

Cancer in families
Blood relatives of cancer patients have an increased risk of developing the same malignancy (see Heston, 1976 for review). It is not possible to exclude absolutely the effect of carcinogens common to members of these families but it is likely the family members possess a heritable susceptibility to cancer *of the appropriate type*, there being no increase in other kinds of cancers. The occurrence, degree and quality of the immune response to any given antigen is heritable and depends upon 'immune responsiveness' (IR) genes, some of which are associated with histocompatibility loci (McDevitt and Benacerraf, 1969). Familial cancer susceptibility may thus be due, at least in part, to genetically determined inadequacy of IR genes.

Multiple primary tumours
The simultaneous occurence of more than one malignancy is rare, but the sequential development of different malignancies is not uncommon. As patients who have had one cancer have an increased likelihood of developing a second, increased therapeutic success will probably lead to more patients developing multiple malignancies. Factors involved include increasing carcinogen exposure, late responses by less carcinogen-sensitive tissues and immunosuppression by carcinogens, tumour or treatment applied to the initial malignancy.

Circulating tumour cells
Tumour cells are identifiable in the blood of cancer patients, even when there is no evidence of metastatic disease. There is little correlation between the number of tumour cells present and prognosis and the number of metastases subsequently established. This suggests that there are materials and cells in the blood capable of destroying tumour cells.

Treatment responses
Some patients with Burkitt's lymphoma or with choriocarcinoma have responded to doses of chemotherapy below those regarded as optimal. It has been suggested that the chemotherapy initiates tumour cell destruction, a process completed by the immune response.

Choriocarcinomas (see Chapter 29)
These remarkable tumours arise in foetal tissues, invade maternal tissues and may kill the mother despite being half allografts which should be rejected on the basis of transplantation antigen disparity. The mechanisms which protect the growing foetus thus appear to cover the less welcome tumour. Other evidence for immunological factors in choriocarcinoma include the favourable significance of lymphocytic infiltration, interesting results from early attempts as immunotherapy with paternal leucocytes or xenoantisera against paternal spermatozoa, and slow rejection of paternal skin grafts which may not be associated with the expected agglutinins.

Experimental studies – in vivo

The immunization and tumour challenge approach of animal tumour immunology is inapplicable to man; data on tumour-directed immunity from *in vivo* studies are therefore limited.

Tumour grafts
Interesting data have been obtained from studies of tumour grafts. Patients have had portions of their own tumours reimplanted (autografts) and a surprisingly

small number of such implants had grown. Tumour autograft acceptance correlates with tumour inoculum size, with skin reactivity to tuberculoprotein (immunological memory) and dinitrochlorobenzene (primary immune response) and with macrophage function. If the autograft cells are mixed with autologous peripheral blood leucocytes the number of tumour cells required to give a growing graft is increased, suggesting that some leucocytes can inhibit tumour cells. Tumour cells have also been transferred between individuals (allografts). Normal recipients or those with non-malignant diseases reject tumour allografts normally and completely. However, immunosuppressed individuals without malignant disease may permit local growth of allogeneic tumour cells and there are reports of metastases and death (e.g. Scanlon *et al.*, 1965). Most cancer patients reject tumour allografts but rejection may be slow. Enthusiasm for the grafting approach has never been high, and has been further reduced by the realization that the graft recipient may receive genome material of oncogenic or other pathogenic viruses. Some recipients of renal allografts have received kidneys which contained tumour; however, such tumour and any metastases which may have developed usually regress when therapeutic immunosuppression is removed. This impressive tumour regression is to be regarded as due to transplantation rather than tumour-associated antigens.

Cutaneous delayed hypersensitivity to tumour materials
Attempts have been made to demonstrate (tuberculin-type) delayed cutaneous hypersensitivity to tumour cells and tumour cell fractions. A proportion of cancer patients react to material from tumours similar to their own but a few normal individuals also react and where appropriate control materials have been employed a somewhat similar selectivity of reaction may be seen, suggesting the observed reactions to be at least in part organ-specific.

Studies employing membrane preparations purified by enzymatic digestion, salt extraction, column separation and electrophoresis, indicate several apparently unique tumour-associated antigens on each tumour which can elicit positive skin tests. Surprisingly there are also membrane-located inhibitor molecules which, when combined with the skin reactive antigens, may abolish their reactivity, which may explain some previous negative results with crude preparations.

Skin window technique
The skin is abraded by fine sandpaper and a glass coverslip applied (Rebuck and Crowley, 1955). Cells from the underlying tissues move on to the coverslip and may be identified and counted after fixation and staining. Serial samples between 6 and 48 hours show

that the cell population changes from initial granulocyte predominance to a mixed population including macrophages, lymphocytes, basophils and occasionally eosinophils. Patients with advanced cancer have reduced macrophage emigration. The technique may be modified by placing cryostat sections of tumour on the coverslip. Lies and Black (1970) reported 'specific' reactions to autologous tissue sections in 40% of cancer patients.

Skin tests with non-tumour antigens
These test the integrity of the immunological mechanisms. Recall antigens, antigens such as tuberculin, candida DHS, mumps, and streptokinase-streptodornase, to which most individuals have previously been sensitized, test immunological memory. Studies of recall antigen reactivity of cancer patients are relatively numerous and although they have yielded somewhat conflicting results when the individual antigens are considered, there is a consensus that early cancer patients have no major deficit of immunological memory but there is a decline of reactivity in patients with advanced cancer.

There is also interest in the use of the new antigens, synthetic or bizarre antigens to which the individual is unlikely to have had previous exposure. If tumour-associated antigens are truly new or have not been 'seen' by the immune system after the end of tolerance the capacity to mount a new immune response is critical and likely to be more important than the memory function. The agents employed have been synthetic contact sensitizing agents such as dinitrochlorobenzene or dinitrofluorobenzene, or biological molecules such as keyhole limpet or horseshoe crab haemocyanin which induce an immune response in virtually all normal individuals. It is claimed that they induce a reaction in a lower proportion of cancer patients or a weaker individual response. Cancer patients who are incapable of being sensitized are said to have a poor prognosis. This approach is limited by the possibility that repeat testing may lead to reimmunization, a problem which may be avoided by *in vitro* assays.

Experimental studies – in vitro

These divide into tests of the integrity of the immunological apparatus, tests for antitumour immunity (antibodies and sensitized lymphoid cells) and tests for evidence of a continuing immune response (antigen–antibody complexes and complement consumption).

Tests of immunological integrity
This approach has the advantage of relative technical simplicity, but as it assesses the components of a complex and sophisticated process in isolation, interpre-

tation of even grossly abnormal results is difficult. If we consider first the cells involved in the immune response, a number of techniques is available to examine the morphology and function of lymphocytes and macrophages.

1. *The assessment of numbers, morphology and behaviour of lymphocytes.* Lymphocyte counting remains important in the haematological evaluation of cancer patients but appears to have a limited place in immunological assessment. Examination of the proportion of lymphocytes of different sizes in peripheral blood has shown abnormalities of distribution in patients with Hodgkin's disease. Such simple assessments have now been replaced by more complex assays of lymphocyte sub-populations. Membrane characteristics of lymphocytes permit their subdivision into thymus-dependent (T) cells, involved in cell-mediated immunity, and thymus-independent (B) cells which produce antibody. There is also a population of cells which lacks the characteristics of B and T cells (null cells) and a population of cells with some characteristics of both. Variations of the conditions under which T-cell identifying techniques are performed has yielded further sub-populations of T-cells (active T-cells, auto-rosetting T-cells and super-rosetting T-cells). Animal studies have shown that T-cells subserve a variety of specific and quite different functions including cell killing (T-killer cells), assistance to B-cells in antibody production (T-helper cells) and limitation of the extent of immune responses (T-suppressor cells). Interest has recently focused on cells which are capable of killing antibody-primed target cells (K-cells) (MacLennan 1976) and NK cells (see above).

The possibility of variations in lymphocyte sub-populations in cancer patients is of interest. There may be variations in the relative proportions and absolute numbers of the different lymphocytes or they may be quantitatively normal, but functionally abnormal. Most results indicate relative minor variations in the classical T- and B-cell populations, except where these have been modified by treatment. However, some patients have a much reduced T-cell count suggesting that, while in the majority of patients the cause of T-cell inefficiency is to be sought in perverted functions, a few suffer from an absolute reduction in these cells. There are also reports of variations in the sub-populations of T-cells between cancer patients and controls, and between cancer patients with limited local disease and those with advanced disease. The techniques for assessing these populations remain cumbersome and it seems unlikely that elucidation of the significance of these variations will be possible until simpler techniques become available. The availability of monoclonal antibodies to lymphocyte subpopulations is especially promising.

To permit clonal expansion after antigenic stimulation, lymphocytes must be capable of mitotic division. In order to investigate this capacity mitogens, materials which are not antigens in a strict sense but which cause lymphocyte to undergo blast transformation, a necessary prelude to mitosis, are widely employed, most commonly phytohaemagglutinin (PHA), pokeweed mitogen (PWM) and concanavalin A (Con A). As these mitogens have selective activity for different lymphocyte sub-populations they provide a further method of categorizing them. While these techniques appear deceptively simple, they require scrupulous control and very experienced technicians to provide reliable results. Mitogen-induced lymphocyte blastogenesis has been found to be reduced in malignant disease by some authors but not by others. The situation probably differs for different malignancies; malignancies of the lymphoreticular system are certainly different from those of non-lymphoid tissues, also lymphocyte transformation may be reduced by a defect intrinsic to the lymphocytes or by materials circulating in the plasma.

Blastogenesis can also assess immunological memory for antigens previously encountered such as tuberculoprotein and brucellin. Other tests such as leucocyte migration inhibition by Bacillus Calmette-Guerin (BCG) may also be used in this way.

The mixed lymphocyte reaction (MLR), generally as a 'one-way' test in which one set of lymphocytes is rendered incapable of replication by exposure to a chemical such as mitomycin C, has also been employed. It assays the capacity of lymphocytes to recognize a new (transplantation) antigen as foreign and to initiate an immune reaction to it. Intrinsic (lymphocytic) and serum-mediated abnormalities of MLR have been reported in cancer patients by a number of groups.

On antigenic stimulation, and to a lesser extent on mitogen stimulation, T-lymphocytes and occasionally B-lymphocytes produce non-immunoglobulin humoral factors known as lymphokines, which are involved in cell-mediated immunity *in vivo*. The capacity to produce them is clearly an important attribute of lymphocytes and there is much interest in techniques which permit the identification and quantification of lymphokines.

2. *Assessment of the activity of macrophages.* It has recently been recognized that, in addition to their phagocytic function, macrophages have an important role in the immune response. Therefore in a complete assessment of the immunology of a cancer patient, consideration should be given to the functional integrity of these cells. Morphological and enzyme histochemical techniques permit the enumeration of macrophages in mixed cell populations although the separation of macrophages in good condition from

solid tissues such as tumours, remains difficult. Established methods exist for the assessment of macrophage phagocytosis, chemotaxis, motility, responsiveness to migration inhibition factor and specific and non-specific cytotoxicity (see Lejeune, 1975 for review). The assessment of macrophage performance in antigen handling and cellular cooperation and the investigation of macrophage products remains at a developmental stage and is not yet applicable in a routine screening role.

3. *The assessment of humoral factors.* The most obvious humoral factor to be assayed is the level of circulating immunoglobulins, most simply by immunodiffusion against calibrated standards. There are many reports of variations in serum Ig levels in cancer patients, but little unanimity concerning the nature and extent of the abnormalities detected. The problem is not the detection of abnormalities but the interpretation of such anomalies as are observed. The immunoglobulin fraction includes molecules with and without antibody specificity and the proportion of molecules with antibody specificity for tumour-associated antigens is likely to be small. Patients with advanced malignancy are prone to infections, a tendency exacerbated by immunosuppressive treatment and alterations in serum proteins may be a consequence of micro-organismal invasion rather than of cancer. Patients unable to eat or retain food as a result of their disease or treatment may be malnourished which will be reflected in the plasma proteins. It is difficult to see how immunoglobulin estimations may be useful in the assessment of cancer patients.

Tests for evidence of a continuing immune response
1. *Assessment of complement components.* If tumour is persistent and there is an immune response against it abnormalities in the complement system should be detectable due to the continued consumption of its components. Techniques are available for assessing the system as a whole and its components, and abnormalities have been detected in cancer patients. The problem is once again one of interpretation. While the abnormalities may indicate a continuing immune reaction to tumour antigens, intercurrent infection, activation of the alternative pathway by endotoxin and the effects of tumour necrosis may be involved. Complement abnormalities in cancer patients, while of interest, remain of unproven value in assessment or monitoring.

2. *Circulating immune complexes.* A continuing reaction between tumour antigens and antibodies to them would produce circulating immune complexes. Studies of blocking factors (see below) suggest that such complexes do exist and that their presence may correlate with tumour growth activity. Immune complexes have been shown to cause nephrotic syndrome in a variety of human malignancies and in some cases these are complexes of tumour antigens and antibodies to them. The methods for the detection of complexes are technically demanding; however simpler tests depending on the physicochemical properties of immune complexes are being developed and seem likely to increase understanding of this important subject.

Studies of tumour directed immunity in vitro
In undertaking studies of this kind, the investigator has three basic questions in mind. Do tumour cells possess molecules which differ from those on comparable mature normal cells; if so, can such molecules function as auto-antigens and induce tumour-directed immune responses? If immune responses do develop against tumour neoantigens, do they contribute to the rejection of the tumour?

Investigations of antibodies and lymphoid cells specifically sensitized against tumour-associated antigens are clearly complementary and it is unfortunate that many studies have been limited to one or other aspect of tumour immunity. Antibodies can most readily be identified in body fluids but may also be sought attached to tumour cells, their natural substrate. Sensitized lymphoid cells may be found in the peripheral blood, in the lymphoid organs and the tumour itself. Since peripheral blood is most readily accessible most studies have examined lymphocytes from this source. To avoid repetition I have dealt with the results of studies of humoral and cell-mediated immunity together, separating them only where there is a disparity of results.

1. *General findings.* The main problem remains the unsatisfactory nature of the techniques available; their multiplicity merely indicating that none is preeminently better than any other. The difficulty of demonstrating and interpreting specificity in these studies is also a problem. We remain unsure as to whether tumour neoantigens are re-expressed embryonic antigens, organ specific markers, differentiation markers or antigens of classes as yet unidentified. Absolute tumour specificity has not yet been demonstrated in any of these systems, and it now seems unlikely that other than relative tumour-specificity exists. From an operational standpoint, this may be sufficient, and allow some techniques to be employed in, for instance, the monitoring of cancer patients to predict metastases at a sub-clinical level. Without knowledge of the carcinogens involved in man, and we are very ignorant of this, it is impossible to identify human tumour-associated antigens as carcinogen-associated.

Many studies have found tumour-directed reactions in the majority of cancer patients, but also in between 15 and 20% of ostensibly normal control individuals. Although possibly artefactual, this finding raises questions about the specificity of the reaction. The simplest concept is of immunogenic neoantigens unique to carcinogen-influenced cells including tumour cells. These would induce reactions in individuals with tumours and in those who had had abortive, or as yet unproductive carcinogen contact. Alternatively, apparently tumour-specific antigens may also exist on normal adult cells at low concentrations, or in a masked state; increased frequency or exposure on tumour cells might suffice to render them immunogenic. Mechanisms other than carcinogenesis may be capable of enhancing the antigenicity of the cells of some tumour-free individuals inducing tumour cross-reactive immunity. Oncofoetal (OF) antigens such as α-foeto protein and carcinoembryonic antigen exist at high concentration on embryonal and tumour cells and are absent or infrequent on normal cells. Reports of spontaneous immune reactions to *known* OF antigens are infrequent but some apparently tumour-directed reactions may in fact be specific for as yet unidentified OF antigens. The pattern of results makes it unlikely that we are detecting reactions to major transplantation antigens. The reactions may be directed to some extent against auto-antigens of, for instance, smooth muscle, nuclear proteins and bile canaliculi perhaps due to carcinogen-induced alteration in antigens or tumour necrosis.

Predictably, reactions may be detected in purely autologous situations but the findings differ from the animal situation in that reactivity at a similar frequency may be seen in combinations of lymphoid cells or serum and allogeneic tumour cells of the appropriate histogenetic type. While reminiscent of the observation that animal tumours induced by the same virus share antigens, the histological specificity observed in man is not seen in all animal tumour-virus systems. It is not excluded that some target antigens are organ-markers or related to passenger viruses.

Some studies of antitumour immunity have reported that as tumour volume and extent increases, the frequency and strength of reactions declines. The simplest explanations are that, as tumour volume increases, antibodies or lymphocytes become involved with the tumour cells and are no longer detectable in the circulating blood or that the tumour is immune-suppressive. In advanced malignancy large amounts of tumour-associated antigen free or complexed to antibody may cause immunological paralysis or high zone tolerance. The reappearance of tumour-directed antibody in patients with advanced melanoma after the injection of autologous irradiated tumour cells is against this hypothesis (Ikonopisov *et al.*, 1970). Lewis *et al.* (1971) suggested that the apparent loss of antitumour antibody might be due to its combination with anti-idiotypic antibodies similar to those occurring in chronic inflammatory diseases. Tumour cells may alter antigenically (modulation) during the course of malignant disease which may favour the emergence of cells with less readily detectable antigens. Selection pressures may also favour the survival of cells with masking of surface antigens. Cells modified in these ways would provide reduced immunogenic stimulus and in the absence of an adequate continuing stimulus, the immune response might decline.

Patients who remain tumour-free after excision of a tumour are of interest. Tumour-directed immunity can be detected in most such patients for about two years after tumour removal, but after this, the reaction frequency declines progressively with increasing length of tumour freedom.

2. Tumour-directed immunity in cancer contacts. A curious and possibly highly significant observation is the finding that family contacts of cancer patients show tumour-directed immunity at a high frequency relative to no-contact control populations. This has been observed with osteogenic sarcoma, neuroblastoma, the leukaemias, Burkitt's lymphoma and breast carcinoma. Professional contacts of neuroblastoma patients also show an increased reaction frequency (Graham-Pole *et al.*, 1976). This is reminiscent of the situation in a feline leukaemia where horizontal transmission of feline leukaemia virus is established. The data available do not prove that viruses are involved, but horizontal transmission of an immunogenic stimulus certainly occurs. While the overall epidemiology of cancer contacts remains to be studied, it would appear that exposure to the immunogenic stimulus merely results in immunization, and that there is no major increase in the risk of cancer development.

3. Tumour cell-associated immunoglobulins. With the exception of B-cell lymphomas, where cell-associated immunoglobulins are part of the cell membrane, immunoglobulins attached to tumour cells are worthy of examination as possible antibodies to tumour-associated antigens. However, non-specific attachment of immunoglobulins can occur and proof of the antibody specificity of attached immunoglobulins is difficult. It is also necessary to explain why only a proportion of tumour cells has immunoglobulin attached. This may be due to reduced antibody production in advanced malignancy making insufficient antibody molecules available to coat each tumour cell, the removal of low avidity antibodies by even gentle preparative techniques, poor antibody penetration into solid tumours or cleavage of antibody molecules by cell-associated lysosomal proteolytic enzymes, leaving only the Fab (antibody fraction) portion attached. In this last situation antisera directed against the Fc (crystalline fraction) portion of the molecule (which has been most commonly employed in these studies) would not detect the attached Fab portion of the molecule. Interest in cell-associated immunoglobulin has increased recently, with the realization that certain antibody molecules (even at low concentration) attached to tumour cells make them sensitive to K-cell attack.

4. *Tumour progression in the presence of antitumour immunity.* Why do tumours continue to grow and spread in the face of demonstrable antitumour immunity? The answer to this central question is not known. At worst it is possible that antitumour immunity may merely be an interesting epiphenomenon with no spontaneous tumour restrictive activity *in vivo*. Data from animal experiments are clearly against this but these have mainly derived from specially chosen situations and the situation in man is less clear. It seems more likely that the relationship between tumour and host is constantly evolving and that the 'face' which tumour cells present to the environment continually alters as a result of antigenic selection or modulation or by the concealment of antigens under masking coats. If the appropriate antigenic targets are withdrawn or hidden it is likely that the antitumour immune response is less effective. There is also the possibility that antitumour immunity may be 'blocked' by antigens shed from tumour cells into the body fluids or complexes of such antigens with anti-tumour antibodies or less likely by non-cytotoxic antitumour antibodies attached to tumour cells. Immune complexes are also known to be immunosuppressive in some situations. There is thus much to be investigated before an answer to the question posed at the beginning of this section may be answered. It is even possible that a weak immune response may enhance tumour growth.

Immunotherapy

While the studies outlined above indicate subtle relationships between tumours and the host response, our understanding of such interactions remains rudimentary. It seems reasonable therefore to continue to probe these relationships in the hope that further understanding of them will permit the development of means of increasing the effectiveness of the host response. The numerous patients with advanced cancer who are beyond conventional therapy has, however, emboldened a number of therapists to attempt, despite our ignorance of the details of the biology of host responsiveness in cancer, various forms of immunological manipulation which have been arbitrarily called immunotherapy. In the majority of animal studies it has proved possible to prevent the development of cancer transplants, or to slow their rate of development and metastasis; however the treatment of established malignancy has proved more difficult. Few animal models bear any real resemblance to the slowly developing widely metastasizing malignancies which comprise the majority of human cancers. The relevance of the findings in such animal models for human cancer is therefore distinctly doubtful.

Types of immunotherapy

Immunotherapy can be divided into *active immunotherapy* in which an attempt is made to stimulate the immune system of the tumour-bearing individual, either non-specifically by immunological adjuvants, or specifically by a vaccine which contains putative tumour-associated antigens with or without an adjuvant. Those employing this approach believe that the cancer patient has a tumour-directed immune response which is either inherently incapable of killing significant numbers of tumour cells, or has become incapable of such killing during tumour growth. Active immunotherapy is designed to augment this response and render it effective. In *passive immunotherapy* antibodies or specifically sensitized lymphocytes raised in another individual of the same species or a member of another species or lymphocyte products, are administered to the tumour-bearing individual. It is argued that as the naturally occuring antitumour immune response seems ineffectual against tumour growth and spread it is unlikely that we will be able to augment it significantly. An extraneous source of immunologically active materials is therefore necessary. More recent attempts at passive immunotherapy have included efforts to transfer 'information' from specifically immunized individuals by the transfer of sub-cellular fractions such as transfer factor or 'immune RNA'.

Logistics of immunotherapy

The design of immunotherapy trials is hampered by ignorance of the optimum routes and timings of administration of reagents in absolute terms and *vis-à-vis* other forms of therapy.

There is some evidence that immunotherapy is maximally effective against relatively small numbers of tumour cells and should therefore be given after tumour reduction by conventional therapy, ideally after excision of the primary or after excision of involved lymph nodes when the tumour cell numbers

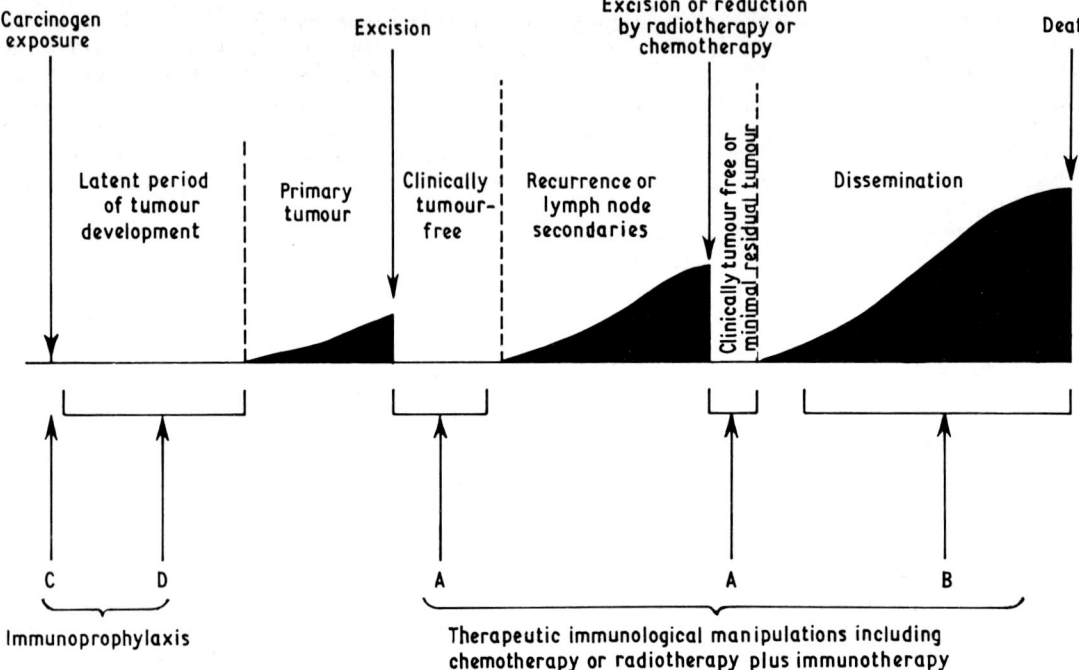

Fig. 7.1   The timing of immunotherapy.

A. Therapeutic immunological manipulation when clinically detectable tumour is absent or minimal; B. Therapeutic immunological manipulation when tumour burden is considerable; A and B may be combined with radiation therapy or chemotherapy; C. Immunoprophylaxis; immune manipulation at time of carcinogen exposure (in animals) at time of tumour transplantation; D. Immunoprophylaxis; immune manipulation during latent period between carcinogen exposure (or tumour transplantation) and emergence of a clinically detectable tumour (from Cochran, 1978). (Reproduced with permission from *Man, Cancer and Immunity*. Copyright by Academic Press Inc. (London) Ltd.)

are minimal (Fig. 7.1). In animal studies, the best results have been with immunoprophylaxis, adjuvants being deployed at the time of carcinogen exposure or tumour transplantation, and it is difficult to see the relevance of this approach in man.

When planning immunotherapy, the periods of immune suppression following radiotherapy, chemotherapy and surgery seem best avoided although it has been claimed that adjuvants may reduce the degree of immune suppression and myelosuppression induced by these other agents. The judicious use of immunological adjuvants may on the one hand reduce the incidence of opportunistic infections and coagulation failure, and on the other permit the use of larger doses of radiation or chemotherapy. Following a course of chemotherapy, there is a period of 'immunological overshoot' in which the immune system is hyper-reactive and at this time would seem especially responsive to stimulation.

In determining the dose, timing and frequency of administration of agents, the general principles devised for the testing of new chemotherapeutic agents must be followed. There is no reason why immunological reagents should be treated any differently from other drugs in this respect (Carter and Slavik, 1975).

The site and route of administration of immunotherapeutic agents remains dependent upon the site and known degree of dissemination of tumour cells and has to be modified in relation to the toxicity of the particular agents employed. Where there is an obvious group of lymph nodes into which lymphatic spread of tumour is likely to occur, immunostimulation of these nodes may assist in containing the tumour.

Therapeutic success with immunotherapy is claimed to be limited to patients who are immunocompetent prior to treatment or who develop competence during therapy. Regrettably, few immunotherapy studies have included immunological competence among the criteria for inclusion. If, as has been suggested, cell-mediated immunity has a good effect against tumours and antitumour antibodies may under certain circumstances have a bad effect, immunostimulants may require to be developed which will selectively stimulate cellular immunity. This view is weakened by the demonstration that tumour cells coated with antibody are susceptible to killing by K-cells. It seems likely that the currently available adjuvants are not ideal and different preparations vary widely in their physical, chemical and cultural characteristics, in their capacity to effect lymphocytes and macrophages *in vitro* and in their capacity to effect tumours in animal models. We need to know more of the significance of these variations and of which parameters measured *in vitro* predict antitumour activity *in vivo*. Reagents to be used for passive immunotherapy need to be as highly specific as is technically possible. In order to obtain interpretable results it is vital to compare the various regimes in concurrently controlled prospective clinical trials.

With the possible exception of local immunotherapy, there is at present no clinical situation where immunotherapy might be accepted as a treatment of choice. The *ad hoc* administration of immunotherapy in an uncontrolled situation has no background of clinical results to commend it and if immunotherapy is to be attempted it must be within the framework of a suitable trial. In order to avoid unnecessary duplication of studies, negative results must be reported, and it is hoped that journals will see the desirability of this. It is also highly desirable that any complications occurring from the various regimes employed be promptly and widely reported.

Active immunotherapy

Active non-specific immunotherapy

The requirement is for a strong stimulant of the immunological system which induces no major side-effects or morbidity. Adjuvants divide into biological agents, whole micro-organisms or materials derived from them and synthetic preparations, such as Levamisole and poly-IC. The use of micro-organisms in immunotherapy goes back to the late 19th century (Coley, 1891). There have been reports over the years of cancer regression associated with bacterial infection and inflammatory processes. Although mainly anecdotal, they indicate an occasional beneficial effect of some infections on malignant disease. An inverse relationship has been claimed between cancer incidence and the frequency of infectious disease, and it is postulated that the reticuloendothelial system activated by micro-organisms may be active in cancer

prevention or the induction of tumour regression. Burchenal (1966) suggested that the response of African Burkitt's lymphoma patients to low dose chemotherapy might be due to a stimulated reticuloendothelial system, although other micro-organismal infections, particularly viruses and plasmodia depress the immune system. The use of BCG, *Corynebacterium parvum* (CP) and vaccinia virus is thus a recrudescence of interest in Coley's approach.

1. *Bacillus Calmette-Géurin.* BCG, an attenuated bovine tubercle bacillus, is the adjuvant which has received most attention. Many studies have shown it to increase the strength of humoral and cell-mediated immunity *in vivo* and *in vitro*. It also increases resistance to infections with unrelated organisms, increases the strength of allograft rejection and increases resistance to tumour challenge. BCG is also reported to increase phagocytosis *in vitro*, bring about the development of macrophages cytotoxic for tumour cells, increase circulating T-cells and increase mitogen responsiveness of lymphocytes.

Early studies showed that BCG had activity against animal tumours, maximal in immunoprophylaxis and when brought into close contact with small numbers of tumour cells. Reports of the use of BCG against human cancer came with studies in leukaemias and 'haematosarcomas' and most strikingly in acute lymphoblastic leukaemia (ALL) (Mathé *et al.*, 1963, 1969). After chemotherapy-induced remission, these individuals were divided into a group which received no further treatment, and a group which received maintenance immunotherapy (BCG or pooled irradiated allogeneic ALL cells or both). The immunotherapy recipients seldom relapsed and some achieved remissions which have persisted to the present. All those in the group receiving no maintenance therapy relapsed. Unfortunately similar studies in a number of centres have not confirmed Mathé's findings. It should however be emphasized that there were real differences between Mathé's study and these more recent studies in terms of reagents, and route of administration. The effectiveness of combination chemotherapy and central nervous system irradiation in ALL has increased so dramatically that most clinical haematologists now rely on this therapy, rather than any form of immunotherapy.

BCG with or without irradiated allogeneic tumour cells has been used in acute myeloid leukaemia after remission induction by chemotherapy. Some studies suggest that immunotherapy patients have longer remissions than those maintained on chemotherapy and that it is simpler to reinduce remission in such patients; however, the case for BCG immunotherapy in this disease remains unproven. Despite a large number of clinical trials currently in progress (Terry and Windhorst, 1978) the role of BCG in solid tumours remains debatable. Some encouraging results have been claimed in tumours as diverse as malignant melanoma, lymphoma, carcinoma of colon, breast carcinoma and sarcomas, but the design of many of the trials does not permit an adequate analysis of their results.

The most impressive recent report of BCG therapy is that by McKneally *et al.* (1976) who gave a single dose of BCG intrapleurally after lobectomy or pneumonectomy for lung cancer. In patients with limited tumour, but not those with advanced tumour, BCG reduced recurrences and improved survival relative to randomized control individuals who had no BCG. A number of trials are in progress which are attempting to repeat this study.

It is a matter of major concern that we still do not know the best preparations of BCG for use in immunotherapy, although we know that preparations vary widely in their characteristics, nor do we know the optima for dose, site and timing. Mathé has suggested an optimum dose for *fresh living Pasteur BCG* which differs for the immunocompetent and the immunoincompetent (to recall antigens). He states that 'septicaemia of given intensity . . . correlated with the anti-tumour reaction'. It appears necessary to establish a symbiosis between cancer patient and mycobacteria. This septicaemia would require careful monitoring and Mathé claims that the dose could best be arranged by intravenous administration. These studies present considerable problems as fresh Institute Pasteur BCG is not readily available to most workers and data on dosage cannot be extrapolated to other strains or preparations of BCG. Better characterization of BCG is urgently required and this may be the main direction of BCG research in the next few years.

The complications of BCG therapy have mainly resulted from its being a living infective organism. Interest has therefore been directed to identifying materials within the organism which mediate the adjuvant effect. Extracts of the mycobacteria such as methanol-extracted residue, water-soluble adjuvant and hydrosoluble adjuvant have shown some effects in animals, but remain at a developmental stage having not yet been extensively tested in man. A related approach has been to use mycobacterial wall skeletons combined with known active materials from mycobacteria (e.g. trehalone dimycolate-cord factor) attached to mineral oil droplets. This has shown activity against animal tumours and is as effective as BCG on intramelanomatous injection.

2. *Corynebacterium parvum.* CP has the advantage that it is employed as a killed vaccine. It is a member of the group of anaerobic corynebacteria, all of which stimulate the reticuloendothelial system producing a remarkable range of effects in experimental animals (see Halpern, 1975), including increased macrophage phagocytosis, chemotaxis and killing of bacteria and tumour cells. It may also stimulate T- and B-lymphocytes and increase antibody synthesis against T-dependent and independent antigens and increase delayed hypersensitivity and lymphocytotoxicity including lymphocytotoxicity against tumour cells. CP also stimulates the precursors of macrophages and lymphocytes.

In vivo CP has been found to have tumour inhibitory activities for a wide range of animal tumours. The observed effects have, however, varied widely depending on the tumour examined, the size of tumour inoculum, the route of administration of CP, and the time between tumour inoculation and the administration of CP. Trials of CP in human malignant disease are in progress, but the results as yet remain insufficient to permit evaluation of the role of CP in oncology. That the agent is associated with unpleasant side-effects will certainly delay evaluation (see below).

3. *Levamisole.* Levamisole* is an anti-helminthic which has effects on the functions of lymphocytes and macrophages restoring these to normal levels where they are initially depressed (immune restoration) but not apparently inducing supra-normal activity in normally functioning cells. Early clinical studies have reported no effect on advanced cancer, but two recent reports have suggested that Levamisole may stabilize less extended bronchogenic carcinoma and breast carcinoma, and reduce the incidence of subsequent metastases. The drug causes skin rashes and granulopaenia which may proceed to agranulocytosis, necessitating its very cautious evaluation.

Many of the problems of biologically derived adjuvants may be overcome by synthetic agents, and it seems likely that this is the source from which future generations of agents will be derived.

4. *Other adjuvants.* Very considerable ingenuity has been displayed in the search for substances with adjuvant properties. These have ranged from yeast extracts to silica and beryllium, extracts of mushrooms, lymphokines, viruses and synthetic substances, filiron and poly-IC, which may act via their activities as interferon inducers. The length of this list indicates the scale of any attempt to evaluate the substances contained on it in a clinical context. We must either develop means of identifying the desirable properties of adjuvants in model systems, or develop more adequate animal models.

*Janssen, Belgium

Active specific immunotherapy

General imunostimulation, regardless of the potency of the adjuvant seems unlikely preferentially to stimulate antitumour immunity which has led to attempts actively to immunize cancer patients against (putative) tumour-associated antigens (TAA). But, why should the administration of relatively small numbers of tumour cells be expected to produce a result when the spontaneous tumour does not induce a significant tumour inhibitory response? The administration of autologous irradiated melanoma cells to patients who lack detectable antitumour immunity induces anti-melanoma antibodies and lymphocytes. This response is transient but can be prolonged by combining the vaccine with BCG. It is possible that the preparative manipulations may remove masking or blocking substances, rendering the cells more immunogenic. Concomitant immunity has to be considered, i.e. the observation that while spontaneous tumours grow apparently unhindered *in vivo*, cells from them implanted in fresh sites in the same animal are rejected unless large numbers are used. Tumour cells may produce immunosuppressive materials and it is possible that the tumour cells modified for immunotherapy may have this undesirable activity diminished. Attempts have been made to render tumour cells more immunogenic by attaching foreign proteins to the membrane, removing masking coats to expose more deeply located antigens or subjecting the cells to viral oncolysis. The most promising of these seems to be the stripping of sialic acid masking coats by neuraminidase.

Unfortunately few trials of active specific immunotherapy in man have involved randomized or concurrently controlled trials and most have involved small numbers of patients. While the vast majority of patients have derived no benefit from this type of treatment, a few individuals in most trials have had (temporary) tumour regressions. However, in a protean disease it is impossible to assess the significance of this in the absence of adequate trial design. There is a slightly more promising situation in the leukaemias. It is claimed that active specific immunotherapy (autologous or allogeneic leukaemia cells with or without an adjuvant), may benefit patients with acute lymphoblastic leukaemia, acute myeloid leukaemia and chronic myeloid leukaemia. Active specific immunotherapy has also been employed in choriocarcinoma with interesting results.

The irritating thing is that from what we know of auto-immune disease active specific immunotherapy should be the correct way to treat cancer. That it has so far been relatively unproductive may be due to technical factors, but raises real concern as to the nature and significance of tumour associated antigens.

Local immunotherapy

There is considerable interest in the application of immunogenic materials directly into contact with accessible tumours either by injection into the tumour (Morton *et al.*, 1970) or by the application of contact sensitizors to the overlying tissues. The agents employed include BCG, dinitrochlorobenzene, vaccinia virus, CP, streptokinase-streptodornase, *in vitro* activated autochthonous lymphocytes and fractions of serum from immunized patients. The findings have been similar regardless of the agent applied: an area of delayed cutaneous hypersensitivity develops in and around the treated area, followed by necrosis and ulceration after which the lesion heals leaving a depressed scar. Microscopy shows infiltration by lymphocytes and macrophages, with poorly formed giant cells containing follicular granulomas in mycobacterial lesions. Tumour cells show necrosis and disintegration; resolution is usually complete in 4–6 weeks. There is considerable debate as to whether the effect is purely a local one, or whether a systemic response develops. A proportion of non-injected tumours regress but these are usually in the same lymphatic area as the injected nodules. By contrast non-injected nodules adjacent to injected tumours may be unaffected. BCG mycobacteria are disseminated after intratumoral injections, as is shown by mycobacterial granulomata in the liver and other organs. Alterations in tumour-directed immunity do occur in patients receiving BCG, even in those with disseminated disease, indicating systemic effects (Cochran *et al.*, 1978). That this systemic effect is weak is suggested by extension of visceral metastases despite regression of locally treated lesions. While local immunotherapy does not cure cancer, it is a simple means of removing obvious lesions which may be distressing to the patient and can be undertaken as an out-patient avoiding anaesthesia and hospitalization.

While most attempts at local immunotherapy have involved treatment of intradermal metastases, some authors have treated primary tumours, either as a preliminary to surgical excision or as a sole form of therapy. With some ingenuity, local immunotherapy can be applied to tumours of extracutaneous sites, such as the vagina, uterine cervix and bladder.

The mechanism of tumour destruction is incompletely understood, the consensus being that tumour is destroyed in a non-specific fashion by the cells involved in the induced delayed hypersensitivity reaction. However, after the breakdown of tumour cells with release of tumour-associated antigens, enhanced specific immunity may develop to complement the initial non-specific effects.

Passive immunotherapy

Passive immunotherapy with antitumour antibodies

The specificity of combining sites should allow effective localization of antibodies at tumour cells, and if the antibodies involved can bind complement or sensitize the tumour cells to K-cell attack this should destroy tumour cells bearing the appropriate antigens. The other side of the coin is that antibodies may act as blocking agents and protect the tumour cells from potentially more effective immunological agencies. A few reports of tumour regression following administration of sera from cured patients, or patients with regressing cancer, do exist and have encouraged some attempts at serotherapy. The results of such studies have been essentially negative although occasional transient remissions have been recorded. The provision of suitable serum donors is difficult and xenogeneic antisera present their own problems which are ameliorated slightly by the fact that antitumour activity survives quite extensive absorption procedures.

It has been considered that non-cytotoxic antibodies might be used to carry cytotoxic drugs or radioactive isotopes which would be preferentially concentrated at the tumour cell site. The problem is to devise antibodies of sufficient specificity and to link them to agents which will not destroy that specificity. Monoclonal antibodies may be very useful in this context, linked to radioisotopes, cytotoxic drugs or toxins such as ricin (Olsnes, 1981). Initial studies with murine leukaemia and lymphoma and the Ehrlich's ascites carcinoma suggested that this approach was valid and there has been a report of responses in patients (Ghose *et al.*, 1972). It has been suggested that the antibody-drug linkage is loose and probably non-covalent and that rapid dissociation occurs *in vivo*. Linkage of antibody and drug may be unnecessary and the administration of drug followed by antitumour antibody is said to achieve effects considerably in excess of either alone. Drug given after antibody does not enhance tumour cell killing. Thus antibody may kill drug-effected tumour cells, but antibody-affected cells are not especially sensitive to drugs (Davies and O'Neill, 1973).

Immunotherapy with lymphocytes

To employ the patient's own lymphocytes in this situation, their performance would have to be improved by 'education' *in vitro* (i.e. exposure to tumour antigens of maximized immunogenicity) and culture to increase their number, a formidable task. Lymphocytes activated by mitogens would provide a technically simpler although non-specific alternative. Lymphocytes from sources other than the cancer patient could also provide specifically sensitized or non-sensitized cells.

The latter, while most readily available, seem unlikely to survive sufficiently long *in vivo* to undergo education, and in any case, the reaction to tumour antigens would probably be only a minor part of a complex reaction to stronger species, strain and organ markers. Allogeneic sensitized lymphocytes could be obtained from patients whose tumours had undergone spontaneous or therapy-induced regression, or from cancer patients' contacts. Cross-immunization with subsequent reverse exchange of lymphocytes and of serum is limited ethically to exchanges between cancer patients. The results of this approach have not been encouraging although a minority of patients have had some benefit. Survival of allogeneic lymphocytes in the recipient is short, due to transplantation disparity although despite their destruction such cells may impart 'information' to the host lymphocytes via transfer factor or immune RNA. Graft versus host reaction is also a problem, especially where bone marrow transplantation is involved. Attempts to employ xenogeneic lymphocytes have not been successful due to problems in achieving immunization against tumour-associated antigens and rapid destruction of donor lymphocytes by the host versus graft reaction.

Immunotherapy with lymphocyte extracts and products

1. *Transfer factor.* Lawrence (1969) has shown that a low molecular weight fraction from lymphocytes of tuberculin-reactive guinea pigs can transfer this reactivity to non-reactive animals. A similar phenomenon has been reported in man and in view of the postulated immune deficiency in malignant disease, there have been attempts to use transfer factor to restore immune competence in cancer patients. Pilot studies have been inconclusive but not entirely negative and a number of trials are currently in progress.

2. *Immune RNA.* This material can be extracted from the lymphoid organs or peripheral blood lymphocytes of sensitized animals and can confer immunity passively. The immune RNA molecule is 3–4 times the size of the transfer factor molecule but its exact nature remains to be elucidated and it is possible that transfer factor may be included within it. Preliminary attempts to employ immune RNA in the therapy of human cancer are in progress.

3. *Lymphocyte products.* Tumour regression after intralesional immunotherapy is largely due to the effects of lymphocyte activation products (lymphokines). There is therefore considerable interest in the production of substances such as immune interferon, migration inhibition factor and lymphotoxin on a scale sufficiently large to allow investigation of the effects of

their systemic administration. Currently developing technological improvement makes this type of investigation more practical.

4. *Interferons.* Interferons are indeed completely new agents for treatment of cancer. They are of course the class of protein (described by Isaacs and Lindenmann in 1957) secreted by virus-treated cells which can then absorb on to other cells and give them resistance to virus infection (Editorial, *Lancet*, 1979). It has been found that interferon restrains the growth of various tumours in mice, even if they are not virus-induced, and this is consistent with knowledge that it has various effects on cells including slowing of cell division, enhancing natural killer (NK) activity and modulation of immune responses.

Interferon is now, at last, being produced in larger quantities by preparation from cultured Namalva strain lymphoblastoid cells and by recombinant DNA techniques. The compound has already been shown to have some affect on human osteosarcoma as an adjuvant to surgery and radiation, on myeloma, or lymphoma, and on breast cancer. Necessarily only few patients have so far been treated and this very promising method, as others, requires statistically valid results in reasonably sized random control trials. (*Interferon I*, 1979; and *Interferon II*, 1980).

5. *Thymic extracts.* The exact means whereby the thymus gland exerts its effect remains unknown although there is evidence that hormones from the epithelial component are important. A major function of such hormones would be to commit lymphocytes to function as T-cells and if this activity were in abeyance, due to ageing or micro-organisms or chemicals including drugs, T-lymphocyte activities including those against tumour cells would be reduced. Various thymic extracts have been prepared and examined in animals and more recently in man. If thymic dysfunction is important in oncogenesis, or cancer progression, replacement therapy with thymic hormones would seem a logical approach (see Editorial in *British Medical Journal*, 1977 for review).

Complications of immunotherapy

The major theoretical problem is that the results of therapy may be deleterious rather than advantageous. Tumour enhancement is unlikely to be detectable other than within the framework of a clinical trial which adds further weight to the argument for confining immunotherapy to such trials. Another theoretical possibility which does not appear to have been encountered in practice is the development of organ-specific autoimmune disease in patients treated with active specific immunotherapy.

The major problems encountered have related to the use of infective organisms, especially BCG. Local problems encountered with BCG include extensive crusting, scarring and occasional depigmentation which make the prospect of prolonged therapy unattractive to some patients. BCG–tumour cell mixtures and intralesional BCG cause abscesses which produce large quantities of pus from which live BCG organisms are readily cultured. Caution must be exercised in handling infected dressings especially in the domestic situation. Some patients receiving BCG develop liver dysfunction and biopsies suggest that many of these patients develop granulomatous hepatitis with mycobacteria in the liver. Such lesions seem likely to persist without anti-tuberculous therapy as Gormsen (1955) found that children dying from other causes years after the administration of BCG for tuberculosis prophylaxis, had a few hepatic granulomata. In the presence of foci of mycobacteria care must be exercised if high doses of steroids or other immunodepressive drugs are being considered. Spread of mycobacteria to the draining lymph nodes seems an inevitable concomitant factor of BCG administration, producing mildly enlarged nodes and occasionally abscesses. Generalized progressive infection with BCG is rare but was a major contributory cause of death in one of our earliest patients to receive BCG (Grant *et al.*, 1974). This patient responded to a limited degree to antituberculous therapy but eventually died of a myocardial infarction, and had mycobacterial bronchopneumonia and granulomata in the lung, liver, kidneys, spleen, and adrenals. This disastrous complication has also been recorded by others and may in part be the result of terminal immune depression. It is predominantly a sequel of intralesional BCG but we have encountered it in two patients who had received BCG only by scarification. Early detection is essential and demands frequent follow-up assessment of patients at risk with radiographic monitoring of the chest and a high index of awareness of the possibility of its occurrence. Antituberculous therapy rapidly resolved the condition in the two patients referred to above.

Deaths have been recorded as a result of anaphylaxis to BCG with high fever and major coagulation failure, non-responsive even to strenuous resuscitation techniques. Rarer complications include lichen scrofulosum and osteomyelitis.

CP is associated with a febrile reaction regardless of its route of administration. This is usually of short duration and may reduce in severity with successive doses. However sub-cutaneous and intralesional injections cause pain which may occasionally be sufficiently severe to necessitate the ending of treatment. Intratumoral injections produce major local inflammation proceeding to suppuration. Intraperitoneal and intravenous injections are said to be well tolerated although systemic reactions may be more severe in patients receiving CP by these routes and hepatotoxicity has been recorded. Mild changes in blood pressure are observed in most CP recipients. Diffuse intravascular coagulation, thrombocytopaenia and nephrotic syndrome may develop in a minority of CP recipients.

Levamisole is well tolerated by most patients but serious problems have been encountered with a few individuals. Side-effects are said to be most common in patients with rheumatoid arthritis and include skin rashes and gastrointestinal symptoms. Granulopaenia has occurred and there is an increasing number of recent reports of agranulocytosis. The requirement for close haematological scrutiny is obvious.

Active specific immunotherapy has not yet been reported to be associated with any major problems. The potential growth of living allogeneic tumour cells in immunosuppressed recipients has dictated that such cells have, in most studies, been rendered incapable of replication prior to the administration, although this may reduce their immunogenicity. Allogeneic tumour cell transfer carries the theoretical risk of introducing oncogenic viruses or oncogenes which would subsequently induce new malignancies, a possibility which cannot be excluded at present.

Passive immunotherapy is associated mainly with anaphylaxis, serum sickness and glomerulonephritis after the administration of allogeneic or xenogeneic serum. Graft versus host disease may also occur when foreign immunocompetent cells are given. There is insufficient experience of other forms of passive immunotherapy to allow any firm statement on problems associated with their use.

Comments

The preceding pages outline the findings from a considerable body of ingenious attempts to employ the immune system in cancer therapy. The returns to date have been limited but are sufficient to warrant the cautious continued evaluation of promising areas by committed specialist groups willing and able to undertake adequately controlled clinical trials. The combination of therapy with immunological adjuvants and chemotherapy or radiation therapy seems especially worthy of careful evaluation. Local immunotherapy also merits continued assessment, perhaps even as a prelude to surgery in accessible tumours. Logically, effective immunotherapy will stem from a full understanding of the host – tumour interaction, an understanding which will probably require many years of effort to achieve. It is likely, therefore, that immuno-

therapy will develop slowly as part of a combined approach to cancer treatment rather than as an isolated form of therapy.

It would be pleasant to have this opinion proved unduly cautious.

Appendix. Immunotherapeutic agents

Recommendations on dosage for the various agents need to be considered with considerable caution. In the present stage of knowledge optimal doses remain to be established in appropriately designed clinical trials and it is probably necessary to tailor doses for individual patients in relation to general immunological status, agent-specific immunity and the type of preparation employed. These recommendations do not indicate that such preparations are ready for 'off the shelf' use. They should only be used in the framework of adequately controlled clinical trials.

Table 7.1 gives indications of the routes of administration, doses, frequency of administration and duration of employment of some of the commoner agents. Those interested in initiating clinical studies with these classes of material will find much useful and salutory information in the recent publications by Terry and Windhorst (1978) and The M.D. Anderson Hospital and Tumor Institute (1978).

Further reading

Castro, J.E. (ed.) (1978), *Immunological Aspects of Cancer.* Medical and Technical Publishers Ltd., London

Cochran, A.J. (1978), *Man, Cancer and Immunity.* Academic Press, London and New York.

M.D. Anderson Hospital and Tumor Institute. Univ. Texas System Cancer Center (1978), *Immunotherapy of Human Cancer.* 22nd Ann. Clin. Conf. Cancer, Raven Press Inc., New York.

Terry, W. and Windhorst, D. (eds) (1978), *Immunotherapy of Cancer: Present Status of Trials in Man.* Raven Press Inc., New York.

Wybran, J. and Staquet, M.J. (eds) (1976), *Clinical Tumour Immunology.* Pergamon Press Ltd., London.

References

Burchenal, J.H. (1966), Geographic chemotherapy – Burkitt's tumour as a stalking horse for leukaemia. *Cancer Res.,* **26**, 2393–405.

Burnet, F.M. (1967), Immunological aspects of malignant disease. *Lancet.* **1**, 1171–4.

Carter, S.K. and Slavik, M. (1975), A chemotherapeutic perspective on clinical trials with *Corynebacterium parvum*. In: *Corynebacterium parvum*

Table 7.1 Ranges of doses, routes of administration, frequency and duration of therapy for various immunotherapeutic agents.

Agent	Route of administration	Dose range	Frequency of administration	Duration of therapy
Bacillus Calmette-Guérin (BCG)	percutaneous	$2 \times 10^6 - 1 \times 10^9$ viable units*	weekly then monthly	once up to five years
	intralesional	$4 - 9 \times 10^5$ viable units	once	–
	intravesicle	$40 - 120$ mg†	once	–
	intrapleural	10^7 viable units‡	once	–
Corynebacterium parvum (CP)	sub-cutaneous	2 mg/m² up to 4.2 mg	weekly then monthly	six months
	intravenous	$0.2 - 5$ mg/m²	weekly	up to three months
	intralesional	$2.8 - 4.2$ mg	weekly	–
Levamisole	oral	150 mg	daily for 3 days – biweekly	up to 2 years
Vaccinia virus	intralesional	not $<10^8$ pock forming units	once	–
Methanol-extracted residue of BCG	intradermal	0.1 mg/m² up to 1 mg (in divided doses)	weekly or monthly	8 months
Poly I: Poly C	intravenous	300 mg/m²	once	–
Interferon	intramuscular	3×10^6 units	daily then twice weekly	up to 17 months
Transfer factor	sub-cutaneous	1 unit (derived from 10^9 lymphocytes)	once to twice weekly	–

* The best means of quantifying BCG dose and permitting comparisons of materials and trial is to state number of 'viable units' employed or number of 'colony forming units'.

† Dry weight.

‡ This single dose regime is covered by anti-tuberculosis therapy (isoniazid) given for 90 days, starting two weeks after BCG.

(ed. B. Halpern), Plenum Press, London and New York, p. 329.

Cochran, A.J. *et al.* (1978), Immunological changes in cancer patients receiving BCG. *Devl. Biol. Stand.*, **38**, 441–8.

Coley, W.B. (1891), Contribution to the knowledge of sarcoma. *Ann. Surg.*, **14**, 199–220.

Davies, D.A.L. and O'Neill, G.J. (1973), *In vivo* and *in vitro* effects of tumour specific antibodies with chlorambucil. *Br. J. Cancer*, **28**, Suppl. I, 285–98.

Editorial (1977), Thymic hormones. *Br. Med. J.*, **i**, 1559–60.

Editorial (1979), Can Interferon cure cancers? *Lancet*, **i**, 1171–2.

Everson, T.C. and Cole, W.H. (1966), *Spontaneous regression of cancer*, W.B. Saunders Co., Philadelphia and London.

Ghose, T. *et al.* (1972), Immunochemotherapy of cancer with chlorambucil-carrying antibody. *Br. Med. J.*, **iii**, 495–9.

Gormsen, H. (1955), On the occurrence of epithelioid cell granulomas in the organs of BCG-vaccinated human beings. *Acta. Path. Microbiol. Scand.*, **111**, 117–20.

Graham-Pole, J. *et al.* (1976), Sensitisation of neuroblastoma patients and related and unrelated contacts to neuroblastoma extracts. *Lancet*, **i**, 1376–9.

Grant, R.M., *et al.* (1974), Results of the administration of BCG to melanoma patients. *Lancet*, **2**, 1096–8.

Halpern, B. (1975), *Corynebacterium parvum*, Plenum Press, London and New York.

Heston, W.E. (1976), The genetic aspects of human cancer. In: *Advances in Cancer Research* (eds G. Klein and S. Weinhouse), **23**, Academic Press, New York and London, p. 1.

Ikonopisov, R.L. *et al.* (1970), Autoimmunisation with irradiated tumour cells in human malignant melanoma. *Br. Med. J.*, **ii**, 752–4.

Interferon I (1979) and *Interferon II* (1980), (ed. I. Gresser), Academic Press, London and New York.

Lawrence, H.S. (1969), Transfer factor. *Adv. Immunol.*, **11**, 195–266.

Lejeune, F.J. (1975), Role of macrophages in immunity, with special reference to tumour immunology; a review. *Biomedicine*, **22**, 25–34.

Lewis, M.G. *et al.* (1971), Possible explanation for loss of detectable antibody in patients with disseminated malignant melanoma. *Nature (Lond.)*, **232**, 52–4.

Lies, H.P. and Black, M.M. (1970), Human breast carcinoma. 3. Cellular responses to autologous breast cancer: skin-window procedure. *N.Y. St. J. Med.*, **70**, 2583–8.

Mathé, G. *et al.* (1963), Demonstration de l'efficacité de l'immunotherapie active dans le leucémie aigue lymphoblastique humaine. *Rev. Franc. Etudes Clin, Biol.*, **13**, 454–9.

Mathé, G. *et al.* (1969), Active immunotherapy for acute lymphoid leukaemia. *Lancet*, **1**, 697–9.

McDevitt, H.D. and Benacerraf, B. (1969), Genetic control of specific immune responses. *Adv. Immunol.*, **11**, 31–50.

McKneally, M.F., Mavor, C. and Kausel, H.W. (1976), Regional immunotherapy of lung cancer with intrapleural BCG. *Lancet*, **1**, 377–9.

MacLennan, I.C.M. (1976), Function and evaluation of human K-cells. In: *Clinical Tumour Immunology* (eds J. Wybran and M.J. Staquet), Pergamon Press, London, p. 47–54.

Morton, D.L. *et al.* (1970), Immunologic factors which influence response to immunotherapy in malignant melanoma. *Surgery*, **68**, 158–64.

Olsnes, S. (1981), Directing toxins to cancer cells. *Nature*, **290**, 84.

Rebuck, J.W. and Crowley, J.H. (1955), Skin window technique. *Ann. N.Y. Acad. Sci.*, **59**, 757–805.

Scanlon, E.F. *et al.* (1965), Fatal homo-transplanted melanoma: a case report. *Cancer*, **18**, 782–9.

Thomas, L. (1959), In: *Cellular and humoral aspects of the hypersensitivity state* (ed. H.S. Lawrence), Hoeber, New York, p. 529.

Woglom, W.H. (1929), Immunity to transplantable tumours. *Cancer Rev.*, **4**, 129.

Part Two: Clinical Practice

8 Lips and oral cavity

R.C.S. Pointon and
E.N. Gleave

Incidence and sex ratio

Lips

Cancer of the lips occurs most frequently in those geographic areas that are subject to long hours of sunlight and in workers who have a long outdoor exposure. In Western Canada, squamous cell carcinoma of the lip accounts for 5% of all new cancers registered (Dick, 1962). Whilst in Saskatoon, Canada, 11.3% of the registrations were cancers of the lip (Burkell, 1950). Such tumours are rare amongst negroes, Eskimos and Canadian Indians (Dick, 1962). In England and Wales the average annual registration of lip cancer between 1962 and 1967 was 618 cases, comprising 548 males and 70 females (Binnie, 1976), thus representing an incidence of 0.6% of all malignant tumours. The registration rates in England and Wales per million of the population for the period 1960 to 1970 are shown in Table 8.1. In Great Britain as a whole, there would appear to be a higher incidence in those of Irish descent. Cancer of the lip occurs most frequently between 50 and 80 years, with a mean age of 64 years. These tumours occur predominantly in males, the ratio of males to females being 12–14:1.

Oral cavity

In Britain oral cancers account for about 2% of all malignant tumours; 2400 new cases are registered annually (Binnie, 1976). Such tumours are much more common in certain other countries, especially those of the Middle and Far East. In Bombay, for example, they account for 13% of all new registrations of malignant tumours (Jussawalla, 1976).

The incidence of cancer of the oral cavity has shown a continuing decline in Great Britain (Table 8.2). This has been due to a striking decrease of the incidence amongst males, whilst the female incidence has remained largely unchanged.

At the Christie Hospital and Holt Radium Institute, Manchester, over the past 40 years, there has been a progressive decline in the number of male patients registered and the present male: female sex ratio is 1.6:1. A detailed examination of the changes in sex ratio for the different sites in the oral cavity is as shown in Table 8.3 (Easson and Palmer, 1976).

In the North-west of England, the modal age group was 70–74 years, with 50% of patients aged between 65 and 79 years. The mean age for males was 68.5 years and for females 67.3 years respectively. An earlier age incidence, by a decade, as well as increased frequency is seen in the countries of the Far East. These differences can be readily attributed to specific aetiological factors.

Table 8.1 Registration and deaths of lip cancer patients in England and Wales 1960–70 (Binnie, 1976) (rates per million per year).

	1960–62 mean		1963–67 mean		1968–70 mean	
	Registrations	Deaths	Registrations	Deaths	Registrations	Deaths
Male	29	3	24	2	18	2
Female	4	0	3	0	2	0

Table 8.2 Oral cancer registrations 1950–70 at the Christie Hospital and Holt Radium Institute.

Years	Male	Female
1950–55	719	298
1956–60	559	239
1961–65	445	245
1966–70	451	254
Total	2174	1036

Table 8.3 Sex ratios (males:females) by site of cancer within the oral cavity.

Site	1932–39	1940–49	1950–59	1960–69
Tongue	7.8:1	3.3:1	2.3:1	1.7:1
Floor	13.1:1	9.7:1	5.6:1	4.1:1
Upper alveolus	1.7:1	2.3:1	2.0:1	1.2:1
Lower alveolus	5.3:1	3.0:1	1.9:1	1.4:1
Cheek	2.8:1	2.2:1	1.6:1	1.2:1
Hard palate	3.1:1	2.4:1	1.9:1	0.9:1

Aetiology

Actinic exposure is the principal aetiological factor in the development of lip cancer whilst other climatic factors are prolonged exposure to wind and cold. It has long been recognized that lip cancer occurs principally in outdoor workers. Clay-pipe smoking used to be an important factor (Wynder and Bross, 1957; Ebenius, 1943) but few patients would now admit to this habit. Industrial exposure to tar or oils would not appear to play a significant role as an aetiological factor.

For the oral cavity, the commonly recognized aetiological factors are tobacco, alcohol, syphilis, dental sepsis, iron deficiency anaemia, betel nut chewing. With the exception of the latter, their respective relevance to the individual patient is often obscure. More recently attention has been drawn to the possible relationship between chronic hyperplastic candidiasis and the development of oral cancer (Cawson, 1969; Pindborg, 1971).

Moss and Lee (1974) have shown there is an increased risk for oral cancer in certain sub-groups of the cotton and woollen textile industries, in particular to those workers exposed to the dust created by internal 'carding' of new cotton and wool.

Anatomy

Lips

The lips consist of not only their vermilion borders, the exposed mucosa between mucocutaneous junction and line of contact between the lips, but also adjacent skin and underlying muscle. The mucosa is non-keratinizing squamous epithelium without sebaceous glands or hairs and transparent, thus accounting for the characteristic red appearance. The upper lip includes centrally its philtrum, extending up to the base of the nose, and laterally the skin and soft tissues as far as the nasolabial folds, whilst the lower lip includes the skin and soft tissues as far down as the mentolabial skin crease. The bulk of the lips is formed by the underlying muscles including orbicularis oris. This complex arrangement of small muscles produces normal eversion and protrusion of the lips as well as their movements during speech, eating and facial expression. The lips have a very good blood supply by means of superior and inferior labial arteries. Motor innervation of the lips is essentially by the buccal and mandibular branches of the facial nerves, whilst sensory innervation is derived from the trigeminal nerve by means of the infraorbital and mental nerves.

For clinical purposes the lips are classified into three anatomical sites:

1. Lower lip.
2. Upper lip.
3. Commissure.

The lower lip is the primary site of cancer in over 90% of cases, approximately 1% occur at the commissure and the remainder on the upper lip.

Oral cavity

The oral cavity is divided into different parts for descriptive purposes thus allowing more accurate localization of tumours (Table 8.4); however, the posterior third of the tongue is not included in this classification since it is considered to be a part of the oropharynx.

The oral cavity is lined throughout by a mucosa of squamous epithelium, hence the predominant type of malignant tumour. Many minor salivary glands, including the paired sublingual glands of the anterior floor of mouth, lie deep to the mucosa of the lips, cheeks, floor of mouth and palate. The ampullae of the ducts draining the major salivary glands can be readily seen. The openings of the submandibular ducts lie on either side of the midline adjacent to the frenulum of the tongue, whilst those of the parotid ducts are found on a level with the upper second molar teeth.

Table 8.4 Anatomical sub-division of the oral cavity.

1. Buccal mucosa   (i) inner surface of the lips
    (ii) lining of cheeks
    (iii) retromolar triangle
    (iv) buccoalveolar sulci, upper and lower
2. Lower alveolus and gingiva
3. Upper alveolus and gingiva
4. Hard palate
5. Tongue   (i) dorsum and lateral borders of anterior two-thirds (i.e. anterior to the valleata)
    (ii) ventral surface
6. Floor of mouth

NB. Posterior third of tongue and soft palate are included as constituents of the oropharynx.

The buccal mucosa is reflected at the buccoalveolar sulci on to the upper and lower alveoli where it is firmly adherent to the bone of the maxilla and mandible, forming the gingivae of the teeth-bearing arches and, in turn, is continuous with the mucosa covering the hard palate and floor of mouth. The inferior dental nerve and vessels occupy the inferior dental canal which passes through the mandible as far as the mental foramen on each side. That part of the oral cavity outside the arches of the maxilla and mandible is known as the vestibule, whilst the oral cavity proper is bounded by the alveoli. Voluntary muscles, including buccinator, pterygoid and masseter muscles, form the thickness of the cheeks. The junctional area on each side between vestibule and oral cavity is the retromolar space which includes the retromolar triangle.

The oral cavity is limited by the anterior pillar of the fauces on each side, the junction of hard and soft palates above and the junction of the middle and posterior thirds of the tongue below. The hard palate and upper alveolus separate the oral cavity from the external nasal passages and maxillary antra.

The bulk of the tongue is formed by intrinsic and extrinsic groups of muscles. The intrinsic muscles, responsible for controlling shape, have transverse, longitudinal and vertical components arranged on each side of the median fibrous septum. The extrinsic muscles, including genioglossus, hypoglossus and styloglossus, control movements of the tongue. The tongue has a very good blood supply which is derived essentially from the lingual arteries. Motor innervation is by the hypoglossal nerves, whilst sensory innervation is by taste fibres from the chorda tympani which accompany the lingual nerves.

The floor of the mouth is formed by a muscular diaphragm covered by mucosa which separates the oral cavity from the neck. The sub-mandibular duct, lingual nerve and a branch of the lingual artery pass between the muscles on each side, whilst the deep lobes of the submandibular salivary glands are found between the mylohyoid and geniohyoid muscles. The submental nodes lie on the superficial surface of mylohyoid bounded laterally by the anterior bellies of the digastric muscle and covered by the platysma and skin of the neck.

Knowledge of the anatomy of the lips and oral cavity is of practical clinical importance to the understanding of the origin and extension of malignant tumours. Extension of tumour from the retromolar fossa can cause progressive trismus whilst involvement of the muscles of the tongue leads to loss of mobility and ultimate fixity. Alveolar tumours may spread rapidly along the periosteal plane of the maxilla and mandible. Erosion of the lower alveolus by tumour with penetration of the inferior dental canal is a cause of severe pain and retrograde extension of the tumour along the canal. Such characteristics may be the cause of presenting symptoms and interference with normal function causing difficulties with speech and nutrition.

Lymphatic drainage

Lymphatic drainage of the lips and oral cavity is essentially to submental, submandibular and deep cervical or internal jugular lymph nodes. Occasionally, however, metastasis may occur to the parotid and lateral pharyngeal lymph nodes. The submental nodes form clusters within the submental triangles, one on each side of the midline, whose boundaries are formed by the anterior belly of the digastric muscles and the body of the hyoid bone. The submandibular nodes lie along the lower border of the horizontal ramus of the mandible. They are arranged in groups both anterior and posterior to the submandibular salivary gland and in relation to the facial artery and vein as they cross the mandible. The deep cervical or internal jugular nodes form a chain lying adjacent to the internal jugular vein throughout its course in the neck. Specific anatomical names have been given to some of these nodes but they do not have particular clinical significance. The submental nodes communicate by efferent lymphatics with the deep cervical chain in the lower part of the neck, whilst those of the submandibular triangle communicate at a higher level. These connections may have an effect on prognosis since metastatic involvement of nodes in the lower part of the neck carries a less favourable outlook. Lateral pharyngeal nodes are found lying on the constrictor muscles of both sides of the pharynx above the level of the styloid and digastric muscles. The parotid lymph nodes are enclosed within the capsule of the parotid salivary gland, some lying superficially and others deeply within the substance of the gland.

Tumours of the lateral thirds of both lips metastasize most commonly to the submandibular lymph nodes although they may spread to the submental nodes. Centrally placed tumours of the lower lip drain to the submental nodes by cutaneous and sub-cutaneous lymphatics whilst some of these lymphatics cross the midline so that bilateral dissemination can occur. Tumours of the central third of the upper lip metastasize to the submandibular nodes although, occasionally, they may spread to submental parotid lymph nodes.

In a series of 59 histologically positive specimens removed at block dissection for cancer of the lips, the submandibular group of nodes was most commonly involved (Table 8.5).

In general terms, lymphatic drainage from tumours of the oral cavity relates to their position within the oral cavity. Anterior tumours of the outer or buccal aspect of the alveoli and buccal surfaces of lips and cheeks may spread to the submental or anterior submandibular nodes, whilst those that are situated farther back go to the submandibular nodes. The inner or lingual surfaces of the alveoli, floor of mouth and hard palate drain to submandibular and upper cervical nodes although there may occasionally be spread to lateral pharyngeal nodes. The tongue has a complex lymphatic drainage again relating to the anterior or posterior position of tumours and whether they are situated centrally or marginally. There are superficial mucosal and deep muscular lymphatic plexuses which join common collecting trunks. The marginal lymphatics of the tongue drain to the submental and submandibular nodes whilst some central lymphatics go directly to the nodes of the ipsilateral cervical chain and others cross the midline so that bilateral spread of tumours not uncommonly occurs.

Natural history and metastasis

Lips

The majority of tumours of the lips present at an early stage as a fissure, nodule or ulcer, but may be superficial and involve much of the lip. As the lesion progresses the typical features of an epithelioma develop with ulceration and proliferation or an admixture of the two. Rarely in neglected cases, the lesion may cause great destruction of tissue with involvement of the adjacent skin, cheek and jaw.

Metastasis to regional lymph nodes by cancers of the lips is a relatively uncommon problem. The percentage of cases presenting with clinically involved nodes is

Table 8.5   Sites of lymph node metastasis from cancer of the lips in 59 positive block dissection specimens.

Site	Number involved
Submental	3
Submandibular	57
Upper deep cervical	1
Middle deep cervical	1

about 8% (Pointon, 1972). An additional 8–10% will develop metastatic nodes within five years of presentation. Distant metastases from cancers of the lips are very uncommon and Ebenius (1943) reported only five cases occurring in a total of 792 patients, three of which were proven at autopsy.

Second primary tumours of the lips are rare, occurring in only 0.7% of cases (Pointon, 1972). The management of the new lesion will be influenced by its proximity to the original lesion. Further radiation may be practical if there is an adequate margin between the two lesions.

Oral cavity

Lymphatic metastasis to regional lymph nodes is a common problem with malignant tumours of the oral cavity. About 24% of patients with squamous cell cancers have metastatic lymphadenopathy at the time of presentation whilst an additional 36% of patients will develop nodal metastases within five years of treatment. Small differences in incidence are seen between the anatomical sites within the oral cavity (Table 8.6). In contrast, distant blood-borne metastasis is a relatively small problem, only occurring in about 4% of patients. However, reports are being made of a changing pattern in metastasis due to the greater use of cytotoxic drugs in sequential management. It would

Table 8.6   Development of metastatic lymphadenopathy in 1730 patients with oral cancers treated by irradiation.

Site	Incidence at 5 years (%)
Buccal mucosa	26.8
Palate	31.5
Alveoli	32.8
Floor of mouth	40.5
Tongue	50.0
Average	36.3

seem that better control of lymphatic metastasis is therefore increasing.

Multiple primary squamous cell cancers within the oral cavity are not a numerically frequent problem, 7.5%, but their management can sometimes be difficult. It would seem that some patients have a generalized instability of the oral mucosa that predisposes to the formation of multiple tumours that are either coexistent or develop over a period of years. Most of these are found in the lips or within the oral cavity; however, it should be remembered that neighbouring anatomical areas are also lined by squamous epithelium and that subsequent tumours may develop in these areas (Table 8.7).

Table 8.7 Incidence of multiple tumours of mouth and adjacent sites.

Site	Incidence of multiple tumours (%)
Mouth	6
Adjacent sites – nasal passages pharynx larynx proximal oesophagus	1.5

Direct extension of tumours to involve adjacent sites leads to unpleasant local manifestations of the primary tumour with progressive interference with function and appearance. Evidence of malnutrition is not uncommon at the time of presentation. This is not only a local effect of the disease but further aggravated by the age and social circumstances of many patients as well as associated infection. Extracapsular spread from regional lymph nodes leads to involvement of and fungation through overlying skin. In addition, infiltration can involve deep and vital structures especially when the deep cervical nodes are involved.

Pathology and histological classification

Squamous cell cancers account for the vast majority of malignant tumours of the lips and oral cavity. They are usually well-differentiated and anaplastic tumours are uncommon, whilst other types of malignant tumours are rare. The ratio of cancers of the lips to those of the oral cavity is 1:4. 96% of oral cancers are squamous cell in type; the remainder includes cancers of minor salivary glands, sarcomas of soft tissues, malignant melanoma, tumours of vascular and neural origin and localized manifestations of the reticuloses (Table 8.8).

Table 8.8 Incidence of different malignant tumours within the oral cavity (469 cases) (%).

Squamous cell cancers	96%
Adenoid cystic carcinoma	3%
Mucoepidermoid carcinoma	0.2%
Fibrosarcoma	0.4%
Malignant melanoma	0.2%
Angiosarcoma	0.2%

Squamous cell cancer

Grading of squamous cell cancers has some relevance to prognosis although it is not as important as other factors. It is done according to the degree of keratinization, frequency of epithelial pearls, mitotic rate, presence of atypical mitoses, numbers of multinuclear giant cells and evidence of nuclear and cellular pleomorphism. Tumours are not necessarily homogeneous so that variations are found between different samples from the same tumour. Factors that have a greater effect on prognosis are stage of disease at the time of presentation and anotomical site or a tumour. Multiple tumours occur in a small percentage of patients. These may be coexistent, when tumurs of different stages may be apparent or develop over a period of time.

Verrucous carcinoma

This tumour is regarded as a variant of squamous cell carcinoma and is characterized by its circumscribed papilliferous appearance (Fig. 8.1). The epithelium is well differentiated and epithelial pearls and small cysts are common although mitoses and cellular pleomorphism are less frequently seen. There is invariably an intense inflammatory infiltration of the stroma and often reactive lymphadenopathy. The behaviour of these tumours is indolent and metastasis occurs late and is therefore uncommon.

Leukoplakia

Leukoplakia is localized hyperkeratosis of mucous membranes which is characterized by white plaques due to the increased deposition of keratin. It may be limited in extent but can be more generalized with multiple lesions on the lips and oral mucosa or there may be larger confluent areas. Associated fissures and ulceration may be apparent with underlying chronic inflammatory reaction.

It is the more florid forms of leukoplakia in which

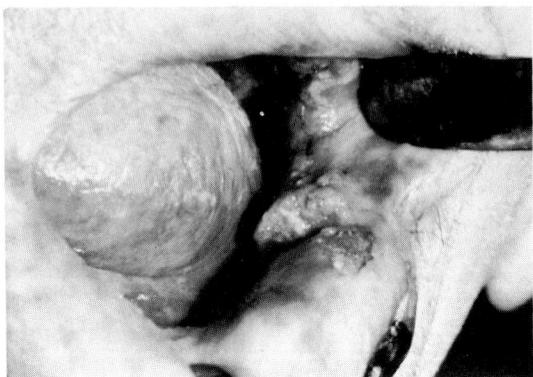

Fig. 8.1 Verrucous carcinoma arising from left buccal mucosa.

there is hyperplasia and dysplasia that must be regarded as pre-malignant (Fig.8.2). There is disturbance of normal maturation with dyskeratosis, increased mitotic rate, cellular pleomorphism and nuclear hyperchromatism. These sinister features cannot be recognized clinically so that biopsy and histological examination is essential in order to make the diagnosis. It is difficult to estimate the statistical association between leukoplakia and squamous cell cancer but, in our experience, it is of the order of 5%.

Symptoms and presentation

Cancers of the lips present in their early stages as asymptomatic fissures, ulcers or nodules. Persistence of such lesions should increase the index of clinical sus-

picion and biopsy is essential in order to make a histological diagnosis. They are initially confined to the vermilion border but progress to involve adjacent skin, the mucosa of their buccal surfaces and underlying muscle. If situated laterally, then extension occurs with involvement of the commissure of the mouth. Involvement of the mental nerve can cause paraesthesiae or numbness of the lower lip. Continued growth leads to deformity and destruction of the lips with loss of lip seal and dribbling of saliva which is aggravated by

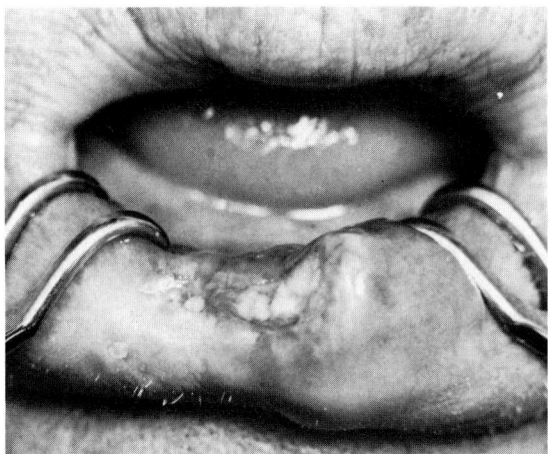

Fig. 8.3 Ulcerating carcinoma of lower lip extending to buccal surface.

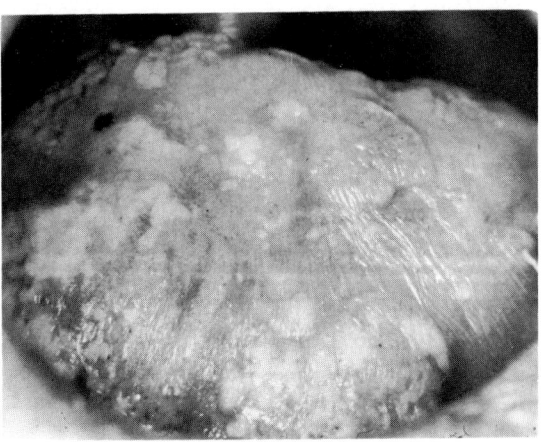

Fig. 8.2 Gross leukoplakia of tongue with multiple hyperplastic plaques.

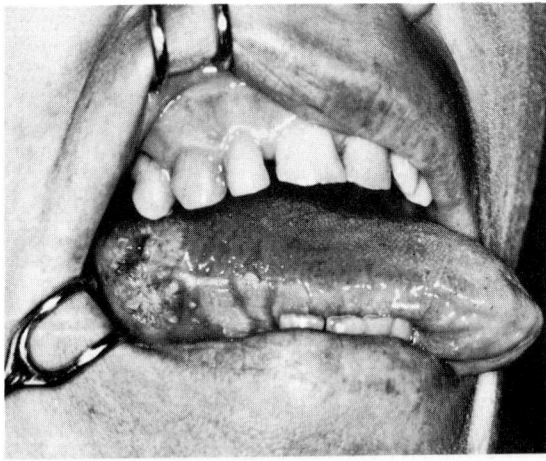

Fig. 8.4 Squamous carcinoma of right lateral border of tongue, junction of middle and posterior thirds; leukoplakic plaques can be seen on ventral surface of adjacent tongue.

eating and speech (Fig. 8.3). Ulcerative lesions, although extensive, may remain superficial. Ulceration and fungation are associated with local infection and the risk of haemorrhage.

The symptoms and presentation of oral cancers depend on their nature and anatomical situation. Squamous cell carcinomas present usually as endophytic or ulcerative lesions which may be associated with local soreness or discomfort although less commonly may have a nodular or papillary appearance (Fig. 8.4). Malignant ulcers have typically irregular, raised and indurated margins whilst the base is either covered by slough or appears granular and red. Persistance of ulceration despite local conservative treatment must be regarded with suspicion and biopsy is again essential in order to make a definite diagnosis. Miscellaneous tumours of the oral cavity tend to present as exophytic or nodular lesions with ulceration tending to occur later in the course of their growth. Tumours of the tongue infiltrate underlying muscles leading to tethering with loss of mobility that interferes with both eating and speech. Invasion of adjacent areas occurs by direct extension to the floor of the mouth, tonsillar fossa or lateral pharyngeal walls. Most of the patients with oral squamous cell cancers are from the later decades of life and are therefore oedentulous so that tumours of the alveoli and hard palate often present due to irritation by or instability of dentures. In such patients, tumours of the upper alveoli tend to present at a more advanced stage than those of the

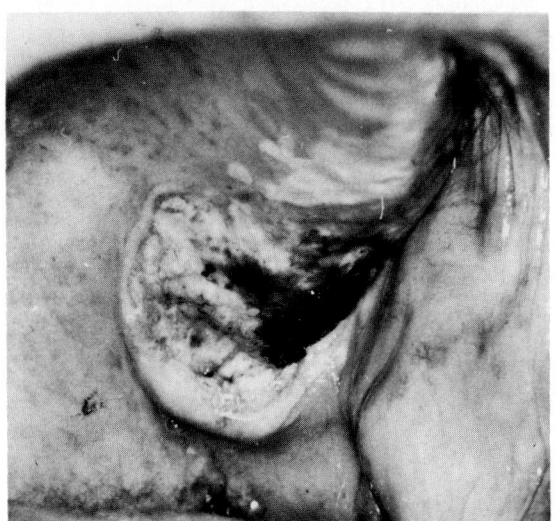

Fig. 8.5 Ulcerating carcinoma of left upper alveolus extending to hard palate.

lower alveoli, presumably due to them being in a less readily visible situation (Fig. 8.5).

Alveolar tumours often spread locally following the periosteal plane of the jaws. Invasion of bone is a cause of severe and sometimes intractable pain, especially when there is invasion of the mandible with involvement of the inferior dental nerve and rapid extension of tumour along the inferior dental canal. Tumours of the buccal mucosa and retromolar triangles may infiltrate adjacent muscles of the cheeks and pterygoid regions causing increasing trismus and difficulty in eating. Obstruction of the outlet of the parotid and submandibular ducts may occur as a local effect of buccal tumours or those of the floor of the mouth associated with non-specific sialadenitis of these major salivary glands and the development of tender painful swellings.

The majority of miscellaneous malignant tumours of the oral cavity tend to present as nodular expanding lesions that may eventually ulcerate and bleed. Malignant melanoma begins as a localized pigmented lesion with increase in size and variability in the degree of pigmentation although, occasionally, the tumours may be amelanotic.

Leukoplakia is sometimes seen in association with squamous carcinoma of the lips and oral cavity. It is characterized by the presence of white plaques due to increased deposits of keratin. There may be associated inflammatory changes or fissuring. Of greater significance are the appearance of hyperplastic plaques of frank ulceration with an increase in tissue bulk. Although there is no recognized increase in association between squamous cell cancer and lichen planus of the oral cavity, these conditions may coexist. Lichen planus is typified by the often generalized inflammatory reaction with an atrophic mucosal appearance and irregular areas of superficial ulceration which may be extensive.

Metastatic regional lymphadenopathy invariably presents with one or more asymptomatic lumps in the neck. Symptoms do not develop until there is extracapsular spread of disease with involvement of overlying skin or fixity to deeper vital structures.

Significant degrees of malnutrition may be readily apparent with obvious weight loss but lesser degrees depend on physical and biochemical measurement for recognition and confirmation. Copeland and his colleagues (1978) have defined malnutrition according to objective criteria and two of their criteria are easily applicable in clinical practice: (*a*) recent loss of 10 lbs or more of body weight; (*b*) serum albumin concentration of less than 3.4 grams %. Supplementary or alternative feeding can make good the deficit thus helping patients to withstand the effects of treatment.

Diagnosis

As an orificial and readily accessible lesion, clinical diagnosis of lip cancer is usually not difficult. A persistent ulcer on the lip should be regarded as malignant and biopsy is therefore essential.

Frank squamous cell carcinoma of the oral cavity should not present difficulty in diagnosis. The principal difficulty arises when there is a general instability of the mucosa or when leukoplakia is present. Adequate biopsy is essential and serial biopsies of any suspicious areas should be undertaken. Where there is the possibility of bone involvement full radiology of the jaw should be carried out, including sinus films for lesions of the palate and upper alveoli.

Every patient should have routine full blood counts and chest X-rays.

Clinical staging

Clinical staging provides accurate assessment of the extent of tumours of the lips and oral cavity at the time of presentation. Such information can be used to determine policies of treatment and analysis of the results of treatment. Using the TNM Classification of the International Union Against Cancer, the assessment of nodal and metastatic disease is common to both sites, but there are differences in assessment of primary tumours (Table 8.9)

Treatment policy

Lips

Cancers of the lips can be cured by any well planned method of radiotherapy or surgery and failure to control the primary tumour occurs only in exceptional circumstances. Irradiation of small and moderate tumours gives a high cure rate whilst maintaining good cosmetic and functional results and it is therefore the initial treatment of choice in the majority of centres in Great Britain. Surgery is used primarily for more extensive tumours, for those developing on a lip that is wholly at risk because of specific aetiological factors and for those of known limited radiosensitivity. It is also used as a second treatment after irradiation has been used but failed.

Oral cavity

The successful management of oral cancer is the product of a multi-disciplinary approach involving radiotherapist, surgeon, oral surgeon, pathologist and chemotherapist. It is not only desirable but sensible that the treating clinicians should see the patient together before definitive treatment is decided upon.

Table 8.9 TNM classification of tumours of the lips and oral cavity.

1. T – *Primary tumour of lip*

T_1S Pre-invasive carcinoma (carcinoma in situ)

T_0 No evidence of primary tumour

T_1 Tumour measuring 2 cm or less in its largest dimension, strictly superficial or exophytic

T_2 Tumour measuring 2 cm or less in its largest dimension, with minimal infiltration in depth

T_3 Tumour measuring more than 2 cm in its largest dimension, or tumour with deep infiltration, irrespective of its size

T_4 Tumour involving bone

2. T – *Primary tumour of oral cavity*

T_1S Pre-invasive carcinoma (carcinoma in situ)

T_1 Tumour 2 cm or less in its greatest dimension

T_2 Tumour more than 2 cm but not more than 4 cm in its greatest dimension

T_3 Tumour more than 4 cm in its greatest dimension

3. N – *Regional lymph nodes*

N_0 Regional lymph nodes not palpable

N_1 Moveable homolateral nodes
N_{1a}: Nodes not considered to contain growth
N_{1b}: Nodes considered to contain growth

N_2 Moveable contralateral or bilateral nodes
N_{2a}: Nodes not considered to contain growth
N_{2b}: Nodes considered to contain growth

N_3 Fixed nodes

4. M – *Distant metastasis*

M_0 No evidence of distant metastases

M_1 Distant metastases present

While each form of treatment will be specific for the individual patient, it is cogent that a sequential treatment policy is followed for otherwise it becomes impossible to treat enough cases similarly to evaluate the chosen treatment policy.

If progress in the results of treatment is to be achieved, periodic review of the roles of each mode of treatment are essential. Whenever possible these reviews should be based on random clinical trials. Such trials should be based on sound statistical principles and adequate numbers of cases.

At present radiotherapy and surgery remain the main effective methods of treatment of carcinoma of the oral cavity. The emphasis on each method will vary from centre to centre and will be influenced by the resources available and the experience of the clinicians involved.

In the treatment of oral cancer both radiotherapy

and surgery should be used almost only when there is a high probability of primary control. Palliative radiotherapy and surgery have generally been found to be of little value and for the majority of patients with advanced disease add to rather than relieve their symptoms.

At the Christie Hospital and Holt Radium Institute, approximately 10% of cases on presentation have disease that is too advanced for any useful radiotherapy or surgery. Modern chemotherapy, however, can often give useful palliation without severe side-effects. The agreed policy of management has been that radiotherapy is the treatment of choice for the majority of squamous carcinomas of the oral cavity and of all cases treated, 95% are treated with radiotherapy and only 5% with primary surgery, although secondary surgery is used more often. At the M.D. Anderson Hospital, Houston, Texas, of 521 cases of oral cancer presenting without nodes, 70% were treated with radiotherapy and 30% with primary surgery (Jesse *et al.*, 1970).

Metastatic nodes

Treatment of mobile metastatic lymphadenopathy of the neck secondary to tumours of the lips and oral cavity is best done by surgical block dissection. However, a holding dose of irradiation may be given to a small field in order to allow completion of treatment of a primary tumour by radiotherapy before clearance of the cervical nodes can be done.

Surgery for cancers of the lips and oral cavity

In Great Britain, surgery for malignant tumours of the lips and oral cavity is more often used after previous irradiation. This approach to treatment is in contrast to that of the United States of America, where surgery is more often the initial choice of treatment. The difference in attitude perhaps reflects the method of referral in the two countries.

Although it is not pertinent to describe surgical procedures in detail, an understanding of basic principles and some knowledge of the variety of surgical techniques and their results is essential for all those concerned in their management regardless of therapeutic background. Such information is especially important in view of the increasing dependence on multidisciplinary collaboration with wider application of carefully selected sequential treatment and the introduction of synchronous treatment using different methods in combination.

Primary surgery

Surgery is used as first treatment for malignant tumours of the lips and oral cavity under special but uncommon circumstances. Some of these are common to both situations whilst others are specific to each.

Common indications for primary surgery
1. Large or extensive tumours – for which irradiation is inevitably bound to fail because of the volume of tumour.
2. Extensive associated leukoplakia – where there is a wide field change requiring treatment as well as the primary tumour.
3. Multiple tumours – when overlapping fields of irradiation would be inevitable and the risk of radionecrosis therefore increased.
4. Tumours of known limited radiosensitivity – e.g. malignant melanomas, soft tissue sarcomas.
5. Radiation-induced tumours – both occupational and therapeutic.

Specific indications for primary surgery
1. *Lips:*
   – young patients, in whom radiation-induced tumours are a real risk at a later point in time.
   – exposure to extreme weather conditions, with persistence of a known contributory factor, e.g. farm workers, fishermen.
2. *Oral cavity:*
   – special anatomical site, e.g. tip of tongue, a difficult site to treat by irradiation because of its lack of support.

Histological confirmation of the diagnosis must always be obtained before definitive surgery and, in most instances, this should be combined with examination under anaesthesia so that proper assessment of the tumour can be made.

Primary surgery can often be relatively limited in extent provided that an adequate margin of tissue is excised for clearance of the tumour. For small or moderate tumours of the lips, wedge-shaped excision with direct closure is done. The wedge is cut through the full thickness of the lip and is shaped like a shield with curved borders so that a smaller block of tissue need only be removed. The lip should always be repaired in three separate layers, mucosa, muscle and skin. Up to 30% of the length of either lip can be excised in this way without significant cosmetic or functional disability. If larger excision is indicated then the defect should be repaired with a local flap (see Table 8.10) from the other lip, an Abbe-Estlander flap, in order to provide lips of equal length although this has an effect on symmetry about the midline.

The Abbe-Estlander flap is a rotational full-thickness flap dependent for its initial viability on the appropriate labial artery which forms a vascular pedicle. It is designed to be slightly smaller than the

Table 8.10 Flaps used for reconstruction.

Local flaps	– used for repair of small defects or for particular purposes, e.g. replacement of vermilion border of lip
	  1. nasolabial skin
	  2. tongue, with or without underlying muscle to provide bulk

Regional flaps	– used for repair of larger defects, either internal or external
	  1. *Simple*, i.e. skin with subcutaneous tissue
	  (*a*) *Axial* – blood supply from named vessels dependent on normal multiple anastomoses (multiple angiotomes)
	    (i) forehead non-hairy skin
	    (ii) deltopectoral suitable for internal or external use
	    (iii) bipolar forehead and scalp – for use in the male with non-hairy forehead skin for lining and hairy scalp skin for cover
	  (*b*) *Random* – random blood supply
	    (i) transverse cervical
	    (ii) nape of neck
	  2. *Compound*, i.e. skin with subcutaneous tissue and underlying muscle with axial blood supply
	    (i) trapezius
	    (ii) pectoralis major
	    (iii) latissimus dorsi

Free flaps	– tissue from a distant site with its blood vessels for direct microvascular anastomosis to appropriate regional vessels of similar calibre
	  1. *Simple*, i.e. skin with subcutaneous tissue and blood vessels of supply
	    (i) dorsalis pedis – thin flap suitable for lining or cover
	    (ii) groin – thicker flap due to depth of subcutaneous tissue suitable for cover rather than lining
	  2. *Compound*, i.e. skin, subcutaneous tissue, muscle and even bone with blood vessels of supply
	    (i) anterior rib – with segments of internal mammary vessels for anastomosis
	    (ii) iliac crest – with circumflex iliac vessels

defect it is going to fill in order to conserve maximal length of both lips. The vascular pedicle is divided after an interval of two weeks by which time the new blood supply has developed and inset can be completed. For patients whose whole lip is at risk, due to leukoplakia or exposure to extreme weather, wedge excision is combined with excision of the whole vermilion border, lip shave. The vermilion can be replaced by either advancing mucosa from the buccal surface of the lip, a procedure that tends to produce an indrawn lip, or by application of a narrow tongue flap so that the mucosa replaces the vermilion border. Ventral mucosa produces a better cosmetic appearance in the female, since it is smoother, but dorsal mucosa will suffice for the male.

Relatively small tumours of the anterior third of the tongue, including the tip, can be excised as a wedge with direct closure of the defect without functional disability. Moderately-sized tumours of the tongue, without significant local infiltration into the underlying muscles, can be excised by partial glossectomy without need for reconstruction (Fig. 8.6). Provided that haemostasis is secured at the time of operation then the cut surface does not need cover and it will re-epithelialize within a short period of time. Transverse or oblique resection of the tongue is accompanied by

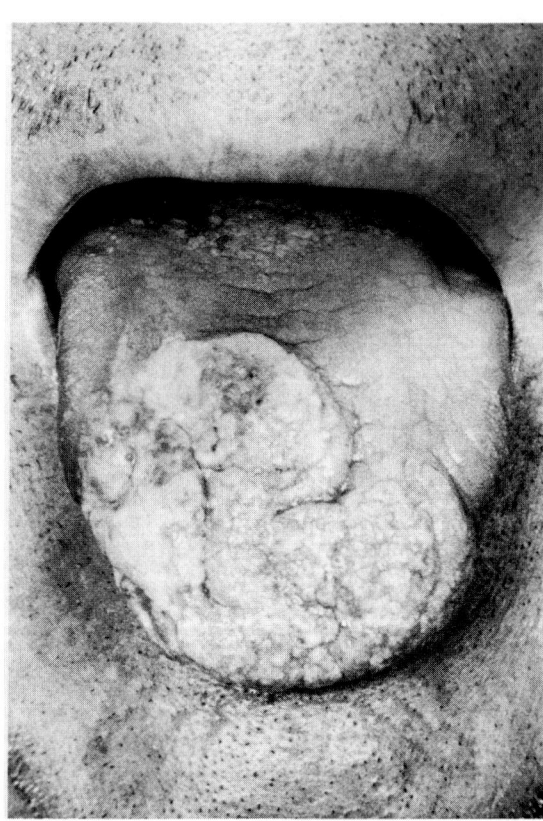

Fig. 8.6 Extensive but superficial ´squamous carcinoma superimposed on syphilitic slossitis.

less functional interference than longitudinal resection when fibrosis during healing can cause tethering with a loss of essential mobility. It is unusual that other intra-oral tumours can be treated by localized surgery although, on occasions, this may be possible. Primary closure of the defect after excision of tumours of the buccal mucosa can sometimes be done provided that this does not lead to a shortage of tissue and produce trismus. Very occasionally, localized alveolar tumours can be excised by marginal or segmental resection but the indications for limited surgery must be carefully assessed.

Secondary surgery

Surgery for cancers of the lips and oral cavity is more often used secondary to irradiation and is then more radical in extent and has become known as 'salvage surgery'. The indications for its use are:

1. Residual tumour – when a tumour has proved, insensitive to irradiation.
2. Recurrent tumour – when a tumour undergoes initial regression but recurs after a of period time, only moderately sensitive to irradiation.
3. Radionecrosis – an uncommon problem, occurring in about 6% of patients but only 2% have major complications that require surgical treatment (Fig. 8.7).

Radical surgery has two components, resection and reconstruction. Resection must include the primary

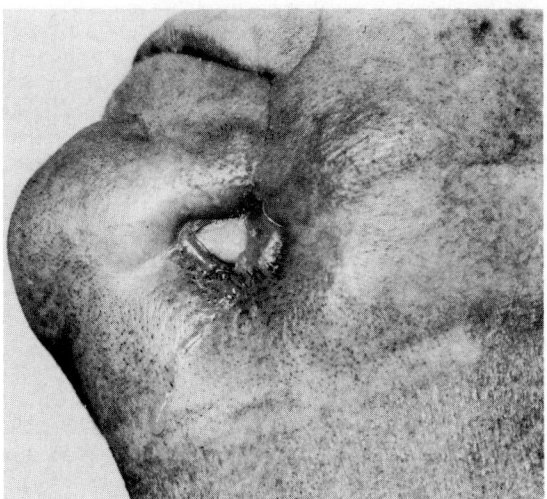

Fig. 8.7 Osteoradionecrosis with an orocutaneous fistula at two years after irradiation for squamous carcinoma of the left lower alveolus.

tumour with an adequate margin of clearance and previously irradiated tissue so that repair is done between normal healthy tissues. It is often necessary during surgery for oral tumours to include block dissection of cervical lymph nodes in continuity. The full extent of resection can only be assessed by appropriate radiological examination in order to look for invasion of adjacent bone and by examination under anaesthesia with geographic biopsy. The adequacy of excision must always be monitored at operation by histological examination with frozen section technique of multiple biopsies from the edges of resection. Reconstruction is designed to replace mucosal lining, provide new external skin cover and give alternative support in place of bone if necessary.

Loss of the middle third of the mandible without replacement of support produces an unacceptable deformity, the 'Andy Gump' deformity, whereas unilateral loss of the lateral third of the mandible is associated with minimal disability provided that there is adequate replacement of soft tissues, although deviation across the midline occurs during movement due to unopposed muscular action. Many types of mandibular prosthesis have been designed but there is no ideal. Immediate reconstruction of the mandible using a segment of clavicle carried on a vascular pedicle formed by sternomastoid muscle (Siemssen *et al.*, 1978), free flap transfer of anterior rib and microvascular anastomosis of its vessels of supply (Arryan, 1978) or delayed free bone graft can be considered in younger patients but are not suited to older edentulous patients who have had previous irradiation. The simplest prosthetic method of mandibular replacement is by use of a twist of stainless-steel wire covered by a sleeve of silastic tubing in order to stop it cutting through overlying soft tissues (Towers and Wilson, 1974) (Fig. 8.8). Sometimes, because of local complications, the prosthesis must be removed but provided that it has remained in position for a period of at least three weeks then it will probably have provoked sufficient fibrous reaction to provide an acceptable cosmetic result.

The choice of methods used for reconstruction of a defect in soft tissue is complex due to the wide variety of flaps that have been designed for such purposes (Table 8.10). Proper selection in order to achieve the best cosmetic and functional result for each patient can only be made providing the surgeon is familiar with all methods. Factors that influence the choice include age and sex of the patient; size, shape and situation of the defect; as well as colour and texture of the tissues to be used. Such surgery is complex and time-consuming, often depending on a series of staged procedures.

When local or regional flaps are used for reconstruction, an interval of three weeks must be allowed

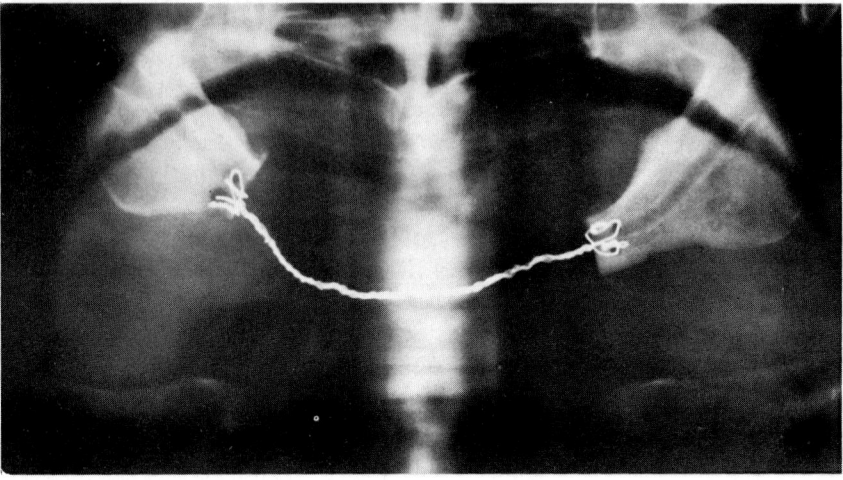

Fig. 8.8   Simple wire twist bridging mandibular defect after resection of middle third of mandible for squamous carcinoma of anterior floor of mouth extending to lower alveolus.

between stages for flaps to establish their blood supply in their new position during which time the feeding vessels are essential for viability. The pedicles of the flaps are divided subsequently, inset of the flap into the defect completed and redundant tissue returned to the donor site. Initial cover of all donor sites is provided by split skin grafts although the eventual grafted area may be quite small in size. It is essential that the design of reconstruction should never prejudice the adequacy of resection and for this reason, in many centres, the surgery is undertaken as collaborative teamwork, one surgeon being responsible for resection and another for reconstruction.

Radical excision of the whole upper or lower lip necessitates reconstruction. This is best done using a forehead flap based on the anterior branch of one superficial temporal artery. The flap is folded longitudinally and inset to the mucosal and cutaneous edges of the defect (Fig. 8.9). After an interval of three weeks, the flap is divided, its inset completed and the redundant portion returned to the temporal region. The folded forehead skin provides rather bulky replacement but initial trimming of subcutaneous tissue would prejudice viability; however, this can be adjusted once the skin has become soft and pliable. After an interval of a few months, the fold is incised and its bulk reduced. The vermilion border can then be reconstituted using a bipedicled mucosal flap from the edge of the anterior tongue which is divided and its inset completed after an interval of two weeks.

Radical resection of the oral tongue should be combined with some form of reconstruction since the functional result is improved if the bulk of the tongue is replaced. A deltopectoral flap, the skin of the upper chest wall supplied by perforating branches of the second, third and fourth intercostal arteries, is well suited for this purpose. It is raised and passed through a dependent salivary fistula in the submental and submandibular regions and inset posteriorly to the mucosal edge of the residual pharyngeal tongue and laterally to the mucosa of the floor of the mouth on either side. The middle part of the flap is converted to a tube pedicle (Fig. 8.10*a*) and the donor site covered with split skin grafts. The flap is divided after three weeks and its intraoral inset completed anteriorly whilst the redundant skin is returned to the chest wall. Slight folding of the portion of the flap used for intraoral repair helps to replace the bulk of the tongue with simulation of the tip of the tongue, allowing improved mobility for eating and speech (Fig. 8.10*b*).

Lateral resection of the mandible with significant loss of mucosal lining for alveolar or retromolar tumours requires reconstruction and this is best done using forehead skin. Since alternative support is not needed to replace the mandible, it is convenient to disarticulate the segment at the tempero-mandibular joint as this will allow more space for passage of the flap. A complete forehead flap is raised using the whole cosmetic unit because it is a more acceptable cosmetic defect than a partial forehead flap. It is tunnelled deep

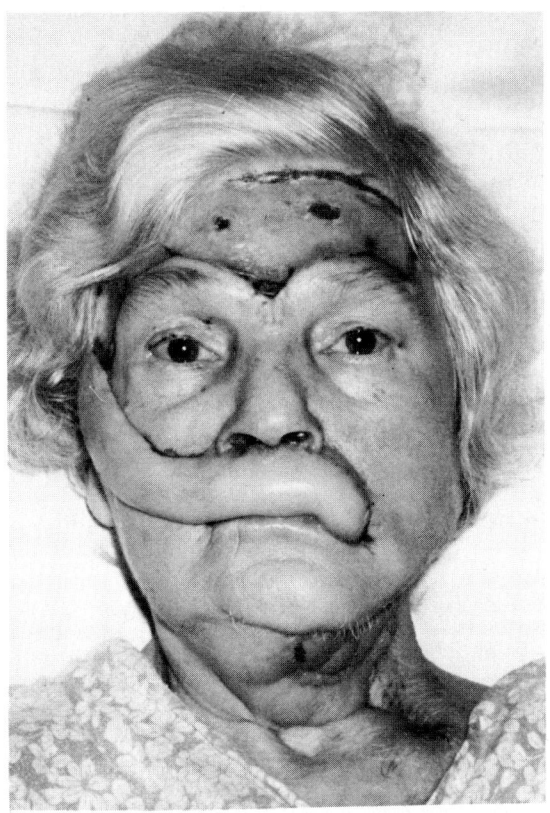

Fig. 8.9 Initial reconstruction of upper lip with folded forehead flap and split skin graft to forehead donor site.

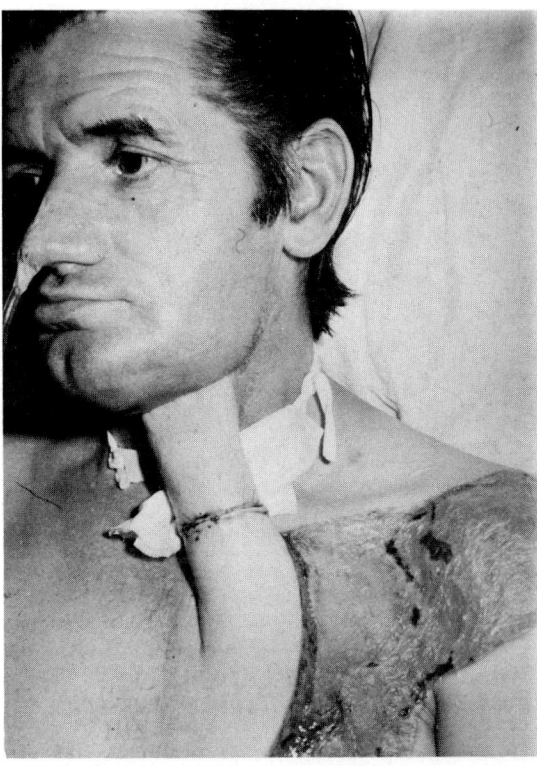

Fig. 8.10(a) Deltopectoral flap passing through dependent salivary fistula for a reconstruction of tongue after sub-total glossectomy.

to the zygomatic arch and through the soft tissues of the cheek into the oral cavity. The flap is trimmed to fit the defect but adequate skin should be allowed to compensate for loss of the mandibular arch and preserve facial symmetry as far as possible (Fig. 8.11). It is inset into the mucosal defect. On occasions, for large invasive tumours, it is necessary to take part of the lateral tongue. If this is done, then the medial edge of the skin flap is better inset to the cut muscle of the tongue rather than to the dorsal mucosa. This produces a step between tongue and the new lining which reduces the amount of lateral tethering with preservation of better mobility. The anterior floor of the mouth is best relined with a forehead flap (Fig. 8.12). If the covering skin of the mental region has to be included within the limit of excision then a second flap will be required in order to provide sufficient tissue for proper reconstruction. Occasionally, it is necessary, for large infiltrating

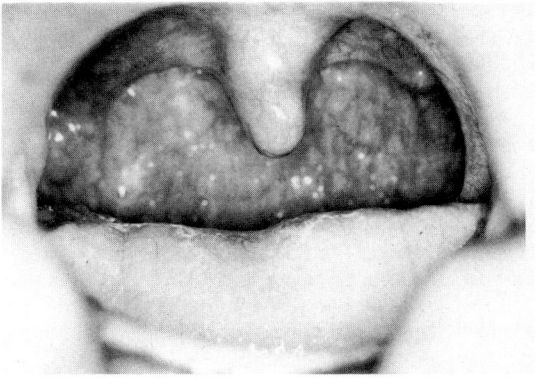

Fig. 8.10(b) Finished intraoral appearance of deltopectoral flap used for replacement of tongue after sub-total glossectomy.

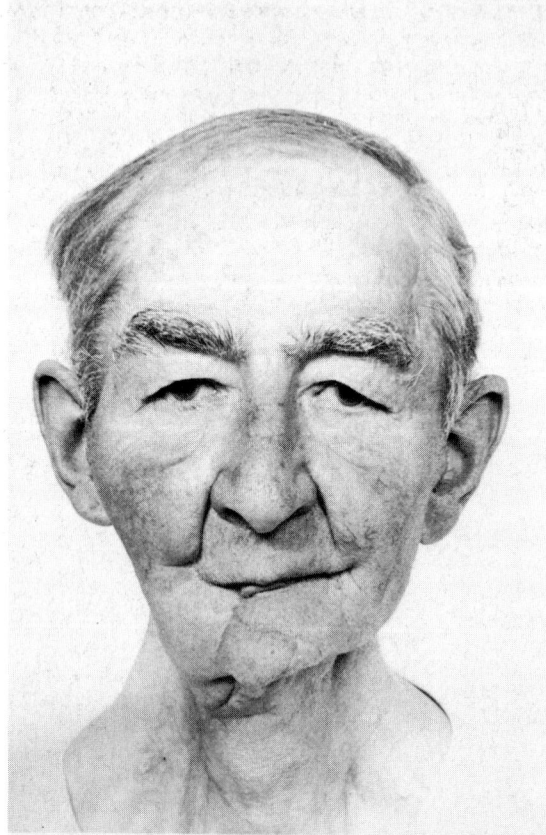

Fig. 8.11 Patient after right hemimandibulectomy and replacement with forehead flap for lining.

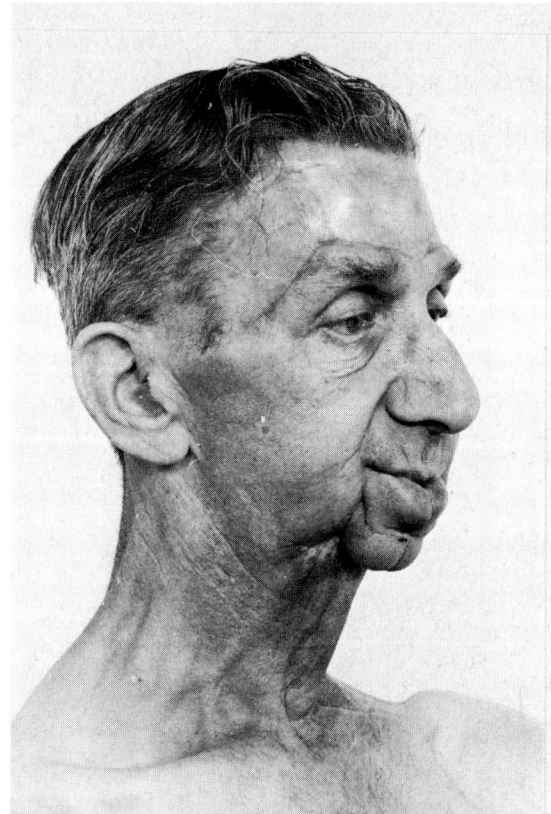

Fig. 8.12 Appearance after resection of middle third of mandible. Forehead flap used for lining and replacement of bony defect by simple wire twist.

tumours, to resect most of the lower third of the face and repair is then more complex needing a forehead flap for lining and bilateral deltopectoral flaps for rebuilding the chin and lower lip (Figs. 8.13 *a, b*).

Cancers of the buccal mucosa spread quickly by local invasion to involve the skin of the cheek. Full thickness excision of the cheek is often therefore needed for clearance of such tumours. If the defect is relatively small, a single forehead flap can be folded transversely to give both lining and cover. The edge of the fold must be shaved since it is to be implanted into the cheek. This technique needs careful assessment of the adequacy of available skin with allowance for contraction during healing in order to prevent a shortage of tissue and ultimate trismus. Usually, two flaps are required for repair of such defects. In the female, for whom non-hairy skin is needed for both lining and cover, a forehead flap is used for lining combined with a deltopectoral flap for cover. In the male, for whom

hair-bearing skin is desirable for use as cover, the bipolar forehead and scalp flap can be used. The forehead flap does not need to be tunnelled through into the oral cavity but is raised and simply turned over on itself for inset into the mucosal defect. The scalp flap, dependent on the posterior branch of the superficial temporal artery, is raised and rotated into position for external cover (Fig. 8.14 *a, b*). The flaps are divided, their inset completed and redundant tissue returned after an interval of three weeks.

Palatal and upper alveolar tumours, depending on their size, necessitate partial or sometimes complete but conservative maxillectomy. Access to the maxilla is obtained by splitting the upper lip and reflecting the soft tissues of the cheek as a flap. Unless these tumours are very large, it is usually possible to preserve the floor of the orbit. Initially, the passages of the external nose and oral cavity are then in free continuity. Relining of

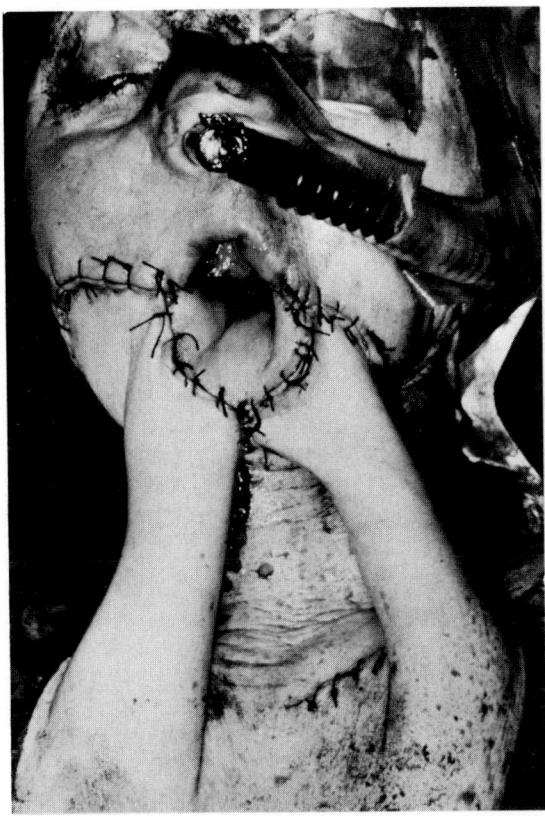

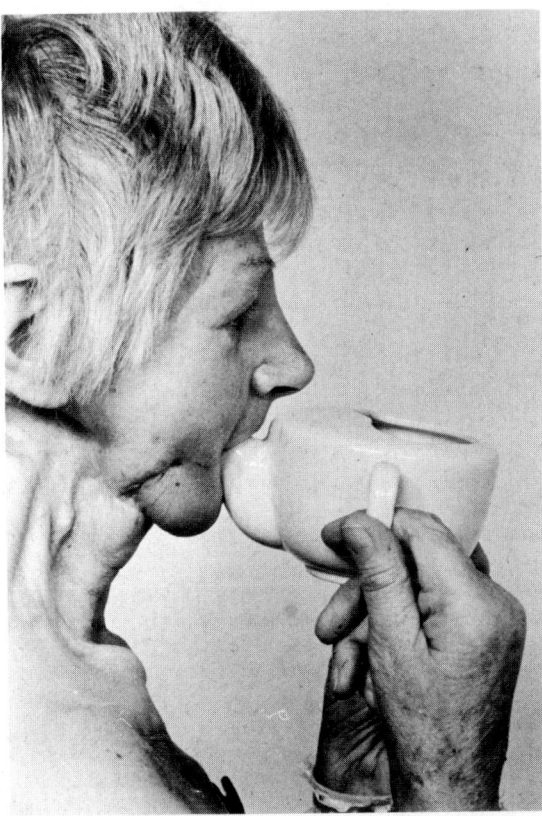

Fig. 8.13(a)   Radical resection and first stage of reconstruction for simulatneous squamous carcinomas of right lower buccal surface of left lower lip necessitating removal of middle third of mandible. Patient had had a previous total glossectomy. Forehead flap used for oral lining and bilateral deltopectoral flaps for external cover.

Fig. 8.13(b)   Patient after completion of reconstruction with acceptable function.

the cavity is most often done with split skin grafts draped over a mould made from dental compound which is supported by an upper dental plate and fixed with wires around the zygomatic arches. The plate and mould are removed after an interval of ten days and the cavity is also inspected. A definitive upper denture with obturator to fill the cavity is then made which prevents communication between nose and oral cavity which is essential for normal speech and swallowing without nasal reflux. Occasionally, bilateral maxillectomy is indicated for extensive infiltrating tumours. The subsequent dental prosthesis with obturator is perhaps the greatest challenge for dental technicians. Usually, the prosthesis is supported by fibrous bands that form in

the cheeks but mechanical support with fine springs attached posteriorly to a lower denture may be needed (Fig. 8.15).

The application of free flaps with microvascular anastomosis for reconstruction after resection of oral tumours has not yet been fully determined. The facial artery and vein, as they cross the lower border of the mandible, are readily available for use as recipient vessels for either internal or external repair. Such techniques reduce the need for multiple staged procedures but total operating time is long and this may be undesirable especially in elderly patients with underlying medical problems. Careful selection of suitable cases for such methods of reconstruction is needed in order to build up sufficient experience to determine their uses and limitations.

Temporary respiratory bypass by tracheostomy is necessary in some cases in order to prevent acute problems after operation due to loss of essential support to the upper airway or obstruction due to oedema or

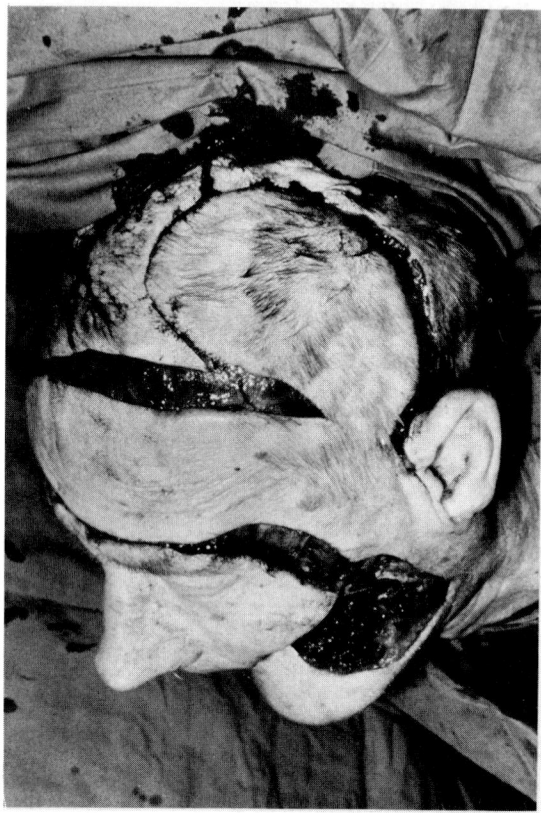

Fig. 8.14(a) Bipolar forehead and scalp flap for reconstruction of full thickness defect of left cheek for second verrucous carcinoma.

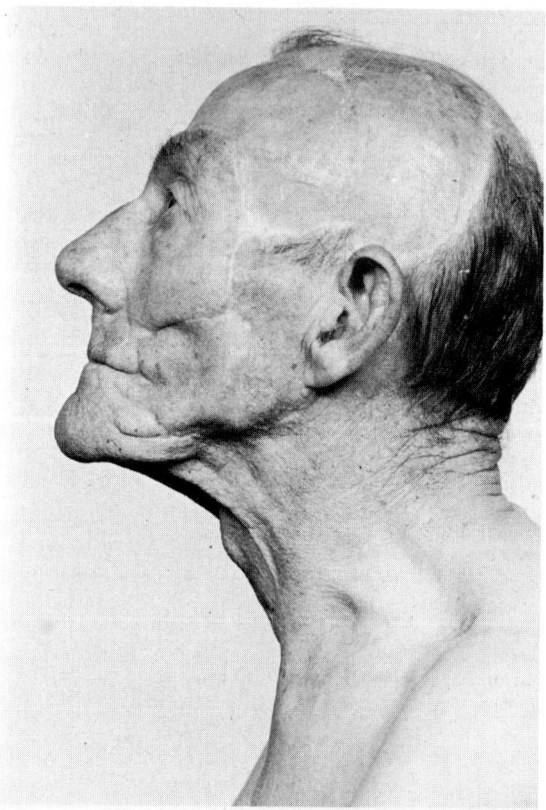

Fig. 8.14(b) Patient at nine months after completion of surgery. Donor sites grafted with split skin.

haematoma. Alternative nutritional support must be given after operation until return to normal oral feeding can be achieved whilst for patients with evidence of malnutrition such feeding should be commenced before operation. High levels of nutrition can be given either by nasogastric tube or intravenous feeding which minimize the catabolic effects of surgery and facilitate wound healing and reaction to infection. Such regimes, however, need careful supervision with regular monitoring of biochemical indices since such methods of feeding can induce temporary hepatic dysfunction (Tweedle *et al.*, 1979).

The complete care of patients demands a high level of nursing with attention to both physical and psychological effects. Many other ancillary departments are also called upon during daily management. Pharmacists are involved in the calculation and preparation of alternative nutrition, whilst dieticians are essential to the supervision of return to oral feeding both during

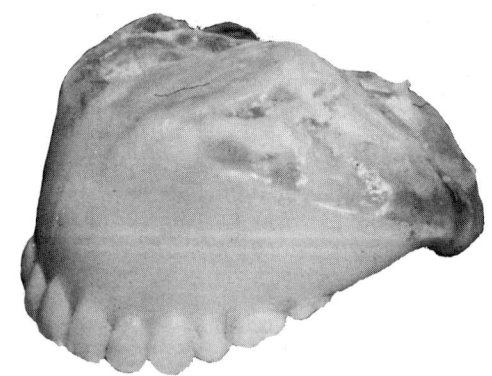

Fig. 8.15 Light hollow upper dental prosthesis with obturator for use after bilateral maxillectomy for mucosal malignant melanoma of hard palate.

the convalescent period and also after discharge from hospital. Because of the average age of patients undergoing this type of surgery, intensive physiotherapy is required for all patients in order to reduce the incidence of significant chest infection and especially in the care of patients with an elective tracheostomy. Dental hygienists are of great help in the early period after operation when a high standard of oral hygiene improves well-being and promotes wound healing. Prosthetic technicians are important to the ultimate result both in the preparation of dental prostheses and when an external prosthesis is needed to supplement surgical reconstruction.

Such radical surgery is complex and its results, in terms of cure and palliation must justify its use. Although acceptable cosmetic and functional results can be achieved within a limited period of time, further additional procedures may become indicated in order to effect the optimum result. The need for these is only determined by careful objective and subjective assessment during long-term follow-up.

Metastic nodes

The management of metastatic nodes is described in Chapter 14.

Cryotherapy for pre-malignant conditions

Cryosurgery is finding a place in the treatment of pre-malignant conditions of the oral cavity. It depends for its success on dehydration and disruption of cells by freezing with liquid nitrogen or nitrous oxide. This may be done with the use of a fine open-ended nozzle or probes of varying size with closed ends or plates for direct application. The latter is the method that has been used more extensively and found greater favour. Control of the open-ended nozzle is difficult due to the cloud of gas that is emitted. A small lesion may be amenable to single application of a closed probe whilst more extensive areas need multiple applications with overlap of the edges. The closed probes produce an approximately hemispherical ice-ball including the abnormal lesion and a margin of normal tissue. A maximum period of application of two minutes and rewarming of five minutes is usually allowed although slightly shorter periods may be used for areas of very superficial change. The lesions suited to this type of treatment are keratoses, leukoplakia and erythroplakia. Careful follow-up should, however, be maintained. Studies are currently in progress and more time is needed to assess the long-term outcome.

Complications of surgery

Early

Haemorrhage
Haemorrhage after operation is usually associated with infection when named or significant blood vessels are affected. Provided that prompt resuscitation and treatment by replacement of blood and control of bleeding is done then the outcome is good. Even when dramatic bleeding occurs from a carotid artery, it is not necessarily fatal, although cerebral ischaemia and hemiparesis may follow. The outcome of a carotid 'blow-out' depends on the level at which it occurs in the carotid arterial tree and adequacy of the collateral circulation from the opposite side.

Wound infection
Wound infections are not uncommon after labial and oral surgery but this is hardly surprising on consideration of the bacterial flora of the oral cavity. Since the consequences can be serious when reconstruction has been done, prophylactic use of broad spectrum antibiotic cover is justifiable and accepted practice. Of particular seriousness is the development of infection of prosthetic replacement of the middle third of the mandible, when it becomes an indication for removal of the prosthesis.

Wound dehiscence
Dehiscence of wounds is due either to wound infection or previous irradiation. Separation occurs most commonly at the junction of incisions, especially when triradiate. If limited in extent, then granulation and re-epithelization can be awaited but, if extensive, then cover by grafts or flaps must be considered especially if a major blood vessel is exposed.

Necrosis of flaps
Necrosis of flaps does occur after reconstruction but it is fortunately uncommon. Age, type of flap and mechanical factors may contribute to the development of this complication. Pressure must never be allowed over the pedicle of local or regional flaps since it can lead to ischaemia. Similarly, twisting or kinking of a vascular pedicle can have a similar effect.

If necrosis does occur and is limited in extent then the flap can often be trimmed, advanced and re-inset to fulfil its original purpose. Should more extensive necrosis occur and there be insufficient length of a flap for advancement then it may be suitable for conversion to and implantation as a tube pedicle.

Late

The late complications of radical surgery are essentially

those of altered appearance and function. Further surgical procedures may become indicated which will improve matters and effect the optimum result. Insufficient replacement of soft tissue and an excess can both lead to a poor functional result but trimming of an excess is a simpler matter than provision of additional soft tissue which is a major procedure. Adjustment of facial scars or other cosmetic deformities relieves embarrassment and give increased confidence.

Loss of lip seal with dribbling of saliva and food may follow total replacement of a lip since the new tissue has no active muscular component. Excision of redundant tissue to tighten the lip or support with a fascial sling can effect marked improvement. The tongue may become fixed due to contraction of scar tissue when remobilization and an inlay graft to the floor of mouth can correct the situation with improved speech and mastication. Trismus may develop after resection of buccal tumours due to the formation of fibrous bands which can be corrected by Z-plasty. Other causes of trismus must be treated mechanically by the use of wedges or a screw.

Correction of such complications improves the quality of life and thereby facilitates rehabilitation. Continuing follow-up is therefore not only of importance to control of disease but also to ensure optimum cosmetic and functional results.

Radiotherapy for cancer of the lip

The selection of the preferred method of treatment will be influenced by the extent of the lesion, i.e. size or thickness, the age and general condition of the patient, technical facilities available and local preference.

The present modes of irradiation employed are:

1. *X-ray therapy*
   (a) Superficial X-ray therapy 100–140 kV.
   (b) Orthovoltage X-ray therapy 300 kV.
2. Electron therapy 8–10 MeV.
3. Surface applicator (double mould radium or ^{60}Co).
4. Interstitial irradiation (radium needle or equivalent, or gold (^{198}Au) grains or seeds).

X-ray therapy

This is the most universal method of radiotherapy. The advantages are:

1. No operative procedure required.
2. Minimum of technical skill required.
3. No handling of radioactive sources by personnel.
4. Treatment may be commenced with minimum of delay.
5. Exposure times are short and out-patient treatment is very feasible.

Superficial X-ray therapy

As the majority of lip cancers are not unduly thick, X-ray energies of 100–140 kV of HVL 2–3 mm Al provide an adequate depth dose. To shield the mouth a suitably moulded lead sheet carried on a 'bite' is slipped behind the lip. This shielding may be combined with an external lead cut-out to reduce the tissue irradiated to an adequate minimum. For this X-ray energy, 1 mm of lead is sufficient. Dosage of 4500 rad is given in 8 treatments over 10 days. Dick (1962) using 140kV gave 3850 rad in 7 treatments over 8 days. In aged subjects with a small lesion exposure of 1750–2000 rad is a simple effective measure.

Orthovoltage X-ray therapy

For lesions too thick for superficial X-ray therapy resort may be made to orthovoltage X-ray therapy, i.e. 300 kV. A single direct field is used which subtends the lesion and an adequate margin. Similar lead shielding is employed as with superficial X-ray therapy, but the lead will need to be 2 mm thick. A dose of 5000–5500 rad is given in 15 fractions over 3 weeks.

Electron therapy

Cancer of the lip may be treated by electron beams of 8–10 MeV energy. The mouth is protected by the use of a lead bite block as described for X-ray therapy. Because of the beam characteristics of the electron beam, a margin of at least 2 cm clear of the lesion should be sustained. The average dose is 4500 rad in 8 exposures over 10 days. Tapley (1976) recommended a dose of 5000 rad in 4 weeks followed by an interstitial implant achieving an additional 2000–2500 rad to avoid late fibrosis.

Electron therapy is, however, an elaborate treatment for lip cancer which can be treated adequately and more simply by conventional forms of radiotherapy.

Surface applicator (double mould)

A surface applicator or double mould affords a very satisfactory method of treatment of cancer of the lower lip giving good results with an excellent cosmetic appearance (Fig. 8.16). The chief merits are that it is a precise and accurately calculated treatment; there is an absence of local high dose areas and a reasonably homogeneous dose is delivered to the treated volume. Originally, radium was used but this has been replaced by radioactive ^{60}Co slugs which give greater flexibility and planning distribution of the sources. To construct a double mould, a fairly high degree of technical skill is necessary. The mould must be removable with ease and replaceable with certainty. It must be closely adapted to the part treated so that relative movement is reduced

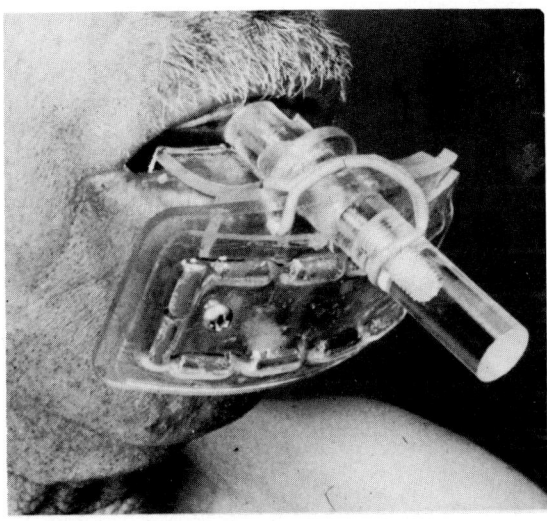

Fig. 8.16 Carcinoma of the lip. Surface applicator (double mould).

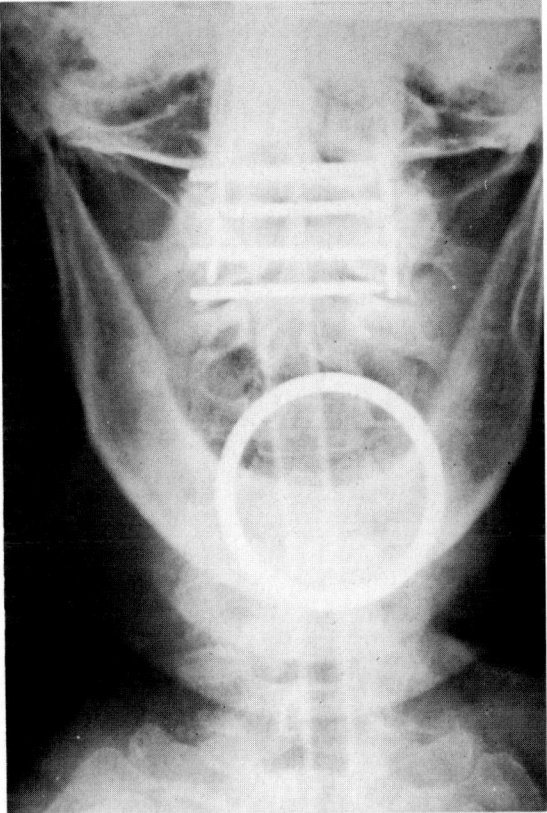

Fig. 8.17 Carcinoma of the lip. Radium needle implant.

to the minimum. It must be comfortable enough to be worn without discomfort throughout the treatment. The materials used should be easy to fashion, be stable at body temperature and resistent to body fluids.

The applicator consists of two parts, an inner and an outer mould, the planes of which are parallel to each other. For the inner mould the surfaces treated are concave and the treating distance is 0.5 cm. The area to be treated should include a margin of 1–1.5 cm of tissue width of lesion. For a lip thickness of 1 cm the treating distance for the outer plane will be 1.5 cm and for a lip thickness of 1.5 cm the treating distance is 2 cm. The incorporation of lead to shield the mouth is impractical and the best protection is distance provided by good design of the mould.

The mould is worn for approximately 6 hours a day for 8 days. The average dose to the mucosa is 7000 rad and 6000 rad on the skin. The mid-lip dose is not less than 5500 rad (Pointon, 1972).

With a double mould it is possible to treat the whole of the lower lip if required; it is of particular value when there is extension of the lesion to the buccal mucosa. If there is extension into the alveolar buccal sulcus, a mould treatment is unsatisfactory as it is not possible to obtain an adequate margin of normal tissue. Cancer of the upper lip cannot be treated satisfactorily with a double mould.

Interstitial irradiation

This affords a very satisfactory method of treating carcinoma of the lip and is the treatment of choice for carcinoma of the upper lip. (Fig. 8.17). The implant is usually carried out under general anaesthesia, but local anaesthesia may be used. A single plane through the base of the tumour is used and the area implanted should include at least 1 cm of healthy tissue around the tumour. A rectangular implant is employed and to avoid uncomfortable splinting of the lip an interleaving implant is preferred. The dose delivered should be 6500 rad at 0.5 cm in 7 days or its equivalent.

Durrant and Ellis (1973) replaced the use of radium needles by steel tubes which were often loaded with iridium-192 wires. The tubes were implanted using a jig and thereafter were loaded with iridium-192 wires cut to the appropriate length. A minimum tumour dose of 5500 rad was given in 5–8 days depending on the activity of the wire used.

[198]Au grains or seeds afford a simple treatment in an elderly subject and requires minimal hospitalization. The implant is carried out under local anaesthesia. The

sources are distributed following the Paterson Parker rules. The aimed dose is 6500 rad at 0.5 cm.

Radiotherapy for cancers of the oral cavity

The methods of radiotherapy used at the Christie Hospital in the treatment of oral cancer are as shown in Table 8.11. The two main forms of treatment of oral cancer are interstitial irradiation and external beam directed megavoltage X-ray therapy.

Table 8.11   Methods of irradiation of oral cancers 1966–1970.

Methods	Number treated	%
Interstitial irradiation	166	30
4 MeV XRT	342	61
kV XRT	17	3
Telecobalt	31	5
Mould	8	1

Interstitial irradiation

Interstitial irradiation is subject to certain limitations: first, only accessible tumours can be treated; second, effective dosage is restricted to a plane of little depth but, because of this, the dose permitted is a high one. A high dose which is strictly confined and accurately placed continues to represent the optimum concept in the treatment of carcinoma of the oral cavity. The numbers of patients treated by the different techniques of interstitial irradiation are shown in Table 8.12.

The fall in the incidence of tongue cancer together with the inherent problems of handling radioactive sources has led to a decline in the use of interstitial irradiation in the treatment of oral cancer. As a result, experience in this method of treatment and the neces-

Table 8.12   Interstitial irradiation 1966–70.

Method	Number treated	%
Single plane implant	87	52.5
Volume implant	27	16.2
Two-plane implant	9	5.3
Gold seed implant	43	26

sary training to gain competence has become more difficult to achieve. This is to be regretted as interstitial irradiation remains the treatment of choice for at least 25% of oral cancers; furthermore when sophisticated X-ray treatments are not available interstitial irradiation will give better results than can be achieved with indifferent external irradiation.

The methods to be described are based on the use of radium but other sources of γ-rays of the same intensity may be used instead. The types of implant used are based on the radium dosage systems described by Paterson (1963). For full details of the physical basis of the system reference should be made to Meredith (1949).

The development of after-loading techniques using flexible ¹⁹²Ir wire has provided an alternative system (Pierquin, 1964; Paine, 1972). This has been further developed into the Paris system in interstitial radiation therapy. For the basic principles of this and its use in clinical practice, reference should be made to Pierquin *et al.* (1978).

The incidence of various types of implant carried out for carcinoma of the oral cavity at the Christie Hospital is shown below (Fig. 8.18).

Single plane implant

The single plane radium needle implant may be termed the classical implant (Fig. 8.18). Its principal use is in the treatment of carcinoma of the tongue, but it may also be used for some carcinomas of the buccal mucosa. The principles and technique of implantation are common to all types of implant within the mouth.

Before the implant is carried out a careful examination of the lesion and surrounding tissue should be made. The selection of the appropriate implant will depend on the shape of the lesion and the ability to place the peripheral needles in normal tissue. Having decided on the type of implant, the dimensions of the implant should be measured. The dose and time having been decided from the appropriate tables, the amount of radiation required can be calculated and the necessary needles ordered.

While the implant may be carried out under local anaesthesia, general anaesthesia with endotracheal intubation is to be preferred. For a typical lateral side of tongue, needles of 3 cm actual length containing 2 or 1 mg of radium are used. Normally the top end only will be crossed and it is usually more convenient to use slightly shorter needles (2.5 cm AL) containing 1.5 mg of radium to avoid splitting of the tongue. Each needle is silked and the strength colour identified. Each needle following implant is sewn individually using chromic catgut. Before the implant is completed, the distribution may be checked by the use of an image intensifier. At the completion of the implant the silks

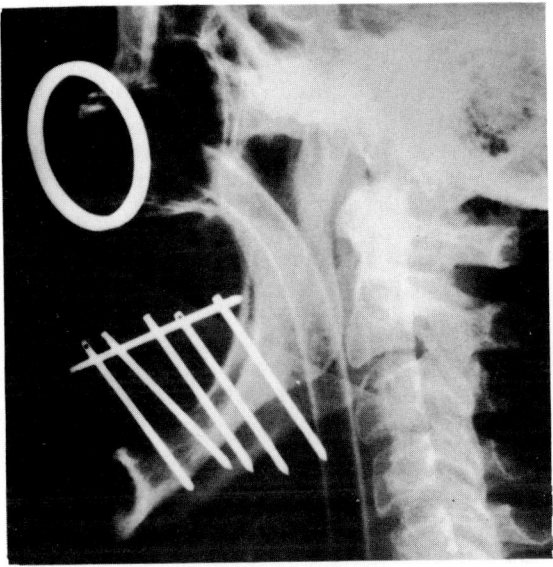

(a)

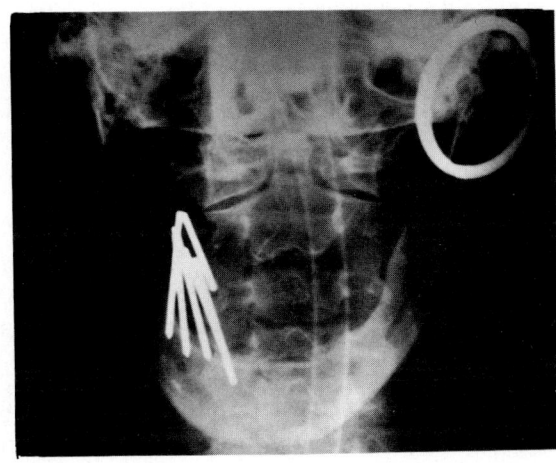

(b)

Fig. 18(a) and (b)   Carcinoma of the tongue. Single plane needle implant.

are collected together and fixed by a single thread suture to prevent any undue tension disturbing the implant. The silks are then lead out through a curved rubber tube to prevent friction on the angle of the mouth. The needles are then counted by the ward nurse. Before the patient returns to the ward, radiographs of the implant are taken. The aimed dose is 7000 rad at 0.5 cm in 7 days.

Volume implant

In the oral cavity the use of a volume implant is confined to lesions arising in the tongue and floor of the mouth. Its usefulness is principally in the tongue for those lesions not suitable for a single plane implant. In practice the volume takes the form of a cylinder with the top end closed by crossing needles. The implant consists of a vertical belt or rind of needles surrounding the periphery of the lesion with a core of needles (half the loading of the belt) evenly spaced in the tumour, the upper end of the implant being crossed by 2–3 horizontal needles. The lower end of the implant may be crossed by the use of Indian club or dumb-bell needles.

In practice, this implant is facilitated if the tongue is fixed to the floor of the mouth by a stay suture. Both ends of the suture are passed through the submental skin then through the tongue and tied over a rubber tube. In the tongue the common volume implant has a mean diameter of about 3.5 cm. The needles used are of 3 cm actual length and the most satisfactory

strengths are 0.75 mg for the periphery (minimum of 7) and 1.5 mg for the core and the crossing needles. The aimed dose is 6500 rad in 7 days.

Two-plane implant

A two-plane implant treats a slab of tissue more than 1 cm thick. In the mouth, its use is limited to the lateral border of the tongue. In the tongue, it is possible for the lateral plane to be clear of tumour; the needles should be as superficial as possible. When the tumour is too friable to hold needles, it may be very difficult to secure the aimed parallelism. Two-plane implants in the mouth are the most difficult form of implantation, even for the most experienced operator, and account for the relative rarity of their use.

Alternative forms of implant to a two-plane implant are:

1. To convert the implant into an elongated oval volume implant
2. Where the lesion is not greater than 1.5 cm thick to convert into a single plane 'thick' implant as described previously.

The aimed dose is 6500 rad at 0.5 cm from the inner aspect inside each radium plane in 7 days.

Even with careful pre-calculation and meticulous care in carrying out the implant, it may be difficult to reproduce the implant as planned. As a result the physical calculations from the past implant radiographs may be found to give a dosage rate greater or less than that intended. It follows that the overall time for the prescribed dose will be different from that planned. It has been accepted that in order to achieve the same effect from implants of varying dose rate there must exist some correlation between high dose rate implants of short duration and low dose rate implants of long duration (Dobbie, 1958). As a result of experience an empiric curve of biological equivalence can be constructed (Paterson, 1963). From this curve the appropriate correlation in time can be applied to produce the effect of 7000 rad in 7 days.

Pierquin *et al.* (1973) using ^{192}Ir wire implants reported that a dose rate of 23–90 rad corresponded to an overall implantation time for 6500 rad between 11 and 3 days. No difference in necrosis or recurrence rates was found in cases treated to the same dose within these limits of overall time. As a result, no correction for variation in dose rate was made.

Barkley and Fletcher (1976) also made no reduction in dose for higher dose rates. Certainly for small implants the difference in dose rates is not likely to vary much and it is doubtful that any correction for dose rate is necessary. Where large volumes are irradiated the dose rate is more critical and corrections are either made using an empiric curve as described, which has the virtue of consistency, or at the discretion of the treating radiotherapist.

Gold (^{198}Au) seeds or grain implant

Permanent implants using ^{198}Au seeds or grains afford a practical substitute for removable implants. The method suffers from the fact that some practice is necessary if an accurate distribution of sources is to be obtained and it lacks the physical control common to removable implants. The sources are small and can be applied to highly curved surfaces; their main use is for small superficial lesions. Normally the implant is carried out under general anaesthesia but can be done under local anaesthesia. The aimed dose is 6000–6500 rad.

The use of an image intensifier will permit the checking of source distribution at the completion of the implant. While it is usually impossible to remove sources, further seeds or grains may be added to correct for defects in distribution. Fortunately, most seed implants are small and will tolerate some overdosage. If the final physical calculation indicates that too low a dose has resulted the defect may be made good by an additional contribution of external X-ray irradiation. A useful rule of thumb to calculate the amount of external irradiation necessary to remedy underdosage is as follows: if it is accepted that an exposure of 2000 rad of X-rays given in a single exposure is cancericidal, then 2000 multiplied by the fraction of underdosage will give the tumour dose in rad to be given in a single exposure of X-rays necessary to rectify the defect.

External irradiation

Two thirds of cases of oral cancer treated by radiotherapy will be treated by external irradiation. A high dose accurately placed represents the ideal concept for the treatment of squamous cell carcinoma of the oral cavity. As a result, normal tissue is spared as much as possible with the advantage that impairment of further surgery, if necessary, is minimized. Modern beam-directed megavoltage X-ray therapy has been developed to fulfil these criteria. The use of wedge filter techniques permit the design of precision treatments allowing homogeneous irradiation of the desired volume with remarkably sharp fall-off outside the treatment volume. The absence of differential absorption in bone makes megavoltage radiation particularly suitable for treatment of oral cancer.

In the choice of machine, the linear accelerator working at 4–6 million volts is to be preferred for routine clinical practice. Telecobalt machines are a practical alternative to the linear accelerator, but cannot with ease reproduce the same degree of precision therapy possible with a linear accelerator. Any beam-directed treatment must proceed through the stages of:

1. Localization – the object is to form the best possible visualization of the lesion and hence the volume to be treated. From this a decision on the field size can be made and the relationship of the lesion to known anatomical structures noted. To facilitate radiographic localization, it is very helpful if the limit of the lesion is marked and this can be done by the insertion of inactive gold seeds or equivalent at noted positions around the lesion.
2. Selection of field size to subtend the lesion and an adequate margin of normal tissue.
3. Verification of localization by means of radiography.
4. Treatment plan and prescription.

For the majority of carcinomas of the oral cavity, two basic techniques suffice:

1. Wedge pair treatment.
2. Two opposed lateral fields in which a wedge filter can be used to compensate for varying tissue thickness.

Wedge pair technique

This technique permits the treatment of eccentric tumours with restriction of the dose to the side of the mouth (Figs. 8.19 and 8.20). The use of wedge filters requires detailed planning representing the best in small field beam-directed X-ray therapy. One of the major advantages of wedge filter techniques is the sharp cut-off outside the subtended treatment volume. As a result the radiation reaction will be sharply demarcated and for lateral lesions the contra-lateral

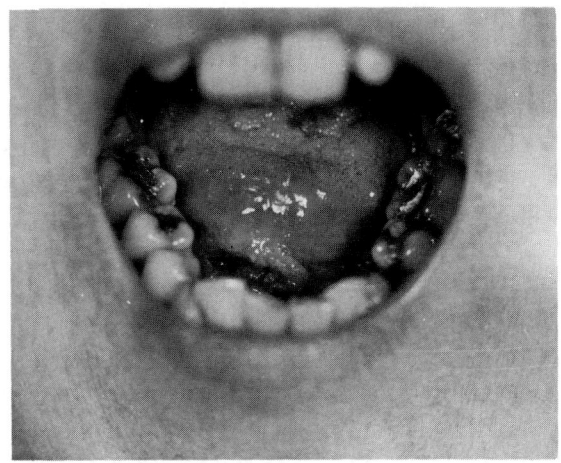

(a)

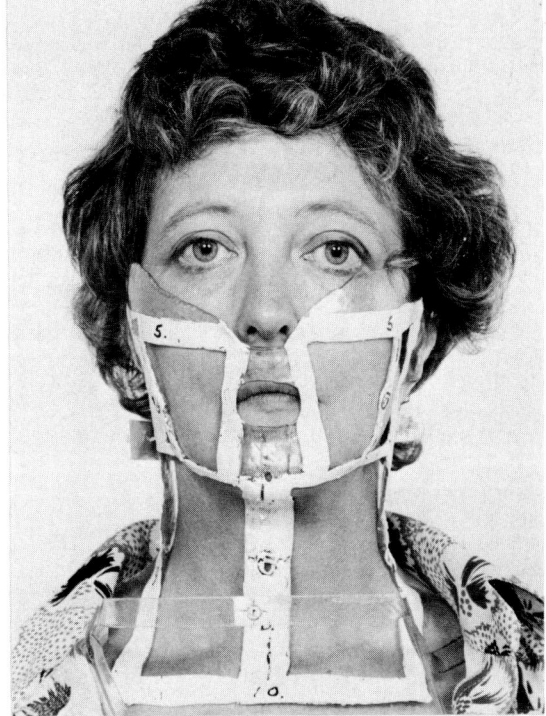

(b)

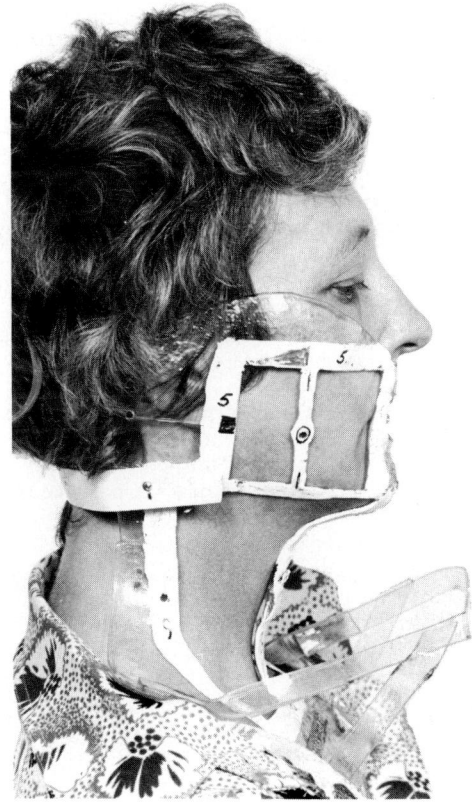

(c)

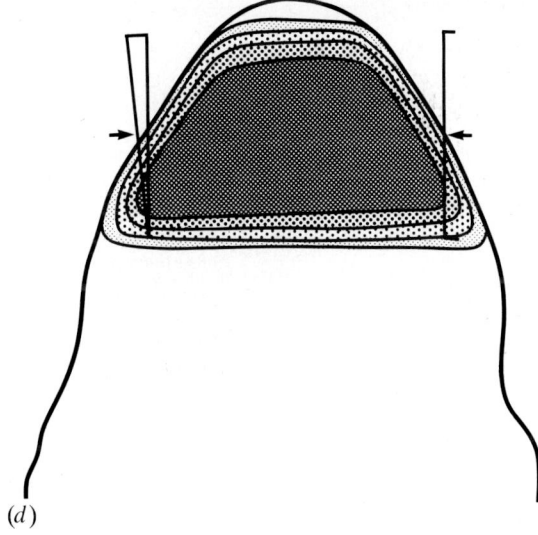

(d)

Fig. 8.19(a) Carcinoma of the floor of the mouth.
(b) and (c) Treatment shell – patient received elective neck irradiation.
(d) 4 MeV X-ray. Dose distribution – wedge filter to overcome oblique incidence.

side of the mouth will be spared any gross reaction. The use of such techniques demands beam direction of a high order of accuracy and reliability. While it is perfectly possible to carry out such treatments by a 'free-hand' set-up, it is no real substitute for a beam direction shell used in conjunction with the mechanical means of beam direction fitted to the machine.

The degree of wedging of a beam is defined by the wedge angle. In practice it is desirable to have a small range of wedge filters of varying steepness of wedge angle to facilitate compensation for oblique incidence. The effect of obliquity in normal use is to undo to some extent the effect of the filter. The normal method of compensation is to use a steeper wedge. The method of compensation applies only to obliquity in the direction of the wedge. Obliquity in the other axis, normally vertically, is either ignored or if it is marked the use of wax or similar material can level out the obliquity.

Field selection and treatment plan
The preliminary decision must be the approximate shape and size of the volume to be treated. Having decided this, the orientation of the treatment fields can be made. For eccentric lesions, e.g. carcinoma of the lower alveolus, a wedge pair affords the optimum treatment. For midline lesions, resort is usually made to a parallel opposed pair frequently wedging one field either to cope with obliquity or as a compensator for varying tissue thickness.

The availability of computer planning may simplify

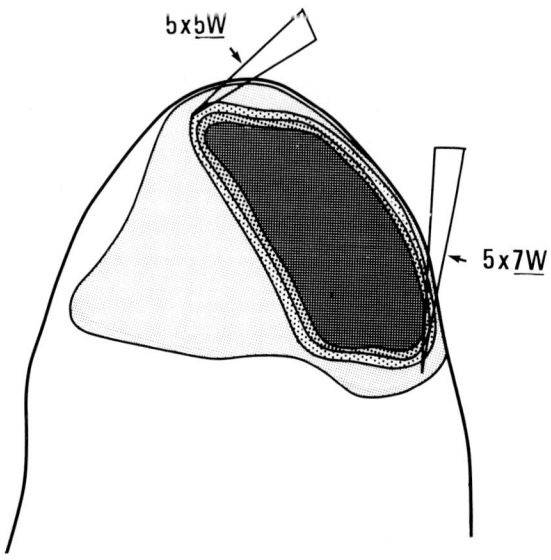

Fig. 8.20 Carcinoma of lower alveolus. 4 MeV X-ray wedge pair dose distribution.

the choice of the optimum field arrangement but only the clinician can make the final decision on its acceptability for the individual case. The influence of computerized transaxial tomography on the treatment planning of oral cancer has yet to be fully explored.

Dose
The average volume treated in cancer of the oral cavity will normally be less than a 6-cm cube. The normal dose for such a volume in an overall time of 3 weeks will be 5250–5500 rad given in 15–16 fractions, or appropriately increased for longer overall times.

Electron therapy

For all practical purposes in clinical use, electrons and megavoltage X-rays can be regarded as identical in radiobiological effect. The shape of the depth-dose curve of electron beams of low energy shows a flat initial plateau in the first few centimetres of tissue followed by a sharp dose fall-off; as the electron energy increases, the fall-off is much less pronounced. The attraction of this sharp dose fall-off characteristic has lead to the use of single field treatment of relatively superficial lesions. With energies in the 15–20 MeV range a fairly even dose distribution in the first 4–5 cm of tissue would be obtained with a moderately rapid fall-off in dose thereafter. In the lower energy range, i.e. up to 10 MeV, the advantagees of electron beam therapy are maximal, and can be used satisfactorily to treat lip and some carcinomas arising from the buccal mucosa.

The beam edge characteristics of electron beam are such that edges are not sharply delineated and as a result it is necessary to take a more generous treatment margin than would be the case with megavoltage X-rays.

The effects of tissue inhomogeneity are of considerable importance in electron beam therapy and as such lead to problems in accuracy of dosimetry. In addition, irregularities of the surface treated will produce variations in dosage (Jackson, 1970).

In cancer of the oral cavity single field electron beam therapy affords a method of treating superficial lesions, particularly if facilities for accurate beam direction of megavoltage X-rays are unavailable. Electrons of low energy, i.e. 10 MeV, may be used to treat involved cervical nodes or usefully to carry out elective neck irradiation if desirable.

The doses used for electron beam therapy are the same as for megavoltage X-ray therapy.

Dental hygiene

In the North-west of England, 85% of patients presenting with oral cancer are edentulous. For patients with teeth receiving radiation for cancer of the oral cavity, the general principles of management are as follows:

1. If the teeth are sound and free from sepsis and present no obstruction to treatment, then they are left in position.
2. If there is gross caries or dental sepsis, then the teeth should be removed under an antibiotic cover before radiation treatment is begun. It is of particular importance in the lower jaw, that following dental extraction, the mucoperiosteum should be sutured back in position for much of the vascular supply of the anterior mandible is derived in the mucoperiosteum. Following extraction, a needle implant may be performed without delay. If external radiation or a radioactive applicator is to be used, an interval of two weeks must be allowed to permit healing of the gums.
3. Following treatment, conservative dental management is to be encouraged and patients should be instructed in simple dental hygiene. If extractions are inevitable then it is desirable that these be carried out in stages to avoid the risk of precipitating necrosis of the jaw.

Complications

Necrosis
Significant soft tissue necrosis is rare following radiation for cancers of the lips. Similarly bone necrosis is very uncommon and has only been seen when there is gross concomitant dental sepsis.

Radionecrosis of any severity is uncommon following a well planned course of radiotherapy for oral cancers. Any persistent breakdown in the irradiated area should always be regarded with suspicion and usually represents residual or recurrent malignancy. Resort to biopsy should not be delayed to confirm this. Superficial ulceration due to high dose usually settles with simple symptomatic measures. If a major soft tissue breakdown should occur, early surgical intervention and repair is indicated.

Bone necrosis is principally confined to the lower jaw. Of 204 consecutive treated cases of oral cancer, 5 or 2.5% developed necrosis of the lower jaw. All 5 cases had been treated for carcinoma of the floor of the mouth and the necrosis was undoubtedly related to the poor vascularity of the anterior third of the mandible. When necrosis is suspected, full radiology of the jaw is essential to establish the extent of bone involved. When the presence of necrosis has been established, early intervention is usually contraindicated as ultimately interference will usually precipitate further

breakdown. A programme of observation and serial radiology is the preferred course. Minor bone necrosis will usually settle following the spontaneous separation of small sequestra. Operative interference should be delayed until there is clear evidence of sequestration. Secondary infection may be a problem and long-term antibiotic therapy may be called for. Occasionally a sinus through the skin may result and dead bone may be visible externally when surgical resection with reconstruction is mandatory.

Recurrence
The recurrence rate for cancer of the lip following a full course of radiotherapy will vary with the technique, but is approximately 5%. Surgical salvage should ensure primary control in all but the most exceptional cases.

Recurrent carcinoma of the oral cavity following radiation occurs for all practical purposes within two years of the initial treatment. In the majority of cases it occurs within the first year. Whilst later recurrences may occur it is more likely that the apparent recurrence represents a new primary malignancy.

While it is possible to treat occasional edge recurrences with further radiation therapy, the subsequent treatment for the majority of cases will be surgery. Where salvage surgery is not practical, then chemotherapy can give useful palliation and an occasional long survivor.

Chemotherapy for cancers of the lips and oral cavity

Chemotherapy is usually considered when recurrent disease has developed which is not amenable to further surgery and/or radiotherapy. Relapse may occur either at the primary site or more frequently in the lymph nodes that drain the primary lesion. The clinician is usually thus confronted with a patient who is concerned about visible deposits of tumour that are causing pain and there may be associated ulceration. The choice of treatment lies between single agent therapy or combinations of different drugs.

The most effective single agent is methotrexate when 40–60% of patients will respond favourably and in a smaller proportion (20–30%) encouraging results may be achieved that last for 12–24 months. Various schedules have been suggested but it is now generally accepted that intermittent intravenous (i.v.) administration is more preferable to chronic oral administration. Initially, doses of 50–150 mg/m² i.v. every two weeks are required to achieve the optimum effect. Doses of 100 mg/m² or more should only be administered when facilities are available to assay the serum concentration at 24 hours after administration as potentially toxic concentrations can then be reversed

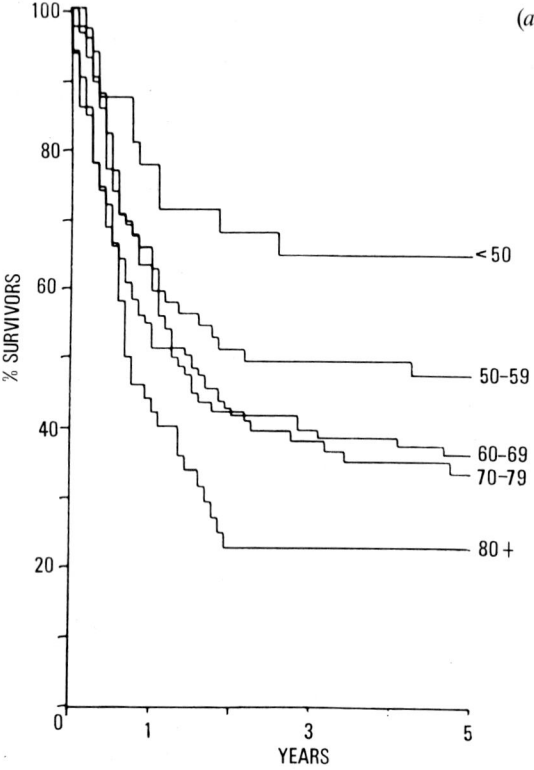

Fig. 8.21 Carcinoma of oral cavity. Survival related to age
(*a*) Male; (*b*) Female.

with citrovorum factor. To achieve the optimum response the dose must be adjusted by monitoring the
serum concentration because of the wide variation in
the handling of methotrexate by individual patients.
When a response has been achieved this can then be
maintained with moderate non-toxic doses of 40–80
mg/m² i.v. at monthly intervals. Much higher doses of
methotrexate followed by leucovorin rescue have been
advocated in this situation but the response rate is no
greater than that achieved by the doses suggested.

Bleomycin, which is preferentially concentrated in
squamous cells, has been used in the management of
head and neck cancer. The drug is normally given by
intramuscular or i.v. injection in doses of 15–30 mg/m²
once or twice weekly. Response rates are, however,
inferior to those of methotrexate and because many
patients are elderly, toxic effects may be more frequent. Thus, particular attention should be paid to the
skin and respiratory system during treatment.

Other single agents that have been used are cyclophosphamide, 5-fluorouracil and adriamycin but the
results are inferior to both methotrexate and bleo-

mycin. Encouraging reports are appearing concerning
the efficacy of cis-platinum but a more careful appraisal
of this drug is required before it is introduced into
general use because of its toxic effects, notably those on
the kidney.

Combinations of drugs have been tried in an attempt
to improve the response rate, but in the majority of
instances the combination does not improve the proportion of patients responding but does increase toxicity. As in this situation there is no possibility of cure,
chemotherapy should be moderated so that minimal
toxicity is experienced by the patient and an acceptable
quality of life therefore maintained

Prognostic factors

Stage

The size of the primary lesion is the most significant
factor, not only because the rate of primary control is
high for T₁ lesions but also because the incidence of
metastatic nodes on presentation is low and the chance

of subsequent development of nodes is also small. Nodal involvement is associated with a rapidly worsening prognosis whilst fixed or bilateral nodes carry a grave outlook.

Site

Patients with cancer of the buccal mucosa would appear to have a better prognosis than other sites in the mouth, but the difference stage-for-stage between sites is not statistically significant.

Sex

Female patients with oral cancer have a slightly better prognosis than males. This difference has narrowed as the sex incidence of the disease has closed and is no longer as marked as it was three decades ago.

Age

The deterioration in survival with increasing age in both sexes is shown in Figs. 21 (*a, b*). The curves show the mortality from cancer of the mouth alone, having been corrected for death from unrelated causes. The hazard rate due to age *per se* is about two and a half times greater in the oldest age group compared with the youngest (Palmer, 1978).

In comparing results from different treatments for oral cancer all these factors must be taken into account and only true random clinical trials with adequate numbers of patients, thus allowing proper stratification, will show whether there is a significant advantage in one method of treatment and another.

Results

Cancer of the lips

The results from treatment of squamous cell cancers of the lips are good relative to tumours at other sites. The majority present at an early stage although a small number of cases that are neglected and more advanced do occur. Between 1970 and 1972, 100 cases were seen at the Christie Hospital and Holt Radium Institute and the corrected survival rate at 5 years for this group was 86%. These patients were treated either by superifical X-ray therapy or with ^{60}Co applicator moulds, the corrected survival rates 5 years being respectively 85% and 89%. The slightly better results obtained with ^{60}Co reflect the smaller, more localized tumours included within the group. Burkell (1950) obtained a 5-year survival rate of 91% for 349 patients treated by radium

implant, whilst Dick (1962) reported a rate of 95% in patients treated by 140 kV radiation comparing this with 82% after primary surgical treatment. In 1973, Durrant and Ellis described local control of tumours less than 3 cm in diameter, in 29/30 patients treated by ^{192}Ir implant after 3 years.

Mortality from squamous cancer of the lips is rarely due to failure to control the primary tumour but more commonly because of regional or occasional distant metastasis.

Cancer of the oral cavity

The overall results of treatment for squamous cell cancers of the oral cavity are less good than those for cancers of the lips, with overall survival rate at 5 years of 42% although patients without metastatic nodes at presentation do slightly better with a survival rate of over 50%. Such overall figures, however, are not very meaningful since variations occur due to stage, anatomical site, sex, age and method of treatment.

More detailed consideration of results is therefore important. In the 5 years between 1966 and 1971, a total of 564 patients with oral cancer was treated. There was a progressive deterioration in survival figures with increasing stage of disease at presentation (Table 8.13). The corrected survival rates at 5 years varied from 76% for T_1N_0 tumours to 5% for T_3N_{1-3}. There are slight differences in local control between different anatomical sites within the oral cavity and stage of disease (Table 8.14) and the earliest tumours obviously do better.

The results of treatment between 1970 and 1972 also show differences according to sex and age. Quite a marked difference exists between patients under the age of fifty years and those from the later decades. A difference is also seen between females and males, the females having a better survival than males. Female

Table 8.13 Number of patients treated and corrected survival rates at 5 years for patients with oral cancer treated between 1966 – 1970.

T N Stage	Number of patients	% 5 year survival
T_1N_0	117	76
T_1N_{1-3}	6	(66.7)
T_2N_0	188	53
T_2N_{1-3}	35	35
T_3N_0	111	17
T_3N_{1-3}	107	5
	——	——
Total	564	42

Table 8.14   Successful control of primary tumours at selected sites within the oral cavity.

Site	Percentage control	
	T_1	T_2
Tongue	86	69
Buccal mucosa	81	71
Floor of mouth	95.5	77

patients with all stages of disease under the age of fifty years having a rate of primary control of 75% whilst males of similar age have a survival rate of 65%. A difference by a factor of three is observed between the youngest and the oldest age group.

In recent years, the degree of interdisciplinary collaboration has improved with a consequent improvement in results. Recent figures show that properly timed sequential treatment has ensured control in all cases with T_1N_0 tumours. The corrected survival rate at 3 years for primary tumours of all stages without nodal metastasis at presentation is 75%

It is unfortunate that, to a large extent, surgeons have been more concerned with improvements in surgical technique rather than the results of treatment. Proper analysis of the results of radical surgery is made difficult by the limited number of cases at each anatomical site that come to surgery and the variations in the procedures that are used for their treatment. The crude results for radical surgery for squamous cell cancers of the oral cavity done at the Christie Hospital and Holt Radium Institute since 1975 show that about one half of the patients accepted for such surgery are helped by it, including those who are alive and free from tumour and those who died from intercurrent disease (Table 8.15). The operative morality reflects the age of patients undergoing radical surgery, a mean of 67.6 years, and their associated acute or chronic medical conditions.

More statistically acceptable results can be found in the published literature for certain specific anatomical sites. Harrold (1975) reported 5-year determinate results for the gingivae and floor of mouth, 42% and

Table 8.15   Crude results of radical salvage surgery for oral squamous cell cancers since 1975.

Alive and well	38.7%	} = 48.3%
Dead from intercurrent disease	9.6%	
Operative deaths, i.e. within one month of operation	9.6%	
Dead from tumour	41.4%	

36% respectively. He related these results to the presence or absence of metastatic cervical nodes. Patients with gingival tumours and positive nodes had only 25% survival whilst those with tumours of the floor of mouth and positive nodes did worse with a 20% survival. Patients with tumours at either site and negative nodes had survival rates of around 63%. Moore and his colleagues (1975) suggested that surgery and radiotherapy for early tumours of the tongue, $T_1N_0M_0$ and $T_2N_0M_0$, were equally good with a 5-year survival rate of 75%. They further suggested that for more advanced tumours, radical surgery alone or sequential surgery and radiotherapy were more advantageous than irradiation alone. For patients with tumours classified as $T_3N_0M_0$ and all N_1 patients, the 5-year survival rate falls to 45% whilst those with more advanced tumours had a survival rate of less than 20%.

Kalnins and his colleagues (1977) have examined the correlation between prognosis for oral cancers and the degree of lymph node involvement as determined at block dissection of the neck. Their observations suggest that useful predictive prognostic factors are the number of nodes involved, the level of involvement and the presence or absence of both capsular involvement and soft tissue infiltration.

Reasons for failure

The main factors that determine prognosis are size of the primary tumour at presentation, presence or absence of regional metastatic lymphadenopathy, site of the tumour and the age and sex of the patient. An excellent account of these prognostic factors has been given by Easson and Palmer (1976) based on the experience accumulated from 8500 patients registered at the Christie Hospital and Holt Radium Institute since 1932. These authors also suggest that further epidemiological surveys could give more information about the aetiology of oral cancer which could then be used in a preventative manner. In addition, they feel that aggressive public and professional education could result in earlier diagnosis, the one factor that could lead to significant improvement in mortality figures.

Size of primary tumour

In common with other malignant tumours, the size of the primary lesion at presentation has a marked effect on survival figures for cancers of the lips and those of the oral cavity. The gradient for survival with advancing stage is steep. Greater size is associated with increased hypoxia and this, no doubt, has a significant effect on the success of treatment by irradiation. It has led to the continuing search for drugs that can increase the oxygenation of tumours and therefore their radiosensitivity. The limits of surgical resection have expanded markedly within the last two decades due to the availability of improved methods of facial reconstruction. Other factors must therefore be identified as reasons for surgical failure of control of the primary tumour such as implantation of tumour at operation or more generalized field change. Tumour volume limits the value of cytotoxic drugs so that combined or adjuvant treatment deserves more attention.

Metastatic lymphadenopathy

Involvement of regional lymph nodes has a significant effect on the success of treatment. Taking both the incidence at presentation and development of nodes within five years of treatment into account, then about 60% of patients develop metastatic lymphadenopathy. The first two years after diagnosis and treatment are the most critical. The high incidence of nodal metastasis has led to the recommendation of prophylactic irradiation of the neck at the time of treatment of the primary tumour but the benefit and saving from subsequent block dissection for metastases is small. Prophylactic cervical block dissection as a part of radical salvage surgery has greater justification on technical grounds at least.

The variability in the patterns of lymphatic dissemination due to alternative and contra-lateral pathways as well as the effects of obstructive lymphadenopathy are responsible in part for failure to control nodal disease. A feature of serious prognostic significance is the presence of transcapsular spread and local infiltration with involvement of adjacent vital structures.

Anatomical site

A progressive gradient in survival is seen with anatomical site of incidence of primary tumours. Cancers of the lip do better than those of the oral cavity whilst those of the buccal mucosa do better than those of the alveoli and tongue. Pathways of tumour spread, including lymphatic and periosteal routes, may be responsible in part for this variation in behaviour. There is no evidence that histological grade has any effect.

Age and sex

The adverse effect of advancing age on survival is more marked in the male than the female although, even in them, there is progressive deterioration. Selective treatment of younger age groups would yield better survival figures than those obtained from a more widely constituted group and range of age must be taken into account when comparing results from different centres.

An overall difference in results between the sexes is apparent when all stages of disease are considered. Analysis by stage shows, however, that this overall difference is due to significant differences in the earlier stages which is lost with more advanced disease.

Therapy

Clinical experience has demonstrated that close interdisciplinary cooperation in the sequential use of radiotherapy and surgery can improve survival figures. It would now seem that adjuvant use of or combination with cytotoxic drugs may bring about further improvements. Failure to observe such principles is reflected in the results from treatment so that management of cancers of the lips and oral cavity demands a multidisciplinary approach.

Advances in therapy

Primary control on T_1 oral cancer may be achieved in almost 100% of cases whilst in T_2 cases approximately 70–75% of tumours will be controlled. However, when the primary lesion is greater than 4 cm in diameter (T_3) control is obtained in a little over 50% of cases under optimum circumstances. In addition, nodal involvement on presentation will be present in 45% of T_3 tumours. If there are bilateral or fixed nodes present then the prognosis is extremely poor with conventional radiotherapy and surgery. In spite of very considerable efforts to improve the methods of irradiation and extend the scope of surgery, survival rates have remained largely unchanged. However, closer multidisciplinary cooperation can bring about improvement by optimal use of sequential or combined treatment.

Radiotherapy

1. High LET particle beam therapy – neutron therapy.
2. The use of hypoxic radiosensitizers.
3. Combined radiotherapy and chemotherapy.

High LET radiation – fast neutron therapy
One approach to overcome the problem of hypoxic cells in tumours is radiation therapy with high LET particle beams. The use of fast neutron therapy in the treatment of head and neck cancer is being extensively investigated following the studies reported by Catterall and Bewley (1979). These studies in advanced carcinoma of the oral cavity have shown that a high degree of local control can be achieved with fast neutron therapy. Of 39 cases of cancer of the oral cavity so treated, persisting control was obtained in 72%. However, it would seem that morbidity may be increased

and further studies are needed with better comparison against more conventional methods (see Chapter 4).

Hypoxic radiosensitizers

The problem of hypoxic cells in tumours has been approached by (a) treatment in hyperbaric oxygen chambers; (b) the use of high LET particle beam therapy and (c) the use of chemical resiosensitizers which are active against hypoxic cells only. Most sensitizers of this type are electron-afinic compounds and mimic the radiosensitizing effect of oxygen (Fowler and Adams 1975) (see Chapter 3).

Pilot studies in patients have been carried out and clinical trials are being started in head and neck cancer but the early results have not shown any significant benefit.

Combined chemotherapy and X-ray therapy

The combination of chemotherapy and low LET radiation has been tried with a number of cytotoxic agents, either singly or in combination. In the majority of studies the agent or agents have been given before radiotherapy and have generally been unable to show any significant improvement in results. O'Connor and his colleagues (1977) used synchronous vincristine, bleomycin and methotrexate (VBM) and radiotherapy in the treatment of poor prognosis squamous cell carcinomas of the head and neck. On average 4–5 pulses of VBM were given during treatment combined with radiotherapy on a cobalt unit; 60 patients were treated with a crude actual survival rate at 24 months of 61%. It is suggested that the potentiation of radiotherapy and an increased therapeutic ratio was obtained by the addition of VBM to radiotherapy. Similarly, Shanta and Krishnamurthi (1976) showed improved results by combining bleomycin with radiotherapy. Methotrexate given synchronously with radiotherapy has also given encouraging response. The studies have been compared with historic controls with their inherent deficiences. Random clinical trials are essential to establish synchronous combination therapy and some have been initiated.

Surgery

Further surgical developments are most likely to be concerned with improving facial reconstruction so that better cosmetic and functional results can be obtained. However, more attention should be given to the treatment and control of recognizable pre-malignant conditions by the use of cryotherapy. This approach to the management of oral cancer is preventative and should be allied to more aggressive programmes of professional and public education.

Microsurgical techniques are beginning to offer the possibility of the use of innervated flaps so that motor and perhaps sensory function can also be replaced. Such surgery is time-consuming and the results must be reliable. It is likely that artificial prosthetic replacement of the mandible will always be needed in some cases and further search is required in order to find better materials for this purpose.

The value of chemotherapy adjuvant to surgery must be explored further. Poor prognostic factors can now be recognized and chemotherapy before or after operation is now being tried.

Further reading

Chambers, R.G., Jansen de Limpens, A.M.P., Jaques, D.A. and Routledge, R.T. (eds) (1975), *Cancer of the Head and Neck, Proceedings of an International Symposium*, Montreux, Switzerland, April 2–4, 1975. Excerpta Medica, Amsterdam and Oxford; Elsevier Publishing Co. Inc., New York.

Conley, J. (1976), *Regional Flaps of the Head and Neck*. George Thieme Publishers, Stuttgart.

MacComb, William S. and Fletcher, Gilbert H. (eds) (1968), *Cancer of the Head and Neck*. The Williams and Wilkins Company, Baltimore.

Paterson, Ralston (1963), *The Treatment of Malignant Disease by Radiotherapy*, (2nd edn). Arnold, London.

References

Arryan, S. (1978), Personal communication.

Barkley, H.T. Jr. and Fletcher, G.H. (1976), Volume and time factors in interstitial gamma-ray therapy. *Am. J. Roentg.*, 126–63.

Binnie, W.H. (1976), A perspective of oral cancer. *Proc. R. Soc. Med.*, **69**, 737–40.

Burkell, C.C. (1950), Cancer of the lip. *Can. Med. Ass. J.*, **62**, 28–33.

Catterall, M. and Bewley, D.K. (1979), *Fast neutrons in the treatment of cancer*. Academic Press, London.

Cawson, R.A. (1969), Leukoplakia and oral cancer. *Proc. R. Soc. Med.*, **62**, 610–5.

Copeland, E.M., *et al.* (1978), In: *Intravenous Hyperalimentation and Cancer*. Univ. Texas System Cancer Center.

Dick, D.A.L. (1962), Clinical and cosmetic results in squamous cancer of the lip treated by 140 kV radiation therapy. *Clin. Radiol.*, **XIII**, 304–12.

Dobbie, J.L. (1958), Methods of applying radium in cancer therapy. In: *Treatment of Cancer and Allied Diseases*. Vol. 1, (ed. Pack and Ariel), Pitman, London, pp.355–78.

Durrant, K.R. and Ellis, F. (1973), The treatment of squamous cell carcinoma of the lower lip by rigid implants. *Clin. Radiol.*, **24**, 502–5.

Easson, E.C. and Palmer, M.K. (1976), Prognostic factors in oral cancer. *Clin. Oncol.*, **2**, 191–202.

Ebenius, B. (1943), Carcinoma of lip. *Acta Radiol.*, (Stockholm) Supplement 43.

Fowler, J.F. and Adams, G.E. (1975), Impact radiosensitizers: hypoxic cells. In: *High Energy Photons and Electrons: Clinical Application in Cancer Management*. (eds S. Kramer, N. Santharalingam and S.F., Zinninger), Wiley, New York, p.309.

Harrold, C.C. (1975), In: *Cancer of the Head and Neck – Proceedings of an International Symposium*, Montreux, Switzerland, April 2–4, 1975. (eds R.G. Chambers, A.M.P. Jansen de Limpens, D.A. Jaques and R. Routledge), Excerpta Medica, Amsterdam, Oxford; American Elsevier, New York.

Jackson, S.M. (1970), The clinical applications of electron beam therapy with energies up to 10 MeV. *Br. J. Radiol.*, **43**, 431–40.

Jesse, R.H. *et al.* (1970), Cancer of the oral cavity: Is elective neck dissection beneficial? *Am. J. Surg.*, **120**, 505.

Jussawalla, D.J. (1976), The problem of cancer in India: An epidemiological assessment. In: *Cancer in Asia*, Gann Monograph on Cancer Research, No. 18. (ed. T. Hirayama), University Park Press, Baltimore, London and Tokyo, pp. 265–73.

Kalnins, I.K. *et al.* (1977), Correlations between prognosis and degree of lymph node involvement in carcinoma of the oral cavity. *Am. J. Surg.*, **134**, 450–454.

Meredith, W.J. (1949), *Radium Dosage: The Manchester System*. E.and S. Livingstone, Edinburgh.

Moore, C., Flynn, M.B. and Scott, R.M. (1975), In: *Cancer of the Head and Neck — Proceedings of an International Symposium*, Montreux, Switzerland, April 2–4, 1975. (eds R.G. Chambers, A.M.P. Jansen de Limpens, D.A. Jaques and R. Routledge). Excerpta Medica, Amsterdam and Oxford; American Elsevier, New York.

Moss, E. and Lee, W.R. (1974), Occurence of oral pharyngeal cancers in textile workers. *Br. J. Indust. Med.*, **31**, 224–32.

O'Connor, A.D. *et al.* (1977), Synchronous VBM and radiotherapy in the treatment of squamous carcinoma of the head and neck. *Clin. Otolaryngol.*, **1**, 347–57.

Paine, C.H. (1972), Modern after-loading methods for interstitial radiotherapy. *Clin. Radiol.*, **23**, 263–72.

Palmer, M.K. (1978), The statistical analysis of survival following treatment for cancer. Ph.D. Thesis, University of Manchester.

Paterson, R. (1963), In: *The Treatment of Malignant Disease by Radiotherapy*. Arnold, London.

Pierquin, R., (1964), *Precis de Curietherapie*, Masson et Cie, Paris.

Pierquin, B. et al. (1973), Clinical observations on the time factor in interstitial radiotherapy using iridium 192. *Clin. Radiol.*, **24**, 506–9.

Pierquin, B. et al. (1978), The Paris system of interstitial radiation therapy. *Acta Radiol.*, **17**, 33–48.

Pindborg, J.J. (1971), Oral leukoplakia. *Aust. Dent. J.*, **16**, 83–93.

Pointon, R.C.S. (1972), Cancer of the lips. In: *Encyclopaedia of Medical Radiology*, Vol. XIX. pp. 405–34. (eds A. Zuppinger and E. Krokowski), Springer Verlag.

Shanta, V. and Krishnamurthi, S. (1976), *Gann Monograph on Cancer Research*, No.19, 159.

Seimssen, S.O., Kirkby, B. and O'Connor, T.P. (1978), Immediate reconstruction of a resected segment of the lower jaw, using a compound flap of clavicle and sternomastoid muscle. *Plast. Reconstr. Surg.*, **61**, 724–735.

Tapley, N. du V. (1976), *Clinical Application of the Electron Beam*, Wiley, New York.

Towers, J.F. and Wilson, J.S.P. (1974), Simple reconstruction of the mandible following resection. *Proc. R. Soc. Med.*, **67**, 607–9.

Tweedle, D.E.F. *et al.* (1979), Nutritional support for patients undergoing surgery for cancer of the head and neck. *Res. Clin. Forums*, **1**, 59–65.

Wynder, E.L. and Bross, I.J. (1957), Aetiological factors in mouth cancer. An approach to its prevention. *Br. Med. J.*, **i**, 1137–43.

9 Eye and orbit

J.M. Henk, J.E. Wright and
M. Ruth Sandland*

Tumours of the orbit

Anatomy

The orbit is a pyramidal space enclosed within bony
walls. The medial walls of the orbits lie anteroposterior, parallel with each other. Each extends from the
anterior lacrimal crest on the frontal process of the
maxilla across the lacrimal bone and the orbital plate of
the ethmoid to the body of the sphenoid and the optic
foramen. The orbital floor consists mainly of the orbital process of the palatine bone at its apex and the
orbital plate of the maxilla. The lateral wall of the orbit
is composed of the greater wing of the sphenoid and
the zygomatic bone. Between the lateral wall and the
floor is the inferior orbital fissure which leads into the
pterygopalatine and infratemporal fossae. The roof is
the orbital plate of the frontal bone with the lesser wing
of the sphenoid. Posteriorly the superior orbital fissure
leads into the middle cranial fossa between the greater
and lesser wings of the sphenoid. The approximate
dimensions of the adult male orbit are height 34 mm,
width 41 mm, length of floor 53 mm. The volume of the
orbital cavity is approximately 30 ml.

The orbit contains the eyeball, the optic nerve, the
extrinsic muscles of the globe, and the vessels and
nerves that supply them. Connective tissue supports
the globe so that it maintains its position within the
orbit.

For practical purposes the orbit can be divided into
four surgical spaces:

1. The sub-periosteal space which is a potential space
   between the walls and the lining periosteum.
2. The peripheral surgical space which lies between
   the muscle cone with its fascia and the orbital
   periosteum.
3. The inner surgical space which lies within the muscle cone.
4. The episcleral space which lies between Tenon's
   capsule and the globe.

* Dr Sandland has contributed the section on retinoblastoma

Recent work by Koornneff (1975) had cast doubt on
this concept. However, for practical purposes the
broad division into four spaces holds true.

Examination

The clinician should examine each orbit noting any
localized or generalized swelling of the eyelids and
looking for a similar change on the contra-lateral side,
since sometimes in unilateral proptosis caused by
dysthyroid eye disease there may be some oedema
present in both orbits. Other signs commonly seen in
dysthyroid eye disease are retraction of the upper
eyelid and lid-lag when the patient looks down. The
affected orbit should be examined to see if proptosis is
present. Relative proptosis exists if there is a forward
movement of the globe in excess of 2 mm compared
with the other eye. The usual method of measuring the
position of the eye is to relate the apex of the cornea to
the lateral orbital margin.

The clinician should palpate both orbits simultaneously, comparing the resistance of corresponding
quadrants. The normal lacrimal gland is often palpable
above a proptosed eye, and can be mistaken for a more
deeply situated tumour. With practice one can ascertain the presence of the tumour even though it lies
fairly deeply within the orbit.

The first seven cranial nerves should be thoroughly
examined. The range of the eye movements must be
checked and any restriction of movements or deviation
of alignment recorded. The general rule is that the
patient has difficulty in looking towards a benign orbital tumour, e.g. if there is a mass on the medial wall of
the orbit the movement of the globe will be reduced
when the patient attempts to look nasally. This is due
to the mass of the tumour placing the muscles at a
mechanical disadvantage. Reduction of movement
because of ocular motor nerve damage is rarely seen
unless an invasive tumour is present or there is a small
mass well back in the orbital apex. The visual acuity
and the visual fields must be charted. If an optic nerve

process. In a high proportion of patients in whom the biopsy shows frank malignancy, evidence of systemic lymphoma is found at the time of presentation, or subsequently. On the other hand disseminated lymphoma or chronic lymphatic leukaemia occurs in only 25% of patients whose biopsy specimens are reported as indeterminate lymphocytic lesions.

Symptoms and presentation
The majority of lymphomatous lesions occur in the anterior part of the orbit. In most cases the mass is noticed by the patient at an early stage. There is usually a swelling of the eyelid and there may be displacement of the eye. On examination a rubbery mass is palpable, and often visible beneath the conjunctiva where it has a characteristic reddish-pink appearance. Pain, or signs of an inflammatory reaction, are usually absent, in contra-distinction to the pseudotumours which constitute the main differential diagnosis.

Diagnosis and investigation
A tissue diagnosis is mandatory. Biopsy material can readily be obtained because of the anterior position of the tumour. It is advisable to perform full investigations for evidence of systematic spread (see Chapter 36) regardless of the histological appearances; an exception can be made in the case of an elderly patient with an indeterminate tumour or a well differentiated lymphocytic lymphoma, where the results of investigations are rarely positive.

Treatment and prognosis
Those patients discovered to have systemic lymphoma are treated as described in Chapter 36. In the majority of patients however investigations are negative, and these are treated by radiotherapy. A tumour dose of 3000 rad in 3 weeks achieves virtually 100% local control regardless of histological type (Kim and Fayos, 1976). Rapid regression occurs and there are rarely any local complications of treatment.

The prognosis depends on the histological type. As mentioned above, the majority of well differentiated lymphocytic lymphomata and indeterminate lymphocytic tumours do not disseminate; those which do often run a protracted and relatively benign course, as chronic lymphatic leukaemia or cutaneous lymphoma.

Of those patients with a histological definite malignant lymphoma, but with no evidence of dissemination on full investigation, approximately 50% develop systemic lymphoma within 5 years. The remainder appear to be cured by local radiotherapy alone (Kim and Fayos, 1976). There seems to be no need to give chemotherapy unless or until dissemination is found.

Lacrimal gland tumours

Pathology
Lacrimal gland tumours are extremely rare. They occur predominantly in young and middle-aged adults, and are commoner in males than females. The most frequently occurring types are the pleomorphic adenoma and the adenoid cystic carcinoma, but all histological types of tumour which affect the salivary glands may also arise in the lacrimal gland (see Chapter 13). The lacrimal gland may be involved by other tumours, e.g. lymphoma and pseudotumour.

Diagnosis and investigation
For the purpose of diagnosis and management, lacrimal gland tumours can be conveniently divided into two groups, the pleomorphic adenoma (benign mixed cell tumour) and the others. This is a convenient classification for it is essential that benign mixed cell tumours are removed *in toto* without a biopsy and with the capsule of the tumour intact. In all other cases a biopsy should be obtained so that the diagnosis can be established at an early stage. The two groups can be distinguished by the history and the physical signs. Investigations such as plain X-rays, CT-scans and ultrasonic scans are of secondary importance in this decision. Over 90% of patients with a benign mixed cell tumour have noticed the mass for a minimum of twelve months. It is extremely rare for these patients to experience any pain referrable to the mass which is hard and expands extremely slowly.

Lesions of the lacrimal gland with a short history, i.e. less than twelve months, are usually either pseudotumours, lymphomas or primary lacrimal gland carcinoma. In all these cases an early decision to obtain tissue for biopsy is imperative so that the appropriate treatment can be given.

Treatment and prognosis
The treatment of pleomorphic adenoma of the lacrimal gland is essentially surgical. The diagnosis is made on clinical grounds and the decision to remove the whole of the lacrimal gland through a lateral orbitotomy should be made. This is the only approach which enables the surgeon to remove the lacrimal gland *in toto* with its capsule intact. An anterior approach, or worse still, a transcranial approach, are doomed to failure for the capsule of the tumour will be broken and eventual recurrence is inevitable. Such recurrences are extremely difficult to treat; radiotherapy to a dose of 5500–6000 rad in 6 weeks may retard growth but is never curative. Occasionally a recurrence shows malignant transformation in which case the prognosis is hopeless.

In most cases of carcinoma of the lacrimal gland the

tumour has spread outside the confines of the orbit at an early stage. Radiotherapy offers the only chance of reducing the size of the tumour and prolonging life. A tumour dose of at least 6 000 rad in 6 weeks should be delivered, accepting a high risk of ocular complications.

In some cases where the histological diagnosis is obtained at an early stage and the tumour can be shown to be confined to the orbit then radical surgery is justified. Such surgery involves *en bloc* removal of the orbital contents together with the roof and lateral wall. The defect in the face and skull is then covered with a large skin flap based on the superficial temporal artery.

The prognosis of malignant lacrimal gland tumours is poor, with a 5-year survival rate of less than 25%.

Other malignant tumours

A wide variety of malignant tumours may arise in the orbit. These include melanoma, teratoma, the various types of connective tissue sarcoma, e.g. fibrosarcoma and liposarcoma, and malignant varieties of haemangiopericytoma, fibrous histiocytoma, neurilemmoma and meningioma. All are very rare. In general the treatment is surgical in the first instance; post-operative radiotherapy may be needed where excision is incomplete.

The orbit may be involved secondarily by direct extension of carcinoma from adjacent structures, especially the paranasal sinuses, nasopharynx and surrounding skin.

Blood-borne metastases to the orbit are not uncommon. The primary tumours most often responsible are, in order of frequency, carcinoma of the breast, carcinoma of the bronchus, carcinoma of the thyroid, and neuroblastoma. Palliative radiotherapy is often indicated to relieve local symptoms, especially pain, in addition to any appropriate systemic therapy. A tumour dose of 3000 rad in 2 weeks is recommended for metastatic carcinoma; 800–1000 rad in 1 week or less is usually adequate for neuroblastoma.

Radiotherapy techniques

A variety of techniques is available for external beam radiotherapy of the orbit. It is not possible to irradiate the entire orbit perfectly homogeneously and effect adequate shielding of the cornea and lens, so an appropriate technique must be chosen to suit the individual patient which minimizes the dose to radiovulnerable structures while giving adequate dosage to the tumour.

Small, anteriorly-placed lesions, e.g. lymphoma, can be treated with a single anterior field on 140–300 kV according to thickness. A diaphragm system and field-defining lamp is preferable to an applicator, to facilitate shielding of the cornea. A small lead disc can be suspended on fine cross-wires and positioned in the beam so that its shadow just covers the cornea.

Most orbital tumours are treated by supervoltage irradiation. The most commonly used technique is an anterior and lateral field as shown in Fig. 9.1. The lateral field is positioned to pass behind the lens of the eye on the affected side and angled 5° or 10° posteriorly so that there is no danger of any dosage to the contra-lateral lens. Care must be taken with this technique to avoid under-dosage anteriorly, especially on the medial side, therefore the anterior field is weighted at least 2:1 compared with the lateral field. Wherever possible the cornea and lens are shielded by a fine lead cylinder positioned along the line of the beam (Fig. 9.2). This however results in some under-dosage of the posterior orbit immediately behind the globe; this under-dosed region tends to be larger from a linear accelerator than from a cobalt machine, because of the penumbra effect from the latter.

When there is involvement of the posterior orbit or where there is considerable proptosis, e.g. with a large rhabdomyosarcoma, it is preferable to use superior and inferior fields as in Figs. 9.3 and 9.4. The cornea may be shielded from one or both fields according to the position of the tumour, e.g. if the tumour is mainly superior in the orbit a shield can be used with the superior oblique field, accepting a small area of under-dosage inferiorly. In any case, where shielding of the cornea is inadvisable, the patient should be asked to keep the eye open during irradiation, making use of the surface-sparing effect of a supervoltage beam which is sufficient to avoid corneal complications; the lens will of course receive the full incident dose so cataract is probable.

In cases where the disease is known to be limited to the posterior orbit, lateral fields alone can be used avoiding dosage to the anterior chamber.

Complications of radiotherapy

Dryness of the eye
The lacrimal gland and secretory glands of the conjunctiva have a sensitivity to radiation similar to that of the major and minor salivary glands. Doses in excess of 3000 rad in 3 weeks cause significant diminution in secretion. Consequently if the lacrimal gland and most of the conjunctival sac receive more than this dose, some dryness of the eye results with consequent corneal irritation. This may be relieved by regular instillation of hypromellose drops. With a severe degree of dryness there is a risk of corneal ulceration, in which case a haptic contact lens is necessary to protect the cornea.

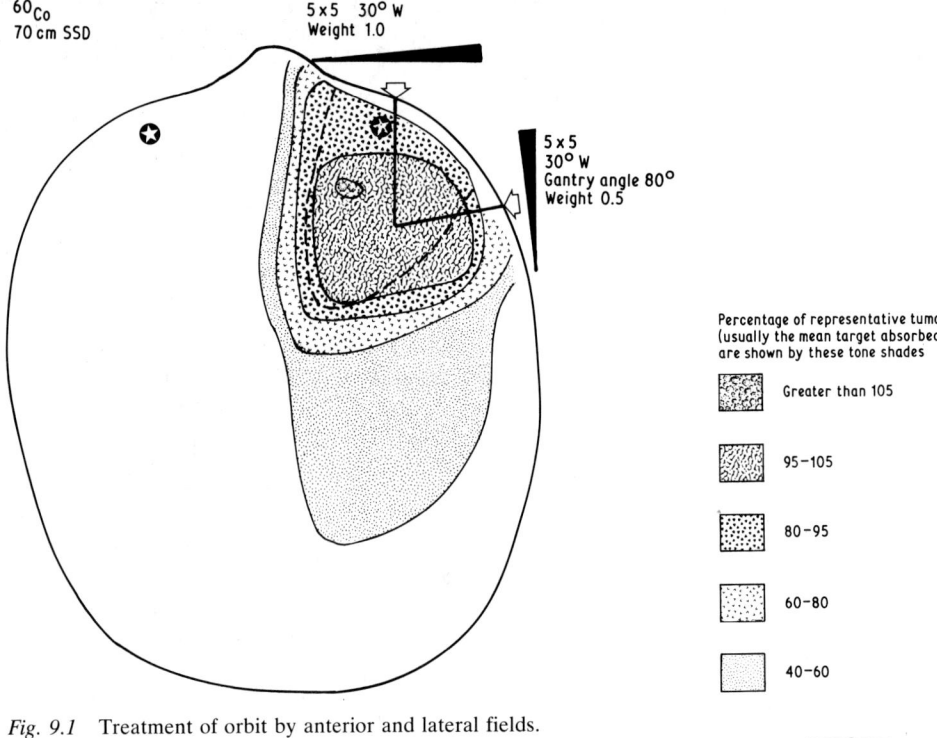

^{60}Co
70 cm SSD

5 x 5   30° W
Weight 1.0

5 x 5
30° W
Gantry angle 80°
Weight 0.5

Percentage of representative tumour dose
(usually the mean target absorbed dose)
are shown by these tone shades

Greater than 105

95–105

80–95

60–80

40–60

Fig. 9.1   Treatment of orbit by anterior and lateral fields.

Corneal damage

Direct radiation injury to the cornea occurs only with doses in excess of 5000 rad in 5 weeks, so in practice it is seen only in those cases where the tumour is so extensive that it is not possible to irradiate it adequately and at the same time shield the cornea. The acute corneal reaction under these circumstances manifests itself as a painful punctate keratitis with hyperaemia of the conjunctiva which may proceed to corneal ulceration. There is often an associated iridocyclitis. Steroid drops are necessary to control the pain. The acute reaction subsides leaving corneal scarring, and secondary glaucoma may supervene. Often the eye gradually becomes phthisic over a period of several months after irradiation.

Cataract

The lens is the most radiosensitive structure in the eye. Opacities have been observed with doses of 200 rad, and progressive cataract impairing vision with as little as 800 rad. In practice, however, the opacities which occur with small doses of irradiation are usually non-progressive and do not impair visual acuity. Many patients whose lenses receive between 1000 and 2000 rad have no impairment of vision, but doses in excess of

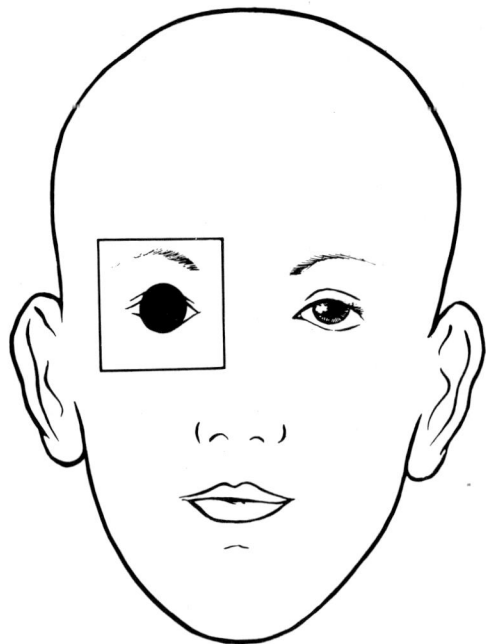

Fig. 9.2   Anterior orbital field, showing position of lead shield.

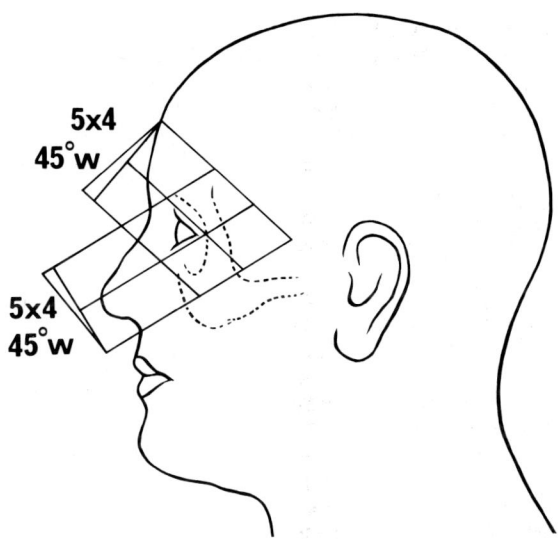

Fig. 9.3 Treatment of orbit by superior and inferior oblique fields.

this level to the whole of the lens are almost certain to cause progressive cataract. Radiation-induced cataract is managed in the same way as other types of cataract; vision can be restored by lens extraction.

Retinal damage

The retina and optic nerve have the same tolerance to radiation as other parts of the central nervous system. Acute effects are not seen with external beam irradiation. Late damage may be seen after high dosage; it rarely occurs unless the dose exceeded 5000 rad in 5 weeks, while the young healthy retina can usually tolerate 6000 rad. The changes which occur in the retina are secondary to vascular damage and include haemorrhages, exudates and degeneration; they progress slowly over a period of several years. Vision is usually only moderately impaired unless there is massive haemorrhage, large vessel occlusion or secondary glaucoma, which lead to complete blindness. Optic atrophy may occur as a result of high dosage to the optic nerve or chiasma.

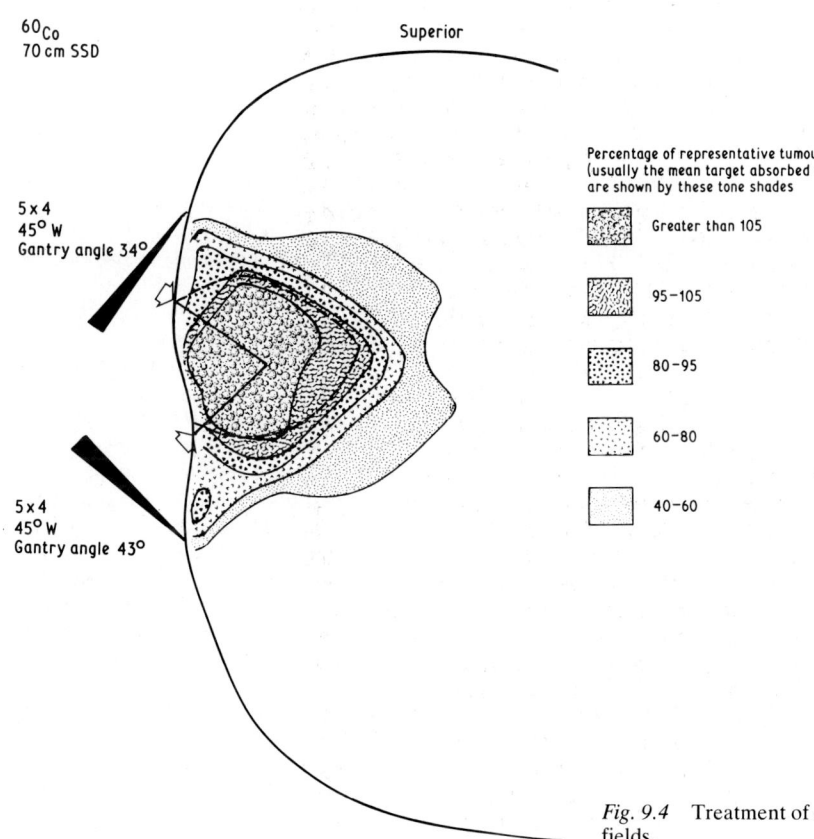

Percentage of representative tumour dose (usually the mean target absorbed dose) are shown by these tone shades

Greater than 105

95–105

80–95

60–80

40–60

Fig. 9.4 Treatment of orbit by superior and inferior oblique fields.

Disturbance of growth

Irradiation of the orbit of a young child suppresses bone growth to some extent. Consequently as the child grows some degree of facial asymmetry appears. This is rarely sufficient to cause noticeable deformity, except in those individuals treated in the first year of life who may be severely disfigured.

Tumours of eyelids

Pathology

Both basal cell and squamous cell carcinomata may arise from the skin of the eyelids, where they have the same aetiological and pathological features as similar lesions arising in the skin elsewhere in the body. The incidence of eyelid tumours in the United Kingdom is approximately 6 per 100 000 per annum. The male/female ratio is about 3:2. The peak age incidence is in the seventh decade.

Basal cell carcinoma

This occurs most frequently on the lower eyelid or at the medial canthus; less than 20% of basal cell carcinomata of the lids occur on the upper lid or at the lateral canthus. The tumour characteristically grows very slowly. Orbital invasion is rare, occurring insidiously in patients who have neglected to seek medical advice for a lesion which has been present for a number of years.

Squamous cell carcinoma.

This accounts for about 10% of tumours of the eyelids. It occurs with equal frequency on the upper and lower lids. It may invade the orbit and metastasize to pre-auricular and upper deep cervical lymph nodes.

Treatment

Most carcinomata of the eyelids may be treated equally effectively by surgery or radiotherapy. It is important to assess which method of treatment is more appropriate for the individual patient, so close collaboration between surgeon and radiotherapist is necessary. Very small lesions not involving the lid margin may be excised with primary skin closure without deformity of the lid; surgery is therefore usually simpler and quicker than radiotherapy.

In most cases, even with lesions as small as 0.5 cm diameter, surgical removal necessitates skin grafting or lid reconstruction. Here the choice between surgery and radiotherapy is controversial, and is often determined by the availability of skill and facilities at the particular centre where the patient is treated. The recurrence and complication rates after either method

of treatment properly applied are negligible. The cosmetic results of both methods depend largely on the skill of the practitioner; there is usually little difference between surgery and radiotherapy, except with larger lesions where the appearance after skilled plastic surgery is often better in the long-term. Surgery is indicated for tumours on the middle third of the upper lid, because of the possible complications of radiotherapy at this site (see below), and is probably preferable for younger patients with larger tumours. For the majority of patients, however, radiotherapy is simpler, safer and less costly than surgery.

In the advanced case with orbital and bone invasion radiotherapy alone is rarely effective. Radical surgery including orbital exenteration is required. Postoperative radiotherapy to 6000 rad in 6 weeks is advisable as it is not usually possible to be certain that excision is complete.

Pre-auricular lymph node metastases from squamous carcinoma are fortunately rare. Provided the patient is fit enough the best chance of cure is gained by radical surgery, which must include parotidectomy and neck dissection, followed by radiotherapy. An elderly patient should be treated solely by radiotherapy using a technique similar to that recommended for parotid tumours.

Radiotherapy technique

Treatment is by superficial X-rays in the 60–140 kV range. The energy should be selected according to the thickness of the tumour, so that the deepest extent receives at least 80% of the incident dose. The area to be treated is defined by a lead cut-out. In the case of squamous carcinoma a 1-cm margin of apparently normal skin round the lesion should be irradiated; in the case of basal cell carcinoma this margin need be no more than 5 mm.

The eyeball and unaffected lid are protected by a spatula-shaped lead shield inserted into the fornix beneath the involved lid (Fig. 9.5). Topical anaesthesia is usually, but not invariably, necessary to enable the patient to tolerate the shield; one drop of an agent such as proxymetacaine 0.5%, is put into the conjunctival sac before insertion of the shield. Care must be taken to avoid trauma to the cornea and infection when the shield is inserted. This method is not suitable if there is extensive destruction of the lid; in these cases indirect shielding of the cornea is necessary, as described above.

Fractionated irradiation probably gives the best cosmetic results, although good results from single doses to small tumours have been reported (Fitzpatrick *et al.*, 1972). An incident dose of 5000 rad in 10 fractions over a minimum of 3 weeks is recommended.

Eyelid tumours have been treated by both intersti-

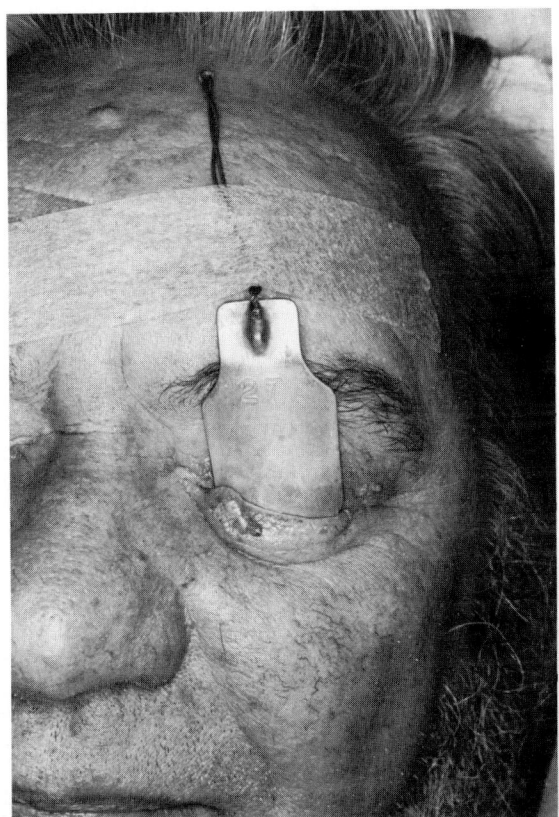

Fig. 9.5 Basal cell carcinoma of lower eyelid. Spatula-shaped eye shield in position ready for treatment with superficial X-rays.

tial and surface applicator techniques in the past and some good results reported, especially with lesions around the medial canthus. However it is more difficult to avoid irradiation of the eye and in virtually all cases external radiation is both simpler and safer.

Complications of radiotherapy

The early literature contained a formidable list of ocular complications of irradiation of the eyelids, including cataract, glaucoma, and complete destruction of the eye. These resulted from plesiotherapy or from failure to shield the globe, and do not occur with present-day techniques. The following complications are seen:

1. *Epiphora.* About 10% of treated patients complain of some degree of watering of the eye. This occurs when the lower canaliculus becomes occluded as a result of the radiation reaction, but is rarely troublesome except when there is lid deformity or other abnormality of the eye causing a reflex increase of lacrimation. Routine syringing of the nasolacrimal apparatus during or after radiotherapy does not reduce the risk of epiphora.

2. *Keratinization of the conjunctival mucosa.* This occurs in about 5% of cases. In the lower lid it causes only minor irritation which can be alleviated by regular removal of the keratin plaque. In the upper lid keratinization of the palpebral conjunctiva, especially the middle third, can cause corneal abrasion, so a haptic contact lens may be needed to protect the cornea.

3. *Dryness of the eye.* Radiation causes diminished secretion of glands within the field. This is an especial problem when the upper lid is irradiated. Minor degrees of dryness of the eye may be alleviated by regular instillation of hypromellose drops. In more severe cases a contact lens may be needed to prevent corneal damage.

4. *Lid deformity.* When the full thickness of the lid is involved by neoplasm, healing after radiotherapy is accompanied by fibrosis and a contraction deformity ensues. This results in ectropion or entropion; the latter is by far the commoner. Alternatively an existing ectropion may be exacerbated by radiation. There is permanent loss of lashes within the irradiated area.

5. *Late skin changes.* Some degree of depigmentation and telangiectasia occurs in most cases. These changes do not usually appear for at least two years after radiotherapy and progress slowly. They are rarely sufficient to cause any noticeable disfigurement except when large areas have been treated.

Skin necrosis is a rare complication. It may occur as a result of trauma or exposure to strong sunlight several years after radiotherapy. Necrosis nearly always heals with removal of the precipitating factor and application of a corticosteroid ointment.

Results and prognosis

1. *Basal cell carcinoma.* Radiotherapy fails to cure the lesion in less than 5% of all cases; most of the failures are deeply infiltrating tumours, especially at the medial canthus. Recurrences after radiotherapy must be treated surgically; about 15–20% recur again after surgery. However, ultimate failure and death from uncontrolled disease is exceedingly rare, only occurring in a small percentage of those patients in whom there was deep penetration of the orbit at the time of presentation. The recurrance rate in most reported

series treated by primary surgery is also less than 5%.

2. *Squamous carcinoma.* The reported radiotherapy failure rate varies between 2% (Fitzpatrick *et al.,* 1972) and 12.5% (Lederman, 1976). Surgical results are similar.

Involvement of lymph nodes occurs in about 15% of patients either at presentation or subsequent to successful treatment of the primary. There is a small mortality, not more than 10%, nearly all due to lymphatic spread.

Tumours of the conjunctiva

All conjunctival tumours are rare. The least rare is the melanoma. Squamous carcinoma also occurs both in its invasive and intraepithelial forms, as does muco-epidermoid carcinoma, and basal cell carcinoma.

Squamous carcinoma-in-situ (Bowen's disease)

Squamous carcinoma-in-situ occurs almost exclusively in middle-aged and elderly men. It is of multifocal origin and may involve, in order of frequency, the bulbar conjunctiva, cornea, palpebral conjunctiva, and eyelids. It tends to arise in sites of chronic infection, or after burns or pannus formation. It is pre-malignant and invasive squamous carcinoma may supervene, often after many years.

Small lesions are treated by local excision. Larger lesions not amenable to simple excision are treated by radiotherapy. Those which are confined to the cornea and bulbar conjunctiva can be treated by β-ray therapy using a strontium-90 applicator; a dose of 6000–10000 rad in 10 fractions is given, depending on the thickness of the lesion. Where there is involvement of the palpebral conjunctiva or lids superficial X-ray therapy is used, shielding as much of the cornea as possible and giving 4500 rad in 10 fractions.

Squamous carcinoma

Squamous carcinoma of the conjunctiva is a disease of the elderly, commoner in males than females. It may arise *de novo,* or from pre-existing in-situ carcinoma. The most common site of origin is the limbus, whence it may spread to the adjacent conjunctiva, over the cornea, and eventually may invade the orbit. Lymphatic spread to the pre-auricular nodes sometimes occurs, but this is usually a late manifestation where there is advanced local disease.

Surgery is the treatment of choice for very small early lesions which can be excised completely without sacrificing the eye, and also for the very advanced disease extending into the orbit. All other cases are

best treated solely by radiotherapy. In the case of limbal and bulbar lesions the main bulk of the lesion should be removed to establish histology and provide a flat surface which can then be irradiated with β-rays from a strontium-90 applicator; a dose of 8000 rad in 8 fractions over 2–3 weeks is advisable. More bulky lesions and those involving the lids can be treated by superficial X-ray therapy, giving 5000 rad in 10 fractions in 3 weeks. Large lesions with orbital invasion are dealt with in the same way as similar tumours arising on the eyelid.

The prognosis is good. Local recurrence and metastases rarely occur unless the lesion was very advanced at presentation. Radiotherapy complications are minimal; occasionally corneal scarring and cataract occur after superficial X-ray therapy when it has not been possible to shield the cornea and lens completely because of the site and position of the tumour.

Conjunctival melanoma

Pathology

Melanoma of the conjunctiva has an annual incidence in the United Kingdom of approximately 0.01 per 100 000 population. It can occur at any age from adolescence onwards. It is approximately twice as common in females as males. It may arise in one of three ways:

1. De novo, on the conjunctiva, usually the bulbar surface. It appears as a pink, brown or black spot, which steadily increases in size.
2. From a pre-existing naevus, again usually on the bulbar surface. There is a long history of a spot on the conjunctiva which may be pigmented or non-pigmented, and then slow increase in size.
3. From 'pre-cancerous melanosis' which is an in-situ melanoma, having the same histological features as lentigo maligna of the skin. This change occurs in middle-aged and elderly people. Invasive melanoma supervenes after a number of years and may be multifocal.

Most conjunctival melanomata grow slowly and are of low grade malignancy, especially those arising in melanoma-in-situ. A minority are of high malignancy with rapid growth and both lymphatic and blood-borne metastases.

Treatment

Most cases can be treated adequately with conservation of the eye.

In the case of small lesions on the bulbar conjunctiva local excision should be performed. This serves to establish the histological diagnosis and also to provide a flat surface with only a thin layer of residual tumour cells which can be effectively treated by β-ray therapy. The base of the lesion is irradiated using a strontium-90 plaque, giving 1000 rad on the surface twice weekly to a total dose of 8000–10 000 rad. In the event of local recurrence without evidence of distant metastases, enucleation is necessary.

In the case of a larger nodular lesion involving the palpebral conjunctiva, lids, canthi, or caruncle, surgery is advisable which usually necessitates exenteration of the orbit. Elderly patients or those considered unfit for major surgery may be treated by radioactive gold grain implants; these achieve local control in over 50% of cases but it is impossible to shield the intraocular structures and loss of vision in the affected eye is probable.

Pre-cancerous melanosis is easily diagnosed clinically; it should be observed carefully but not biopsied or treated unless raised nodular areas appear indicating change to invasive melanoma – 'cancerous melanosis'. Melanoma arising in this way is relatively radiosensitive and usually can be managed satisfactorily by radiotherapy. Bulbar lesions are treated by shaving flat and β-ray therapy as above. Where there is involvement of the lids or canthi, superficial X-ray therapy can be used with corneal shielding; large individual dose fractions appear to give better results and an incident dose of 4500 rad in 8 fractions over 4 weeks is effective.

Results and prognosis

In general the prognosis of conjunctival melanoma is relatively good with a 5-year survival of around 75% overall.

Lesions confined to the bulbar conjunctiva are controlled by conservative measures in over 90% of cases. Most recurrences can be successfully treated surgically, and there is only a very occasional death from distant metastases.

The further from the limbus the lesion, the worse the prognosis. When the eyelids or caruncle are involved there is an approximately 30% incidence of lymphatic and blood-borne metastases.

Radiotherapy technique

Beta irradiation is given by a strontium-90 applicator (Fig. 9.6). The isotope is incorporated in a rolled silver sheet coating the convex inner surface of the applicator. Active discs of either 12 mm or 18 mm diameter are used, according to the area to be irradiated. The activity should be sufficient to give a surface dose-rate of approximately 1000 rad per minute so that treatment times can be tolerably short. The eye is anaesthetized with a topical anaesthetic, and the patient asked to fix his gaze on a suitable point. The applicator is then inserted into the conjunctival sac and

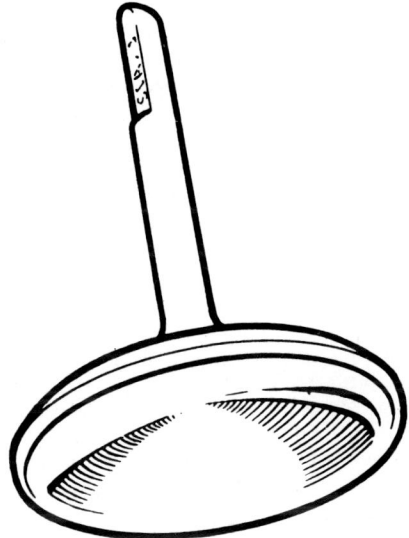

Fig. 9.6 Strontium-90 applicator for irradiation of corneal and conjunctival lesions (Reproduced by courtesy of The Radiochemical Centre, Amersham).

held in position over the area to be treated for a time calculated to give the required dose.

The dose falls to 40% of the surface dose within 1 mm of tissue, therefore lesions thicker than 1 mm cannot be treated satisfactorily by this method. The dose falls to zero within 6 mm, therefore no radiation reaches the equator of the lens so there is no risk of cataract.

Applicators are available with active coating on both convex and concave surfaces so that β-irradiation can be given to both bulbar and palpebral conjunctiva. This method may be used for some cases of carcinoma-in-situ, but there is difficulty in obtaining an adequate dosage in the fornices, so superficial X-rays are generally preferable.

Retinoblastoma

Incidence

Retinoblastoma is a rare tumour of childhood making up approximately 3% of the cases recorded annually in the Manchester Children's Tumour Registry. Its incidence throughout the world seems to be uniform. Nevertheless a steadily increasing number has been noted by many observers, the rate having doubled from about 1/34 000 live births in 1930 to about 1/15 000 live births in 1975. Males and females are approximately equally affected.

The increasing incidence is largely explained by the survival of more patients able to transmit the genetic abnormality to their children.

Aetiology

This tumour may occur unexpectedly as a somatic mutation or be inherited as an autosomal dominant characteristic due to a germinal mutation (Francois, 1977)

The apparently sporadic cases are mostly unilateral and there is then a small risk of their offspring having either unilateral or bilateral disease. If the sporadic case is bilateral there is a 50% chance of the offspring being involved; 70% of hereditary cases are bilateral and in unilateral cases the second eye must be watched for possible later involvement.

A family history may not always be obtainable as a parent may be an unaffected carrier due to the incomplete penetrance of the dominant gene.

The risk to the offspring in the hereditary type is almost 50%. Where at least two siblings are affected, further siblings have a high chance of being affected also, in spite of the absence of the tumour in previous generations.

Five per cent of cases have a demonstrable deletion of the long arm of chromosome 13 and such children commonly have other abnormalities including mental retardation. Other defects at the same chromosome locus may be responsible for the tendency for some bilateral cases to develop second malignant tumours unrelated to radiation or other treatment, especially osteogenic sarcoma.

Pathology and histology

Previously, retinoblastoma was considered a gliomatous tumour but electron microscopy has confirmed its origin in the photoreceptor cells (Ts'O *et al.*, 1970). On light microscopy these tumours are of a 'small round cell' type, their cells having dense nuclei and scant cytoplasm and being arranged in solid sheets or pseudorosettes.

Natural history and metastases

Retinoblastoma may present as a single tumour but in hereditary cases there may be multiple discrete tumours in one or both eyes. This feature is quite distinct from seeding which can occur as tumour fragments break off a lesion growing out into the vitreous.

Spread of a tumour may also occur in the sub-retinal space giving rise to a retinal detachment. Large tumours may penetrate the choroid, and vascular invasion with subsequent blood-borne metastases then becomes likely. Penetration through the sclera gives the risk of extrascleral involvement, and in the untreated case disruption of the global anatomy and fungation.

The optic nerve may become directly involved if the tumour grows into the nerve head and through the lamina cribrosa. If the extension occurs back to where the central retinal artery and vein leave the nerve, about 1 cm behind the globe, access to the subarachnoid space is possible, resulting in dissemination of tumour cells around the base of the brain and within the cerebrospinal fluid.

Most common sites of metastases are bones, bone marrow, lymph nodes and liver. The lungs are affected infrequently. Where there is extrascleral extension or orbital recurrence cervical lymph node involvement may occur.

Symptoms and presentation

Most commonly a child presents under the age of two years with a white pupil ('cat's eye') and this is a sign of a large tumour. Smaller tumours situated posteriorly may prevent visual fixation and give rise to strabismus as the presenting sign.

Other less common presentations are of glaucoma, a pseudohypopyon due to the presence of free tumour cells in the anterior chamber, or a hyphaema due to a rupture of a new vessel on the iris, or an endophthalmitis.

Diagnosis and investigation

By far the most important investigation is the examination of both eyes under general anaesthetic by the experienced ophthalmologist using the intense light of the binocular stereoscopic ophthalmoscope worn on his forehead. With scleral indentation the whole retina can thus be checked for abnormalities. With this technique, tumours of less than 0.5 mm diameter can be detected, and treatment administered under the same anaesthetic. The screening of children in affected families from birth is thus exceedingly accurate.

In both symptomatic and asymptomatic cases this procedure will include assessment of tumour site and size and the observation of any vitreous seeding, as well as an estimate of possible optic nerve infiltration or extrascleral extension. Both eyes must be evaluated similarly.

The diagnoses with which a retinoblastoma can most readily be confused are a larval granulomatosis due to *Toxocara canis,* Coats' disease, primary hyperplastic vitreous and unclassifiable retinal dysplasias. Biopsy of a suspected retinoblastoma is unwise as the requisite puncture of the globe will provide a pathway for extension of tumour and this can decrease chance of cure. Other investigations may sometimes be of help in the more advanced cases especially where tumour cannot be seen because of cloudy vitreous. However, these do not influence subsequent management substantially. They include ultrasonic and CT-scanning as well as measurements of urinary catecholamines and serum lactic dehydrogenase isoenzymes. A cerebrospinal fluid examination, including cytology, may be performed where there is a suspicion of central nervous system (CNS) involvement and other tests may be done in selected cases to screen for metastases, including chest X-ray, and bone scan.

Clinical staging

The classification of retinoblastoma suggested by Reese and Ellsworth (1964) is an attempt to relate tumour extent in the eye to treatment alternatives and prognostic criteria and thus to aid in comparison of results:

Stages

I   Single or multiple tumours of size less than 4 disc diameters at or behind the equator.
II Single or multiple tumours of size 4 to 10 disc diameters at or behind the equator.
III Tumours anterior to the equator or a single tumour larger than 10 disc diameters at or behind the equator.
IV Multiple lesions some greater than 10 disc diameters. Any lesion extending anterior to the ora serrata.
V   Large lesions involving more than half the retina. Vitreous seedings.

Treatment

The modern treatment of retinoblastoma has shifted away from the earlier policy of enucleation of the worse or only affected eye and conservative treatment, if possible, for the remaining eye.

Rather, the aim is now two-fold, namely to eradicate tumour and to preserve maximum vision. This is feasible so long as the attempts to achieve the latter are not inconsistent with saving the patient's life.

Each eye must be assessed by an experienced ophthalmologist, using indirect ophthalmoscopy with the patient anaesthetized and pupils dilated as detailed above. Information concerning the number, site, and size of tumours is noted precisely and the treatment policy is determined for each eye on this basis.

Small tumours

If a tumour is detected of less than 3 mm in size and is accessible to the scleral depressor, it is quick and effective to use cryosurgery (Tolentino and Tablank, 1972). If such a tumour is situated more posteriorly, light coagulation using the xenon arc may be used (Höpping *et al.*, 1964).

However, if such a tumour is near the optic disc or macula, light coagulation could damage vision seriously and so external beam irradiation by a single lateral field is commonly advised.

For a tumour of 3–10 mm in size focal radiation with a radioactive cobalt plaque is most suitable. But if the lesion is near the macula or optic disc, vascular complications are frequent and again lateral beam irradiation is preferable.

For a tumour larger than 10 mm, irradiation to the whole eye is recommended. Whether the field applied is anterior or lateral depends on the site of the tumour and the presence of vitreous seedings. The use of lateral beam therapy can only be considered if the lesion is posterior and there is no suspicion of vitreous seedings or of other tumours anteriorly. Otherwise, in an effort to avoid the lens and subsequent radiation cataract, inadequate treatment may be given. In addition, the lens of the contra-lateral eye is put at risk.

If there is anteriorly sited tumour or vitreous seeding, it is only by a direct anterior field that one can safely encompass the tumour-bearing tissue without giving unacceptable doses of radiation to the contra-lateral eye. If after a course of external radiation one is still in doubt about the presence of tumour activity, it may be possible to follow with focal treatment to the residue.

Multiple tumours

If there are more than two tumours present in one eye, radiation should be given to the whole eye by external beam. With only two tumours it may be possible to treat both by focal methods so long as the larger is not greater than 10 mm. It is often possible to treat one by light coagulation or cryosurgery and the other by focal radiation using a cobalt plaque. However it is not advisable to use cobalt plaques for both because of the increased risk of vascular complications.

Large tumours

Where tumours extend anteriorly beyond the limit of ophthalmoscopy or where they involve more than half the retinal area, the whole eye should be treated. Where the optic nerve is obviously infiltrated, enucleation of the eye should be done, as the risk of spread along the nerve is not inconsiderable and useful sight is unlikely with conservative measures. Similarly, enucleation should be performed on suspicion of such involvement where adequate assessment is difficult due to a clouded vitreous. In all other circumstances, large tumours may be treated by external radiation via an anterior field, with the possibility of enucleation later.

Bilateral tumours

It has already been stated that each eye should be treated on its merits, and this means that enucleation of one eye will not be required in all cases. If it is required, the efforts to preserve vision in the remaining eye are all the more important. The use of a lateral beam will then only be limited by its ability to encompass the existing tumour, and not by the possibility of the divergent beam producing a radiation cataract in the contra-lateral eye. Thus lens damage in the remaining eye could be avoided in a few cases.

Residual orbital tumour

If histological examination of the enucleated specimen reveals evidence of extrascleral extension or of optic nerve infiltration, post-operative radiation to the whole orbit and optic foramen should be given. In these cases, the risk of tumour dissemination by the blood stream or into the central nervous system via the sub-arachnoid space is very high and consideration should be given to chemotherapy and whole CNS irradiation.

Metastatic disease and the role of chemotherapy in its prevention and treatment

The presence of metastases at diagnosis or their subsequent development is always a grave prognostic sign, as there are no reports of long-term survivors in such circumstances.

In specialized centres where large experience in these rare tumours has been obtained and in countries where referrals occur early in the disease, a cure rate of 85–90% is usual, using the methods of treatment outlined above. Adjuvant chemotherapy as a means of eradicating microscopic disease at distant sites would therefore seem inappropriate except if a group where local treatment alone has a significant chance of failure could be identified.

Such cases are those in stage V where choroidal invasion is common and with it the possibility of extrascleral extension. Some centres are now evaluating combination chemotherapy and the most commonly used drugs are cyclophosphamide, vincristine, and actinomycin D given by intravenous pulses every two or three weeks as the patient's bone marrow allows and their disease status dictates (Lonsdale *et al.*, 1968). Where the risk of CNS involvement is high, consideration should be given to the use of irradiation to the whole neuraxis as well as intrathecal methotrexate and systemic combination chemotherapy.

Follow-up and treatment of tumour recurrence

Because of the natural history of this disease, especially in cases with a positive family history, it is essential that examinations under anaesthesia should be repeated every 4–6 weeks for up to 2 years after the last evidence of tumour.

The detection of new tumour may mean further light coagulation or cryosurgery if it is small and suitably situated. Larger tumours or those in which previous treatment has failed to achieve control may require external beam irradiation or, if this has already been given, enucleation. In the past it was not uncommon in some centres to give a second course of external beam radiotherapy if the first failed. Because of the long-term effects of high dosage in young children such a policy should be avoided, though in some circumstances external beam treatment may follow a previous cobalt plaque treatment in the same eye.

The difficulty that even an experienced observer has in assessing tumour recurrence should be stressed. After successful treatment a 'cottonwool mass' or calcified cluster may remain visible on ophthalmoscopy. Recurrence at the edge of such a mass is relatively easily recognized, but it is more difficult to detect in the centre of the chorioretinal scar.

Treatment techniques

Cobalt plaque

This method of local irradiation is most useful for tumour up to 10 mm diameter and a little distance from the macula and nerve head (Stallard, 1962).

The cobalt is vacuum-sealed in a platinum casing with projecting lugs for the scleral sutures. The discs come in a range of sizes from 5–15 mm active diameter and are shaped as a portion of a sphere such that the inner radius approximates the radius of a child's globe.

Within a disc, the cobalt is arranged as a single annulus in the two small sizes and as a central source with one or two concentric annuli in the larger sizes. The tumour is localized from the scleral surface of the globe by three or four punctures whose position internally can be checked ophthalmoscopically. Its diameter is measured and a disc chosen whose active diameter is 1–2 mm greater. The disc is then sutured against the sclera and left in position for 7 days in which time it is planned to give the apex of the tumour at least 4000 rad while the base of the tumour may receive 25 000–35 000 rad.

External beam therapy

This should be administered with megavoltage apparatus using either a telecobalt unit or linear accelerator to minimize scattered radiation and reduce bone absorption. The cobalt beam can be further sharpened by the use of special applicators of a range of field sizes which fit the treatment head and penumbra trim up to the 80% isodose level. The young child will need to be sedated, but for reliability in administering irradiation accurately ketamine anaesthesia is frequently preferred, with the child's head steadied between sandbags for treatment.

1. *Anterior field.* By this approach the whole globe is irradiated, including any vitreous seedings and all parts of the retina. (Fig. 9.7). Field sizes will range from 2 × 3 cm to 3 × 4 cm. Treating 3 times per week, 3500 rad at 2.5-cm depth is given in 12 fractions over 4 consecutive weeks.

2. *Lateral (temporal) field.* The child is in the supine position as for an anterior field. In order to protect the lens of the affected eye, the anterior limit of the field is just in front of the bony rim of the orbit and additional lead is positioned at this edge for trimming of the penumbra. A field size of 4 × 3 cm is usually adequate.

In the case where the tumour is posteriorly situated and there is no suspicion of vitreous seeding, slight angulation of the field posteriorly (approx. 3–4°) may make a significant reduction in the dose the lens of the

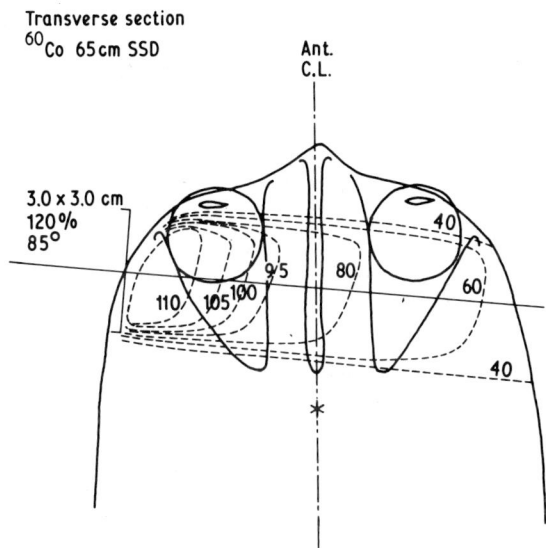

Fig. 9.8   Treatment of posteriorly situated tumour by a lateral field.

opposite eye receives. If the opposite eye has been enucleated, this need not be done (Fig. 9.8). The dose given to the posterior retina is 3500 rad in 12 fractions over 4 weeks, treating 3 times per week.

3. *Bilateral treatment.* Occasionally both eyes need to be irradiated simultaneously. A single anteriour field is then used with the central portion between the inner canthi shielded by a lead block 1 cm wide.

4. *Postoperative irradiation.* Where the eye has been enucleated and there is orbital residue the whole orbit and optic foramen should be included. A similar approach is required for orbital recurrence after enucleation. For a satisfactory dose distribution a pair of wedged fields is usually required and a dose of 4500–5000 rad is given in 15 fractions over 5 weeks, treating 3 times a week with the child anaesthetized (Fig. 9.9).

Complications of treatment

In the early years of radiation for retinoblastoma, the complication rates were high and it is noteworthy that loss of vision was more often due to radiation damage than to uncontrolled tumour. High doses were used, but it is now recognized that lower doses may still control the tumour and result in less complications.

Fortunately a dose of 3500 rad in 4 weeks is adequate to control most intraocular retinoblastomas and a

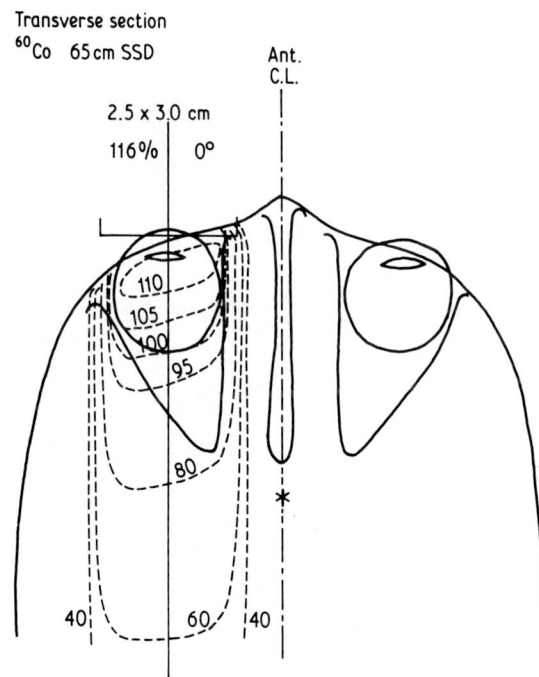

Fig. 9.7   Treatment of whole globe by a single anterior field.

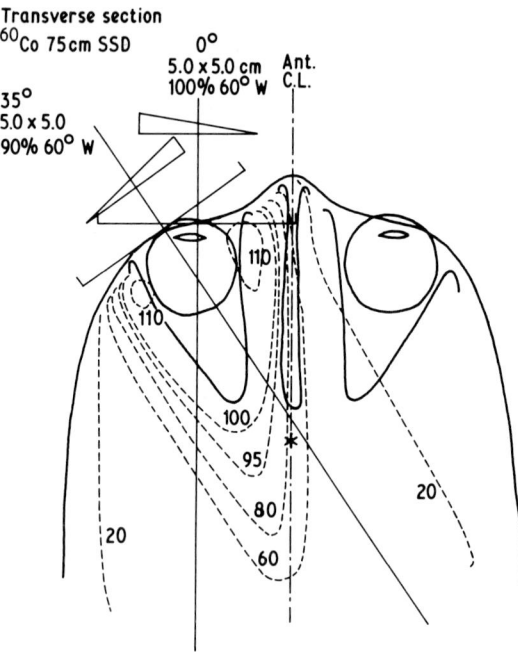

Transverse section
^{60}Co 75cm SSD

0°
5.0 x 5.0 cm Ant.
100% 60° W   C.L.

35°
5.0 x 5.0
90° 60° W

110
110
100
95
80
60
20
20

Fig. 9.9   Treatment of orbit after enucleation.

complication rate of less than 10% is expected at this level. The four main complications which concern us are discussed below.

Cataract formation
All eyes treated with an anterior radiation field will develop some degree of cataract. However this risk may be overstated. Not all cataracts impair useful vision and not all are progressive. If they are, they can be treated adequately by modern aspiration techniques. One practical difficulty of cataract formation however, is its interference with good visualization of the retina at follow-up examination.

Vascular complications
Lesions near the macula and nerve head are best treated by methods other than cobalt plaque because of the risk of the high radiation dose damaging the large blood vessels near the optic disc with later vitreous haemorrhage or haemorrhagic retinitis (MacFaul and Bedford, 1970).

Bone growth
In the young child, one is concerned that delayed growth of the orbital bones due to radiation may result in deformity. It is likely that the socket will be smaller if irradiated, but this effect is much less marked with megavoltage than with orthovoltage therapy.

Radiation-induced tumours
After radiotherapy, the occurrence of sarcomas around the orbit, and especially osteogenic sarcomas, has been reported in several series. Most cases however, were treated with high dosage and using orthovoltage with its even higher bone absorption dose. It must also be remembered that there is a genetic tendency to the formation of osteogenic sarcoma in a proportion of retinoblastoma patients.

Follow-up

With the risk of recurrence being greatest for the first two years after treatment ophthalmoscopic and general examinations should be done every four to six weeks. In the pre-school child anaesthesia will be required. In the older cooperative child examination may be undertaken in the out-patient clinic.

Once the high risk period is over, long-term follow-up is still desirable in all cases because of the need for observation of long-term effects of treatment, for genetic counselling and checking of offspring. Six to twelve monthly checks are adequate.

Results

Published results vary greatly from country to country depending on the stage of disease at presentation and the availability of specialized facilities and experienced personnel.

In western countries cure rates of 85% are usual, with specialized centres achieving higher than 90% cure. From St. Bartholomew's Hospital and Moorfields Hospital London, Bedford reports 100% cure of stage I and II cases and a 75% cure in the less common stage IV and V cases, with an overall cure rate of 90% (Bedford *et al.*, 1971).

Future trends

The incidence of this tumour is likely to increase and the need for careful genetic counselling and early examination of the offspring of patients will become increasingly important. With such good cure rates with local methods of treatment, adjuvant chemotherapy for all cases cannot be justified. However, identification of cases at high risk of developing metastatic disease should be improved and adjuvant chemotherapy and the use of CNS radiation in these cases studied.

Other intraocular tumours

Melanoma of the uveal tract

Incidence
Primary melanoma of the uveal tract is the commonest

malignant tumour of the eye. In the United Kingdom its incidence is approximately 0.2 per 100 000 population per year. The sexes are equally affected. Nearly all cases occur after the age of thirty, with a peak incidence in the sixth decade.

Aetiology
There are no known causative factors. The majority arise *de novo* in an apparently normal eye. It is very rare for a benign pigmented tumour of the uveal tract to undergo malignant change.

The majority of malignant melanomata arise in the choroid; approximately 9% arise in the ciliary body; 6% arise in the iris, nearly always from a pre-existing benign lesion.

Natural history and metastasis
Melanoma begins as a mass in the choroid. As it grows it causes retinal detachment and encroaches on the vitreous cavity. Extraocular extension may occur by one of two pathways; lesions involving the posterior pole can infiltrate through the emissaria, while large lesions may infiltrate directly through the sclera. In most cases growth is characteristically slow. There are reports of untreated cases surviving for many years with very slow growth of the primary tumour and no evidence of metastases (Gass, 1977).

Blood-borne metastases occur in approximately 50% of cases. The time interval between diagnosis and appearance of metastases varies between one month and twenty years, the mean being about four years, reflecting the normally slow growth of this tumour. Nearly all patients who develop metastases have liver involvement; the liver is the presenting site of metastases in over half the patients. Other sites of metastases include lung, bone, skin, breast, and central nervous system.

Symptoms and presentation
The tumour is symptomless in the early stages unless it is close to the macula. Occasionally it is detected at routine ophthalmological examination. The first symptom is disturbance of vision, the nature of which depends on the site of origin of the tumour and its size. There may be a scotoma, field defect, or total loss of vision. Pain is not normally a feature unless an anteriorly placed lesion causes a secondary glaucoma.

Diagnosis and investigation
The diagnosis is established on the physical findings by the ophthalmologist. The principal sign is a mass in the fundus, usually globular and pigmented. The differential diagnosis includes serous detachment, pigmented intraocular cyst, scleritis, disciform exudative senile macular degeneration, haemangioma of the choroid,

and choroidal metastases. Fluorescein angiography and ultrasound help to distinguish melanoma from these simulating lesions.

The only useful investigations for detection of blood-borne metastases are general physical examination, chest X-ray, liver scan and liver function tests.

Treatment
The approach to the management of uveal melanoma has changed considerably in recent years. Formerly enucleation was performed immediately in nearly all patients with a clinical diagnosis of melanoma, in the belief that it gave the best chance of survival. It is now realized that many smaller melanomata can be safely watched for many years, especially in older patients, while others can be managed by conservative measures with preservation of the eye. It has even been suggested that enucleation may shorten survival time because of dissemination of tumour cells at operation (Zimmerman, McLean and Foster, 1978).

Small tumours of less than 3 disc diameter should be observed carefully, and not treated until there is definite evidence of growth. They may then be suitable for photocoagulation. Larger lesions which are remote from the macula and not involving the optic nerve may be treated by radioactive cobalt applicators in a similar manner to retinoblastoma (Stallard, 1966). A higher dose is needed than in the case of retinoblastoma; 8000 rad in 2 weeks at the apex of the tumour is recommended. Tumours of the iris present early, and can usually be removed by iridectomy.

A promising alternative method of irradiation of choroidal melanoma is by particle beams, making use of the Bragg peak to confine the high dose of radiation to the tumour and a small margin of surrounding normal tissue, thus avoiding the very high scleral dose which is a disadvantage of the cobalt discs. Both protons (Suit *et al.*, 1977) and helium ions (Castro *et al.*, 1980) have been used in this way, and preliminary follow-up data show good local control.

Enucleation remains the treatment of choice for those patients with large lesions and poor vision due to involvement of the macula or optic disc, or due to an extensive retinal detachment. It is also indicated where there is pain, secondary glaucoma, or extrascleral extension. If extraocular extension is found at enucleation a partial exenteration is advisable, preserving the lids and conjunctival sac. Post-operative radiotherapy should be given to the orbit in an attempt to prevent local recurrence. A high dose is required, so 6000 rad in 6 weeks using the 2-field technique (Fig. 9.1) is usually given. There is some evidence that the relative radioresistance of melanoma is due to a high capacity for intracellular repair of radiation damage, so that an equivalent biological dose in fewer fractions may give better results, for example 3000 rad in 6 fractions.

Results and prognosis

The overall survival for choroidal melanoma is 70% at 5 years, declining to 50% at 10 years. Survival rates for melanoma of the ciliary body appear similar from the small number of patients available for review. Malignant melanoma of the iris has a much better prognosis with only about 5% of patients succumbing from the disease. The prognosis of uveal melanoma is related to histological type, the spindle cell type having a better prognosis than the epitheloid and mixed cell types.

The prognosis of small lesions treated by photocoagulation or local irradiation is excellent with less than 10% developing metastatic disease. Of patients requiring enucleation, approximately half eventually succumb from metastases. Local recurrence in the orbit is not common, occurring in about 20% of patients in whom extraocular extension was found at enucleation; it is very rare when no extraocular extension has been found. Post-operative radiotherapy to the orbit probably reduces the incidence of local recurrence, but no controlled clinical trials have been performed, so clear evidence of its value is lacking. All patients who develop blood-borne spread eventually succumb to the disease. The mean survival after presentation of metastases is one year.

Intraocular metastases

The eye is an uncommon but well recognized site of metastasis from malignancy elsewhere in the body. The majority of intraocular metastases occur in the choroid at the posterior pole. Metastases in other parts of the uveal tract, in the retina, and in the conjunctiva have been described, but are exceedingly rare.

More than half of all choroidal metastases arise from carcinoma of the breast. Patients developing choroidal metastases from carcinoma of the breast usually have other soft tissue metastases, especially in the lungs. Occasionally the choroidal metastasis is the presenting sign of dissemination, but in such a patient other unsuspected metastases can usually be detected at the same time.

About one-third of choroidal metastases arise from carcinoma of the bronchus. Metastases from most other types of malignant tumour have been reported from time to time, but all are rare.

The patient complains of defective vision and sometimes pain in the affected eye. Examination reveals a solid-looking retinal detachment in the posterior pole, the elevated area appearing pale in colour, often with haemorrhagic areas. There may be raised intraocular pressure. The lesion must be distinguished from primary malignant melanoma and other causes of retinal detachment; usually this is quite easy because of the history of a malignancy elsewhere.

The prognosis of all patients with choroidal metastases is serious and few survive more than a year or so. Nevertheless palliative treatment is indicated to relieve symptoms and maintain morale. Nearly all cases respond to radiotherapy with regression of the tumour leading to relief of pain if present and preservation of the remaining useful vision in the affected eye; in some cases there can be quite marked improvement of vision. Treatment can be given by a single lateral field or by opposed lateral fields where there are bilateral lesions, taking care to avoid both lenses. A fairly high dose should be given to avoid regrowth of the tumour during the patient's remaining life-span, so 3500–4000 rad tumour dose in 3 weeks is recommended.

Further reading

Henderson, J.W. (1973), *Orbital Tumours*. W.B. Saunders and Co., Philadelphia.

References

Bedford, M.A., Bedotto, C. and MacFaul, P.A. (1971), Retinoblastoma. A study of 139 cases. *Br. J. Ophthal.*, **55** 19–27.

Castro, J.R. *et al.* (1980), Current status of clinical particle radiotherapy at Lawrence Berkeley Laboratory. (in press).

Fitzpatrick, P.J. *et al.* (1972), Tumours of the eyelids and their treatment by radiotherapy. *Radiology*, **104**, 661–5.

Francois, J. (1977), Genetics of retinoblastoma. *Mod. Prob. Ophthal.*, **18**, 165–72.

Gass, J.D. (1977), Problems in the differential diagnosis of choroidal nevi and malignant melanomas. The XXXIII Edward Jackson Memorial Lecture. *Am. J. Ophthal.*, **83**, 299–323.

Höpping, W. and Meyer-Schwickerath, G. (1964), Light coagulation treatment in retinoblastoma. In: *Ocular and Adnexal Tumours*, (ed. M. Boniuk), Mosby, St. Louis. pp. 192–6.

Kim, Y.H. and Fayos, J.V. (1976), Primary orbital lymphoma; a radiotherapeutic experience. *Int. J. Radiat. Oncol.*, **1**, 1099–105.

Koornneff, L. and Los, J.A. (1975), A new anatomical approach to the human orbit. *Mod. Prob. Ophthal.*, **14**, 49–56.

Lederman, M. (1976), Radiation treatment of cancer of the eyelids. *Br. J. Ophthal.*, **60**, 794–805.

Lederman, M. and Wybar, K. (1976), Ocular malignant diseases. *Proc. R. Soc. Med.*, **69**, 895–903.

Lonsdale, D. *et al.* (1968), Chemotherapeutic trials in patients with metastatic retinoblastoma. *Cancer Chemother. Rep.*, **52**, 631–4.

MacFaul, P.A. and Bedford, M.A. (1970), Ocular complications after therapeutic irradiation. *Br. J. Ophthal.*, **54**, 237–47.

Morgan, G. and Harry, J. (1978), Lymphocytic tumours of indeterminate nature; a five year follow-up of 98 conjunctival and orbital lesions. *Br. J. Ophthal.*, **62**, 381–3.

Reese, A.B. and Ellsworth, R.M. (1964), Management of retinoblastoma. *Ann. N.Y. Acad. Sci.*, **114**, 958–62.

Sagerman, R.H., Tretter, P. and Ellsworth R.M. (1972), The treatment of orbital rhabdomyosarcoma of children with primary radiation therapy. *Am. J. Roentg.*, **114**, 31–4.

Stallard, H.B. (1962), The conservative treatment of retinoblastoma. *Trans. Ophthal. Soc. U.K.*, **82**, 473–534.

Stallard, H.B. (1966), Radiotherapy for malignant melanoma of the choroid. *Br. J. Ophthal.*, **50**, 147–55.

Suit, H.D. *et al.* (1977), Clinical experience with protons and heavy ions. *Int. J. Radiat. Oncol. Biol. Phys.*, **3**, 115–25.

Tolentino, F.I. Jr and Tablante, R.T. (1972), Cryotherapy of retinoblastoma. *Arch. Ophthal.*, **87**, 52–5.

Ts'O, M.O., Fine, B.S. and Zimmerman, L.E. (1970), The nature of retinoblastoma. 11. Photoreceptor differentiation; an electron microscopic study. *Am. J. Ophthal.*, **69**, 350–9.

Zimmerman, L.E., McLean, I.W. and Foster, W.D. (1978), Does enucleation of the eye containing a malignant melanoma prevent or accelerate the dissemination of tumour cells? *Br. J. Ophthal.*, **62**, 420–5.

10 Central nervous system

Arthur Jones and John Currie

The variety and behaviour of tumours occurring in the central nervous system (CNS) reflect the complexities both of the nervous system and of the tumour processes involved. These complexities involve several clinical disciplines, and the full investigation and treatment of patients so affected requires at various times the close and informed collaboration of

Table 10.1 Classification of main types of primary brain tumour.

---

1. *Maldevelopmental*
   Teratoma
   Dermoid cyst
   Craniopharyngioma
   Ectopia and hamartoma

2. *Neuroglial*
   Astrocytoma
   Oligodendroglioma
   Ependymoma

3. *Neuronal*
   Medulloblastoma
   Neuroblastoma
   Ganglioneuroma

4. *Meningeal*
   Meningioma
   Sarcoma

5. *Blood vascular*
   Angioma
   Haemangioblastoma

6. *Reticular*
   Microgliomatosis
   Reticulum cell sarcoma

7. *Pineal*
   Pineocytoma
   Pineoblastoma
   Teratoma

8. *Optic nerve and chiasmal*
   Glioma

---

neurosurgeons, neurologists, neuropathologists, neuroradiologists, endocrinologists, and radiation oncologists. This chapter is concerned with such collaboration in the management both of intracranial and of spinal tumours.

CNS tumours account for about 9% of all primary tumours, and for authoritative and concise discussions of their pathology the reader is referred to the monograph by Rubinstein (1972). In the present discussion of treatment the authors have concentrated on the commoner disorders and on those of current interest to clinical oncologists (Tables 10.1 and 10.2). Tumours arising mainly in childhood are discussed in Chapter 37, and those of the pituitary gland in Chapter 17. Reasons of space prevent consideration of a number of conditions such as craniopharyngioma, haemangioblastoma and chordoma in which combinations of surgery and radiotherapy have a place in management.

Intracranial tumours

Clinical features

The clinical features of an intracranial tumour depend principally upon the combination of three factors. First, the expansion of the tumour causing raised intracranial pressure; secondly epilepsy and finally the occurrence of focal neurological defects. The nature of the tumour and its site contribute to its characteristic presentation.

Raised intracranial pressure

Any expanding lesion within the skull will eventually cause raised pressure. Initial growth of the tumour displaces cerebrospinal fluid (CSF) from the ventricles and subarachnoid space, the convolutions being flattened against the inner table. This may in children increase the convolutional markings on the inner table of the skull, cause separation of the sutures and

Table 10.2 Classification* of Gliomas.

Type	Synonyms and related terms	
I. *Astrocytoma*		
Astrocytoma Grade 1	Protoplasmic, fibrillary,	
Astrocytoma Grade 2	pilocytic and gemistocytic astrocytomas.	} Differentiated astrocytoma
Astrocytoma Grade 3	Anaplastic astrocytoma	} Malignant astrocytoma
Astrocytoma Grade 4	Glioblastoma multiforme	
II. Oligodendroglioma		
III. Ependymoma (Grades 1–4)	includes ependymoblastoma	
Choroid plexus		
papilloma		

* 'Classifications must be regarded as providing merely arbitrary pockets into which we can place tumours in order they may be more easily considered . . . . No two gliomas are identical'. (Bucy and Gustafson, 1939.)

enlargement of the head. When the fluid reserve within the pathways is taken up displacement of cerebral tissue follows, and this distorts and finally causes often dramatic loss of function in the brain stem and medulla. Slowly growing lesions may cause gross displacement with remarkably little neurological disturbance. More rapidly expanding lesions do not allow time for this adjustment to take place. Unilateral cerebral hemisphere lesions cause herniation beneath the falx of the pericallosal gyrus and displacement of the pineal (recognized radiographically when calcified). As expansion continues the medial inferior portion of the temporal lobe (hippocampal gyrus) is forced through the tentorial opening adjacent to the brain stem on one or both sides. This tentorial pressure cone causes congestion and numerous, usually fatal haemorrhages in the brain stem. Concomitant with the brain stem compression the oculomotor nerve and the posterior cerebral artery are trapped giving rise to pupillary and oculomotor paralysis and infarction of the occipital lobe. Similarly raised pressure within the posterior fossa, due to a tumour or secondary to pressure from above, causes displacement of the cerebellar tonsils through the foramen magnum which may cause fatal medullary compression.

In addition to the growth of the tumour itself two further changes may occur to aggravate the raised pressure. One of these is cerebral oedema, the other the development of hydrocephalus. Many intracranial tumours are associated with swelling of the surrounding brain and often this is extremely extensive. Hydrocephalus is most likely to accompany tumours sited in the third ventricle, brain stem or posterior fossa. Both cerebral oedema and the formation of hyd-

rocephalus may occur suddenly, causing a dramatic rise in pressure with rapid deterioration in the clinical state of the patient.

The symptoms of raised intracranial pressure, headache, vomiting, and visual disturbance as papilloedema develops, are seen with most tumours but are usually more marked in those of the posterior fossa. In some tumours certain symptoms predate the development of the full clinical picture and may even be misleading, as is often the case with early persistent vomiting in children with medulloblastoma.

Epilepsy
An epileptic attack may occur at any stage during the growth of a tumour and may dramatically herald its onset. Usually the lesion is supratentorial, but posterior fossa tumours giving rise to hydrocephalus may cause an attack. The most frequent episodes are grand mal in type but focal seizures may occur and assist in clinical localization.

Neurological deficit
Pressure, infiltration and oedema of cerebral tissue at the site of a tumour result in focal loss of function. In addition there may be non-specific effects, the so called non-localizing signs, the bilateral sixth nerve palsies associated with raised intracranial pressure being an example. The degree of neurological change produced by a tumour varies enormously depending upon the nature of the tumour, its rate of growth and destruction of infiltrated cerebral tissue. Some tumours, such as the low grade astrocytomas in the brain stem, may be very extensive yet remarkable for the continuing normal function of the infiltrated tracts and nerve nuclei.

Other tumours growing rapidly – with a tendency to undergo necrosis, form cysts or cause haemorrhage with much surrounding oedema – may rapidly interfere with function, sometimes dramatically if bleeding and sudden local destruction occur.

Investigational methods

The diagnosis and localization of an intracranial tumour depends upon clinical assessment and the use of modern diagnostic techniques which may also give an indication as to the type of tumour present.

A clinical history noting the mode of onset and evolution of symptoms, together with examination of both the nervous and general systems forms the basis of management. The initial investigation should, in so far as is possible, exclude systemic disease and then proceed to define the site and nature of the lesion.

Skull and spinal radiography – plain films
Routine skull and spinal radiographs are indispensable and may reveal congenital and acquired abnormalities. Tumours may erode or destroy bone, give rise to raised intracranial pressure causing skull enlargement, suture separation in the young, or sellar erosion in the adult. If calcified, pineal and choroid plexus displacement may be observed, and calcification may be present in a tumour (demonstrable on skull X-rays in 10% of all tumours) (Fig. 10.1 *a–d*).

Contrast studies
Investigation of tumours by invasive techniques may sometimes be required to attempt to define and localize a lesion. Angiographic studies will demonstrate the presence of vascular tumours (Fig. 10.2) and displacement of vessels due either to a tumour mass or cerebral hernia. Display of the ventricles and subarachnoid pathways is possible by introduction of air or contrast media, either at ventriculography or lumbar puncture. A ventriculogram is performed after making a burr hole and is the safest procedure of the two in the presence of papilloedema or suspected sub-tentorial lesion. By either route, air, myodil or a water-soluble contrast medium may be introduced, and in this way tumours may be outlined, displaced ventricles shown and hydrocephalus revealed (Fig. 10.3).

Computerized tomography
Computerized axial tomography (CAT- or EMI-scanning) gives a greater display of intracranial detail, with evidence as to the consistency of a tumour and an indication of surrounding cerebral oedema. When combined with the use of contrast enhancement a high rate of tumour detection is obtained (Fig. 10.4 *a, b*). The uptake of the contrast medium in a tumour is related to its vascularity and to a defect in the blood brain barrier causing an extravascular leak and accumulation of contrast. Fusion between vascular endothelial cells is normally sound but in gliomas it becomes increasingly less so the higher the grade of malignancy.

In supratentorial gliomas there is a close correlation between the malignancy of the tumour and the degree of enhancement, it being greatest with high grade tumours and least with the Kernohan grades 1 and 2. This relationship, however, is not seen in posterior fossa gliomas where even low grade tumours enhance (Butler *et al.*, 1978).

Surgical measures in management

The aim of surgery should be to excise the tumour where possible and establish a definitive pathological diagnosis. In certain situations, frontal, occipital, anterior temporal and cerebellar, a radical excision of tumour is possible by lobectomy. Tumours sited in areas not amenable to radical surgery, because of the subsequent unacceptable neurological deficit, may in some cases be locally excised if well demarcated from surrounding tissue, or 'sub-totally' removed. The presence of a cyst may assist such a partial excision. More limited surgery may be restricted to open or burr hole biopsy to obtain a diagnosis. In those tumours in the posterior fossa obstructing the outlet of the fourth ventricle, sufficient mass of tumour should be removed to free the obstruction to the CSF flow. Surgery for patients with cerebral tumours has become a safer and less hazardous procedure. The improvements which have brought this about have been largely due to better and safer anaesthesia together with the means of controlling the dangerous complications of cerebral oedema and hydrocephalus.

Cerebral oedema
Swelling of the surrounding brain, sometimes very extensive, is seen around the site of a tumour. Likewise it may occur during or after surgery and during postoperative radiotherapy. The oedema present in these conditions is due primarily to increased fluid in the extracellular spaces in the white matter and, to a much less extent, swelling of the cells in the white and grey matter. Rapid deterioration in a patient's condition may require equally rapid control of cerebral oedema. In order to achieve this, an osmotic dehydrating agent should be given intravenously, either urea or mannitol.

Urea is administered as a freshly prepared solution in 5% dextrose in a strength of 30%. The total dose is 1–1.5 g/kg body weight, and the infusion should be given slowly at 4 ml per minute. A rapid diuresis fol-

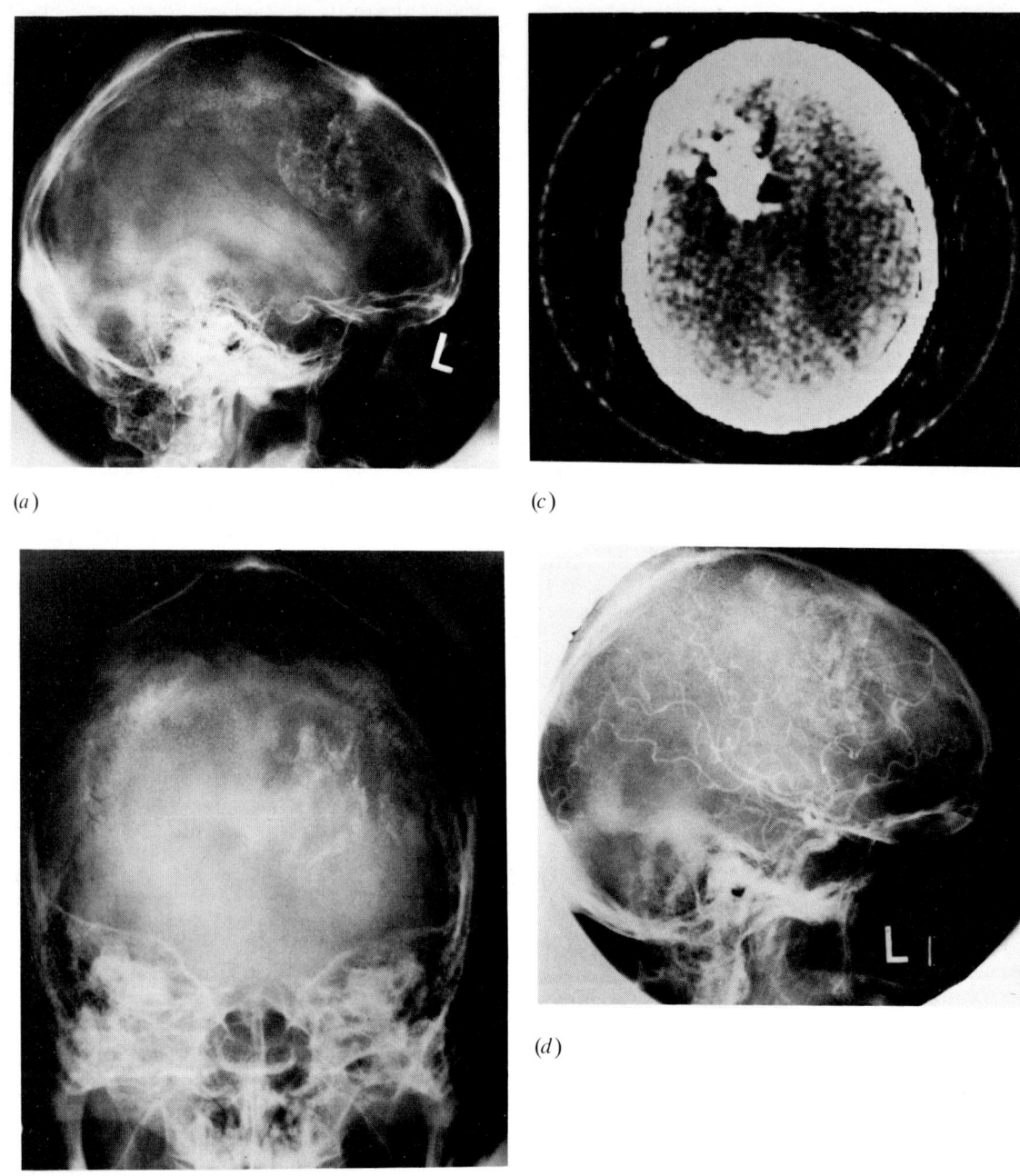

(a)

(c)

(b)

(d)

Fig. 10.1 Astrocytoma of left frontal lobe (Grade 2 gemistocytic) with intracerebral calcification shown in plain radiographs (*a*) and (*b*) and in CAT scan (*c*), and displacing
anterior cerebral artery in carotid arteriogram (*d*).

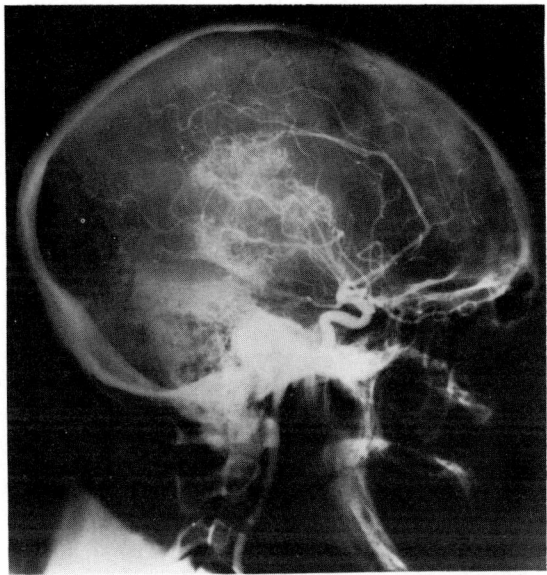

Fig. 10.2 Intense tumour blush of malignant astrocytoma (Grade 4) shown in parieto-temporal area on carotid arteriography.

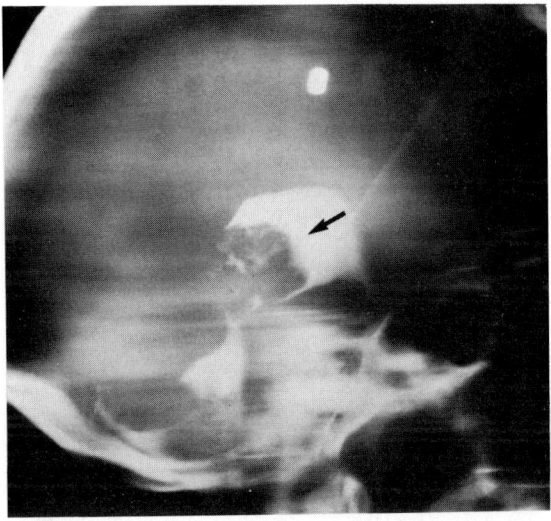

Fig. 10.3 Pineal tumour delineated by contrast ventriculography (metrizamide). Partial obstruction of the aquaduct by tumour, causing dilatation of the third ventricle which in turn produces pressure erosion of the dorsum sellae.

lows and an indwelling catheter is advised. Clinical improvement is dramatic and any definitive treatment should then be instigated.

Mannitol has similar but less rapid effects. It is given as a 20% solution in a dose of 2–3 g/kg body weight. Though less dramatic than urea it has the advantage of the treatment being more readily repeatable to control brain swelling.

Corticosteroids have proved very effective for long term control of cerebral oedema. The benefit of steroid therapy in post-operative cerebral swelling was first observed by Ingraham in 1952; French in 1961 introduced dexamethasone as a powerful synthetic anti-inflammatory substance with low mineralocorticoid activity, specifically to control cerebral oedema. It effectively reduces and controls swelling around a tumour in a most remarkable manner for long periods, safely preparing a patient for investigation or surgery and it can maintain a patient fit for radiotherapy throughout a course of irradiation. Finally, it has a most useful place in the palliation of distressful symptoms during the terminal stages of the disease. In addition to the anti-oedema effect of dexamethasone, it is possible that there may be some direct anti-tumour action which improves the survival of treated patients.

Dexamethasone may be given by mouth or by either intravenous or intramuscular injection. Absorption via

the intramuscular route is slower than by the oral or intravenous injection method. For cerebral oedema an initial dose of 10 mg is advised followed by 4 mg every six hours until symptoms of brain swelling subside. Response is quite rapid, i.e. in 24–48 hours and well established usually in 3–4 days, after which time a maintenance dose of 2 mg three times a day can be continued. The lowest dose compatible with a good response should be used. In addition antacids and cimetidine, to reduce the risk of gastrointestinal ulceration and bleeding, are advised. Of the other side-effects produced by long-term use of dexamethasone the development of a Cushingoid state is the complication most troublesome, but has to be tolerated by the patient during therapy.

Hydrocephalus
Hydrocephalus may require treatment prior to or following definitive surgery. Ventricular drainage is required if there is sudden acute obstruction. For long-term control of hydrocephalus a bypass shunt, either ventriculoatrial or ventriculoperitoneal is carried out, and this is frequently an important step in the management of third ventricular tumours. Filters designed to reduce the risk of tumour cells passing through the shunt are available and may be incorporated into the system. Such a safeguard should be considered in neoplasms like medulloblastoma and

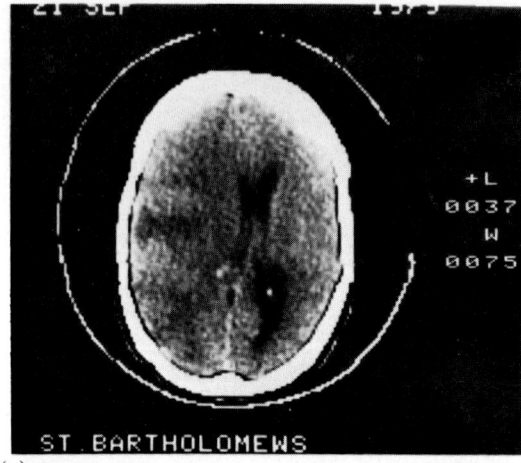

(a)

(b)

Fig. 10.4 Malignant astrocytoma (Grade 4) of left parietal lobe shown on CAT scan by (*a*) mass effect with surrounding oedema and midline shift and (*b*) contrast enhancement mainly of the periphery of the tumour which has central necrosis of low attenuation.

pineal tumours, shunt-produced metastases having been well documented.

Radiotherapy

Radiotherapy has for fifty years been known on clinical grounds to be of value in a variety of neurological tumours, but only in the last ten years has it been possible to assemble series of cases truly representative of the natural history of each tumour type for compara-tive assessment of the results of treatment. The poten-tialities are quite clear. Clinical and special methods of neurological investigation are precise and capable of a degree of sophistication in diagnosis and tumour delineation well beyond that obtaining in many other malignant disorders. The malignant cell burden is in general terms relatively small (even if not in relation to the focal area of brain or spinal cord involved). Few CNS tumours metastasize, and then only rarely outside the nervous system. Modern methods of radiotherapy can usually ensure adequate and uniform irradiation of the tumour-bearing volume, and the physical proper-ties of megavoltage radiation can be turned to good advantage in minimizing the dose outside this volume.

Despite these potential advantages the benefits of present methods of radiotherapy, while substantial in some tumours, are strictly limited. It has become apparent that these limitations are due mainly to the growth-pattern of tumours so that their limits are ill-defined, to the limited sensitivity of the highly malig-nant gliomata, to the inability of nervous tissue to reject and absorb the mass of sterilized cells deep within the brain, and to the limited radiation tolerance of the CNS itself. Of these factors the radiosensitivity of normal nervous tissue is of major importance in a discussion of the place of radiotherapy in the manage-ment of these disorders.

Responses and tolerance of the CNS to irradiation

The brain and spinal cord are both 'critical organs' in that their radiosensitivity limits the dose of radiation permissible to a level below that of connective tissue tolerance. While CNS responses have been extensively documented over the last thirty years and the clinical syndromes are well recognized, the determination of actual tolerance limits has been fraught with substan-tial difficulties. The important limiting responses of the CNS are *late* effects, with latent periods varying from about six months to over five years, and four factors contribute to the difficulties of determining critical dose-response relationships. The first is diagnostic: when brain tumours are irradiated the pathological changes of radiation damage are often rendered dif-ficult to recognize by the predominance of persisting tumour, and also by radiation changes themselves simulating the appearance of glioma. Secondly because of the latent interval many patients do not survive long enough from their neoplastic disease to enter the period of risk: whether it be malignant glioma in relation to brain tolerance, or bronchial carcinoma in relation to that of the thoracic spinal cord. Thirdly in historical published cases of radiation damage there is rarely an indication of the size of the pool of patients irradiated and their survival pattern to provide a reli-able denominator of incidence. Finally as radiation oncologists have become increasingly aware of limited CNS tolerance, the knowledge has been incorporated into routine radiation treatment planning, so that cases of overt damage for study are less common. Nevertheless with higher doses being advocated for malignant gliomata, and with increasing efforts being made for the control of many tumours near the cerebrospinal axis, the radiation tolerance of the nervous system (both intrinsic, and in relation to the natural history of the diseases irradiated) has become increasingly important.

The delayed radiation responses of the CNS within the therapeutic dosage range are of two varieties: those, usually transient in nature, occurring relatively early after periods of a few weeks or months, and the true late and progressive damage manifest after periods of from six months to over five years. Although all nervous elements are *sequentially* affected by irradiation the neurones are incapable of division, and cell turnover in the CNS is confined to neuroglia and vascular endothelium; the pathogenesis of delayed effects whenever they may occur has to be considered against this cell kinetic background. Early and late delayed effects can be manifest either in the spinal cord or in the brain.

1. *Radiation responses and tolerance of the spinal cord.* While the most important spinal effects of irradiation are the late progressive myelopathies, the commonest response is in fact an early and transient syndrome which occurs at dosage well below that of cord tolerance.

(*a*) *Transient radiation myelopathy.* In clinical neurology the phenomenon of an abnormal sensation of electrical discharge down the spine and limbs on neck flexion is well recognized; known as 'Lhermitte's sign' it indicates an organic lesion of the cervical cord, and while commonly due to cervical spondylosis or multiple sclerosis it may be caused by any intrinsic or extrinsic disorder which gives rise to demyelination. A similar syndrome is now recognized (Jones, 1964) occurring two weeks to seven months after therapeutic irradiation, with electrical paraesthesiae as its sole manifestation. The distribution of paraesthesiae varies from patient to patient, but most commonly affects the lumbosacral segments and it is precipitated or aggravated by neck flexion and by fatigue. The symptoms are transient and abate spontaneously within a few weeks or months without physical signs appearing. While commoner with higher radiation doses, the dose responsible may be as low as 2000 rad in 20 fractions in 4 weeks. This early benign form of radiation myelopathy is to be distinguished from the later and progressive disorder which usually appears after a longer latent period of about eighteen months, for transient radiation myelopathy does not, unless the evocative dose is above accepted tolerance level, herald later and progressive myelopathy. The explanation postulated for the syndrome was that irradiation inhibits the activity of a proportion of oligodendroglia along the axons of neurones in the irradiated zone. The clinical latent interval corresponds with the normal survival of myelin, but when replacement is needed the turnover is defective. As the oligodendroglia recovers myelin synthesis is resumed but during a period corresponding with the clinical duration of Lhermitte's sign the axons remain denuded and sensitive to physical distortion. Experimental confirmation has recently been provided by the elegant studies of Mastaglia *et al.* (1976) who demonstrated (in the cords of rats, by single fibre teasing and electron microscopy), breakdown of paranodal myelin and nodal widening as early as two weeks after doses as low as 500 rad. In relation to Lhermitte's sign it should be noted that: (i) it is commonly due to a transient myelopathy which is benign and self-limiting providing that the evocative dose is below the accepted level of cord tolerance and such patients can thus be reassured; it occurs in 1/6th of cases of Hodgkin's disease treated by mantle irradiation; (ii) it can nevertheless occur in patients with progressive radiation myelopathy, both at an early stage and later, but only after doses beyond accepted cord tolerance; (iii) if other symptoms or physical signs appear, investigation is then necessary for possible extradural deposits, particularly in the lymphomata.

(*b*) *Progressive radiation myelopathy.* This condition which results in severe and often irreversible morbidity after latent periods of months or years was first described by Ahlbom in 1941 following treatment of hypopharyngeal carcinoma, and it has attracted increasing attention since Boden's (1948, 1950) classical studies. Three syndromes have since been delineated:

(i) An *acute paraplegia* or *quadriplegia*, presumably the result of spinal cord infarction secondary to vascular changes (Boden, 1950). After a latent interval of about six years there is rapid progression to completion of neurological deficit over a period of a few hours or days, after which the condition may stabilize. It appears to be exceedingly rare.

(ii) A *motor neurone disorder* of the lower (or rarely the upper) limbs, presumably due to selective anterior horn cell damage, and which is also rare. As a flaccid paralysis of the legs without sensory loss it has been reported following radiotherapy for testicular tumours (Maier *et al.*, 1969).

(iii) The important condition is however *chronic progressive radiation myelopathy* occurring after latency of five months to five years but usually of about eighteen months. The pathology of earlier cases (Jellinger and Sturm, 1971) showed spongy demyelinization and astroglial reaction with loss of oligodendroglia, without definite vascular lesions; while later cases showed radionecrosis with focal or diffuse demyelination, astroglial response and vascular lesions ranging from fibronoid wall necrosis to hyalinization and telangiectasia. Despite a great deal of histopathological study in man and experimental work in rats the exact pathogenesis of the lesions is far from clear (particularly the mechanism of the prolonged latent period), but recent work supports the hypothesis that its development is a dose-dependent effect in relation to the degree of cellular depopulation both of neuroglia and of vascular endothelium. The clinical features are those of a progressive cord lesion affecting particularly the lateral columns and manifest first by numbness and paraesthesia of the lower limbs (often initially unilateral) followed by weakness and loss of sphincter control; many patients present with a Brown-Séquard syndrome. Over a period of months the disability gradually develops into a spastic paraparesis which in half the cases is fatal within two years. Incomplete lesions, particularly those arising asymmetrically in the cervical region, may however stabilize with varying degrees of permanent disability. The diagnosis turns on recognition of a neurological lesion coincident with a level of high-dose cord irradiation, and the myelographic demonstration of the absence of an extrinsic or intrinsic spinal deposit. In relation to the level, Reagan *et al.* (1968) has shown that the neurological deficit from radiation damage may initially suggest a lesion located at a lower level than that of the cord segment irradiated and so be misleading. While myelography (which is essential) may show an atrophic segment of cord, in a number of instances of proven myelopathy the appearance has been that of cord *swelling* simulating an intramedullary tumour. The differential diagnosis includes: conditions related to neoplasia – both extramedullary and intramedullary metastasis, and also 'necrotizing carcinomatous myelopathy' (which is a remote effect of cancer on the CNS); and independent cord disorders.

(c) *Spinal cord tolerance.* The first attempt at establishing the limits of cord tolerance was that of Boden (1948, 1950) who related the incidence of myelopathy not only to the evocative dose but also to the length of cord irradiated. He suggested that the dose to the cord in 17 days should not exceed 3500 R with large and 4500 R with small (less than 10 cm) fields, and he used Strandqvist's type of log–log plot with a slope of 0.22 to extrapolate these doses to other overall periods of time; so that at 42 days Boden's two critical doses become 4100 rad and 5200 rad respectively. For such overall periods and daily irradiation these have in large measure withstood the test of time as safe dose levels in treatment planning. The difficulty lies in extrapolating to different fractionation schedules and to shorter overall times; for with increased numbers of cases reported it is apparent that the curve has variable slopes and that fraction number may be more important than overall time. Strandqvist's curve was based on skin tolerance data, and there is no reason why cell renewal and partly non-cell renewal systems should behave identically. Similar difficulties arise from applying the Ellis formula (total dose = NSD $\times$ $N^{0.24}$ $\times$ $T^{0.11}$) developed for connective tissue tolerance to that of the spinal cord. Wara *et al.* (1975a) in their study related fractionated regimes to their own formula of equivalent dose (ED) by total dose = ED $\times$ $N^{0.377}$ $\times$ $T^{0.058}$, and from this concluded that the 1% incidence level of myelopathy in the thoracic cord was 1015 ret (ED) and the 50% incidence level 1476 ret (ED).

While frequency diagrams can provide indications of the minimum dose likely to evoke myelopathy, the actual dose-response curve is sigmoidal, and what the clinician needs to know is the probability of damage with each increment of dosage. With the short survival of many patients, and doubt as to the size of the 'at risk' denominator, this cannot yet be accurately estimated. The steepness of the curve is suggested by the discrepancy between the Boden 'safe' level and recent estimates of Abbatucci *et al.* (1978) of 'practically no risk' with doses lower than 5500 rad in 27 fractions in 37 days but complications 'almost inevitable' following dosage greater than 7000 rad in 30 fractions in 49 days; and the estimate of Reinhold *et al.* (1976) of 50% incidence at 6500 rad in 26 fractions in 40 days. Until sufficient data are available for 'probit analysis', the statistical prediction of the probability of inducing this major complication for each level of dosage, it is necessary to proceed empirically, and particular caution should be exercised when using small numbers of fractions or much reduced overall treatment times. Recent experimental findings of dose vs fraction number slopes of about 0.4 (instead of the 0.22 Strandqvist value) should at present be more a warning against the possible effects of small numbers of fractions than an encouragement to proceed to abnormally high doses in protracted treatments. Wara *et al.* state that 2000 rad in 5 fractions, 3000 rad in 10 fractions and 5000 rad in

25 fractions appear to be safe, but point to the cluster of positive cases in the literature treated with approximately 4000 rad in 15 fractions.

Hypertension has been shown experimentally to potentiate radiation damage to the spinal cord, but while it may be responsible for some instances of idiosyncratic response at relatively low dosage its significance has not been established in larger series. In practice the important factors predisposing to late cord damage are those conducive to high dosage and aberrant fractionation: particularly overlap from contiguous fields, failure to appreciate that the cord dose may be higher than that in the target volume (e.g. in bronchial carcinoma irradiated with opposed megavoltage fields especially in the presence of kyphosis), faulty set-up and immobilization, the rapid application of booster doses of another modality (e.g. electrons) near to the spinal axis, and repeated courses of treatment. Until further probability data are available the present authors regard dosage of 5000 rad in 30 fractions in 42 days to short lengths of cord to be relatively safe in the curative treatment of malignant disease. But this figure cannot reliably be extrapolated to shorter times or fraction numbers by present nomograms, and caution is necessary in high dosage treatment of neoplasia with treatment times as short as 3 or 4 weeks.

2. Radiation responses and tolerance of the brain. As with the spinal cord, early and transient disturbances are not uncommon following cranial irradiation but it is the syndrome of late radiation damage which is dose-limiting.

(a) *Early responses.* During X-irradiation of gliomata episodes of headache, vomiting, drowsiness and disorientation may occur, and their incidence is related to the degree of pre-existing raised intracranial pressure. They respond to dexamethasone and fluid restriction which usually enable radiotherapy to be continued. These episodes may occur both early and at the end of a course of irradiation, when they may be aggravated by a too rapid reduction in dexamethasone dosage often after the patient has left hospital. Boldrey and Sheline in 1966 drew attention to a post-irradiation response which occurred during the second month after treatment, consisting mainly of headache, malaise and increase in symptoms and signs of the pre-existing lesion, and which subsided spontaneously after a few days or weeks; such changes are however difficult to distinguish from those arising in the tumour itself.

(i) *Somnolence syndrome.* A transient cerebral disturbance characterized by somnolence was described by Freeman *et al.* (1973) in children after cranial irradiation given as part of CNS prophylaxis for acute lymphoblastic leukaemia in remission. Consisting of drowsiness, lethargy, anorexia and irritability it occurred in about 60% of children some six weeks after irradiation, and was associated with EEG abnormalities. The symptoms lasted for about three weeks and subsided without sequelae. This benign syndrome is regarded as a transient radiation-induced disturbance of myelination (having parameters similar to those of the Lhermitte phenomenon), and its occurrence has no effect on the prognosis of the treated leukaemia. It is important to recognize its existence so as to reassure the parents and prevent unnecessary investigation.

(ii) *Early demyelination syndrome.* Rider in 1963 described three cases of a syndrome of cerebral disturbance occurring about ten weeks after completion of telecobalt therapy for tumours in and around the middle ear. The patients suffered from nausea and vomiting, followed by ataxia, dysarthria and dysphasia, with nystagmus, Rombergism and in one case an abducent palsy and extensor plantar response. Over a period of eight weeks two patients made a complete recovery; but the third died after four weeks, and autopsy revealed patchy demyelination confined to the irradiated volume; the maximum evocative dose was of the order of 5500 rad in 20, 27, and 16 fractions in each case. This syndrome is clearly rare, and few instances have subsequently been reported, but with its early demyelination and absence of vascular degeneration it is important in the understanding of radiation effects, and possibly relevant to the late effects of neutron therapy on the brain.

(b) *Late radiation necrosis of the brain.* Late radiation damage is manifest clinically by progressive neurological deficit originating in a volume of brain previously irradiated, and occurring without evidence of raised intracranial pressure some three months to five years after irradiation. The lesions consist particularly of areas of necrosis, demyelination and gliosis with haemorrhage, vascular hyalinoid necrosis, endothelial proliferation and extravasation of fibrin into the neural parenchyma. The changes have a predilection for the subcortical white matter. While the evidence is against a direct neuronal effect of irradiation, the problems of impaired turnover of vascular endothelial and neuroglial cells and of their consequent interaction in precipitating necrosis after a prolonged latent interval are still far from solved. Breakdown of the blood-brain barrier is an important link in this chain of events, and is particularly important in the hypothalamus which with its rich capillary bed is the most vulnerable part of the CNS.

The pathological changes of late radionecrosis may simulate the appearances of glioma and this, together with the brief survival and paucity of autopsies, makes cases of glioma less suitable for the assessment of true radiation tolerance. Lindgren (1958) found that the minimum dose to produce necrosis was between 4500 and 5000 R in 30 days when delivered through medium-sized fields with orthovoltage radiation. More recent megavoltage data, derived from collateral evidence when the brain was incidentally irradiated, suggests that the tolerance of *cortical* white matter is of the order of 5500 rad in 30 fractions in 42 days. For shorter periods and fractionations the data are too incomplete for extrapolation; 4500 rad in 20 fractions in 28 days is usually considered safe in the treatment of malignant disease, but on the other hand there are distinct advantages for brain tolerance in prolonging the overall period to 5 or 6 weeks.

The limited tolerance of the *brain stem* was described by Boden (1950) when using orthovoltage radiation with multiple small fields; but for modern megavoltage methods the tolerance of this area should be regarded as similar to that of the spinal cord (i.e. some 10% less than that of cerebral white matter).

The late responses of the *hypothalamus and optic pathways* are of particular importance in the radiotherapy of pituitary adenomas and craniopharyngiomas, both conditions which are compatible with prolonged survival after treatment. Disturbances of the hypothalamic-pituitary axis are considered in Chapter 17. Visual loss following irradiation of pituitary tumours has been described on several occasions, and the possible causes are tumour expansion, the 'empty sella' syndrome (with chiasmal traction), and radiation damage to the optic pathways. For elucidation of this problem it is therefore necessary to have recent air encephalography and full details of radiation dosage and of its fractions and spatial distribution. Visual pathway damage which can lead to blindness has been reported after intervals of about six months to three years after high dose irradiation, and two recent studies have revealed the importance both of total dosage and of the fractionation pattern in its causation. Harris and Levene (1976) described five such cases (out of a series of 55 patients with pituitary adenomas or craniopharyngiomas irradiated) and found that *within their dosage range* no patient who received less than 250 rad per day fractions showed such visual loss. Aristizabal *et al.* (1977) reviewed 122 patients treated over a 20 year period by a variety of techniques, but usually over periods of about 4.5 weeks, and found five instances of radiation damage to optic pathways; and in the analysis this complication began to appear only above a dose level of 4600 rad. Clearly the isodose distribution is also of importance, and taking only the minimum tumour dose can lead to problems from high spots. The risks from techniques of pituitary irradiation which employ less than daily fractions are difficult to estimate in relation to the total dosage which should be prescribed, and so are preferably to be avoided. Isodosimetry is necessary in all cases, and the present authors employ a total pituitary dosage of 4500 rad in 26 fractions in 35 days, at which level no cases of optic pathway damage have been encountered.

3. Modification of CNS tolerance by other agents. Compared with other critical organs relatively few agents are known to augment radiation response in the CNS. There is a suggestion that irradiation in hyperbaric oxygen increases the risk of later myelopathy (Coy and Dollman, 1971). The main problems concern the use of methotrexate which is itself toxic to the nervous system. Leucoencephalopathy (Price and Jamieson, 1975) has followed CNS prophylaxis of acute leukaemia by intrathecal methotrexate with and without cranial irradiation, and multifocal pontine lesions have similarly been described (Breuer *et al.*, 1978) in various tumours both after methotrexate and methyl-CCNU. Blindness as a possible complication of multimodal therapy has been described by Margileth and Poplack (1977) in two patients eight months after CNS prophylaxis by irradiation and cytosine arabinoside. The roles of the neoplastic process, the toxic agent and the irradiation are difficult to separate: while irradiation may play a part, it is unlikely that at the radiation dosage levels employed there can be increased permeability from radiation-induced breakdown of the blood–brain barrier.

Astrocytoma

The important CNS tumours are those arising from the neuroglia, particularly the astrocytic series. The classical studies of Bailey and Cushing emphasized that the longest survivals were associated with the best differentiated tumours, but what they also emphasized – a correlation with embryonic development – may now be seen as merely an expression of genetic derepression during oncogenesis. Nevertheless their classification and descriptive approach so influenced pathologists throughout the world that some experienced workers have been reluctant to employ a quantitative approach to tumour grading, arguing that it engenders a spurious sense of accuracy. Sampling errors may occur with small needle biopsies, and the kinetics of the heterogeneous cell populations of a glioma may produce different static pictures at different times, corresponding with increasing histological gradings during periods of sub-clinical and clinical growth. But Kernohan and Sayre (1952) who introduced the grading system 1–4 found clear cut differences in post-operative survival times for astrocytoma, particularly for Grades 1 and 4. Neuropathologists may differ in designating a glioma as 1–2 or 3–4, but there is generally uniformity of opinion in separating low grade from high grade gliomas. It should be noted that the use of the term glioblastoma multiforme, a characteristic clinical and pathological entity, has different connotations depending on whether it is regarded as a highly malignant neoplasm *de novo*, or the end-result of anaplastic growth of a pre-existing astrocytoma. From the point of view of therapeutic trials attempts at stratification, albeit within a continuum of histopathological appearances, are to be encouraged so that clinical oncologists may be more confident that they are comparing like with like.

Differentiated astrocytomas (Astrocytomas Grades 1 and 2)

These tumours are found throughout the brain and spinal cord, relatively slowly growing and occurring most commonly in the frontal, temporal and parietal lobes of adults and in the brain stem and cerebellum of children. In the cerebral hemispheres they usually form an infiltrating tumour mass deep to the cortex, rather tough and rubbery in consistency and which may be associated with cyst formation. In the basal portions of the hemispheres and brain stem they infiltrate and expand the normal structure causing the appearance of diffuse hypertrophy. Characteristically function may be preserved because the tumour cells displace rather than destroy, except in the hypothalamus where interference with the visual and endocrine pathways occurs. The more deeply placed and central tumours frequently obstruct the third ventricle or aqueduct and give rise to hydrocephalus. Astrocytomas of the cerebellum characteristically occur in early life, are usually cystic and rarely undergo malignant change, so that in contrast to other tumours the prognosis after surgery is exceptionally good.

Differentiated astrocytomas are of two types, the more common having the typical stellate *fibrillary* cell and the less common a larger so-called *protoplasmic* cell type restricted to the cerebral cortex. Both may in certain circumstances undergo degenerative changes, perhaps a reaction to the site in which the tumour occurs, giving rise to *pilocytic* and *gemistocytic* variants. However, histological variation within a tumour is extremely common, and such a classification is a guide only to the predominant type of cell present. Moreover during the development of an astrocytoma its overall nature may alter, there being a strong tendency for more malignant changes to occur after many years of slow growth. The gemistocytic variant is particularly prone to change into glioblastoma multiforme.

Well-differentiated cerebral astrocytoma is typically a disorder of long duration, with average post-operative survival times of 73 months for Grade 1 and 24 months for Grade 2 tumours (Kernohan and Sayre, 1952). While surgical excision may often encompass the visible tumour, particularly if cystic and with a mural nodule, in the cerebrum the neoplastic process is often diffuse. Nevertheless a prolonged period of symptomatic relief may be achieved before gradual increase or rapid anaplastic growth become apparent. It has therefore been difficult to assess the possible role of post-operative radiotherapy, for while there were instances of occasional clear clinical responses statistical evidence was lacking. Sheline (1977) has compared the survivals of two similar groups of patients, with and without irradiation after incomplete surgical excision. The 5-year survival rate for Grade 1 lesions was 58% with irradiation but only 25% without; for Grade 2 the survival rate was 25% with irradiation and nil without. Gemistocytic astrocytomas, however, fare badly as so many undergo frankly malignant changes.

Clearly patients with astrocytomas that can be totally resected do not require additional radiotherapy, but it is our policy to post-operatively irradiate those incompletely excised, especially in young people. Fibrillary tumours are often diffuse gliomatous processes, so that the volume irradiated may occupy half or even two-thirds of a hemisphere. By a megavoltage technique which depends on the tumour configuration, a tumour dose of 5000 rad in 30 fractions in 6 weeks is prescribed (Fig. 10.5).

Malignant astrocytomas (Astrocytomas Grades 3 and 4)

The malignant astrocytomas are highly invasive and often diffuse processes. The median survival of patients with these tumours is about 5.5 months; about 20% of patients are alive at the end of 1 year and less than 10% at the end of 2 years (Walker, 1973). Young patients fare better, and the age composition of a series is often significant. Variations in published survival data are mainly due to differing series' compositions and to the differing criteria for histological grouping. In the United States the term 'glioblastoma multiforme' may be synonymous with Grades 3 and 4, while in this country its use is confined to Grade 4; and a varying mixture of these grades can produce significantly different series results.

Biologically the important features, apart from anaplasia, are the widespread degenerative and vascular changes which are characteristic of glioblastoma. The

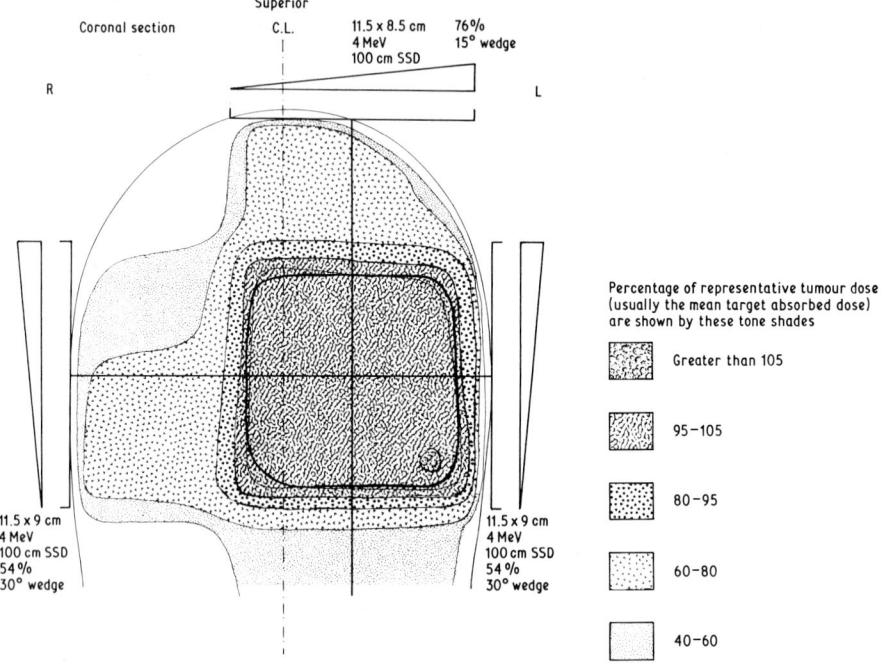

Superior
Coronal section   C.L.   11.5 x 8.5 cm   76%
                              4 MeV   15° wedge
                              100 cm SSD

R   L

Percentage of representative tumour dose
(usually the mean target absorbed dose)
are shown by these tone shades

Greater than 105

95–105

80–95

60–80

40–60

11.5 x 9 cm
4 MeV
100 cm SSD
54%
30° wedge

11.5 x 9 cm
4 MeV
100 cm SSD
54%
30° wedge

Fig. 10.5 Isodose plan of 4 MeV X-irradiation for differentiated astrocytoma (Grade 2) of the left temporal lobe. (Note different 'weighting' of plain and wedged fields).

areas of degeneration and necrosis may vary from microscopic foci to large cavities recognizable on needle biopsy. The vascular changes consist not only of thromboses, with multiple areas of tumour infarction and haemorrhage, but also the development of new vessels having small calibre, thin walls and endothelial proliferations; this vascular hyperplasia may be of such intensity as to resemble an angioma. Folkman and his colleagues in Boston (Brem *et al*., 1974) have applied his quantitative method of grading endothelial proliferation – the microscopic angiogenesis grading system (MAGS) – to astrocytomata, and for each consecutive grade the average MAGS score paralleled the malignancy of the tumour. Of the various histological features studied, the endothelial cytology (e.g. mitoses) correlated best with tumour cell anaplasia while capillary density correlated least.

Cell kinetics
The brain is unique in that neurones are incapable of cell division after birth, while glial cells of the supportive tissue retain their proliferative capacity with a low proliferation rate. Much of the work on brain cell kinetics in relation to tumours has been done by Hoshino and Wilson (1975) in San Francisco. While investigating cell kinetics of different human gliomas, they found that the labelling index (the percentage of cells in *S*-phase) varied among gliomas and among different areas of the same tumour, and while it correlated reasonably well with histological characteristics, the relationship was not a strict one. Glioblastomas had an average labelling index of 5–10%, well differentiated astrocytomas 1% or less, and the anaplastic astrocytomas were somewhere in between. In contrast to this variability of labelling index in different types, the duration of *S*-phase (DNA synthesis) remained within 7–10 hours. Turnover time – relating duration of *S*-phase to labelling index – gives values for malignant gliomas of a few days to a week, and for astrocytomas it approaches two months. Calculations based solely on cell production would give doubling times of less than five days for glioblastoma: to accord with clinical observations of a possible doubling time of five to six weeks there must be a high cell loss factor

which has been estimated at 80% and this accords with the large areas of necrosis which are a feature of the more malignant tumours. What is important, of course, is the growth fraction (the ratio of the proliferating cells to the total of tumour cells), for this is an index of the proportion of the tumour cell population susceptible to 'cell cycle' or 'phase specific' drugs. Again the data come from Hoshino and Wilson who found growth fractions of 0.3–0.4 for glioblastoma multiforme, with cell cycle times of 2–3 days. As the labelling data came from intact areas of tumour, the growth fraction would be smaller for the whole tumour which contained necrotic areas, and if these occupied half the tumour the growth fraction might be as low as 15–20%. Cell cycle times for these tumours were about 57 hours (Hoshino *et al.,* 1975).

Radiotherapy
Clinically, the value of radiotherapy in individual cases in selected series of malignant glioma has long been recognized, but it proved difficult to assemble series truly representative of the natural history of the tumours for comparative evaluation of surgery and post-operative irradiation. However, Sheline (1976, 1977) combined data from various sources, classifying the tumours as either Grade 3 or Grade 4 astrocytoma, and compared the results of 'resection only' and 'resection with post-operative irradiation'. Patients with Grade 3 astrocytoma who were irradiated had greater 1–5 year survival rates than those unirradiated – the average 5-year survival without irradiation being 2% compared with 16% for those having radiotherapy. For Grade 4 tumours, the weighted averages of these data again showed a marked difference in favour of the irradiated groups. At 1 year the survival rates were 24% with irradiation and 8% without; at 3 years 6% of the irradiated were living but none of the unirradiated; but by 5 years there were no survivors in either group. From Sheline's review the importance of distinguishing between Grades 3 and 4 stands out clearly. Treatment of Grade 3 lesions may, in about a fifth of cases, be actually curative, but while post-operative irradiation appears to increase survival for Grade 4 up to about 3 years, very few survive beyond this point.

Anaplastic astrocytomas tend to spread widely within the brain: they also seek a route of escape from the confines of the space-occupying lesion, and this is often provided by the corpus callosum. As long ago as 1957 Bull and Rovit showed that a quarter of their cases of glioblastoma had bilateral involvement of the brain, and this 'butterfly distribution' in the fronto-temporal region clearly demands an appropriate technique of irradiation (Fig. 10.6 *a–c*). Nevertheless such tumours were in the past often subjected to over-localized radiotherapeutic techniques, and the pen-

dulum has now tended to swing in the other direction, based on studies ranging from those of Kramer (Concannon *et al.,* 1960) to those of Salazar and Rubin (1976) which have shown that glioblastomas have been more extensive at autopsy than was expected on diagnostic assessment. Salazar and Rubin showed that only infrequently was glioblastoma confined to one lobe (35% of cases); usually it involved another adjacent lobe (45%) or the entire hemisphere (25%) and about one in four tumours crossed to the opposite hemisphere. In their series the diagnostic methods employed gave only 14% accuracy for determining tumour extent, and Salazar and Rubin therefore advocate whole-brain irradiation with boosting of a suitable target volume to higher dosage. Whole-brain irradiation is both simple and time-saving, but certain points have to be considered. First, diagnostic methods of tumour delineation are fast improving, and the pathological studies mentioned were done before the advent of CAT scanning. Secondly, and probably most important, in none of these studies was there evidence that the primary tumour had been sterilized, so that in practice the omission of small remote tumour foci has not been a deciding factor in the ultimate result. (In the limit Erlich and Davis (1978) have recently demonstrated spinal leptomeningeal metastases at autopsy in a quarter of cases of glioblastoma: but until control of the primary tumours becomes feasible these findings do not modify treatment policy, and there is no suggestion that the *spine* should also be irradiated.) Thirdly, the brain stem is only at risk of invasion from temporal lobe tumours, and as this and the hypothalamus are particularly vulnerable to irradiation they should not be unnecessarily subjected to very high doses. The present authors employ techniques which irradiate a 'tumour volume' at least 2 cm clear of all evidence of neoplastic involvement in each direction (it must be remembered that the actual field sizes will be some 2 cm larger than this, to allow for beam-edge fall off) and in practice it amounts to about half of each hemisphere. Opposed fields are always used so as to encompass any 'butterfly extension'.

With regard to radiation dosage, Salazar *et al.* (1976*a*) again analysed retrospectively the patterns of failure in the radiotherapy of 148 astrocytomas, and recognized that the most important factors influencing survival were both tumour dosage and treatment volume. On the basis of this study they proposed that the whole brain should be treated to 5000–6000 rad and that the target volume be boosted to 7000–8000 rad. In a preliminary report (Salazar *et al.,* 1976*b*) on such high dose radiation therapy, in which 38 patients were compared with a previous 70 patients who had received 'standard dosage' of 5000–6000 rad, the high dose group had a significant increase in survival. For

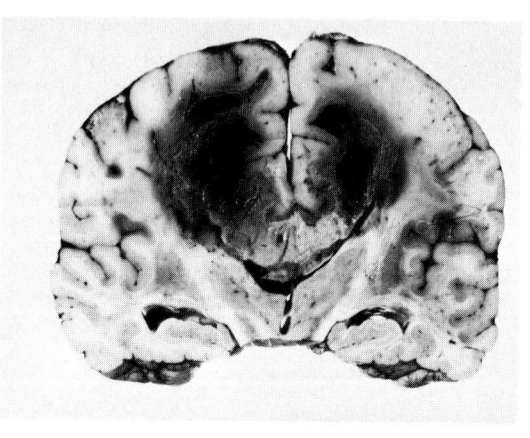

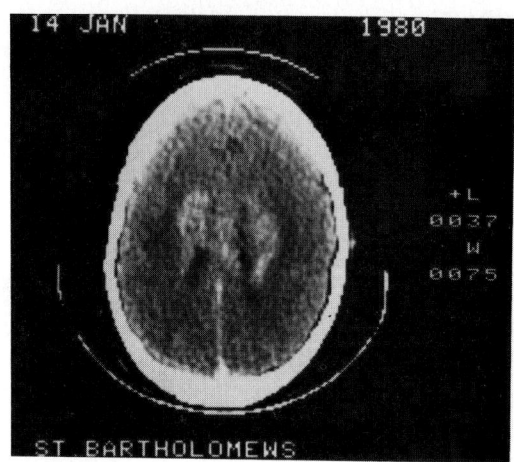

(b)

(c)

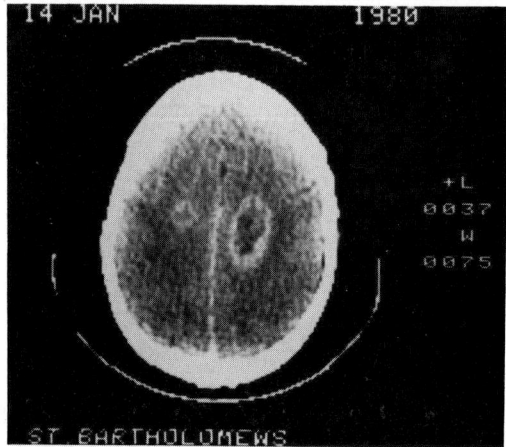

Fig. 10.6 (a)The so-called 'butterfly distribution' of malignant astrocytoma (Grade 4) (glioblastoma multiforme), with tumour extension into the opposite hemisphere through the corpus callosum. (b) and (c) CAT scans of another patient showing appearances of extension of right hemisphere glioblastoma through the corpus callosum into the left hemisphere.

the Grade 4 astrocytomas the median survival was 50 weeks compared with 34 weeks for the standard dose group; 56% were alive at 1 year compared with 29%. This difference in survival persisted for 2 years only; the cause of death in the high dose group was in every case recurrence of tumour, and gross radiation necrosis was not seen although the microscopic vascular and neuronal changes were still being studied. The Grade 3 cases were few in number and 4 out of 6 were still surviving.

The responsiveness of Grade 3 cases has been seen in a number of previous series. In an early 1 MeV series (Jones, 1960), the median survival was 46 months, while in the series studied by Kramer (1973), 5 out of 23 patients survived 5 years and almost three-quarters returned either to normal performance status or self-care. If the very high dosage method for irradiating malignant gliomata should become widely applied or

be subjected to randomized trial of large numbers of patients, it will become even more important to recognize Grade 3 tumours, for in those of Grade 4 high dosage merely increases the immediate survival, and if it proves to have undue late effects it may be advisable to reserve this treatment for the most malignant group only. All the patients in Salazar and Rubin's (1976) high dose series had recurrence of tumour in fully irradiated volumes, with high doses of from 1590 ret or 6000 rad to 2000 ret or 8000 rad and this emphasizes that tumour control is impossible by this means alone. The radiation dosage used by the present authors is 5000 rad in 27 fractions in 37 days to the main irradiated volume, with an additional 500 rad in 3 fractions to a localized tumour area in selected cases (e.g. in young patients in good condition with focal neurological deficit) (Fig. 10.7).

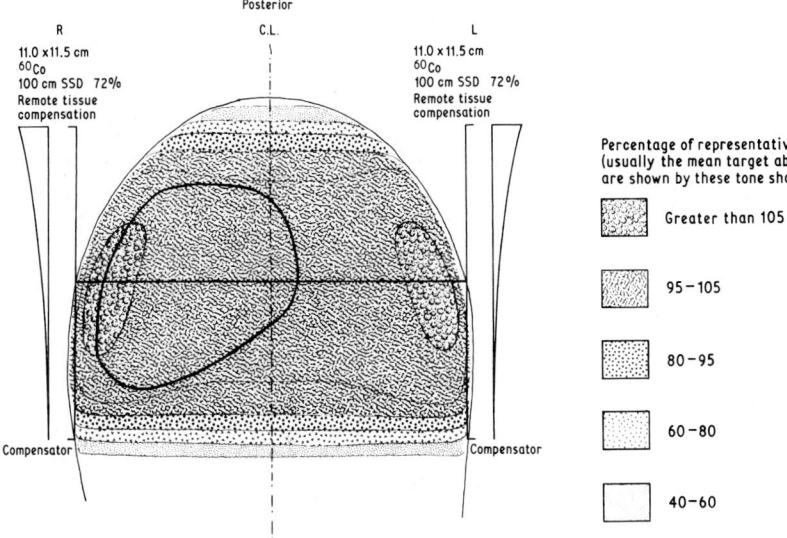

Fig. 10.7 Isodose plan for radio-cobalt therapy of right posterior parietal malignant astrocytoma (Grade 3) using two opposed fields: tissue compensation is required because of skull curvature in the parieto-occipital region.

The widespread degenerative and vascular changes of glioblastoma multiforme, with necrosis and diminished blood flow, suggest that hypoxia may be an important factor in its radioresistance. Attempts to overcome such an 'oxygen effect' in glioblastoma have been made by irradiation in hyperbaric oxygen, by using another type of radiation having high linear energy transfer (LET) and less dependence on the oxygen effect, and by using chemical radiosensitizers of hypoxic cells.

A controlled clinical trial with hyperbaric oxygen was undertaken by Chang (1977) in New York with slight improvement in terms of survival. Fast neutrons, much less dependent than are photons on the oxygen effect, have been extensively investigated by the MRC team at Hammersmith Hospital, and a controlled comparison with photons (Catterall and Bloom, personal communication) has produced interesting results. For while neutron dosage of 1560 rad in 12 fractions in 26 days was in fact able to sterilize glioblastomatous tumours, there was no improvement in survival because of a demyelinating syndrome in the normal brain reminiscent in some ways of that described by Rider (1963) for photons. Rather than its being a manifestation of the diminished oxygen effect, this may well be related to the different 'relative biological effectiveness' and the lesser capacity for repair of cellular sublethal damage from neutrons.

When we turn to chemical radiosensitization of hypoxic cells there are promising possibilities. The proposal in 1963 by Adams and Dewey that a relationship exists between the ability of a few chemical compounds to sensitize hypoxic bacterial cells and the electron-affinity of these compounds led to the discovery of the radiosensitizing properties of the group of nitroimidazoles – particularly, in 1973, of metronidazole (Flagyl) and later, of the more effective Ro-07-0582 or misonidazole. A controlled trial of γ-radiation alone and radiation plus high dose metronidazole was carried out in Edmonton, Alberta, by Urtasun *et al.* (1976) and the radiation regime should be noted – a tumour dose of only 3000 rad in 9 fractions in 18 days (1288 ret) given by large parallel fields to two-thirds of the brain. The preliminary results indicated that patients receiving metronidazole 4 hours before brain irradiation had a significant delay in the time of tumour recurrence, presumably due to a higher degree of inactivation of the radioresistant hypoxic cell population. A later report (Urtasun *et al.*, 1977), when nearly all these patients had died, confirmed without change what was predicted when most of the patients were still alive, and the difference between the two groups is striking. The control group receiving only this relatively low radiation dosage produced survivals inferior to those of conventional X-ray therapy, but with metronidazole the results were as good as those of the American BTSG's study. A limiting factor in this promising approach is the incidence of sensory peripheral neuropathy from misonidazole related to the total dose of drug used. A full-scale controlled study of misonidazole in conjunction with radiotherapy for the treatment of astrocytomas Grades 3 and 4 has now been organized (1978) under the auspices of the Medical Research Council. Eligible patients are randomized as follows:

Grade 3 and 4 cerebral astrocytoma
— 4500 rad in 4 weeks (225 rad × 20 fractions) each radiation dose preceded 4–5 h by oral placebo

— 4500 rad in 4 weeks as above, each radiation dose preceded 4–5 h by 600 mg/m^2 oral misonidazole

The study will continue until 400 patients have been admitted, which will give a 9 in 10 chance of detecting an improvement from a 10% survival rate to a 20% survival rate at 2 years, and the results of this trial will clearly be of great interest.

Chemotherapy
Chemotherapy has been under investigation for over a decade and from the variety of drugs tested only the nitrosoureas have been shown to have significant activity. In relation to other situations in cancer chemotherapy, the malignant cell burden is small, by a factor of 1 or 2 log-fold compared with common intrathoracic or abdominal tumours. The factors influencing the outcome of chemotherapy have been analysed by Ausman (1973) and these range from the route of administration, the blood flow and drug distribution in the tumour and the microenvironment, to the tumour cell kinetics and sensitivity and the brain reaction to both tumour and drug.

Brain tumours do not have the same capillary barrier (BBB) which protects the brain from water-soluble drugs of more than 200 mol.wt. and Ausman and Levin (1969) have shown that water-soluble molecules may enter experimental intracerebral tumours. Nevertheless, lipid solubility favours the entry of drugs into the central nervous system, and clinically the most effective drugs for treating intracerebral tumours have been the lipid-soluble ones, such as the nitrosoureas. Two special features of tumour spread and microcirculation may be important: (a) the infiltrative cells usually appear in advance of a histologically apparent induced neovasculature and, while these cells have a higher growth fraction, they are, from the pharmacokinetic viewpoint, at a disadvantage since fewer drugs can penetrate (Levin, 1975); and (b) in glioblastoma multiforme vascular shunts are present towards the centre of the tumour which may allow the drug to bypass some of the tumour cells (Ausman, 1973). While cell kinetic

studies may help by indicating, for instance, that there is likely to be very limited benefit from cell-cycle-specific (CCS) drugs, the heterogeneity of cell population in malignant gliomas tends to nullify any detailed application, and more help in planning treatment is likely to come from pharmacokinetic studies.

The most successful of the clinically effective agents (Levin and Wilson, 1975) are the nitrosoureas: BCNU, which is probably the most active, CCNU and methyl-CCNU – known in the USA as carmustine, lomustine, and semustine respectively. The toxicity of these is considerable, mainly haematological and cumulative. The leucopenia from a single dose is delayed to about six weeks and lasts one to two weeks, so that the spacing of doses must be at intervals of at least six weeks. Procarbazine, a methyl-hydrazine compound, is oxidized to a lipophilic azo intermediate which crosses the blood brain barrier. DTIC, an imidazole carboxamide, and epipodophyllotoxin (PTG) have also recently been shown to have clinical activity. The responses in these studies of single drugs, based on clinical improvement, varied between 25% and 50%, and they encouraged systematic evaluation in controlled trials, ultimately of multimodal therapy.

The best known of these trials was organized at the National Cancer Institute – with major participating neurosurgical services throughout the United States (the Brain Tumor Study Group) (Walker and Gehan, 1972; Walker, 1975) – in order to determine the degree of efficacy of chemotherapy with and without radiotherapy. Patients in this four-arm study were randomized after surgery between BCNU (80 mg/m^2/day intravenously for 3 days every 6–8 weeks) with or without radiotherapy (whole brain 6000 rad/6 weeks) concurrently, or to the best conventional care. An interim report (Walker, 1975) showed that the control group had a median survival of 17 weeks, BCNU 25 weeks, above 5000 rad radiotherapy 37 weeks, and BCNU plus radiotherapy 40 weeks. This was the first investigation to show a significant increase in survival as the result of adjuvant chemotherapy; the side-effects in the radiotherapy and adjuvant groups were identical, with platelet counts of about 95 000/mm^3 on day 25.

While the increased survival of patients treated fully by irradiation and BCNU has been substantiated in a later (1979) evaluation, a new late toxic effect of chemotherapy has also become apparent. This is chronic interstitial nephritis noted in patients having a cumulative dose of 1500 mg/m^2 of BCNU. No urinary changes herald the appearance of focal tubular necrosis which leads to glomerular sclerosis and this is likely to be a limiting toxicity of nitrosourea therapy. High dose corticosteroids may have some protective effect against this nephrotoxicity.

A valuable outcome of the BTSG trial was the recognition of prognostic features for patients with malignant astrocytoma which will dictate stratification variables for the design of future trials. Gehan and Walker (1977) have reported that when therapeutic considerations (radiotherapy or chemotherapy) were *not* included the characteristics most related to survival were age (the older the patient the poorer the survival), biopsy only (unfavourable), and parietal location (also unfavourable), but the presence of fits as a presenting symptom and ocular palsy were recognized as 'favourable'.

Oligodendroglioma

This is an uncommon tumour often of characteristic appearance and long natural history which accounts for only 5% of CNS tumours and 10% of all gliomata in man, but in dogs it actually accounts for half. The histological appearance of small cells closely packed, with perinuclear haloes in a honeycombed arrangement 'like the cross-section of a plant' may be very characteristic, but mixed forms of oligo/astrocytoma are not infrequent, and tumour grading is not feasible. Tumour calcification is common, 70% recognized on histology and 40% on radiography. While oligodendroglioma may occur at any age, the tumours commonly present in the fourth and fifth decades, sometimes with a long history especially if epilepsy is the presenting feature, but a history of raised intracranial pressure may be quite brief. While most common in the frontal lobes, it is one of the few tumours which may arise in the occipital lobes; it usually originates and spreads in the white matter and may be very extensive at presentation.

The treatment of choice is as radical a surgical removal as is possible. The prognosis with surgery alone is uncertain, and in the series analysed by Roberts and German the average post-operative survival was 5.6 years and the longest 36 years. With the long natural history it is difficult to judge the effect of post-operative X-irradiation, but Sheline (1977) reported 10-year survival rates of 55% with post-operative radiotherapy and only 25% without this adjunctive treatment.

It is now customary to prescribe post-operative irradiation by megavoltage X-rays, to a tumour dose of 5000 rad in 30 fractions in 42 days, given to a moderately large volume which amply encompasses the tumour-bearing area.

Thalamic tumours

Tumours originating deeply in the thalamus account for only 1% of intracranial tumours, and occur mainly in two age groups: in the first two decades and in the fifth and sixth. In childhood these tumours are commonly well differentiated astrocytomata, but in the older group glioblastoma multiforme predominates, while some thalamic tumours are ependymomas, oligodendrogliomas or, occasionally, angiomatous malformation. The presenting symptoms are commonly those of raised intracranial pressure, but hemiparesis is frequently present especially in young patients and often associated with a small pupil on the side of the lesion. In general such tumours are inaccessible and inoperable, and as even a needle biopsy may produce neurological deterioration the diagnosis has often to be based on neuroradiology, particularly CAT-scanning and air encephalography, the useful features in diagnosis being the appearance of elevation of the floor of the lateral ventricle, and displacement and bowing of the third ventricle with varying degrees of obstruction.

Surgery for thalamic gliomata is confined to the relief of raised intracranial pressure by providing a shunt, and radiotherapy is the mainstay of treatment. The technique of megavoltage X-irradiation depends on the size and distribution of the disease, a tumour dose of 5000 rad in 30 fractions in 42 days being suitable for adults. In the series reported by Cheek and Taveras (1966) 6 of 11 cases survived more than 3 years after irradiation alone, the longest survivor being at 17 years.

Tumours of the pineal and third ventricle

Although uncommon (with tumours of the pineal accounting for only 0.5–1% of intracranial tumours) this group of third ventricular tumours is of particular interest both because of the clinical syndromes encountered and the response to treatment with potential for cure of certain types. If *'pinealoma'* is rare, almost identical syndromes can be caused by a number of teratomatous or glial tumours at the *posterior end* of the third ventricle, while at its *anterior end* a variety of space-occupying processes can produce obstruction or pituitary-hypothalamic dysfunction. The work of Russell established that the important tumour in this area was in fact a variant of teratoma. In 1944 she defined two main groups of pineal tumour: those derived from pineal parenchymal cells (pineocytomas and pineoblastomas) and a group which she termed 'atypical teratoma of the pineal'. Some years later she described the relationship between atypical teratoma and 'pinealoma occurring in the infundibulum and suprasellar region', where nests of pineal tissue are not found, and the term 'ectopic pinealoma' came into use. However, Friedman (1947) had in the meantime introduced the term 'suprasellar germinoma' for this group of tumours whose histological picture was identical with that of seminoma of the testis or dysgerminoma of the ovary. A current classification of tumours of the pineal region (after Russell and Rubinstein) is set out in Table 10.3.

As already noted tumours arising in the pineal gland itself or in the posterior third ventricle produce similar neurological syndromes, and because of their deep midline location histological diagnosis of pineal tumours was in the past seldom possible during life. Among patients treated by bypass surgery and radiotherapy there were however several long-term survivors, and it became apparent that their tumours were mainly in the group of germinoma. Both pineal and suprasellar germinomas present early in life, mainly in the second decade, and males predominate with tumours in the pineal area. These rare tumours appear to be more prevalent in Japan than elsewhere. Germinoma is composed of two distinct populations of cells – large rounded germ cells with prominent nuclei, and lymphocytic aggregates. Usually about three centimetres in diameter at the time of diagnosis, the tumour obstructs the aqueduct or third ventricle, and often infiltrates the quadrigeminal plate and subarachnoid space. Focal invasion of the wall of the third ventricle and rostral midbrain is common, and seeding may occur throughout the ventricular system and in the subarachnoid space to the spinal cord and cauda equina. Rarely, blood-borne spread may occur following surgical removal. In contrast, the true pinealoma resembles the pineal gland at various stages of development, and only occasionally invades the ventricular system. The anaplastic variety – pineoblastoma – resembles medulloblastoma both in appearance and propensity for spread.

Whatever the histological nature of a tumour of the *posterior* third ventricle, the initial effects are those of CSF pathway obstruction; compression of the tectum of the midbrain and cerebellar dysfunction by interference with the superior cerebellar peduncles and dentatorubrothalamic tracts; and disturbance of hypothalamic function from obstruction and growth

Table 10.3   Third ventricular tumours: posterior end.

1. *Teratomas*
    (a) typical and less differentiated
    (b) germinoma or 'atypical teratoma'
2. *Pinealomas*
    (a) pineocytoma
    (b) pineoblastoma
3. *Gliomas* (astrocytoma, ependymoma)
4. *Cysts*

Table 10.4   Third ventricular tumours: anterior end.

1. *Pituitary tumours*
    Chromophobe
    Eosinophil
    Basophil
2. *Hypothalamic or stalk tumours*
    Craniopharyngioma
    Meningioma
    Optic chiasm glioma
    'Ectopic pinealoma' – germinoma
    Glioma
    Metastases
    Hamartoma
3. *Granulomas*
    Histiocytosis-X
    Sarcoidosis
    Tuberculosis
    Syphilis
4. *Miscellaneous* – including reticulosis

into the floor of the third ventricle. The clinical picture is of headache, vomiting, and papilloedema or consecutive optic atrophy, often with restriction of eye movements known as Parinaud's syndrome (paralysis of upward gaze and dilated pupils fixed to light). Nystagmus is common, and there may be ataxia, central deafness, ptosis, internal strabismus, and bilateral spasticity. Manifestations of endocrine dysfunction include abnormalities of sexual maturation; anterior pituitary insufficiency; and diabetes insipidus which is in fact by far the commonest endocrine abnormality. Diabetes insipidus is less common in tumours of the posterior third ventricle than in those arising anteriorly, so that when it occurs it is usually due to anterior extension or metastasis of tumour rather than to simple ventricular obstruction.

Tumours affecting the *anterior* end of the third ventricle are more diverse in origin and type, and the main varieties are listed in Table 10.4. The characteristic initial presentation differs from that in posteriorly placed lesions – with the triad of diabetes insipidus (often preceding other symptoms by months or years), visual disturbance from chiasmal compression, and hypopituitarism – dominating the picture. While these may be caused by any of the disorders listed, Rubin and Kramer (1965) drew attention to ectopic pinealoma (germinoma) as a 'radiocurable neuroendocrinological entity', and they stressed that diabetes insipidus of unexplained aetiology should be carefully followed during the first and second decades of life for associated visual disturbances and hypopituitarism. Craniopharyngioma, despite a greater frequency of raised pressure and hemianopia, less commonly causes diabetes insipidus (unless it has been subjected to surgery). With growth and extension of the tumour hypothalamic involvement results in pyrexia, somnolence and electrolyte imbalance, together with symptoms of obstructive hydrocephalus.

The diversity of clinical features of third ventricular tumours calls for a wide variety of diagnostic measures to establish the nature and extent of the disease. In addition to detailed and repeated clinical assessment and routine radiology, the methods include CAT-scanning (Fig. 10.8), air encephalography, and contrast ventriculography (Fig. 10.3) and the CSF should of course be examined by ultracentrifuge for malignant cells. The association of endocrine dysfunction with pineal and chiasmal tumours is important both from a diagnostic and a therapeutic viewpoint, for some other component of dysfunction may occur while the patient is under observation. The successful management of such cases depends on collaboration between physicians from several disciplines, and the endocrine function needs to be assessed by those fully familiar with the methods involved.

Every effort should be made to assess quantitatively the reserve function of each component; it is generally unwise to start treatment on the basis of suggestive symptoms without careful assessment and laboratory confirmation (especially as the therapy of diabetes insipidus and anterior pituitary insufficiency are generally life-long undertakings) (Axelrod, 1977). When the situation is life-threatening and treatment urgent, specimens for laboratory studies should be obtained before therapy is initiated. The main investigations required are those for assessment of neurohypophyseal and of adenohypophyseal reserve.

While a tissue diagnosis would be desirable for planning management, the mortality and morbidity of surgery of the *pineal region* have in the past been such that primary excision of these lesions at the time of diagnosis has not been warranted, particularly as over 80% are highly malignant tumours. Stereotactic biopsy and even excision are now however being more widely investigated. At the *anterior end* of the third ventricle the situation is very different, and exploratory craniotomy is the important final step in establishing the diagnosis. In the case of germinoma a radical removal is not justified, and diagnostic biopsy and decompression of the optic chiasm are the objectives. Surgery is thus usually confined to providing tissue diagnosis and to relieving the effects of pressure. In the case of ventricular obstruction this was originally achieved by Torkildsen's operation of ventriculo-cisternostomy, a procedure now superseded by the provision of a ventriculoatrial shunt.

The high radiosensitivity of pineal and suprasellar germinomas is well-known (Fig. 10.8). The essential

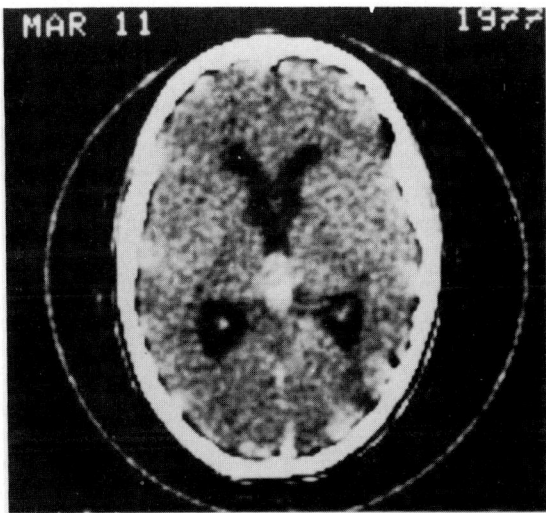
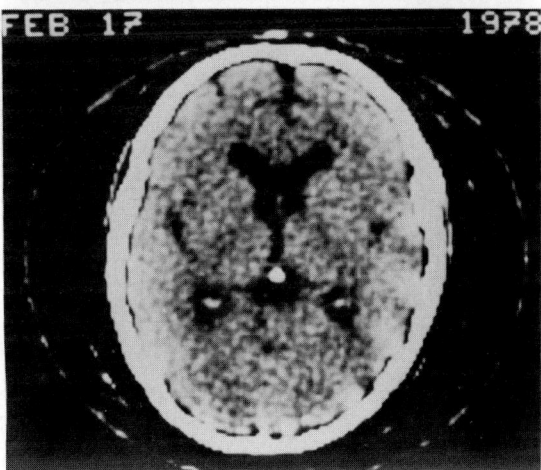

Fig. 10.8 Regression of pineal germinoma following X-irradiation, monitored by serial CAT-scanning.

considerations are therefore the level of radiation dosage required for high probability of local control, and the volume to be irradiated as determined by the propensity for spread in the ventricles and subarachnoid space. In an important study Sung *et al.* (1978) from the Columbia-Presbyterian Medical Center, New York, reviewed 61 patients with midline pineal tumours and 16 patients with suprasellar germinomas treated by surgical docompression and relatively high dose radiotherapy to the primary site. It was found that 10% of the midline pineal tumours and 37% of the suprasellar germinomas metastasized to the ventricular of spinal subarachnoid space within six months to five years. Irradiation of the entire neuraxis is therefore recommended for locally extensive tumours, for simultaneous pineal and hypothalamic lesions, and for all biopsy-proven germinomas. Regarding dosage, of the patients given 3800–4500 rad in 4–5 weeks, 47% recurred at the primary site, while of those given 5000–5500 in 5–6 weeks only 10% recurred locally. Although these dose levels are high, radiotherapeutic complications involving the hypothalamic–pituitary axis following 5000–5500 rad in 6 weeks were regarded as less of a threat than was treatment failure due to inadequate dose. The results of Sung *et al*. were excellent – the 5-year survival rate was 79% for midline pineal tumours and 77% for suprasellar germinomas – and there were no long-term complications. A different view was taken in a report from the US Childrens Cancer Study Group (Wara *et al.*, 1979) who reviewed 118 patients treated at CCSG member institutions from 1960–1975. Two-thirds of the biopsied patients had germinomas and the survivals of patients in the biopsied and unbiopsied groups were identical. As only 8% of patients developed spinal metastases, in the CCSG's view this did not warrant routine prophylactic irradiation of the spine which could cause significant morbidity in a growing child. They did however raise the question of whether aggressive surgical techniques in the future may result in a higher spinal seeding rate, for 14% of the biopsy-proven germinomas had spinal metastases compared with 1.7% in the unbiopsied group.

The present authors adhere to the view that spinal irradiation as part of whole cerebrospinal axis treatment is usually indicated in all biopsy-proven germinomas.

The technique advocated for tumours of high metastatic potential (whether germinomas or pineoblastomas) is therefore whole brain irradiation to a dosage of 3500 rad in 20 fractions in 28 days, followed by local third ventricular irradiation (by a 3-field planned technique) to an additional 1500–2000 rad in 15 fractions in 21 days; the spinal axis being irradiated to 3500 rad in 23 fractions in 32 days, starting after 17 days of the whole brain irradiation (Fig. 10.9). A high standard of precision is required for planning and execution of the treatment, with plastic shell immobilization and great care in the apposition of junctions. A careful watch is kept on the blood counts, and the progress is assessed clinically, by repeated CAT-scans and by hormonal estimations of human chorionic gonadotrophin (HCG) sometimes present in blood and CSF as a tumour marker. Surgery is attempted only in patients who show clinical and radiographic evidence of recurrent, slowly growing, relatively benign lesions after radiotherapy. Chemotherapy has been little used, but drugs known to be efficacious in testicular germ cell tumours (daunorubicin, vincristine, and bleomycin) have been reported to be active in recurrent pineal germinoma.

Brain stem tumours

Because of their site these tumours are inoperable, and as biopsy is also usually hazardous the diagnosis depends on a combination of history, clinical findings, CAT-scans and radiographic contrast studies. The majority occur in children with a peak incidence at between 4 and 8 years, but they may occur at any age and particularly in early adult life. Commonly arising in the upper pons, the histological diagnosis in cases subsequently autopsied is usually of astrocytoma, and in childhood this is frequently anaplastic.

While some patients may require a decompressive shunting procedure, radiotherapy is the mainstay of treatment and the initial response of this group of tumours is often gratifying, even in the presence of severe brain stem deficit. Whyte *et al*. (1969) reported clinical or subjective improvement in 84% of 61 patients irradiated at the Mayo Clinic, with a 38% 5-year survival rate; and more recently Sheline (1975) at the University of California, San Francisco, described definite improvement in 19 of 27 patients, with survival at 5 and 10 years of 41% and 33% respectively.

In the technique of megavoltage irradiation the irradiated volume usually extends to include from the midbrain to the upper cervical cord, either by opposed lateral fields or by a 3-field and wedge arrangement, both with tissue compensating filters. Radiation dosage is determined by the particular vulnerability of the brain stem, and a lesion dose of 5000 rad in 30 fractions in 6 weeks is usually employed; some authors advocate a higher dosage in adults, of 5500 rad, for which the overall time must be extended to 7 weeks.

Ependymoma

Ependymoma, the second most common form of glioma, is predominantly a disease of children and young adults with an average age of 23 years at presentation. Ependymal cells are normally found lining the ventricular system, the central canal of the spinal cord, and the terminal ventricle of the conus medullaris and also scattered in the filum terminale and as rests deep in cerebral hemispheres. Tumours of such origin may therefore occur at any of these sites. Intracranially some 60% are infratentorial, usually in the midline. In the spinal canal 60% of gliomas are ependymomas, usually arising in the lumbosacral areas (page 215).

While ependymomas are usually slowly growing tumours (and are in fact the only gliomas which can show purely concentric growth) they should always be

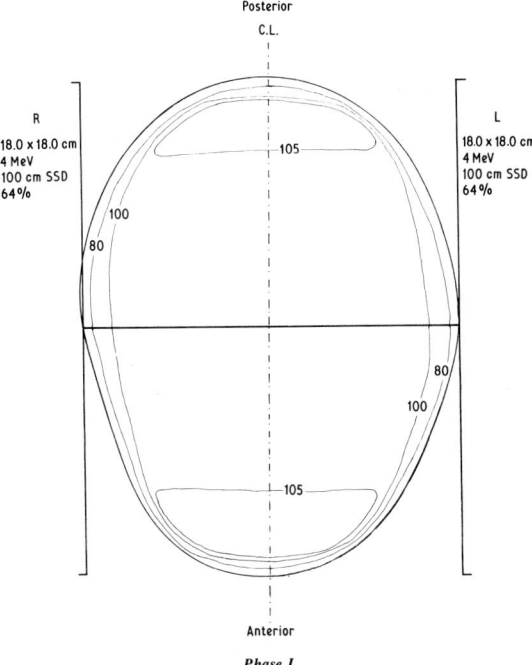

Posterior
C.L.

R
18.0 x 18.0 cm
4 MeV
100 cm SSD
64%

L
18.0 x 18.0 cm
4 MeV
100 cm SSD
64%

105

100

80

80

100

105

Anterior

Phase I

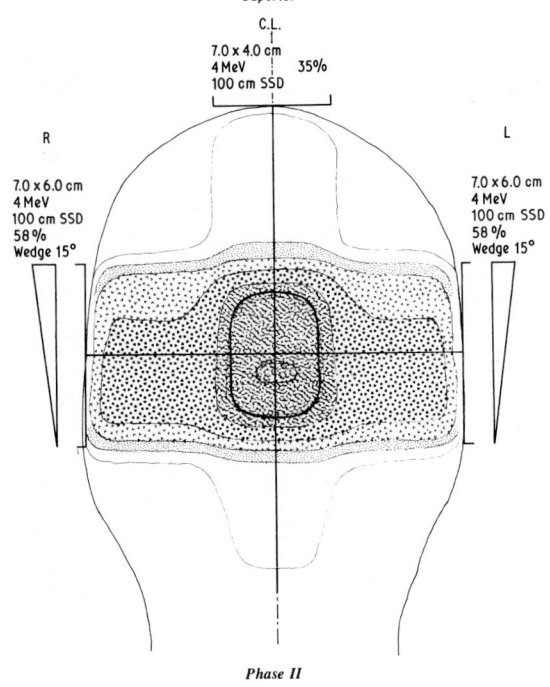

Superior
C.L.
7.0 x 4.0 cm
4 MeV   35%
100 cm SSD

R

L

7.0 x 6.0 cm
4 MeV
100 cm SSD
58%
Wedge 15°

7.0 x 6.0 cm
4 MeV
100 cm SSD
58%
Wedge 15°

Phase II

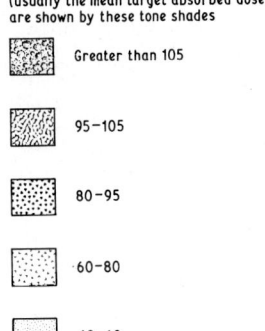

Percentage of representative tumour dose
(usually the mean target absorbed dose)
are shown by these tone shades

Greater than 105

95—105

80—95

60—80

40—60

Fig. 10.9 Isodose plans for radiotherapy of pineal tumour by 4 MeV X-rays. Treatment is carried out in two phases. I. Whole brain irradiation by lateral fields, followed by II. localized irradiation of third ventricle. For germinoma, spinal irradiation is also given, and it is important that the initial cranial irradiation shall be planned with the correct degree of neck flexion, immobilization and angulation of the lateral cranial fields to facilitate keying-on of spinal fields.

regarded as malignant with varying degrees of aggressiveness. Their clinical behaviour is closely correlated with their degree of anaplasia, and the value of the Kernohan system of grading was first shown by Mabon *et al.* (1949) who reported a 79% 3-year survival for Grade 1 cases, and only 9% for those of Grade 4. Of intracranial ependymomas 65% are of low grade. Tumour spread is both by local expansion and invasion, but CSF seeding may also occur and this is of course commoner with high-grade tumours. Particularly following incomplete surgical removal, invasion of dura, bone and scalp may occur, and distant metastasis to lungs, bone, and cervical lymph nodes has also been recorded.

The recurrence-free 5-year survival for historical series is about 20% for surgery alone, but this proportion rises to 30–40% if surgery is followed by irradiation of the primary site (Sheline, 1975). In view of the recognized radiosensitivity of ependymomas and the known tendency to CSF seeding in certain cases, there has in the past been controversy as to the need for whole cerebrospinal axis irradiation in these cases. The question turns essentially on the incidence of seeding in relation to tumour grade and site, and the evidence has been well marshalled by Bloom (1975) and by Sheline (1975). Discrepancies in reported incidence depended on whether the evidence was clinical, myelographic or pathological; for with a clinical incidence of 3% and pathological incidence of 30% it is clear that with uncontrolled growth of the primary tumour such implants may remain symptomless during the remainder of the patient's lifetime. In contrast to the low incidence reported by Sheline, Bloom in the Royal Marsden Hospital series found the risk of seeding to be greatest in high-grade posterior fossa tumours (4 out of 7). In these cases there is often a tongue of tumour passing downwards from the fourth ventricle into the spinal sub-arachnoid space which may predispose to dislodgement of tumour cells. Bloom has therefore evolved a treatment policy (to which we subscribe) in which, for low-grade supratentorial tumours, local large volume irradiation is prescribed: but for high-grade supratentorial tumours and for all infratentorial tumours the whole CNS is irradiated, with a maximum dose localized to the primary area. A lesion dose of 5000 rad in 30 fractions in 42 days (in adults) is given to the primary area, and if the whole cerebrospinal axis is also to be irradiated the dose to the remainder is 3000–3500 rad in 25 fractions in 5 weeks by a technique identical to that used for medulloblastoma (Fig. 10.10). It must be stressed that only exceptionally is whole cerebrospinal axis irradiation required for ependymoma in adults, for these tumours are usually well differentiated. While the 5-year survival for low-grade tumours in adults is now about 80%,

it is still low in the high-grade infratentorial tumours of childhood, and attempts are being made to improve this by adjuvant chemotherapy. A current international trial of such adjuvant chemotherapy in medulloblastoma and ependymoma Grade 3 and 4 in childhood (under the auspices of the International Society of Paediatric Oncology) utilizes X-irradiation as above, with or without chemotherapy in the form of vincristine and CCNU given in 8 to 9 courses over 48 weeks.

Medulloblastoma

Medulloblastoma, from primitive neuroepithelial cells originating from the roof of the fourth ventricle, accounts for about 6% of all intracranial tumours. But in childhood the proportion is much higher, 50% of cases occurring in the first decade; this tumour is therefore considered in Chapter 37. It should nevertheless be remembered that about one-third of cases occur in adolescence and early adult life, between the ages of 15 and 35. The clinical problem is almost always that of a posterior fossa tumour, and although the disease has the same propensity for dissemination by the CSF, it unfolds more slowly than in childhood. The principles of multimodality treatment of medulloblastoma in adults, by the combination of surgery, craniospinal irradiation and chemotherapy, are identical with those in children.

Meningioma

Meningiomas, which account for about 15% of all primary intracranial tumours, arise from meningeal cell elements and particularly from those packing the arachnoid villi in the walls of dural veins and sinuses. While most frequently arising in the parasagittal region, other important sites are the sphenoidal ridge, the olfactory groove, and the basicranium from the sella to the foramen magnum; rarer sites of origin are the ventricles and the optic nerve sheath within the orbit. Whereas most meningiomas are benign and well defined tumours exhibiting histologically the uniform appearances to which the descriptive *syncytial, transitional* or *fibroblastic* labels are attached, an *angioblastic* type is well recognized as having potential for rapid growth. Invasion of the dura and marrow spaces, sometimes stimulating osteoblastic proliferation and hyperostosis, does not however indicate malignancy in a meningioma.

Malignant meningiomas are quite rare, and while malignant change may occur in any of the varieties it is seen most frequently in the angioblastic type. Malignant tumours are soft and grey in appearance, widely infiltrating the brain meninges, skull and scalp; in the

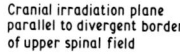

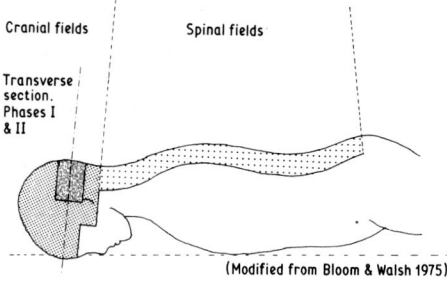

Cranial irradiation plane
parallel to divergent border
of upper spinal field

Cranial fields   Spinal fields

Transverse
section.
Phases I
& II

(Modified from Bloom & Walsh 1975)

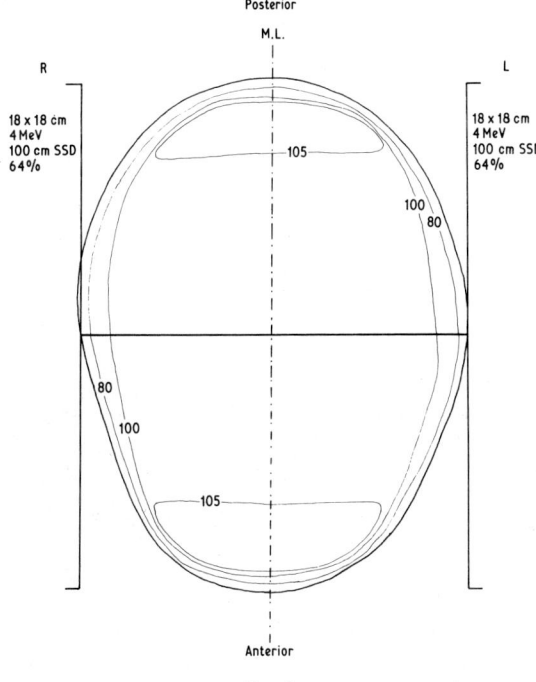

Posterior

M.L.

R   L

18 x 18 cm
4 MeV
100 cm SSD
64 %

105

100
80

18 x 18 cm
4 MeV
100 cm SSD
64 %

80
100

105

Anterior

Phase I

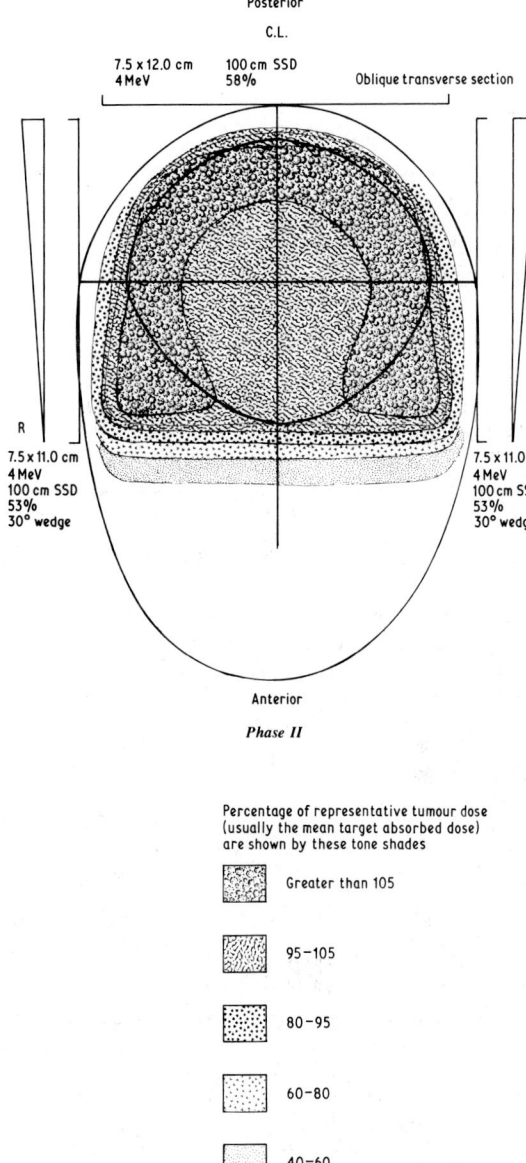

Posterior

C.L.

7.5 x 12.0 cm
4 MeV

100 cm SSD
58%

Oblique transverse section

R
7.5 x 11.0 cm
4 MeV
100 cm SSD
53%
30° wedge

L
7.5 x 11.0 cm
4 MeV
100 cm SSD
53%
30° wedge

Anterior

Phase II

Percentage of representative tumour dose
(usually the mean target absorbed dose)
are shown by these tone shades

Greater than 105

95–105

80–95

60–80

40–60

Fig. 10.10 Isodose plans for radiotherapy of posterior fossa
ependymoma of high malignancy (4 MeV X-rays) (modified
from Bloom and Walsh, 1975). Cranial treatment is carried
out in two phases. I. Whole brain irradiation by lateral fields
followed by II. localized irradiation of the posterior fossa by a
3-field technique: one posterior and two lateral wedged
fields. The angle of the section is such that the inferior limit of
the posterior field should (allowing for beam divergence) exit
above the orbits. Using a plastic immobilization shell the
spinal irradiation is carried out simultaneously, by posterior
fields with carefully calculated gaps.

brain the tumour and normal tissues become indistinguishable at operation. The cells in these tumours are spindle shaped with many mitotic figures and at the margin of the growth there is a proliferation of glial tissue. Very rarely distant metastases may occur. An important variant, *papillary meningioma*, is recognized as occurring often early in life and as being particularly prone to recurrence and metastasis after surgery.

Meningiomas are of limited radiosensitivity so that total surgical removal should whenever possible be carried out. As the natural history of these tumours is prolonged and variable the role of radiotherapy given post-operatively for those incompletely excised has been difficult to establish. However Sheline and his colleagues, in a review of 213 cases of meningioma from the University of California, San Francisco (Wara *et al.*, 1975*b*) found that the overall recurrence rate after subtotal removal of the tumour was 22% for patients given post-operative irradiation to a tumour dose of at least 5000 rad, in contrast to an overall recurrence rate of 74% for such patients not irradiated. These authors concluded that (a) if a meningioma can be totally resected, surgical excision is the treatment of choice; (b) if resection is incomplete, radiation therapy may prevent or markedly delay recurrence; (c) some previously non-irradiated recurrent meningiomas may be controlled by irradiation for extended periods of time; (d) the resectability of certain highly vascular meningiomas may be increased by pre-operative irradiation; and (e) the value of radiation therapy appears unrelated to the histologic type. With tumours having such a long natural history it is important that the radiation tolerance of normal brain should not be exceeded, and the present authors employ a tumour dose of 5000 rad in 30 fractions in 42 days given by an individually isodosed technique depending on the distribution of the tumour. Irradiation may be particularly valuable in cases of inoperable sphenoidal ridge tumours (Fig. 10.11) where the technique employed must carefully avoid both eyes.

The problems of management of truly malignant meningioma are similar to those of *meningeal sarcoma*, the features and pathology of which are excellently discussed by Rubinstein (1972). These sarcomas arise from the dura (most frequently in the early years of life) though occasionally the lesion is situated in the brain without apparent meningeal attachment. The infiltrating mass grows rapidly undergoing degenerative changes, necrosis, haemorrhages and cyst formation. The cells are predominantly spindle shaped but most of these tumours contain polymorphic cells in addition.

The treatment policy adopted by the present authors for meningeal sarcoma is excision of as much tumour as

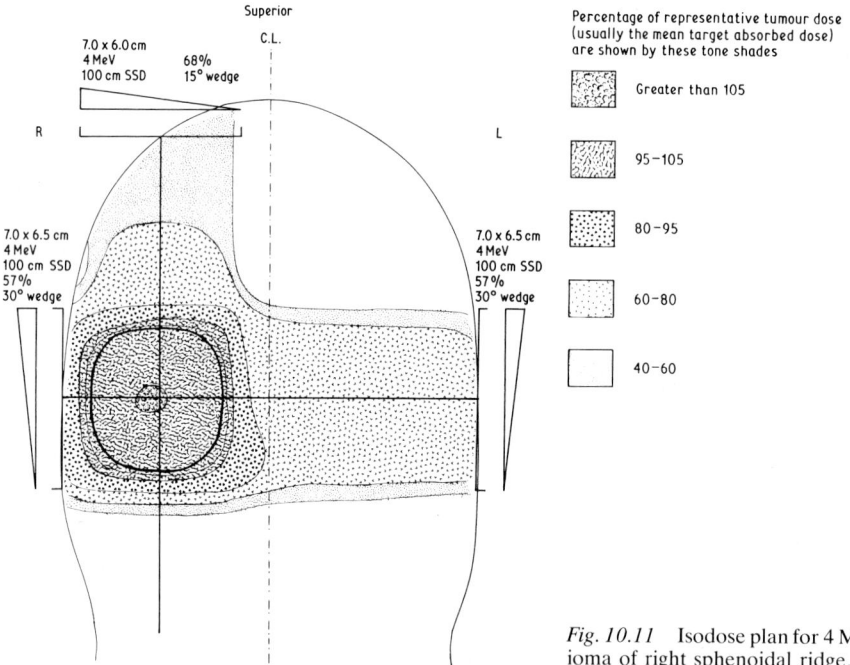

Percentage of representative tumour dose (usually the mean target absorbed dose) are shown by these tone shades

- Greater than 105
- 95–105
- 80–95
- 60–80
- 40–60

Fig. 10.11 Isodose plan for 4 MeV X-ray therapy of meningioma of right sphenoidal ridge. Avoidance of irradiation of both eyes is particularly important.

is possible, followed by full X-irradiation of a tumour volume having generous margins, up to brain tolerance dosage according to the age of the patient.

Spinal tumours

Primary *intraspinal* tumours account for about 15% of all primary tumours of the nervous system and its coverings, and they are predominantly disorders of adult life. In a series of some 1300 cases from the Mayo Clinic, Slooff *et al.* (1964) found the incidence of Schwannomas to be about 30%, meningiomas 25%, gliomas 22%, sarcomas 12%, vascular tumours 70%, chordomas 4% and epidermoid and other tumours 1%. Among the intraspinal gliomas the ependymomas form the largest group, partly due to their high incidence in the filum terminale where about 60% of the spinal ependymomas originate. In the *cord* itself ependymomas account for two-thirds of intramedullary gliomas, the remainder being mainly astrocytomas two-thirds of which are well differentiated. There is a regional gradation of incidence with, in the cervical segments a preponderance of astrocytoma, in the thoracic segments astrocytoma and ependymoma equal, but below this level ependymomas are in the majority and they are virtually the only tumours to arise within the cauda equina.

The differential diagnosis of an expanded *cord* lesion shown on myelography includes cystic conditions such as syringomyelia; benign tumours such as lipoma and vascular malformations; glioma; very rarely metastatic carcinoma; and late radiation myelopathy. That of a space-occupying lesion in the *lumbosacral canal* includes a large variety of disorders, ranging from prolapsed intervertebral disc to epidermoid tumours, meningioma, ependymoma, lymphoma and metastatic carcinoma, as well as primary tumours of the vertebrae and sacrum such as chordoma.

Surgical exploration by laminectomy is therefore usually an essential step in management of intraspinal tumours, to exclude a non-malignant tumour or other disease, to remove tumours such as ependymomas having mainly an expansile (as opposed to an infiltrative) growth pattern, and to obtain pathological diagnosis of the tumour type and its differentiation.

While intradural tumours may be excised if they arise from the filum terminale, intramedullary cord tumours cannot easily be removed in this way and surgery may be limited to decompression, aspiration of cysts in relation to the growth, or obtaining a small piece for histology. But not uncommonly gliomas of the cord form an apparently well defined greyish mass which can be separated from the normal tissue. In such cases, after incising the cord longitudinally over the tumour, the margin of the growth is dissected free using microsurgical techniques. In this way tumours extending over several segments may be separated from the normal tissue.

In many cases of cord astrocytoma, however, radiotherapy is the only possible treatment, and its efficacy is limited by the radiation tolerance of the spinal cord itself. Well-differentiated astrocytoma in young people is often extensive over several segments of cord, but still compatible with several years of survival albeit with increasing neurological deficit. It is therefore important in these cases not to exceed cord tolerance and add to the patient's disability in a forlorn hope of cure. The mean survival of differentiated astrocytoma is about six years; the uncommon Grade 3 and 4 tumours (which account for less than 10% of spinal gliomas) run a much shorter course despite temporary response to irradiation taken to cord tolerance dosage of 5000 rad in 30 fractions in 6 weeks (Fig. 10.12 *a–c*).

In the lower end of the dural canal occupied by the cauda equina and the conus medullaris, very large tumours (giant meningeal and epidermoid) may be found or the entire canal may be filled with a glioma or an ependymoma. It is surprising what size these tumours, both those of developmental origin and others, can attain without compressing the structures enclosed in the dura to the point of preventing function.

Ependymomas account for the large majority of gliomas arising in the *conus medullaris* and *filum terminale,* and are usually well-differentiated. A distinct clinicopathological variant – myxopapillary ependymoma – occurs exclusively in this area; it contains mucin from connective tissue in the filum terminale and appears slimy to the surgeon's touch. Although encapsulated these tumours which grow slowly ultimately deform and erode the lumbosacral canal. Massive extension into the paravertebral soft tissues can occur, to be followed occasionally by extraneural metastasis.

The highly vascular ependymoma of the cauda equina can be macroscopically removed in the majority of cases. The difficulties are the thin fragile capsule, adherence to nerve roots, involvement of the conus by upward extension, and haemorrhage. Damage to the nerve roots may result in paralysis of the lower limbs, sphincter disturbances and impotence, and it is often better therefore to rely on post-operative irradiation than to carry out extensive dissection among the roots of the cauda equina. Post-operative radiotherapy is given routinely in ependymoma to diminish the incidence of local recurrence, and as the tumours are well differentiated, and spread by the CSF is very unusual, radiotherapy is confined to the area of the tumour bed. Megavoltage X-ray therapy by a single posterior field

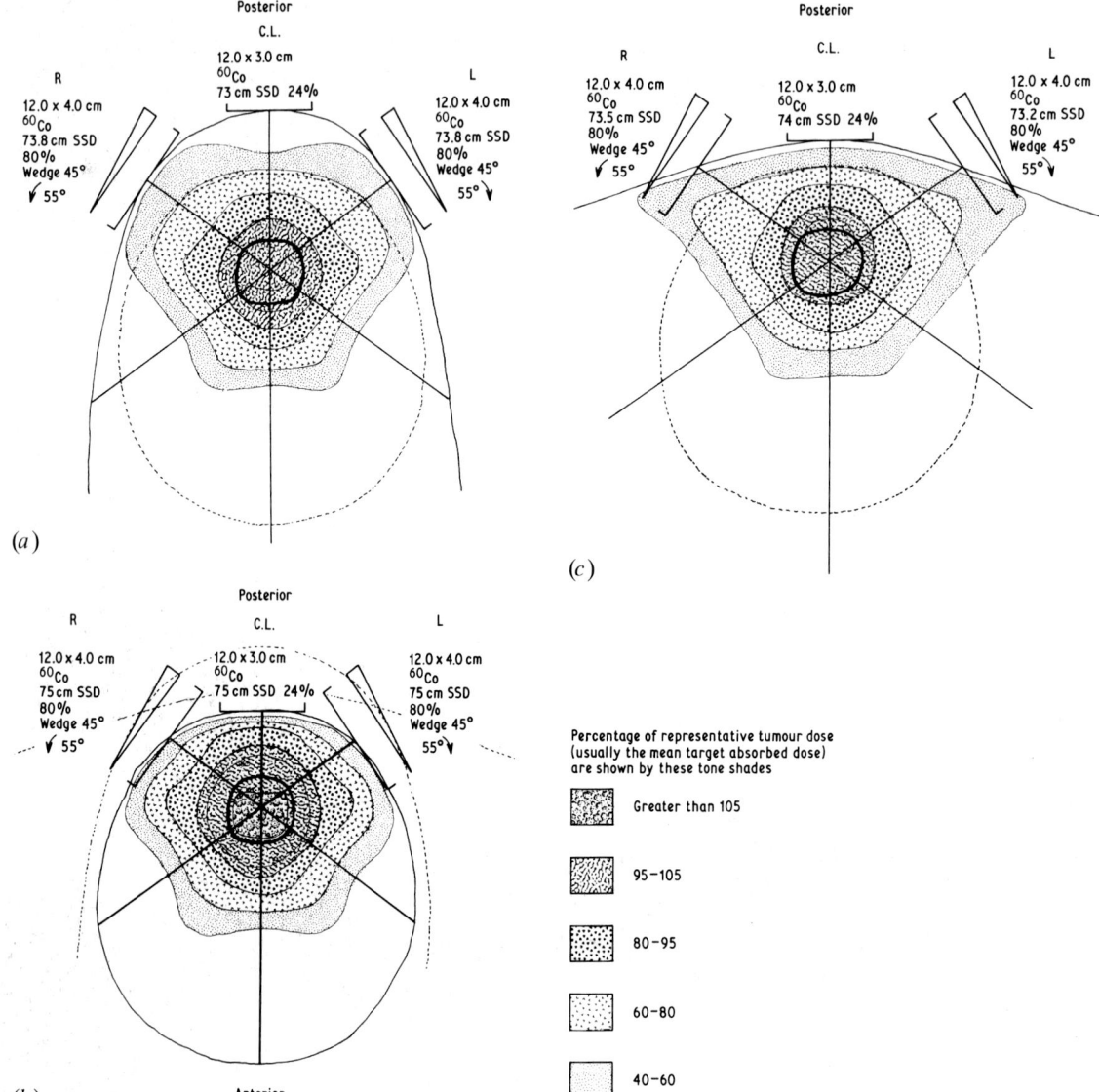

Posterior
C.L.
12.0 x 3.0 cm
^{60}Co
73 cm SSD 24%

R
12.0 x 4.0 cm
^{60}Co
73.8 cm SSD
80%
Wedge 45°
55°

L
12.0 x 4.0 cm
^{60}Co
73.8 cm SSD
80%
Wedge 45°
55°

(a)

Posterior
C.L.
12.0 x 3.0 cm
^{60}Co
74 cm SSD 24%

R
12.0 x 4.0 cm
^{60}Co
73.5 cm SSD
80%
Wedge 45°
55°

L
12.0 x 4.0 cm
^{60}Co
73.2 cm SSD
80%
Wedge 45°
55°

(c)

Posterior
C.L.
12.0 x 3.0 cm
^{60}Co
75 cm SSD 24%

R
12.0 x 4.0 cm
^{60}Co
75 cm SSD
80%
Wedge 45°
55°

L
12.0 x 4.0 cm
^{60}Co
75 cm SSD
80%
Wedge 45°
55°

(b)

Anterior

Percentage of representative tumour dose
(usually the mean target absorbed dose)
are shown by these tone shades

Greater than 105

95–105

80–95

60–80

40–60

Fig. 10.12   Isodose plan for radio-cobalt therapy of glioma of cervical spinal cord (well-differentiated ependymoma). Note that because of variation of contours three separate sections are taken, orthogonally to the spinal cord axis, at (a) superior end, (b) middle, and (c) inferior end of the field.

is given to a *lesion* dose of 4000 rad in 25 fractions in 5 weeks. (Because of the proximity of the kidneys wedge-field arrangements are inappropriate at this site.) The late results in cases of ependymoma of the cauda equina are very good, over 90% being free from disease at 5 years.

Metastatic deposits in the nervous system

The central nervous system is frequently affected by metastatic neoplastic disease, the location of which is chiefly determined by blood stream spread. Involvement of the brain is mainly parenchymatous, but increasing attention is now being paid to meningeal involvement, both in solid tumours as well as in reticuloendothelial disorders in which it more typically occurs. Medullary involvement of the spinal cord, on the other hand, is rare and the common spinal syndromes are those produced by extradural pressure or subarachnoid seeding. Currently there is a two-fold interest in CNS metastatic disease. Firstly, from the clinical view point, because of its frequency, its serious influence on prognosis, and the variety and complexity of the syndromes encountered; and secondly from the investigational and therapeutic aspects, centered on the role of the CNS as a 'sanctuary' in protecting tumour cells from the effects of systemically administered agents.

Intracranial deposits

The incidence of intracranial deposits of metastatic carcinoma in reported series varies widely, from 4% to 37%, depending on whether the data are obtained from neurosurgical services, from departments of clinical oncology, or from pathological practice: in the latter it accounts for 15%–25% of cases of tumour. Most commonly (in some 65%) the site of origin is bronchogenic carcinoma, with breast carcinoma about half as frequent: but other important sites of origin are kidney, colon, pancreas, and testis; and in some series malignant melanoma accounts for 15% of cases. While intracranial metastases usually present during the clinical course of established malignant disease, not infrequently in neurosurgical practice it may be the presenting feature and rarely this may precede the discovery of the primary by several years. Blood-borne metastases to the brain are rarely solitary, although one lesion may dominate the clinical picture at presentation. There are, however, instances in which detailed investigation fails to reveal any other focus in the brain or elsewhere, either initially or perhaps long after the successful treatment of the primary tumour: hypernephroma is a notable example. In these cases surgical excision of the metastasis followed by radiotherapy may be justifiable

and sometimes rewarding. In most instances however the treatment of intracranial metastatic carcinoma is palliative and part of the management of the systematized disorder.

The most potent agents for the relief of symptoms of intracranial metastases are corticosteroids, usually administered as dexamethasone. Improvement in symptoms, particularly headache and the level of consciousness and cerebration, is usually rapid and can often be maintained for several weeks by this agent alone. The dosage needs to be regulated carefully to minimize Cushingoid and other side-effects during what is often long-term use.

Radiotherapy has been shown to be a valuable agent of palliation, the response of intracranial metastases depending more on the anaplasia of the tumour than on its histological type. As intracranial metastases of even well-differentiated squamous cell bronchial carcinoma frequently respond, it may be that the metastases arise from dissemination of the more primitive clones of the primary tumour. Symptoms of headache, obtundation, dysphasia and hemiparesis frequently improve, but a dense hemiplegia seldom responds to treatment. The selection of cases for treatment is thus essentially a clinical decision, depending on the general condition of the patient and on the extent of other lesions and their possible management. It is no kindness to a patient suffering from uncontrollable and relentless metastatic or visceral disease to have the development of intracranial metastases temporarily reversed, when they are not the main cause of his suffering.

As intracranial metastases are seldom solitary, whole brain irradiation is the standard method of treatment, by megavoltage X-irradiation from two large opposed lateral fields (which include, in addition to the cerebral hemispheres, the posterior fossa and the meninges). For radio-cobalt no bolus or tissue compensation is required (Fig. 10.13), for the possible dosage heterogeneity is largely corrected by the shape of the skull; the eyes are of course carefully protected from both beams. While a midline dose of 3500 rad in 20 fractions in 28 days is usually effective, there are real advantages to the patient and his family in completing radiotherapy in as short a period as possible, providing adequate and equivalent palliation can be achieved. Two consecutive studies have therefore been carried out by the Radiation Therapy Oncology Group in the United States (Kramer *et al.*, 1977) on the management by different dose/time fraction schemes, with about 1000 patients entered into each trial. From the first trial (1971–1973) it was concluded that 3000 rad in 10 fractions in 2 weeks was as efficacious as 4000 rad given over 3 weeks; moreover in this trial in 40% of the treated patients the ultimate demise was not due to

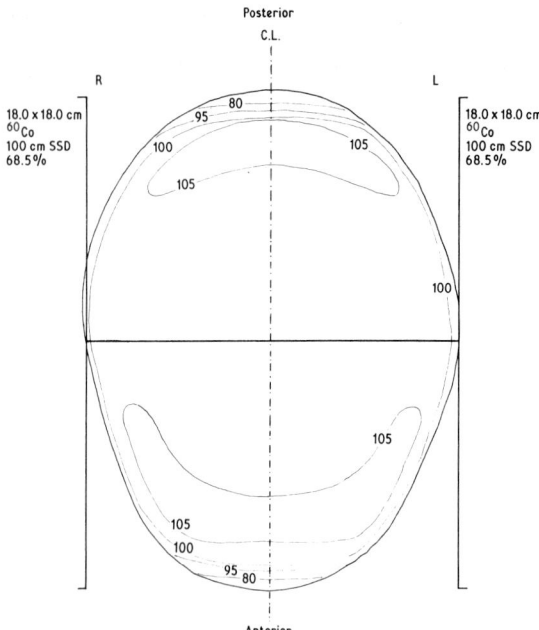

Fig. 10.13   Isodose plan for radio-cobalt therapy of cerebral metastases by two large opposed fields.

brain metastasis. Following the results of this trial the RTOG studied in 1973–75 even shorter overall treatment times, comparing the best arms of the previous trial with 2000 rad in 5 fractions in 1 week, or 1200 rad in 2 days.

The preliminary results suggest that short treatment times of a week or less give poor results, and it seems that the treatment regimen of 3000 rad in 10 fractions in 2 weeks to the whole head is at present the best for most patients with brain metastasis. There are however occasions when more protracted radiotherapy is advisable, especially when a well-differentiated and ostensibly solitary deposit has been excised – in this case additonal localized irradiation of the target volume is indicated. In the case of breast carcinoma the adequate treatment of brain metastasis is just one part of the general management of the systematized disease by hormonal and chemotherapy.

Spinal metastases

While blood-borne deposits within the spinal cord are rare, it is frequently affected by metastatic tumour growth in the vertebrae and extradural tissues or in the subarachnoid space. Spinal deposits may compress the cord or cauda equina by extension of tumour or by actual vertebral collapse, and relief of such pressure constitutes one of the emergencies of oncology. The management will entail a prompt assessment of the general condition of the patient, of the rapidity of onset and severity of the neurological deficit, of the presence of multiple spinal lesions and of the prognosis of the generalized disease. The considerations are very different from those relating to cerebral metastases, and the relief of cord compression usually takes precedence over other aspects. For the majority of solid tumours emergency myelography and laminectomy are the essential measures, followed as soon as possible by localized irradiation of the affected spinal segments. Megavoltage X-irradiation by a single posterior field to a lesion dose of 3000 rad in 15 fractions in 3 weeks is commonly used; but shorter overall treatment times may be indicated in cases of poor prognosis, and conversely an ostensibly 'solitary' spinal lesion may on occasion justify treatment on the lines of a primary tumour.

In the lymphomata (other than leukaemia), neurological involvement is predominantly by growth in the extradural space. It occurs most often in the course of established disease, when the patient is being followed up in a radiotherapy department or oncological centre. As the neurological effects are most readily reversible when they are detected early, it is essential for all seeing such patients to have a 'high index of suspicion' for these complications, and to be alerted by complaints of back pain and paraesthesiae before ataxia, paraparesis, or sphincter disorder dominate the picture. Myelography is essential, for plain X-rays are normal in 60% of the cases. Because of the space available for growth, a deposit in the lumbosacral canal may be large before neurological deficit ensues. But in the upper thoracic spine the converse is true and there may be considerable ataxia from a posteriorly placed lesion before the myelograms become abnormal by showing a complete block. The differential diagnosis of a cord lesion in these circumstances is usually between extradural tumour compression, paraneoplastic neuromyopathy, vincristine neuropathy, and radiation myelopathy. The recognition of root pain is important, for if a patient with established vincristine neuropathy and absent reflexes becomes more ataxic, this time it may be due to extradural metastases.

The relief of extradural compression when it presents is a matter of urgency, and while for most tumours emergency laminectomy is the first treatment of choice, in the lymphomata a number of factors complicate the situation. While the neurological level may be well defined, the myelogram often shows more extensive involvement and pathologically the longitudinal extent may be even greater; there may also be multiple deposits. The relief obtainable by laminectomy may therefore be very restricted, and even with departments close together neurosurgery inevitably means some delay in starting irradiation. As many of these tumours are highly radiosensitive there would, in the past, have been less hesitation in starting immediate irradiation had it not been for a lurking spectre of post-irradiational oedema. To prevent this the initial doses of irradiation were often greatly reduced and the beneficial effect restricted. These problems have been elucidated by experimental and clinical work carried out by Rubin in the United States (Rubin and Miller, 1969; Rubin *et al.*, 1969), who showed that the achievement of prompt tumour regression was more important than the slight possibility of oedema, so that there is every justification for applying the requisite radiation dose initially. Our experience with a series of lymphomata suggests that the patients likely to benefit from immediate laminectomy rather than urgent irradiation are mainly those with severe neurological deficit, often of rapid onset, with progressive motor and sphincter disturbance when the previous history and histology suggest that the response to irradiation may be delayed. These include localized lesions of nodular sclerosing Hodgkin's disease; and some cases of diffuse histiocytic lymphoma (reticulosarcoma) in which the responses of other deposits (for instance cervical nodes) have *in that patient* previously been inadequate. Corticosteroids in the form of dexamethasone often result in dramatic improvement, and radiotherapy is now always covered by this drug in sufficient dosage. An adequate length of spinal canal (often as much as 20 cm) is irradiated by a megavoltage method to a dose of 3500 rad in 20 fractions in 4 weeks, at the end of which time chemotherapy is given if blood count and bone marrow picture permit.

In the leukaemias spinal involvement is essentially by subarachnoid spread, which may also involve the nerve roots, and its management, both prophylactic and therapeutic, is considered in Chapters 33 and 37.

Carcinomatous meningitis

Leptomeningeal invasion has in the past been regarded as a rare complication of systemic cancer, but improved techniques for identifying malignant cells in the CSF, and the possibilities for management by radiotherapy and chemotherapy, have stimulated interest in this not uncommon condition which may be difficult to diagnose both clinically and pathologically. Commonly due to carcinoma of the bronchus, stomach, or breast the pathological changes may be slight, consisting of leptomeningeal thickening, tumour nodules along the cord and cauda equina, and sometimes hydrocephalus. As the microscopic changes are multifocal rather than diffuse, extensive sampling

of the leptomeninges may be necessary to establish the diagnosis at autopsy. Haematogenous spread was regarded as the probable route to the CNS, but Gonzales-Vitale and Bunuel (1976) have produced evidence that the malignant cells reach the cerebrospinal leptomeninges via perineural, endoneural and perivascular lymphatics and sheaths, through the foramina. As leptomeningeal carcinomatosis is the only sign of spread beyond the regional lymph nodes in about 40% of cases, this implies that radiotherapy or intrathecal chemotherapy may be helpful if the diagnosis can be made early.

Clinically the patients usually present with symptoms or signs at more than one CNS site. After a period of vague ill-health, headache, cranial nerve palsies, changes in mental state, and neck stiffness occur; in the spinal form, pain, paraparesis and sphincter disturbances dominate the picture so that myelography is necessary to exclude a focal compressive lesion. Clinically the CSF pressure is increased, the protein raised and the sugar reduced; but the diagnosis turns essentially on the recognition of malignant cells in the fluid. Repeated cytological examination by ultracentrifuge (the slides being examined by an experienced observer) is often necessary to establish the diagnosis. The disease is usually inexorably progressive over several weeks, but useful palliation has been achieved by whole cerebrospinal axis irradiation and intrathecal chemotherapy. The agents usually employed are methotrexate (12.5 mg) and cytosine arabinoside (50 mg) once every 5 days over a period of 3 weeks. In bronchial carcinoma good temporary palliation is obtainable, in breast carcinoma useful survival for even a year is possible, but in malignant melanoma any relief of symptoms is difficult to attain.

Acknowledgement

The authors are indebted to D. Doughty, M.Sc. for advice and illustrations of radiation treatment planning.

Further reading

Northfield, D.W.C. (1973), *The Surgery of the Central Nervous System*. Blackwell Scientific Publications, Oxford.

Paoletti, P. (ed.) (1979), *Multidisciplinary Aspects of Brain Tumor Therapy*. Elsevier Associated Scientific Publishers, Amsterdam.

Rubinstein, L.J. (1972), *Tumors of the Central Nervous System*. Second Series, Fascicle 6, Armed Forces Institute of Pathology, Washington, DC.

US Dept. of Health, Education and Welfare (1977), *Modern Concepts in Brain Tumor Therapy: Lab-*

oratory and Clinical Investigations. National Cancer Institute Monograph 46 NCI Bethesda.

Yarbro, J.W. (ed.) (1975), Brain Tumors. *Sem. Oncol.*, **2**, (1), Grune and Stratton.

References

Abbatucci, J.S. *et al.* (1978), Radiation myelopathy of the cervical spinal cord: time, dose and volume factors. *Int. J. Radiat. Oncol. Biol. Phys.*, **4**, 239–48.

Aristizabal, S., Caldwell, W.L. and Avilla, J. (1977), The relationship of time-dose fractionation factors to complications in the treatment of pituitary tumors by irradiation. *Int. J. Radiat. Oncol. Biol. Phys.*, **2**, 667–73.

Ausman, J.I. (1973), Factors influencing the outcome of chemotherapy of brain tumors. In: *Cancer of the Central Nervous System*, Proc. 7th Nat. Cancer Conf., Lippincott, Philadelphia, pp. 805–9.

Ausman, J.J. and Levin, V.A. (1969), Intra- and extra-vascular distribution of standard drug molecules in brain tumour and brain. Fourth International Congress of Neurosurgery – Ninth International Congress of Neurology, *Excerpta Medica*, New York.

Axelrod, L. (1977), In: *Pineal Tumors* (ed. H.H. Schmider), Masson Publ. U.S.A. Inc. New York. p. 61–78.

Bloom, H.J.G. (1975), Combined modality therapy for intracranial tumours. *Cancer*, **35**, 111–20.

Bloom, H.J.G. and Walsh, L.S. (1975), Tumours of the central nervous system. In: *Cancer in Children* (ed. H.J.G. Bloom *et al.*), UICC, Springer-Verlag, Berlin.

Boden, G. (1948), Radiation myelitis of the cervical spinal cord. *Br. J. Radiol.*, **21**, 464–9.

Boden, G. (1950), Radiation myelitis of the brain stem. *J. Fac. Radiol.*, **2**, 79–94.

Brem, S.S., Cotran, R.S. and Folkman, M.J. (1974), Angiogenesis in brain tumors: a quantatitive histological study. *Surg. Forum.*, **25**, 462–3.

Breuer, A.C., Blank, N.K. and Schoene, W.C. (1978), Multifocal pontine lesions in cancer patients treated with chemotherapy and CNS radiotherapy. *Cancer*, **41**, 2112–120.

Bucy, P.C. and Gustafson, W.A. (1939), Structure, nature and classification of the cerebellar astrocytomas. *Amer. J. Cancer*, **35**, 327–53.

Butler, A.R. *et al.* (1978), Computed tomography in astrocytomas. *Radiology*, **129**, 433–9.

Chang, C.H. (1977), Hyperbaric oxygen and radiation therapy in the management of glioblastoma. In: *Modern Concepts in Brain Tumor Therapy*, National Cancer Institute Monograph No. 46.

Cheek, W.R. and Taveras, J.M. (1966), Thalamic tumors. *J. Neurosurg.*, **XXIV** (2), 505–13.

Concannon, J.P., Kramer, S. and Berry, R. (1960), The extent of intracranial gliomata at autopsy and its relationship to techniques used in radiation therapy of brain tumors. *Am. J. Roentg. Rad. Ther. Nucl. Med.*, **84**, 99–107.

Coy, P. and Dolman, C.L. (1971), Radiation myelopathy in relation to oxygen level. *Br. J. Radiol.*, **44**, 705–7.

Erlich, S.S. and Davis, R.L. (1978), Spinal subarachnoid metastasis from primary intracranial glioblastoma multiforme. *Cancer*, **42** (6), 2854–64.

Freeman, J.E., Johnstone, P.G.B. and Voke, J.M. (1973), Somnolence after prophylactic cranial irradiation in children with acute lymphoblastic leukaemia. *Br. Med. J.*, **4**, 523–5.

Gehan, E.H. and Walker, M.D. (1977), Prognostic factors for patients with brain tumors. In: *Modern Concepts in Brain Tumor Therapy*, National Cancer Institute Monography No. 46, pp. 189–95.

Gonzales-Vitale, J.C. and Garcia-Bunuel, R. (1976), Meningeal carcinomatosis. *Cancer*, **37**, 2906–11.

Harris, J.R. and Levene, M.B. (1976), Visual complications following irradiation for pituitary adenomas and craniopharyngiomas. *Radiology*, **120**, 167–71.

Hoshino, T. and Wilson, C.B. (1975), A review of basic concepts of cell kinetics as applied to brain tumors. *J. Neurosurg.*, **42**, 123–31.

Hoshino, T. *et al.* (1975), Chemotherapeutic implications of growth faction and cell cycle time in glioblastomas. *J. Neurosurg.*, **43**, 127–35.

Jellinger, K. and Sturm, K.W. (1971), Delayed radiation myelopathy in man. *J. Neurol. Sci.*, **14**, 389–408.

Jones, A. (1960), Supervoltage X-ray therapy of intracranial tumours. *Ann. R. Coll. Surg. Engl.*, **27**, 310–54.

Jones, A. (1964), Transient radiation myelopathy. *Br. J. Radiol.*, **37**, 727–44.

Kernohan, J.W. and Sayre, G.P. (1952), Tumors of the central nervous system. *Atlas of Tumor Pathology*. Section X. Armed Forces Institute of Pathology, Washington, F.35 p.23.

Kramer, S. (1973), Radiation therapy in the management of malignant gliomas. In: *7th National Cancer Conference Proceedings*, Philadelphia, Lippincott, pp. 823–6.

Kramer, S. *et al.* (1977), Therapeutic trials in the management of metastatic brain tumors by different time/dose fraction schemes of radiation therapy. In: *Modern Concepts in Brain Tumor Therapy: Laboratory and Clinical Investigations*, National Cancer Institute Monograph 46.

Levin, V.A. (1975), A pharmacologic basis for brain tumor chemotherapy. *Sem. Oncol.*, **2**, (1), 57–61.

Levin, V.A. and Wilson, C.B. (1975), Chemotherapy:

the agents in current use. *Sem. Oncol.*, **2**, (1), 63–7.

Lindgren, M. (1958), On tolerance of brain tissue and sensitivity of brain tumours to irradiation. *Acta Radiol.*, Suppl. No. 170.

Mabon, R.F. *et al.* (1949), Ependymomas. *Proc. Staff Meet., Mayo Clin.*, **24**, 65–71.

Maier, J.G. *et al.* (1969), Radiation myelitis of the dorsolumbar spinal cord. *Radiology*, **93**, 153–60.

Margileth, D.A. *et al.* (1977), Blindness during remission in two patients with acute lymphoblastic leukaemia. *Cancer*, **39**, 58–61.

Mastaglia, F.L. *et al.* (1976), Effects of X-radiation of the spinal cord: an experimental study of the morphological changes in central nerve fibres. *Brain*, **99**, 101–21.

Price, R.A. and Jamieson, P.A. (1975), The central nervous system in childhood leukaemia. II. Subacute leukoencephalopathy. *Cancer*, **35**, 306–18.

Reagan, T.J., Thomas, J.E. and Colby, M.Y. (1968), Chronic progressive radiation myelopathy. *J. Am. Med. Ass.*, **203**, (2), 128–30.

Reinhold, H.S., Kaalen, J.G.A.H. and Unger Gils, K. (1976), Radiation myelopathy of the thoracic spinal cord. *Int. J. Radiat. Oncol. Biol. Phys.*, **1**, 651–7.

Rider, W.D. (1963), Radiation damage to the brain – a new syndrome. *J. Can. Ass. Radiol.*, **XIV**, 67–9.

Rubin, P. and Kramer, S. (1965), Ectopic pinealoma: a radiocurable neuroendocrinologic entity. *Radiology*, **85**, (3), 513.

Rubin, P., Mayer, E. and Poulter, C. (1969), Extradural spinal cord compression by tumour. Pt.II. High daily dose experience without laminectomy. *Radiology*, **93**, 1248.

Rubin, P. and Miller, G. (1969), Extradural spinal cord compression by tumor. Pt. I: Experimental production and treatment trials. *Radiology*, **93**, 1243.

Russell, D.S. and Rubinstein, L.J. (1977), *Pathology of Tumours of the Nervous System*. 4th edn, Edward Arnold, p. 283.

Salazar, O.M. and Rubin, R. (1976), The spread of glioblastoma multiforme as a determining factor in the radiation treated volume. *Int. J. Radiat. Oncol. Biol. Phys.*, **1**, 627–37.

Salazar, O.M. *et al.* (1976a), Patterns of failure in intracranial astrocytomas after irradiation: analysis of dose and field factors. *Am. J. Roentg.*, **126**, (2), 279–92.

Salazar, O.M. *et al.* (1976b), High dose radiation therapy in the treatment of glioblastoma multiforme: a preliminary report. *Int. J. Radiat. Oncol. Biol. Phys.*, **1**, 717–27.

Sheline, G.E. (1975a), Radiation therapy of primary tumors. *Sem. Oncol.*, **2**, (1), 29.

Sheline, G.E. (1975b), Radiation therapy of tumors of the central nervous system in childhood. *Cancer*, **35**, 957–64 (Suppl.).

Sheline, G.E. (1976), The importance of distinguishing tumor grade in malignant gliomas: treatment and prognosis. *Int. J. Radiat. Oncol. Biol. Phys.*, **1**, 781–6.

Sheline, G.E. (1977), Radiation therapy of brain tumors. *Cancer*, **39**, 873–81.

Sloof, J.L., Kernohan, J.W. and MacCarty, C.S. (1964), *Primary intramedullary tumours of the spinal cord and filum terminale*. Saunders, Philadelphia.

Sung, D.II, Harisiadis, L. and Chang, C.H. (1978), Midline pineal tumors and suprasellar germinomas: highly curable by irradiation. *Radiology*, **128**, (3), 749.

Urtasun, R. *et al.* (1976), Radiation and high-dose metronidazole in supratentorial glioblastomas. *New Engl. J. Med.*, **294**, 1364–67.

Urtasun, R.C. *et al.* (1977), Radiotherapy pilot trials with sensitizers of hypoxic cells: metronidazole in supratentorial glioblastoma. *Br. J. Radiol.*, **50**, 602.

Walker, M.D. (1973), Nitrosoureas in central nervous system tumors. *Cancer Chemother. Rep.*, **4**, Pt.3, 21–6.

Walker, M.D. (1975), Chemotherapy: adjuvant to surgery and radiation therapy. *Sem. Oncol.*, **2**, (1), 69–72.

Walker, M.D. and Gehan, E.A. (1972), An evaluation of 1–3-bis (2-chloroethyl)-1-nitrosourea (BCNU) and irradiation alone and in combination for the treatment of malignant glioma. *Proc. 63rd Ann. Meeting Am. Ass. Cancer Res.*, **13**, 67.

Wara, W.M. *et al.* (1975a), Radiation tolerance of the spinal cord. *Cancer*, **35**, 1558–62.

Wara, W.M. *et al.* (1975b), Radiation therapy of meningiomas. *Am. J. Roentg.*, **123**, 453–8.

Wara, W.M. *et al.* (1979), Tumors of the pineal and suprasellar region: Childrens Cancer Study Group treatment results 1960–1975. *Cancer*, **43**, 698–701.

Whyte, T.R., Colby, M.Y. and Layton, D.D. (1969), Radiation therapy of brain-stem tumors. *Radiology*, **93**, 413–6.

11 Ear, nose and throat

J.M. Henk and
David E. Whittam

Oropharynx

Anatomy

The oropharynx is the central portion of the pharynx, extending from the level of the palate above to the hyoid bone below. It contains the tonsillar fossae, the soft palate, the posterior third of the tongue, the vallecula and the anterior surface of the epiglottis.

The lymphatics of the tonsillar region drain into the adjacent jugulodigastric node. The remainder of the oropharynx has a bilateral lymphatic drainage, the posterior third of the tongue drains into the jugulo-omohyoid nodes, while the soft palate and posterior wall drain into the retropharyngeal and anterosuperior deep cervical nodes.

Incidence and aetiology

Squamous carcinoma of the oropharynx in the United Kingdom is now predominantly a disease of the elderly, with a peak age incidence at about 65 years. It is about four times as common in males as females. There is often an association with smoking and high alcohol intake and this is almost invariably the case where the disease occurs under the age of 60.

By contrast, both lymphoma and mucous gland carcinoma have a much wider spread of age incidence and are nearly as common in women as men.

The relative incidence of carcinoma of the various sites in the oropharynx is as follows: tonsil 60%, base of tongue 25%, soft palate 10%, posterior wall 5%.

Pathology

The commonest malignant tumour of the oropharynx is the squamous cell carcinoma, usually poorly differentiated with little or no keratinization. The anaplastic type with a lymphoid stroma is sometimes described as 'lympho-epithelioma', but this term has become obsolete with the realization that this tumour is merely a variety of squamous carcinoma.

The second commonest tumour of the oropharynx is the malignant lymphoma. Where this arises primarily in the oropharynx, it is of the 'non-Hodgkin's' type and classified accordingly. Waldeyer's ring may be involved in all types of systemic lymphoma and leukaemia.

Mucous gland carcinoma occasionally occurs in the oropharynx but is quite rare.

Symptoms and presentation

Carcinoma of the base of tongue usually presents with diffuse pain, often referred to both ears, and dysphagia. Infiltration of the muscles causes fixation of the tongue and consequent slurring of speech. Some 70% of patients have palpable lymph node metastases at presentation which are bilateral in about 25%.

Carcinoma of the tonsil often produces no symptoms or only a mild discomfort in the throat in its early stages. Pain in the ear and dysphagia occur with advanced lesions, especially when there is infiltration of the base of tongue. There may be evidence of direct extension to the sub-mandibular triangle or parapharyngeal space.

Lymph node metastases are palpable in about 60% of patients at presentation. Contra-lateral nodes are involved in less than 15%. A lump in the neck may be the first symptom, especially with the more rapidly growing anaplastic tumours.

Malignant lymphoma of the tonsil characteristically produces a large, painless, non-ulcerated mass, which may give rise to no symptoms until its bulk causes dysphagia or respiratory obstruction. Lymph nodes in the neck are frequently involved and systemic spread occurs in approximately 50% of cases.

Carcinoma of the soft palate usually presents as discomfort on swallowing, followed by pain referred to the ear and the side of the face and head. Destruction or fixation of the soft palate causes severe dysphagia with regurgitation of food down the nose.

Diagnosis and investigation

The diagnosis of oropharyngeal cancer is made from the history and clinical examination. The primary tumour is usually visible on direct inspection, or on mirror examination. Biopsy may be performed under local anaesthetic, but in most cases a general anaesthetic is advisable in order to carry out a full examination of the upper respiratory tract, including the nasopharynx, and to assess the extent of the tumour by both direct inspection and palpation. The neck must be palpated for evidence of lymph node involvement, and a chest X-ray performed.

In a case of malignant lymphoma full investigation must be performed for evidence of systemic disease, i.e. bone marrow aspiration, lymphogram, etc. (see Chapters 35 and 36).

Staging

The UICC T-staging is as follows:

T_{is} Pre-invasive carcinoma (carcinoma-in-situ).
T_0 No evidence of primary tumour.
T_1 Tumour limited to one site.
T_2 Tumour extending into two sites.
T_3 Tumour extending beyond oropharynx.

As this classification is based on the position, rather than the size of the tumour, it correlates poorly with prognosis and is not particularly useful for reporting results. An alternative system proposed by the M.D. Anderson Hospital is often used (MacComb and Fletcher, 1967).

Treatment

Radiotherapy remains the treatment of choice for the primary tumour. The local cure rates are high, especially for early disease. In recent years the development of new reconstructive techniques has led to a renewed interest in surgical treatment. However, the extensive operations necessary still carry an appreciable morbidity and some mortality, while many of the more advanced lesions cannot be removed completely. Some authorities recommend a combined approach with pre-operative radiotherapy and surgery, but there is as yet no evidence that the combined treatment is superior to radiotherapy alone; in fact retrospective comparison of the different treatment techniques within individual centres has shown an advantage to radiotherapy alone, in terms of better local control and

fewer complications (Pierquin *et al.*, 1966; Perez *et al.*, 1976). The rare radioresistant mucus and salivary tumours should be treated surgically, but those of squamous origin are best treated by radiotherapy.

Mobile unilateral (N_1) lymph node metastases are best treated either by radiotherapy alone or by a combination of radiotherapy and block dissection, as the local recurrence rate after block dissection without radiotherapy is high. Surgery is often recommended where the primary is well differentiated, and radiotherapy where it is anaplastic. However, there is no evidence that lymph node metastases are more radioresistant than the primaries from which they are derived, and if radiotherapy controls the primary, it usually also controls mobile node metastases, regardless of the histological differentiation.

The high incidence of lymph node metastases suggests the advisability of elective irradiation of lymphatic drainage areas where microscopic metastases are considered likely. It is now standard practice in many radiotherapy departments to include clinically uninvolved lymphatic drainage area in the irradiated volume; this procedure certainly reduces the incidence of recurrence in the neck but there is as yet no clear evidence that survival rates are improved.

Bilateral or fixed nodes are unsuitable for surgery and should be treated by radical radiotherapy in the first instance. Local removal of residual masses can be considered in cases where the primary disease is controlled.

Malignant lymphoma confined to the oropharynx should be treated by wide field radiotherapy.

Radiotherapy technique

Tonsil

Small lesions without lymph node involvement are best treated by a pair of wedged, oblique fields from the same side, including the primary site and the adjacent upper deep cervical nodes (Fig. 11.1). Larger lesions involving the soft palate or the base of the tongue, and all cases with lymph node involvement should be treated by parallel-opposed fields (Fig. 11.2). A two-to-one weighting is helpful to boost the dose to the primary site (Fig. 11.3). This field arrangement serves to give prophylactic irradiation to the contra-lateral upper deep cervical nodes. Where there is involvement of homolateral upper deep cervical nodes, it is advisable to irradiate the whole of that side of the neck by the addition of an anterior field below the volume treated by the parallel-opposed pair.

Other sites

Carcinomata of the base of tongue, soft palate and

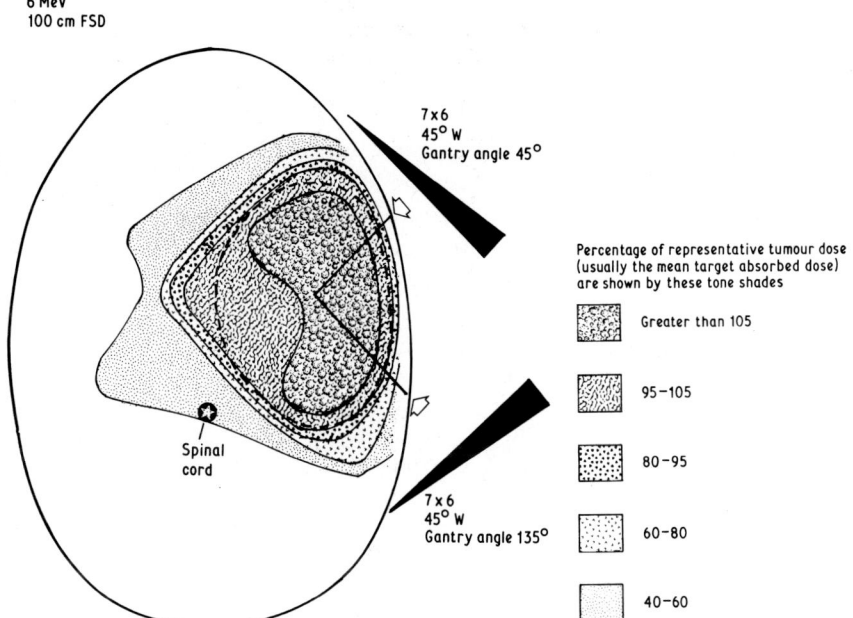

6 MeV
100 cm FSD

7 x 6
45° W
Gantry angle 45°

Percentage of representative tumour dose
(usually the mean target absorbed dose)
are shown by these tone shades

Greater than 105

95 – 105

80 – 95

60 – 80

40 – 60

Spinal
cord

7 x 6
45° W
Gantry angle 135°

Fig. 11.1   Carcinoma of tonsillar fossa. Small wedged field technique.

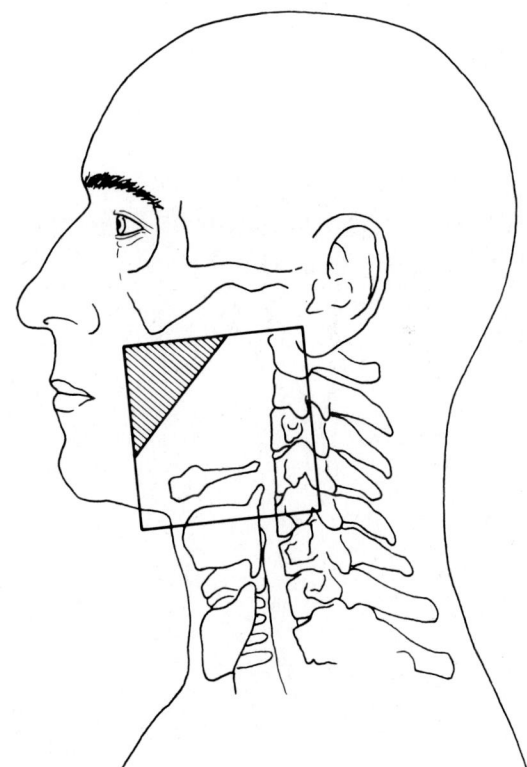

Fig. 11.2 Carcinoma of oropharynx. Treatment by parallel-opposed fields, to include upper deep cervical and sub-mandibular nodes bilaterally.

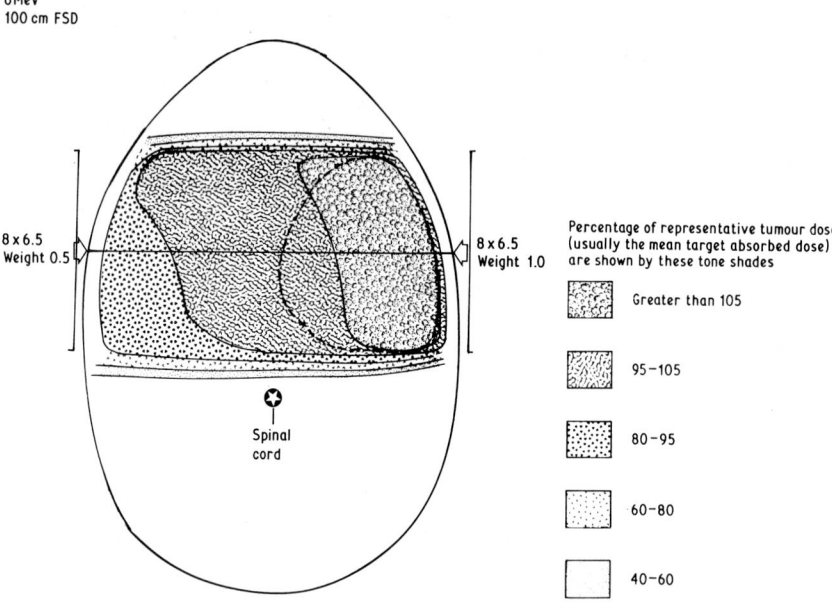

6MeV
100 cm FSD

8 x 6.5
Weight 0.5

8 x 6.5
Weight 1.0

Spinal
cord

Percentage of representative tumour dose
(usually the mean target absorbed dose)
are shown by these tone shades

Greater than 105

95–105

80–95

60–80

40–60

Fig. 11.3 Carcinoma of tonsillar fossa. Treatment by parallel-opposed fields with 2:1 weighting.

posterior wall are treated by parallel-opposed fields to cover the primary site and upper and midcervical nodes on both sides. In patients with lymph node involvement, the lower part of the neck can be treated with an anterior split field, shielding the midline structures. In patients with extensive bilateral lymph node involvement, it is often impossible to include the nodes in a parallel-opposed pair of fields without also including most of the cervical spinal cord. There is no really satisfactory technique available for treating the nodes and primary site homogeneously while avoiding the spinal cord. The best compromise is to treat any nodes not included in the parallel-opposed fields shown in Fig. 11.2 by an additional lateral field using 10–14 MeV electrons.

Dose
Small volumes with field sizes up to 50 cm² can be treated satisfactorily over a 3-week period to a tumour dose of 5000 rad in 15 fractions. Where larger volumes are treated more prolonged fractionation is advisable to minimize acute reactions and possibly late effects also; a tumour dose of 6500 rad in 6.5 weeks is recommended. Doses above this level probably give higher local control rates but there is a steep rise in the incidence of late complications.

Lymphoma
The whole of Waldeyer's ring and the lymph nodes of both sides of the neck must be irradiated. The pharynx and upper half of the neck are treated by lateral fields; the lower half of the neck and supra-clavicular fossae are treated by an anterior field shielding the midline structures. For recommended doses see Chapter 36.

Complications of treatment
Mucositis, followed by dryness, is an inevitable consequence of irradiating the oropharynx. The mucosa gradually returns to normal over a period of several months after treatment. Necrosis of the soft tissue occurring months or years after radiotherapy is seen occasionally and is related to dose; it is rarely seen where doses below 6500 rad in 6.5 weeks, or the equivalent in shorter times, have been used. Necrosis of the mandible is another occasional late complication, also dose-related, but normally only occurs when it has been necessary to extract teeth immediately before or some time after radiotherapy; it is rarely seen in patients who are edentulous at the time of presentation.

Prognosis

This depends on the size and stage of the tumour. In carcinoma of the tonsil, for example, cure rates vary from nearly 100% for T_1 N_0 tumours under 2 cm in diameter to zero for large, deeply infiltrating tumours with trismus. It is difficult to compare results from different centres because of the variety of staging systems used. Table 11.1 below shows average figures for radiotherapy control and survival from a number of publications from various parts of the world.

Table 11.1

Site	Crude 5-year survival	Two-year local control by radiotherapy
Tonsil	40%	60%
Base of tongue	25%	30%
Soft palate	40%	50%
Posterior wall	30%	40%

Nearly all local recurrences occur within the first two years, therefore the 2-year local control rates are a good index of the success of radiotherapy. Distant metastases are found in about one third of patients dying of their disease, but the majority of these also have uncontrolled local disease in the head and neck. Only about 10% of patients die of distant metastases after successful treatment of the local disease. Crude 5-year survival figures are a poor indication of the success of treatment because of the high age incidence, especially in the United Kingdom, and the association with alcoholism, heavy smoking and poor nutritional status.

Larynx

Anatomy

For the purpose of description and classification of tumours, the larynx is divided into three regions:

1. Supra-glottis
   (*a*) Epilarynx, including the 'marginal zone' which was formerly classified as part of the hypopharynx. This consists of the posterior surface of the supra-hyoid epiglottis, the aryepiglottic folds and the arytenoids.
   (*b*) Supra-glottis excluding epilarynx, i.e. the infra-hyoid epiglottis, the ventricular bands or false cords, and the ventricular cavities.
2. Glottis, the true vocal cords, joined by the anterior and posterior commissures.

3. Sub-glottis, the region below the vocal cords which adjoins the trachea at the level of the inferior border of the cricoid cartilage.

The true vocal cords have very sparse lymphatics. The supra-glottic region has a rich lymphatic drainage; lymphatic vessels pass to the pre-epiglottic space and pierce the thyrohyoid membrane to drain to the upper cervical nodes. The sub-glottis also has a rich lymphatic drainage downwards through the cricothyroid ligament to lower deep cervical nodes, and to nodes in front of and alongside the trachea which extend down into the superior mediastinum.

Pathology

Pre-malignant lesions

These are quite common in the larynx. Their management may present considerable problems.

The simple *keratosis* consists of hyperplasia of the prickle cell layer and downgrowths of the basal layer with an intact basement membrane; it is not normally pre-malignant but may be difficult to distinguish from a keratinizing squamous carcinoma histologically if only part of the lesion is presented to the pathologist.

Dysplasia consists of hyperplasia of the basal and prickle cell layers with 'atypia', i.e. pleo-morphism, hyperchromatic nuclei, variable nuclear cytoplasmic ratio and an increase in mitosis; there is however maturation on the surface of the epithelium. This is definitely a pre-malignant condition and frank carcinoma develops eventually in up to 20% of cases.

In *carcinoma-in-situ* the epithelium is largely replaced by malignant type cells; there is no stratification or maturation on the surface, but the basement membrane remains intact. This change often, but not invariably, progresses to invasive carcinoma of non-keratinizing type.

Malignant tumours

These are nearly all squamous carcinoma, usually well differentiated; about 50% show keratinization. Verrucous carcinoma is a rare variant of squamous carcinoma. Anaplastic carcinoma is uncommon. Other rare tumours of the larynx include mucous gland adenocarcinomata of the various types, oat-cell carcinoma, and sarcomata.

Incidence and aetiology

Carcinoma of the larynx accounts for approximately 1.5% of malignancy in the United Kingdom. Between 1930 and 1970 the incidence steadily declined but in the past five years an increased incidence in the younger age groups has been reported, suggesting the beginning of an upward trend.

Primary sub-glottic carcinoma is rare and occurs with approximately equal frequency in men and women; 90% of glottic and supra-glottic cancer occurs in men. The relative frequency at these two sites varies in different parts of the world; in the United Kingdom glottic carcinoma is approximately three times as common as supra-glottic.

Cancer of the larynx is commoner in smokers, and associated with excessive consumption of alcohol, but a clear-cut causal relationship has not been established.

Symptoms and presentation

Supra-glottic carcinoma normally presents as a feeling of discomfort on swallowing, progressing to dysphagia with pain referred to the ear. Hoarseness is occasionally the first symptom in tumours of the ventricular band, but it normally occurs rather late in the course of the disease. Haemoptysis is an occasional presenting symptom. There may be a complaint of a lump in the neck; approximately 30% of patients with supra-glottic carcinoma have unilateral nodes, and a further 15% bilateral nodes, palpable at presentation. Symptoms tend to be slight in the early stages of the disease so unfortunately the majority of patients present with advanced disease.

Glottic carcinoma presents as persistent hoarseness, which occurs with very small lesions and therefore early diagnosis is possible. Stridor may occur as the disease becomes more advanced causing obstruction of the glottis. Pain and dysphagia are late symptoms indicating spread beyond the glottis.

Sub-glottic carcinoma presents with stridor in over half the cases. The remainder present with hoarseness.

Diagnosis and investigation

Most laryngeal carcinomata are visible on indirect laryngoscopy. The neck must be examined for evidence of lymph node involvement and expansion or distortion of the laryngeal framework.

A chest-X-ray and a plain lateral view of the neck should be performed in all cases. Xerography, tomography and double contrast laryngography may also yield useful information about the site and spread of the disease. A barium swallow should be performed where dysphagia is a prominent symptom, as a simultaneous second primary sometimes occurs in the hypopharynx or oesophagus.

Direct laryngoscopy and biopsy is mandatory in all cases. Laryngomicroscopy helps greatly in the recognition of early lesions and should be performed wherever possible. The exact limits of the tumour in three dimensions must be accurately recorded. Several biopsies from various parts of the tumour are advisable.

Staging

Accurate delineation of the extent of a tumour in the larynx is exceedingly difficult, even with the best microendoscopic and radiological techniques. Consequently any descriptive staging is only approximate, so that it is difficult or impossible to make valid comparisons of the results of different methods of treatment between centres or from retrospective surveys.

The current TNM classification is as follows:

T — Primary tumour
1.   Supra-glottis

T_{is} Pre-invasive carcinoma (carcinoma-in-situ).
T_1 Tumour limited to the region with normal mobility.

    T_{1a} Tumour confined to the laryngeal surface of the epiglottis or to an aryepiglottic fold or to a ventricular cavity or to a ventricular band.

    T_{1b} Tumour involving the epiglottis and extending to the ventricular cavities or bands.

T_2 Tumour of the epiglottis and/or ventricles or ventricular bands, and extending to the vocal cords, without fixation.

T_3 Tumour limited to the larynx with fixation and/or destruction or other evidence of deep invasion.

T_4 Tumour with direct extension beyond the larynx, i.e. to the pyriform sinus, or the post-cricoid region or the vallecula or the base of tongue.

2. Glottis

T_{is} Pre-invasive carcinoma (carcinoma-in-situ).
T_1 Tumour limited to the region with normal mobility.

    T_{1a} Tumour confined to one cord.

    T_{1b} Tumour involving both cords.

T_2 Tumour extending to either the sub-glottic or the supra-glottic regions (i.e. to the ventricular bands or the ventricles), with normal or impaired mobility.

T_3 Tumour limited to the larynx with fixation of one or both cords.

T_4 Tumour extending beyond the larynx, i.e. into cartilage or the pyriform sinus or the post-cricoid region or the skin.

3. Sub-glottis

T_{is} Pre-invasive carcinoma (carcinoma-in-situ).
T_1 Tumour limited to the region with normal mobility.

  T_{1a} Tumour limited to one side of the sub-glottic region and not involving the under surface of the cords.

  T_{1b} Tumour extending to both sides of the sub-glottic region and not involving the under surface of the cords.

T_2 Tumour involving the sub-glottic region and extending to one or both cords.
T_3 Tumour limited to the larynx with fixation of one or both cords.
T_4 Tumour extending beyond the larynx, i.e. to the post-cricoid region or the trachea or the skin.

N – Regional lymph nodes

N_0 Regional lymph nodes not palpable.
N_1 Movable homolateral nodes.

  N_{1a} Nodes not considered to contain growth.
  N_{1b} Nodes considered to contain growth.

N_2 Movable contralateral or bilateral nodes.

  N_{2a} Nodes not considered to contain growth.
  N_{2b} Nodes considered to contain growth.

N_3 Fixed nodes.

M – Distant metastases

M_0 No evidence of distant metastases.
M_1 Distant metastases present.

Stage-grouping

Stage I	T_1 N_0 or N_{1a} or N_{2a}	M_0
Stage II	T_2 N_0 or N_{1a} or N_{2a}	M_0
Stage III	T_3 N_0 or N_{1a} or N_{2a}	
	T_4 N_0 or N_{1a} or N_{2a}	M_0
	Any T N_{1b} or N_{2b}	
Stage IV	Any T with N_3	M_0
	Any T Any N with M_1	

Treatment

The principles outlined below must be regarded as guide lines only. Every patient with laryngeal cancer should be seen jointly by a surgeon and radiotherapist before definitive treatment is begun. The patient's age, sex, occupation and social habits must be taken into account when deciding upon the treatment policy most appropriate for that individual. For example, the disease tends to respond better to radiotherapy in women than men, whereas men are better at learning oesophageal speech after laryngectomy. The alcoholic or anyone who is unlikely to attend regularly for follow-up, may be better treated by surgery than radiotherapy, whereas a professional man may wish for every possible effort to be made to preserve his larynx.

Glottic carcinoma

In-situ carcinoma is treated initially by stripping of the vocal cords, with regular follow-up examinations. Radiotherapy need be given only if histological evidence of invasion is found.

An early lesion confined to one vocal cord with full mobility (T_{1a}) should be treated by radiotherapy. The operation to remove the vocal cord by laryngo-fissure is now scarcely ever practised. It can however, be done in some cases with a small recurrence after radiotherapy. Where there is involvement of the anterior commissure (T_{1b}), there is no need to perform laryngectomy as the results of treatment by radiotherapy are very good; in these cases however a careful watch must be kept for recurrence which may occur in the sub-glottic space and regular direct examination is advisable after radiotherapy. In T_2 lesions where there is a minimal spread beyond the glottis but without complete fixation of the vocal cord, the results of radiotherapy are good so this is the treatment of choice; good results have been claimed for partial laryngeal surgery from some centres, especially in the United States, but this operation is not popular in the United Kingdom. In general the quality of the voice is better in successfully irradiated cases than after partial laryngeal surgery. Where recurrence occurs after radiotherapy partial laryngeal surgery is difficult and carries a high morbidity, so laryngectomy is advisable.

The treatment of more advanced (T_3) glottic carcinoma is especially controversial. The choice lies between immediate laryngectomy, or initial radical radiotherapy with careful follow-up reserving laryngectomy for those cases where there is persistent or recurrent disease. There is no evidence that either policy gives a better survival rate (Marshall, 1972); the advantage of a policy of initial radiotherapy is that approximately 60% of the survivors retain the larynx. The disadvantage of radiotherapy is the need for very close follow-up, and problems may arise with the subsequent management of the patient. It is usual for the mucosa to heal after radiotherapy but the larynx rarely returns completely to normal, so it may be difficult to detect recurrence in the deeper tissues of the larynx. Persistent slight oedema and limitation of vocal cord movement are quite common after radiotherapy and do not necessarily indicate persistent tumour: in fact approximately 25% of recurrence-free 5-year survivors still have a fixed vocal cord. Whenever recurrence is suspected direct laryngoscopy and deep biopsies must be performed. Occasionally, in the very oedematous larynx, it is not possible to obtain positive histology and it may be advisable to perform laryngectomy without confirmation of recurrence; the occasional removal of a larynx which on subsequent histological examination shows only radiation changes is inevitable if this treatment policy is adopted.

In very advanced glottic carcinoma where there is significant respiratory obstruction necessitating tracheostomy, or where there is extension beyond the larynx (T_4), surgery is advisable, as radiotherapy usually fails, especially if a preliminary tracheostomy has been done. The commonest site of recurrence after laryngectomy is around the tracheostome. Such recurrences are rarely curable by subsequent radiotherapy, so in these advanced cases it is advisable to give immediate post-operative radiotherapy to the neck including the stoma.

Supra-glottic carcinoma
In the United Kingdom supra-glottic carcinoma rarely presents in the early stages, i.e. T_1 or T_2, N_0; when it does so, it is usually treated by radiotherapy. Where supra-glottic carcinoma is commoner and more early cases are seen, e.g. in North and South America, horizontal partial laryngectomy is popular, removing the tumour but preserving the vocal cords. In the post-operative period the patients experience difficulty with swallowing and a long period of rehabilitation is often necessary; the procedure is only applicable to younger, fitter patients, and good results are only obtained in centres where a large number of these operations can be done.

Where there is evidence of unilateral mobile lymph node involvement (N_1) with an early primary, radiotherapy is usually equally successful in controlling the node as in controlling the primary and so it is doubtful whether a block dissection needs to be performed as part of the initial treatment unless the primary is also treated surgically.

In-situ carcinoma of the supra-glottis cannot be treated by stripping, and invasive changes can usually be found at some points, so radiotherapy is advisable.

Unfortunately the majority of patients with supra-glottic carcinoma present with an advanced primary tumour (T_3 or T_4). Many are in poor general condition, with other diseases and poor nutrition, associated with heavy smoking and drinking. Where the disease is staged N_0 or N_1, and the patient is considered fit enough, surgery is the treatment of choice. The incidence of local recurrence after surgery can be reduced by the addition of radiotherapy; pre-operative radiotherapy has been popular in a number of centres for many years, both in high dose (Goldman *et al.*, 1972) and low dose (Hendrickson and Liebner, 1968). However, more recent studies suggest that post-operative radiotherapy is at least as effective, and carries a lower morbidity (Cachin and Eschwege, 1975).

High dose pre-operative radiotherapy may be an advantage in patients with large lymph node metastases of doubtful operability. Otherwise low dose radiotherapy is preferable which can be combined with additional dosage post-operatively, or the entire treatment may be given post-operatively.

Patients staged N_2 and N_3 are unsuitable for surgery and are normally treated by radiotherapy, but the results are poor.

Advanced supra-glottic carcinoma has a rather similar natural history and presents similar problems in management to pyriform fossa cancer (see below).

Sub-glottic carcinoma
Early cases where there is an adequate airway may be treated by radical radiotherapy with quite good results, reserving laryngectomy for recurrence. Where there is obstruction of such a degree that tracheostomy is necessary it is preferable to perform laryngectomy initially, with post-operative radiotherapy. In all cases the lower cervical and upper mediastinal lymph nodes must be included in the irradiated volumes.

Rare tumours
Mucus gland carcinoma is best managed surgically if possible. However, local control is often obtained by radiotherapy, especially in the case of the adenoid cystic type, so these tumours should not be regarded as totally radioresistant. Where surgery is considered inadvisable, because of the general condition of the patient or the extent of the disease, a radical course of radiotherapy should be given, with a reasonable prospect of success.

Sarcomata should be treated surgically, with post-operative radiotherapy if removal is thought to be incomplete, and adjuvant chemotherapy as described in Chapter 31.

The management of verrucous carcinoma is controversial. Reports of recurrences after radiotherapy with an undifferentiated histological pattern have led to the belief that radiation induces 'anaplastic transformation', and therefore surgery is the treatment of choice. However, similar undifferentiated recurrences have been reported after cryosurgery to oral verrucous carcinoma, and it seems likely that the tumours contain anaplastic cells prior to treatment. The largest reported series of verrucous carcinoma of the larynx suggests that the behaviour and response to radiotherapy of this tumour is no different from that of other types of squamous carcinoma, and should be treated in the same way (Burns *et al.*, 1976).

Radiotherapy technique

Glottic

There is no need to irradiate lymph nodes electively as the incidence of nodal metastases is so low. In T_1 and T_2 cases the irradiated volume can be kept small (Fig. 11.4). A T_1 lesion confined to one cord can be treated very suitably by a single lateral field from a 4–6 MeV Linear Accelerator (Fig. 11.5). The whole larynx must be treated where there is involvement of both cords or the anterior commissure; this can be done by parallel-opposed fields or a pair of anterior oblique wedged fields (Fig. 11.6). Slightly longer fields should be used for T_3 tumours, and in particular where there is sub-glottic spread the treatment volume should be extended downwards to at least 2 cm below the cricoid cartilage.

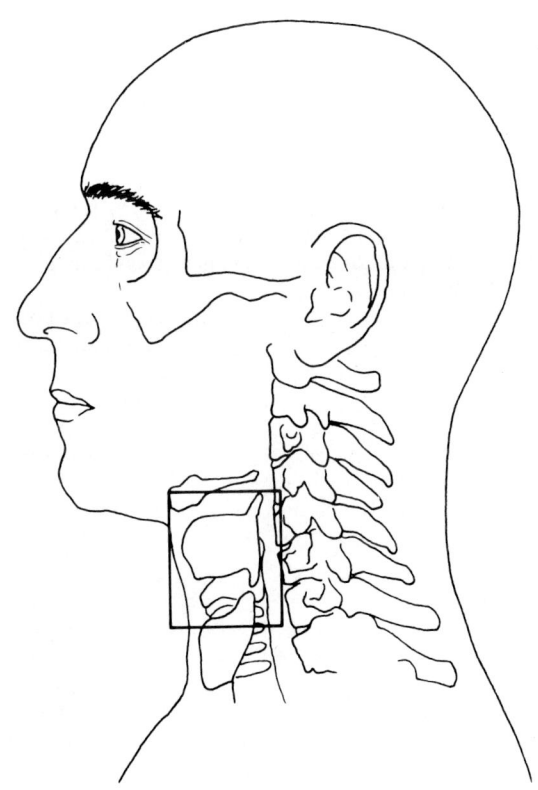

Fig. 11.4 Volume to be irradiated in a patient with glottic carcinoma. The fields should be centred on the vocal cord, 1 cm below the promontory of the thyroid cartilage.

A wide range of fractionation schemes is in current use from as short as three weeks to as long as eight weeks, with very similar results. A clear-cut relationship between dose and tumour control has not been established, but there is no doubt that higher doses cause an increased incidence of late complications, such as persistent oedema and perichondritis, and also increase the difficulty and morbidity of salvage laryngectomy in cases where this is necessary. A dose level should be chosen at which there is a negligible risk of cartilage necrosis; this is particularly important in T_3 cases, of whom at least 50% will require subsequent laryngectomy; these patients should not be subjected to an increased operative risk. There is some evidence, for example from hyperbaric oxygen trials, that survival is lower where high doses are used. A maximum tissue dose of 5500 rad in 4 weeks gives satisfactory results.

Supra-glottic

Supra-glottic carcinoma should be treated by parallel-opposed lateral fields. It is advisable in all cases to include the jugulodigastric and jugulo-omohyoid nodes (Fig. 11.7). Where there is lymph node involvement the entire deep cervical chain should be irradiated. Wedge filters or some other form of compensation is necessary to ensure a homogeneous dose (Fig. 11.8).

Several reports suggest that local control of supra-glottic carcinoma is strongly dose-related, but high doses lead to increased morbidity; 6500 rad in 6 weeks is probably optimum.

Sub-glottic

The primary site, lower deep cervical nodes and superior mediastinum must be irradiated homogeneously en bloc. This can be achieved by an anterior T- or cross-shaped field and two lateral neck fields angled inferiorly (Fig. 11.9).

Care of patient during radiotherapy

Most patients develop some degree of mucositis towards the end of a course of radiotherapy; where large volumes are irradiated, this can be quite severe with pain, dysphagia and increasing hoarseness. The patient must be encouraged to maintain an adequate fluid and calorie intake. Aspirin mucilage is very useful before meals to relieve pain and dysphagia. Local irritants to the mucosa, especially smoking, should be discouraged. Most patients can be treated as out-patients, except where there is impairment of the airway when observation in hospital during radiotherapy is necessary. Tracheostomy is best avoided if at all possible. Oedema occurring during radiotherapy usually subsides rapidly if treated by bed rest, antibiotics and a few

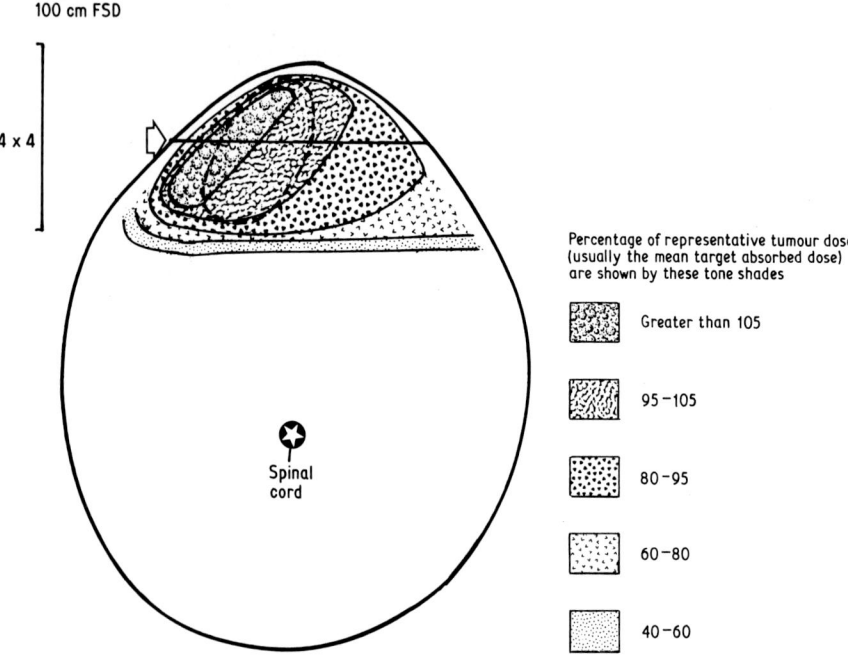

6 MeV
100 cm FSD

4 x 4

Spinal
cord

Percentage of representative tumour dose
(usually the mean target absorbed dose)
are shown by these tone shades

Greater than 105

95 – 105

80 – 95

60 – 80

40 – 60

Fig. 11.5 Treatment of early vocal cord carcinoma by a single field.

days' course of high dose steroids, e.g. dexamethasone 4 mg three times daily.

Results

Glottic

T_{1a}: the mortality is negligible with determinant 5-year survival rates over 95%. About 10% recur after radiotherapy; of these recurrences, approximately two-thirds occur in the first two years after treatment, the remainder occur at any time later and have been recorded at over fifteen years; many of these late recurrences are probably new primary cancers.

T_{1b}: the mortality is again low with determinant 5-year survival rates exceeding 90%. Local recurrence after radiotherapy occurs in approximately 20% of cases.

T_2: 5-year determinant survival rates are approximately 80% with some 25–30% recurring after radiotherapy.

T_3: most reports give 5-year survival rates of around 60%, whether the initial treatment is laryngectomy or radical radiotherapy. Radiotherapy fails in over 50%. Hyperbaric oxygen significantly reduces the failure rate.

Supra-glottic

In Stage 1 (T_1 N_0) carcinoma, reported 5-year survival rates vary between 70% and 80%. Local recurrence occurs after radiotherapy in approximately 20% of cases. As the disease becomes more advanced the success rates fall sharply, on average radiotherapy fails in about 40% in T_2 and 80% in T_3 cases. The 5-year survival rate falls from about 60% in Stage 2 to less than 10% in Stage 4. Overall the 5-year survival rates for supra-glottic carcinoma are around 40%, 60% where the nodes are free, and 15% where they are involved. A number of authors have reported that the prognosis is better in females than males.

Sub-glottic

Sub-glottic carcinoma has the poorest prognosis, with reported 5-year survival rates rarely exceeding 30%.

Hypopharynx

Anatomy

The hypopharynx is the lower part of the pharynx, extending from the level of the hyoid bone to the lower border of the cricoid cartilage. It surrounds the larynx

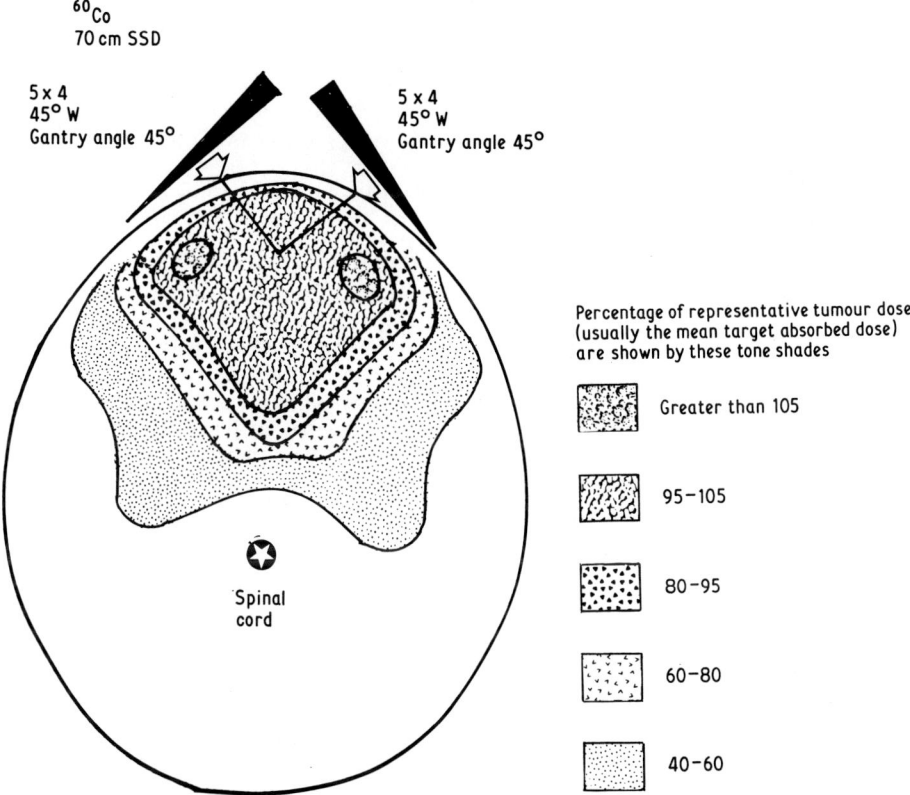

^{60}Co
70 cm SSD

5 x 4
45° W
Gantry angle 45°

5 x 4
45° W
Gantry angle 45°

Spinal
cord

Percentage of representative tumour dose
(usually the mean target absorbed dose)
are shown by these tone shades

Greater than 105

95−105

80−95

60−80

40−60

Fig. 11.6 Wedged field technique for carcinoma involving the anterior commissure or both vocal cords.

posteriorly and laterally. For the purpose of classification of tumours it is divided into three sites, the pyriform fossae, the posterior wall, and post-cricoid space, which forms the central part of the anterior wall of the hypopharynx and the posterior wall of the larynx.

There is a rich lymphatic drainage which passes mainly through the thyrohyoid membrane to the deep cervical nodes of both upper and lower groups.

Incidence and aetiology

Carcinoma of the pyriform fossa occurs predominantly in men over 40 years old: the peak age incidence varies between geographical regions and is now around 65 years in the United Kingdom. The majority of patients have a history of excessive use of tobacco and alcohol.

Carcinoma of the post-cricoid space and posterior pharyngeal wall occurs predominantly in women between 40 and 60 years old, and is particularly common in Northern Europe, especially Scandinavia and Wales. There is an association with iron deficiency and between a third and a half of women with carcinoma of the hypopharynx have the Paterson-Kelly syndrome.

Pathology

Almost all malignant tumours of the hypopharynx are squamous carcinoma, usually poorly differentiated. Mesenchymal tumours also occur but are very rare.

Symptoms and presentation

Carcinoma of the pyriform fossa first gives rise to a sensation of irritation in the throat, followed by pain on swallowing referred to the ear on the same side. As the tumour enlarges dysphagia and weight loss occur. A tumour on the medial wall may invade and fix the larynx causing hoarseness. A tumour on the lateral wall rapidly invades the thyroid cartilage, and may

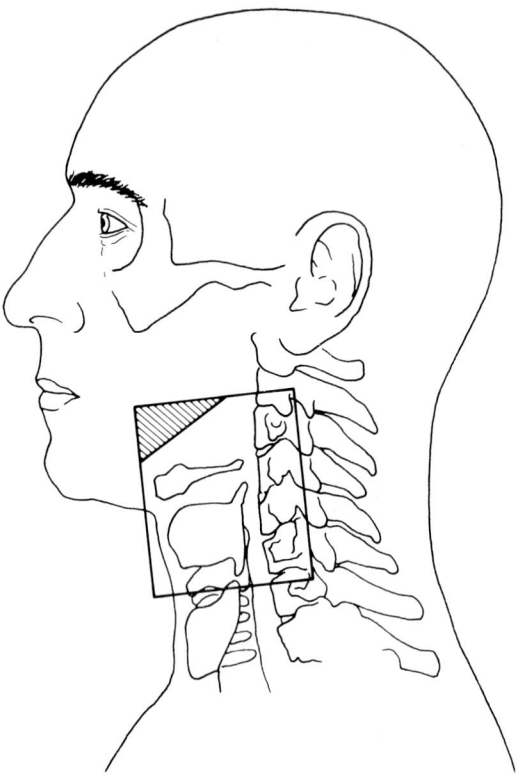

Fig. 11.7 Volume to be irradiated in a patient with supraglottic carcinoma. N.B. Whenever the neck is irradiated with lateral or oblique fields it is advisable to position the patient so that the spinal canal is as straight as possible.

produce a palpable mass. Involved homolateral lymph nodes are palpable in about 75% of patients at presentation, and bilateral nodes in about 25%. A lump in the neck may be the only symptom and it is not uncommon to find massive lymph node involvement with only a small asymptomatic primary which may be difficult to detect.

Carcinoma of the post-cricoid region and posterior pharyngeal wall almost invariably present as progressive dysphagia. In many cases there is a long history of dysphagia, associated with the Paterson-Kelly syndrome or a post-cricoid web, and the significance of the increasing dysphagia may not at first be recognized, hence these patients often present with quite advanced tumours. There is often downward spread to the cervical oesophagus; post-cricoid carcinoma in particular rapidly becomes annular. Involvement of the larynx causes hoarseness and dyspnoea. Lymph nodes are palpable at presentation in about 20% of cases of post-cricoid carcinoma, with inferior lymphatic spread of paratracheal nodes and the mediastinum in about 15%. The incidence of involved neck nodes is even higher in carcinoma of the posterior wall, occurring in 50% of patients at presentation, in half of whom the nodes are bilateral.

Diagnosis and investigation

Carcinomas of the pyriform fossa and posterior pharyngeal wall are usually visible on mirror examination. Those of the post-cricoid region are not normally visible unless they extend above the arytenoids, but pooling of saliva and mucus can be seen in the hypopharynx. The neck must be examined for palpable

6 MeV
100 cm FSD

7 x 6
15° W

7 x 6
15° W

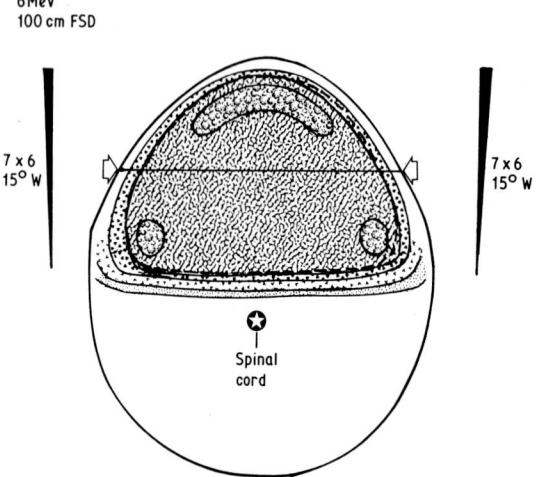

Spinal cord

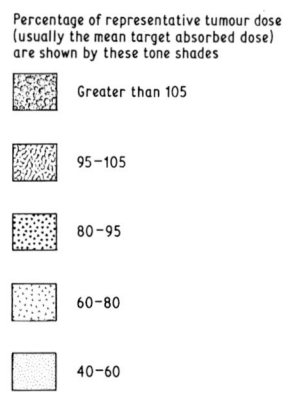

Percentage of representative tumour dose (usually the mean target absorbed dose) are shown by these tone shades

Greater than 105

95–105

80–95

60–80

40–60

Fig. 11.8 Treatment of supra-glottic carcinoma by parallel-opposed fields, using wedge filters to compensate for the curvature of the neck.

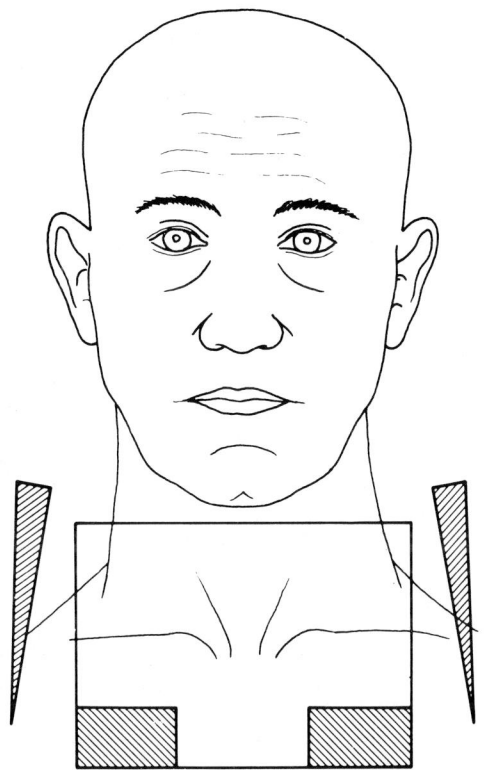

Fig. 11.9 Three-field technique for irradiation of sub-glottic carcinoma, suitable for a cobalt unit or linear accelerator.

lymph nodes, and for direct extension of the tumour which can be distinguished from nodes by its movement on swallowing.

A lateral soft tissue X-ray of the neck is valuable in delineating the extent of posterior pharyngeal wall tumours. In post-cricoid tumours, widening of the space between the trachea and the vertebral column is seen, and in the case of pyriform fossa tumours destruction of the thyroid cartilage may be seen. Valuable additional information may be obtained from the barium swallow, especially with the use of a cine-video recording. Chest X-ray must be performed to exclude mediastinal node involvement and pulmonary metastases, and to demonstrate pulmonary infection due to spill-over into the trachea.

Endoscopy is mandatory to examine the pharynx, larynx and trachea fully and to facilitate the taking of material for biopsy. It is especially important to delineate the lower border of the tumour.

Staging

The current classification is as follows:

T – Primary tumour
1. *Pyriform sinus*

T_{is} Pre-invasive carcinoma (carcinoma-in-situ).

T_0 No evidence of primary tumour.

T_1 Tumour confined to the pyriform sinus and without fixation to the surrounding structures.

T_2 Tumour extending from pyriform sinus to posterior pharyngeal wall or to post-cricoid area and without fixation to surrounding structures.

T_3 Tumour invading larynx or thyroid cartilage or soft tissues of the neck.

2. *Pharyngo-oesophageal junction (post-cricoid area)*

T_{is} Pre-invasive carcinoma (carcinoma-in-situ).

T_0 No evidence of primary tumour.

T_1 Tumour confined to the post-cricoid area without fixation to the surrounding structures.

T_2 Tumour extending into pyriform sinus or to the posterior pharyngeal wall and without fixation to the surrounding structures.

T_3 Tumour invading larynx or prevertebral muscles.

3. *Posterior pharyngeal wall*

T_{is} Pre-invasive carcinoma (carcinoma-in-situ).

T_0 No evidence of primary tumour.

T_1 Tumour confined to the posterior pharyngeal wall and without fixation to the surrounding structures.

T_2 Tumour extending into the pyriform sinus or to the post-cricoid region and without fixation to the surrounding structures.

T_3 Tumour invading prevertebral muscles or extending to neighbouring structures.

Treatment

Carcinoma of pyriform fossa

An early lesion confined to the medial wall of the pyriform fossa can often be treated initially by radical radiotherapy and careful follow-up. In the event of recurrence, there is a good chance of successful laryngectomy. Early lesions on the lateral wall are best treated by surgery initially because of the likelihood of involvement of the thyroid cartilage.

More advanced lesions, Stages T_2 and T_3, N_0 and N_1, should be treated by extended laryngectomy and radical neck dissection, provided the patient is fit enough to tolerate surgery. Some authorities have claimed from retrospective data that low dose pre-operative radiotherapy, 1500–3000 rad in 2–3 weeks, improved local tumour control and survival. There are conflicting reports on the value of higher dose radiotherapy. Van den Brouck *et al.* (1977) compared the same dose of radiotherapy, namely 5500 rad in 5.5 weeks, given pre- and post-operatively. The group selected for post-operative radiotherapy had a significantly higher survival rate, fewer post-operative complications and spent a shorter period in hospital. The overall picture suggests that if combined treatment is used, a high dose of radiation should not be given pre-operatively. Low dose pre-operative radiotherapy can be followed by additional post-operative treatment, or the radiation can be given entirely post-operatively.

Very advanced lesions with bilateral nodes or fixed masses in the neck are unsuitable for surgery. In younger, fitter patients, radiotherapy is worth trying and occasionally a good result is obtained. In general, however, the results are very poor, and there is a place for trying new methods of improving the effectiveness of radiotherapy, such as neutron therapy, radiosensitizers, or concomitant cytotoxic drugs. Radiotherapy of large lesions is associated with a high morbidity, due to the acute mucosal reaction and impaired nutrition, and in many patients, especially the elderly, may increase suffering and hasten demise. The surgeon and radiotherapist must judge each patient as an individual problem and decide whether or not treatment is justified.

Post-cricoid carcinoma

The patient presenting with post-cricoid carcinoma invariably has lost weight and is usually anaemic and in negative nitrogen balance. The extent of the disease must be accurately assessed as described above, to determine whether any curative treatment should be attempted. A patient with detectable disease in the mediastinum, or with bilateral or fixed nodes in the neck, virtually never survives more than one year, however treated. Neither surgery nor radical radiotherapy should be attempted in such a patient and only minimal palliative measures employed. If there is absolute dysphagia with regurgitation of saliva a low dose of radiation to the primary site may help, but this is unlikely, and insertion of a Celestin tube usually gives better palliation. Gastrostomy should be avoided because although it may prolong survival, it adds to the patient's distress without relieving any symptoms.

The physical, psychological and spiritual aspects of terminal nursing care described in Chapter 39 are particularly relevant to the patient with advanced post-cricoid carcinoma.

In a patient where there is no clinical evidence of lymphatic spread or where there is only a mobile unilateral node in the neck, curative treatment can be attempted so the approach is entirely different. It is imperative to bring the patient into positive nitrogen balance and to correct anaemia before embarking on radical treatment. To achieve this, blood transfusion and hyperalimentation via a nasogastric feeding tube are usually necessary; in some cases it is not possible to pass a feeding tube through the obstructed upper oesophagus and so a gastrostomy may be necessary. The chances of successful extirpation of the tumour are slightly higher by surgery than by radiotherapy, so in younger fitter patients where the primary disease is not fixed to the pre-vertebral fascia, surgery is the treatment of choice. Laryngopharyngectomy is performed with restitution of the alimentary tract by the use of a skin tunnel, the stomach or the colon. For shorter, higher lesions, the pharynx can be reconstructed with a skin tunnel; for the more usual, longer lesions involving the upper oesophagus, the oesophagus must be removed and a viscus used for reconstruction. However performed the operation of laryngopharyngectomy carries an appreciable mortality and morbidity (Griffiths and Shaw, 1973).

In the patient with an inoperable primary, or considered unfit for laryngopharyngectomy, a radical course of radiotherapy is given to the hypopharynx, upper oesophagus, and the immediate lymphatic drainage in the superior mediastinum and both sides of the neck.

Posterior wall

The posterior wall is the least common site for a carcinoma of the hypopharynx, therefore the numbers in all reported series are small and it is difficult to compare the results of various methods of treatment. Surgical removal is possible if there in no upward extension to the oropharynx or fixation to the pre-vertebral fascia: laryngopharyngectomy is necessary with the associated morbidity described above. The reported results of radical radiotherapy for N_0 lesions are as good, if not better, than those of surgery; therefore within the limits of our present knowledge radiotherapy seems the treatment of choice. Where there is a unilateral mobile node, this should be included in the radiation field and a radical neck dissection performed three weeks after completion of radiotherapy. Unfortunately lymph node involvement is often bilateral, in which case the prognosis is virtually hopeless, but occasionally long-term control by radiotherapy to the pharynx and both sides of the neck may be effected.

Radiotherapy technique

Early carcinoma of the pyriform fossa should be treated by parallel-opposed fields, using a technique simi-

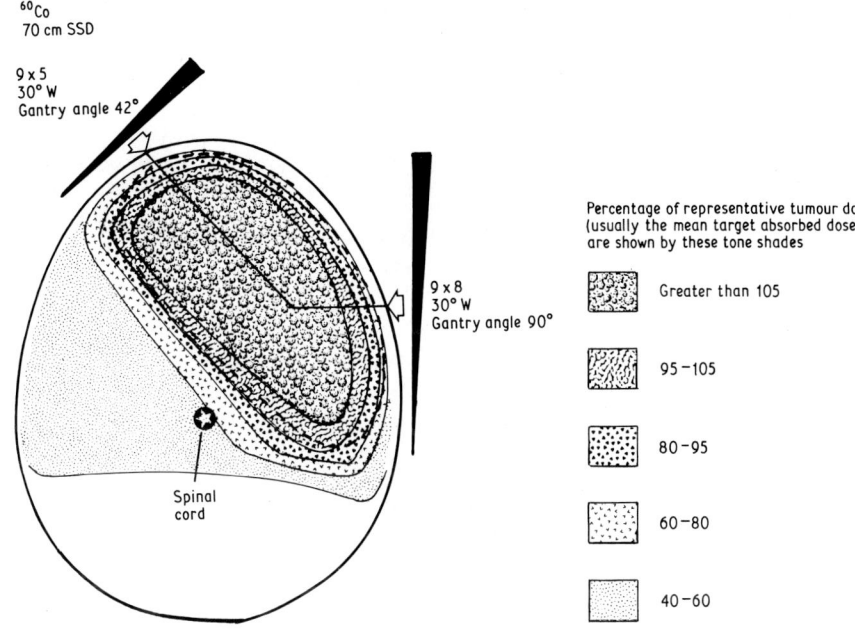

⁶⁰Co
70 cm SSD

9 x 5
30° W
Gantry angle 42°

9 x 8
30° W
Gantry angle 90°

Spinal
cord

Percentage of representative tumour dose
(usually the mean target absorbed dose)
are shown by these tone shades

Greater than 105

95 – 105

80 – 95

60 – 80

40 – 60

Fig. 11.10   Field arrangement for treatment of advanced carcinoma of the pyriform fossa with unilateral node involvement.

lar to that recommended for supra-glottic carcinoma. The fields should encompass the upper and lower deep cervical lymph nodes and extend from the lower border of the mandible to the lower border of the cricoid cartilage. A dose of 5000 rad in 5 weeks is given to this volume, which should be adequate to control microscopic lymph node metastases; the fields are then reduced to cover the primary site alone and a further 1500 rad given in 10 days. In the case of more advanced disease with unilateral node involvement, the treatment volume must extend more posteriorly on the involved side of the neck and so an oblique field arrangement is necessary (Fig. 11.10). This large volume will not tolerate more than 6000 rad in 6 weeks by daily fractionation, following which an extra 500 rad may be given by small fields to any residual disease, either at the primary site or in the nodes.

In the treatment of post-cricoid carcinoma it is important that the lower edge of the tumour in the cervical oesophagus be defined accurately. The treatment volume should extend at least 2 cm and preferably 3 cm, below this lower border in order to cover potential submucosal lymphatic spread. To achieve this and also irradiate the lymphatic drainage in the neck, two lateral fields angled inferiorly are recommended, with the addition of an anterior mediastinal field if necessary to deliver an adequate dose to the inferior margin of the volume (Fig. 11.11).

Posterior pharyngeal wall carcinoma is treated by a simple parallel-opposed pair of lateral fields. Some inferior angulation of the fields may be necessary to cover the lower border of the tumour, especially in short-necked individuals.

Results

Results of treatment of hypopharyngeal carcinoma vary greatly between different reported series because of geographical differences in the relative incidence of tumours at the various sites, differences in age incidence and stage of disease at presentation, and selection of patients for different modes of treatment. The overall 5-year survival for carcinoma of the pyriform fossa is about 15%. Some series have reported 5-year survivals as high as 50% in selected patients suitable for surgical treatment, but in general only about 1 in 3 patients is suitable for surgery (Cachin, 1969). In the late or inoperable patient treated by radiotherapy alone, the 5-year survival rate is less than 10%.

The prognosis of post-cricoid carcinoma is even worse. The overall 5-year survival is less than 10%. Pearson (1966) reported a 5-year survival of 25% from

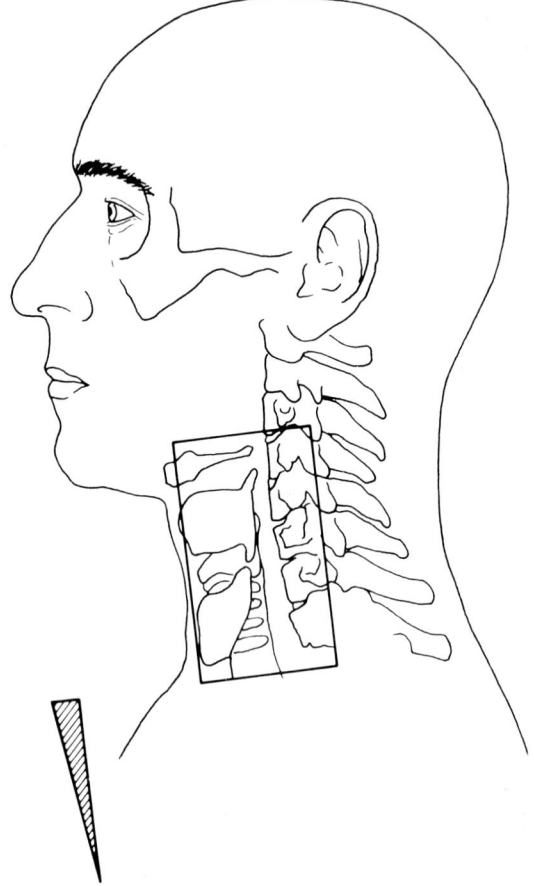

radiotherapy alone, but most other series fail to achieve such a high figure. Five-year survivals of up to 35% from surgery have been reported. N_2 and N_3 disease carries a hopeless prognosis, with virtually no 2-year survivors.

It is difficult to assess prognosis for carcinoma of the posterior pharyngeal wall because of the small numbers in all reported series. Wang (1971) reported 7 out of 15 N_0 patients alive at 3 years, treated by radiotherapy alone: only 4 out of 21 who had involved nodes were alive at 3 years.

Complications of treatment of carcinoma of the hypopharynx and larynx

The severity of 'post-radiation' changes in the larynx is related to the dose of radiation given, and to the extent of the original tumour. A slight persistent oedema after radiotherapy is common when infiltrating tumours have been treated, but rare after treatment of early disease. Damage to laryngeal cartilage causes marked oedema, pain, tenderness and intermittent low grade fever; it occurs after treatment of tumours which have already invaded the cartilage, or may be the result of overdoses of radiation, especially where hyperbaric oxygen or neutrons are used, presumably because normal cartilage is a hypoxic tissue. The symptoms and signs may subside with long-term antibiotic therapy and short courses of steroids, but some cases progress to frank cartilage necrosis, with a useless larynx and chronic ill health, for which laryngectomy may be the only solution.

Fibrous strictures commonly occur after successful radiotherapy of tumours which have encircled the pharynx and frequent dilatations may be necessary. Myxoedema has been reported in a small proportion of

6 MeV
100 cm FSD

6 x 11.5 wedged
Gantry angle 90°
Couch angle 10°

6 x 11.5 wedged
Gantry angle 90°
Couch angle 10°

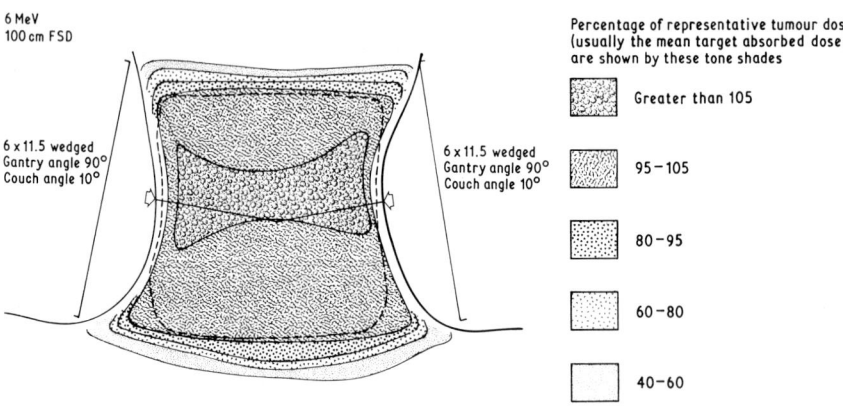

Percentage of representative tumour dose (usually the mean target absorbed dose) are shown by these tone shades

	Greater than 105
	95 – 105
	80 – 95
	60 – 80
	40 – 60

Fig. 11.11   Field arrangement for irradiation of post-cricoid carcinoma.

patients after irradiation of the lower anterior part of the neck.

The risk of post-surgical complications is increased when major resections are performed after high-dose radiotherapy. These include delayed healing, wound infection, fistulae and, most catastrophic of all, carotid artery rupture. They may be minimized by ensuring adequate nutrition, and by the use of correctly placed neck incisions. If the skin of the neck shows radiation changes it is better to excise the skin and replace it with a deltopectoral flap. Scrupulous attention to closure of the pharynx, with removal of redundant mucosa in order to achieve a water-tight seal, will help prevent the formation of a fistula. The carotid artery may be protected by rotating the levator scapulae as a flap anteriorly to cover it.

Post-operative nutrition is of vital importance. This may consist of intravenous feeding initially followed by nasogastric tube feeding until the patient is able to swallow adequately. Post-operative haemoglobin should be maintained at 12 g or higher by transfusion if necessary.

Ear

Anatomy

External ear
The external ear consists of two parts, the auricle and the external auditory canal. The latter is about 2.5 cm in length and is made up of an outer one-third, a cartilaginous portion, and the inner two-thirds which is the bony portion. The lymphatic drainage of the external ear flows anteriorly into the parotid lymph nodes, posteriorly into the post-auricular nodes, and below into the external jugular nodes.

Middle ear and mastoid
The middle ear cleft is situated between the tympanic membrane laterally and the medial wall which separates it from the bony and membranous labyrinth. It communicates posteriorly with the mastoid antrum and the mastoid air cells. It contains the bony ossicles and the facial nerve.

Pathology

Malignant lesions of the external auditory canal are rare. They occur in females more than males, usually in the middle decades. The two commonest types of tumour are the basal cell carcinoma and squamous cell carcinoma; the latter is the commoner. Squamous cell carcinoma tends to spread outwards to the auricle or inwards to the middle ear, and bony invasion may occur early. Basal cell tumours do not normally metastasize, but the squamous cell tumours metastasize to regional nodes in 10–15% of cases.

The malignant tumours occurring in the middle ear and mastoid are squamous carcinoma, adenocarcinoma, rhabdomyosarcoma, and malignant melanoma. Although rare, the squamous carcinoma is the commonest primary malignant tumour of the middle ear. Males and females are affected equally. It tends to occur most commonly in the fifth decade in pre-existing chronic infected mastoid air cells. It may spread laterally into the meatus, forwards into the parotid gland, superiorly into the middle cranial fossa, posteriorly into the mastoid bone, inferiorly into the jugular bulb region, medially into the inner ear and facial nerve, and occasionally anteriorly around the eustachian tube and into the post-nasal space. Extension into this area may occur from tumours of the external ear, the parotid gland, the nasopharynx or more rarely the paranasal sinuses.

Glandular tumours arise from ceruminal glands. A small proportion resemble adenoid cystic tumours of salivary origin. They tend to behave in a malignant fashion metastasizing to adjacent lymph nodes and to the lungs.

Symptoms and presentation

Carcinoma of the external auditory canal and middle ear give rise to very similar symptoms. Over 70% of the patients have long-standing chronic suppurative otitis media. Suspicion of malignant change should be aroused by an increase in otorrhoea which may become blood-stained, and the development of deep boring pain. There is increasing deafness, conductive initially, which may become perceptive if the inner ear is involved.

On inspection of the external auditory canal there is usually a profuse discharge and there are often polyps and granulations which bleed readily on touch. Facial palsy of lower motor neurone type may be present; eventually the lower cranial nerves may become involved by direct extension.

Diagnosis and investigation

Clinical examination must include the ear, the parotid region, the neck for enlarged lymph nodes, and the cranial nerves. X-rays of the skull and mastoid region, including tomograms, should be performed. Occasionally subtraction arteriograms and retrograde venograms are useful. The place of the latter is now declining as computerized axial tomography (CAT) becomes available and is proving of increasing value in delineating lesions in and around the base of the skull.

Examination under anaesthetic and biopsy is necessary finally to establish the diagnosis.

Treatment

Carcinoma of the middle ear and external auditory canal will be considered together as the natural history, prognosis, and management are very similar. In many cases both these structures are involved and it is impossible to determine exactly where the lesion arose. There are three alternative approaches to treatment.

1. Mastoidectomy, followed by radiotherapy. This is the most often practised method but only very small lesions can be removed completely. In the majority of cases only a partial removal is possible; if so this method of management gives the lowest survival rate and often fails to relieve the pain.
2. Radical temporal bone resection. Large lesions can be removed by this method, provided they do not extend medially as far as the internal carotid artery. Nevertheless the procedure is somewhat mutilating and carries a high morbidity and an appreciable mortality (Lewis, 1973).
3. Radiotherapy with no surgical procedure other than biopsy. This is the simplest method of treatment with the lowest morbidity; it appears to give survival rates as high as those of aggressive surgery. The main disadvantage of this method is that where the tumour is not controlled by irradiation there is usually little or no relief of pain.

Radiotherapy technique

The entire petrous bone must be irradiated so that in transverse section the high dose volume is triangular with its apex just anterior to the brain stem (Figs. 11.12 and 11.13). This is achieved by anterolateral and posterolateral wedged fields. The treatment plane must be inclined so that the exit dose from the posterolateral field avoids the eyes. Preferably the patient should be treated supine with the posterolateral field directed from below the horizontal plane, because if the patient is positioned on his side it is very difficult to avoid some lateral curvature of the cervical spine with a consequent risk of the spinal cord being included in the inferior part of the high dose volume. The best reported results are from tumour doses of 5000–5500 rad in 3 weeks.

Complications

During radiotherapy skin reaction behind the pinna may be troublesome and epilation occurs. Antibiotic cover is advisable to prevent increasing infection. Late

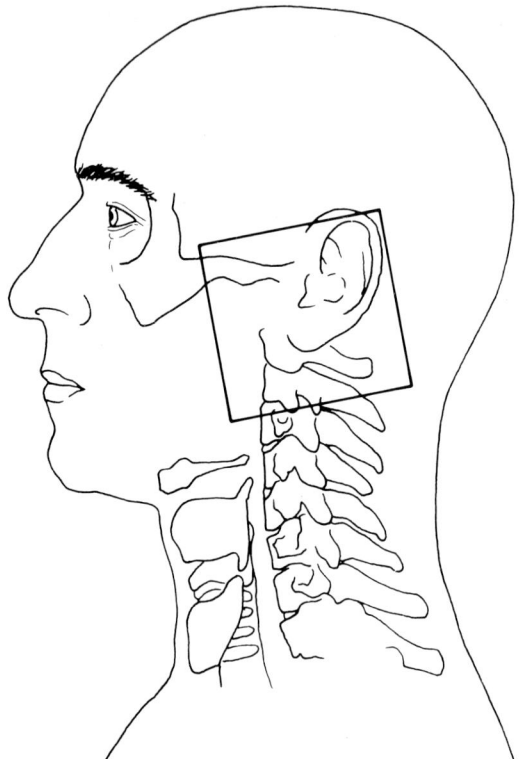

Fig. 11.12 Lateral view of volume to be irradiated in a patient with carcinoma of the middle ear or external auditory canal.

complications are few if the disease is controlled. Osteoradionecrosis should not occur if the irradiation is given homogeneously, avoiding areas of high dose. Radiation effects on the inner ear are negligible; sensineural threshold elevation may be detectable but there is rarely any significant hearing loss.

Results

Five-year survival rates for squamous carcinoma of the middle ear and external auditory canal are around 25%, regardless of the method of treatment. A small series reported by Holmes (1965), treated solely by radiotherapy with a 4 MeV linear accelerator, showed a 5-year survival rate of 54%, but this is unusually high. The prognosis for basal cell carcinoma and most glandular tumours is rather better.

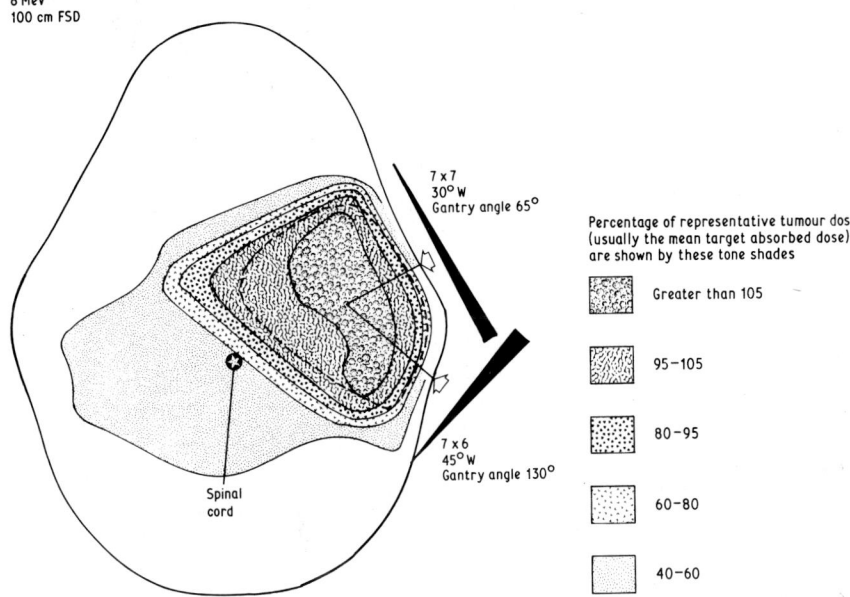

8 MeV
100 cm FSD

7 x 7
30° W
Gantry angle 65°

7 x 6
45° W
Gantry angle 130°

Spinal cord

Percentage of representative tumour dose
(usually the mean target absorbed dose)
are shown by these tone shades

Greater than 105

95 – 105

80 – 95

60 – 80

40 – 60

Fig. 11.13 Field arrangement for irradiation of carcinoma of the middle ear, or external auditory canal. A similar plan is used for a glomus jugulare tumour.

Glomus jugulare tumours

Pathology

The glomus jugulare tumour is benign or of low grade malignancy. It arises from non-chromaffin paraganglionic chemoreceptor tissue situated in or in close relationship to the middle ear. It occurs mainly over the age of 40 years and is commoner in females than males.

It may arise from one of three sites:

1. In the tympanic cavity from the paraganglion on the tympanic branch of the ninth cranial nerve.
2. The glomus bodies in the adventitia of the jugular bulb.
3. The paraganglion related to the ganglion nodosum of the tenth cranial nerve.

Histologically the glomus tumour is a chemodactoma, therefore it is similar to a carotid body tumour. The cells are long and polygonal, appearing in columns, clusters or cords, surrounded by a vascular network containing non-myelinated nerves. The size of the vessels varies from capillary to cavernous spaces, and fibrosis may be present.

Growth is slow with local invasion of surrounding structures. Metastases are rare, occurring in approximately 4% of cases.

Symptoms and presentation

Most patients have a long history of aural symptoms before the diagnosis is made. Deafness is the commonest presenting symptom, conductive at first but may later become perceptive. Tinnitus often occurs, described as a swishing sound synchronous with the pulse. Pain and vertigo occasionally occur but are not usually severe. Some patients present with facial palsy or bulbar palsy due to involvement of cranial nerves.

The tumour is visible on examination of the ear if the tympanic cavity is involved. It appears as a red flush of the tympanic membrane without bulging, a pulsating mass, or a vascular, fleshy red polyp. A bruit is sometimes audible. In very advanced cases a pulsating tumour may be felt over the mastoid or seen in the nasopharynx. There may be multiple cranial nerve palsies, the nerves most commonly involved being the seventh and the ninth to twelfth.

Diagnosis and investigation

Wherever possible a specimen should be obtained for biopsy in order to distinguish the tumour from a simple inflammatory polyp, a haemangioma, or a meningioma. However, great care is needed as massive haemorrhage may result. Biopsy is particularly hazardous in the case of lesions of the jugular bulb, where the diagnosis may rest upon clinical and radiological features only.

X-rays, including tomography of the temporal bone, should be performed in all cases. Arteriography shows the tumour as a characteristic blush, but is not normally necessary except in those cases where the diagnosis cannot be established by clinical examination and biopsy.

Treatment

Small, purely tympanic lesions can be excised with good results. For large lesions and those in the jugular bulb, radiotherapy is the treatment of choice as surgery is hazardous. A fairly high dose is needed: 5000 rad in 4 weeks with daily fractionation is recommended, using the same technique as for squamous carcinoma of the middle ear (see above).

Results

Where complete excision is possible, the prognosis is excellent. In those cases treated by radiotherapy there is usually slow shrinkage of the tumour and symptoms are gradually relieved over a period of several weeks. Clinical and radiological evidence of the tumour persists indefinitely but it rarely causes further trouble (Maruyama *et al.*, 1971). Less than 20% of the tumours show evidence of regrowth within 20 years, and the mortality from the disease is less than 10%.

Nasal fossa

Anatomy

The nasal fossa is defined as the interior cavity of the nose. It is bounded above by the inferior margin of the ethmoid air cells, below by the hard palate, and laterally by the medial wall of the maxillary sinuses.

The lymphatic vessels arise in the superficial part of the mucous membrane. The external nose and anterior part of the nasal fossa drain into the sub-mandibular lymph nodes and occasionally into a small facial node. The remainder of the nasal fossa drains into the upper deep cervical glands either directly, or indirectly through the retropharyngeal nodes.

Incidence and aetiology

Malignant tumours of the nose form 0.3% of all cancers in the United Kingdom. The commonest malignant tumour in the nasal fossa is a carcinoma arising in the paranasal sinuses and reaching the nasal fossa by direct extension. A variety of primary malignant tumours arise in the nasal fossa but are all rare. Squamous carcinoma is mainly a disease of the elderly, commoner in males and white people. Aesthesioneuro-epithelioma occurs at all ages. There is an association between adenocarcinoma and certain occupations, as seen in cases of tumours of the paranasal sinuses (see below).

Pathology

The inverted papilloma is benign but should be followed carefully as occasionally malignant transformation arises.

The squamous carcinoma is the commonest malignant tumour, arising usually from the middle or lower turbinate, the septum, or the vestibule. It tends to grow slowly and metastasize late, with the reported incidence of lymph node metastases at presentation being only 10%.

Tumours may arise from mucous glands, mainly in the olfactory epithelium. These may be adenocarcinoma, sometimes mucin-producing, or of the adenoid cystic type.

The nasal cavity is the commonest site for solitary plasmacytoma. Melanoma and glioma occasionally occur.

The aesthesioneuro-epithelioma is a rare tumour arising from the olfactory epithelium. It consists of small round cells, some of which may be in rosettes, and therefore it sometimes goes by the name of 'olfactory neuroblastoma'. However, this is a misleading term as this is not an embryonic tumour and its behaviour is very different from that of the neuroblastoma of childhood. It grows slowly and infiltrates widely but rarely metastasizes.

Symptoms and presentation

The first symptoms are nasal obstruction which may be unilateral or bilateral, a unilateral nasal discharge, and epistaxis. More advanced disease may cause swelling of the nose, pain or anaesthesia in the side of the face, post-nasal discharge, malocclusion due to involvement of the hard palate, and enlarged nodes in the neck.

Diagnosis and investigation

Most tumours of the nasal fossa are visible on anterior or posterior rhinoscopy, particular attention being paid to areas of ulceration or increased pigmentation. The examination should include the face for evidence of asymmetry, and the oral cavity for signs of involvement. Plain X-rays of skull and sinuses should be performed, and in addition, tomography may yield useful information. Examination under anaesthetic is normally necessary to assess the exact extent of the lesion and to obtain a specimen for biopsy. In the case of plasmacytoma full investigation for evidence of disseminated desease is mandatory (see Chapter 34).

Treatment

Most cases of squamous carcinoma are best treated by radiotherapy with good results, although some authorities prefer surgery for small anterior lesions, especially of the nasal septum, where healing after radiotherapy is sometimes poor. There is no need for prophylactic block dissection or neck irradiation.

Plasmacytoma localized to the nose is treated solely by irradiation. Chemotherapy is indicated only if there is evidence of disseminated disease.

Melanomas are treated by wide excision. Preoperative radiotherapy is sometimes recommended because of the poor results, but there is no real evidence of its value.

In the case of aesthesioneuro-epithelioma, small lesions are probably best excised. Larger, infiltrating lesions are treated by radiotherapy.

Radiotherapy technique

Squamous carcinoma of the nasal fossa and aesthesioneuro-epithelioma is treated by a similar technique to that used for the antrum and ethmoid (Fig. 11.14). A small lesion of the nasal vestibule can be treated by two anterior oblique wedged fields or by electrons at 10–14 MeV.

In the case of plasmacytoma it is advisable to use wide fields treating the whole nasal fossa and paranasal sinuses on both sides. A tumour dose of 4000 rad in 3 weeks or the equivalent in a longer time is sufficient to achieve local control (Todd, 1965).

Results

The prognosis of squamous carcinoma is quite good with local cure in about 70% of cases. Melanoma, on the other hand, has a very poor prognosis. Radiotherapy achieves local control in virtually all cases of plasmacytoma but dissemination occurs eventually in between 30% and 40% which is inevitably fatal eventually. Approximately 75% of patients with aesthesioneuro-epithelioma survive 5 years after treatment.

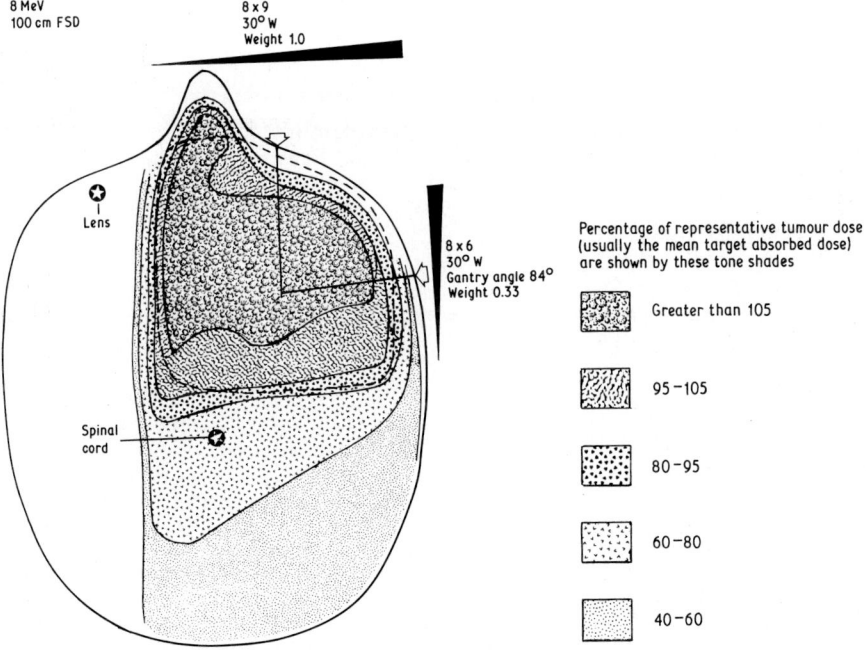

Fig. 11.14 Field arrangement for irradiation of carcinoma of the maxillary antrum.

Complications

An acute radiation reaction occurs in the nasal mucosa towards the end of a course of radiotherapy, leading to soreness, discharge and obstruction. As this subsides, it leaves the mucosa dry and atrophic. Fibrous adhesions between the septum and lateral wall occasionally occur.

Cartilage necrosis is very rare after radiotherapy, except where the cartilaginous portion of the septum was initially invaded by tumour. In these cases healing may be delayed and recurrent infections become a problem.

The paranasal sinuses

Anatomy

The paranasal sinuses are spaces within the maxilla, ethmoid, frontal and sphenoid bones. They are lined with a mucous membrane continuous with that of the corresponding nasal cavity through their ostia.

The maxillary sinus is related above to the floor of the orbit and the infraorbital nerve. Its medial wall separates it from the nasal cavity. The floor is formed by the alveolar process and hard palate. The anterior wall is covered by the skin of the cheek. Posteriorly it is related to the pterygoid plates and pterygopalatine fossa.

The ethmoid sinuses consist of a number of thin-walled cavities within the lateral masses of the ethmoid bones. These cells may be divided into anterior and posterior groups. The anterior cells drain into the middle meatus of the nose and the posterior cells into the superior meatus. They are related superiorly to the anterior cranial fossa and laterally to the orbit and lacrimal sac.

The lymphatic vessels of the paranasal sinuses arise from a continuous network in the superficial part of the mucous membrane. They drain into the upper deep cervical nodes either directly or after traversing the retropharyngeal nodes.

Incidence and aetiology

Of the malignant tumours involving the paranasal sinuses over half arise in the maxillary antrum, and about one third in the ethmoid air cells. Malignant tumours of the frontal sinus and sphenoid sinus are extremely rare.

Males are affected more than females in the ratio of 2:1, and the average age at diagnosis is 54 years. A higher incidence of malignant tumours in the paranasal sinuses has been found in certain occupations, e.g. in the chrome and nickel industries. Adenocarcinomas have a higher incidence in the furniture and boot and shoe industries.

Pathology

The commonest malignant tumour of the paranasal sinuses is the squamous carcinoma, usually well differentiated, but occasionally anaplastic forms occur. Adenocarcinoma is less common except in certain occupationally exposed persons as mentioned above. Rarer tumours include the various types of mucous gland carcinoma, sarcomata, and lymphomata.

Carcinoma of the paranasal sinuses usually grows slowly and spreads by invasion of surrounding structures. Lymphatic spread occurs at a late stage and only about one in six of patients have involved lymph nodes in the neck palpable at presentation.

Symptoms and presentation

Tumours confined within a sinus usually give rise to no symptoms, therefore late presentation is the rule. Symptoms occur when there is spread beyond the sinus to surrounding structures. There is often spread from the ethmoid to the maxillary sinus or vice versa, and then it may not be possible to determine the exact site of origin. The presenting symptoms may be classified as follows:

Facial
Swelling of the cheek and a palpable mass may occur when a maxillary sinus carcinoma spreads anteriorly; pain in the face and numbness of the cheek occur when the infraorbital nerve is involved.

Nasal
The nasal cavity may be involved by direct spread from any of the paranasal sinuses. There may be unilateral obstruction, bleeding and discharge.

Orbital
Ethmoid carcinoma frequently involves the orbit by direct local extension. Maxillary carcinoma may also do so by upward extension. Unilateral proptosis, epiphora, diplopia, or loss of vision may occur.

Oral
Carcinoma of the maxillary antrum may spread inferiorly through the hard palate or superior alveolus to involve the mouth. This may present as an ulcer on the palate or gum, loosening of the teeth, toothache, or malocclusion. Posterior spread to the pterygoid fossa may cause trismus.

Diagnosis and investigation

Full clinical examination of the face, nose, eyes, oral cavity, neck and cranial nerves is necessary. Plain X-ray of the sinuses may reveal only a diffuse opacity which is not diagnostic of malignancy. There may be destruction of bone which can be better seen by tomography. CAT-scanning is a useful method of delineating the extent of the tumour, especially posteriorly.

Examination under anaesthetic and biopsy are necessary to establish the diagnosis. Access to the maxillary antrum for biopsy can be obtained by an intranasal antrostomy or the Caldwell-Luc incision. The former is recommended as safer and disturbing the tumour less.

Staging

There is no internationally agreed TNM staging for carcinoma of the paranasal sinuses. The M.D. Anderson Hospital system is used in many centres in the United States (MacComb and Fletcher, 1967).

Treatment

The management of malignant disease in the paranasal sinuses requires the combined efforts of ear, nose and throat surgeon, oral surgeon and radiotherapist. In all cases presenting with advanced disease combined treatment is essential.

The initial treatment is radical radiotherapy. This is not pre-operative in the accepted sense as complete removal of the entire area involved may not be possible, and the upper jaw is a site where surgery is possible after high dose radiotherapy without an unacceptable morbidity; therefore a full radical dose is given.

Intra-arterial infusion of cytotoxic agents is sometimes performed before or during radiotherapy. Good initial regression of the tumour is often obtained by this method, but vascular complications are not infrequent. This technique is now declining in popularity because of the technical difficulties, and the realization that systemic chemotherapy has a similar effect (see below). However, there is as yet no clear evidence that the addition of chemotherapy to radiotherapy improves the therapeutic ratio; for example, intra-arterial infusion of fluorouracil was reported by Shigematsu *et al.* (1971) to give a significant increase in local control, but was reported by Chan and Shukovsky (1976) to give a significant increase in late complications.

After radiotherapy, radical surgery is performed. The aim should be to remove the entire volume of tissue originally involved by tumour if at all possible. The surgeon should not be tempted to perform a limited resection in those cases where there is considerable tumour regression during radiotherapy (Harrison, 1973). Maxillectomy is always necessary with orbital exenteration if the orbital periosteum is involved.

Following removal of the maxillary antrum the cavity is filled with a mould attached to the patient's own dental plate if present, or a new one if the patient has normal dentition. This is then moulded to conform with the normal contours of the patient's face. If, following surgical removal, there is histologically proven residual disease the cavity produced by carrying out a maxillectomy provides an adequate space for intracavitary radiotherapy.

Contra-indications to surgery include the age and the general condition of the patient and the extent of the disease. If it is evident from the pre-operative investigations that there is involvement of the dura, surgical removal is not usually attempted. However, dural involvement may only become apparent at operation; should it not be too far through the procedure, this is usually an indication to abandon the operation. Involvement of the pterygoid fossa again is difficult to establish prior to surgery, but usually the majority of the contents of this region can be removed satisfactorily. In those rare cases with fixed cervical lymph nodes, surgery is contra-indicated.

If local recurrence occurs after radical combined therapy, further treatment usually has little effect on the course of the disease. However, a small superficial recurrence in the maxillectomy cavity may sometimes be amenable to intracavitary radiotherapy.

Radiotherapy technique

Carcinoma of the maxillary antrum and ethmoid sinus is most commonly treated by anterior and lateral wedged fields (Fig. 11.14). It is important to avoid any dosage at all to the eye on the unaffected side, so if a cobalt unit is employed fields must be well trimmed. An alternative is to use a single anterior field with an electron beam of energy of 25–35 MeV (Bataini and Ennuyer, 1971), but this gives a more severe skin reaction than photon treatment.

The treatment volume must include the maxilla, the pterygoid fossa, the whole of the ethmoid bone on both sides, and the homolateral lateral pharyngeal lymph nodes. The cornea, lens, and lacrimal gland on the affected side can be shielded (Fig. 11.15), provided there is no gross involvement of the orbit, in which case the eye must be sacrificed anyway and no ocular protection should be used.

Similar results have been reported from tumour doses varying from 5000 rad in 3 weeks up to 7000 rad in 8 weeks.

Acute reactions during treatment are rarely troublesome. If the eye is not shielded there may be a painful corneal reaction; the pain can be relieved by steroid drops. If there is persistent pain and swelling of the cheek during radiotherapy indicating infection in the

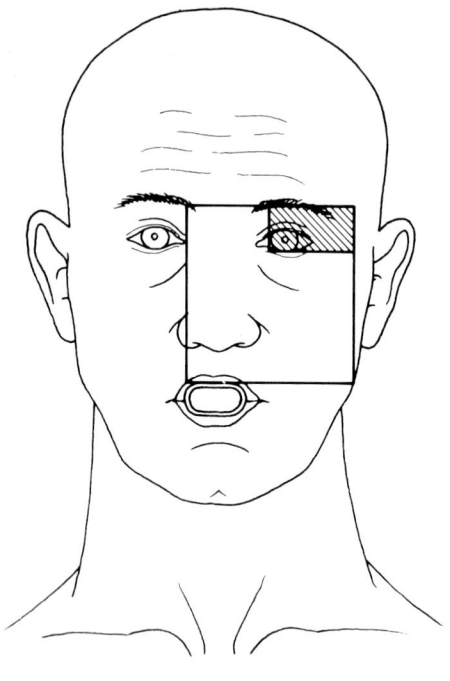
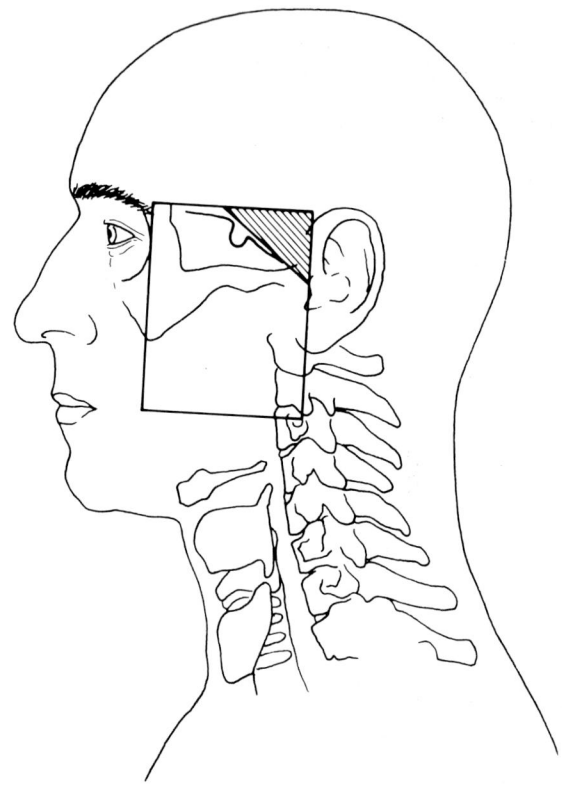

Fig. 11.15 Treatment of carcinoma of the maxillary antrum, anterior and lateral fields.

antrum, antibiotics should be given. A drainage procedure is now rarely, if ever, needed before or during radiotherapy.

A variety of techniques are available for intracavitary irradiation after maxillectomy. An obturator can be loaded with small radioactive sources of radium, cobalt or caesium to provide local irradiation of the suspected parts of the cavity, or the whole cavity can be packed with ovoids (Barley *et al.*, 1976). Postoperatively a dose of 4000 rad in 3 days at a depth of 0.25 cm is recommended. In the case of frank recurrence this can be increased to 6000 rad in 5 days.

Results

Most series reported in the past ten years show 5-year survival rates for squamous carcinoma of the paranasal sinus between 25% and 40%. The prognosis depends on size, site and histology of the tumour, being more favourable in the case of early anteroinferior well differentiated lesions. Most recurrences occur within three years, but occasionally later; a 10-year survival rate of about 20% is usual. Adenocarcinoma is usually slow-growing, and late recurrence is quite common;

consequently the 5-year survival rate tends to be somewhat higher, and the 10-year survival rate rather lower, than for squamous carcinoma.

Ethmoidal carcinoma is generally regarded as having a poorer prognosis than maxillary antral carcinoma, but published series are small, and survival rates do not differ significantly between the two sites.

Local recurrence is present in the majority of fatal cases. Death from distant metastases in the absence of local disease is unusual, except in the case of the rare anaplastic carcinomata in younger adults.

Future trends

There now seems only a limited scope for improvement in techniques of surgery and radiotherapy, and significant future developments of combinations of these two methods of treatment seem unlikely. However better results may be expected from existing methods of treatment if a greater proportion of patients are seen and managed in specialized combined clinics, where all disciplines involved in the management of the patient are represented.

There is some hope that application of knowledge

gained in the radiobiology laboratory may reduce the incidence of failure of radiotherapy. There is now little doubt that the hypoxic tumour cell is one of the factors militating against successful radiotherapy of ear, nose and throat cancer. Hyperbaric oxygen has been shown to reduce radiotherapy failure by at least 20%, with a particularly pronounced effect in moderately advanced disease (Henk, Kunkler and Smith, 1977). Unfortunately hyperbaric oxygen involves a time-consuming, unpleasant and potentially hazardous procedure; it is applicable to only a limited proportion of patients and therefore seems unlikely ever to be adopted as a routine method of treatment, or to make a significant contribution to improvement of overall results. Other methods of tackling the problem of the hypoxic tumour cell do, however, show promise. Fast neutron therapy (Catterall *et al.*, 1977) has been shown to improve radiotherapy control of advanced tumours but so far without influencing survival: this method of treatment is at present limited by the expense and technical constraints of the apparatus needed. Another approach under investigation is the use of electron-affinic chemicals which mimic the radiobiological effect of oxygen (see also Chapters 3 and 4).

The role of cytotoxic chemotherapy has yet to be clearly defined. Several drugs are effective in causing temporary tumour regression, especially methotrexate and bleomycin. The combination of vincristine, bleomycin, high dose methotrexate and fluorouracil (Price *et al.*, 1978) is more effective, with approximately 70% of advanced and recurrent tumours showing at least 50% regression. In 40% of responders remission lasts for at least a year. The response rate is higher in untreated than in previously treated patients, so the use of combination chemotherapy as an adjuvant before and after radical treatment is now under investigation.

Simultaneous treatment with radiotherapy and cytotoxic drugs as single agents has been disappointing (Bertino *et al.*, 1975). The administration of a combination of vincristine, bleomycin, and methotrexate during radiotherapy shows more promise (O'Connor *et al.*, 1977), but clear evidence of increase in therapeutic ratio is still awaited and random controlled trials are desirable.

Acknowledgements

Miss A.M. Bidmead, Mr. M. Chow and Miss M. Viljoen, Physics Department, Royal Marsden Hospital, for isodose plans. Mr. A.R. Jones, Department of Educational Technology, St George's Hospital, for drawings.

References

Barley, V.L., Ellis, F. and Paine, C.H. (1976), Carcinoma of the maxillary antrum. *Proc. R. Soc. Med.*, **69**, 697–700.

Bataini, J.P. and Ennuyer, A. (1971), Advanced carcinoma of the maxillary antrum treated by cobalt teletherapy and electron beam irradiation. *Br. J. Radiol.*, **44**, 590–8.

Bertino, J.R., Boston, B. and Capizzi, R.L. (1975), The role of chemotherapy in the management of cancer of the head and neck; a review. *Cancer*, **36**, 752–8.

Burns, H.P., Van Nostrand, A.W. and Bryce, D.P. (1976), Verrucous carcinoma of the larynx. Management by radiotherapy and surgery. *Ann. Otol.*, **85**, 538–43.

Cachin, Y. (1969), Le traitement des cancers du sinus pyriforme. *Presse Med.*, **77**, 1072.

Cachin, Y. and Eschwege, F. (1975), Combination of radiotherapy and surgery in the treatment of head and neck cancers. *Cancer Treat. Rev.*, **2**, (3) 177–91.

Catterall, M., Bewley, D.K. and Sutherland, I. (1977), Second report on results of a randomised clinical trial of fast neutrons compared with x-or gamma-rays in treatment of advanced tumours of head and neck. *Br. Med. J.*, **i**, 164.

Chan, R.C. and Shukovsky, L.J. (1976), Effects of irradiation on the eye. *Radiology*, **120**, 673–5.

Goldman, J.L. *et al.* (1972), High-dose pre-operative radiation and surgery for carcinoma of the larynx and laryngopharynx, a 14-year program. *Laryngoscope*, **82**, 1869–82.

Griffiths, J.D. and Shaw, H.J. (1973), Cancer of the laryngopharynx and cervical oesophagus. Radical resection with a repair by colon transplant. *Arch. Otolar.*, **97**, 340–6.

Harrison, D.F.N. (1973), The management of malignant tumours affecting the maxillary and ethmoid sinuses. *J. Lar. Otol.*, **87**, 749–72.

Hendrickson, F.R. and Liebner, E. (1968), Results of pre-operative radiotherapy for supra-glottic larynx cancer. *Ann. Otol.*, **77**, 222–9.

Henk, J.M., Kunkler P.B. and Smith, C.W. (1977), Radiotherapy and hyperbaric oxygen in head and neck cancer. Final report of first controlled clinical trial. *Lancet*, **ii**, 101–3.

Holmes, K.S. (1965), Carcinoma of the middle ear. *Clin. Radiol.*, **16**, 400–4.

Lewis, J.S. (1973), Squamous carcinoma of the middle ear. *Arch. Otolar.*, **97**, 41–2.

Marshall, H.F. *et al.* (1972), The management of advanced laryngeal cancer. *J. Lar. Otol.*, **86**, 309–15.

Maruyama, Y., Gold, L.H.A. and Kieffer, S.A. (1971), Radioactive cobalt treatment of glomus jugulare tumours. Clinical and angiographic investigation. *Acta Radiol.*, **10**, 239–47.

O'Connor, A.D. *et al.* (1977), Synchronous VBM and radiotherapy in the treatment of squamous cell carcinoma of the head and neck. *Clin. Otolar.*, **2**, 347–57.

Pearson, J.G. (1966), The radiotherapy of carcinoma of the oesophagus and post-cricoid region in south east Scotland. *Clin. Radiol.*, **17**, 242–57.

Perez, C.A. *et al.* (1976), Non-randomised comparison of pre-operative irradiation and surgery versus irradiation alone in the management of carcinoma of the tonsil. *Am. J. Roentg.*, **126**, 248–60.

Pierquin B. *et al.* (1966), Etude comparative des resultats concernant les épithéliomas de la région amygdalienne traités à l'Institut Gustave-Roussy et à la Fondation Curie. *Annls. Radiol.*, **9**, 815–24.

Price, L.A. *et al.* (1978), Improved results in combination chemotherapy of head and neck cancer using a kinetically-based approach. *Oncology*, **35**, 26–8.

Shigematsu, Y., Sakai, S. and Fuchihata, H. (1971), Recent trials in the treatment of maxillary sinus carcinoma, with special reference to the chemical potentiation of radiation therapy. *Acta Otolar.*, **71**, 63–70.

Todd, I.D.H. (1965), Treatment of Solitary Plasmocytoma. *Clin. Radiol.*, **16**, 395–9.

Van Den Brouck, C. *et al.* (1977), Results of a randomized clinical trial of preoperative irradiation versus postoperative in treatment of tumors of the hypopharynx. *Cancer*, **39**, 1445–9.

Wang, C. C. (1971), Radiotherapeutic management of carcinoma of the posterior pharyngeal wall. *Cancer*, **27**, 894–6.

12 Nasopharynx

John H. C. Ho

Incidence

There are wide ethnic differences in the morbidity of nasopharyngeal cancer. It is highest in Chinese originating from the southern province of Guangdong, formerly known as Kwangtung, intermediate in Alaskan and Canadian Eskimos, native Greenlanders, an Eskimo population with some admixture of Caucasian blood, Malays in South-east Asia and Tunisians, and lowest in Caucasians (Table 12.1). The cancer is not associated with the mongoloid race per se, because mongoloid northern Chinese, Koreans and Japanese all have a low frequency of the disease.

Aetiology

The predominant tumour of the nasopharynx is a carcinoma of the epidermoid type. Current epidemiologi-cal and experimental data suggest that its aetiology involves (a) a genetically determined susceptibility, (b) an abortive infection of some nasopharyngeal epithelial cells by the ubiquitous Epstein-Barr virus (EBV) at an early period of life, and (c) an environmental factor, which may vary from one population group to another. In the case of southern Chinese the most probable environmental factor is the inclusion of salted fish and deficiency in vitamin C in their diet during early life (Ho, 1978).

Anatomy

The nasopharynx is a space behind the nasal fossae and above the oropharynx. Although developmentally it is a part of the pharynx, functionally it is a part of the upper respiratory passage. It is bounded in front by the

Table 12.1 Age-adjusted incidence rates* for nasopharyngeal carcinoma for selected population groups.

	Period	Male	Female	Reference
Hong Kong†	1970–74	29.0	12.1	Ho (unpublished data)
Singapore Chinese	1968–72	18.7	7.1	Waterhouse et al. (1976)
Cantonese	1968–70	29.4	10.8	Shanmugaratnam (1973)
Hokkiens	1968–70	13.7	4.0	Shanmugaratnam (1973)
California				
Bay Area Chinese‡	1969–73	19.1	6.4	Waterhouse et al. (1976)
Greenland Eskimos	1965–76	12.3	8.5	Nielson et al. (1977)
Taiwanese		5.9	2.8	Lin et al. (1971)
Singapore Malays	1968–72	4.8	0.6	Waterhouse et al. (1976)
USA Connecticut	1968–72	0.6	0.1	Waterhouse et al. (1976)
Sweden	1966–70	0.5	0.3	Waterhouse et al. (1976)
Japan, Osaka	1970–71	0.4	0.2	Waterhouse et al. (1976)
UK, Oxford	1968–72	0.4	0.2	Waterhouse et al. (1976)

* All rates standardized to the world population age distribution (Doll, 1970).

† 98.3% of the population classified as Chinese and 92.3% of them originated from Guangdong (Census and Statistics Department, Hong Kong Government, 1971).

‡ Predominantly Cantonese.

choanae and the nasal septum and below by the soft palate and the pharyngeal isthmus. Its superoposterior wall lies subjacent to the body of the sphenoid with its sinus, the basisphenoid, basiocciput, the pharyngeal aponeurosis, the upper attachments of the capitis anterior and longus capitus muscles and the anterior arch of atlas with its anterior tubercle where the superior constrictor is attached posteriorly. Its lateral wall is formed by the pharyngeal tubercle or Eustachian cushion with its Eustachian tubal orifice and a collection of lymphoid tissue commonly referred to as the Eustachian tubal tonsil, and the fossa of Rosenmuller (lateral pharyngeal recess). The fossa is in fact the corner between the lateral and posterior walls. It is related above to the internal carotid canal within the petrous bone and the petro-occipital fissure, both being common sites of upward spread of the tumour from the fossa of Rosenmuller. On the superior wall is another collection of lymphoid tissue, the adenoids, which usually undergo atrophy with age, but occasionally it may persist to late adult life. There is a weak spot in the lateral wall, where the cartilaginous portion of the Eustachian tube enters. It is through here that a lateral spread of the tumour to involve the palatal and pterygoid muscles readily occurs.

The nasopharynx is supplied by three arteries – the ascending pharyngeal, the artery of the pterygoid canal and the sphenopalatine, which freely anastomose with one another and with the same arteries of the opposite side. They are all branches of the external carotid artery, thus allowing direct infusion through this artery or its superficial temporal branch.

The nasopharyngeal plexus of veins communicate with the internal jugular vein, but there is also a pathway leading to the orbital veins through the inferior orbital vein traversing the inferior orbital fissure. The posterior part of this fissure is a common avenue of direct spread to the orbit from a carcinoma entering the nasal fossa and spreading laterally through the perpendicular plate of the palatine bone or the sphenopalatine foramen at its upper part to gain entry to the apex of the orbit through the pterygopalatine fossa situated immediately below the inferior orbital fissure.

Lymphatic drainage

The nasopharynx has a rich plexus of lymphatics, the efferent channels of which either drain directly to the jugular and spinal accessory chains of nodes or via the lateral parapharyngeal nodes in the retrostyloid space and the retropharyngeal node. There are also lymphatics crossing the midline, accounting for contra-lateral nodal involvement.

Pathology and histological classification

By far the commonest malignant tumour of the nasopharynx in all races is epidermoid carcinoma, but peculiarly this tumour appears frequently in an undifferentiated form under light microscopy and this includes the so-called lymphoepithelioma. If differentiated, it is more often poorly than well differentiated. Tumour cells ranging from undifferentiated to poorly and well differentiated may be found in different parts of the same tumour, and difference in the degree of differentiation may be found between the primary tumour and its metastases. Consequently, it is not possible to sub-classify the tumour on the histological appearance of a biopsy specimen, which is no more than a tiny fraction of the whole. In any case we have not found such subclassification offers any useful guide to the management of the patient.

Of the other malignant tumours occurring in the nasopharynx, malignant lymphomas (Hodgkin's and non-Hodgkin's) are the next commonest. Occasionally, adenocarcinomas (classical and adenocystic), malignant melanoma, chordoma, malignant teratoma and various soft tissue sarcomas have been encountered.

Natural history

There are 3 clinical types: (a) the mainly invasive, (b) the mainly metastatic and (c) mixed. In the mainly invasive types cervical nodal metastases are either absent or insignificant throughout the course, but haematogenous metastases to spine, lungs and liver may occur when tumour extension reaches a basal venous sinus.

In the mainly metastatic type there is early spread to the cervical nodes. Usually, but not always, haematogenous metastases appear after the appearance of cervical nodal metastases. The progress of this type in an untreated or inadequately treated patient may be very slow extending over ten years or more or very rapid spreading to the lymph nodes in various regions of the body and other organs within a year of onset of symptoms. The sites of metastases are bone (50% of cases), lung (30%), liver (30%), lymph nodes below the clavicles, especially the superior mediastinal and hilar (10%). The brain is apparently immune to haematogenous but not contiguous spread from meningeal metastasis or the primary tumour.

In the mixed type both invasion of adjacent organs and metastases may occur concurrently or one after the other with a varying interval in between.

Symptoms and presentation

The presenting symptoms may be classified as cervical nodal, nasal, aural, neurological, headache and miscellaneous.

Cervical nodal

As a rule the upper nodes enlarge before the lower, and the supra-clavicular nodes are never the first ones involved. The enlargement is unaccompanied by pain except when there is concurrent infection and it is unilateral initially in the majority of cases. In most reported series cervical nodal enlargement is the most frequent first symptom.

Nasal

The complaints range from nasal obstruction and persistent nasal discharge following what was thought to be a common cold, blood-stained discharge, epistaxis to hawking and coughing up of blood-stained sputum in the morning due to post-nasal discharge dripping down the tracheobronchial tree during the night.

Aural

Impairment of hearing of the conductive type, usually unilateral, with or without tinnitus is a common presenting symptom. It is due to the obstruction of the Eustachian tube by the primary tumour. The obstruction may lead to serous otitis media, which will not respond to the usual remedies. Consequently, if it does not clear up in two to three weeks of treatment, a thorough examination of the nasopharynx including biopsies should be carried out to exclude nasopharyngeal carcinoma as the cause.

Neurological

Any of the cranial nerves, the upper cervical sympathetics, the lesser occipital and greater auricular nerves may be involved. Fig. 12.1 shows the relative frequency of the various cranial nerves as the earliest nerve involved either alone or in combination with other cranial nerves. The lesser occipital and greater auricular nerves are usually involved in late disease.

Of the ocular nerves the sixth is invariably the first nerve involved. The patient may voluntarily close one eye to avoid diplopia, and this must not be mistaken for genuine ptosis. If the third nerve is involved first, nasopharyngeal carcinoma is unlikely to be the cause. Horner's syndrome usually occurs together with paralysis of the last four cranial nerves, but occasionally it may occur alone due to involvement of the sympathetic

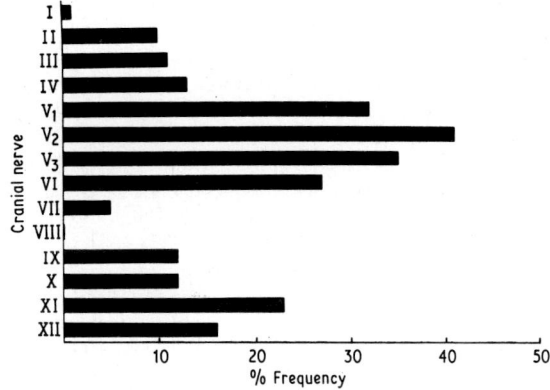

Fig. 12.1   Relative frequency of various cranial nerves as the first nerve involved alone or with other nerves in NPC in 513 consecutive cases.

plexus surrounding the internal carotid artery in the carotid canal.

Headache

It is usually unilateral and the most frequent site is temporoparietal. The other sites are frontal, vertical, occipital with or without radiation down the back of the neck. It is neuralgic in character and due to irritation of the meningeal branches of the maxillary division of the fifth nerve.

Miscellaneous

These include trismus due to the involvement of the pterygoid muscles, and this can be distinguished from temporomandibular disease by the patient's localization of the site of tightness to a point 3–4 cm below the temporomandibular joint at the insertion of the pterygoid muscles at the ascending ramus of the mandible. The other symptom is frequent hawking of phlegm from the back of the throat due to excessive post-nasal discharge from an ulcerated tumour in the nasopharynx.

Diagnosis

Examination of the nasopharynx should be left to the experts. It is usually done with a post-nasal mirror with or without spraying the throat with a topical anaesthetic, but such an examination will not be possible in the presence of trismus, and when the pharyngeal reflex is hyperactive, general anaesthesia is required. Direct nasopharyngoscopy suffers from the fact that the instrument has to be introduced through the nasal passage to enter the nasopharynx and in its passage the optical system may be smeared with discharge or blood from a traumatized haemorrhagic tumour. The fossa of Rosenmuller may be very spacious or very narrow. In the case of the latter it should be inspected by the use of a Yankauer speculum, which also allows the fossa to be swabbed clean of mucus, topically anaesthetized and biopsied under direct vision which is not possible by other means. With practice the whole procedure takes less than one minute for one side.

Radiography has the advantage over posterior rhinoscopy in that it is not only unrestricted by the presence of trismus or a hyperactive pharyngeal reflex, but also provides a permanent record for following progress. The initial examination should include five projections (Ho, 1967) and not just a lateral and an axial, which alone are inadequate for studying the nasopharynx or the detection of involvement of adjacent bones and paranasal sinuses. The five projections are:

1. Lateral with the beam centred on a point 1 cm below the orbitomeatal line and 2 cm in front of the external auditory meatus.
2. Axial (the classical submentovertical).
3. Occipito submental taken with the head extended until the orbitomeatal line is at an angle of about 55 degrees to the film, and the beam angled 25 degrees rostrally and centred midway between the external auditory meati. This projection demonstrates the jugular foramina and the basiocciput and petro-occipital fissures parallel to the film, hence unforeshortened, and also the nasopharyngeal cavity as a different angle from the axial.
4. Occipitomental with a 25-degree tilt and mouth fully opened to show the pterygoid plates and foramina ovale above the petrous bones.
5. Occipitomaxillary (occipitofrontal with 25-degree tilt) to demonstrate the orbits and foramina rotundum above the petrous bones.

Radiography has, however, its limitations. Small tumours, especially those in the form of a granular plaque, and situated on the anterior part of the roof of the nasopharynx close to the choana, are obscured by the nasal septum and the pterygoid plates in the lateral view and not demonstrable by the other projections. Consequently, the absence of radiographic abnormality does not exclude the presence of a nasopharyngeal tumour. The nasopharynx has within its cavity a highly satisfactory natural contrast medium, air, for demonstrating the soft tissue outlines and the fossae of Rosenmuller without obscuring the neighbouring bones. Contrast radiography with an opaque medium is, therefore, not required, and so far, computed tomography has not been found to be superior to conventional tomography in the examination of the nasopharynx and its adjacent bones, but the former is useful in demonstrating brain involvement.

The close association between EBV and nasopharyngeal carcinoma irrespective of geography has provided a useful marker for the diagnosis of the tumour. Raised serum IgA antibodies to the viral capsid antigen (VCA) of EBV were reported in 93% of untreated patients from East Africa, Hong Kong and California (Henle and Henle, 1976; Ho et al., 1976) and their titres were usually high, although some patients with other cancers of the head and neck also had raised IgA antibodies to VCA, but their titres were usually low and this applies also to two other EBV-related diseases, Burkitt's lymphoma and infectious mononucleosis. None of the 89 healthy subjects without a family history of nasopharyngeal carcinoma reported by Ho et al. (1976) had titres of ≥10, but among 133 sibs of the patients 28 (21%) had such titres and one of them, who had a titre of 10, nine months before clinical onset, showed a 16-fold increase in the titre at onset (Ho et al., 1978). Furthermore, three instances have been encountered in which patients who had elevated serum IgA antibodies to VCA from 30–61 months before onset (Ho et al., 1978). Consequently, EBV-specific serum IgA reactivity is not only a useful aid to the diagnosis or exclusion of nasopharyngeal carcinoma in those patients with suggestive symptoms but an occult primary tumour, but also may be of value in screening individuals with a high risk of the cancer such as apparently healthy members of the families of such patients of southern Chinese origin (Ho, 1972). Huang et al. (1978) found three other EBV-specific antibodies to be of diagnostic value, and they are IgA to the diffuse component of the early antigen complex, EA(D), and IgG to VCA and EA(D). Serum antibodies to the nuclear antigen of the virus (EBNA) have not been found, however, to be discriminating, but EBNA-positive carcinoma cells in biopsy specimens have so far been reported in only nasopharyngeal carcinoma and some undifferentiated carcinoma of the nasal fossa. The search for these cells in cervical nodal metastases from an occult primary tumour should be, therefore, of help in the differential diagnosis.

The diagnosis of nasopharyngeal carcinoma is established on the demonstration of a primary tumour in the nasopharynx with a positive biopsy. However, the tumour may not be clinically demonstrable, in which case adequate specimens should be taken from at least three sites for biopsy. These are the middle region of the superoposterior wall of the nasopharynx and the dorsal wall of two fossae of Rosenmuller. If they are all negative and there is no suggestive evidence from the results of the EBV-specific serological studies, then nasopharyngeal cancer can be considered to have been excluded. If, however, the serological findings are suggestive, an enlarged cervical node should be examined histologically and for the presence of EBNA-positive cells. If both examinations are in favour of nasopharyngeal cancer then further biopsies of other sites of the nasopharynx, including the Eustachian orifice, and the posterior part of the nasal fossa, through a split palate if necessary, should be performed. As a rule, there is a wide zone of sub-mucosal infiltration around the macroscopic primary focus and there may be another occult primary on the apparently normal opposite side with the midline specimen showing no histological evidence of tumour. Very occasionally, however, the primary tumour may be so small that of many specimens biopsied only one revealed the disease.

In the differential diagnosis, it is well to bear in mind that:

1. Close to 80% of nasopharyngeal carcinomas are eccentrically situated.
2. An eccentrically located nasopharyngeal tumour accompanied by radiographic evidence of bone involvement is almost always due to nasopharyngeal carcinoma as bone involvement in lymphomas is very rare.
3. Undifferentiated or poorly differentiated epidermoid carcinomas is common in nasopharyngeal carcinoma, but rare in other head and neck carcinomas except in the case of carcinoma of the posterior part of nasal fossa.
4. The third cranial nerve is practically never the first ocular nerve involved.
5. Lymphatic spread to the spinal accessory chain of nodes is common, but rare in other carcinomas of the head and neck.
6. The supraclavicular nodes are never the first nodes involved.

A carcinoma from the posterior part of the nasal fossa, arising usually from the ethmoidal region, frequently protrudes backwards to enter the nasopharynx through the choanal orifice, and nasopharyngeal cancer frequently extends forwards to involve the posterior part of the nasal fossa. Only when the major part of the tumour is in the nasal fossa and it regresses towards the fossa during a course of radiation therapy could we be sure that it is a nasal carcinoma and not nasopharyngeal carcinoma. It is important to differentiate between the two because the treatment plans for the two will be different. It is also important to determine whether an anteriorly situated nasopharyngeal carcinoma has extended to the nasal fossa, because such an extension will present special problems in planning radiation therapy. In case of doubt the posterior part of the nasal fossa should be biopsied.

The following studies are recommended for all patients diagnosed with malignant primary neoplasms of the nasopharynx:

1. A full physical examination to determine the local, regional and distant extent of the tumour.
2. The five routine radiographs of the nasopharynx mentioned earlier supplemented by special views such as the reversed Stenver's for the petrous bones and the hypoglossal canals, the reversed Towne's for the pterygomaxillary and inferior orbital fissures, and tomograms (parasagittal, paracoronal and transverse) when required.
3. Posteroanterior and lateral chest radiographs.
4. Bone scans in patients with N_2 or N_3 cervical nodal involvement.
5. Liver scan when the liver is palpably enlarged.
6. Routine blood counts and urinalysis.
7. EBV-specific serology: titration of IgA and IgG antibodies to VCA and EA(D).
8. Pre-radiation therapy dental check up and treatment.

Clinical staging

For cancers of the nasopharynx this author disagrees with UICC's 1974 staging of T and N (Ho, 1978), and as yet UICC has not produced a grouped TNM staging. The main objection to UICC's N staging is that it was designed primarily to guide block dissection and indicate prognosis when surgery is the definitive treatment. For instance, N_1 (homolateral mobile) node(s) would require at least a block dissection on the involved side, N_2 (contra-lateral or bilateral mobile) node(s) bilateral block dissections and N_3 (fixed) node(s) are probably not dissectable and hence are considered to carry the worst prognosis irrespective of the level of nodal involvement. It must be said, however, that UICC in 1974 recognized that the level of involvement has a bearing on both treatment and prognosis, and recommended that they should always be recorded. Since nasopharyngeal cancers are treated mainly by radiation therapy it is only logical to have an N stage classification based on the radiotherapy results of nasopharyngeal cancer and not on the results of surgery on other head and neck cancers. As the involvement of cervical nodes is usually from above downwards and nodal fixation does not restrict radiotherapy, its N involvement should, therefore, be staged according to the level of involvement, which has been shown to determine the prognosis regardless of the mobility of the nodes and the laterality of the involvement (Ho, 1978).

The following stage classification, based on that described by Ho (1970), has evolved from successive analysis of results of treatment obtained in our institute since 1965. It gives a good indication of the prognosis by the stage of the tumour and also a good guide to treatment planning.

T. Primary Tumour

T_1 Tumour confined to the nasopharynx (space behind the choanal orifices and nasal septum and above the level of the posterior margin of the soft palate in its resting position).

T_2 Tumour extended to the nasal fossa, oropharynx or adjacent muscles or nerves below the base of the skull.

T_3 Tumour extended beyond T_2 limits and sub-classified as follows:

T_{3a} Bone involvement below the base of the skull. (Floor of the sphenoid sinus is included in this category).

T_{3b} Involvement of the base of the skull. (The lateral and posterior walls of the sphenoid sinus are included in this category).

T_{3c} Involvement of cranial nerve(s).

T_{3d} Involvement of the orbits, laryn-gopharynx (hypopharynx) or infratem-poral fossa.

N. Regional Lymph Nodes (Figs. 12.2 and 12.3):

N_1 Node(s) wholly in the upper cervical level bounded below by the neck crease extending laterally and backward from or just below the thyroid notch (laryngeal eminence).

N_2 Node(s) palpable between the crease and the supra-clavicular fossa, the upper limit being a line joining the upper margin of the sternal end of the clavicle and the apex of an angle formed by the lateral surface of the neck and the superior margin of the trapezius.

N_3 Node(s) palpable in the supra-clavicular fossa and/or skin involvement in the form of carcinoma en cuirasse or satellite nodules above the clavicles.

Grouped TNM staging:

I.   Tumour confined to the nasopharyngeal mucosa: $T_1 N_0$

II.   Tumour extended to nasal fossa, oropharynx, or adjacent muscles or nerves below the base of skull (T_2) and/or N_1 involvement: $T_1 N_1$, T_2, N_0 and $T_2 N_1$.

III.   Tumour extended beyond T_2 limits or bone involvement (T_3) and/or N_2 involvement: $T_1 N_2$, $T_2 N_2$, $T_3 Np$ and $T_3 N_1$.

IV. N_3 irrespective of the primary tumour: $T_{1, 2 \text{ or } 3}$ N_3.

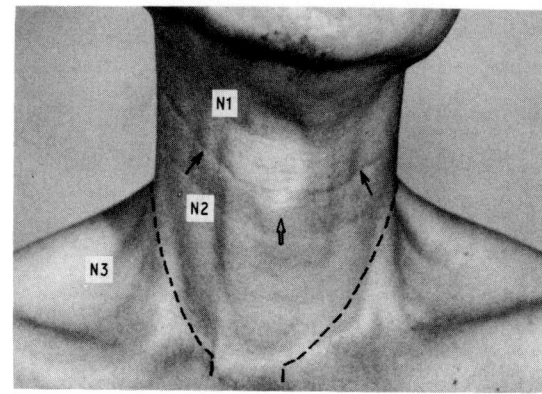

Fig. 12.2   Front view of neck showing the N levels. Neck crease indicated by solid arrows and the thyroid notch by an open arrow.

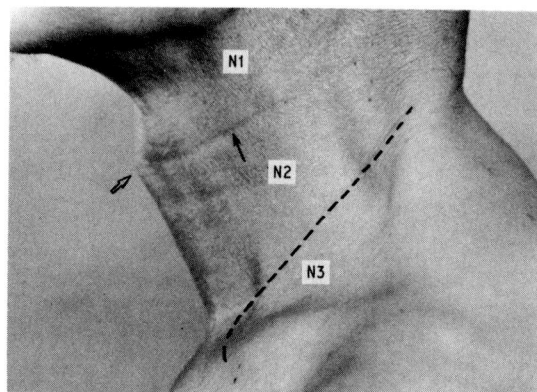

Fig. 12.3   Side view of neck showing the N levels.

V.   Haematogenous metastasis and/or involvement of skin or lymph node(s) below the clavicles (M).

Treatment of nasopharyngeal carcinoma

Policy

For Stages I–IV the treatment is radical radiation therapy with chemotherapy given either prior to radiotherapy to reduce the size of some very large nodes or as an adjuvant after radiotherapy in Stage III with N_2 involvement and Stage IV patients, in whom the major cause of treatment failure is distant metas-tases. For Stage V disease the main treatment is chemotherapy with radiotherapy reserved for palliative purposes, such as relief of pain or pressure symptoms caused by skeletal or lymph nodal metastases. Hormones are not known to have any place in the management and immunotherapy is yet untried. Palatal fenestration may be required to facilitate the inspection of the posterior parts of the nasal fossae and the anterior part of the nasopharynx during follow-up examinations for tumour recurrence after radiotherapy in patients with a hyperactive pharyngeal reflex, but the operation is contra-indicated in advanced disease or when there is trismus due to involvement of the pterygoid muscles. The cervical nodal metastases are usually effectively controlled by radiotherapy in the absence of a persistent primary tumour, and the cause of treatment failure is usually either due to this or distant metastases. There is however, the occasional residual node that persists after a full course of radiotherapy. As long as it is resectable it is best excised in order to avoid further radiation. Since prophylactic irradiation of cervical nodes has not been found to improve treatment results in Stage I cases, it should be withheld until nodal involvement becomes clinically evident. (Ho, 1978). This policy may be extended to Stage II and III cases without nodal involvement, because the main cause of treatment failure in these cases is uncontrolled primary tumour. If, however, cervical nodal metastasis is present, the cervical nodes on both sides should be treated even if the involvement is ipsilateral because the nasopharynx has a bilateral lymphatic drainage.

Radiation therapy technique

In the treatment of nasopharyngeal carcinoma we are confronted with a target volume related to the primary tumour and another to the cervical nodes. The former is situated in front of the brain stem and the latter have the spinal cord sandwiched in the middle. Consequently, the two volumes cannot be irradiated throughout *en bloc* without either overdosing the brain stem or the spinal cord depending on whether opposed anterior and posterior or lateral fields are employed. The two volumes should, therefore, be treated throughout or at least part of the course by split fields. The primary tumour should be treated with parallel-opposed lateral facial fields with the brain stem, a part of the tongue and the posteroinferior corner of the field shielded to avoid an overlap between the corner and the superior margin of the anterior cervical field. These two are supplemented by an anterior facial field with the eyes shielded. The purpose of the anterior facial field is to reduce the dose to the temporomandibular joints and the middle ears which lie outside the region irradiated by the anterior beam. The central

axis of this beam must be directed slightly upwards so that the shadows of the eye-shields are cast above the highest point of the maxillary sinus (the junction of its superior, medial and posterior walls), the tip of the petrous bone and the petro-occipital fissure on both sides. They are potential sites of direct spread from the primary tumour. In the absence of pharyngeal involvement below the nasopharynx or high upper nodes, the cervical nodes are most conveniently treated by an anterior cervical field with the head extended and the larynx and spinal cord shielded. We have not found a gap between the posteroinferior margins of the lateral fields and the superior margin of the anterior cervical beam necessary to avoid overdosing the junctional zone when a 4.5 or 5.6 MeV photon beam with isodose curves flattened at 10 cm depth from our linear accelerators was used. With such a beam treating the anterior cervical field, the supraclavicular nodes and most of the nodes in the anterior cervical triangle will be within the 90% isodose region, where the target dose is reckoned. Those furthest back are at the apex of the posterior cervical triangle and within the 70% isodose region. For residual nodes at this and other sites we normally give two booster doses of 375 rad of 10 MeV electrons reckoned at the 90% isodose level 3 days apart commencing a week after the last weekly anterior cervical dose has been given. These two doses are given by a direct field applied over the residual nodes. In the absence of 10 MeV electrons, photons from a short-distance telecobalt or tele-caesium unit or an orthovoltage X-ray machine can be used to give a biologically equivalent dose. A posterior cervical field parallel and opposed to the anterior cervical is not recommended because it is difficult to set up such a field with the patient in the prone position with the head extended. The position causes much discomfort and shielding of the spinal cord could be inaccurate. If the beam is directed from under the couch with the patient supine, there will be no radiation sparing at the skin because the neck has to rest on something.

The nasal fossa presents special problems in treatment planning when it is involved by the anterior extension of the nasopharyngeal tumour. Its upper part is situated between the two orbits. From experience we have found that the anterior margin of the opposed lateral facial fields must be at least 1.5 cm behind the outer orbital margin to avoid optic neuropathy or retinopathy. This would leave the anterior part of the nasal fossa outside the field of irradiation. To treat this part of the fossa without overdosing the brain stem, a high energy electron beam applied through an anterior nasal field is necessary. This field could be enlarged to cover the maxillary sinus on the affected side. In fact, all the ipsilateral paranasal sinuses except the frontal, the sphenoid sinus

Table 12.2 Nasopharyngeal carcinoma: treatment technique A.

Radiation	Field no.	Name of field	Wedge	Figure	Prescription	Remarks
4.5 MeV	I	L. lateral facial	–	12.7	*NP*: For T₁, T₂ or T₃ₐ cases	Figs. 12.7 and 12.9: for case
photons	II	R. lateral facial	–	}	give 420 rad at 100% IL (Fig.	with involvement of posteri
S.S.D.	Ia	L. lateral facial	30°		12.8) per fr. through I and II	cranial fossa the brainsten
100 cm	IIa	R. lateral facial	30°	12.9 and	twice weekly to 2520, then	shield should be 1 cm fro
	III	Anterior facial	–	12.10	420 rad at 100% IL (Fig.	the base of the dorsum sell
	IV	Anterior cervical	–	12.12	12.11) through Ia, IIa and III	and 2 cm from the anteric
	IVa	Upper anterior cervical	–	12.12	daily twice weekly to another	margin of the foramen
10–15 MeV	V,VI	Residual nodes	–		2520. Total: 5040 rad/12	magnum
electrons	etc				fr/6 weeks	Fig. 12.10: during the last
					For T₃ᵦ or T₃c cases give	quarter of the course exten
					instead 250 rad at 100% IL	one eye-shield from 1.75
					per fr 4 times a week	1 cm of ML to reduce tot
					to total of 6000 rad/24	dose to contra-lateral opti
					fr/6 weeks through same	nerve if tumour eccentric
					fields	nerve of the better eye if
					Neck: give 560 rad at 90% IL	tumour in ML, and no
					per fr through IV weekly	extension if sphenoid sinu
					times 6, then through IVa the	invaded
					7th fr. For residual nodes add	
					a week later 2 fr of 375 rad at	
					90% IL 3 days apart through	
					direct small fields	

NP = Nasopharynx   ML = midline   IL = isodose level   fr = fraction

Table 12.3 Nasopharyngeal carcinoma: treatment technique B.

Radiation	Field no.	Name of field	Wedge	Figure	Prescription	Remarks
4.5 MeV	I	L. lateral facial	30°		*NP*: give 250 rad at 100% IL	Figs. 12.9 and 12.10: for
photons	II	R. lateral facial	30°	12.9 and	(Fig. 12.11) per fr through I,	shielding brain see remark
S.S.D.	III	Anterior facial	–	12.10	II and III daily 4 times a week	on Fig. 12.7 in Technique
100 cm	Ia	L. lateral facial	30°		to 3000, then 250 rad at	
	IIa	R. lateral facial	30°	12.13	100% IL (Fig. 12.14) per fr	
15 MeV	IIIa	Anterior facial	–		daily 4 times a week through	Figs. 12.13 and 12.14: no
electrons					Ia, IIa and IIIa to another	change in eye-shields
4.5 MeV	IV	Anterior cerival	–	12.12	3000	throughout
photons	IVa	Upper anterior cervical	–	12.12	Total: 6000 rad/24 fr/6	
					weeks	
					Neck: same as in Technique	
					A	

on it the wax compensator, the eye and ipsilateral pinna shields. A wax tongue depressor is held in the mouth when an anterior facial field is irradiated to displace the anterior two-thirds of the tongue and the sub-mandibular and sub-lingual salivary glands downward below the field. This depressor is removed when the anterior cervical field is irradiated so that they can return to their original position above the photon beam. This move is to reduce post-radiation xerostomia.

If prophylactic irradiation is to be carried out for Stages II and III disease, we recommend the neck should be irradiated only down to the level of the lower margin of the cricoid cartilage. For N₁₋₃ involvement it should be irradiated down to the level of the sternal notch.

Table 12.4 Nasopharyngeal carcinoma: treatment technique C.

Radiation	Field no.	Name of field	Wedge	Figure	Prescription	Remarks
4.5 MeV photons	I	L. lateral facial	30°	12.9	*NP*: give 250 rad at 100% IL (Fig. 12.15) per fr through I, II and III daily 4 times a week to 3000, then 250 rad at 100% IL (Fig. 12.16) per fr through Ia, IIa and IIIa daily 4 times a week to another 3000	Figs. 12.9 and 12.13: remarks as Technique B Figs. 12.13 and 12.16: III and IIIa should cover all ipsilateral (left in this case) paranasal sinuses, except frontal unless involved, and also see remarks on Fig. 12.10 in Technique A for IIIa
	II	R. lateral facial	30°			
	III	Anterior facial	–			
	Ia	L. lateral facial	30°	12.13		
15 MeV electrons	IIa	R. lateral facial	30°			
	IIIa	Anterior facial	–			
4.5 MeV photons	IV	Anterior cervical	–	12.12	Total: 6000 rad/24 fr/6 weeks *Neck*: same as in Technique A	
	IVa	Upper anterior cervical	–	12.12		

Table 12.5 Nasopharyngeal carcinoma: treatment technique D.

Radiation	Field no.	Name of field	Wedge	Figure	Prescription	Remarks
4.5 MeV photons S.S.D. 100 cm	I	L. lateral facio-cervical	–	12.17	Give *NP* and upper neck 200 rad CD through I and II daily 5 times a week to 4000, and to *lower neck and SCF* 5 weekly fr of 560 rad at 90% IL through IVb. Then give *NP* 250 rad at 100% IL (Fig. 12.11) per fr through Ia, IIa and III daily 4 times a week to 2000, *neck and SCF* one weekly fr of 560 rad at 90% IL through IV, and *upper neck only* one weekly fr of 560 rad at 90% IL through IVa Thus total dose to *NP* = 6000 rad/6 weeks, *upper neck* = 4000 rad/4 weeks + 560 rad weekly × 2, and *lower neck and SCF* = 560 rad/ week × 6 (5 fr through IVb and 1 fr through IV)	Figs. 12.17 and 12.9: see remarks in technique A regarding brain-stem shielding Fig. 12.10: one eye-shield to extend from 1.75 to 1 cm from ML during the last 6 fr
	II	R. lateral facio-cervical	–			
	IVb	Lower anterior cervical	–	12.17		
	Ia	L. lateral facial	30°	12.9 and		
	IIa	R. lateral facial	30°			
	III	Anterior facial	–	12.10		
	IV	Anterior cervical	–	12.12		
	IVa	Upper anterior cervical	–	12.12		

CD = central dose   SCF = supra-clavicular fossa

Since vital and important organs are in the immediate vicinity of the primary and secondary target volumes it is essential that verification films should be taken with the actual treatment beam to ensure that such organs are accurately shielded.

Chemotherapy

The best results from this modality are seen in the treatment of visceral metastases which had no previous radiotherapy. For treating tumour recurrence after radiotherapy the benefit derived is usually slight due to the impaired blood supply to the region reducing the

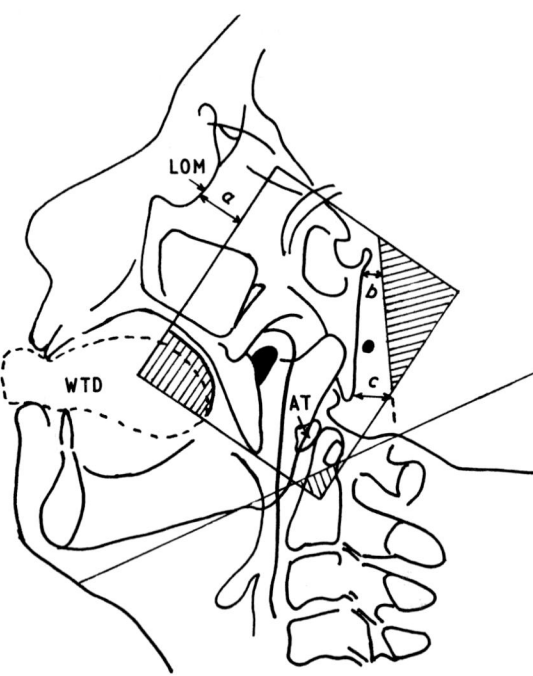

Fig. 12.7 Lateral facial field with the various shielded areas shaded. LOM lateral orbital margin; WTD wax tongue depressor; AT: atlantoid tubercle; *a:* 1.5 cm; *b:* 0.75 cm and *c:* 1.5 cm.

amount of chemotherapeutic agents reaching the tumour cells.

We have found cyclophosphamide to be as effective as any other drug now available. It is economical to use and has no serious side-effects. For reducing the size of large cervical nodes before radiotherapy we normally give 1 g intravenously weekly twice, and for treating metastases 1 g intravenously weekly to a total of 10 g followed by 50 mg orally t.i.d. for maintenance.

The value of adjuvant chemotherapy after a course of radiotherapy in Stage III patients with N_2 involvement and Stage IV patients has not yet been fully investigated, but it is worth considering because the major cause of failure in these cases is distant metastases.

Side effects and complications of radiation therapy

Swelling of the parotid salivary glands invariably occurs following the first treatment given to the nasopharynx because the radiation from the lateral fields has to pass through the highly radiosensitive parotid glands. The swelling always subsides within 24 hours. Patients must be forewarned of this side effect to avoid unnecessary anxiety. The degree of nausea and vomiting varies considerably from patient to patient, but seldom an interruption of treatment is necessitated. They are readily controlled by anti-emetics, but the worst cases may require small doses of corticosteroids in addition.

4.5 MeV
100 cm FSD

8 x 7   8 x 7

Percentage of representative tumour dose (usually the mean target absorbed dose) are shown by these tone shades

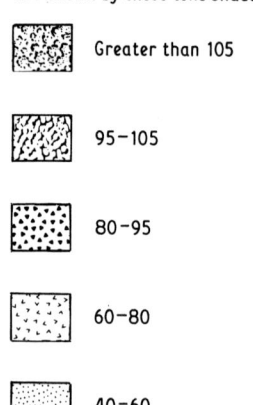

Greater than 105

95–105

80–95

60–80

40–60

Fig. 12.8 Isodose contours at level of the superior nasopharyngeal wall. Left or right lateral facial field: 8 × 7 cm; 4.5 MeV photons; souce-to-skin distance 100 cm; given relative dose: 71.4%; compensator: nil; shield brain, tongue and overlapping area between lateral facial and anterior cervical fields (Fig. 12.7); orientation angle: 9°; Stationary field.

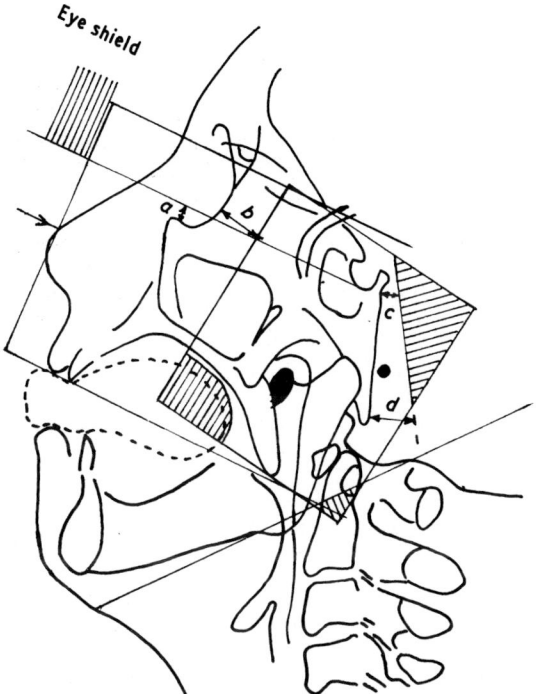

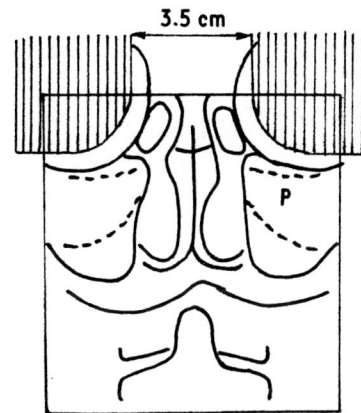

Fig. 12.10 Anterior facial field with eye-shields. P: petrous bone.

Fig. 12.9 Diagram showing the position of the lateral and anterior facial fields and the upper margin of the anterior cervical beam with the shielded area shaded; a: 0.5 cm; b: 1.5 cm; c: 0.75 cm, and d: 1.5 cm.

4.5 MeV
100 cm FSD

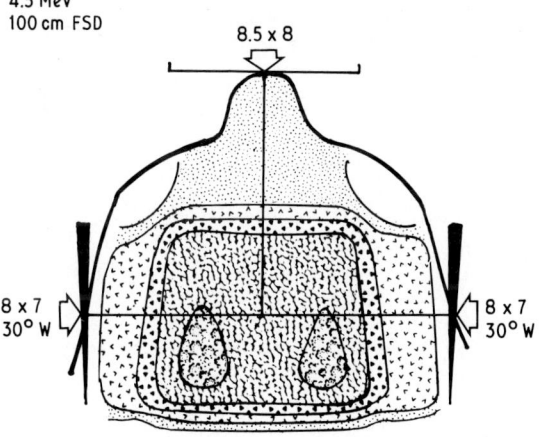

8.5 x 8

8 x 7
30° W

8 x 7
30° W

Percentage of representative tumour dose
(usually the mean target absorbed dose)
are shown by these tone shades

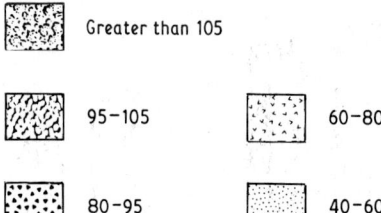

Greater than 105

95–105   60–80

80–95   40–60

Fig. 12.11 Isodose contours at level of superior nasopharyngeal wall. Anterior facial field: 8.5 × 8 cm; 4.5 MeV photons; source-to-skin distance 100 cm; given relative dose: 48.5%; compensator: nil; shield both eyes (Fig. 12.10); orientation angle: 0°, stationary field. Left or right lateral facial field: 8 × 7 cm; 4.5 MeV photons; source-to-skin distance 100 cm; given relative dose: 48.5%; wedge orientation: anterior; wedge angle: 30°; compensator: nil; shield brain, tongue and overlapping area between lateral facial and anterior cervical fields (Fig. 12.9); orientation angle: 9°; stationary field.

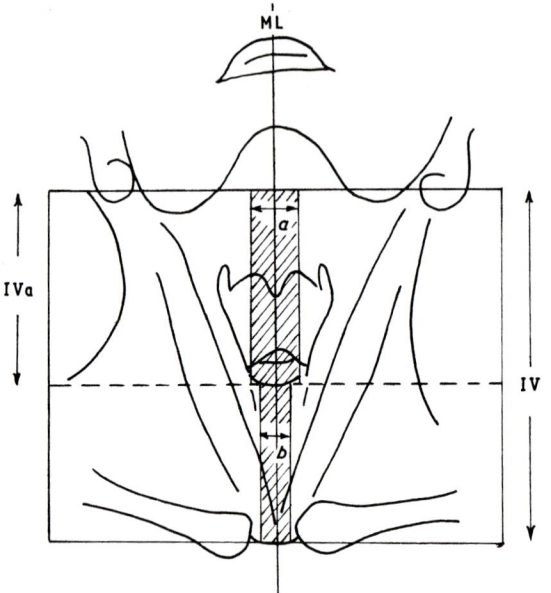

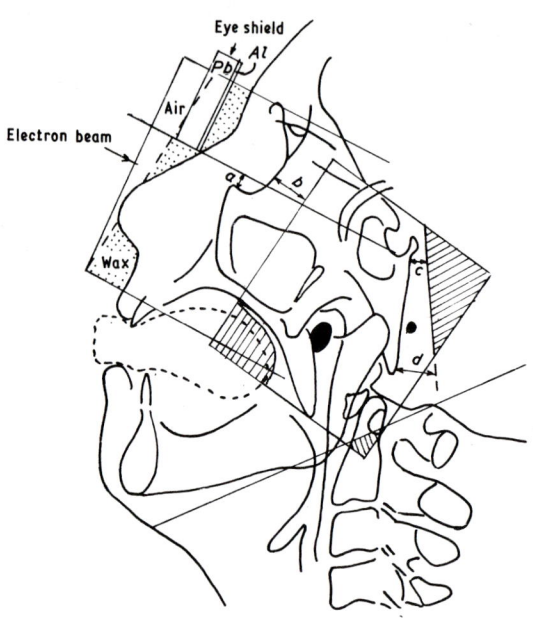

Fig. 12.12 Anterior cervical field. ML: midline; a: 3 cm, and b: 2.0 cm. Dotted line at level of lower margin of cricoid cartilage.

Fig. 12.13 Diagram showing the positions of the lateral and anterior facial fields with shielded area shaded; a: 0.5 cm; b: 1.5 cm; c: 0.75 cm, and d: 1.5 cm.

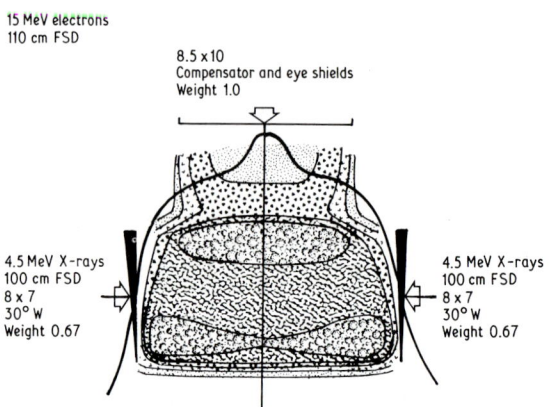

Percentage of representative tumour dose (usually the mean target absorbed dose) are shown by these tone shades

▦	Greater than 105
▨	95–105
▩	80–95
░	60–80
░	40–60

Fig. 12.14 Isodose contours at level of head 1 cm above the superior nasopharyngeal wall. Anterior facial field: 8.5 × 10 cm; 15 MeV electrons; source-to-skin distance 110 cm; given relative dose: 100%; presence of wax compensator (Fig. 12.13); shield both eyes; orientation angle: 0°; stationary field. Left or right lateral facial field: 8 × 7 cm; 4.5 MeV photons; source-to-skin distance 100 cm; given relative dose: 66.7%; wedge orientation: anterior; wedge angle: 30°; compensator: nil; shield brain, tongue and overlapping area between lateral facial and anterior cervical fields (Fig. 12.13); orientation angle: 9° (central axis of lateral field 1 cm below this cross-section); stationary field.

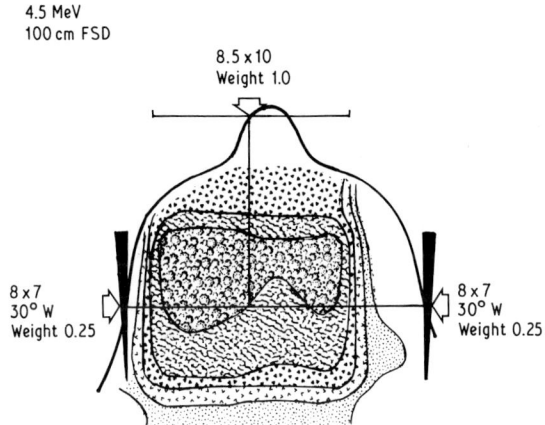

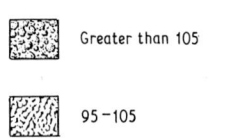

Percentage of representative tumour dose
(usually the mean target absorbed dose)
are shown by these tone shades

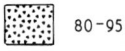 Greater than 105

95 – 105

80 – 95

60 – 80

40 – 60

Fig. 12.15 Isodose contours at level of superior nasopharyngeal wall. Anterior facial field: 8.5 × 10 cm; 4.5 MeV photons; source-to-skin distance 100 cm; given relative dose: 100%; compensator: nil; shield both eyes; orientation angle: 0°; stationary field. Left or right lateral facial field: 8 × 7 cm; 4.5 MeV photons; source-to-skin distance 100 cm; given relative dose: 25%; wedge orientation: anterior; wedge angle: 30°; compensator: nil; shield brain, tongue and overlapping area between lateral facial and anterior cervical fields (Fig. 12.9); orientation angle: 9°; stationary field.

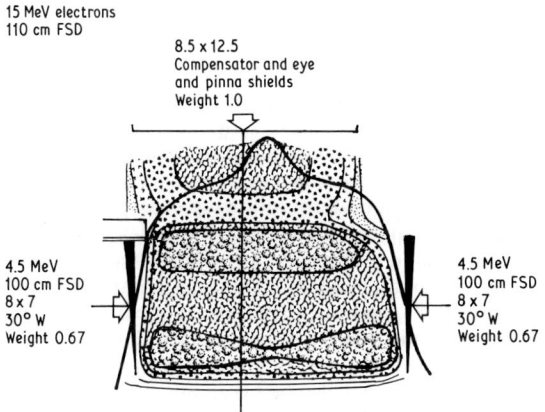

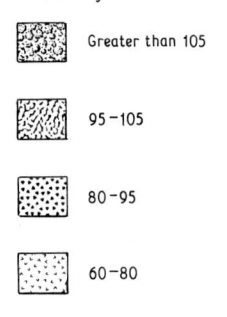

Percentage of representative tumour dose
(usually the mean target absorbed dose)
are shown by these tone shades

Greater than 105

95 – 105

80 – 95

60 – 80

40 – 60

Fig. 12.16 Isodose contours at level of head 1 cm above the superior nasopharyngeal wall. Anterior facial field: 8.5 × 12.5 cm; 15 MeV electrons; source-to-skin distance 110 cm; given relative dose: 100%; presence of wax compensator (Fig. 12.13); shield both eyes and ipsilateral pinna; orientation angle: 0°; stationary field. Left or right lateral facial field: 8 × 7 cm; 4.5 MeV photons; source-to-skin distance 100 cm; given relative dose: 66.7%; wedge orientation: anterior; wedge angle: 30°; compensator: nil; shield brain, tongue and overlapping area between lateral facial and anterior cervical fields (Fig. 12.13); orientation angle: 9°; (central axis of lateral field 1 cm below this cross-section); stationary field.

Soon after the completion of a course of radiation therapy when the whole neck has been irradiated slight puffiness of face and sub-mental oedema may develop, and they may take six to eight months to subside completely. Transient episodes of cramps in the neck muscles occasionally occur and may persist for one to two years. Neither Lhermitte's sign nor radiation neuropathy has been encountered in our patients who have had only one radical course of radiotherapy. Following a second course for primary tumour recurrence temporal lobe radiation neuropathy may occur and presents problems in differential diagnosis from tumour extension to the inferior surface of the lobe through the middle cranial fossa causing softening and oedematous swelling of the lobe. Radiation-induced cranial nerve palsies have been reported by Cheng and

13 Salivary glands

S. Rafla

Salivary tumours whether affecting major or minor salivary glands are rare, forming less than 3% of all tumours and affecting 1.5/100 000 population (US whites) to 2.5/100 000 population (US black females) (Dorn and Cutler, 1958). Yet they have disproportionate interest principally because of their frequent occurrence in the parotid and prevalence in middle aged females, significant since the cosmetic effect of the lesion or its treatment has sometimes been poor and complicated by facial nerve damage, turning a case of a superficial tumour into that of human tragedy.

The scientific curiosity caused by salivary tumours was particularly intense in the first half of this century when their histogenesis was a point of great debate. This question was almost fully settled in the fifties when recent authors such as Willis (1948) and McFarland (1943) proved that the early theories first advanced by Verneuil (1869) of the epithelial adult glandular origin are correct. Willis's term 'pleomorphic adenoma' indicating a benign epithelial tumour has been gradually gaining grounds over the old descriptive term of 'mixed tumour'.

The controversy of histogenesis gave ground to another one related to the natural history of various histologic types. The relative malignancy of some of the more common tumours such as pleomorphic adenoma (mixed tumour) or cylindroma is now generally understood. On the other hand, mucoepidermoid carcinomas were only identified by Stewart *et al*. in 1945 and recently recognized to be aggressive. Tumours like acinic cell carcinomas are still claimed by some to be only 'locally malignant'. This continuing controversy over the natural history of the disease is accompanied by an equal one related to treatment and especially to the role of radiotherapy.

This chapter will summarize the major aspects of these tumours and discuss in some detail the place of radiotherapy in their management.

The bulk of the clinical material upon which this study is based was treated in the Royal Marsden Hospital, London, UK by Dr. M. Lederman who was kind enough to allow me free access to his cases.

Anatomy

Of the three paired major salivary glands the parotid is the most important, not only by virtue of its size and rather complicated anatomical structure but it is also the gland most commonly involved with neoplasia (90% of cases: Skolnik *et al.*, 1977). The submandibular gland is affected to a much lesser extent (9%) and the sub-lingual is much smaller and less frequently afflicted. However, salivary glandular tissue may be found in many other sites, mainly the mucous membrane of the upper air and food passages forming minor salivary glands which are, as a rule, much less complex structurally as compared to the major ones. Other secretory glands such as the lacrimal and ceruminous glands share with minor salivery glands common features of neoplastic processes, though embryologically and functionally are distinctly different.

The three major salivary glands share a number of common features: a similar embryological origin as active epithelial invaginations into adjacent mesoderm; all have secretory and conducting portions and all have dual autonomic innervation in addition to a general afferent visceral innervation. The facial capsule which separates the glandular tissue from surrounding structures varies in thickness and development among the three. Minor salivary glands rarely display a capsule. Important differences among the three major salivary glands exist, however: the parotid is composed predominantly of serous secretory cells, the sub-mandibular has equal proportions of serous and mucin secreting cells; while the sub-lingual gland and all minor salivary glands are composed almost exclusively of mucin secreting cells. A description of the morphology and anatomy of major glands is at best only schematic since variations almost always exist.

Parotid gland

The parotid gland lies in its own fascial compartment wedged in the space between the mandible and mastoid process resting upon the styloid process and, on a

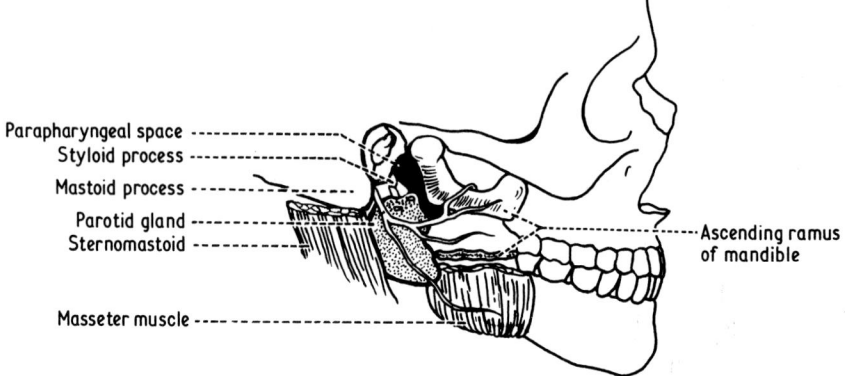

Parapharyngeal space
Styloid process
Mastoid process
Parotid gland
Sternomastoid

Masseter muscle

Ascending ramus
of mandible

Fig. 13.1 Relations of parotid gland to surrounding structures. (Redrawn from Rafla-Demetrious, 1970).

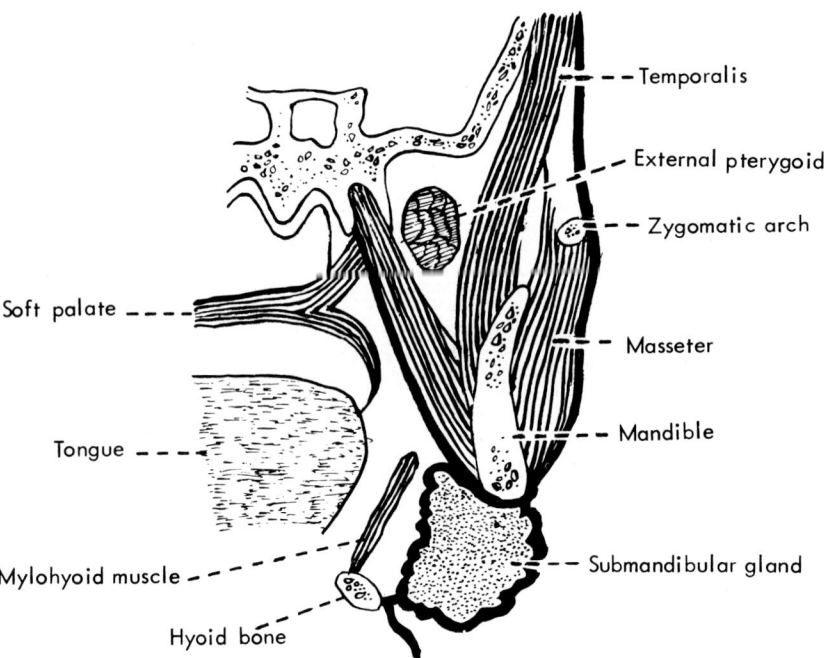

Temporalis

External pterygoid

Zygomatic arch

Soft palate

Masseter

Mandible

Tongue

Mylohyoid muscle

Submandibular gland

Hyoid bone

Fig. 13.2 Coronal section at the angle of mandible showing connections of the deep fascia about the sub-mandibular salivary gland and parpharyngeal space. (Redrawn from Hollinshead, 1956).

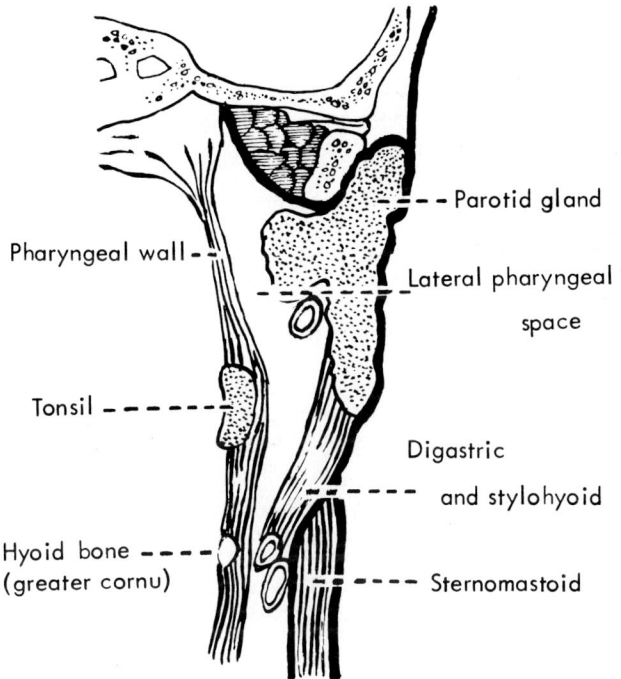

Pharyngeal wall

Tonsil

Hyoid bone
(greater cornu)

Parotid gland

Lateral pharyngeal
space

Digastric
and stylohyoid

Sternomastoid

Fig. 13.3 Relations of the parapharyngeal space to the parotid and sub-
mandibular salivary gland. (Redrawn from
Hollinshead, 1956).

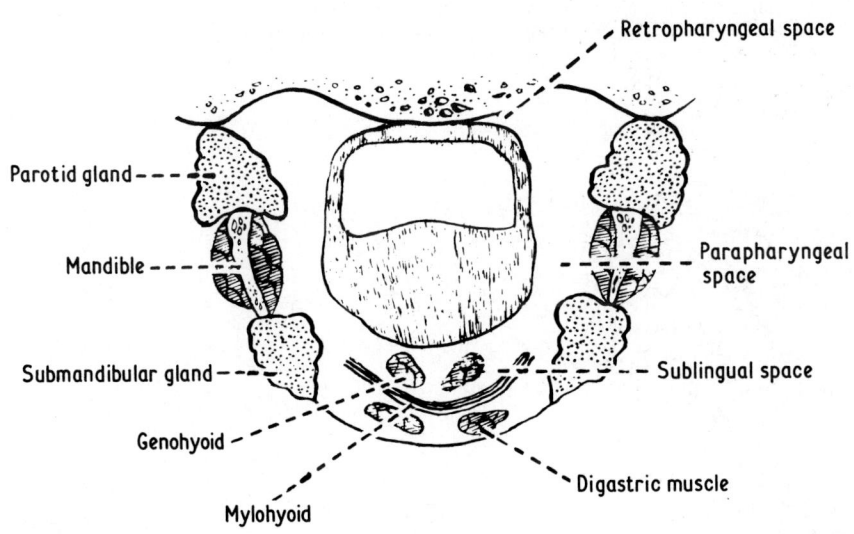

Retropharyngeal space

Parotid gland

Mandible

Submandibular gland

Genohyoid

Mylohyoid

Parapharyngeal
space

Sublingual space

Digastric muscle

Fig. 13.4 Relations of the parapharyngeal space to the parotid and sub-
mandibular salivary gland. (Redrawn from
Hollinshead, 1956).

deeper plane, on the transverse process of the second cervical vertebra (Fig. 13.1). The gland overflows its confines both superficially on the masseter muscle and deeply to come to be directly related to the lateral pharyngeal wall and the parapharyngeal space, a proximity enhanced by the relative looseness of the medial layer of the fascial compartment. The parotid facial compartment is limited superiorly by the zygomatic arch to which it is attached and anteromedially by the stylomandibular ligament which forms an occasional partial barrier between the parotid and the submandibular compartments (Figs. 13.2, 13.3, and 13.4).

The unique anatomical interest of the parotid gland comes from its relation to the facial nerve, which is the main nerve supply of the structures arising from the second branchial cleft. This nerve also exercises a physiological effect on gland function. The facial nerve sends some secretory fibres to the gland via the otic ganglion and is also a medium for proprioception. Maloney and Kennedy (quoted by Hollinshead, 1956) concluded that the facial nerve transmits pressure pain from various facial components.

The facial nerve leaves the skull through the stylomastoid foramen, typically situated slightly posterolateral to the styloid process and hence between this and the mastoid process. It almost immediately comes to lie on the deep and posterior aspect of the parotid gland. The nerve enters the substance of the parotid gland and splits into two main divisions: an upper temporofacial and a lower cervicofacial. Thereafter, a plexus forms within the gland from which five main branches emerge: temporal, zygomatic, buccal, mandibular, and cervical.

The relation between the facial nerve and the parotid gland is complex. The embryological development of the gland confirms its unitary single lobed nature as demonstrated recently by Gasser (1970), who described clearly the encirclement of the facial nerve (appearing in the fourth or fifth foetal week) by an ingrowth of the later developing parotid primordium (Fig. 13.5). McKenzie's (1948) results indicate that parotid tissue, ducts, and facial nerve are intimately interwoven. This demonstrates the difficulties of a conservative parotidectomy (with sparing of facial nerve) which cannot therefore be considered a truly radical cancer operation.

Lymphatic drainage (Fig. 13.6)
Most of the lymphatics of the parotid gland drain into the parotid lymph nodes which are divided into three groups:

1. Superficial pre-auricular nodes, situated superficial to the fascial capsule of the parotid gland.
2. Sub-fascial nodes, found deep to the fascial covering of the parotid. Two subgroups are identified: the deep pre-auricular nodes and the sub-auricular nodes.
3. Deep intraglandular nodes, usually grouped along the external jugular and the posterior communicating facial veins.

Most of the lymphatics from the parotid gland drain in the second and third groups. The efferent lymphatics from all groups usually terminate in the upper deep cervical nodes. On rare occasions, a lymphatic trunk drains directly into the middle cervical nodes.

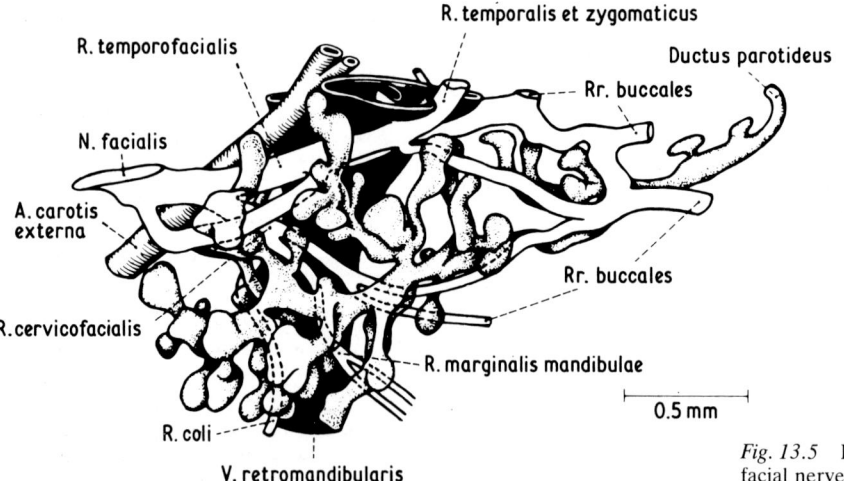

Fig. 13.5 Embryological relations of the facial nerve and the parotid gland. (Redrawn from Gasser, 1970).

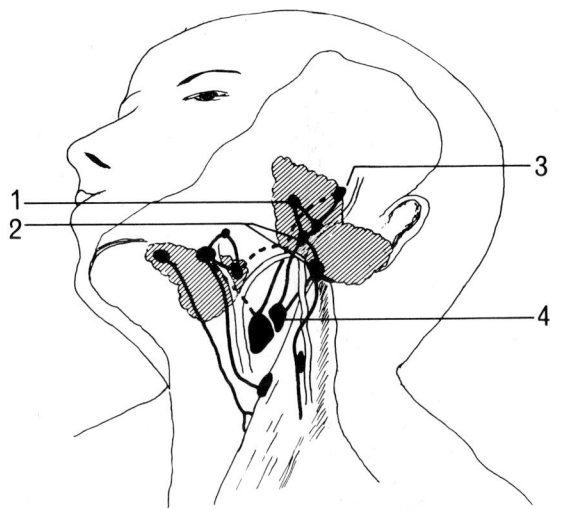

Fig. 13.6 Lymphatic drainage of parotid and sub-mandibular glands. 1 and 3: deep superficial pre-auricular nodes; 2: intraglandular nodes; 4: upper deep cervical nodes (jugulo-digastric). (Redrawn from Rouvière, 1932).

Sub-mandibular gland

The sub-mandibular gland occupies most of the sub-mandibular triangle and expands beyond it, over the superficial surfaces of the anterior and posterior bellies of the digastric. Superiorly, the gland extends over the mylohyoid line, along its duct above the mylohyoid muscle. Inferiorly, the gland reaches the level of the hyoid bone. Its posterior border is close to the lower part of the parotid gland at the angle of the jaw, where it is separated from this gland by the sphenomandibular and stylomandibular ligaments (Fig. 13.7).

A deep portion of the sub-mandibular gland lies along its duct, around the posterior border of the mylohyoid muscle in direct relation to the genioglossus and hyoglossus muscle. The terminal portion of the sub-mandibular duct is in immediate contact with the sub-lingual gland.

The nerves related to the sub-mandibular gland are the mylohyoid, and the hypoglossal. Above the level of the gland runs the lingual nerve. The sub-maxillary ganglion with its roots and branches forms a connection between the gland and lingual nerve, a relation which may expose the nerve to injury during removal of the gland by pulling the nerve down to the field of the operation.

The sub-mandibular gland, together with other structures, occupies the sub-mandibular fascial space which is limited above by the mucous membrane of the tongue, and inferiorly by attachment of the fascia to the hyoid bone.

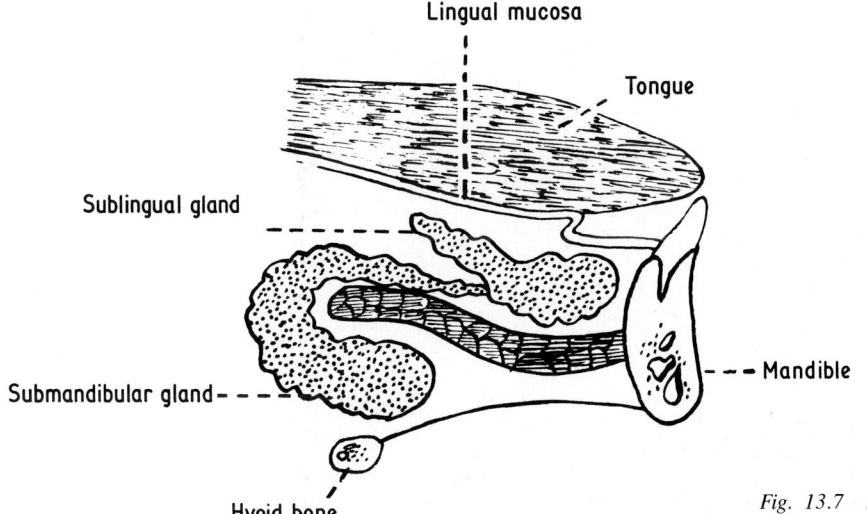

Fig. 13.7 Anatomy of sub-mandibular and sub-lingual salivary gland. (Redrawn from Rafla-Demetrious, 1970).

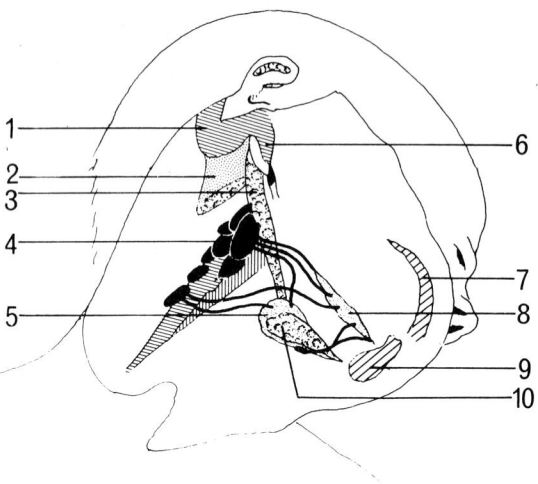

1
2
3
4
5
6
7
8
9
10

Fig. 13.8 Lymphatic drainage of sub-mandibular and sub-lingual salivary gland. 1 and 2: mastoid process and ster-namastoid muscle; 3: jugulo-digastric; 4: upper deep cervical nodes (jugulo-digastric); 5: submaxillary salivary gland; 6 and 7: styloid and mandible; 8: sub-lingual salivary gland; 9 and 10: hyoid bone and mylohyoid muscle. (Redrawn from Rouvière, 1932).

The deep aspect of the sub-mandibular gland is situated lateral to the parapharyngeal space. The gland is innervated by the lingual nerve, the sympathetic plexus (surrounding the facial artery) and the sub-mandibular ganglion. The latter supplies the parasympathetic secretory fibres derived from the chorda tympani.

Lymphatic drainage (Fig. 13.8)
Lymphatic drainage of the sub-mandibular gland follows two routes:

1. Lymph vessels which end in the sub-mandibular lymph nodes and drain mainly the surface and lateral aspects of the sub-mandibular salivary gland.
2. Lymphatics which drain directly into the deep cervical nodes. This route is more constant than the first one and usually drains the deep portion of the gland. These vessels usually follow the path of the facial artery, ending in the upper cervical nodes.

Sub-lingual gland

The sub-lingual gland is the smallest of the three major salivary glands and is often regarded as an accumulation of several mucous glands. It lies in the floor of the mouth beneath the mucous membrane, which may be raised into a sub-lingual fold. It rests above the mylohyoid muscle in contact with the sub-lingual fossa

on the inner surface of the mandible (Fig. 13.7). Anteriorly, the gland is contiguous to the opposite one and, posteriorly, to the deep portion of the sub-mandibular gland.

The lingual nerve descends lateral to the posterior end of the gland, while, further forward, the nerve, in conjunction with the sub-mandibular duct, curves round the lower border of the gland to reach its medial surface. More anteriorly still, the lingual nerve in conjunction with the hypoglossal nerve lies medial to the gland, between it and the genioglossus muscle.

The sub-lingual gland occupies the sub-lingual portion of the sub-mandibular fascial space; thus it is related to the parapharyngeal space (Fig. 13.8) but it is separated from the sub-mental space by the mylohyoid muscle. Thus, a tumour of the sub-lingual gland has to penetrate the myohyoid muscle before it can present as a distinct sub-mental swelling.

Lymphatic drainage (Fig. 13.8)
Lymphatics draining the sub-lingual glands have two routes, one anterior and the other posterior. The anterior route arises mainly from the anterior part of the gland, traverses the mylohyoid muscle ending in the sub-mandibular lymph node. The posterior channels usually drain the posterior two-thirds or three-quarters of the sub-lingual gland ending in the jugulodigastric nodes.

Generally lymphatics draining the three major salivary glands end ultimately in the upper deep cervical nodes. An occasional trunk drains into the middle deep cervical nodes. The frequency of lymph node metastases corresponds to this pattern.

Clinical pathology and natural history

The pathology and natural history of salivary tumours is complicated by the variety of histological types and the multiplicity of sites of origin (Spiro *et al.*, 1973). When describing the histological picture of these tumours, the author will draw on the experiences of Penner and Lauchlin.

The classification which follows relies heavily on differences in the natural history (and consequently prognosis and methods of management), rather than microscopic and staining characteristics alone.

Primary
  Benign:
    Pleomorphic adenoma (mixed tumour)
    Monomorphic adenoma (oncocytoma)

  Malignant:
    Adenocystic carcinoma (cylindroma)

Mucoepidermoid carcinoma
Pleomorphic adenocarcinoma (malignant mixed tumours)
Adenocarcinoma (including alveolar and papillary)
Acinic cell adenocarcinoma
Squamous cell carcinoma
Anaplastic carcinoma
Others

Lymphoepithelial lesions:
Benign (Warthin's) (adenolymphoma)
Malignant

Lymphomas

Secondaries (metastatic)
It appears that 80% of salivary tumours occur in the parotid and that pleomorphic adenomas (mixed tumours) form 75% of parotid tumours; 5–10% of salivary tumours occur in the sub-mandibular gland and 10–15% in minor salivary glands. Sub-lingual gland tumours form about 1% of the whole group.

Benign tumours

Pleomorphic adenoma (mixed tumour)
The term 'mixed tumour' was introduced in the latter half of the nineteenth century by Broca in 1866 to suggest a dual origin of these tumours (epithelial and mesenchymal), but its use has been maintained as a descriptive term rather than for its histogenetic connotation. The epithelial origin of the tumour and its pleomorphic histological appearance lead to the present term popularized by Willis (1948).

Incidence. Pleomorphic adenomas form between 55% and 60% of salivary tumours of major salivary glands, and about 40% of tumours affecting minor glands, with the palate being the site most commonly affected where it forms 22–56% of its salivary tumours (Spiro *et al.*, 1973). The incidence in sub-mandibular gland occupies an intermediate position between these two figures (40–60%). Only sporadic cases are reported affecting the sub-lingual gland. However, since the parotid gland is the one most commonly involved with any salivary tumour, about 84% of pleomorphic adenoma occur in the parotid as reported by Rauch (1959) in a review of some 4000 pleomorphic adenomas.

Age and sex. Pleomorphic adenoma can occur in children very rarely in about 1%. Generally it is a disease of adult age with a zenith in the fifth decade of life for tumours of major salivary gland and the sixth decade

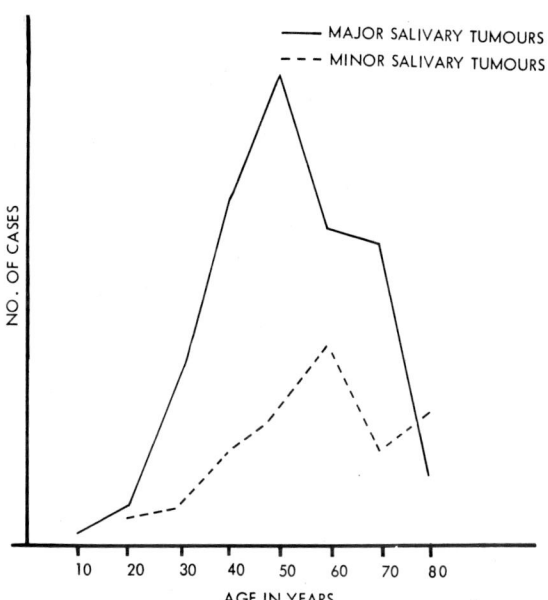

Fig. 13.9   Age incidence of pleomorphic adenoma.

for those affecting a minor gland (Fig. 13.9).

Women are more commonly affected than men with a ratio of almost 2:1. This preponderance is more pronounced, however, in major salivary tumours as compared to tumours affecting minor glands (Table 13.1).

Histology. The tumour displays a superficially mixed amalgam in almost infinitely varying proportions, of sheets and cords of epithelial cells with a stroma which may be myxoid, as in Wharton's jelly of the umbilical cord, cartilaginous or hyalinized. On occasion, osteoid tissue may be present. The cellular component of mixed tumours shows a greater variability than in any other salivary tumour, ranging from almost acellularity to crowded, cellular specimens, the latter not to be confused with malignant tumours.

The epithelial component of salivary mixed tumours is commonly in the form of small, dark, polyhedral cells lining acini or forming slender, anastomosing cords or solid epithelial sheets. A single nucleolus is often prominent. A pattern resembling adenoid cystic adenocarcinoma is found in some areas of about 10% of benign mixed tumours. This finding does not carry the prognostic significance of true adenoid cystic carcinoma. More frequently, some epithelial cells take on squamous characteristics, including intercellular bridges. Myoepithelial patterns may be present focally or as the dominant feature of an individual tumour.

Table 13.1   Sex incidence of pleomorphic adenoma.

	Major salivary glands tumours	Minor salivary tumours	Total
Males	49	20	69
Females	80	24	104
Total	129	44	173

The stromal component is usually composed of a loose myxoid matrix enclosing scattered elongated or stellate cells. The stroma usually has a faint basophilia, accentuated when pre-cartilaginous or cartilaginous changes supervene, but it may show a strong eosinophilia in hyalinized 'mature' areas. Calcification and ossification may be superimposed on well hyalinized areas.

Attempts to establish the aggressiveness or otherwise of mixed tumours on the basis of microscopic appearance have proved largely fruitless. Of greater significance than the cellular characteristics is the nature of the surgical specimen received and the degree of circumscription of the tumour itself. A mixed salivary tumour is not encapsulated. A compressed pseudocapsule of greater or lesser thickness is usually present, but this is frequently imperfect, and even in its denser parts is commonly traversed by fingerlike processes ('pseudopods') or segregated islands of tumour tissue. Enucleation or narrow excision under these circumstances is an open invitation to single or, commonly, multiple areas of continued tumour growth.

Natural history. The slow *rate of growth* of the tumours is well recognized with an average interval of about five years delay between first symptoms and presentation for treatment (Rafla-Demetrious, 1970). Much longer intervals (up to forty years) are not unknown. The lag period before presentation is shorter in tumours of minor salivary gland with a mean of 2.8 years.

The *clinical presentation* of pleomorphic adenomas is usually that of a mass and since the tumour is essentially benign with little invasive characteristic, pressure symptoms are rare occurring in less than 3% of parotid tumours. However, some authors (Rauch, 1959) reported a higher incidence of a 'pressure sensation'. Presentation with pressure symptoms, pain or mechanical effects is more common in minor salivary gland tumours amounting to 25% of palatal tumours, 50% of tonsillar tumours, and 75% of pharyngeal lesions (Rafla-Demetrious, 1970).

In the parotid the tumour usually affects the superficial lobe but the deep lobe is affected in about 4% of cases. The pre-auricular and retromandibular portions of the gland are the sites of origin in 84% of cases. It is rare for the tumour to involve more than one portion of the gland and almost unknown to involve the skin except in recurrent cases. Nerve paralysis and bone involvement do not occur.

In the palate which is the most common site among minor salivary glands, ulceration of the mucous membrane is noted in about one fifth of the cases, probably due to pressure. Palatal tumours are more common in the hard than soft palate (2:1) and rarely spread from one to the other.

The *course* of pleomorphic adenoma is usually benign without metastases to nodes or haematological spread, though local recurrences can occur. Such repeated recurrences have persuaded some early authors that these tumours are unpredictable and may indeed undergo malignant degeneration (Ahlbom, 1935). However, since a more aggressive therapeutic approach has resulted in a drastic reduction of repeated recurrences, the benign nature of the lesions is now accepted. Malignant degeneration of pleomorphic adenoma must be a rare incident; only one of 172 cases in our experience underwent such a change after two recurrences and three excisions. Multiple operative procedures were blamed by some for malignant degeneration (Ahlbom 1935).

Oncocytoma
The oxyphil adenoma is the salivary gland homologue of a number of similar tumours in such organs as the parathyroids, thyroid, pituitary, known collectively as oncocytoma.

Structurally, the oncocytoma is made up of cells with finely granular, brilliantly eosinophilic cytoplasm and small, usually fairly dense nuclei. Columns and occasional sheets of these cells form a well circumscribed uninodular or multinodular tumour which is fleshy in consistency. Infiltration is not seen. On occasion, lymphocytes may be sprinkled or aggregated in the tumour. The salivary oncocytoma is almost always a benign tumour.

Sebaceous cell tumours
Sebaceous cells are occasionally present in normal

salivary glands. Pure tumours of such cells are rare, though from time to time, fat-containing sebaceous cells are present as minor and occasionally major components of other salivary gland tumours.

It was formerly believed that most sebaceous tumours were benign, but Silver and Goldstein (1966) have reported a sebaceous cell carcinoma of the parotid, and other malignant tumours in which sebaceous cells were a dominant component have been reported. At the time of publishing their case, four instances of association of sebaceous cysts and lymphoid tissue (sebaceous lymphadenoma) were noted by Pheek and Pitcock (1966).

Malignant lesions

The multiplicity of the pathalogical types of malignant salivary tumours has led to a considerable degree of confusion. It is a prudent policy to recognize malignant salivary tumours as potentially lethal. All of them display a spectrum of varying growth, spread and response to treatment.

The characteristics common to all malignant salivary tumours are described first.

Malignant tumours account for about 30% of all salivary tumours but for 46% of all minor salivary tumours (Conley, 1957; Hayes, 1948). Well differentiated adenocarcinomas are the more prevalent type in the parotid (Rafla-Demetrious, 1970), with pleomorphic adenocarcinoma and cylindroma next (Table 13.2). Sub-mandibular gland tumours display almost the same pattern (Rafla, 1970). On the other hand, palatal tumours (the site most commonly involved by minor salivary tumours) display a different pattern, with cylindroma and epidermoid carcinomas the most prevalent.

The zenith of age incidence is the sixth decade of life, but the disease may affect children on very rare occasions. Both sexes seem to be almost equally affected with slight preponderance in the males (Table 13.3).

Except for anaplastic carcinoma and squamous cell carcinoma, malignant salivary tumours are slow-growing, presenting after long periods of delay (about three years), especially when originating in the parotid.

About 80% of patients suffering from malignant salivary tumours present with a lump and the remaining fifth present with symptoms related to neurological involvement – pain in 80% of cases and frank nerve

Table 13.2 Incidence of malignant salivary tumours.

	Major salivary gland tumours	Minor salivary tumours	Total
Cylindroma	14	43	57
Malignant mixed tumour	13	7	20
Mucoepidermoid tumour	9	6	15
Anaplastic carcinoma	16	5	21
Miscellaneous adenocarcinoma	34	37	71
Squamous cell carcinoma	8	–	8
Total	94	98	192

Table 13.3 Sex distribution of malignant salivary tumours.

	Male	Female	Total
Malignant mixed	11	9	20
Cylindroma	30	27	57
Mucoepidermoid	13	2	15
Differentiated carcinoma	38	33	71
Anaplastic tumours	7	14	21
Squamous cell carcinoma	5	3	8
Total	104	88	192

Table 13.4 Presenting symptoms of malignant salivary tumours (Major salivary glands).

	Mass	Pain	Nerve palsy
Cylindroma	12	2	–
Adenocarcinoma	32	2	–
Anaplastic carcinoma	13	3	1
Malignant mixed tumour	13	1	–
Mucoepidermoid tumour	9	3	1
Squamous cell carcinoma	8	–	–
Total	87	11	2

paralysis in 20% (Table 13.4). Nerve involvement occurs in about 25% of tumours of minor salivary glands (Table 13.5). Secondary lymph nodes may be the presenting feature on very rare occasions in the posterior tongue or pharynx.

Spread is probably more related to tumour sites than histological types. Generally malignant salivary tumours behave no differently from other malignant tumours. They involve the surface integument in about one quarter of the cases in the parotid (skin) and more often in tumours originating in palate or oral cavity. However skin involvement in parotid tumours is a sign of advanced disease and will be accompanied in about one third by other signs of spread such as lymph node metastases. Skin involvement in parotid tumours is more frequent than in the other two major salivary glands, because of the sub-cutaneous position of the parotid and the relatively more protected deep situation of the sub-mandibular salivary gland.

Deeper and wider infiltration of parotid tumours is characterized by its late occurrence, paucity of bone invasion and frequency of nerve involvement. While the parotid and its tumours are virtually wedged bet-

ween three bones, the mandible anteriorly, the mastoid posteriorly and the styloid medially, bone changes are rarely demonstrated – only in about 10% of cases (Rafla, 1977). Factors such as the dense parotid fascia, difficulties of demonstrating changes in these bones radiologically and the relative superficial positions of most of these tumours may help to explain this rarity. The incidence of nerve involvement by malignant parotid tumours varies from 8 to 33% depending on individual tumour types with cylindroma displaying a particularly high incidence. Conley and Hamaker (1975) reported an average of 12% in a series of 279 cases. While the facial nerve is in a particularly hazardous position other nerves such as cranials nine, ten, eleven and twelve may be affected in advanced cases which may reach the base of the skull. The prognosis of patients presenting with this finding is usually very poor with salvage only possible after a radical approach and only when the treatment volume is limited enough to make such a line of management feasible.

Malignant parotid tumours involve more than one region of the gland (divided arbitrarily into pre-

Table 13.5 Presenting symptoms of malignant salivary tumours (Minor salivary glands).

	Mass	Pain	Nerve palsy
Cylindroma	31	9	3
Adenocarcinoma	26	9	2
Anaplasic carcinoma	5	–	–
Malignant mixed tumour	5	2	–
Mucoepidermoid tumour	6	–	–
Total	73	20	5

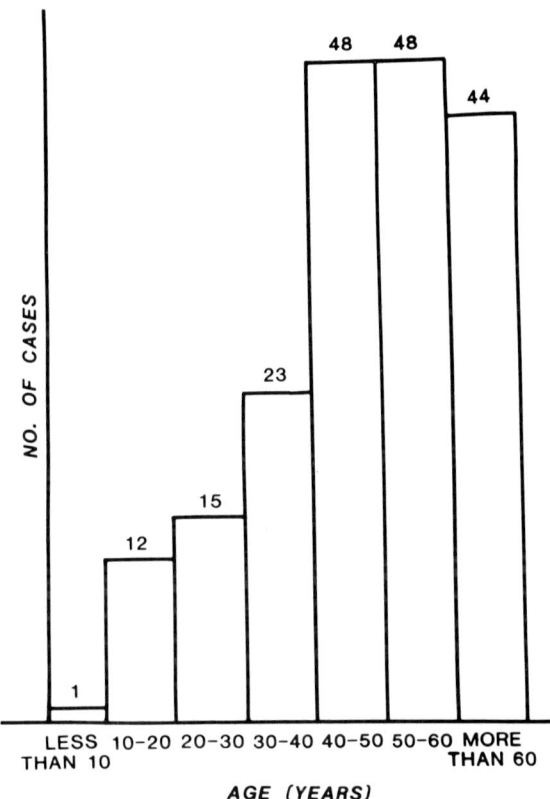

Fig. 13.10 Age distribution of patients with malignant salivary tumours.

auricular, retromandibular and sub-mandibular portions) in over a third of cases. In another third the retromandibular region only is involved. Extension to soft structures surrounding the parotid such as the pinna of the ear (2%), auditory meatus, and external canal (7%) and the sub-mandibular salivary gland (7%) is rather rare (Rafla, 1977).

Local spread of sub-mandibular tumours is rather limited. Skin is rarely involved except in recurrent cases, and nerve palsy is rarely encountered, because of the anatomy. Deeper extension through the parapharyngeal space to involve the faucial region or palatal arches and soft palate occurs in about one fifth of cases.

Lymphatic spread of malignant salivary tumours is controlled primarily by site of origin whereas tumours originating in regions with rich lymphatic supply such as the oral cavity and tongue involve nodes more readily than parotid tumours, 50% and 24% respectively. Tumours of minor salivary glands as well as certain cell types such as squamous cell carcinoma show a relatively higher incidence of nodal metastases as compared to the average. Generally lymphatic spread occurs in about one quarter of cases (Table 13.6).

Distant haematogenous spread of malignant salivary tumours used to be considered very rare (Ahlbom, 1935). However, it is now accepted that metastases occur initially in about a quarter of all cases with half of those who die having widespread metastases. More than half occur in the lungs with bone involvement next. Bone metastases have a particular affinity for flat bones (skull, clavicles, ribs, mandible) and the spine (Table 13.7). Some metastatic deposits reproduce the slow pattern of growth in the parent tumours in some patients surviving for several years untreated. (Fig. 13.11).

Table 13.6 Incidence of lymph node metastases.

	No. of cases	No. of cases with lymph nodes	Percentage
Cylindroma	57	11	19%
Mucoepidermoid tumours	15	2	13%
Malignant mixed tumours	20	6	30%
Anaplastic carcinoma	21	5	24%
Squamous cell carcinoma	8	4	50%
Adenocarcinoma (differentiated)	71	18	25%
Total	192	47	24%

categories can be increased to take account of assumed clinical significance. For example, N_{1a} describes palpable mobile nodes that are considered to be free from tumour whilst N_{1b} describes palpable mobile nodes that are considered to contain tumour. Such assessment, based on purely clinical grounds, is difficult and open to a considerable margin of error. Updating of the clinical stage can also be done in the light of histological diagnosis by use of additional cyphers. Minus $(-)$ and plus $(+)$ being used to designate the absence or presence of tumour.

Staging of tumours at all sites in the head and neck must take account of lymphatic drainage to the nodes of both sides of the neck since bilateral disease occurs in a small percentage of the total number of cases. The incidence is greater in association with midline or adjacent tumours, e.g. tongue and larynx. The basic classification for the description of cervical nodes is:

N_0 no palpable lymph nodes.
N_1 mobile homolateral lymph nodes.
N_2 mobile contralateral or bilateral lymph nodes.
N_3 fixed lymph nodes.

The same system is used for staging of nodal metastases from skin tumours at all sites with the exception of malignant melanoma. Metastases from the lower vagina and penis are also classified in this way. Tumours of the limbs, however, do not give rise to bilateral metastasis and the category N_2 is not therefore applicable. The TNM classification of anal tumours issued in 1966 and 1967 has been withdrawn and no other classification has yet been proposed. The classification of malignant melanoma before treatment is currently under review and awaiting further analysis of data collected by the Collaborating Centre of the World Health Organization before definite recommendations are made.

Treatment policy

From the point of practical management, cases fall into three main clinical groups:

1. No clinical evidence of involved lymph nodes (N_0).
2. Mobile discrete involved nodes in the immediate lymph drainage (N_1, N_2).
3. Fixed nodes or nodes beyond the immediate lymph drainage (N_3).

Prophylactic treatment of regional lymph nodes (N_0)

Elective treatment of the clinically negative neck either by surgery or by irradiation has been the subject of discussion for many years. The advent of better radiotherapeutic techniques which permit satisfactory irradiation of the neck has focused attention on the value of elective X-ray treatment in N_0 disease in the head and neck, the concept followed being the early treatment of potential sub-clinical metastases. As yet, no random clinical trial to evaluate elective neck irradiation has been published.

N_0 represents by far the largest group of cases of tumours of the oral cavity at all stages, 74% presenting without clinically involves nodes. The incidence of metastatic nodes for each T-stage of oral cancer is shown in Table 14.1.

Table 14.1 Node incidence on presentation.

	Number	*No(%)*
T_1	123	95
T_2	223	84
T_3	218	51

Long term follow-up of oral cancer (Figs 14.1a and b) clearly indicate that for practical purposes, secondary nodes develop mostly within two years of primary treatment. This was confirmed by a study of a large number of block dissections (Pointon and Jelly, 1976) where only a small number of cases developed nodes more than two years after their primary treatment and in some of these cases the metastases were undoubtedly due to the development of a second primary tumour. As it is in this initial two year period that the state of control of the primary and nodes will become apparent, maximum attention must be concentrated during this period of time.

Prophylactic treatment of regional lymph nodes in the presence of malignant melanoma has been a subject of controversy for many years. Attempts have been made to rationalize the argument by relating indications to the depth of penetration by a primary tumour. Although reports have favoured elective block dissection in some anatomical sites, the only prospective randomized trial provided no supportive evidence for this approach (Veronesi *et al.*, 1977).

Mobile involved nodes (N_1, N_2)

When mobile involved nodes are a presenting feature then the primary tumour and metastatic nodes should be treated *en bloc*, wherever possible, either by irradiation or surgery. Failing this the primary should be treated first and the nodes treated by block dissection. The interval between the primary treatment and block

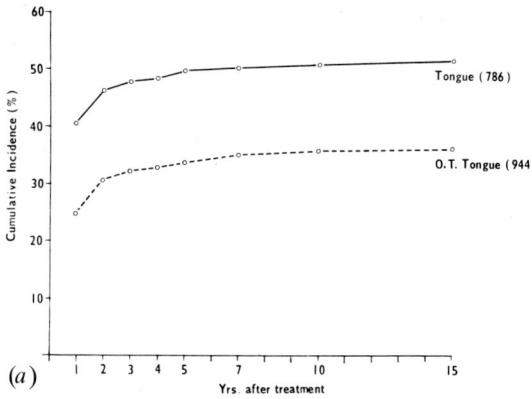

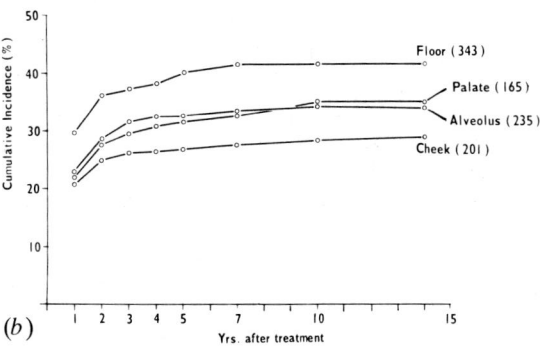

Fig. 14.1 The cumulative incidence of metastatic lymphadenopathy secondary to squamous cell cancers of the oral cavity related to time from treatment of the primary tumour. (*a*) Primary tumours of tongue (786) and those other than tongue (944).

(*b*) Primary oral tumours other than tongue according to site.

dissection will vary according to the method used for treatment of the primary tumour and the site involved but the interval should be kept to the minimum. Occasionally, a single localized X-ray treatment is justified as a holding dose for a large metastatic node in the interval before surgical clearance can be done.

Mobile nodes that develop subsequently are best managed by appropriate block dissection providing that the site of the primary tumour remains well and there are no general contra-indications to surgery.

Advanced nodal disease (N₃)

The control of fixed nodes remains very disappointing in spite of extensive trials of combined therapy. The policy of management must be influenced by the state and extent of the primary lesion. Fixed nodes are normally associated with an advanced primary lesion and are far less commonly the result of 'explosive' growth of nodal metastasis. If there is no real chance of primary control then palliative radiotherapy or surgery offers very little hope of significant benefit.

In spite of this pessimism, in head and neck cancer, there is evidence to suggest that fixed nodes have a better prognosis than bilateral mobile significant nodes. Dobbie (1954) and Henk (1975) reported perceptible cure rates with advanced nodal disease treated by radiotherapy.

From a surgical point of view, individual discretion must be used in interpretation of fixed nodes. If fixity is to overlying skin, then an appropriate area can be excised whilst, if there is fixity to mandible, a segmental resection can be done and Stell and Green (1976)

achieved a survival rate of 12% at five years with such extended cervical block dissection. However, it would never seem justifiable to consider resection of major blood vessels in an attempt to clear disease.

Inoperable secondary squamous cell carcinoma nodes in the axilla carry a very poor prognosis although useful growth restraint may be obtained with X-ray therapy but cure is rarely obtained. Occasional regression may be obtained with chemotherapy but generally the response is poor and relatively short-lived. Similarly, inoperable inguinal nodes respond poorly to X-ray therapy and so far fast neutron therapy has shown no significant advantage. Chemotherapy has proved to be disappointing and, with the available agents, it has not been found worthwhile. Useful growth restraint may be obtained by single field X-ray therapy giving 400 rad once weekly until skin tolerance is reached.

Recurrence following block dissection

Recurrence following block dissection (Fig. 14.2) usually occurs within six months of the operation and, in the neck, no cases have presented more than twelve months after surgery. The histological findings of extra nodal deposits in the soft tissues carry a very poor prognosis and histological evidence of extracapsular spread is invariably associated with recurrence. Strong (1969), in a controlled prospective study, gave preoperative radiation to the entire neck delivering a dose of 2000 rad given as 5 equal fractions on successive treatment days and compared this regime with surgery alone. He concluded that low dose radiation to the

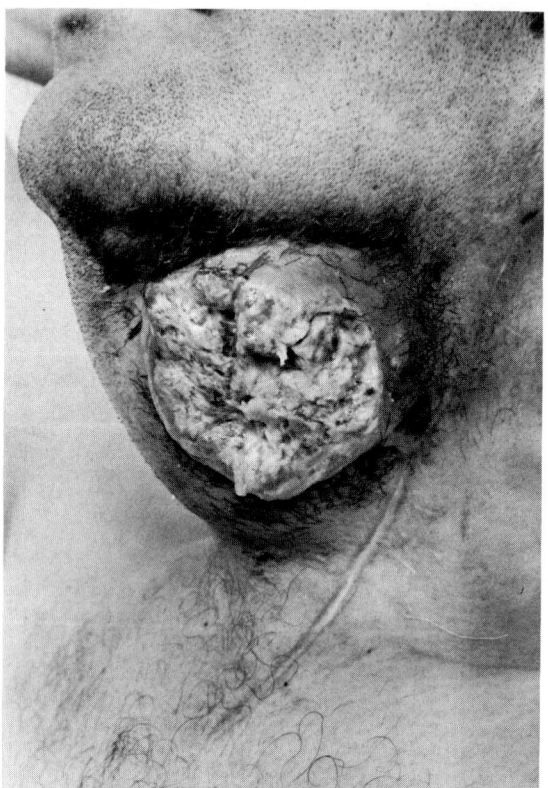

Fig. 14.2 Failed block dissection of the neck with fungation of a residual lymph node. Transient palliation was achieved with cytotoxic drugs.

neck followed promptly by radical neck dissection produced a significant reduction in the subsequent cervical recurrence rate without increasing morbidity or mortality. Occasionally, an isolated recurrence may be excised with success but the recurrences are usually multiple and involve much of the previously dissected area.

The response to radiotherapy of such recurrences is poor and regression is rarely obtained. Chemotherapy, using a high dose methotrexate regime, can give good palliation and is the present treatment of choice but the ultimate prognosis is extremely poor.

Metastatic nodes secondary to an unknown primary tumour

Secondary nodes in the upper and midcervical regions are usually undifferentiated epidermoid carcinoma. The common primary sites are the post-nasal space,

vallecula and pyriform fossa. A very careful examination of these sites is mandatory before accepting that the site of the primary is unknown. Occasionally, the presence of a node may be the only clinical evidence of a carcinoma arising in the thyroid but histological examination of the node should indicate the primary site. Metastatic malignant melanoma may also rarely present in this manner. In patients with secondary adenocarcinoma in cervical nodes, where routine clinical examination and investigation have failed to identify the primary site, extensive investigations are rarely justifiable (Stewart *et al.*, 1979).

The management of secondary nodes from an occult primary varies with the individual patient. Establishment of the diagnosis requires a biopsy. If the histological diagnosis is that of squamous cell carcinoma and the node is solitary, consideration must be given to block dissection of the neck. If the metastatic tumour is undifferentiated and the nodes are large and multiple, as is frequently the case, the primary site is presumed to be in the pharynx and treatment by X-ray therapy of the pharynx and nodes *en bloc* would seem to be a justifiable therapeutic approach. If this is not feasible, then palliation or growth control by irradiation or chemotherapy can be used.

Surgery

The rationale for block dissection of regional lymph nodes is based on the principles that (a) dissemination of tumour is still confined to the regional nodes and (b) the lymph nodes are accessible to surgical excision.

Even the most intensive clinical and investigative search cannot give confirmation of the first of these two principles and failure of treatment occurs because disease is already beyond the scope of surgery at the time that it is done. Block dissection of the neck encompasses a wider anatomical field of clearance than operations on the groin and axilla. The inguinal and axillary lymph nodes, with the exception of rare cases of involvement of popliteal and epitrochlear nodes, are the first station of lymphatic spread from the limbs. When multiple nodes are involved at these two sites, the chance of more proximal disease, in the iliac and supraclavicular nodes, is high.

Despite such considerations, surgical clearance of operable metastatic lymph nodes is the treatment of choice. Operability is determined by clinical assessment. When nodes are considered significant, solitary or few in number and mobile then their operability is not open to question. Tethering or fixity are open to individual interpretation. Tethering to major blood vessels does not preclude excision but arterial resection and replacement, although technically possible, are not justifiable. Using the TNM classification, N_1 and N_2 are considered operable whilst N_3 is open to individual interpretation.

Block dissection of groin

There is a choice of incision that can be used for block dissection of the inguinal lymph nodes and this can be left to individual preference although multiradiate incisions are better avoided since they are associated with a higher incidence of dehiscence and necrosis because of interference with cutaneous blood supply. Thin flaps are reflected in order to expose the whole femoral triangle. The inguinal ligament should be exposed throughout its length by dissecting the subcutaneous tissues off the external oblique aponeurosis. Mobilization of the block of tissue containing the inguinal lymph nodes is continued by clearing the medial margin of the sartorius muscle as far as the apex of the femoral triangle. The femoral vessels and femoral nerve with its branches are exposed as they lie in the deepest part of the gutter of the femoral triangle, from its apex to near the middle of its base. Superficial branches of the femoral artery must be divided as they are encountered. The long saphenous vein is divided and ligated at its junction with the femoral vein and again distally as it passes from the middle to the upper third of the thigh. Sacrifice of cutaneous sensory nerves has to be accepted in the interests of clearance but subsequent sensory recovery is usually good due to dermatomal overlap. Dissection of the groin is completed by clearing the surface of the adductor longus muscle with removal of the whole block of tissue.

Extension of the block dissection to include the lower iliac nodes can be done after retraction or division and repair of the inguinal ligament. Such dissection is indicated in the presence of significant lymphadenopathy although the ultimate prognosis is often poor and salvage rates are small.

Protection of the femoral vessels can be obtained by transposition of the upper end of the sartorius muscle. The muscle is detached from the anterior superior iliac spine and adjacent notch. The muscle is mobilized with preservation of the blood supply from its deep surface. It is swung medially and sutured to the inguinal ligament as well as approximated with sutures along its medial border to adductor longus. Good drainage should be established before skin closure with vacuum suction drains, one to the medial and the other to the lateral part of the dissection. Pressure dressings are best avoided so as to prevent further interference with blood supply to the skin flaps.

Block dissection of axilla

An incision along the anterior axillary fold is recommended for the approach to the axillary lymph nodes. Provided that early mobilization of the shoulder joint is instituted, such an incision does not usually cause significant restriction of movement. The axillary fascia arising from the lower border of the pectoralis major muscle is incised providing access to the axillary contents.

The dissection is begun laterally by clearing the fibro-fatty tissue off the coracobrachialis and biceps muscles. It is continued along the axillary vein in order to remove the lateral chain of lymph nodes up to the apex of the axilla at the start of the cervico-axillary canal. The posterior wall of the axilla, formed by the subscapularis muscle is cleared with removal of the posterior group of lymph nodes, whilst making every effort to preserve the nerves and vessels to the subscapularis and latissimus dorsi muscles although these can be excised, with appropriate loss of function, if they are adherent to involved nodes. The medial wall of the axilla is cleared down to the serratus anterior muscle with preservation of its nerve supply thus clearing the anterior lymph nodes tucked under pectoralis major.

In the female, the lowermost nodes in this group are associated with the tail of the breast which must be amputated at its junction with the upper outer quadrant. Dissection is completed by stripping the axillary fascia off the posterior skin flap and dividing the fibrous strands that normally support the axillary skin. Good drainage should again be established with a vacuum drain in order to prevent collection of fluid and thus facilitate leaking.

Block dissection of neck

Many different skin incisions have been described for cervical block dissection and the choice is according to individual preference. However, two principles should be observed; firstly, the incision should not follow the line of the carotid arteries and, secondly, areas of previous irradiation should, if possible, be avoided. The author's preference is for a goblet-shaped incision with a curved limb extending from mental symphysis to mastoid process with a downward extension from the apex of the curve to the clavicle. The skin flaps are reflected with platysma which helps to maintain cutaneous circulation.

Greater anatomical sacrifice must be accepted in the neck than at other sites in order to effect clearance of the sub-mental, sub-mandibular, anterior cervical and posterior cervical triangles. The sternomastoid and omohyoid muscles are removed as part of the standard operation, whilst the digastric muscle may also be removed if nodes are adherent to it. The internal jugular vein is divided and ligated both below and again above whilst its tributaries are controlled as they are encountered. The contents of the supraclavicular fossa are mobilized laterally as far as the anterior border of the trapezius muscle. The whole block of tissue is dissected upwards exposing the scalene fascia in the floor of the posterior triangle. It should be remembered that the thoracic duct reaches its termination on the left side.

The cervical cutaneous nerves are divided in turn both medially and laterally, also the spinal accessory nerve near the apex of the posterior triangle. The phrenic nerve is seen in relation to the common and internal carotid arteries and also preserved. The ansa hypoglossi is excised as it lies in proximity to the internal jugular vein. Providing the digastric muscle is not removed then the hypoglossal nerve is unlikely to be subject to injury but it may, on occasions, have to be removed in the interests of clearance.

The contents of the submental triangle are cleared in continuity with the submandibular gland and lymph nodes. In order to mobilize the submandibular gland, the facial vessels are divided and ligated as they cross the lower border of the mandible whilst the facial artery is again divided and ligated near its origin. The deep lobe of the submandibular gland is dissected from under the mylohyoid muscle with preservation of the lingual nerve whilst the duct is divided and ligated. The lower pole of the parotid gland is amputated with sacrifice of the mandibular and cervical branches of the facial nerve (Fig. 14.3). Block dissection is completed by dividing the sternomastoid muscle near its upper attachment. Careful haemostasis must be completed and two good drains should be placed in position, one to the submental and the other to the mastoid region, before closing the cervical incisions.

Indications for modifications in technique in order to preserve nerve function must be assessed critically in relation to the number and level of nodal involvement. The effects of paralysis of the lower lip due to sacrifice of the mandibular branch of the facial nerve can be reduced by wedge resection and support formed by a sling of muscle fibres of orbicularis oris (Fig. 14.4). On anatomical grounds and analysis of results of treatment there is no place for limited supra-hyoid dissection in the presence of clinically significant nodes.

Occasionally, synchronous bilateral block dissection of the neck must be done and a horizontal H-shaped incision gives good access. If sequential bilateral block dissection is to be done, then standard unilateral incisions may be used. For reasons of morbidity, preservation of one jugular vein is advisable otherwise cerebral

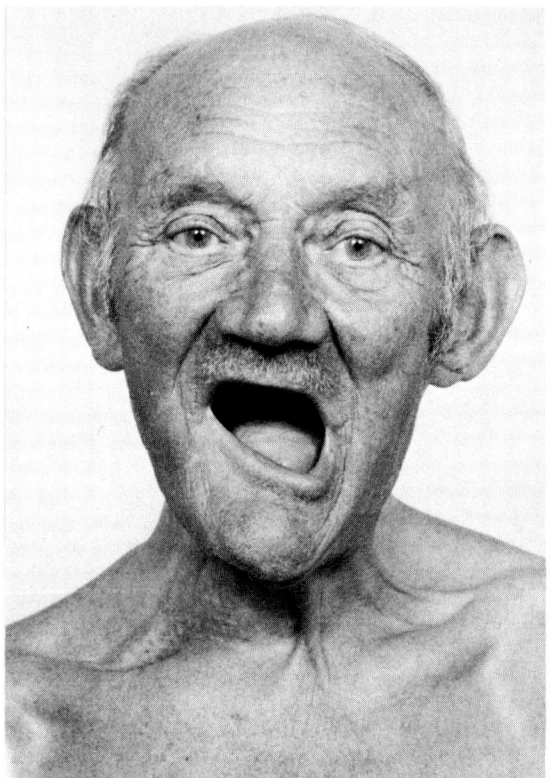

Fig. 14.3   Facial appearance after standard block dissection of the right neck with unilateral paralysis of the contra-lateral lower lip and depression of the shoulder.

oedema or thrombosis are likely complications.

Complications of surgery

The overall incidence of complications after block dissection is low although variable according to site. Beahrs (1973) quoted an operative mortality of 1% for block dissection of the neck and a total incidence of complications of 14.5% in a series of 110 consecutive block dissections of the neck of which 10 were synchronous bilateral procedures. Morbidity after inguinal and axillary operations is not well documented.

Fluid collection

Formation of haematomas should be prevented by proper haemostasis at operation. Collections of lymph should not occur provided that good drainage is established before closure of wounds. Drainage is usually significant in quantity during the first few days after operation and drains should be retained until the

Table 15.11 Typical plasma β-radiation from ^{131}I treatment.

Tumour uptake	Maximum protein-bound ^{131}I	Plasma rad per 100 mCi ^{131}I
50%	0.6%	80
5%	0.06%	30
0.5%	0.01%	35

group referred to on p. 318 (Table 15.9). Decision on whether to give treatment after the first 'ablation' dose will depend upon the presence of adequate uptake, assessed if possible by concentration rather than only total uptake. Even for the patients in whom surgical excision seems complete, but who have not had a total thyroidectomy, radioiodine treatment may give benefit. There is some slight evidence to support this but a controlled trial would be helpful (Mazzaferi *et al.*, 1981). Radioiodine treatment will be of no value for undifferentiated tumours.

Endocrine treatment

It has been known for many years that some well differentiated tumours, usually in young adults, are hormone dependent and that in the absence of thyrotrophic hormone (TSH) they will atrophy, just as the normal thyroid does in Sheehan's disease. There is no doubt that this occurs but there is doubt about the reliability of this as sole treatment and the length of time it persists. Clinical experience (e.g. Thomas and Burns, 1961) suggests that it is unwise to rely on hormone treatment as the sole method except in some children with multiple metastases. Hormone treatment is however simple and virtually harmless and should therefore be given to all patients with differentiated tumours *in addition* to whatever other treatment is indicated.

There are of course two main hormones – sodium L-thyroxine, with slow effect and slow metabolism at average adult daily dosage 0.2–0.3 mg and sodium L-triiodothyronine 80–120 μg daily, much more quickly effective. Clinical experience and experimental studies both show that it is correct to discontinue administration of thyroxine at four weeks, and triiodothyronine at two weeks, before radioiodine tests or treatment. When serum TSH levels are low, because of continued thyroid hormone administration or iodine medication, TSH administration can be tried. TSH is effective within hours and its effect can be built up, usually by 3 to 5 successive daily injections of 10 IU of bovine TSH. This will need to be given for both test

and therapy doses, the last injection being given on the day the dose is administered.

Generally, however, prolonged continuous tumour stimulation by endogenous TSH (secreted because of hypothyroidism) is the best method of ensuring maximum ^{131}I uptake.

Chemotherapy

Experience of the response of thyroid cancer to cytotoxic chemotherapy is at present meagre, but analogy with current results on other adenocarcinomas such as breast, and with other lymphomas, suggests that chemotherapy is of great potential value, though there is less promise so far for the worst prognostic group, the anaplastic carcinomas, that are not 'small cell' or lymphoma.

There is only one single drug that can be said to have been clearly shown of benefit in thyroid cancer itself, adriamycin (doxorubicin). Other drugs of potential value include cyclophosphamide, nitrosoureas, 5-fluorouracil, vincristine, methotrexate, and cisplatinum. Few attempts have been made at successful combination treatment, though Durie *et al.* (1981) in Tucson have had initially encouraging results in small numbers of patients with adriamycin, bleomycin, vincristine and melphalan. There is clearly a very good case to be made for adjuvant chemotherapy to treat micrometastases after surgery and X-ray therapy for undifferentiated carcinoma.

Thyroid lymphoma should be treated similarly to non-Hodgkin's lymphoma in other sites (see Chapter 36).

The endocrine diarrhoea of advanced medullary carcinoma should be mentioned; it may be caused by prostaglandins and it has been claimed that nutmeg (up to 25 g per day) will prevent it (Barrowman *et al.*, 1975).

Finally immunotherapy should be mentioned since lymphocytic infiltration correlates with prognosis in thyroid cancer and autoimmune thyroiditis is so familiar; no trials have yet been reported however.

Tumour markers

There are already two tumour markers of great value in thyroid cancer – serum thyroglobulin (Tg), and calcitonin or carcinoembryonic antigen (CEA) may also sometimes be of value.

Tg is present with various benign thyroid diseases, adenomas especially, as well as with differentiated carcinoma. However, after total thyroid ablation by surgery and/or radioiodine it will then be a marker or index to residual or metastatic thyroid tumour. Good correlation can be found with radioiodine scans and with response to treatment, radioiodine especially quantitative whole body assessment.

The ablation dose may cause minimal side-effects of very slight nausea or loss of appetite and tenderness for a few days in the thyroid region; there will be a slight and temporary fall in the white blood cell count. Hypothyroidism will then begin to develop, with few signs or symptoms becoming apparent until at least four weeks later, including mild deafness, constipation, non-specific muscle and joint pains, dryness of the skin, slight loss of hair, mental slowness, tiredness and apathy; objective signs will include raised blood cholesterol, prolonged electrocardiographic P–R interval and radiological evidence of enlargement of the heart. Most of these features of hypothyroidism will be difficult to detect and hypothyroidism will not be a serious hardship for the patient. Very exceptionally there may be mild psychotic symptoms such as of persecution or phobias which will clear soon after adequate thyroid hormone is given. Biochemical monitoring of thyroid function should be done with serum TSH levels rising, preferably to over 30 mU/l (Edmonds *et al.*, 1977). No thyroid hormone at all should yet be given. A further test dose of ^{131}I of up to 2 mCi should be given at about six weeks after the ablation dose and abnormal concentration in primary or secondary tumour sites should now be demonstrable. If so the first treatment dose can now be given, of 200 mCi. Scanning and uptake measurements should be repeated after this treatment dose. The patient should now also be given thyroid hormone (see below) and this can be initiated 48 hours after the dose. Any hypothyroid symptoms will rapidly disappear. There will be no side-effects to this large dose of the radioiodine usually, because both the whole-body and local radiation dosage will be lower than after the ablation dose given when there is considerable radioiodine uptake in normal thyroid, followed by substantial secretion of labelled thyroid hormone.

Further radioiodine treatment will depend upon both the clinical progress of the patient and the measurement of radioiodine uptake in tumour. It will usually be appropriate to stop administration of thyroid hormone and to do radioiodine uptake scanning and measurements about three months later, followed by a second therapy dose of 200 mCi. If there is adequate uptake up to four or five similar therapy doses can be given but if more than 1000 mCi are given in total dosage there may be significant risks of pancytopenia, aplastic anaemia, or even of leukaemia.

Radiation dosage and hazards from radioiodine (Halnan, 1964)
Very careful thought needs to be given to the absorbed dose (in rad or Gray) from radioiodine treatment, difficult though the calculation may be. Concentration of radioiodine is the important factor, rather than total uptake. A normal thyroid concentrates about 1–2%/g (25–50% in 25 g). At this level β radiation would be 31 000–62 000 rad for 100 mCi iodine-131, assuming an average biological half-life of three days (average for carcinoma). At a concentration of 0.1%/g the radiation dose will still be substantial, 6200 rad from 200 mCi (Table 15.10). It should be remembered that with this concentration a patient with minimal residual post-operative tumour, say 5 g, will only have 0.5% uptake; and conversely a patient with considerable and large metastases, say 250 g, will have a 25% uptake, which will have the same radiation dosage. Gamma dosage from ^{131}I is only small and not worth considering unless the tumour is large.

Whole body or plasma dosage will limit the maximum safe dose and will be mainly determined by the relatively long half-life of protein bound ^{131}I (Table 15.11). Gonadal dosage will be about half this level and will not therefore usually result in sterilization unless, exceptionally, there is a very large bone metastasis in the pelvis close to the ovaries (normal thyroid and thyroid tumour dosage with good uptake will be 100 to 1000 times that of plasma dosage, and the salivary glands, stomach, and lactating breast will receive about 30 times plasma dosage).

Hazards and side-effects are small. Leukaemia or aplastic anaemia has never been seen except after high total dosage of ^{131}I of considerably more than 1000 mCi, usually when there has also been other radiotherapy.

One minor frequent side-effect is stenosis of the parotid ducts resulting in painful parotid swelling at meal times, caused by the concentration of iodine in saliva. This is of minor importance, not to be confused with metastases, and usually self-limiting, subsiding with time.

Radioiodine treatment should be attempted for all patients with well differentiated thyroid cancer (papillary or follicular) except those in the good prognostic

Table 15.10 Typical β-radiation dosage to thyroid cancer from ^{131}I.

Concentration of ^{131}I	Biological half-life (days)	Rad per 100 mCi ^{131}I
1%/g (high)	1.5	18 000
	3	31 000
0.1%/g (average)	7	53 000
	3	3 000
0.01%/g (low)	3	310

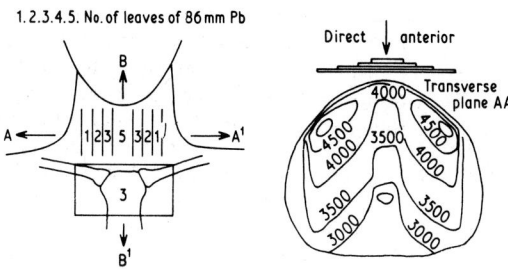
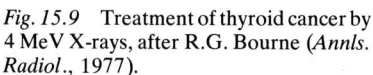
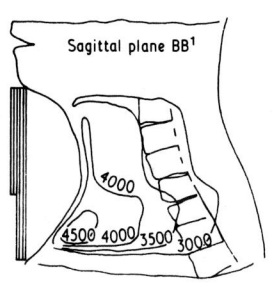

Fig. 15.9 Treatment of thyroid cancer by
4 MeV X-rays, after R.G. Bourne (*Annls.
Radiol.*, 1977).

for all primary carcinoma other than lymphoma and
may therefore vary from say 6000 rad or more in 25
fractions over 5 weeks for a small anaplastic tumour
confined to the thyroid, through to 5000 rad in 25
fractions over 5 weeks to many tumours with lymph
node involvement but confined to the neck, down to
3500 rad in 20 fractions over 4 weeks where virtually
the whole neck and mediastinum is being treated for
lymphoma.

The value of X-ray therapy is often underestimated.
Well differentiated carcinoma will be as sensitive as is
breast carcinoma, and post-operative treatment normally applicable to sterilize microscopic residue and
prevent local recurrence. Anaplastic carcinoma (large
or spindle cell) is less sensitive but growth restraint can
be obtained, and even occasionally cure. Small cell
carcinoma, probably really lymphoma, is as sensitive as
other lymphoma. Medullary carcinoma is sensitive too
but because of the very slow cell turnover clinical evidence of tumour response – shrinkage and disappearance of palpable mass or relief of pain from bone
metastases – will take many months, perhaps even as
long as a year or more.

Radioiodine treatment
Radioiodine is an extremely valuable method of
treatment of potential value for any well differentiated
tumour, papillary, follicular, or mixed and is still insuf-
ficiently understood. Its rationale is simple – the normal thyroid gland, and to a lesser extent many
tumours, will concentrate and retain iodine to such an
extent that a large dose of radioiodine will give lethal
self-destructive radiation to thyroid tissue, while other
tissues will be spared.

The first step will be histological identification of the
tumour as follicular (preferably) or papillary (in which
there will often be sufficient functioning follicular elements). This will often be from a thyroidectomy but

can also be from biopsy of a metastasis in a lymph node
or even from a bone metastasis.

The initial investigation will then be a radioiodine
scan of the neck or whole body. Pre-operatively it will
often seem that there is relatively low uptake in the
primary tumour as compared with the normal thyroid,
a 'cold' area or nodule, but this is to be expected and
should *not* deter one from continuing with treatment.
On the other hand it will also sometimes be the case
that radioiodine concentration can be shown in a
metastasis from the beginning, especially if it be
reasonably large and in a distant site such as the lumbar
spine or pelvis. When the whole body scan is reviewed
it will be important to remember the physiological
pattern of radioiodine distribution in the neck,
stomach, colon and bladder, with concentration building up over the first few days in the liver from labelled
hormone, when there is residual normal thyroid. In the
athyroid patient one will also see more clearly salivary
gland concentration in minor oral salivary glands as
well as in the more obvious parotid and sub-
mandibular glands. A test dose of at least 200 μCi of
[131]I will be required.

However, it is necessary in any case to destroy first as
much as possible of the normal thyroid, by surgery if
practicable, or by an 'ablation' dose of 75 mCi. Before
any test or treatment dose is given it will be necessary
to check that the patient has not been given thyroid
hormone (see below) or iodine-containing drugs, such
as X-ray contrast media especially. Scans and measurement of uptake in key sites should be done twenty
four hours later, and if there is low uptake it will be
easier to detect and measure it about five days after the
dose when most of the surplus radioiodine will have
been flushed out of the body. Daily measurements to
establish biological half-lives will be needed if radiation dosage is to be calculated exactly. Profile measurements of uptake are a good and simple method of

supraclavicular, mediastinal and other lymph nodes, makes it likely that lymph node dissection will seldom be complete. Furthermore, the conservative of French 'functional' dissection seems to give as good results as more radical and mutilating operations and it is rarely correct to remove the sternomastoid muscle. Prophylactic lymph node dissection is not worthwhile.

Radiotherapy

When considering radiotherapy it is very important to know the histological appearance of each individual tumour, this knowledge will be essential for decision not only on radiosensitivity but also, equally importantly, on the natural history of the tumour, the likely microscopic spread, and the scope and value of other methods of treatment. It will be simplest therefore to describe techniques first and after discussing radioiodine, endocrine treatment, and chemotherapy then to outline combined management of the different histological groups and clinical stages.

X-ray therapy

The primary tumour in the neck and neighbouring immediate lymphatic spread make up a U-shaped volume wrapped around the vulnerable spinal cord (Fig. 15.7). Irradiation of this volume uniformly is not easy and the best technique uses high energy electrons by a single anterior field, with bolus over the centre to bring out the dosage in front of, and to spare, the spinal cord (Fig. 15.8). Megavoltage X-rays can also be used to give similar treatment volumes with compensators or wedges and the plan described by Bourne of Brisbane, Australia (*Annls. Radiol.*, 1977) is a good sophisticated example (Fig. 15.9). Most often, however, especially for the most advanced cases, the treatment plan applicable will be a parallel pair of anterior and posterior fields including the neck and upper mediastinum, with partial spinal cord shielding from the posterior field. A good review of techniques has recently been given by Harmer (*Annls. Radiol.*, 1977).

Isolated metastases, in bone especially, will be treated by a simple single field or parallel pair technique as are other metastases, for example from breast carcinoma. Regional treatment, as for Hodgkin's disease, may be required for thyroid lymphoma.

Dosage will usually need to be maximum tolerated

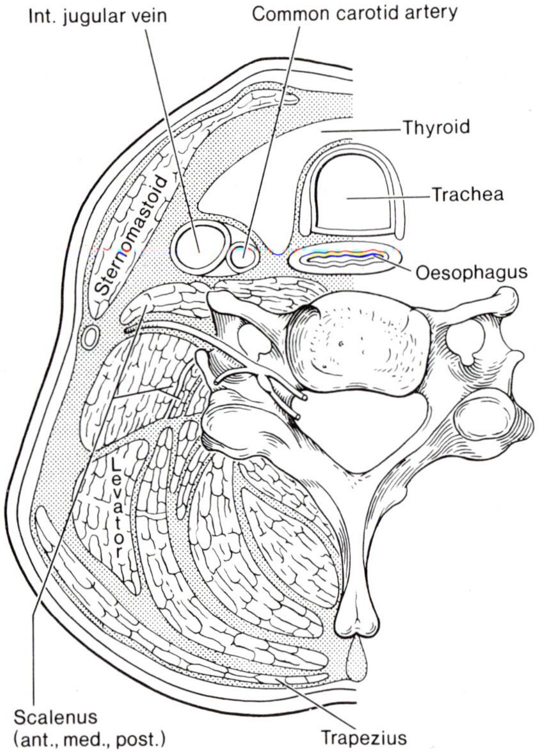

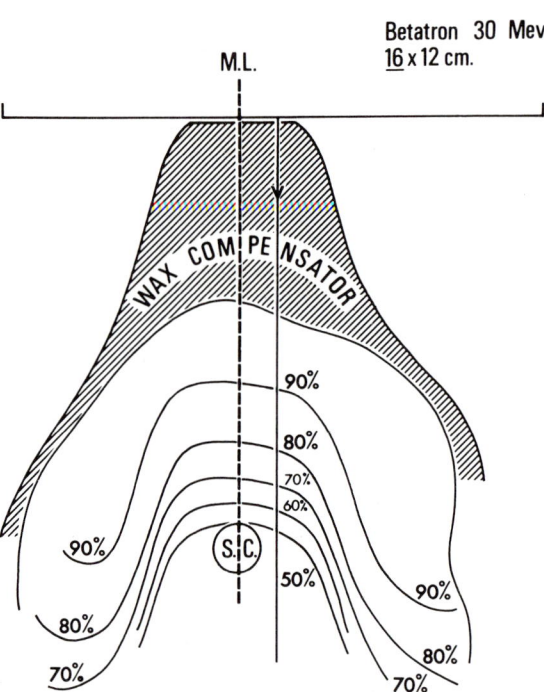

Fig. 15.7 Anatomy of the neck – transaxial section through C6.

Fig. 15.8 Treatment of thyroid cancer by high energy electrons (J.C. Ho, personal communication).

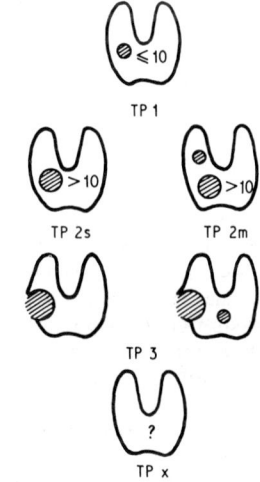

(a) TNM 1976 — Primary tumour: T

(b) TNM 1976 — Histological extent: TP

Fig. 15.6 1976 TNM classification for primary tumours: (*a*) clinical; (*b*) histological.

The very good EORTC analysis, supported by the long-standing Mayo Clinic survival data, suggests that there *is* a good prognostic group and that minimal treatment – usually adequate surgical excision plus hormone treatment – is sufficient for these and these *only* (Table 15.9).

All other cases will need full and adequate treatment planned jointly from the beginning as soon as the diagnosis is certain, with adequate decision made regarding the time and planning for possible chemotherapy, hormones, X-ray therapy and radioiodine. There will

Table 15.9 Minimal treatment good prognosis group

All these criteria together.

Age < 35 years
Papillary or follicular histology
Primary tumour T_1 or T_2 (not penetrating capsule)
No distant or lymph node metastases

---

be a few very advanced, usually elderly, patients for whom attempted curative treatment would be unwise and unkind, but these should be very few and one should always have a biopsy. Unexpectedly good results can be achieved, for example long-standing paraplegia from a spinal metastasis can sometimes be completely reversed.

Surgery

Good histological diagnosis is essential in thyroid cancer. Preliminary evidence can be obtained by biopsy. Fine needle aspiration cytology is possible and can be helpful (Gershengorn *et al.*, 1977) and if the nodule or tumour is solid drill biopsy is practicable (Hawk *et al.*, 1966; Wang *et al.*, 1974). In general, however, these methods are of little value if negative and an open biopsy will be preferable. If lymph node metastasis is evident, excision of a whole lymph node will be very helpful. If adequate diagnosis of lymphoma is then made, no further surgery is necessary but with all other tumours either radical excision or palliative bulk removal should be considered.

If biopsy has not been done frozen section examination during the operation can be very helpful in deciding on the extent of surgery.

There are substantial arguments for total or near total thyroidectomy being the standard operation for all cancers except for lymphoma. When total thyroidectomy is done multiple sections and careful microscopic examination will show unsuspected microscopic clones of cells very frequently in the contralateral lobe. Some experienced surgeons will practise a true total thyroidectomy but two important hazards will be present, hypoparathyroidism because of removal of all four parathyroid glands, and bilateral recurrent laryngeal nerve damage with vocal cord paralysis. Radioiodine scanning almost always shows some residual uptake after 'total' thyroidectomy and it is suggested therefore that it is sufficient to do a complete lobectomy on the affected side and sub-total on the contra-lateral, leaving a tiny residue containing a parathyroid.

Knowledge of the very extensive lymphatic drainage of the thyroid (see above, Fig. 15.3) to paraoesophageal,

Results of treatment

The results for treatment of accessible metastatic lymph nodes must be considered according to histological and anatomical site of the primary tumour. There are many reports of the results obtained from treatment of cervical nodes but information about other sites is scanty.

Squamous cell carcinoma
1. *Head and neck.* Jesse *et al.* (1970) in a pertinent analysis of 624 cases concluded that there was no significant benefit from elective irradiation or surgery for the negative neck in carcinoma of the oral cavity and faucial arch. Subsequently, Million (1974), in a series of 43 patients of carcinoma of the tongue and floor of the mouth, concluded that there was a definite reduction in the incidence of node involvement following elective irradiation of the neck. Bagshaw and Thompson (1971) adduced that elective neck irradiation was of value in patients with primary sites in the head and neck which are known freely to metastasize to the cervical lymph nodes.

Long-term studies indicate that in patients with oral cancer kept under close surveillance the percentage proceeding to block dissection for involved nodes has remained remarkably constant (Table 14.2). If there was to be an improvement in the control of secondary nodes from oral cancer then a trial of elective neck irradiation was justifiable. A randomized prospective clinical trial of elective neck irradiation in N_0 oral cancer has been carried out and although entry into the trial has closed, longer follow-up is needed. However, initial conclusions suggest that elective neck irradiation does reduce slightly the incidence of cervical lymphadenopathy but does not improve survival. It has therefore been decided that routine neck irradiation in oral cancer is not justified although when close surveillance was not found to be practical or where coincidental medical conditions would preclude block dissection then irradiation of the neck as part of initial treatment was a useful and practical measure.

Anderson *et al.* (1978) reported a series of 74 patients with primary malignant tumours of the head and neck treated by *en bloc* irradiation of the primary and lymphatics. They concluded that the technique used was of value in the treatment of nasopharyngeal carcinoma but was poor for carcinomas of the hypopharynx. In the majority of hypopharyngeal lesions the primary lymph drainage will be included in the volume irradiated. The decision to extend this volume to include the whole neck must be balanced against reduction in dose and subsequent failure to control the primary. The principal primary site to benefit from elective neck irradiation would appear to be the post-nasal space.

The general policy for those cases presenting with no clinical evidence of involved nodes is meticulous follow-up. The first year following primary treatment is critical and the interval between visits should not exceed one month.

Churchill-Davidson and his colleagues (1973) reported the results of treatment of 102 patients with secondary squamous carcinoma in cervical lymph nodes from head and neck primary tumours by means of radiotherapy combined with hyperbaric oxygen and compared them with previously reported results from conventional radiotherapy, also with surgery in the case of operable nodes. The conclusion was that with the use of hyperbaric oxygen as an adjuvant to radiotherapy, the nodal clearance rate was doubled but there was no improvement in survival rate for the group of patients. 125 Cases of advanced head and neck cancer with lymph node metastasis treated by megavoltage radiotherapy to primary nodes *en bloc* were reviewed by Henk (1975). The local tumour control rates after treatment were: primary and nodes controlled 31%, primary and nodes recurrent 39%, primary controlled nodes recurrent, 16% and primary

Table 14.2 Numbers of patients undergoing cervical block dissection for metastatic squamous cell cancer of the oral cavity and lips (1950–1970).

Period	Males		Females	
	Number of cases	% Block dissection	Number of cases	% Block dissection
1950–55	719	14.6	298	15.8
1956–60	559	12.5	239	19.7
1961–65	445	15.7	245	15.1
1966–70	451	14.0	254	14.6
Total	2174	14.2	1036	16.2

dehiscence or necrosis of overlying skin and is more likely in the presence of previous irradiation. Provided cover of vessels with healthy tissue is obtained then this complication is unlikely. The outcome after arterial rupture depends on the level of rupture and ligation. If the blowout occurs in the superficial femoral artery then viability of the lower limb is usually maintained by circulation via the profunda femoris artery, providing that there is no obliterative arterial disease, but if it is localized to the common femoral artery then gangrene of the limb is inevitable. Rupture and ligation of the internal or common carotid artery is not necessarily fatal, depending on the contralateral circulation, but is a possible cause of hemiplegia. If localized to the external carotid artery then the effects can be minimal due to the supply from the opposite side.

Chylous fistula
Significant loss of lymph can occur if there is unrecognized damage to the thoracic duct during block dissection of the left side of the neck and a chylous fistula may then develop. Sometimes this condition resolves spontaneously and a pressure pad over the supraclavicular fossa will control it in some cases. The fluid can become locculated due to coagulation and evacuation is then difficult. Occasionally, the neck has to be reopened and oversewing or packs used to control leakage since identification and control of the source is difficult. Serial monitoring of serum protein levels in the presence of this complication is important since the loss of protein may necessitate replacement by parenteral means.

Pneumothorax and mediastinitis
These conditions are rare complications of block dissection of the neck. They are sometimes slow to be recognized. If these two complications are combined as pneumomediastinitis then they are invariably fatal.

Salivary fistulae
Salivary fistulae have been reported after block dissection of the neck due to amputation of the lower pole of the parotid gland. Almost invariably, such fistulae heal without surgical intervention.

Venous thrombosis
Thrombosis of the axillary vein has occasionally followed block dissection of the axilla due to severe handling or trauma at operation. The effects are usually transient due to the good potential collateral venous drainage and early recanalization.

Radiotherapy
The principles of management are:

1. Treat *en bloc* with the primary tumour whenever possible.
2. Whole neck irradiation is practical with megavoltage X-ray therapy provided that the larynx and spinal cord are shielded.
3. Isolated nodes should be treated as radically as possible.
4. Where palliation only is feasible, then the aim should be to obtain growth restraint for as long as is possible.

Radiotherapy methods
A total dose of 4500–5000 rad in 5 weeks given as 5 fractions per week, is adequate to eradicate more than 90% of sub-clinical aggregates of epithelial cancer cells (Fletcher, 1972).

Whole neck irradiation
Irradiation of the whole neck is perfectly practical with megavoltage X-ray therapy provided that the larynx and spinal cord are shielded. Using 4 MV X-rays, a single anterior field will treat the deep cervical chain of lymph nodes either unilaterally or bilaterally and a dose of 4500–5000 rad in 15 fractions in 3 weeks is well tolerated with minimal reaction. If unilateral neck irradiation only is indicated, a practical alternative is to use a single field of 10 MeV electrons, delivering a dose of 4500–5000 rad in 15 fractions over 3 weeks. These treatments may be given concurrently with treatment of the primary lesions or, in cases for which interstitial treatment of the primary has been used, immediately after removal of the sources of irradiation.

Isolated nodes
When a solitary cervical node is involved and surgery is not practical, a localized radical treatment should be attempted. The volume to be irradiated should be kept to a minimum thus permitting a high local dose. Depending on the general condition of the patient, the following dosages, using either X-rays or 10 MeV electrons, may be employed:

1. 2000 rad in 1 exposure;
2. 5000 rad in 10 days;
3. 5500 rad in 15 fractions over 3 weeks; or
4. 6000–7000 rad in 30–40 fractions over 6–7 weeks.

Interstitial irradiation was used in the past to treat secondary cervical nodes but has no advantages over X-ray therapy except perhaps in the rare presence of an isolated preauricular node. In this situation, a small single plane implant is a useful treatment method.

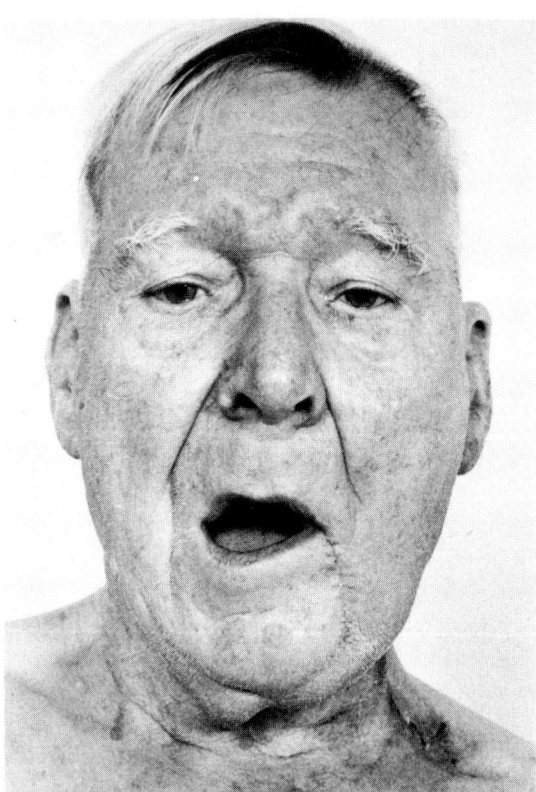

Fig. 14.4 Improvement in appearance and function obtained by lateral wedge resection of the paralysed lower lip and suspension with a muscular sling derived from the orbicularis oris muscle after block dissection of the left neck.

amounts are minimal. Subsequent fluid collection is then unlikely but, if it occurs, it is better left to reabsorb since coagulation often occurs due to the high protein content and aspiration is unfruitful. If, however, there is continuing increase and symptoms due to it, then proper drainage should be re-established.

Wound dehiscence
Wound dehiscence is not uncommon after block dissection of lymph nodes and is more common after operations on the groin or neck. Conservative treatment is usually successful, but if major blood vessels are exposed then cover with skin grafts or flaps is indicated in order to prevent arterial rupture.

Necrosis
Necrosis of skin flaps does sometimes occur after inguinal or cervical clearance and may be related to the design of incision or previous irradiation. Acute angles

should be avoided when making incisions since this predisposes towards ischaemic necrosis. Small areas of loss may be managed by trimming and resuture of viable skin edges but larger areas may require skin grafts or flaps to fill the defect.

Wound infection
Wound infection should be treated with specific antibiotics according to culture and sensitivity of purulent material. Local cleansing or irrigation with bactericidal solutions is of value and treatment with local heat or ozone can expedite resolution and healing.

Loss of nerve function
Loss of sensory or motor nerves may be necessary in the interests of clearance of metastatic disease. If this can be anticipated then it should be explained fully to the patient before operation. Sensory recovery is usually good due to overlap or supply to adjacent dermatomes and ultimate areas of sensory loss are small and not of significant disability. Loss of motor function has a more profound effect. This is seen most typically after standard block dissection of the neck when sacrifice of the accessory nerve causes denervation of trapezius and sagging of the shoulder and paralysis of the ipsilateral lower lip due to division of the mandibular branch of the facial nerve. Shoulder and neck exercises can improve adaptation to denervation of trapezius whilst wedge resection of the lip reduces the functional disability due to salivary loss during eating and speech.

Distal oedema
It is not uncommon to see distal oedema in the early period after block dissection. This is usually a temporary effect and resolves as collateral lymphatic pathways develop and cope with increased flow. However, lymphoedema of the upper limb is aggravated considerably if thrombosis of the axillary vein should occur as a result of handling during dissection. Exercises, massage and elevation of a limb at rest are of benefit in reducing distal accumulation of fluid. Support stockings are of particular value in controlling oedema of the lower limb.

The same effect is seen in the face after block dissection of the neck and the visible asymmetry is aggravated by the concave appearance that results from clearance of the sub-mental and sub-mandibular regions. Collateral compensation usually occurs within a few months of operation.

Arterial rupture
Rupture of the femoral and carotid arteries can occur occasionally after block dissection of the groin and neck. It is usually the result of associated infection with

(Van Herle and Uller, 1975; Gerfo *et al.*, 1977).

Calcitonin is a highly specific and sensitive index or marker for medullary carcinoma, so easily measurable that one is already sometimes confronted with the difficult decision on treatment for microscopic metastases secreting calcitonin after total thyroidectomy whose anatomical site cannot be detected, even by radiology and isotope scanning of chest and bones, CT-scanning and ultrasonics, and liver scanning. Good chemotherapy for medullary cancer needs development and is indeed being investigated.

Calcitonin screening of affected patients and their relatives can now lead to preventive and curative treatment. The best example of this reported so far is the 'J kindred' investigated in Boston, USA – 83 members of the family of 107 have been studied; 12 patients with carcinoma were found before 1970, 12 more cases of carcinoma discovered by initial calcitonin screening in 1970-71 and 21 more patients being found to have raised calcitonin and having thyroidectomy between 1971 and 1978, 13 having pre-carcinomatous C-cell hyperplasia and 8 early carcinoma (mean diameter only 2 mm) with no lymph node metastases (Graze *et al.*, 1978).

It has also been found that CEA is secreted by carcinoma but *not* by C-cell hyperplasia (De Lellis *et al.*, 1978). The tumour has also been much investigated in Sweden and in some families the disease may be relatively benign (Telenius-Berg, 1976).

Special cases

Children have thyroid cancer very rarely, their prognosis is very good indeed and there needs to be a careful balance between treatment benefits and hazards, both being very long term. Curative surgery is of obvious benefit, and even if metastases are present removal of the primary tumour is of value. Hormonal treatment will present no long term hazards and may often establish tumour control, even of lung and other distant metastases. Radioiodine treatment should be given with discretion if there be measurable and sufficient uptake for useful treatment of residual tumour, the ablation and treatment doses can often be smaller than for adults, reduced in proportion to weight and if treatment is clearly ineffective further doses should not be given. X-ray therapy to residual primary tumour and to metastases should also be given with discretion, as with other paediatric tumours (Winship and Rosvoll, 1970).

Pregnancy will only rarely coexist and termination or early delivery of the child should be undertaken before radioiodine treatment. Previous radioiodine treatment should not necessarily be a bar to later successful pregnancy, providing the patient has had no evidence of

disease for two years or more; genetic risks will not be high.

Paraplegia from undiagnosed thyroid carcinoma metastases can occur. Energetic treatment is indicated, surgical decompression, X-ray therapy, and radioiodine can all sometimes be of great value (Halnan and Roberts, 1967).

Ectopic thyroid cancer can sometimes occur in the tongue or thyroglossal duct and should be treated as if in the thyroid, though surgical excision will not usually be practicable; there can be very good results to treatment. The 'struma ovarii', thyroid tissue in ovarian teratomas, are almost always benign (Smithers, 1970).

Summary of treatment policies

Histological confirmation of the diagnosis is essential because (1) thyroiditis and benign thyroid adenomas can mimic cancer, (2) correct treatment varies considerably between the different histological varieties.

STAGING – a simple staging (for *treatment* decisions) is suggested:

$T_0 T_1 T_2 N_0 M_0$	I	Primary 'operable'. No lymph node or distant mestastases.
$T_0 T_1 T_2 N_1 N_2 M_0$	II	Primary 'operable'. Lymph node metastases operable. No distant metastases.
$T_3 N_3 M_0$	III	Primary or lymph node metastases inoperable. Lymph nodes may be present in mediastinum. No distant metastases.
M_1	IV	Distant metastases.

TREATMENT STRATEGY

1. *Papillary or follicular adenocarcinoma* – localized treatment, assess with serum thyroglobulin measurement.
   Stage I and II. Surgery followed by radioiodine and hormones.
   Stage III. Radioiodine, radical X-ray therapy and hormones.
   Stage IV. Radioiodine and hormones, limited symptomatic palliative X-ray therapy, consider chemotherapy if other treatment is ineffective.

2. *Medullary carcinoma* – localized treatment, assess with calcitonin measurement.
   Stage I and II. Surgery, followed by X-ray therapy if full excision doubtful.
   Stage III. Radical X-ray therapy.

Stage IV. Palliative X-ray therapy, consider chemotherapy.

3. *Undifferentiated carcinoma* – regional treatment, wide margins, consider trial of adjuvant chemotherapy.
   Stage I and II. Surgery, always followed by X-ray therapy.
   Stage III. Radical X-ray therapy, bulk removal by surgery if possible.
   Stage IV. Limited palliative X-ray therapy, consider chemotherapy.

4. *Malignant thyroid lymphoma* – regional and prophylactic treatment (as for other lymphoma).
   Stages I, II and III. Radical X-ray therapy, consider chemotherapy.
   Stage IV. Palliative X-ray therapy, chemotherapy.

TREATMENT TECHNIQUES

1. *Surgery*
   (a) Biopsy best by open surgery, needle or drill as second choice.
   (b) Primary tumour preferably removed by near total thyroidectomy in almost all cases, leaving parathyroid gland on contra-lateral side.
   (c) Lymph node metastases should be fully dissected but do not need 'block' dissection with removal of muscles and other tissues.

2. *External irradiation* – spinal cord should be shielded as far as is practicable without shielding tumour.
   (a) Stages I and II – Radical treatment, maximum tolerable dose (say 5000 rad in 20 fractions over 4 weeks). Best is single field electron treatment. Planning is difficult with cobalt or megavoltage therapy. Three fields sometimes helpful but parallel pair treatment may be necessary.
   (b) Stages III and IV – Parallel pair or single field treatments (say 4500 rad in 20 fractions over 4 weeks).
   (c) Regional treatment for lymphoma – as for non-Hodgkin's lymphoma (say 3500 rad in 20 fractions over 4 weeks).

3. *Radioiodine treatment*
   (a) Ablation dose of 80 mCi ^{131}I: give *no* thyroid hormone yet.
   (b) Radioiodine tests 6–8 weeks later.
   (c) Treatment dose of 200 mCi ^{131}I if there is adequate uptake or concentration (about 0.1% per g of tumour).
   (d) Thyroid hormone (see below).

(e) Further test and treatment doses according to clinical progress and iodine uptake.

Note

(a) Negative uptake tests or scans are valueless until at least six weeks after ablation of all normal thyroid. Thyroid hormone and iodine containing drugs, such as X-ray contrast media, must be avoided.

(b) A total cumulative dosage of 1000 mCi should usually not be exceeded.

(c) X-ray therapy can be given at the time of the ablation dose or first therapy dose (the X-ray dosage will not need to be reduced by more than 500 rad, if at all), and may usefully add to the radiation dose from radioiodine, both for the primary tumour and for bone metastases. X-ray therapy will not usually inhibit radioiodine uptake.

4. *Hormones*
   (a) Papillary and follicular carcinoma may be hormone-dependent, though usually only temporarily, if at all. All cases should, therefore, be given hormone treatment in maximum tolerable doses *in addition* to other treatment.
   (b) Other thyroid tumours are never hormone-dependent and thyroid hormone should only be given in the dose that will relieve symptoms of hypothyroidism.
   (c) The only two reliable hormones are:
       (i) Sodium laevo-thyroxine (Eltroxin, T4) – first choice. Maximum adult dosage 0.4 mg per day by mouth. Administration should be discontinued 4 weeks before radioiodine tests or treatment.
       (ii) Sodium laevo-triiodothyronine (T3) may be used when radioiodine treatment is being given. Maximum adult dosage 125 μg per day by mouth. Administration should be discontinued 2 weeks before radioiodine tests or treatment. Action is much quicker than that of thyroxine.

5. *Chemotherapy*
No drug or regime is yet of proven substantial value for any type of thyroid tumour. Doxorubicin adriamycin) may be worth further trial for various types as may also intermittent combination chemotherapy for undifferentiated carcinoma and for lymphomas. Adjuvant or prophylactic treatment is worth careful trial in anaplastic carcinoma.

FOLLOW-UP

Following of thyroid cancer should be close and meticulous, as for other cancer. Radioiodine treatment and chemotherapy may both last a year or two. Special attention should be given to hormone treatment, this may easily lapse and the hypothyroid or even myxoedematous patient become apathetic and deteriorate at home, as after treatment for thyrotoxicosis. Biochemical measurement of thyroid hormone and TSH is a helpful routine. Thyroglobulin, calcitonin, and CEA should be measured in patients with well differentiated and medullary tumours. Bone scans and radiology will be helpful for follicular carcinoma especially, and examination of the lungs also, especially for undifferentiated tumours. Regular annual radioiodine scanning is usually advocated for patients with well differentiated carcinoma, but this may well not be essential, especially if serum thyroglobulin can be measured.

Parotitis, often bilateral, may arise in patients who have had radioiodine treatment; it is more correctly parotid duct stricture, surgical interference or investigation is not needed and the symptoms usually subside without treatment.

Endocrine diarrhoea can occur in patients with medullary cancer, especially if they have escaped follow-up, and will indicate extensive recurrence or metastases, commonly in mediastinum or liver.

Prognosis and results of treatment

Knowledge of the prognosis for thyroid cancer in general depends upon adequate histological diagnosis (since this governs results so much) and equally well upon adequate follow-up of substantial numbers of patients. For many years the best information came from the Mayo Clinic and this remains one of the classic sources (Woolner *et al.*, 1968). The important

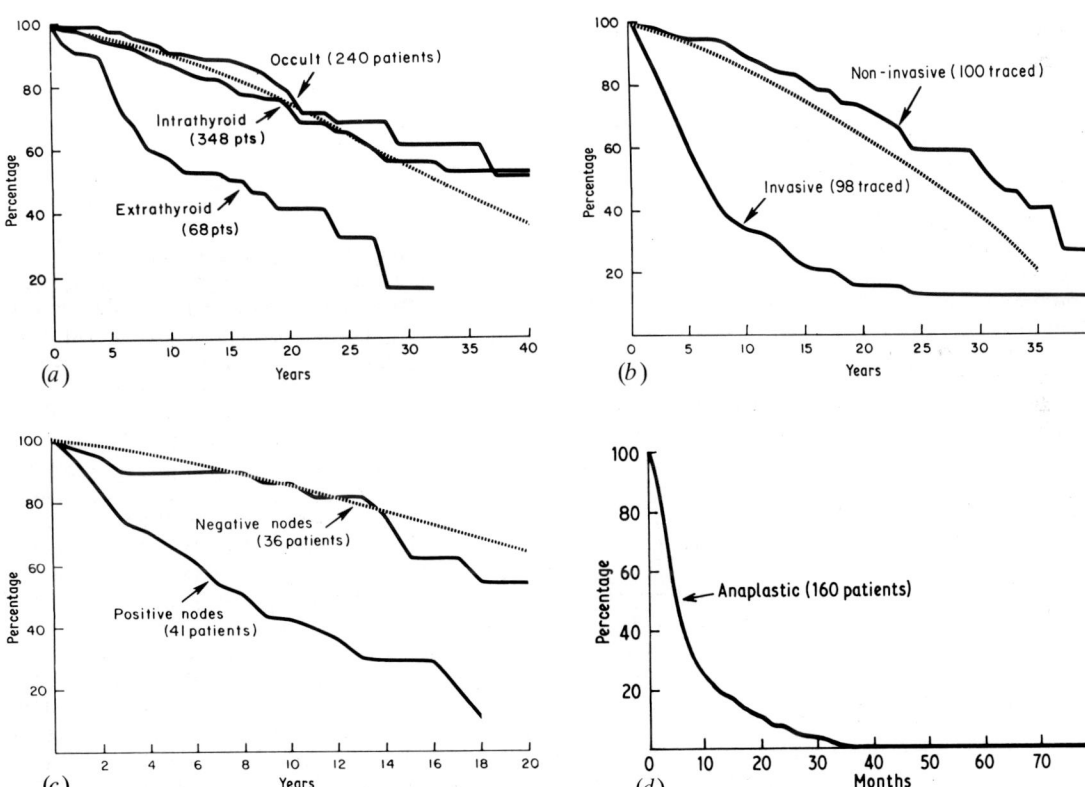

Fig. 15.10 Mayo Clinic survival data for thyroid cancer (dotted lines show survival of normal persons of comparable age and sex). (*a*) papillary carcinoma; (*b*) follicular carcinoma; (*c*) medullary carcinoma; (*d*) anaplastic carcinoma.

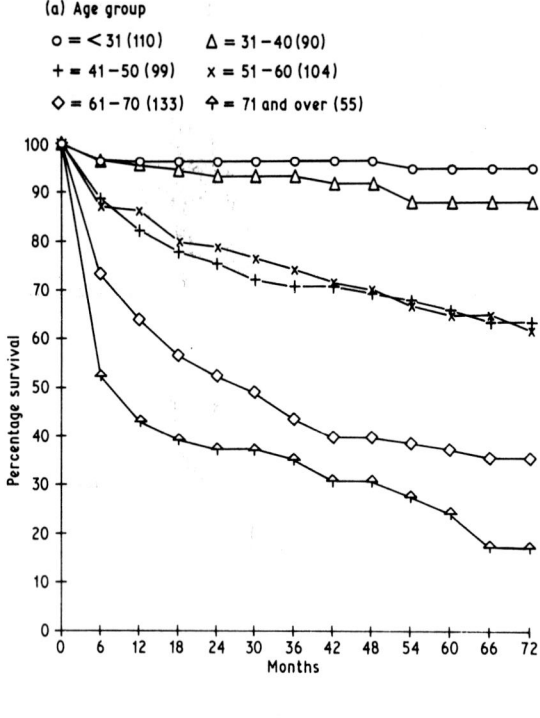

(a) Age group

o = < 31 (110) Δ = 31–40 (90)
+ = 41–50 (99) x = 51–60 (104)
◇ = 61–70 (133) ⟡ = 71 and over (55)

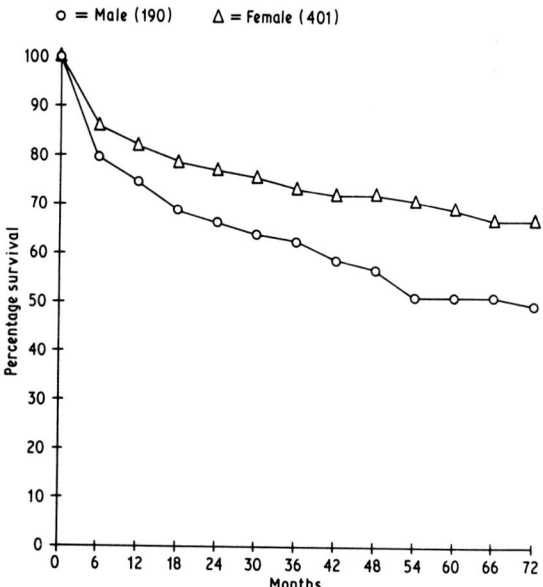

(b) Sex

o = Male (190) Δ = Female (401)

(e) N classification

o = N0 (290) Δ = N1 (163)
+ = N2 (55) x = N3 (38)

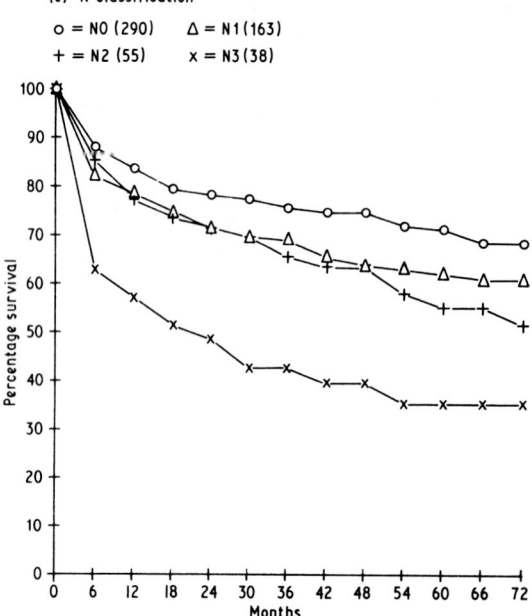

Fig. 15.11 EORTC Thyroid Cancer Data (Byar *et al.*, 1979) (*a*) age groups; (*b*) sex; (*c*) cell type; (*d*) T classification; (*e*) node classification.

points brought out were that anaplastic carcinoma seemed to be universally lethal within three years; that non-invasive follicular, occult and intrathyroid papillary, and medullary carcinoma without nodal involvement all had almost normal expectations of life; but that invasive follicular carcinoma, medullary carcinoma with nodal involvement, and extrathyroid papillary carcinoma had a bad prognosis, 10-year survival being about 35%, 40% and 55% respectively (Fig. 15.10).

The importance of age and sex in prognosis has been stressed since 1966 (Halnan, 1966). It was confirmed by Doll (1969) and more recently has been very well shown by the European Organisation for Research on the Treatment of Cancer Thyroid Study Group. This EORTC group has collected over 1400 cases all with histological review and follow-up (Byar *et al.*, 1979) (Fig. 15.11). It is shown that there is a steady fall in survival as age increases, from over 90% at six years for children, down to under 25% for the over 65 year age group; and that women survive conspicuously better than men. Similar weight is given to histological classification as suggested by the Mayo Clinic but in addition follicular carcinoma can be usefully subdivided into well and less well differentiated. It is also shown that the prognosis for mixed tumours depends upon the presence of the worst prognostic category cells, whether those be the majority or minority cell

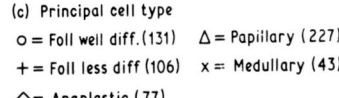

(c) Principal cell type
o = Foll well diff.(131)   Δ = Papillary (227)
+ = Foll less diff (106)   x = Medullary (43)
◇ = Anaplastic (77)

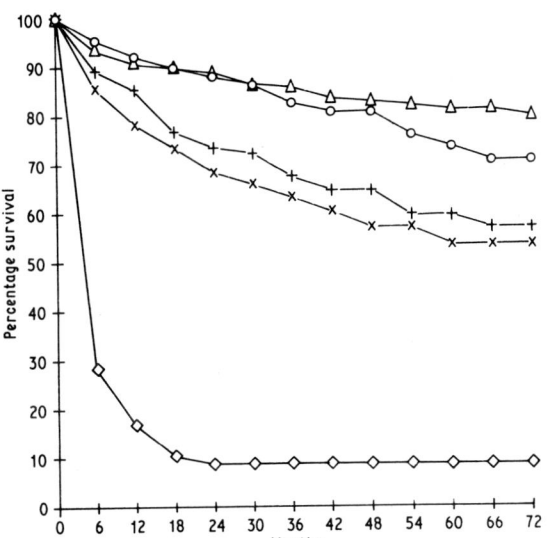

(d) T classification
o = T0 (71)   Δ = T1 (125)
+ = T2 (212)   x = T3 (110)

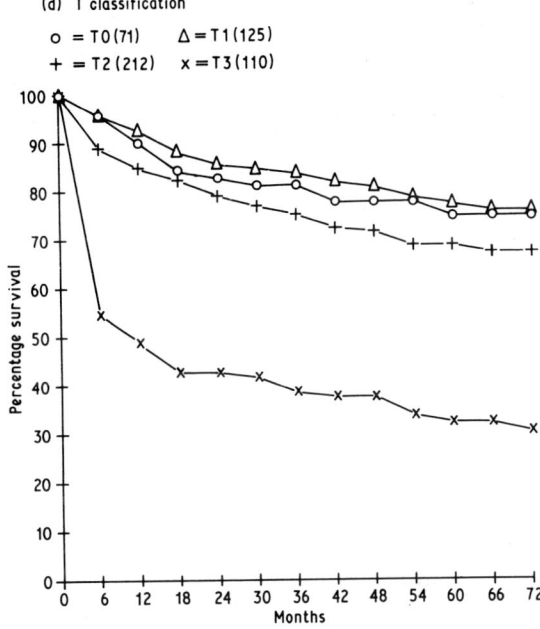

component of the tumour. T_0, T_1 and T_2 primary tumours can be grouped together for prognosis, but node involvement does worsen prognosis successively from N_0 to N_3. The presence of distant metastases will obviously worsen prognosis. A prognostic index can be constructed and this is given in detail in the full EORTC report, which is worth further study.

Future trends

Thyroid cancer as an uncommon highly specialized tumour repays referral and study in specialized centres with adequate long-term follow-up. Improvement in the immediate future would seem to come from continued good surgery, and radiotherapy (including radioiodine treatment) but even more from better localization and control from thyroglobulin and calcitonin measurement. The worst prognosis tumour, anaplastic carcinoma, has no useful tumour marker but may benefit from adjuvant chemotherapy, the field of treatment with perhaps most promise. Immunotherapy is as yet an unexplored field.

Prevention of thyroid cancer will gain from two small contributions – further reduction of unnecessary radiation to the thyroid in infants and children, and the detection of medullary carcinoma in the pre-malignant stage by calcitonin screening in affected families. However, it could be said that this will encourage the spread of the gene responsible for the disease, preventing natural selection.

Prevention in the wider sense does not at present seem practicable when we are not even certain of the role of iodine in causation, though the wider use of iodized salt seems to be elementary harmless good preventive medicine that should have been introduced years ago; it may on the other hand be increasing the proportion of papillary carcinoma. It remains likely that if we could cure or prevent all thyroid cancer we should be able to control all cancer.

Further reading

Duncan, W. (ed.) (1980), *Thyroid Cancer*. Royal College of Radiologists Symposium, Springer, London and Berlin.

Halnan, K.E. (1964), The metabolism of radio-iodine and radiation dosage in man. *Br. J. Radiol.*, 37, 101-7.

Hedinger, C. (ed.) (1959), *Thyroid Cancer*. UICC Monograph 12, Springer, Berlin.

Meissner, W.A. and Warren, S. (1969), Tumours of the Thyroid Gland. *Atlas of Tumour Pathology*, Second series, Fascicle 4. Armed Forces institute of Pathology, Washington, DC, USA.

Smithers, D.W. (ed.) (1970), *Tumours of the Thyroid Gland*. Livingstone, London.

Taylor, S. (ed.) (1981), Progress in the treatment of

thyroid cancer. *World J. of Surg.*, **5**, 1-84.

Werner, S.C. and Ingbar, S.H. (eds) (1978), *The Thyroid*. 4th edn, Harper and Rowe, New York and London.

References

Annls. Radiol. (1977), Symp. Thyroid Cancer, **20** (8), 695-866.

Barrowman, J.S. *et al.* (1975), Diarrhoea in thyroid medullary carcinoma, *Br. Med. J.*, **1**, 11-12.

Byar, D.P. *et al.* (1979), A prognostic index for thyroid carcinoma – an EORTC study. *Eur. J. Cancer*, **15**, 1033-42.

De Lellis, R.A. *et al.* (1978), CEA as a tissue marker in medullary thyroid carcinoma. *New Engl. J. Med.*, **299**, 1082.

Devine, R.M. *et al.* (1981), Primary lymphoma of the thyroid. *World J. of Surg.*, **5**, 33-8.

Doll, R. (1969), Results of treatment of thyroid cancer. In: *Thyroid Cancer* (ed. C.E. Hedinger), Springer, Berlin, p. 309-12.

Durie, B.G.M. *et al.* (1981), High risk thyroid cancer: prolonged survival with early multimodality therapy. *Cancer Clin. Trials*, **4**, 67-74.

Edmonds, C.J., Hayes, S., Kermode, J.C. and Thompson, B.D. (1977), Measurement of serum TSH and thyroid hormones in the management and treatment of thyroid carcinoma with radio-iodine. *Br. J. Radiol.*, **50**, 799-807.

thyroid nodules. *Ann. Intern. Med.*, **87**, 265-9.

Gerfo, P.L. *et al.* (1977), Serum thyroglobulin and recurrent thyroid cancer. *Lancet*, **1**, 881-2.

Gershengorn, M.C. *et al.* (1977), Fine needle aspiration cytology in the pre-operative diagnosis of thyroid nodules. *Ann. Intern. Med.* **87**, 265-9.

Graze, K. *et al.* (1978), Natural history of familial medullary thyroid cancer. *New Engl. J. Med.*, **299**, 980-5.

Halnan, K.E. (1966), Influence of age and sex on thyroid cancer. *Cancer*, **19**, 1534-6.

Halnan, K.E. and Roberts, P.H. (1967), Paraplegia caused by spinal metastases from thyroid cancer. *Br. Med. J.*, **3**, 534-6.

Hawk, W.A. *et al.* (1966), Needle biopsy of the thyroid gland. *Surgery, Gynec. Obstet.*, **122**, 1053-5.

Hedinger, C. and Sobin, L.H. (1974), Histological typing of thyroid tumours. *International Histological Classification of Tumours*, No. 11. WHO, Geneva.

Mazzaferi, *et al.* (1981) Papillary thyroid carcinoma: 10 years follow up of the impact of therapy in 576 patients. *Am. J. Med.*, **70**, 511-8.

Meissner, W.A. and Warren, S. (1969), Tumours of the Thyroid Gland. *Atlas of Tumour Pathology*, Second series, Fascicle 4. Armed Forces Institute of Pathology, Washington DC, USA.

Schimke, R.N. (1976), Multiple endocrine adenomatous syndrome. *Adv. Intern. Med.*, **21**, 249-65.

Schottenfeld, D. and Gershman, S.T. (1977), Epidemiology of thyroid cancer. *Cancer Bull.*, **7** (2), 47-54 and (3), 98-104.

Smithers, D.W. (ed.) (1970), *Tumours of the Thyroid Gland*. Livingstone, London.

Telenius-Berg, M. (1976), Diagnostic studies in medullary thyroid carcinoma. *Acta Med. Scand.*, Supplement 597.

Thomas, C.G. and Burns, S.D. (1961), Studies on the dependency of thyroid cancer. In: *Advances in Thyroid Research* (ed. R. Pitt-Rivers), Permagon, London, p.350.

Van Herle, A.J. and Uller, R.P. (1975), Elevated serum thyroglobulin, a marker of metastases in differentiated thyroid carcinoma. *J. Clin. Invest.*, **56**, 272-7.

Wang, C.A., Vickery, A.L.Jr. and Maloof, F. (1974), Needle biopsy of the thyroid. *Surgery, Gynec. Obstet.*, **143**, 363-5.

Werner, S.C. (ed.) (1955), *The Thyroid*. P.B. Hoeber, New York.

Williams, E.D. *et al.* (1977), Thyroid cancer in an iodide rich area. *Cancer*, **39**, 215-22.

Winship, T. and Rosvoll, R.V. (1970), Thyroid carcinoma in childhood: final report on a 20 year study. *Clin. Proc.*, Children's Hospital, Washington, **36**, 327-48.

Woolner, L.B. *et al.* (1966), Primary malignant lymphoma of the thyroid. *Am. J. Surg.*, **4**, 502-23.

Woolner, L.B. *et al.* (1968), Thyroid carcinoma: general considerations and follow-up data on 1181 cases. In: *Thyroid Neoplasia* (eds I. Young and D.R. Inman), Academic Press, London, pp. 51-76.

16 Breast

William Duncan

Incidence

Cancer of the breast is the most common form of malignant disease occurring in women over the age of 40 years in the Western world. In the United States each year over 90 000 women are found to have breast cancer. About 6% of women in the United Kingdom will develop breast cancer, the present incidence being about 50 per 100 000 population. The prevalence of the disease is reported to be low in developing countries and is relatively uncommon in China and Japan, and certain communities such as the Parsi in Bombay. The incidence of the disease increases to a maximum at about 45 years of age, decreasing rapidly after the age of 65 years.

Breast cancer is rare in men, the incidence being 1% of that of women, and accounts for only 0.2% of all cancer in men.

Aetiology

In spite of its prevalence the definitive causes of breast cancer remain elusive, in part because of the many interrelated factors that contribute to its development (Bulbrook et al., 1980).

Race may be of importance, for the mortality rates from breast cancer are amongst the highest in the Western world (Segi et al., 1969) whereas in Japan the mortality is only about 30% of that in the United Kingdom. In the United States, female breast cancer is more common in whites than non-whites, and in Jews rather than non-Jewish races (Wynder, 1968).

Breast cancer is more common among higher social classes, and the relative incidences in different races may reflect variations in socioeconomic factors and perhaps their diet.

Endocrine influences have also been carefully considered in the aetiology of breast cancer. The increased risk in nulliparous women is well recognized. Significant protection against the disease is apparent only in women with larger than average families, that is over four children, in the study of MacMahon et al. (1968).

It was thought that the low incidence of breast cancer associated with high parity may primarily be related to prolonged breast feeding, but this has not been borne out by more detailed studies. There seems no doubt that an extremely important factor is the age at first pregnancy (MacMahon et al., 1970). Women who have their first child when over the age of 30 years have a threefold increased risk of developing breast cancer than women who have their first child under the age of 20 years.

The incidence of disease increases until about the time of the menopause, when it levels off and then declines. Premature induction of the menopause would seem to protect against the development of breast cancer. The administration of exogenous hormones, such as contraceptive pills, has been studied in some detail in relation to the subsequent development of breast cancer. At present there is no evidence that women who take the contraceptive pill have an increased risk (Kay, 1981; Vessey et al., 1981). Indeed there may be some protective effect, possibly akin to the protection thought to be afforded by early pregnancy. It is now accepted that breast size does not have any influence on the probability of developing the disease.

There is a strong familial tendency to develop the disease. Daughters of women with breast cancer have a probability of developing the disease some fifteen times greater than the general population. Other female relatives also carry an increased tendency to develop breast cancer. It is now thought that these familial factors may be mediated through hormonal mechanisms (Henderson et al., 1974).

There is no evidence that a viral agent transmits breast cancer in the human population.

Male breast cancer is much less common (100-fold); its incidence may be related to hormonal changes and is particularly high in patients with Klinefelter's syndrome (47XXY).

Anatomy and lymph drainage

The female breast lies superficial to the pectoralis

major and serratus anterior muscles, from the second to the sixth ribs, and from the lateral border of the sternum to the mid-axillary line. The axillary tail of Spence is an extension of breast tissue superolaterally up to the level of the third rib in the axilla. It enters the axilla through the foramen of Langu in the axillary fascia.

The breast is a modified sebaceous gland which consists of 12 – 20 lobules. From each lobule runs a duct leading to an ampulla situated deep to the nipple and from which minute ducts lead to the nipple. The gland is normally an irregular hemisphere supported by fibrous septa (ligaments of Cooper) which join the superficial fascia and the lobules of the breast to the deep fascia.

The glandular tissue consists of cuboidal epithelium and the ducts of columnar epithelium. Both are enclosed by two fibrous layers, an inner periductal or periacinar layer and an outer perilobular tissue. The whole gland is surrounded by varying amounts of fat which usually increase with age.

The lymphatic vessels drain the breast substance and the overlying skin, including the areola and nipple (Fig. 16.1). The skin lymphatics are arranged radially and end in surrounding groups of nodes. The vessels on the lateral aspect go to the principal axillary lymph nodes. Those of the skin of the upper part may also proceed directly to the supra-clavicular nodes. From the skin of the medial aspect of the breast the lymph vessels run to the internal mammary nodes and also across the midline to join those overlying the opposite breast. It is invasion of these superficial lymphatics that commonly gives rise to discrete nodular cutaneous recurrences of

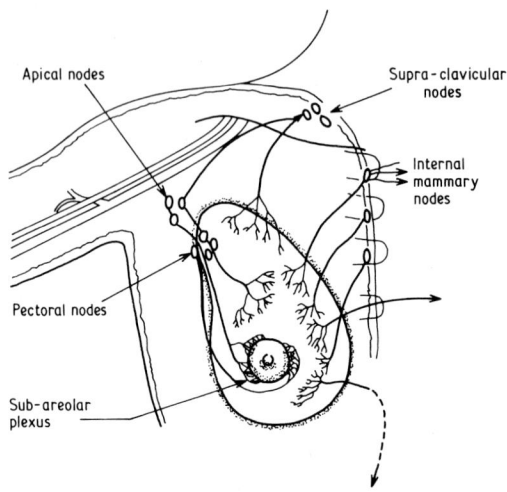

Fig. 16.1　Schematic diagram of the lymphatic drainage of the breast.

tumour. The lymphatic vessels of the nipple and areola join the sub-areolar lymph plexus of Sappey, which then drains to the axillary lymph nodes.

Most lymph vessels from the glandular tissues of the breast lobules drain laterally through the substance of the breast to the axillary lymph nodes, passing to sub-pectoral nodes in the axillary tail. Lymph vessels from the deep surface of the gland also pass through the pectoralis major muscle to the axillary or internal mammary groups of lymph nodes. Lymph vessels from the whole breast enter the internal mammary nodes by following the internal mammary artery and branches of the intercostal blood vessels. At the superior ends of the internal mammary groups of nodes there are fine lymphatic vessels which link the two sides together.

Lymph vessels from the lower and inner quadrant of the breast may pass inferiorly and join the sub-peritoneal lymph plexus in the abdomen. This lymphatic pathway has been suggested to explain the observed clinical spread of breast cancer, rather than being based on conventional anatomical descriptions.

Natural history and metastases

Most patients with breast cancer become aware of a painless lump in the breast. The tumour is more common in the left breast than the right, and more frequently in the outer than the inner half of the breast. The disease may be found to be multifocal in the breast, but usually presents as a single tumour mass. Slow enlargement and local infiltration of the breast substance, ligaments of Cooper and deep fascia are features of progression of disease.

Lymphatic spread is common and up to 75% of patients with apparently 'early' disease will have axillary lymph nodes involved. The number of axillary lymph nodes involved by tumour has an important relation to prognosis. Patients with less then four nodes involved have a better survival rate than when more are invaded (Fisher *et al.*, 1976). The degree of involvement is a good indication of the presence of distant metastases and of internal mammary node involvement. Metastases may also occur to the internal mammary nodes and, if the skin overlying the upper half of the breast is involved, directly to the supra-clavicular nodes.

Haematogenous spread is also common, often occurring early in the natural history of the disease. Recognition of this fact frequently determines the treatment policy in so-called early disease. The most commonly involved distant sites are the skeleton, lungs and the liver, but of course most other organs can at some time be the site of metastases.

Bone is the commonest site of metastases, most often the pelvis and lumbar spine. Other sites in relative frequency are the thoracic spine, sacrum, humerus, scapula and clavicle. These metastases are usually osteolytic, but 5–10% may be osteoblastic. However, widespread intertrabecular metastases in the bone marrow can occur without any radiological changes.

Lung metastases from breast cancer may be demonstrated radiographically in two forms. The more common is the appearance of discrete nodular metastates in the lung fields. The second appears as diffuse infiltration, caused by retrograde infiltration of disease into the peribronchial lymphatics, i.e. lymphangitis carcinomatosis.

Pathology and classification

The World Health Organisation classification by Scarff and Torloni (1968) is the one most commonly used. Carcinoma of the breast arises usually from the epithelium of the ducts, but occasionally can originate within the epithelium of the acini of the lobules.

Non-invasive breast cancer

A number of non-invasive carcinomas are recognized and are of obvious clinical importance. Intraduct carcinoma usually distends the lumen of the duct. A variant is the comedocarcinoma in which the central mass of tumour cells has degenerated leaving a peripheral zone of viable cells. The lumen is filled mainly by debris which can often be expressed from the ducts. Two other forms of intraduct carcinoma are described – the adenoid cystic carcinoma and the papillary carcinoma. The latter may have a vascular core that sometimes shows evidence of infiltration by tumour cells. Lobular carcinoma is extremely rare and arises in the breast lobules as an epithelial overgrowth showing marked cellular pleomorphism.

Invasive breast cancer

Most breast cancers (80–90%) can be described as scirrhous adenocarcinomas. Characteristically, on palpation, the tumour is very hard with an irregular outline. The scirrhous carcinoma is so-called because of its dense fibrocollagenous stroma, in which are embedded strands of malignant epithelial cells. Elastosis may be a prominent feature in the stroma – this is positively correlated with prognosis. The tumour cells are usually uniform, round or polyhedral with small nuclei and few mitoses.

Medullary carcinoma is uncommon, accounting for only 4 or 5% of breast cancers. It tends to be seen in younger women and presents commonly as a large but well circumscribed tumour. It has a soft consistency, often with areas of haemorrhage and necrosis. Microscopically it is composed of highly cellular areas of tumour with little fibrous stroma. The areas of large polygonal tumour cells are frequently surrounded by varying degrees of lymphocytic infiltration.

Mucoid or colloid carcinoma of the breast is also an uncommon form of breast cancer (2 or 3%). It usually presents as an extremely bulky, well circumscribed, and sometimes fluctuant tumour. Microscopically it is a well differentiated adenocarcinoma in which there are large cystic spaces. The small cancer cells have a signet-ring appearance because of mucinous material filling the cytoplasm and pushing the nucleus aside.

Squamous cell carcinoma is a rare tumour of the breast, but when present is usually well differentiated.

Paget's disease is an ulcerated lesion of the nipple, which later becomes indurated and may be eroded by tumour. A tumour is often palpable deep to the nipple, and Paget's disease is always associated with either an infiltrating duct carcinoma or an *in-situ* duct carcinoma.

Sarcoma of the breast is also very rare (1%). It is commonly a spindle-cell tumour, but it can have a wide range of appearances. About 40% arise from a pre-existing fibroadenoma, and the age of incidence is similar to that of carcinoma. However, the prognosis is very much better than for adenocarcinoma of similar clinical stage, deaths from sarcoma being unusual more than 5 years after treatment.

Oestrogen receptors in breast cancer

It has been recognized for many years that breast cancer may localize injected oestrogens, and more recently that hormone-dependent tumours concentrate oestrogens more than tumours unresponsive to hormones. The present understanding of these findings is that a cytoplasmic protein known as an oestrogen receptor is responsible for the specific uptake of oestrogens in normal breast and in breast cancer tissue.

Evaluation of the activity of hormone receptors as an index of response of treatment with either hormone administration or endocrine ablation is clearly of clinical importance. A number of *in vitro* tests have been developed and their value is beginning to be demonstrated (McGuire *et al.*, 1975).

The concentration of oestrogen receptors in human breast cancer varies greatly from 0 to over 1000 fmol/mg cytoplasmic protein. Variations may be due to heterogeneity in the tumour cell population, or to high circulating oestrogen levels which may saturate existing receptors. Certainly oestrogen receptors are less commonly found in pre-menopausal women (30%) compared to post-menopausal patients (60%) who have reduced oestrogen levels. It is now considered that the higher the oestrogen receptor assay the greater the probability of hormone dependence. However, about one-third of patients with oestrogen receptor-positive tumours will not respond to hormone therapy. It is now recognized that differences in the concentration of oestrogen receptors reflect biological differences in breast cancers, such as growth characteristics, and may be an important prognostic variable. It has, for example, been reported that recurrences after primary surgery for breast cancer, with or without involved axillary nodes, are more frequent in patients with oestrogen receptor-negative tumours. It has also been claimed that oestrogen receptor-negative tumours respond better to cytotoxic chemotherapy, but conflicting reports have been published and the correlation remains controversial.

Other steroid hormone receptors, such as progesterone, may be assayed and the definitive clinical role of hormone receptor assay requires to be carefully evaluated. Endocrine therapy has been discussed in more detail in Chapter 6, as well as below.

Breast screening

There is no doubt that the earlier the diagnosis can be made the better the prognosis in breast cancer (Duncan and Kerr, 1976). The acceptance of this principle provides the rationale for establishing screening clinics for women at most risk, to increase the likelihood of detecting the disease at an early stage. Essentially this means the diagnosis of breast cancers less than 3 cm in diameter with no evidence of spread beyond the breast.

Evidence of the benefit of organized community-based screening has been provided by the study of the Health Insurance Plan (HIP) in Greater New York (Strax, 1977). In this study 62 000 women aged between 40 and 64 years were randomly selected into a control (unscreened) group, and a study group. Over two-thirds of the women selected for the screening programme agreed to cooperate, which involved the first examination and three annual follow-up assessments. The assessments included physical examination of the breast and mammography. It is important to note that 33% of cancers detected by mammography were not found on palpation, and 40% of the cancers found by palpation were not recognized by mammography. Obviously both should be used. It is interesting also to note that mammography, when compared with palpation to detect axillary node involvement, showed that the percentage of patients with negative findings in both groups (about 76%) were statistically equivalent. Another important finding of the HIP study was that about 15% of the cancers detected occurred within twelve months following a screening examination.

The result of this screening programme has been a reduction of the mortality rate from breast cancer in the study group by one-third, but this improvement has been seen only in the population of women over the age of 50 years. Other studies have confirmed the benefits of breast screening and provided results that are closely similar to the HIP programme (Strax, 1978). Very large numbers of women have now been screened, and the fact that almost 14% of the growths detected were under 1.0 cm in diameter must surely eventually be reflected by excellent long-term survival rates.

The results of the HIP screening programme obviously raise the question as to whether it is justifiable to screen women under the age of 50 years by physical examination and mammography. Certainly women under the age of 35 years have a low probability of having breast cancer, and 35 years should be the lower age limit for entry to screening programmes. At the present time it would seem that between 35 and 50 years only those women with a strong family history or with previous breast cancer should be screened in this way.

A major source of concern is the possible carcinogenic risk from use of mammography, because of the X-ray exposure of the breast. Recognition of this small but potential hazard has led to the development of new techniques. The radiation dose to the skin over the breast has been reduced to about 0.3 rad, and to the centre of the breast about 0.03 rad for each examination. It has been estimated that 1 rad to the breast tissue of a million women would produce 6 cancers of the breast per year after a latent period of about 6–10 years (Upton, 1978). Therefore if 10 million women in the age group at risk over a span of 25 years were to be screened by mammography using the best techniques now available, (giving about 0.025 rad to the breast each year) the risk would amount to about 36 induced breast cancers. This very small theoretical increase in incidence has to be compared with the 25 000 breast cancers that one would expect to detect in that population of women over the same period of time. But most importantly there is also the possible saving of about 3000 additional lives by the reduction in death rate, providing the results of the Hospital Insurance Plan study can be reproduced.

The possible benefits of mammography seem clear enough, but one has to ensure that women can be motivated to attend screening clinics regularly. Patients at risk for breast cancer are concerned not only with the diagnosis, but also with the mutilating effects of treatment and its efficacy. It would seem that greater evaluation of techniques that conserve the breast in early breast cancer, and the confirmation that they provide as good survival rates as mastectomy, may well contribute greatly to obtaining the continuing cooperation of women in screening campaigns. Self-examination of the breast should also be encouraged. The fact that most women have a palpable lump in the breast at diagnosis, must indicate that self-examination should not be ignored while the development of breast screening clinics is promoted.

Clinical staging of breast cancer

The TNM classification and stage grouping proposed originally in 1954 by the Union Internationale Contre le Cancer (UICC) should be used. In 1978 the latest UICC classification of breast cancer was published (Tables 16.1, 16.2) and this version should apply for at least the next ten years.

The system applies only to histologically confirmed invasive carcinomas of the breast. The T-categories are normally determined by physical examination, but mammography should be used in addition to clinical assessment of size. The N-category (the lymph nodes) are assessed by clinical palpation. Clinicians are

Table 16.1 TNM classification of breast cancer.

Primary tumour mass

T_1	$\leq$ 2 cm	(a) without fixation to pectoral fascia or
T_2	> 2–5 cm	muscle
T_3	> 5 cm	(b) with fixation
T_4	Any size with extention to chest wall/skin	
	(a) chest wall; (b) skin	

Regional (ipsilateral) lymph nodes

N_1	Mobile axillary (a) not considered malignant
	(b) considered metastatic
N_2	Fixed axillary, to each other or other structures
N_3	Supra-clavicular or infra-clavicular or internal mammary or oedema of the arm

Distant metastases

M_0	No evidence of distant metastases
M_1	Evidence of distant metastases

Table 16.2 TNM stage grouping of breast cancer.

Stage I	T_1	N_0, N_{1a}		M_0
Stage II	T_1		N_{1b}	M_0
	T_2	N_0, N_{1a}, N_{1b}		M_0
Stage IIIa	T_3	N_0, N_{1a}, N_{1b}		M_0
	T_1, T_2, T_3	N_2		M_0
Stage IIIb	T_1, T_2, T_3	N_3		M_0
	T_4	Any N		M_0
Stage IV	Any T	Any N		M_1

required to guess, or judge as some may prefer, whether or not enlarged nodes are involved by tumour. This is a highly inaccurate exercise that hardly seems justified except in advanced disease.

The M-categories, indicating the presence or absence of distant metastases, may be assessed by the use of diagnostic radiographic techniques in addition to physical examination. No guidance is given about what radiological investigations should normally be undertaken. It is clear that the thoroughness of investigation and sophistication of the techniques employed will vary considerably, and this may introduce important differences in the stage grouping of patients in different centres.

In addition, more detailed classification may be undertaken after surgery, and the T N M symbols should then be prefixed at pT_1 and so on. If the tumour has been histologically graded the classification G_1, G_2 or G_3 may be added, indicating well differentiated, moderate and poorly differentiated tumours respectively.

It is essential that clinicians who intend to use this system should study the UICC booklet, reading first the principles and general rules before considering the section providing the detailed classification of breast cancer.

Pre-treatment assessment

A complete physical examination is necessary with detailed care being given to the clinical examination of the breast and regional lymph nodes. Classification and stage grouping according to the International Staging System should be completed when histology has confirmed the diagnosis of carcinoma. Biopsy may be successfully carried out using a needle biopsy or drill. This allows paraffin sections to be prepared, and on confirmation of the diagnosis the patient can be told if mastectomy is necessary. If out-patient biopsy fails then open biopsy should be performed with frozen section before mastectomy.

Clinical assessment of axillary lymph node involvement is difficult and highly unreliable. It has been demonstrated from several series of patients treated by radical mastectomy that about 40% of those with no palpable nodes will have histological evidence of axillary metastases. By comparison about 20% of patients with palpable axillary nodes will have histologically negative nodes. It is only when axillary nodes are large and hard (perhaps by fixation showing evidence of extracapsular spread as well) that metastatic involvement can be reliably assumed. Otherwise confirmation of axillary node involvement requires to be made by biopsy and histological examination (Forrest *et al.*, 1976).

Table 16.3 Relationship of axillary and internal mammary lymph node involvement to clinical features of breast cancer (from Hughes and Forbes, 1978).

Clinical features	Percentage histologically positive	
	Axillary nodes	Internal mammary nodes
Axillary nodes		
Impalpable	36	20
Palpable	79	33
Large ± fixation	97	50
Primary tumour		
Less than 5 cm	43	19
Greater than 5 cm	61	45
Inner quadrant	–	30
Outer quadrant	–	15

The examination of the supra-clavicular nodes is of more value. When enlarged the chances of metastatic involvement are high, but biopsy should be considered when significant doubt remains. The internal mammary nodes cannot of course be examined clinically, but the probability of involvement may be assessed from the site and size of the primary tumour and from confirmation of axillary node involvement (Table 16.3). It may be possible to visualize the internal mammary node chain by lymphoscintigraphy, but this technique is not yet of established value.

As the clinical T and N stage increases, the probability of occult distant metastases increases from about 20% in patients with Stage I disease to over 70% in patients with Stage III disease. As the most common sites of metastases from breast cancer are the bones, lungs and liver, pre-treatment assessment must particularly be directed to identifying metastases in these organs.

Radiographic examination of the pelvis and chest are part of the minimum pre-treatment assessment. Bone scintigraphy may be highly desirable, but there is no general agreement about its value in patients with T_1 and T_2 cancers. There is a wide range of positive bone scans, from 2% to over 35% in such patients, and these differences are disturbing. There is no uniform opinion as to how any evidence of abnormal focal increase in activity should influence management of the 'operable' tumour if conventional radiographs do not confirm metastases. Certainly some areas of abnormal uptake may be due to benign disease. Many clinicians would discount the positive bone scan if radiology showed no abnormality and would decide

management accordingly. It has to be recognized too that bone scintigraphy will fail to show a number of small bone defects under 2 cm in diameter. Excretion of nuclide in the urine may also obscure metastases in the pubis, ischium and sacrum and be a source of error.

In an attempt to define the presence of bony metastases more accurately, estimations of the urinary excretion of hydroxyproline or the hydroxyproline/creatinine ratio may be measured (Cuschieri, 1975). This is laborious and although the significance of abnormal excretion ratios has been confirmed, the estimation is too complicated to be accepted as a routine clinical investigation.

It would seem prudent for bilateral mammography to be performed in all patients, since the disease is bilateral at presentation in about 0.5%. Liver scan and ultra-sonography are normally not advised, since the detection rate of metastases is low. CT brain scanning cannot be advised for routine screening since only about 2% of women with advanced disease, but without neurological features, show cerebral abnormalities by this technique.

Treatment of early breast cancer

In the last few years there has been increasing emphasis on more conservative forms of local treatment of the primary tumour, and a more radical approach to adjuvant systemic management of occult metastatic disease.

The number of possible therapeutic approaches is extremely large, and many clinical trials have been conducted or are presently designed to attempt to define optimum management (Stewart, 1977). Many of these studies have failed to provide conclusive answers, because of the diversity of treatment combinations, the complexity of prognostic factors involved, and because of the long natural history of the disease. The limited contribution of clinical trials to influence management has been ably assessed by Fisher (1973) and by Hughes and Forbes (1978). It is essential to employ well established techniques of local management in the care of a patient with an early tumour (primary under 3.0 cm and no involvement of axillary nodes).

Surgery of operable disease

Lumpectomy *alone* for invasive breast cancer must carry a high probability of local recurrence because of the frequent multifocal nature of the disease. One cause for concern is the claim that recurrence after this operation will be deep and thus present as inoperable disease fixed to the chest wall (Hughes and Forbes, 1978). The addition of post-operative radiotherapy is considered advisable, and the technique and dose must be adequate to produce a low probability of recurrence in the breast and in the axilla (*vide infra*). Adjuvant chemotherapy has been given following lumpectomy, but one small study was discontinued because of the high local recurrence rate (Hancock *et al.*, 1976).

Simple mastectomy also carries a high risk of recurrence in the axilla. About one-third of patients with impalpable axillary nodes will have histologically positive nodes. The King's/Cambridge Trial in the United Kingdom has demonstrated to date, in patients treated by simple mastectomy alone, a 28% local/axillary recurrence in Stage I cases and 53% in those with Stage II disease (Hughes and Forbes, 1978). It is acknowledged that recurrent lymph node disease in the axilla is often much more difficult to control than axillary lymph node metastases at first presentation. The outstanding deficiency of the simple mastectomy technique is that sampling of the axillary nodes is not normally undertaken. Forrest *et al.* (1976) have recommended that a group of pectoral nodes in the axillary tail of the breast should routinely be dissected, excised and sent for histology.

Radical mastectomy has for a long time been performed as the standard operation for early breast cancer since first used by Halsted (1894). Certainly recurrence in the axilla is less than 3% for all stages of operable disease, and is lower than following other techniques. The recurrence rates in the chest wall should be no greater than 10% for Stage I and II cases, but in patients with operable Stage III disease over 25% may have breast flap recurrences in the first five years. It has of course been shown that the routine addition of post-operative radiotherapy following radical mastectomy does not improve survival rates. The morbidity after radical mastectomy alone is not inconsiderable, and Patey and Dyson (1948) many years ago proposed a useful modification in which the pectoralis major muscle is preserved. This gives a much improved cosmetic result, but dissection of the axilla is more difficult and the probability of axillary recurrence is higher than after a standard radical mastectomy.

A supra-radical surgical approach has been advocated in which the internal mammary node chain is dissected in addition to radical axillary clearance. This extended operation has been shown to benefit significantly, in terms of increased survival, patients with Stage I and II cancers, but only in the 13% of tumours situated in the inner quadrant of the breast (Lacour *et al.*, 1976). In the group of patients treated by supra-radical mastectomy (of whom 32% had histologically involved internal mammary nodes) the 5-year survival was 71% compared with 52% following the standard radical mastectomy. However, the supra-radical operation has a much higher morbidity than radical mastectomy, and

these results may not be easily repeated; the use of adjuvant radiotherapy may well be more advisable for patients with inner quadrant tumours.

Breast reconstruction after surgery

Many surgeons now consider using a reconstructive procedure after mastectomy to improve the emotional well-being of the patient. These techniques are usually offered only to patients with Stage I disease. Some surgeons would advise waiting twelve months after primary treatment before undertaking reconstruction. Reconstruction involves elaborate plastic surgery using myocutaneous flap techniques and nipple formation or a more simple rhomboid flap rotation. Plastic prosthesis may be implanted sub-pectorally or subcutaneously quite simply, and provides remarkably good cosmetic end-results. Such implants may extrude in about 10% of cases, and other complications of reconstructive surgery can occur. Patients obviously must be selected very carefully for reconstruction or prosthetic replacement and a critical evaluation of these procedures is still required.

Psychiatric problems after mastectomy

It has been demonstrated that the emotional disturbances of women after mastectomy can be considerable. Indeed about 25% of women one year after mastectomy have been found to be seriously depressed or anxious (Maguire *et al.*, 1978). This is not surprising when one considers the recognized loss of femininity, self-esteem and security that a women suffers in accepting mastectomy for breast cancer. There is a need for the medical and nursing team to be aware of and take account of these serious problems during the follow-up period.

Primary treatment by irradiation

In 1936 Baclesse began studies of the management of primary breast cancer by irradiation at the Foundation Curie in Paris (Baclesse, 1949). Calle *et al.* (1978) have recently reviewed their experience over the last ten years using radiotherapy. The policy has involved lumpectomy followed by radiotherapy, when the primary tumour is staged T_1 or T_2 N_0 and is no larger than 3.0 cm in diameter. Patients with larger (T_2 or T_3) primary cancers and clinically significant nodes (N_{1b}) were managed by radiotherapy alone.

The radiation used is mainly cobalt-60 γ rays, with the addition of smaller electron fields in selected patients. The breast and regional lymph node area is given 5000 rad over 6 weeks with an additional 1500 rad to the lumpectomy site, and 1000 rad to the lower axilla in the same overall time. In the more advanced cases, in whom the primary tumour has not been removed, the tumour mass is given a total of 7500–8500 rad at 1000 rad per week. If there are palpable nodes in the axilla they too are given an additional dose to about 7000 rad over 7 weeks. It is claimed that this treatment gives excellent cosmetic results in 60% of patients as well as good tumour control in the earlier cases. The excellent survival rates also compare favourably with the results of primary surgery (Table 16.4). The results of radiotherapy in the larger T₂, T₃ tumours are not so good. The cancer persisted in about 60% of cases and only 30% survived with the breast retained and free of tumour. Of these the cosmetic effect was considered to be good in less than one-third of patients.

Similar trials are now in progress which will soon provide data to indicate better the place of primary radiotherapy in early breast cancer (Veronesi *et al.*, 1981; Levine *et al.*, 1978), promising early results have been reported (Veronesi *et al.*, 1981).

Adjuvant radiotherapy

In order to reduce the morbidity associated with radical mastectomy, McWhirter (1948) introduced the combined technique of simple mastectomy and radical radiotherapy. The objective of radical adjuvant radiotherapy is to irradiate the involved breast and chest wall together with the axillary, supra-clavicular and ipsi-lateral internal mammary lymph nodes. When there is evidence of involved axillary nodes there is a high probability of chest wall recurrence and of involvement of the internal mammary lymph nodes (see Table 16.3). Recognition of these facts requires that all these areas at risk should usually be included in the irradiated volume.

Most centres now employ megavoltage irradiation in an energy range of 1 to 4 MV (which includes tele-caesium and telecobalt γ-rays). In Edinburgh the original technique of McWhirter (1948), which employed 250 kV X-rays, has been modified for application with

4 MV X-rays (Fig. 16.2). By this regime the internal mammary lymph nodes and chest wall are included in one volume. The medial tangential field (usually 15 x 10 cm) is placed 1.0 cm across the midline so that the ipsi-lateral internal mammary nodes are included in the high dose volume. The lateral tangential field is placed with its posterior edge on the mid-axillary line. The interfield distance (or separation) is usually 16–20 cm.

The axillary and supra-clavicular nodes are treated by two parallel semi-opposed fields positioned anteriorly and posteriorly. The anterior field should have its medial edge on the midline and the posterior field has its superior and medial edges placed so that the spinal cord is not included in the irradiation. The field sizes are normally 20–25 × 10 cm.

A maximum dose of 4250 rad is given in 10 fractions over 4 weeks to the cervicoaxillary fields. On alternate days a maximum dose of 4500 rad is given in 10 fractions in the same overall treatment time to the tangential fields. These are high radiation doses equivalent to NSD values of 1800 and 1700 respectively, and some centres recommend lower doses. It is claimed (Fletcher and Montague, 1978) that an NSD of 1600 will control over 95% of sub-clinical nodal disease in the supra-clavicular fossa. In the axillary region, however, where the probability of involved nodes is on average three times greater than in the supra-clavicular fossa, a dose higher than 1600 rad (NSD) would be advised and 1700 rad (NSD) would seem to represent a generally acceptable maximum tissue dose.

It has been suggested (Fletcher and Montague, 1978) that the dose to the internal mammary nodes is uncertain and may be inadequate using this technique. It is however accepted that even in the most unfavourable circumstances, associated with a medially placed primary tumour and histologically positive axillary nodes, parasternal node recurrences occur in less than 19% of patients. In the Edinburgh clinical trial series no parasternal recurrence has been recorded to date in those treated by simple mastectomy and irradiation. Høst and Brennhovd (1977) have reported a statisti-

Table 16.4 Assessment of results at 5 years of primary radiotherapy for early breast cancer (from Calle *et al.*, 1978).

Primary management	Number	Local recurrence	Survival NED	Survival NED no mastectomy
Lumpectomy and irradiation	120	16 (13.3%)	102 (85%)	96 (80.0%)
Irradiation alone	394	234 (59.4%)	268 (68%)	120 (30.5%)

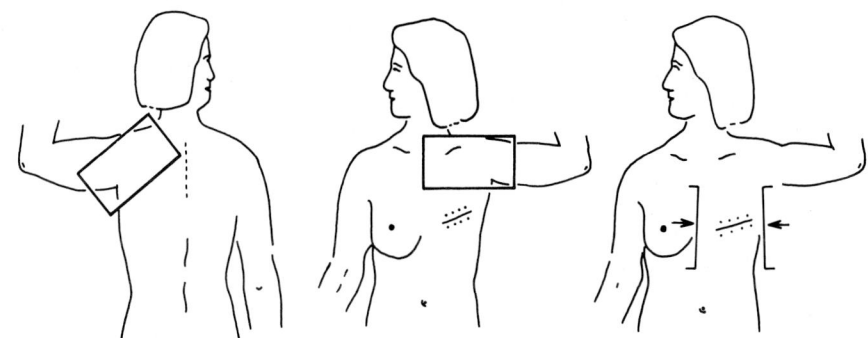

Fig. 16.2 Arrangements of fields employed in the Edinburgh radiotherapy technique.

cally significant improvement in the disease-free survival rates following mastectomy with the addition of post-operative telecobalt radiotherapy to the node areas alone.

Many other techniques have been described; one common variant is to irradiate the internal mammary region by a direct field, sometimes using high energy electrons. Extreme care should be used in treatment planning and dosage should be checked by dosemeters if necessary.

When the breast tumour has not been removed and particularly when the axillary lymph nodes are heavily involved with tumour, it is advisable to irradiate the breast and axillary and supra-clavicular fossa in one volume, and so avoid a junction of irradiation fields in the lower axilla. This may be done by a jig of tissue equivalent plastic through which the shoulder may be passed and on which two parallel opposed fields (usually 30 x 12 cm) may be applied. The jig is filled with bolus material and a maximum tissue dose of 4250 rad may be delivered in 10 fractions over 4 weeks. This dose will control about one-third of these large primary tumours for about one year on average. Some of these patients may later be suitable for simple mastectomy.

Single plane implants of radium needles or iridium wire are used in selected patients. Normally small residual primary tumours have implants to supplement the dose of wide field external beam therapy. The technique may be used in the primary management of early disease (Levine *et al.*, 1978) or to improve local control of locally advanced disease (Pierquin, 1978).

It has frequently been suggested that radiotherapy may unfavourably influence survival rates by depressing the immune system and this hypothesis was developed by Stjernsward (1974). However, the method of analysis has been seriously criticized and the claim is unsubstantiated (see *Cancer* (1977), **39**, 924–40). Indeed in the NSAB trials (Fisher *et al.*, 1978) and the Edinburgh trial comparing radical mastectomy with conservative surgery and radical radiotherapy, the incidence of metastatic disease has been shown to be similar in both groups. Dissemination of disease is not promoted by post-operative radiotherapy.

Adjuvant chemotherapy for early breast cancer

The recognition that many women with apparently early breast cancer, but with axillary nodes involved with tumour, have occult metastatic disease, has led to the introduction of adjuvant chemotherapy for these patients. The first trials evaluated the use of single cytotoxic agents, originally thiotepa and then cyclophosphamide, given as a short course after surgery for the primary tumour (Fisher *et al.*, 1977). Nissen-Meyer *et al.* (1978) have shown in a randomly controlled trial, improved survival rates up to ten years with a reduction in recurrences after a single 6-day course of cyclophosphamide (30 mg/kg total dose). L-phenylalanine mustard (L-PAM) has been given by mouth 0.15 mg/kg/day for 5 days every 6 weeks, for 2 years after mastectomy in 'node-positive' cases. In a randomly controlled trial the recurrence rate was significantly reduced, particularly in pre-menopausal women (Fisher *et al.*, 1977). Increasing evidence suggested that cytotoxic chemotherapy was significantly reducing recurrence rates rather than delaying their appearance. Disease-free survival was increased, the clinicians were encouraged to be more aggressive in their management (Edelstyn, 1978).

Bonadonna *et al.* (1977) then introduced a relatively high dose three-drug regime (CMF) to be given normally in 12 cycles every 28 days:

CMF Regime

Cyclophosphamide	100 mg/m² days 1 to 14	p.o.
Methotrexate	40 mg/m² days 1 and 8	i.v.
5–Fluorouracil	600 mg/m² days 1 and 8	i.v.

The toxicity of this regime was considerable. About 70% of patients suffered hair loss and marked fall in peripheral white blood count or platelets. Only 20% of patients had no toxicity. In this trial of the CMF regime, patients had a radical mastectomy and were found to have positive axillary nodes. The most recent analysis (Rossi *et al.*, 1981) shows a highly significant increase in the relapse-free survival rate at five years in the CMF treated group (55.5%) compared with controls (44.6%). However this difference was accounted for by the improvement seen in pre-menopausal women, there being no significant difference in the results in post-menopausal women. Subsequent analysis has shown that the benefit to pre-menopausal women is not related to CMF-induced amenorrhoea. The efficacy of the regime is dose-related and a higher proportion of pre-menopausal patients received the optimum dose schedule. When optimum doses are given it is claimed post-menopausal women have a relapse-free survival similar to that of the pre-menopausal group (Bonnadonna and Valagussa, 1981).

Endocrine ablation

The recognition of the problem of occult metastatic disease in apparently early cases of breast cancer led to the evaluation of ovarian ablation in pre-menopausal patients. It would seem that radiation ablation of the ovaries is as effective as surgical removal in these patients (Nissen-Meyer, 1976). Nissen-Meyer has also shown in a randomly controlled trial that 'prophylactic' castration gave significantly better tumour-free survival rates than the control group at 15 years and a prolonged tumour-free interval. However the crude survival was the same in both groups. Cole (1976) also conducted a randomly controlled trial of 'prophylactic' X-ray castration in which the crude survival rates in the irradiated group and the control group were similar. There were, however, significantly fewer patients with metastatic disease in the castrated group, and there was a longer disease-free interval after X-ray castration. Meakin *et al.* (1977) have suggested that ovarian irradiation in the pre-menopausal women may prolong survival or delay recurrence but this is not of statistical significance. It is important to note, however, that pre-menopausal women over the age of 45 years who had an X-ray artificial menopause and were also given oral prednisone (2.5 mg t.i.d. for 5 years) had a significant delay in recurrence and an improvement in survival (Fig. 16.3).

Ovarian ablation performed either by surgery or by irradiation after primary management of early breast cancer does influence the course of the disease. The influence is small and the therapeutic benefits of ovarian ablation may be obtained if performed when recurrence is detected. Most clinicians do not advise the use of 'prophylactic' ovarian ablation, although the possible benefit of the addition of prednisone indicated

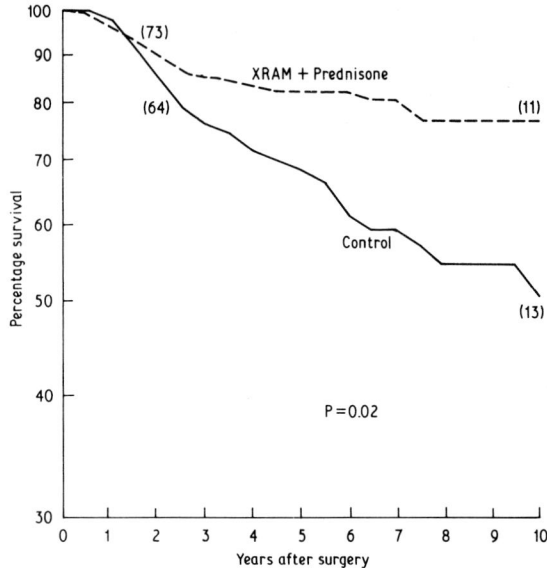

Fig. 16.3   Actuarial survival rates of pre-menopausal patient aged 45 years or more treated by mastectomy and postoperative radiotherapy. Upper curve represents survival of patients randomly selected to have ovarian ablation and oral prednisone; lower curve survival of control patients (from Meakin *et al.*, 1977).

by Meakin *et al.* (1977) requires further evaluation.

It has been proposed that 'prophylactic' adrenalectomy should be considered in some post-menopausal women with unfavourable prognostic features and with high oestrogen receptor activity in the tumour (Dao *et al.*, 1975). This concept requires much more detailed evaluation before it can be advocated as a regular practice.

Adjuvant immunotherapy

Immunotherapy of many cancers is now being evaluated and at present properly controlled trials are not sufficiently advanced to provide any indication about the possible advantages or disadvantages of these methods.

Studies have been initiated by the North American Surgical Adjuvant Group to test the effect of addition of *Corynebacterium parvum* to L-PAM in patients after mastectomy for breast cancer. Another study is comparing the response to CMF + Bacille Calmette-Guerin (BCG) injection and injected tumour autografts in patients with early breast cancer (Haskell, 1977). Other studies have used the methanol extractable residue (MER) of BCG together with cytotoxic chemotherapy, but no benefit was shown. Agents such as 'immune' RNA, transfer factor and the synthetic immune stimulant, levamisole, are also being evaluated in the management of breast cancer, but the results so far would not encourage their use in patients with early breast cancer.

Results of treatment

The overall survival rates of patients managed in Edinburgh over the last 15 years is given in Table 16.5. The results are shown as rounded figures as management was not uniform during this period, and in operable cases they reflect the results that can be obtained following both radical mastectomy and simple mastectomy with post-operative radiotherapy. In addition, at this time most patients under the age of 59 years with operable disease also underwent ovarian ablation as part of the primary management.

Table 16.6 shows the relative incidence of local recurrence and of distant metastases within 5 and 10 years of the primary treatment. The accumulative local recurrence rates are high but in the majority of patients local recurrence presents at the same time as the first clinical manifestation of distant metastases. Indeed the synchronous appearance of local recurrence and distant metastases occurs four times more commonly than local recurrence alone. In our experience local recurrence alone occurred in only 4% of patients with operable disease in the first five years, and in an additional 1% of patients in the subsequent five years after primary treatment. Local recurrence alone then is not a major problem after standard management of operable cases, and it has been established that it does not prejudice survival if adequate treatment is subsequently given. In women with operable breast cancer the development of cancer in the other breast occurred in 4% within the first five years, and in 6% within the first ten years after treatment. It is now hoped that long-term improvements in survival rates and in the reduction of recurrence rates will follow the introduction of systemic therapy in the management of patients with early disease.

The management of advanced and recurrent breast cancer

The management of advanced breast cancer is essentially palliative, but much can be done to improve the quality of life, and many patients will enjoy prolonged survival following skilled treatment. The decisions on optimum management depend on two factors, the menopausal status of the patient, and whether there is operable breast disease or local recurrence, or distant metastases, or a combination.

Locally advanced breast cancer

In most pre- and post-menopausal women, if there is no evidence of blood-borne metastases, management should be directed to control of the primary tumour, usually together with involved lymph nodes. A suitable radiotherapy technique has been described using a large jig which allows inclusion of the breast and regional lymph node area by two parallel opposed fields. A maximum tissue dose of 4250 rad is delivered in 10 fractions on alternate days over 4 weeks using megavoltage irradiation. Others would employ a technique of parallel opposed fields to the breast with or without parallel opposed fields to the cervicoaxillary nodes, and prescribing radiation doses given above.

In patients with extensive soft tissue disease,

Table 16.5 Survival rates by stage of breast cancer (Edinburgh series).

UICC staging 1968	Survival rates	
	5 years	10 years
Stage I	80%	65%
Stage II	70%	60%
Stage III (operable)	60%	50%
(inoperable)	25%	10%
Stage IV	9%	3%

Table 16.6 Local recurrence and distant metastases rates in patients treated for operable breast cancer (Edinburgh series).

Follow-up period	Number of patients	Local recurrence	Distant metastases
5 years	498	93 (18.7%)	144 (28.9%)
10 years	276	61 (22.1%)	101 (36.6%)

cytotoxic chemotherapy will provide excellent results. In the elderly post-menopausal patient it often is preferable to begin by administering Tamoxifen 10 mg b.i.d. or, less commonly because of side effects, stilboestrol 5 mg t.i.d., which will (in up to 50% of patients) result in very satisfactory tumour regression and growth restraint.

Locally advanced disease with blood-borne metastases

In pre-menopausal women the treatment of choice is normally surgical oophorectomy. If the operation is not considered justifiable or is refused, ovarian ablation may be achieved by pelvic irradiation. A dose of 2000 rad megavoltage irradiation, given in 5 equal daily fractions to parallel opposed fields (15 × 10 cm) covering the pelvis, is normally adequate. The effect of X-ray ablation is much less dramatic than after surgical ablation, for it takes up to three months for ovarian function to be lost after irradiation.

In post-menopausal women with locally advanced disease and metastases, the choice of management depends on the detailed features of the disease, but does involve the administration of hormones, cytotoxic drugs, or alternatively either hypophysectomy or adrenalectomy. The relative roles of these forms of management may now be discussed in more detail.

Radiotherapy of metastatic disease

It should be remembered that focal areas of metastatic disease may be very effectively managed by radiotherapy. Bone metastases commonly present as problems of this kind. They are a frequent cause of pain and disability, and improvement usually follows a short course of X-ray therapy. About 80% of lesions respond well to irradiation, although radiographic appearances may not show much change. Pathological fractures in the limbs are often best managed by irradiation after internal fixation. Megavoltage irradiation is preferred for most sites, and a dose of 2500 rad in 5 fractions over 1 week is effective. If the patient's general condition indicates, an even shorter treatment, a single exposure of 1250 rad or 1500 rad, depending on field size, can be equally effective.

When there is widespread skeletal disease continuing to cause distressing symptoms after other forms of management have failed, half-body irradiation has been given (Fitzpatrick and Rider, 1976). Large single doses, usually under 700 rad to avoid pulmonary complications, are delivered by megavoltage X- or γ-rays to the upper and lower half of the body with an interval of about six weeks between treatments. Excellent palliation has been claimed, but this technique requires

further evaluation and comparison with other methods of management before it should be used routinely.

Spinal cord involvement may result by extension from vertebral metastases or by extradural deposits. If there is evidence of motor tract impairment, surgical decompression is usually indicated. Surgery should then be followed by a course of X-ray therapy, although in less urgent cases irradiation can be tried without surgery. A single field is applied and 3000 rad can be given in 10 fractions over 2 weeks.

Symptoms and signs of brain metastases can be most distressing but they can often be alleviated by a short course of radiotherapy. A parallel opposed pair of fields should enclose the whole brain, and a dose of 3000 rad given in 10 fractions over two weeks. Occasionally metastases present in the retina, choroid or in the retro-orbital space. If early treatment is given, usually a single field giving 3000 rad in 10 daily fractions, excellent results can be achieved and vision will often be preserved.

Hormone therapy

Oestrogens are usually administered orally as diethylstilboestrol (5 mg t.i.d.) or ethinyloestradiol (0.1 mg t.i.d.). Oestrogens were for a long time the treatment of choice in women more than five years post-menopausal. Worthwhile remissions are obtained in about one-quarter of these patients with generalized disease, and importantly in about one-third of those with locally advanced or recurrent disease associated with minimal disseminated disease. Side-effects, however, are common (> 50% of patients). Nausea and vomiting may be helped by enteric coated tablets. Other side-effects are urgency of micturition, vaginal bleeding, fluid retention and cardiac failure. Consequently oestrogens have largely been supplanted by the use of Tamoxifen.

The anti-oestrogen triphenylethylene compound, Tamoxifen, is an important addition to oral hormone preparations. It is the hormone of first choice in post-menopausal women. The recommended dosage is 10 mg b.i.d. and at this level clear-cut remissions may be observed in about 36% of patients, particularly in post-menopausal women with localized disease. It is also of value in post-menopausal patients with widespread metastatic disease and is also active in pre-menopausal women. It is remarkably free from side-effects, although it may produce menopausal flushings, fluid retention and gastrointestinal upset. It may rarely cause thrombocytopoenia, which· can remit without discontinuing the drug.

Androgen therapy has commonly been used for patients in the early post-menopausal period.

Androgens are also much more effective than oestrogens in controlling generalized disease in all post-menopausal women. Localized disease in the breast or chest wall responds very poorly (about 15% of cases), and androgens are not to be advised. Several androgen preparations are available, but mention will be made of only two that are commonly prescribed.

19-Nor-androstanolone decanoate is a long-acting preparation which is given intramuscularly 100 mg every two to three weeks – a major advantage. Fluoxymesterone (5 mg t.i.d.) is a form of male hormone that is effective when taken by mouth. Side-effects such as virilization (hirsutism, acne, vocal change and increased libido) may be very upsetting to these patients, and careful enquiry must be made of their acceptability at follow-up assessments. An important tumour-related complication of androgen therapy in patients with bony metastases is hypercalcaemia, which may occur in as many as 10% of patients.

Progestogens are used occasionally in the management of advanced breast cancer, but the response rate is low for localized disease and very poor indeed in respect of generalized metastases. Other agents such as clomiphene, chemically closely related to Tamoxifen, may at times give a satisfactory response, but are usually employed for otherwise refractory clinical problems. Adrenal corticosteroids have been tried in advanced breast cancer as a sole agent with very doubtful benefit. High-dose prednisolone (10 mg t.i.d.) may be tried when all other methods have failed, to manage patients with hepatic, cerebral or pulmonary metastases.

It is common practice to use the appropriate hormonal agent or cytotoxic drugs before advising endocrine ablative surgery. It has been shown that the benefits of adrenalectomy or hypophysectomy are not prejudiced by previous administration of hormones (Stewart, 1970).

Chemotherapy of advanced breast cancer

In common with experience in general of cytotoxic chemotherapy of cancer, it has been found that the combination of three, four or five agents gives better results than any single cytotoxic drug. The use of phenylalanine mustard, adriamycin and cyclophosphamide has been tested as single agents against multiple drug regimes in randomly controlled trials, and shown to be much inferior compared to combination chemotherapy. It has also been demonstrated that the intermittent administration of high doses of a multiple drug regime gives improved results when compared to continuous therapy (Canellos *et al.*, 1974, 1976).

In 1969 a 90% response rate in patients with advanced breast cancer to a combination of cyclophosphamide, methotrexate, 5–fluorouracil, vincristine and prednisone (CMFVP) was reported. Others have not been able to achieve such high remissions, but a response rate of about 60% is often obtained. Several groups have modified this CMFVP regime to reduce its toxicity while retaining a high response rate (Canellos *et al.*, 1976). Adriamycin has also been included in a number of highly effective regimes, the most successful of which (CAF) may achieve an 82% response rate (Bull, 1977):

Cyclophosphamide	100 mg/m^2 day × 14	p.o.
Adriamycin	30 mg/m^2 days 1 and 8	i.v.
5–Fluorouracil	500 mg/m^2 days 1 and 8	i.v.

Priestman *et al.* (1977) have reported a comparative trial of a regime similar to CAF against oral hormone therapy. The complete response rate to chemotherapy was 49%, compared to only 21% to endocrine therapy. The chemotherapy regime was considered to be particularly good for pre-menopausal women with soft tissue disease. Post-menopausal women with similar locally advanced or recurrent disease responded well to Tamoxifen and chemotherapy, and Tamoxifen was preferable in view of the ease of administration, comparative freedom from side-effects and relative cost.

A controversial report (Powles *et al.*, 1980) suggests that even though chemotherapy is of considerable symptomatic value, it may *not* prolong survival in patients with advanced cancer.

Endocrine ablative surgery

Therapeutic ovarian ablation is the treatment of choice for advanced, recurrent or metastatic disease in pre-menopausal patients. The procedure may be advised with an 80% certainty of a beneficial response by measuring oestrogen receptors. It is unlikely that any benefit will occur in patients with no oestrogen receptors in the tumour, and in these circumstances ovarian ablation is not advised.

Adrenalectomy and hypophysectomy are both palliative procedures used in the management of post-menopausal women with disseminated breast cancer. Their application is normally reserved for the control of progressive metastatic disease in patients who relapse after a good initial response to other forms of hormonal management. It is accepted that hypophysectomy is the more effective procedure provided it is complete. The procedure is both difficult and dangerous unless undertaken in specialized departments, and so adrenalectomy may often be preferred.

The most reliable indication for adrenalectomy is oestrogen receptor assay, and if positive there is a 60% probability of response. The mean duration of remission is about two years. In the absence of an oestrogen receptor assay, a good response to oral hormone administration, ovarian ablation, or a long disease-free interval, would suggest that adrenalectomy may also be beneficial in about 40% of patients following relapse. Patients with predominantly skeletal metastases tend to show the best response. The presence of large liver metastases or ascites are usually regarded as contra-indications.

Hypophysectomy, if undertaken as a transcranial operation, is more effective than bilateral adrenalectomy. However, it is doubtful if transethmoidal hypophysectomy or yttrium-90 seed implantation of the pituitary gland gives any better control of metastatic disease than adrenalectomy. The problem is that residual pituitary function remains after yttrium-90 implantation in about 20% of patients, and so its efficacy is reduced. However yttrium-90 implantation is by far the safest procedure with negligible morbidity or mortality, and results in good objective remission in 20% of suitable patients, the average length of which is about one year. The correlation with previous response to ovarian ablation is very good indeed and in patients with oestrogen receptor positive tumours about 40% show a good response to hypophysectomy.

Breast cancer and pregnancy

The association of pregnancy and breast cancer is fortunately rare. It has been estimated that pregnancy may be a complicating factor in at most 3% of patients with breast cancer at child-bearing age (0.5% of breast cancer patients). Delay in diagnosis may be a problem since the incidence of breast cancer is perhaps only 3 per 10 000 pregnancies.

The pathology of breast cancer in pregnancy is similar to that seen in non-pregnant women and inflammatory carcinoma is no more common. The overall prognosis is no worse in pregnant women, although women who present in the second half of pregnancy have a much less favourable outlook. There is no justification for an unduly pessimistic attitude.

Management should follow an accepted policy for breast cancer in general. Survival is not improved by termination of pregnancy and need only be advised if the disease is very advanced. In the main the decision of termination should be made in accordance with the wishes of the parents. When the stage of the disease allows a choice of management, radiation is best avoided in patients with Stage I and II and operable Stage III disease, particularly in the first half of pregnancy. A modified radical mastectomy would seem advisable. In patients with histologically involved nodes adjuvant chemotherapy may be started after delivery. If the cancer is discovered close to full term,

mastectomy may be performed and radiotherapy given after delivery. With more advanced disease termination of pregnancy should be seriously considered. If abdominal hysterectomy is required oophorectomy should be performed at the same time for patients with Stage IV disease. Inoperable Stage III disease may be treated usually after termination by radiation or chemotherapy depending on the features of the disease. Breast cancer associated with lactation presents a special problem. Bromocriptine should be administered to suppress lactation and in the following week a decision may be taken about management dependent on the stage of the disease.

Pregnancy occurring after successful primary management of early breast cancer does not adversely affect prognosis. Honest advice must be given to patients whose prognosis is not good so that unfortunate social consequences of untimely pregnancy can be avoided. In many pre-menopausal patients mechanical contraception of some kind should be advised.

Conclusions

In the last decade there have been continuous improvements in the more rational management of patients with breast cancer. The importance of determining by histological examination whether or not the axillary lymph nodes are involved by tumour has been clearly established. The decision to advise systemic management of apparently early breast cancer depends principally on this assessment. Cytotoxic chemotherapy has been shown to have a role in the early management of pre-menopausal patients with breast cancer and involved axillary nodes. Chemotherapy has now a recognized place in the treatment of advanced disease. The anti-oestrogen, Tamoxifen, has been a most useful addition to effective oral hormone therapy for advanced disease in post-menopausal women. Its contribution to the improved management of early disease in post-menopausal women awaits evaluation.

In patients with Stage I and II disease radical mastectomy alone has good survival rates and low axillary and chest wall recurrence rates, and may be preferred to simple mastectomy and radiotherapy. In patients with operable Stage III disease, simple mastectomy with radical radiotherapy should always be advised. In pre-menopausal women with Stage II disease, multiple cytotoxic chemotherapy given monthly for six months may be indicated. Systemic chemotherapy if tolerated in full dosage may also benefit post-menopausal women with Stage II disease, but Tamoxifen therapy for two to five years should be considered. Many new forms of management are being evaluated, and consideration should be given to participating in one of the many collaborative randomly controlled trials being conducted.

For patients with inoperable Stage III disease local radiotherapy is often the simplest and most effective form of therapy. However, in the pre-menopausal patient cyclical combination chemotherapy should be considered if advanced soft tissue disease is present. Tamoxifen would be recommended initially for a post-menopausal patient with similar disease.

In the management of metastatic disease oophorectomy remains the treatment of choice in pre-menopausal women and usually Tamoxifen initially in older patients. Increased availability of hormone receptor assays may better define the indications for systemic therapy before too long. Endocrine ablative surgery, apart from oophorectomy, is usually reserved for secondary or tertiary management. The valuable contribution of focal irradiation of metastatic lesions should not be forgotten in the control of troublesome symptoms of disseminated disease.

The follow-up of patients with breast cancer has no generally agreed pattern. After management of early disease the patient may be seen every two months in the first year, three monthly in the second and annually for ten years thereafter. However, many of these patients require sympathetic support and skilled counselling, particularly in the early period of follow-up. More frequent visits may be reassuring and very important for their general well-being. The long term care of patients with breast cancer is time-consuming and demanding in many ways, but such a commitment must be accepted by oncologists if adequate support and expert management are to be given to these patients.

Management and rehabilitation are much more satisfactory if patients are able to discuss openly their problems with the oncologist. Most patients who present with a lump in the breast realize that it might be cancer, and if this is confirmed the patient is usually best told the nature of the disease, preferably before mastectomy if it is indicated. Almost always this improves the confidence and trust of the patient in the doctor, and enhances their mutual respect.

Our urgent need is to increase the proportion of patients with breast cancer diagnosed when the tumour is confined to the breast. If the disease is treated when the primary tumour is less than 3.0 cm in diameter, excellent long-term survival rates can be achieved (Duncan and Kerr, 1976) (Fig. 16.4). Early diagnosis in this sense does improve the prospect of cure. It can no longer be accepted that early diagnosis simply improves survival by antedating the primary treatment. The medical profession still requires to be convinced of this fact and to become more positive in promoting breast cancer screening clinics. This

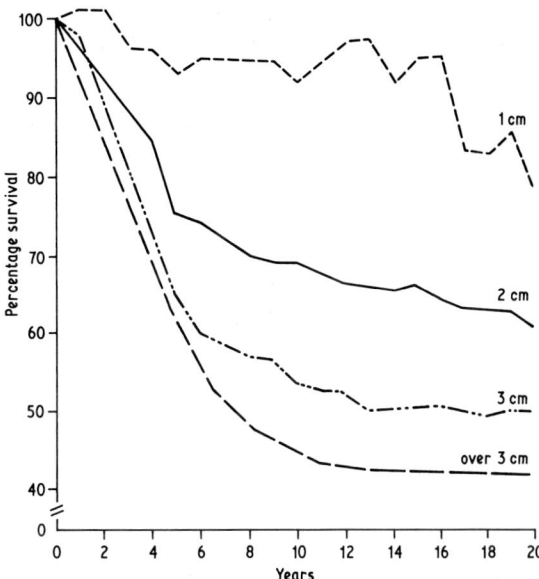

Fig. 16.4 Age-corrected survival rates by tumour size for patients treated for breast cancer apparently confined to the breast.

development is the most sure method at present of minimizing the morbidity and reducing the high mortality of this common form of cancer.

Further reading

Cancer (1977), Supplement on Breast Cancer, **39** 2697-963.

McGuire, W.L. (ed) (1977), *Breast Cancer. Advances in Research and Treatment*, Churchill Livingstone, Edinburgh.

Montague, Eleanor, (ed) (1977), *Breast Cancer*, Liss, New York.

Salmon, S.E. and Jones, S.E. (eds) (1981), Adjuvant Therapy III. Grune and Stratton, New York.

Staquet, M.J. (ed) (1978), *Randomised Trials in Cancer. A Critical Review by Sites*. EORTC Monograph Series No. 4, Raven Press, New York.

Surg. Clinics N. Amer. (1978), Breast Cancer **58**, (4), 657-876.

Wld. J. Surg. (1977), Breast Cancer, **1** (3), 281-360.

References

Baclesse, F. (1949), Roentgen therapy as the sole method of treatment of cancer of the breast. *Am. J. Roentgnol.*, **62**, 311-9.

17 Apudomas, pituitary and other endocrine tumours

Stephen N. Joffe

A multidisciplinary approach to endocrinology including radioimmunoassay of polypeptide hormones, electron microscopy and immunocytochemistry has advanced the diagnosis and management of these rare endocrine neoplasms. This chapter covers a wide spectrum of clinical syndromes and pathological entities. It includes the apudoma concept, carcinoma of pancreatic islet cells, parathyroid gland, adrenal cortex and medulla, carcinoid tumour and carcinoid syndrome, pituitary gland, paraendocrine and ectopic hormone producing tumours and finally multiple endocrine neoplasia. The TMN classification for malignant endocrine tumours at present applies only to the thyroid, but could be used for other endocrine tumours. Immunocytochemistry and serum estimations of the various polypeptide hormones and amines will indicate hormone production by the tumour.

Apudomas

Amine- and peptide-secreting cells are widely distributed in the body. Pearse (1968) proposed the name *apud* for these cells from the initial letters of their common cytochemical characteristics which include a high content of amine, a capacity for amine precursor uptake and the presence of the enzyme decarboxylase (Table 17.1). Apud cells may be considered in two groups, namely those which are known to secrete polypeptides and those whose polypeptide product (if there is one) has not been identified. The first includes most of the endocrine cells of the alimentary tract, including the islets of Langerhans, cells of the anterior pituitary, pineal and thyroid (Table 17.2). The second group (Table 17.3) includes cells in many parts of the body, the most important probably being in the adrenal medulla.

The structural and chemical similarity of apud cells

Table 17.1 Properties of apud cells and apudomas.

1. Fluorogenic amine content
   e.g. catecholamine, 5-hydroxytryptamine
2. Amine precursor uptake
   e.g. dopa or 5-hydroxytryptophan
3. Amino acid decarboxylase
4. High content of
   (i) side chain carboxyl groups
       (masked metachromasia)
   (ii) non-specific esterases and/or cholinesterase
   (iii) α-glycerophosphate dehydrogenase
5. Characteristic ultrastructure (endocrine granules)
6. Specific immunofluorescence

to nerves suggests a neural crest origin. Apud cells of the adrenal medulla, carotid body, thyroid, alimentary tract and melanocytes are of neuroectodermal origin.

The body has a system of chemical messengers comprising an inter-related group of peptides and hormones, many acting as neurotransmitters. A triple control system of peptide hormones and amine function has been proposed: neurocrine implying peptidergic transmitters, paracrine meaning locally acting paracrine substances and endocrine referring to circulating hormones. This simple concept explains the major mechanisms for coordinating bodily activities as a unified system.

Apudomas are tumours or hyperplastic lesions of apud cells usually secreting amines or peptides. They may secrete normal products of their cells of origin, e.g. insulinomas (orthoendocrine), those characteristic of other cells of tissues (paraendocrine) or they may form part of a syndrome of multiple endocrine neoplasia. Szijj *et al.* (1969) suggested the term apudoma to

Table 17.2   Apud cells with known polypeptide and amine and their related orthoendocrine apudomas and syndromes.

Organs	Cells	Polypeptides	Amines	Apudomas	Syndromes
Alimentary tract					
Islet of Langerhans	Small granules				
	B	Insulin			Hypoglycaemia
	A	Glucagon	Dopamine	Hyperplasia	Diabetes, dermatitis
	D	Somatostatin	or	Adenoma	Diabetes
					? hypochlorhydria
		Gastrin	5-HT[1]	Carcinoma	Zollinger-Ellison
	Large granules				
	D₁	VIP[2]			WDHA
	D₂ (PP)	PP[3]			? Diarrhoea
Stomach	G	Gastrin	–	Hyperplasia / Carcinoma	Zollinger-Ellison
	AL (A-like)	Enteroglucagon	–	–	–
	D	Somatostatin	–	–	–
Duodenum and	S	Secretin	–	–	–
small intestine	D₁	GIP[4]	–	–	–
	EC	Motilin	5-HT	Carcinoid	Malignant
		? Substance P			carcinoid
		Somatostatin			
Large intestine	D	VIP[2]	–	–	–
	EG	Enteroglucagon	–	–	–
Other sites					
Anterior pituitary	c (corticotroph)	ACTH[5]	(Tryptamine)	Hyperplasia	Cushing's
	m (melanotroph)	MSH[6]	(Tryptamine)	Adenoma	Pigmentation
	s (somatotroph)	GH[7]		Carcinoma	Acromegaly or
					gigantism
	l (lactotroph)	Prolactin	–	–	Forbes-Albright
Pineal	P	Melantonin	5-HT	Pinealoma	Hypogonadism
Thyroid	C	Calcitonin	5-HT	Medullary Ca.	Medullary Ca.

1. 5-Hydroxytryptamine; 2. Vasoactive intestinal polypeptide; 3. Pancreatic polypeptide; 4. Gastric inhibitory polypeptide; 5. (Adreno) cortico-trophin; 6. Melanocyte stimulating hormone; 7. Growth hormone.

describe a medullary carcinoma of thyroid secreting ACTH. There is little etymological justification for the word apudoma, but it emphasizes the common neoplastic characteristics. Biologically and apudoma is a neoplastic lesion derived from the apud cells, neuroectodermal in quality and secreting normal or modified peptide hormones and/or amines. Hyperplasia, adenoma, adenomatous hyperplasia or carcinoma are seen pathologically and possess apud cytochemical qualities often with greater clarity than their presumptive precursor cells. Endocrine storage granules are present on ultrastructure. More than half the apud cells recognized give rise to apudomas and new ones are frequently being discovered.

Apudomas may be studied in various ways. The concentration of polypeptides and amines may be measured by radioimmunoassay and bioassay in peripheral and venous blood draining the tumour. Tumours may be examined by conventional light mic-

roscopy, histochemistry, electron microscopy and immunocytochemistry and tumour extracts analysed. The full secretory property of an apudoma is elucidated only if every suspected tumour is investigated for as many hormones as possible. Clinically 'silent' hormones may predominate as calcitonin in medullary carcinoma of thyroid.

Apudomas are named after their endocrine product. For single hormone tumours, the term insulinoma is well established but others such as gastrinomas, calcitoninomas and vipomas may also be applied. Avoiding hybrids with multihormone producing apudomas, the combined pathological/histological description used is an 'apudoma secreting ACTH/MSH'.

Apudomas are classified as:

I.   Orthoendocrine – (a) tumours secreting normal polypeptides of their cells of origin and, (b)

Table 17.3   Apud cells without known polypeptide products with amine and possible polypeptide products.

Organs	Cells	Amines	Possible polypeptides	Apudomas	Syndromes
Stomach	EC	5-HT	Substance P	Carcinoid	Atypical carcinoid
Duodenum and small intestine	I	–	VIP	–	–
	K	–	GIP	–	–
	D₁	–	–	–	–
	G	–	Gastrin	–	–
Large intestine	EC	5-HT	Substance P	Carcinoid	–
	H	–	VIP	–	–
Other sites					
Carotid body	Type 1 (glomus)	Catecholamines and 5-HT	–	Carotid body tumour (chemo-dectoma)	–
Skin	Melanocyte	–	–	–	–
Adrenal	A (E)	Adrenaline	–	Phaeochromo-cytoma	Hypertension etc.
	NA (NE)	Noradrenaline	–		
Lung	P (Feyrter)	–	VLP[1]	–	–
	EC	5-HT	–	Carcinoid	Atypical carcinoid
Urogenital tract	U	–	Urogastrone	–	–

1. VLP – Vasoactive lung peptide.

tumours secreting normal amines of their cells of origin.

II.   Paraendocrine – (a) tumours of endocrine glands secreting hormones or humoral agents characteristic of other glands or cells and (b) tumours of organs or tissues not usually regarded as endocrine in nature, secreting hormones or humoral agents.

III.   Multiple endocrine neoplasia in which more than one endocrine gland in the same individual is the site of neoplasia, often an apudoma either orthoendocrine or paraendocrine as listed in Tables 17.2 and 17.3.

Many apparently unrelated endocrine tumours can be classed into the family of 'apudomas', a useful unifying concept. Many apudomas, such as carotid body tumours, need more investigation and there are likely to be as yet unrecognized tumours secreting hormones such as secretin, motilin and urogastrone.

Pancreatic islet cell carcinoma

These tumours occur in less than 1 per 100 000 population (Moldow and Connelly, 1968), but at autopsy the incidence of islet cell adenomas may be as high as 1.5%.

Pancreatic islets are composed of apud cells which give rise to both orthoendocrine and paraendocrine secreting tumours following distinctive clinical syndromes, with characteristic biochemical and physiological abnormalities. Excessive hormone production may be due to hyperplasia, adenoma, adenomatous hyperplasia, or carcinoma of either one or more of the specific islet cell types or by a combination of these (Schein *et al.*, 1973).

As with all endocrine neoplasms, it is often impossible to evaluate malignant potential from histology and pathologists must rely on evidence of blood vessel invasion, lymph node or distant metastases for an unequivocal diagnosis of carcinoma. Routine histological stains cannot differentiate various islet cell tumour types. Histochemical tests are related to properties of the apud cells (Table 17.1) and the final characteristic of specific immunofluorescence is assessed by the indirect or sandwich technique. Ultrastructural analysis by electron microscopy is useful in defining the various tumour cells.

Insulinoma

This commonest islet cell tumour causes periodic hypoglycaemia due to excessive production of insulin.

More than 2000 cases have been reported (Stefanini *et al.*, 1974; Filipi and Higgins, 1973; Creutzfeldt *et al.*, 1978) of which 80% are benign and single and 10% multiple or islet cell hyperplasia.

Moss and Rhoades (1960) reviewing 653 proven cases of insulinomas reported a 10% rate of malignancy and Stefanini *et al.* (1974) in 951 cases found metastases in 5%. Careutzfeldt *et al.* (1978) more recently found only two patients with metastasizing carcinoma in their 50 patients.

Malignant insulinomas tend to be softer, more haemorrhagic and less well encapsulated than benign lesions and as with other endocrine tumours, the usual histological criteria for malignancy (e.g. the presence of mitosis and cellular pleomorphism) are unreliable. Perineural invasion is thought to be diagnostic of malignancy (Laroche *et al.*, 1968), but the most reliable criterion is metastases to regional lymph nodes and liver (Robins, 1967). Benign adenomas do not undergo malignant transformation.

Specific staining granules are present in only two-thirds of the insulinomas but 90% react immunohistochemically with anti-insulin serum. Ultrastructurally four cell types including atypical granules have been found (Creutzfeldt, 1978). Other hypoglycaemic-producing tumours, such as hepatomas and mesotheliomas, are not apudomas secreting insulin.

Some insulinomas histologically suggestive of malignancy behave in a relatively benign fashion and frankly malignant cases with proven metastases occasionally survive for many years. However, without treatment most functioning islet cell carcinomas grow rapidly and cause death usually one to two years after diagnosis. Metastases may be functioning or non-functioning and if functioning continue secreting insulin or pro-insulin even after excision of the primary tumour.

Insulinomas occur in every age group with a peak incidence in the fourth to sixth decades. The main clinical features are attacks of hypoglycaemia occurring during periods of fasting and therefore commonest in the early morning and late afternoon. These attacks are aggravated by exercise, relieved by the consumption of carbohydrates, are often mild and infrequent in the early stages but later become severe and frequent. Manifestations include neuropsychiatric, cardiovascular and gastrointestinal symptoms and the diagnosis is strongly suggested by Whipple's triad consisting of hypoglycaemic symptoms provoked by fasting, accompanied by low blood sugar with rapid symptomatic relief after glucose administration.

In diagnosing an insulinoma, the single most important step is to think of it. The diagnosis is confirmed by the measurement of immunoreactive insulin and several tests are available which depend on the relationship between blood glucose and insulin. In nearly all patients with organic hyperinsulinism this relationship is lost, and high or normal instead of low levels of insulin accompany the hypoglycaemia. Pro-insulin (A and B chains) linked to C-peptide is found in abnormal quantities and fish-insulin helps in the diagnosis. Provocation tests using tolbutamide, leucine or glucagon are rarely used now.

Pre-operatively, localization of the tumour would include selective pancreatic arteriography which can show 5 mm tumours. Additional techniques include stereoscopic serial filming, magnification and subtraction. The tumours are highly vascular, round and well defined on angiography, both in the pancreas and metastases in liver or omentum. Pancreatic scanning and ultrasonography are valueless unless the tumour is large. Percutaneous transhepatic pancreatic and portal venous sampling for insulin may identify the tumour site (Ingemansson *et al.*, 1975; Turner *et al.*, 1978).

Treatment aims at total removal of the tumour remembering that at least 90% are benign adenomas. Improved results of surgery for pancreatic adenocarcinoma means that similar principles can apply to malignant insulinomas. For carcinoma localized to the body or tail, a distal pancreatectomy is advocated and a pancreaticoduodenectomy if the tumour is in the head. A total pancreatectomy is unnecessary unless there are multiple tumours. If lymph node metastases are present, a radical *en bloc* pancreaticoduodenectomy can be performed, with resection and direct repair of portal and mesenteric blood vessels (Fortner *et al.*, 1977). In patients with hepatic metastases, the primary pancreatic lesion should be resected and as much liver tumour as possible. This may include a hepatic lobectomy or enucleation of tumour tissue. The object is removal of as much functioning tumour tissue as possible. Cytotoxic or drug therapy is indicated if the tumour is partially or completely irresectable. Patients may survive for many years with malignant insulinomas as the tumour may be slow growing. Hypoglycaemia is the usual cause of death and every effort should be made to control it. Diazoxide, the thiazide derivative, causes hyperglycaemia and can be used pre-operatively and in patients with metastatic or irresectable tumours. Although the mode of action is uncertain, diazoxide inhibits the secretion of insulin, stimulates catecholamine production and hepatic glycogenolysis. The dose is 100 mg increasing gradually to 500 mg twice daily by mouth. The final dose depends on the therapeutic and toxic effects. Patients becoming refractory to initial diazoxide therapy may respond to larger doses. Toxicity includes anorexia, nausea, vomiting, fluid retention, skin rashes, pigmentation, hirsutism and hyperuricaemia.

Frequent consumption of sugar is effective in controlling hypoglycaemia but causes severe obesity. Protein ingestion, although promoting gluconeogenesis, also stimulates a further secretion of insulin. Glucagon (1 mg subcutaneously or intramuscularly) is useful in emergencies, especially if given by the patient's relatives, but should be followed by glucose intravenously or by mouth. Hydrocortisone (80 mg/day) is also often effective but causes Cushing's syndrome.

Streptozotocin is the only drug which has been meaningfully evaluated in the chemotherapy of islet cell carcinomas. Broder and Carter (1973) at the National Cancer Institute reviewed 52 cases treated with streptozotocin. In 41 functional tumours, a biochemical response was observed in 64% with tumour regression in 50%. All patients with biochemical responses had amelioration of their hypoglycaemic symptoms. The average duration of a biochemical response was 10 months and 13 months for a measurable tumour decrease. The median onset time for the insulin response was 17 days with a maximum response at about 35 days. The dose of streptozotocin is 1 g/m² given slowly intravenously at weekly intervals for 4 weeks and continued if a response is observed. Mechanism of drug action is at present unknown. Side-effects include gastrointestinal, haematological, metabolic and renal toxicity. Nausea and vomiting occurs in most patients within one to two hours after the injection. The hepatotoxicity tends to be transient, mild and usually reversible. Anaemia, leucopenia, rarely thrombocytopenia, alopecia and occasional hypoglycaemia have been seen following the drug infusion and renal toxicity is very common and includes renal tubular acidosis, glycosuria, aminoaciduria and uraemia (Gagel *et al.*, 1976; Carter *el al.*, 1977).

Service *et al.* (1976) at the Mayo Clinic reports a successful response in six of eight patients treated with intravenous 5-fluorouracil (12 mg/kg) and streptozotocin (500 mg/m²) daily for 5 days. Toxicity produced by streptozotocin included stomatitis, nausea, vomiting, diarrhoea and renal complications whereas the side-effects related to 5-FU were bone marrow depression and proteinuria. During therapy, insulin, glucose, haematological, renal and hepatic functions must be carefully monitored. For liver metastases, streptozotocin may be infused into the hepatic artery or adriamycin given (Eastman *et al.*, 1977).

Radiotherapy may temporarily relieve pain or jaundice. The concomitant use of chemotherapy and radiotherapy needs assessment. Intra-arterial embolization of functional hepatic metastases is a useful palliative technique.

Gastrinoma (Zollinger-Ellison Syndrome; ZES)

Zollinger and Ellison (1955) described two patients with a triad of fulminant peptic ulceration which recurred despite gastric operations, gross gastric hypersecretion and a non-β-islet cell tumour of the pancreas. Within the next few years many more patients were reported and it was later established that many had multiple endocrine adenopathy, that the tumours secreted gastrin (or sub-species of gastrin) and were therefore gastrinomas. In a collective study preceding the gastrin immunoassay, 61% of the tumours were malignant but this is probably an underestimate. Metastases and/or a primary lesion are often overlooked at the time of surgery and even at post-mortem. Only if an elevated serum gastrin decreases to normal levels after excision of a gastrinoma can metastases be excluded. The serum gastrin returned to normal in only 1 out of 30 patients after excision of the tumour with total gastrectomy. Even in this patient a lymph node metastasis had been excised together with a duodenal gastrinoma (Creutzfeldt *et al.*, 1978).

The pre-operative diagnosis of gastrinomas is relatively easy by radioimmunoassay (RIA) measurement of gastrin and is occasionally not elevated until stimulated by calcium or secretin. High levels of gastrin may occur in other conditions such as pernicious anaemia (Isenberg *et al.*, 1973).

Five different types of apudomas may produce excessive gastrin and cause a variant of the Zollinger-Ellison syndrome: in the stomach, G-cell hyperplasia or carcinoma; in the pancreas, an islet cell tumour (adenoma or carcinoma) or D-cell hyperplasia; and similarly a carcinoma or adenoma in the duodenum or splenic hilum.

In patients presenting with gastric hypersecretion associated with duodenal, jejunal or recurrent peptic ulceration, basal and stimulated serum gastrin should be measured, and selective angiography, ultrasound and computerized axial tomography (CAT) carried out with an attempt at localization of the tumour by selective venous sampling (Burchard *et al.*, 1979) and immunofluorescent staining of antral biopsies for G-cell hyperplasia. The heterogeneity of gastrins can be determined by Sephadex gel filtration studies.

Since gastrinomas are nearly always malignant and have metastasized at the time of diagnosis, complete surgical excision of the tumour is rarely possible. Therefore, until recently, removal of the end organ, i.e. a total gastrectomy, has been the treatment of choice. This major operation did not cure the patient but gave symptomatic relief. Reports of the primary or metastatic tumours regressing following a total gastrectomy have not been substantiated. The tumour and metastases continue to grow causing abdominal masses, hepatomegaly and jaundice (Hardy and Doolittle, 1977).

Advances in pre-operative investigations, tumour localization, surgical techniques and newer pharmacological agents require a more defined policy for the management of ZES. If associated with primary hyperparathyroidism, parathyroidectomy may cure the hypergastrinaemia and gastric hypersecretion. Since pancreatic gastrinomas are frequently metastatic, multiple, and occult, the preferred surgical treatment remains a total gastrectomy. No residual gastric parietal cells must remain as the patient will develop a recurrent stomal ulcer with bleeding, perforation and possible death. The oesophagogastric anastomosis is performed using a loop of jejunum with an enteroanastomosis or a Roux-en-Y loop anastomosed either end-to-end or preferably end-to-side to the oesophagus. A reservoir or miniature stomach can be created from the jejunum. The serious metabolic and malnutrition problems can be largely prevented by careful observations. If a solitary tumour is found in the body or tail of the pancreas, a distal pancreatectomy can be carried out. The serious metabolic consequences following combined major pancreatic resection such as a pancreaticoduodenectomy with a total gastrectomy outweigh the chance of removing a single tumour.

Approximately half of duodenal wall tumours are solitary and good long-term results are obtained following local tumour excision or a pancreaticoduodenectomy without total gastrectomy. If the serum gastrin does not fall early post-operatively, then either a total gastrectomy or medical treatment is required. This avoids the severe and sometimes rapidly fatal recurrent ulceration after inadequate removal of an apparently solitary lesion. If G-cell hyperplasia is found on antral biopsies without evidence of any other tumour, an antrectomy usually combined with vagotomy is adequate.

In 260 cases reviewed by the ZES tumour registry (Ellison and Wilson, 1964) the overall initial survival for patients treated by total gastrectomy was 100%; by sub-total gastrectomy 50%; and if no gastrectomy, only 20% survived. The survival rates in over 800 patients treated by total gastrectomy at 5 and 10 years were 55 and 42% respectively and with liver metastases 42 and 30% respectively. Most early deaths (30%) after total gastrectomy were due to bleeding or an anastomotic leak, and this reflects the poor general condition of many patients (Fox *et al*., 1974). A total gastrectomy is well tolerated nutritionally and in only 10% are weight losses of over 25 lb a problem. Long-term follow-up is necessary regarding calorie intake, body weight, vitamin B_{12} injections and iron supplementation.

The H_2-receptor antagonist, cimetidine, a potent inhibitor of basal and stimulated gastric secretion, is being used with increasing success in gastrinomas, both pre-operatively and for long-term treatment. The dose used for treating chronic duodenal ulcers (1.2 g/day) appears inadequate for the majority of Zollinger-Ellison patients. The response is assessed by measuring gastric secretion and the dose adjusted for each patient, varying from 2.4 to 10 g of cimetidine daily. The drug, by inhibiting the parietal cell production of gastric secretion, has no effect on the natural history or progressive growth of the primary gastrinoma or its metastases. A French study shows that in 7 ZES patients presenting with duodenal ulcers, cimetidine treatment failed in 2, was satisfactory in 3 and has been continued for over 15 months in a further 2 cases. Cimetidine infusion (2.4 mg/day) controlled the gastric secretion and was used in 6 patients prior to total gastrectomy.

A multicentre USA study of 62 patients with ZES (McCarthy, 1978) showed that two-thirds responded to 300 mg of oral cimetidine 6 hourly but some required higher doses. The drug effectively controlled pain and dyspepsia, restored weight, abolished the diarrhoea and allowed ulcer healing. When a dose was missed or reduced, there was a rapid return of symptoms and the basic neoplastic process progressed unimpeded. All patients tolerated the drug and apart from gynaecomastia (5 cases) and minor transient liver dysfunction (3 cases), no serious side-effects were seen. At follow-up (1–2 years) 48 patients were still on the drug, 3 were treated surgically, 5 died from unrelated reasons and 5 patients had problems. McCarthy (1978) suggests that the drug provides an alternative to total gastrectomy in suitably selected patients. Cimetidine has a definite place pre-operatively and in patients unsuitable for total gastrectomy. The addition of anti-cholinergics increases its efficacy. In patients in whom a tumour cannot be found at laparotomy, we are currently performing a vagotomy with antrectomy, and placing the patients on long-term H_2-receptor antagonists (cimetidine, ranitidine).

Somatostatin is an effective inhibitor of many polypeptide hormones including gastrin but must be given parenterally with few long-acting preparations available. Other effective anti-secretory agents, some being hormones, will become availabe in the future.

Streptozotocin, either alone or in combination with other cytotoxics, is given intravenously and/or intra-arterially. In the acute form of ZES, if there has been no inhibition of gastric secretion using cimetidine or by total gastrectomy, then it is unlikely that patients will survive long enough for the beneficial effects of streptozotocin. The dose and complications of streptozotocin are as for treatment of insulinomas. Cytotoxic therapy should be given to patients with multiple hepatic metastases and symptomatic pancreatic tumours. Radiotherapy is reserved for large inoperable pancreatic tumours causing pain or jaundice.

Verner-Morrison syndrome (WDHA syndrome, pancreatic cholera or vipoma)

Verner and Morrison (1958) reported two patients with a pancreatic non-β-islet cell tumour causing watery diarrhoea without peptic ulceration, subsequently named WDHA after the initial letters of its main characteristics namely *w*atery *d*iarrhoea, *h*ypokalaemia and hypo- or *a*chlorhydria. The syndrome is rare, being about one-tenth as common as the ZES, and sometimes part of multiple endocrine neoplasia.

A non-β-islet cell tumour of the pancreas is usually present (D_1 cells), and about half these tumours are malignant. Tumours occur elsewhere such as bronchial (probably oat-cell) carcinoma or retroperitoneal neuroblastoma and secrete vasoactive intestinal polypeptide (VIP), a polypeptide humoral agent normally produced by the gut. In large dose VIP causes vasodilatation with facial flushing, increases intestinal blood flow, induces watery diarrhoea and inhibits gastric secretion which causes the clinical features. The diarrhoea is explosive, up to 20–30 stools per day and does not respond to simple measures. This causes a hypokalaemia (1–3 mmol/1). The associated hypercalcaemia is unexplained.

Bloom's (1978) 24 cases had either a pancreatic or neural tumour and high concentrations of VIP in the blood and/or in the tumour. Larsson *et al*. (1976) failing to find elevated VIP in some patients suggest that another unknown humoral agent is responsible. Occasionally patients present with the syndrome and elevated levels of pancreatic polypeptide.

The diagnosis is made by eliminating the common cause of watery diarrhoea and hypokalaemia. Hypochlorhydria is found on gastric secretion tests and the diagnosis confirmed by measuring elevated blood levels of immunoreactive VIP (Ebeid *et al*., 1978). A characteristic tumour blush of dilated vessels due to the local action of VIP is found on selective arteriography. The pseudo-Verner-Morrison syndrome refers to patients with watery diarrhoea, hypokalaemia and achlorhydria who have normal serum VIP levels and no obvious tumour.

Pre-operatively the electrolytes and dehydration need to be corrected and if the diarrhoea is severe and continuous, steroids (prednisone 60 mg/day) or somatostatin may be given. Treatment requires early and aggressive surgery to remove both the primary and as much metastatic tumour as possible. For tumours in the body or tail of the pancreas, a distal pancreatectomy and a pancreaticoduodenectomy if in the head, with excision of any enlarged lymph nodes may be carried out. Liver metastases can be shelled out quite easily from adjacent liver tissue.

When surgery fails to cure the diarrhoea, therapy becomes more difficult. Steroids occasionally reduce the diarrhoea. Palliative therapy such as irradiation or cytotoxic drug therapy have been associated with only short symptomatic-free remissions. Streptozotocin may prove effective for metastatic disease but there have been reports of cardiac and nephrotoxicity associated with hepatic intra-arterial perfusion.

Verner-Morrison by 1974 had collected 55 patients with the WDHA syndrome. Eighty percent had a pancreatic tumour and in half these tumours there was evidence of malignancy with metastatic spread. The diagnostic delay was over three years and as a result one-third with metastases died in the early post-operative period due to dehydration and electrolyte problems. Two-thirds were to die in a few months of the diarrhoea. The average length of survival for all patients with malignant disease was only one year. The object therefore is early diagnosis and aggressive surgical treatment which is associated with an improved prognosis (Devine *et al*., 1978). Following excision, serial serum VIP determinations are an effective tumour marker to detect occult metastases.

Pancreatic glucagonoma

Glucagon secreting tumours arise from pancreatic islet α-cells. Earlier reports of islet cell tumours containing hyperglycaemic substances, could not be fully investigated until the development of a radioimmunoassay for pancreatic glucagon. McGavran *et al*. (1966) reported the first patient with diabetes, skin rash and a high concentration of plasma and tumour pancreatic glucagon. The characteristic necrolytic migratory erythematous rash led Mallinson *et al*. (1974) to diagnose nine cases. Eight were post-menopausal females with symptoms for more than one year and in two exceeded ten years. Mild to moderate diabetes was present in seven and a pancreatic tumour was found in eight of which six were malignant with metastases. The pancreatic tumours, in the body and tail of seven of nine were 4–10 cm in diameter, and contained glucagon.

A glucagonoma is suspected by the characteristic rash and diabetes and confirmed by estimation of pancreatic glucagon in the blood with selective angiography and pancreatic venography. Treatment is surgical excision of the tumour with remission, at least temporarily in most patients. No data are available regarding the use of radiotherapy or cytotoxics.

Somatostatinoma

Two middle aged diabetic females with D-cell metastatic pancreatic islet cell carcinomas producing somatostatin, have been reported. One had hyperchlorhydria and steatorrhoea attributable to somatostatin excess. Treatment would appear to be surgical excision when possible.

Pancreatic polypeptide-producing tumours (PPoma)

Pure pancreatic polypeptide producing apudomas (PPomas) are rare, although pancreatic polypeptide is found in one-third of pancreatic apudomas. The three patients with pure PPomas had no consistent clinical features, especially not diarrhoea (Welbourn *et al.*, 1978). One patient presented with watery diarrhoea, hypokalaemia and achlorhydria (WDHA syndrome) with a normal serum VIP but grossly elevated PP concentration (Larsson *et al.*, 1977).

Hyperplasia of insular and extrainsular PP cells (hyperplasia type II) are seen in many patients with insulinomas or glucagonomas and in diabetics. Treatment of PPoma should be surgical excision. An elevated plasma PP concentration can occur postoperatively in the absence of residual tumour due to PP cell hyperplasia (Floyd *et al.*, 1975).

Mixed pancreatic islet cell carcinomas

Mixed tumours are of clinical importance as the spectrum of symptoms may change with time and metastases may contain only some of the primary tumour cell types. Since raised plasma concentration of hormones may originate either from the primary or metastatic tumour tissue or from hyperplastic extratumoural cells, immunocytochemical studies are necessary. Ideally the plasma concentration of as many hormones and polypeptides as possible should be measured, tumour tissue investigated by immunocytochemistry and hormones measured post-operatively to confirm removal of all tumour tissue. Apudomas have been described secreting a combination of several polypeptides, e.g. ACTH, MSH and gastrin (Joffe *et al.*, 1978) and Larsson *et al.* (1975) found more than one polypeptide-producing cell in 7 out of 24 pancreatic tumours.

The aim of treatment is radical surgical excision. If inoperable, the symptoms of the major secreting hormones need to be controlled, e.g. cimetidine if excess gastrin and diazoxide or streptozotocin for hyperinsulinaemia.

Parathyroid carcinoma and hyperparathyroidism

Carcinoma of parathyroid glands occurs in 2–3% of primary explorations and up to 7% in recurrent disease. The tumours are either chief or a mixed cell

variety and the majority are left inferior and palpable (30–70%). The tumour is firm and lobulated with invasion of the thickened capsule, surrounding structures and vascular spaces. The majority are well differentiated but one-third have spread to cervical lymph nodes, lungs, liver and bones (Esselstyn, 1977). As most parathyroid carcinomas produce parathyroid hormone, they present clinically as primary or recurrent hyperparathyroidism (Ackerman and Winer, 1974; Dozois and Beahrs, 1977). This diagnosis is being made earlier and prior to an advanced stage of the disease due to a high index of suspicion, and the availability of routine serum calcium estimations. Three distinct forms of clinical presentation are bone disease without renal stones, renal stones without bone involvement and asymptomatic individuals with hypercalcaemia.

Parathyroid carcinoma has been described with multiple endocrine neoplasia syndrome (Type I or II), peptic ulceration and pancreatitis. Diagnosis of hyperparathyroidism depends on a series of biochemical tests which include serum and urinary calcium, phosphorus and magnesium estimations, tubular reabsorption, cortisone suppression test and cyclic AMP. Immunoassay of parathyroid hormone with selective neck vein cannulation helps to differentiate primary hyperparathyroidism from hypercalcaemia of other causes. The treatment recommended previously was total thyroidectomy with a radical ipsilateral neck dissection. The earlier diagnosis (Stage I) and relatively low malignant potential has led to less radical surgical procedures. If at operation a firmly adherent parathyroid mass is found which on frozen section shows carcinoma, then an *en bloc* local excision with removal of any involved structures is adequate primary treatment. Cervical node metastases require a radical neck dissection. Post-operative serum calcium and PTH determinations help to detect recurrent or distant metastases. These can usually be managed successfully by repeated local excision or palliative resection of functioning metastases. In patients with bone changes 1, α-hydroxy-vitamin D$_3$ (1–2 mg/day) given for several days pre- and post-operatively prevents severe hypocalcaemia. Metastases develop slowly and first appear in the cervical lymph nodes.

Seven of eight parathyroid carcinomas reported by Jarman *et al.* (1978) had a local excision of the tumour and five patients were well 3–7.5 years after operation. One patient had two recurrences within 3.5 years, one died of a myocardial infarction and one patient died of the disease 4 years after surgery. Other reports are of one patient dying 2 years after local excision of a parathyroid carcinoma and three of the five patients being free of disease at 4, 12 and 16 years after surgery. In a collective series, Schantz and Castleman (1973) found a 30% recurrence rate with less than one-half of the patients dying within 5 years of the disease. Cooke's study found 3% with carcinoma which caused intractable hypercalcaemia. Attempts to control the disease by surgery and cytotoxic chemotherapy were unsuccessful and the patients died 2–7 years after presentation (Cooke *et al.*, 1977). Hypercalcaemic crisis may occur and requires adequate hydration, forced diuresis and correction of electrolytes. Inorganic phosphate, steroids, calcitonin and mithramycin can be used.

Adrenal gland

Adrenal tumours may be either non-functional or functional, producing excessive hormones which result in a variety of clinical syndromes. Specific methods for diagnosis are determined by the functional characteristics of the particular adrenal tumour involved. A non-functioning tumour may present as an abdominal mass, and arteriography alone is needed to confirm the diagnosis, whereas the commoner small functioning adenoma produces a clinical syndrome requiring hormonal measurements.

Tumours arising from the adrenal gland are subdivided into:

Cortical	Hyperplasia	Functioning
	Adenoma	Non-functioning
	Carcinoma	

Medullary	Ganglioneuroma
	Neuroblastoma
	Phaeochromocytoma
	Ganglioneuroblastoma

Tumours of adrenal cortex

These tumours may be functioning or non-functioning and either benign or malignant. The incidence of cortical carcinomas is approximately 2 per million population and the percentage of each tumour would be as in Table 17.4.

Table 17.4 Pathology and hormone production of adrenal cortical tumours.

	Functioning	*Non-functioning*
Benign	65%	1%
Malignant	19%	15%

Functioning adrenal tumours produce a variety of syndromes depending on their hormone secretion. These include: (1) Cushing's syndrome due to excess glucocorticoids; (2) virilism due to excess androgens; (3) feminization due to excess oestrogens; (4) aldosteronism due to excess mineralocorticoids and (5) mixed syndromes.

The distinction between functioning and non-functioning tumours is made clinically, since gross or microscopic features do not indicate hormonal status. Larger tumours tend to be malignant and arbitrarily 100 g divides benign from malignant tumours. Well differentiated cortical carcinomas can be difficult to distinguish from adenomas unless there is vascular invasion and metastases, whereas histology usually diagnoses the poorly differentiated variety.

Survival rates correlate with the degree of malignancy and clinical staging (Table 17.5). Metastases to regional lymph nodes occur in 25% of cases, liver in 30–70%, lungs in 50% and bones in 20–40% (Greenberg and Marks, 1978; Geelhoed *et al.*, 1980).

Cushing's syndrome
Clinical and metabolic manifestations result from an excessive production of cortisol by the adrenal cortex. The cause may either be an excess ACTH stimulation of the adrenal cortex or autonomous tumour secretion. In 308 cases of Cushing's syndrome, 75% were found to have 'normal' or hyperplastic glands, 12% were adenomas and 13% a carcinoma (Symington, 1969).

Table 17.5 Clinical staging system for carcinoma of the adrenal cortex (from Bradley, 1975).

T – extent of primary tumour
    1 – 5 cm and confined to adrenal gland
    2 – 5 cm to 10 cm or adherence to kidney
    3 – 10 cm or invasion of surrounding structures including renal vein

M – presence and type of metastases
    0 – no demonstrable metastases
    1 – regional lymphatics
    2 – distant metastases, for example, liver, lung, bone

R – tissue remaining after resection
    0 – tumour completely excised
    1 – tumour entered at operation
    2 – tumour tissue remaining after resection

D – degree of histological differentiation
    1 – differentiated, no capsular or vascular invasion
    2 – moderately undifferentiated, either capsular or vascular invasion
    3 – anaplastic, both capsular and vascular invasion

Stage 1–3 or fewer; for example T_1, M_0, R_0, D_1

Stage 2–4 and 5; for example T_2, M_0, R_1, D_2

Stage 3–6 and 7; for example T_3, M_1, R_1, D_2

Stage 4–8 or more; for example T_3, M_2, R_2, D_3

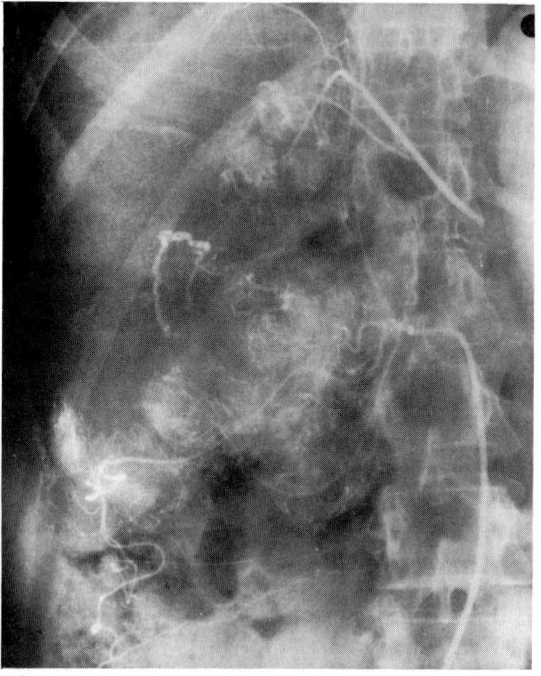

(a)

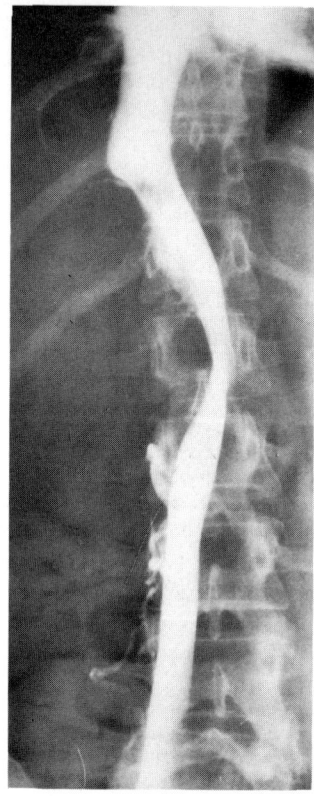

(b)

Fig. 17.1 (*a*) Arteriogram showing a large vascular right-sided adrenal tumour in a patient with a rapid onset of Cushing's syndrome. (*b*) On venography the tumour was both compressing and infiltrating the inferior vena cava. A 650 g well differentiated adrenal carcinoma was excised together with the infiltrated segment of vena cava. A right hepatic lobectomy was carried out for multiple liver metastases and the patient was treated post-operatively with mitotane.

Cushing's syndrome occurs at any age but commonly between 20 and 50 years and is 2–3 times as common in females. Length of history before diagnosis is variable from weeks to years with a mean of three years.

Investigations are designed to answer three main questions: 1. Is Cushing's syndrome present? If so, 2. what complications are there? and 3. what is the underlying lesion? The diagnosis is usually suggested by the clinical features. Steroid examinations in urine and plasma provide the objective evidence and adrenal carcinomas fail to stimulate or be suppressed. Abdominal X-rays show a patchy calcification in 25% of adrenal carcinomas. Retroperitoneal pneumography has been replaced by arteriography which reveals a vascular primary tumour and may also demonstrate liver secondaries. Other investigations include venography with selective adrenal venous sampling, grey scale ultrasonography, CAT and radioisotopic scanning with iodocholesterol (Fig. 17.1*a* and *b*).

The treatment of choice for a functioning adrenal cortical carcinoma causing Cushing's syndrome is surgical resection. The operative techniques have been adequately described through a thoracoabdominal or a wide transabdominal incision (Edis *et al.*, 1975).

It is desirable to remove as much tumour tissue as possible, even when curative resection is not feasible. For large tumours infiltrating the right lobe of the liver, an *en bloc* resection can remove the right kidney and adrenal tumour with a right partial hepatic lobectomy or shelling out or of the liver metastases. The inferior vena cava is usually invaded by tumour and can be resected and grafted.

Radiotherapy is of questionable value due to a lack of well documented data. In Percarpio and Knowlton's (1976) report of 14 patients treated with radiotherapy, 11 had distant metastases and 3 had residual local tumour following resection. Although 8 were functioning tumours, only 2 patients had Cushing's syndrome. Radiotherapy was given in a dose of 3000 to 4000 rad delivered over 2–3 weeks. The median survival from the time of diagnosis was 12 months and only 2 patients survived beyond 5 years. Bone metastases were responsive to palliative doses of irradiation by relieving pain and promoting healing. Chemotherapy, usually with ortho-para-DDD (o-p-DDD) was given to 9 of these patients as well with varying results. In 32 patients treated by radiotherapy at the M.D. Anderson Hospital, there was no demonstrable effect on the primary tumour or its metastases.

Chemotherapy with o-p-DDD (mitotane, lysodren or ortho-para-DDD) is of value in treating inoperable or recurrent adrenocortical carcinoma. Related to the insecticide DDT, it causes necrosis of both normal and adrenocortical tumour tissue, especially affecting the zona fasciculata and reticularis. The oral dose is progressively increased from 2 g/ day (500 mg q.i.d.) to 8 or 10 g/day, if tolerated. Unfortunately due to toxicity only 10% of patients are able to take the full dose. The commonest side-effects include anorexia, nausea, vomiting and diarrhoea, lethargy, depression, vertigo and skin rashes. Replacement therapy is usually necessary whilst on treatment. Either hydrocortisone or dexamethasone (1–2 mg/day) and fludrocortisone (0.1 mg/day) are used, and the response assessed by urinary steroid measurements. The results of 138 patients treated by Hutter and Kayhoe (1966) showed a steroid response in 72% and a measurable disease response in 34% with a response time of 5–10 months. Steroid response meant a 30% or more decrease over pre-treatment values. Lubitz *et al*. (1973) reported a 61% measurable tumour response and a 54% steroid response, without serious side-effects. Objective response differs in men and women (21% versus 60%) and the 4-year survival rate was 52% for women and 38% for men with a median survival of 56 and 19 months respectively.

Another therapeutic agent of possible benefit in carcinoma of the adrenal cortex is aminoglutethimide. First marketed as an anti-convulsant (Eliptin) it was withdrawn because of adrenal insufficiency. Aminoglutethimide inhibits the enzymatic conversion of cholesterol into Δ-5-pregnenolone and in contrast to o-p-DDD has a reversible effect on adrenal steriodogenesis. The side-effects are mainly of central nervous system and thyroid depression with 10% developing skin rashes. Clinical experience is limited but Schteingert *et al*. (1966) reported a good steroid suppression response for six months in a patient with adrenal cortical carcinoma. Plasma and urinary corticosteroids monitor the hormonal response (Wells *et al*., 1978). The dose of aminoglutethimide is 1 to 1.5 g/day and with further experience, its importance will increase.

Non-functioning adrenal carcinomas tend to be highly malignant with a poor prognosis as compared to the well differentiated functioning tumours. Patients with highly malignant tumours die within several months, moderately differentiated live for 0.1–6 years and those with a low grade malignancy can live up to 18 years (Lewinsky *et al*., 1974). Cushing's syndrome because it occurs in functioning adrenal carcinomas, has a slightly better prognosis, especially in females. Recurrence or late metastases may appear in spite of the benign growth and histological characteristics of the primary tumour. It is therefore important to review patients and measure urinary and plasma steroids at regular intervals after surgical excision. Any increase in hormones, irrespective of manifest Cushing's syndrome, should be extensively investigated. Treatment depends on the nature of the recurrence but includes surgery, o-p-DDD, aminoglutethimide and-/or metyrapone.

Virilism due to excess androgens
The adrenogenital syndrome resulting from an excess of adrenal androgens, causes virilism in females and precocious isosexual development (pseudo-puberty) in boys. Both Cushing's and adrenogenital syndrome can occur simultaneously. Congenital bilateral adrenal hyperplasia is the commonest lesion and rarely is an adrenal carcinoma found.

Malignant tumours should be removed surgically if possible. Many are inoperable or recur with metastases soon after removal. In localized recurrences after previous removal, benefit may be obtained from re-exploitation and further excision with adjuvant chemotherapy. This is especially effective if the tumour has previously responded to either radiotherapy or chemotherapy with o-p-DDD. However, the overall prognosis is poor.

Feminization due to excess oestrogens
This is an exceptionally rare condition caused by an oestrogen-secreting tumour of the adrenal gland or of ectopic adrenal tissue. These tumours develop most frequently in adult life, usually in males, are frequently large, malignant and palpable. Histology is similar to other hormone-secreting adrenal tumours but other features of adrenocortical excess such as Cushing's syndrome are unusual.

The clinical features result from the over-production of oestrogens or perhaps gonadotrophin which can be measured in blood and urine. Inhibition of pituitary gonadotrophins leads to testicular atrophy, loss of libido, impotence and gynaecomastia in males. Pre-pubertal girls develop isosexual precocious puberty.

Treatment is surgical removal of the tumour whenever possible and steroid replacement is not required. The prognosis is poor since in most cases the malignancy is advanced by the time the tumour is diagnosed. Chemotherapy with o-p-DDD and radiotherapy may be used.

Primary aldosteronism due to excess mineralocorticoids (Conn's syndrome)

Three patients were independently reported in 1955 with hypokalaemic alkalosis and hypertension, hyperaldosteronism and an adrenal tumour (Conn, 1955 a and b), and an adrenocortical carcinoma (Foye and Feichtmeir, 1955). Primary aldosteronism occurs in under 3% of hypertensive patients and not 20% as originally suggested by Conn *et al.* (1964). In 90%, a single small (0.3–3 cm) benign, well encapsulated cortical adenoma is found. Left-sided occur twice as commonly and the uncommon bilateral form consists of either a single adenoma or hyperplastic nodules. Carcinoma is so rare that it is reported as single cases and tends to encompass large well encapsulated tumours, up to a kilogram in weight. Histologically the cells may be either zona glomerulosa or zona fasciculata in type.

Hyperaldosteronism from sodium retention, expands the plasma volume causing hypertension and cardiovascular lesions. The severity of the hypertension is variable and although the malignant form is rare, headaches are frequent and severe. Chronic hypokalaemia causes postural hypotension with episodes of muscular weakness and even flaccid paralysis. The commonest symptoms in 145 cases included muscular weakness (73%), polyuria or nocturia (72%), headaches (51%), polydipsia (46%), paraesthesia (24%) and visual disturbance, intermittent paralysis, tetany, fatigue and muscle discomfort (Conn *et al.*, 1964).

Routine investigations show a hypokalaemia (3.8–<2.0 mmol/l) but normal values may be found on occasion. The plasma sodium is often slightly raised and the urine is persistently alkaline, of low osmolality with a very high urinary potassium (>25 mmol/day). An adequate sodium intake of 120 mEq/day for a week still maintains an elevated plasma and urinary excretion of aldosterone which is not inhibited by deoxycortone acetate. Other urinary steroids are often elevated in cases of carcinoma. After various biochemical tests, the most important investigation is adrenal angiography and venous sampling which may indicate the site and extent of the tumour.

The treatment of choice in primary aldosteronism is surgical removal. Since it may not always be possible to distinguish pre-operatively between a carcinoma, adenoma or hyperplasia an intraoperative decision may be necessary. If pre-operative localization shows a very large unilateral tumour, then a loin or abdominothoracic incision is used, especially as carcinomas tend to be extremely large. The incidence of bilateral tumours, e.g. carcinoma on one side and adenoma on the other is exceptionally rare. Since there are no problems of hypertensive crises, wound healing or obesity in this syndrome, the surgical complication

rate is low. Removal of the tumour relieves the symptoms and reduces the diastolic blood pressure. Pre-operatively the hypokalaemia is corrected by oral potassium supplementation and after removal of an aldosterone-producing carcinoma, a tendency towards hyperkalaemia occurs due to suppression of mineralocorticoid output from the remaining adrenal cortex. Fludrocortisone (0.1–0.2 mg/day) effectively replaces the temporary deficiency in aldosterone secretion.

Spironolactone is extremely useful in the pre-operative correction of hypokalaemia, in the long-term treatment of poor risk surgical patients and in irresectable or widespread recurrent carcinoma. The primary action is to antagonize the aldosterone effect on the distal renal tubules. This results in a urinary loss of sodium and a conservation of potassium and the lowering of blood pressure is due to its natriuretic activity. The usual dose of spironolactone is 200–300 mg/day. This may be increased to much higher doses or thiazide diuretic may be supplemented. Side-effects include gynaecomastia and impotence in men, and dysmenorrhoea in women. Dyspepsia is minimal if the drug is taken after meals but it may also cause constipation and excessive sweating.

Aminoglutethimide (0.1–1.5 g/day) in divided doses, blocks the synthesis of both cortisol and aldosterone and may be tried as an alternative. Steroid replacement is not required because ACTH secretion is increased which maintains a nearly normal secretion of cortisol. Occasionally patients may require anti-hypertensive drugs added to their regime including a salt-restricting diet.

The survival rate in adrenocortical carcinomas secreting aldosterone appears similar to other hormone-secreting adrenal carcinomas with similar considerations regarding local extent and distant metastases. No follow-up results are available, as compared to Cushing's syndrome.

Mixed syndromes due to multisteroid secretion

It is not uncommon to find some features of both Cushing's and adrenogenital syndrome in the same patient. For example, virilism may be accompanied by hypertension or diabetes and hirsutism may be present in Cushing's syndrome. These mixed lesions are most common in adrenocortical carcinoma. Three out of the 15 patients (Bradley, 1975) with adrenocortical carcinomas had both Cushing's syndrome and virilization. Two were females with left-sided tumours. Patients may initially present with a non-functioning primary tumour and later secrete steroids from a local recurrence or metastases, e.g. 17-keto and 17-hydroxysteroids. In Cushing's syndrome and a feminizing adrenocortical carcinoma with hypokalaemic alkalosis, excessive secretion of several other corticosteroids have been shown.

The treatment is an adrenalectomy with removal of as much tumour tissue as possible. In the one case (Bradley, 1975), this involved a left adrenalectomy, splenectomy and a distal pancreatectomy. In two cases no post-operative adjuvant therapy was given but the third patient received o-p-DDD (6 g/day) which reduced the urinary 17-ketosteroid and 17-hydroxysteroid levels. Further radical surgery may be necessary especially if there are liver metastases. Patients may survive for up to 11 years by careful observation and further radical surgery, e.g. of liver metastases by hepatic resection. Treatment with o-p-DDD, aminoglutethimide (1 g/day) and radiotherapy to involved bones helps considerably in the management of these patients.

Non-functioning adrenocortical carcinoma

Neoplasms of the adrenal cortex with no clinical endocrine abnormality are rare. Rapaport *et al*. (1952) reviewing adrenocortical tumours from 1930 to 1949 found only 37 patients with non-functioning cortical tumours in 277 adrenal tumours which was similar to Dix's (1963) 40 in 277 adrenal tumours. Shons and Gamble (1974) in an extensive literature search found a total of 120 patients with non-functioning adrenal carcinomas reported by 1974. Lewinsky *et al*. (1974) suggested that these tumours should be called non-hormonal rather than non-functional, as they are capable of forming precursor steroids without hormonal activity and added 20 new cases to the literature. Most patients were between the ages of 45 and 60 years with non-specific symptoms of weakness, weight loss, low grade fever implying tumour necrosis, loin pain and occasionally a palpable abdominal mass. The diagnosis is usually suggested by intravenous and retrograde pyelography and confirmed by angiography. The diagnosis of malignancy is once again extremely difficult purely on histological criteria and may require metastases to be present. Ultrastructural characteristics of the nuclei often suggest malignancy.

Surgical excision is the treatment of choice but studies report a high operative mortality and a poor prognosis (Rapaport *et al*., 1952). From the surgical data available in 61 patients (total 178 cases), 42 died within a year and 24 survived only 2 years. In advanced cases, chemotherapy using o-p-DDD was shown to be of some value. Although these tumours are presumed to be radioresistant, combined o-p-DDD and radiotherapy should be tried. Urinary steroid estimations are important, for although patients may present with no clinical syndrome, they can be used to monitor the progress of treatment and the development of any tumour recurrences.

Adrenal medulla

The malignant neuroblastomas arise from the primitive sympathogonium cell, whilst the differentiated ganglion cells, phaeochromocytes and paraganglion cells give rise to the relatively benign ganglioneuromas, phaeochromocytomas and paraganglionomas respectively (Fig. 17.2). Phaeochromocytomas, 75% of ganglioneuromas and neuroblastomas, are orthoendocrine apudomas secreting catecholamines, adrenaline and/or noradrenaline. A few are paraendocrine producing polypeptides as ACTH and VIP.

Phaeochromocytomas

Phaeochromocytomas arise from phaeochromocytes in the adrenal medulla (over 80%) or in sympathetic ganglia from the neck to pelvis, the majority (99%) being intra-abdominal. In adults, tumours are bilateral and multiple in 5–10%, higher in children (25%) and greatest in hereditary syndromes (50–70%). Most adrenal medullary tumours secrete adrenaline whereas extra-adrenal secrete noradrenaline.

The reported incidence of malignant adrenal phaeochromocytomas is conflicting due to a lack of accepted diagnostic criteria. This incidence varies from 7–15% but if diagnosed by the presence of metastases, then it is only 1–2.5% (Goodall and Symington 1953; Hume, 1960). Histologically, benign and malignant phaeochromocytomas may have a similar appearance regarding mitotic figures, nuclear pleomorphism, and even capsular and intravascular invasion (Symington, 1969).

The only absolute criterion for malignancy is the presence of metastases in sites where chromaffin tissue is not normally found, such as lung, liver, lymph nodes and bone (Table 17.6).

Malignant phaeochromocytomas may also arise in extra-adrenal sites. In satisfying malignant criteria only 4 have been described in the organ of Zuckerkandl, 1 out of 23 intrathoracic and 4 of 27 tumours in the urinary bladder, although these sites may be involved with benign multicentric tumours. Sizes vary from small to very large (1000 g) with a mean weight of 100g. The large tumours are metabolically less active and are often missed.

Phaeochromocytomas have been described as 'the great mimic', but important symptoms are paroxysmal or sustained arterial hypertension and sweating. When associated with pregnancy they carry a high mortality both for mother and child unless diagnosed promptly and treated. Patients with phaeochromocytomas are usually thin, but the tumours can rarely be felt. Pressure on the tumour may provoke a hypertensive attack and must be avoided.

Investigations are orientated towards establishing or

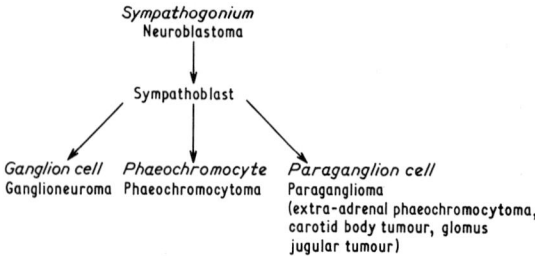

Fig. 17.2 Cells of origin of adrenal medulla and related structures including their associated tumours.

Table 17.6 Site of metastases from malignant phaeochromocytoma (n = 39 cases).

Site	%
Liver	46
Lymph nodes	38
Lung	28
Vertebra	26
Ribs	21
Cranium	15

excluding by biochemical and pharmacological tests the presence of a tumour with subsequent radiographic localization. Pharmacological tests include phentolamine intravenously, a short-acting α-receptor blocking agent, which lowers the blood pressure. Pressor agents such as histamine, tyramine or glucagon are not used any more because of their potential danger. Measurement of 24-hour urinary VMA or metadrenaline on three occasions will be high in 95% of cases and in malignant tumours the urinary dopamine and HVA are also elevated. Serum adrenaline and noradrenaline can also be measured. The majority of tumours can be demonstrated radiologically and selective arteriography and venous sampling will reveal tumours in both the usual and extra-adrenal sites. All patients must be prepared with an α-blocking agent for four to seven days before these investigations and phentolamine is kept available for a hypertensive crisis.

Surgical removal of a phaeochromocytoma is the most effective form of treatment. Medical measures are required for emergencies prior to operation, preoperative preparation and for the few patients whose tumours cannot be removed. With proper attention to the risks of surgery, the morbidity and mortality have been considerably decreased. Phenoxybenzamine is

given for at least seven days pre-operatively at an initial dose of 10 mg t.i.d., which is increased by 10 mg increments until the supine diastolic blood pressure falls below 100 mm Hg without disabling postural hypotension; β-blockers such as propranolol need only be given for cardiac arrhythmias. The α-blockade probably helps restore the lowered blood volume and hydrocortisone is only given if there are bilateral adrenal tumours.

The usual anaesthetic agents are halothane or nitroprusside because of their hypotensive effect and lignocaine is available to treat arrhythmias. Arterial blood pressure is measured continuously and an intravenous phentolamine drip (5–10 mg) is available for the hypertension caused by induction and palpation of the tumour. Operative blood losses are replaced quantitatively with an additional transfusion of up to 2 l of plasma. For unilateral large carcinomas the incision is thoracoabdominal or transabdominal with full exploration of the whole abdomen including aortic region, pelvis, both adrenal glands and liver. Adrenal areas and any other suspicious masses within the abdomen are squeezed gently and the effect on the blood pressure noted. The post-operative course is usually uncomplicated. Biochemical tests are repeated early and if positive the presence of a further tumour or metastatic disease should be considered. Malignant tumours tend to grow very slowly and may recur locally or metastasize as long as ten years after operation, causing a return of symptoms and signs. Operations for recurrent tumours may be difficult and radiotherapy is sometimes effective.

The clinical features of malignant, inoperable or recurrent tumours can be controlled satisfactorily by the long-term treatment with phenoxybenzamine and if necessary, a β-blocker. α-Methyl-P-tyrosine, by blocking the synthesis of catecholamines can also be used, but has unpleasant side-effects.

The survival time following diagnosis of malignant phaeochromocytomas varies and in part depends on the extent of spread at the time of operation. Generally recurrences occur within one year and survival is rare after three years. The period of survival depends on the ability of the surgeon to remove not only the primary but also the secondary lesions. There have been reports in the literature of patients being alive and well for several years following removal of malignant phaeochromocytoma and solitary metastatic lesions such as in the ribs or liver.

Neuroblastoma and ganglioneuroma

Neuroblastomas probably arise from the primitive sympathogonia and are highly malignant, while ganglioneuromas are related to mature ganglion cells and are benign. There are, however, many intermediate forms and the cells of a frankly malignant tumour, which has metastasized, may occasionally mature into a benign form or even disappear altogether. About 75% of tumours secrete catecholamines or their precursors.

The treatment of ganglioneuromas is surgical excision and the tumours can usually be shelled out without difficulty. Neuroblastomas are best treated by radical excision if there is no evidence of metastases. Operation should be undertaken with the same precautions as used for a phaeochromocytoma because of the pressor effects. Neuroblastomas are radiosensitive and irradiation of the operative field after total or incomplete removal is probably beneficial. Radiotherapy may also cause localized secondary deposits to regress. If the disease has spread beyond the primary site, chemotherapy using a combination of vincristine, cyclophosphamide and daunomycin is continuously given for at least two years. Several treatment schedules are available and the possible value of immunotherapy is being evaluated. The course of the disease may be followed by radiology and measurement of urinary catecholamine metabolites.

Prognosis for ganglioneuromas is excellent but extremely poor for neuroblastomas. About two-thirds of the patients with relatively benign tumours and without evidence of metastases are alive and well three years after surgical removal followed by radiotherapy but only 10–15% of those with distant metastases are in remission. After three years' treatment, a small proportion of highly malignant tumours undergo spontaneous cure with the best prognosis in the first year of life.

Malignant carcinoid tumour (argentaffinoma) and the carcinoid syndrome

Carcinoid, implying a benign tumour resembling a carcinoma, is now recognized as being potentially malignant. The appendix is the commonest site and most tumours, especially if small, are benign. However, extra-appendiceal carcinoids are probably all malignant (MacDonald, 1956). The small intestine being the second commonest site of carcinoid tumours, is the most frequent origin of metastasizing carcinoids and the most common source of the classical carcinoid syndrome. These tumours are multicentric (25–33%) and often there is an unrelated malignant tumour (33%) such as a colonic adenocarcinoma (Table 17.7). Occasionally the tumour forms part of the multiple endocrine neoplasia syndrome. Malignant carcinoids (argentaffinomas) secrete 5-hydroxytryptamine (5-HT) and kinins in large amounts into the portal circulation which are normally inactivated by the liver. When large hepatic metastases develop and secrete these hormones and enzymes, they directly enter the systemic circulation and cause the malignant carcinoid syndrome. Carcinoids have been described in sites draining directly into the systemic circulation (e.g. ovary) and cause the syndrome in the absence of metastases. Motilin and substance P are produced by intestinal EC cells but the other substances secreted include prostaglandins, insulin and ACTH.

Clinical features of carcinoid tumours depend on the site, size and presence of metastases. Symptoms of the syndrome include flushing, diarrhoea and asthma and the most sinister is tricuspidal or pulmonary stenosis with congestive cardiac failure. The most helpful initial investigation is measurement of urinary excretion of 5-hydroxyindole acetic acid (5-HIAA), the major metabolite of 5-HT (Anon., 1975). Investigations of the gastrointestinal tract include barium studies, fibreoptic endoscopy, angiography, ultrasound and CAT-scanning.

Treatment is influenced by the fact that most carcinoid tumours do not metastasize and those which do, grow very slowly. Patients with liver metastases have survived in reasonable health for many years. Surgical resection is the treatment of choice for the primary tumour but the extent depends upon the site of origin (Welch and Malt, 1977). Most appendiceal carcinoids are not diagnosed clinically, are often an incidental pathological finding and the further management is therefore controversial. Some advocate reoperation depending on the size, site or invasion of the tumour. In a review of over 1000 appendicular carcinoids treated by appendicectomy alone, only two developed a post-operative recurrence. It appears that simple appendicectomy is adequate treatment regardless of the local stage of the disease. If there is lymph node involvement or the tumour is at the margin of excision or greater than 2 cm, then several authors also advocate a right hemicolectomy. The prognosis for appendicular carcinoids is excellent with 97% survival rate at 5 years and 75% at 10 years.

The approach to carcinoid tumours of the small intestine is completely different as these tumours commonly metastasize causing the malignant carcinoid syndrome. Surgical treatment should therefore be radical with a wide *en bloc* resection of the small intestine and mesentery (Sworn *et al.*, 1978). Involved lymph nodes are removed and a careful search made for multiple carcinoid tumours and a second malignancy. The survival at 5 years in operable cases is 70%, where irresectable 40% and in patients with liver metastases is 20%. Overall survival is 33–40% with the average duration from onset of symptoms to death being 8 years.

A carcinoid tumour in the rectum, less than 2 cm, confined to the mucosa and histologically benign may be treated by local excision but larger tumours require

Table 17.7 Site of gastrointestinal carcinoid tumours (collected series of over 4000 cases).

		Percentage of total number		
		Incidence	Metastases	Carcinoid syndrome
Foregut (6.5%)	Stomach	2.5	23	9
	Duodenum	3.5	20	3
	Pancreaticobiliary	0.5	30	8
Midgut (75%)	Jejuno-ileal	28	34	9
	Meckel's	1	19	7
	Appendix	46	2	0.4
Hindgut (18.5%)	Colon	2.5	60	5
	Rectum	16	18	0.2

an abdominoperineal or anterior resection of the rectum. Patients with malignant rectal carcinoid tumours rarely survive more than three years after radical operation. Colonic carcinoids tend to be the most malignant with a 60% incidence of metastases. The majority tend to be in the caecum, large in size and treatment is a right hemicolectomy. Tumours in the biliary tract and pancreas, if large, tend to be inoperable with metastases, but formal operative procedures such as pancreaticoduodenectomy should be attempted although prognosis is poor. Bronchial carcinoids may present with a carcinoid syndrome which does not necessarily indicate metastases. Resection gives a good prognosis with a 5-year survival rate of 65%.

Treatment of the malignant carcinoid syndrome

The objective is destruction or surgical removal of functioning tumour mass and drug therapy to antagonize or suppress the release of the humoral substances. Bronchial and ovarian carcinoids have a venous drainage directly into the systemic circulation and resection of the primary tumour may cure the syndrome. This is rare and most tumours have metastasized to regional lymph nodes and the liver. It is worthwhile resecting as much tumour tissue as possible, for reduction of the secreting mass temporarily reduces the symptoms. Radiotherapy has very little place. Since the primary tumour and metastases usually grow slowly, patients will have several years of distressing symptoms.

Cytotoxic drugs may be administered systemically or by local infusion into the hepatic vessels. At the Mayo Clinic a good response was obtained with streptozotocin alone in three out of six patients and in six out of nine cases when combined with 5-FU. During and immediately after treatment there may be an acute exacerbation of symptoms. The dose of 5-FU is either 12.5 mg/kg intravenously for 3–5 days every 4 weeks or 15 mg/kg weekly for 6 weeks. The dose is adjusted in patients with abnormal liver, renal or bone marrow function. The dose of streptozotocin is 1 g/m^2 intravenously for 4 weeks which is continued if there is a response. When using the combination, the daily intravenous dose of 5-FU is 12 mg/kg and streptozotocin 500 mg/m^2 for 5 days. Cyclophosphamide can also be used either alone or in combination with 5-FU and streptozotocin. Other procedures include portal vein infusion of 5-FU after ligation of the common hepatic artery. This may decrease the size of the liver secondaries with regression of the syndrome.

Two patients with hepatic metastases were treated by selective hepatic artery embolization using absorbable gelatin sponge. Pre-treatment consisted of steroids, antibiotics and aprotinin. The flushing disappeared immediately and the liver metastases reduced in size (Allison, 1978; Zammit et al., 1978). In localized liver tumours, either a formal hepatic lobectomy or enucleation can be carried out. This helps considerably in patients with fever and abdominal pain. Response to therapy is monitored clinically, using isotopic and CAT-scanning and by a fall in urinary excretion of 5-HIAA after successful treatment. Serial 5-HIAA measurements give early information about recurrent tumour. Since the carcinoid syndrome is caused by more than one humoral agent, no single drug is effective in suppressing all symptoms. Therefore, serotonin antagonists such as methysergide and cyproheptadine block the serotonin-related symptoms of watery diarrhoea, abdominal colic and malabsorption. Parachlorophenylalanine, by inhibiting trypto-

Table 17.8 Drugs available for the treatment of the malignant carcinoid syndrome.

Drugs	Dose	Mode of action	Use
Cytotoxic chemotherapy			
5-Fluorouracil (5-FU)	15 mg/kg i.v. weekly × 6		Metastases
Streptozotocin	1 g/m² i.v. weekly × 6		Metastases
5-FU + streptozotocin	12 mg/kg i.v. daily for 5 days 500 mg/m² i.v. daily for 5 days		Metastases
Cyclophosphamide	40 mg/kg i.v. or oral as single dose or 2–4 mg/kg oral for 10 days		Metastases
Anti-humoral			
Methysergide	2 mg 8 hourly orally	5-HT antagonist	Bronchospasm Diarrhoea
p-Chlorophenylalanine	1–8 g daily	5-HT inhibitor	Diarrhoea
Cyproheptadine	4 mg 8-hourly orally	5-HT antagonist Bradykinin antagonist	Flushing Bronchospasm Diarrhoea Abdominal colic
Chlorpromazine	25–300 mg 8-hourly orally	Antikinin 5-HT antagonist	Flushing
α-Methyldopa	125–1000 g 8-hourly orally	Inhibits 5-HTP decarboxylase	Flushing
Aprotinin	50 000 U i.v.	Antikinin	Bronchospasm Vasodilation
Phenoxybenzamine	10–30 mg daily	Antikallikrein	Diarrhoea Bronchospasm
Others			
Isoprenaline aerosol			Bronchospasm
Prednisone	5–50 mg 12-hourly		Flushing Facial oedema
Codeine phosphate	5–10 mg 6-hourly orally		Diarrhoea
Diphenoxylate hydrochloride (Lomotil)	2–4 tablets 6-hourly		Diarrhoea
Spironolactone (diuretics)			Oedema

phan 5-hydroxylase may control gastrointestinal symptoms and kinin inhibitors such as phenothiazines can be used to control flushing. Codeine phosphate or diphenoxylate hydrochloride (Lomotil) is given for the diarrhoea. Oedema responds usually to diuretics or spironolactone and patients with right heart lesions may require operation for the pulmonary or tricuspid stenosis (Table 17.8).

Pituitary tumours

Tumours may be classified according to their functional state and cell of origin:

1. Inactive endocrine tumours are chromaffin adenomas and craniopharyngiomas.
2. Active endocrine tumours are acidophil, basophil (mucoid cell), chromophobe and mixed chromophil–chromophobe adenomas. These tumours are occasionally associated with adenomas or hyperplasia of other endocrine glands, especially pancreatic islet cells and parathyroid glands in the MEN syndromes. Pituitary tumours, especially chromophobe adenomas, previously described as 'functionless' are frequently associated with hypersecretion of prolactin causing reproductive disorders.

Anterior pituitary tumours cause clinical features by excessive hormone secretion and by local pressure effects on adjacent normal pituitary and hypothalamic tissue. The lesions are nearly always benign but invade surrounding structures as they grow larger with a tendency to local malignancy. In Cushing's syndrome with pituitary enlargement, 25–50% have a tendency to local malignancy, representing about 5% of Cushing's patients. The cells of origin of the apudomas and the various clinical syndromes are given in Table 17.2.

Investigations include skull X-rays with pituitary fossa tomography, pneumoencephalography and CAT to determine tumour extension. Carotid arteriography and cavernous sinus venography assess lateral extension.

Functioning pituitary tumours are treated by a variety of ablative techniques which depend upon the particular circumstances in the individual patient and local availability of facilities. Tumours producing primarily pressure effects require relief, and preservation of normal pituitary function is a secondary consideration. Endocrine-secreting pituitary tumours, on the other hand, are often slow growing and may not cause local effects. Treatment is aimed at curing the endocrine syndrome without, if possible, compromising normal pituitary function.

Non-invasive techniques

Conventional external radiation
Current practice is to give 4000–5000 rad of either X-ray or γ-rays from a linear accelerator or cobalt-60. Two or three narrow converging beams are used over a 3–6 week period. Treatment is usually well tolerated with pituitary function being retained. The visual defects may improve and serious complications, which are dose-related, are rare. As with surgery, it is justifiable to accept a small risk of complications in the interests of a good response rate (see Fig. 17.3).

Heavy particle irradiation (see Chapter 4)
This allows greater penetration and using the Bragg peak effect, a single beam can be used to increase the energy on the target area without absorption by other tissues. Doses of 6000–8000 rad are used which can be doubled to produce total pituitary destruction. Treatment is restricted to centres with a cyclotron and is not suitable for tumours with supra-sellar extension. External irradiation reduces the recurrence rate of surgically treated chromophobe adenomas. As chromophobe adenomas are moderately radiosensitive, external irradiation can be used as the initial treatment of choice. Approximately one-third of the patients treated initially by radiotherapy require subsequent surgery, either because of rapid deterioration of vision or recurrence of the tumour (Chang and Pool, 1967).

Invasive techniques

Surgery
Transphenoidal route is now widely used for small to medium sized tumours. Microsurgical techniques allow selective removal of the tumour (Wilson and Dempsey, 1978). Transfrontal surgery may damage the frontal lobes or optic chiasma. Operative mortality varies from 5 to 20% and is especially high (17%) for large tumours but vision improves in 55–80% of patients (Elkington and McKissock, 1967). Although radical excision reduces tumour recurrence, it increases the operative mortality. The advantages of surgery are that lesions can be seen, biopsied and the treatment response is rapid.

Pituitary implantation
Pituitary implantation of radioactive sources is usually undertaken by the transphenoidal route and allows a much greater dose of pituitary irradiation. Yttrium-90

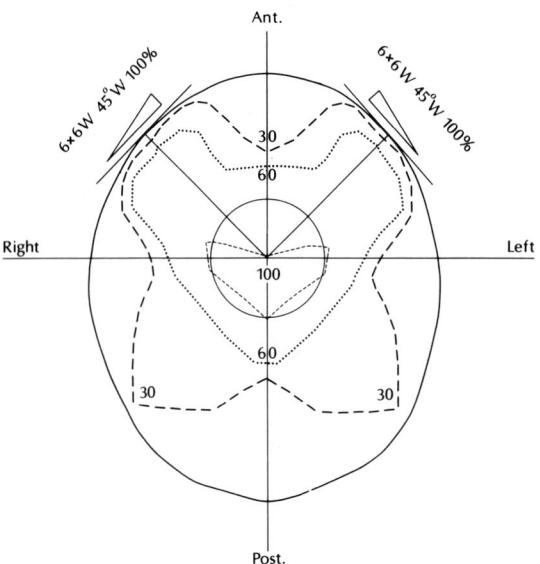

Fig. 17.3 Radiotherapy technique for pituitary tumours. Schematic diagram of the transverse section of skull at level of the pituitary gland showing two anterior oblique radiotherapy beams (6 × 6 cm) converging (45°C) on the pituitary fossa. The numerals 100, 60 and 30 refer to the radiation dose at the various sites.

in doses up to 300 000 rad from a high density β-irradiation causes an intense local necrosis. Gold-198, a γ-emitting isotope, gives a more diffuse irradiation to the pituitary and therefore may cause damage to the surrounding structures depending on the dose given. This is usually 10 000 rad. Pituitary implants may result in damage to the optic or occular motor nerves but with experience of bone landmarks, these complications have now been nearly eliminated. The main complication is a cerebrospinal fluid rhinorrhoea and meningeal infection.

Cryohypophysectomy

Cryohypophysectomy is achieved by circulating liquid nitrogen through a transphenoidal probe inserted into the pituitary gland. Transient external occular muscle paresis may occur and cerebrospinal rhinorrhoea.

In summary surgery is the initial treatment of choice for pituitary tumours with marked extrasellar spread, when there is a large visual defect, and in cases of diagnostic uncertainty. Surgery is mandatory if vision rapidly deteriorates which indicates the probable occurrence of haemorrhage into the tumour (pituitary apoplexy) and the need for urgent decompression. All surgically treated patients should be considered for post-operative irradiation. After treatment, hypopituitarism is common and must not be missed. Elkington *et al.* (1967) found 78% of 152 patients followed for 1–25 years after treatment, to have clinical hypopituitarism, less than half of whom were receiving replacement therapy. Occasionally pituitary function may improve after ablative therapy for chromophobe adenomas (Joplin *et al.*, 1975).

Prognosis is difficult to assess because many large 'benign' adenomas tend to be locally invasive although metastases are rare. The prognosis for non-functioning tumours is better than for large GH- or ACTH-secreting tumours. In patients requiring operation for visual defects or other serious complications, about 75% are alive at 2 years and 50% at 20 years. After hypophysectomy and external radiotherapy about 10–20% show signs of recurrence, usually within 5 years. Invasive adenomas are incurable and usually cause death within 2–3 years of diagnosis.

Medical treatment is aimed at either suppressing the release or production of hormones or preventing their peripheral action. This varies according to the hormones being produced. In acromegaly, oestrogens, progesterone and chlorpromazine have been advocated but recent reports have not been encouraging. The dopamine antagonist, bromocriptine is effective in suppressing growth hormone secretion and analogues of somatostatin may be available in the future. Prolactinomas tend not to be malignant or locally invasive and medical treatment includes the use of dopaminergic drugs.

In 1921 Cushing wrote: 'It is certain that no one method is applicable for all conditions of the pituitary tumour'. The variety of clinical problems and the different aims of treatment for the various types of pituitary tumours, makes it essential that centres concerned with their management should have several forms of therapy available.

Follow-up after treatment requires measuring the plasma and urinary level of the various hormones. After surgical hypophysectomy, the hormone values fall abruptly but the decline is more gradual after irradiation. The initial hormone level gives some indication of prognosis. However, there is a poor correlation between the clinical response and alteration in hormone levels.

Multiple endocrine neoplasia (adenopathy, MEA, MEN) and the paraendocrine syndromes (PES)

These closely related syndromes impinge on all aspects of endocrinology and the clinical features may sometimes provide the only clues to an underlying cancer. Even when tumours cannot be eradicated, correction of metabolic disturbances may provide symptomatic relief.

Multiple endocrine neoplasia

This describes a group of syndromes, often familial, in which two or more endocrine glands undergo hyperplasia or tumour formation in the same individual, either at the same time or consecutively. The hyperfunctioning glands secrete their normal major hormones (orthoendocrine syndromes) and/or abnormal hormones (paraendocrine syndromes). There are two main varieties.

Multiple endocrine neoplasia Type I (MEN I or MEA I) (Wermer, 1954)

This manifests from the second decade into old age with an equal sex distribution. In 85 patients reviewed by Ballard *et al.* (1964), the glands involved in order of frequency were parathyroids (88%), pancreatic islets (81%), anterior pituitary (65%), adrenal cortex (38%) and thyroid follicular cells (19%). Pairs of glands, any two of the first four, were involved in 60% and all of the first three endocrine glands in 40%.

The parathyroids usually undergo chief cell hyperplasia or less commonly multiple adenoma formation. The islet cells may be involved by an adenoma (multiple or single), carcinoma and very rarely a generalized hyperplasia. In the pituitary an adenoma, or rarely a carcinoma or hyperplasia may involve any of the different cell types. The adrenal cortices usually show bilateral diffuse or nodular hyperplasia, but adenomas have been reported. The changes in the thyroid are very variable and occasionally carcinoid tumours are present in the lungs, pancreas or intestine. Peptic ulceration, especially duodenal, is a common feature in some families and may affect more than half the patients. Some members of such families have peptic ulceration without evidence of endocrinopathy. The peptic ulcers are often multiple and liable to serious complications and may form part of the Zollinger-Ellison syndrome due to an associated pancreatic gastrinoma or due to hyperparathyroidism. Many of these lesions are apudomas and the syndrome may result from a widespread dysplasia of the apud cells.

Each feature of the syndrome should be treated on its merits. If more than one syndrome is present at the same time, that presenting the most urgent features should be treated first. Peptic ulceration should initially be treated by medical measures or standard surgical procedures. If due to a gastrinoma, then either H_2-receptor antagonists or a gastrectomy are required. On the other hand, parathyroidectomy occasionally reduces gastrin production. Post-operatively the patient should be followed carefully so that other features of the syndrome may be detected early and relatives should be examined.

Multiple endocrine neoplasia Type II (MEN II or MEA II) (Sipple, 1961)
This syndrome is usually inherited, affects sexes equally and may manifest itself from the first decade onwards, especially between 20 and 40 years. Three forms of the syndrome are recognized. The commonest is medullary carcinoma of the thyroid with a phaeochromocytoma in one or both adrenals. Hyperparathyroidism due to hyperplasia or adenoma may be present and is probably due to hypercalcitoninaemia. Another variant is a medullary carcinoma of thyroid and phaeochromocytoma with multiple small subcutaneous and sub-mucous neuromas of the eyelids, tongue and buccal mucosa with a diffuse hypertrophy of the lips. These lesions are present from birth. In the last type, all these features are present together with autonomic ganglioneuromatosis and various other congenital abnormalities. These include intestinal diverticula, sugarloaf skull and features suggestive of Marfan's syndrome. These syndromes are probably due to a dysplasia of neural crest cells (Carney and Hayles, 1977).

The phaeochromocytoma is the lesion which requires the most urgent treatment, because investigation or treatment for other lesions may precipitate a fatal hypertensive crisis. The possibility of MEN II should be considered in all patients with a medullary carcinoma of the thyroid or hyperparathyroidism and patients should be routinely screened for a phaeochromocytoma, Measurements of calcitonin in the blood in patients and their families may reveal the presence of medullary carcinoma in a pre-cancerous form. (see Chapter 15 on Thyroid Cancer)

Paraendocrine syndromes
Paraendocrine tumours usually contain small amounts of hormones, compared with normal endocrine glands, but the plasma hormone concentration is often very high. Secretory activity may exhibit a cyclical pattern. The following paraendocrine syndromes (PES) are recognized most frequently and have been conveniently divided into three main groups.

In PES I, tumours of endocrine glands secrete hormones or humoral substances which are foreign to their presumptive cells of origin, but characteristic of others, e.g. non-pituitary tumours secreting ACTH causing Cushing's syndrome. Tumours may secrete normal hormones or synthesize several hormones which are not necessarily released into circulation.

In PES II, tumours or other lesions of organs or tissues, which are not usually regarded as endocrine, secrete natural hormones or similar substances characteristic of endocrine tissues, e.g. oat-cell carcinoma of bronchus secreting ACTH or GH. PES I and II are sometimes said to reflect 'ectopic' or 'inappropriate' secretion of hormones.

In PES III, clinical or biochemical features usually attributable to hormone excess, are present in the absence of any recognizable endocrine abnormality.

Cushing's ectopic syndrome
Ectopic ACTH syndrome is the commonest form of the paraendocrine syndrome (PES I and II). The common causative lesions are bronchial oat-cell carcinoma and carcinoid tumours, thymic epithelial carcinoma, pancreatic islet cell tumours, phaeochromocytomas and ovarian carcinomas. If a bronchial carcinoma is the cause, it is usually far advanced and effective therapy impossible. Carcinoid tumours, especially of the bronchus, may be benign and their removal cures the syndrome. Adrenalectomy is rarely justified, except if the tumour is slow growing and cannot be eradicated.

Schwartz-Bartter (ectopic ADH) syndrome
The most frequent cause of anti-diuretic hormone (ADH) secretion is an advanced oat-cell carcinoma of the bronchus, but several other tumours and nontumerous conditions may be responsible (PES I and II).

If the primary tumour can be removed or eradicated

successfully, the patient will excrete large amounts of dilute urine until the hyponatraemia is corrected. Symptomatic treatment includes fluid restriction and fludrocortisone (0.2–0.4 mg daily).

Hypercalcaemia

Hypercalcaemia may be due to secondary deposits in the bone (PES III) but some patients with cancer have hypercalcaemia and hypercalciuria without evidence of skeletal metastases (PES I and II). Some tumours, e.g. kidney, bronchus or ovary, contain immunoreactive human PTH. Surgical removal of the tumour but not parathyroidectomy alone, may abolish the hypercalcaemia.

Miscellaneous PES syndromes

Tumours have been described secreting erythropoietin, gonadotrophins and hypoglycaemic agents causing erythrocythaemia, precocious puberty and gynaecomastia. Removal of the causative tumour usually leads to remission. Often, however, due to an advanced stage of the tumour and poor prognosis, symptomatic therapy only is given.

Conclusion

The realization that many apparently unrelated endocrine tumours can be classed as apudomas provides a convenient unifying concept which increases the understanding and may in time lead to more effective methods of treatment. Many of the tumours discussed are rare and represented often as case reports and assessment and evaluation of treatment and prognosis is difficult. However, with an increasing understanding, better methods of investigation and earlier diagnosis, more effective treatment can be planned and the overall prognosis should improve. Wider knowledge of these tumours may lead to realization that they are more common than at present seems likely; better assessment of the value of modern radiotherapy and chemotherapy is needed.

Further reading

Edis, A.J., Ayala, L.A. and Egdahl, R.H. (1975), *Manual of Endocrine Surgery*. Springer-Verlag, New York.

Friesen, S.R. (1978), *Surgical Endocrinology: Clinical Syndromes*. Lippincott, Philadelphia.

Hartog, M. (1978), Pituitary Tumours. In: *Recent Advances in Endocrinology and Metabolism* (ed. J.L.H. O'Riordan), Churchill-Livingstone, Edinburgh, p. 17.

Montgomery, D.A.D. and Welbourn, R.B. (1975). *Medical and Surgical Endocrinology*. Arnold, London.

Paloyon, E., Lawrence, A.M. and Strauss, F.H. (1973), *Hyperparathyroidism*. Grune and Stratton, New York.

Welbourn, R.B. and Joffe, S.N. (1977), The apudomas. In: *Recent Advances in Surgery* (ed. Selwyn Taylor) No. 9, Churchill-Livingstone, Edinburgh, p. 311.

References

Ackerman, N.B. and Winer, N. (1974), The Differentiation of primary hyperparathyroidism from the hypercalcaemia of malignancy. *Ann. Surg.*, **181**, 226–31.

Allison, D.J. (1978), Therapeutic embolization. *Br. J. Hosp. Med.*, December 1978, 707–15.

Anon. (editorial) (1975), Diagnosis of malignant carcinoid syndrome. *Br. Med. J.*, **2**, 122–3.

Ballard, H.S., Frame, B. and Hartstock, R.J. (1964), Familial multiple endocrine adenoma-peptic ulcer complex. *Med.*, **43**, 481–516.

Bloom, S.R. (1978), The VIP Controversy. *Digestive Diseases*, **23**, 370–1.

Bradley, E.L. (1975), Primary and adjunctive therapy in carcinoma of the adrenal cortex. *Surgery, Gynec. Obstet.*, **141**, 507–11.

Broder, L.E. and Carter, S.K. (1973), Pancreatic islet cell carcinoma: Results of therapy with streptozotocin in 52 patients. *Ann. Intern. Med.*, **79**, 109–18.

Burchard, F., Strange, J.G., Stadil, F., Jensen, L.I. and Fischermann, K. (1979), *Localisation of gastinomas*, **77**, 444–50.

Carney, J.A. and Hayles, A.B. (1977), Alimentary tract manifestations of multiple endocrine neoplasia, Type 2b. *Mayo Clinic Proc.*, 533–48.

Carter, S.K., Bakowski, T. and Hellman, K. (1977), *Chemotherapy of Cancer*. Wiley Medical, New York.

Chang, C.H. and Pool, J.L. (1967), The radiotherapy of pituitary chromophobe adenomas. *Radiol.*, **89**, 1005–16.

Conn, J.W. (1955a), Painting background: Part I. Primary aldosteronism. *J. Lab. Clin. Med.*, **45**, 3–17.

Conn, J.W. (1955b), Progress Report: Primary aldosteronism. *J. Lab. Clin. Med.*, **45**, 661–4.

Conn, J.W., Knopf, R.F. and Nesbit, R.M. (1964), Clinical characteristics of primary aldosteronism from an analysis of 145 cases. *Am. J. Surg.*, **107**, 159–72.

Cooke, T.J.C. *et al.* (1977), Parathyroidectomy: extend of resection and late results. *Br. J. Surg.*, **64**, 153–7.

Creutzfeldt, R. Arnold and Frerichs, H. (1978), Insulinomas and Gastrinomas. In: *Gut Hormones* (ed. S.R. Bloom), Churchill Livingstone, Edinburgh, pp.589–98.

Devine, B.L. *et al.* (1978), Cyclical release of vasoactive intestinal polypeptide (VIP) from a pancreatic islet cell apudoma. *Postgrad. Med.*, **54**, 566–70.

Dix, V.W. (1963), Tumours of the adrenal cortex. *Br. J. Urol.*, **35**, 356–66.

Dozois, R.R. and Beahrs, O.H. (1977), Surgical anatomy and techniques of thyroid and parathyroid surgery. *Surg. Clinics N. Amer.*, **57**, 647–61.

Eastman, R. C. *et al.* (1977), Adriamycin therapy for advanced insulinoma. *Am. J. Surg.*, **131**, 352–6.

Ebeid, A.M., Murray, P.D. and Fischer, J.E. (1978), Vasoactive intestinal peptide and the watery diarrhoea syndrome. *Ann. Surg.*, **187**, 411–6.

Elkington, S.G., Buckell, M. and Jenkins, J.S. (1967), Endocrine function following treatment of pituitary adenoma. *Acta endocrinol.*, **55**, 146–52.

Elkington, S.G. and McKissock, W. (1967), Pituitary adenoma: results of combined surgical and radiotherapeutic treatment of 260 patients. *Br. Med. J.*, **i**, 263–6.

Ellison, E.H. and Wilson, S.D. (1964), The Zollinger-Ellison Syndrome: Reappraisal and evaluation of 260 registered cases. *Ann. Surg.*, **160**, 512–30.

Esselstyn, C.B. (1977), Parathyroid pathology: its relation to choice of operation for hyperparathyroidism. *Wld. J. Surg.*, **1**, 701–8.

Filipi, C.J. and Higgins, G.A. (1973), Diagnosis and management of insulinoma. *Am. J. Surg.*, **125**, 231–9.

Floyd, J.C. Jr. *et al.* (1975), Concentrations of a newly recognised pancreatic islet polypeptide in plasma of healthy subjects and in plasma and tumours of patients with insulin-secreting islet cell tumours. *Clin. Res.*, **23**, 535A.

Fortner, J.G. *et al.* (1977), Regional Pancreatectomy: en bloc pancreatic portal vein and lymph node resection. *Ann. Surg.*, **186**, 42–50.

Fox, P.S. *et al.* (1974), The influence of total gastrectomy on survival in malignant Zollinger-Ellison tumours. *Ann. Surg.*, **180**, 558–66.

Foye, L.V. Jr. and Feichtmeir, T.V. (1955), Adrenal cortical carcinoma producing solely mineralocorticoid effect. *Am. J. Med.*, **19**, 966–75.

Gagel, R.F. *et al.* (1976), Streptozocin-treated Verner-Morrison Syndrome. *Arch. Intern. Med.*, **136**, 1429–35.

Geelhoed, G.W., Dunnick, N.R. and Doppman, J.L. (1980), Management of extensions of endocrine tumours, *Am. J. Surg.*, **139**, 844–8.

Goodall, A.L. and Symington, T. (1953), Studies in phaeochromocytoma: clinical aspects: Diagnosis by adrenergic blocking drugs and treatment. *Glasgow Med. J.*, **34**, 95–7.

Greenberg, P.H. and Marks, C. (1978), Adrenal cortical carcinoma: a presentation of 22 cases and a review of the literature. *Am. Surg.*, **44**, 81–5.

Hardy, J.D. and Doolittle, P.D. (1977), Zollinger-Ellison syndrome. *Ann. Surg.*, **185**, 661–71.

Hume, D.M. (1960), Phaeochromocytoma in the adult and in the child. *Am. J. Surg.*, **99**, 458–96.

Hutter, A.M. Jr. and Kayhoe, D.E. (1966), Adrenocortical carcinoma. *Am. J. Med.*, **41**, 572–81.

Ingemansson, S. *et al.* (1975), Portal and pancreatic vein catheterization with radioimmunologic determination of insulin. *Surgery, Gynec. Obstet.*, **141**, 705–11.

Isenberg, J.I., Walsh, J.H. and Grossman, M.I. (1973), Zollinger-Ellison syndrome. *Gastroenterology*, **65**, 140–65.

Jarman, W.T., Myers, R.T. and Marshall, R.B. (1978), Carcinoma of the parathyroid. *Archs. Surg.*, **113**, 123–5.

Joffe, S.N. *et al.* (1978), Clinically silent gross hypergastrinaemia from a multiple hormone-secreting pancreatic apudoma. *Br. J. Surg.*, **65**, 277–80.

Joplin, G.F. *et al.* (1975), The effect of Yttrium-90 implantation on endocrine function and visual fields in patients with 'functionless' pituitary tumours, with biopsy and radiological findings. *Clin. Endocrinol.*, **4**, 139–63.

Laroche, G.P. *et al.* (1968), Hyperinsulinism. *Arch. Surg.*, **96**, 763–72.

Larsson, L.-I., Grimelius, L. and Hakanson, R. (1975), Mixed endocrine pancreatic tumours producing several peptide hormones. *Am. J. Pathol.*, **79**, 271–84.

Larsson, L.-I. *et al.* (1977), Pancreatic somatostatinoma – clinical features and physiological implications. *Lancet*, **i**, 666–8.

Larsson, L.-I. *et al.* (1976), Occurrence of human pancreatic polypeptide in pancreatic endocrine tumours. *Am. J. Pathol.*, **85**, 675–82.

Lewinsky, B.S. *et al.* (1974), The clinical and pathological features of non-hormonal adrenocortical tumours. *Cancer*, **33**, 778–90.

Lubitz, J.A., Freeman, L. and Okun, R. (1973), Mitotone use in inoperable adrenal cortical carcinoma. *J. Am. Med. Assoc.*, **223**, 1109–12.

McCarthy, D.M. (1978), Report on the United States experience with cimetidine in Zollinger-Ellison syndrome and other hypersecretory states. *Gastroenterology*, **74**, 453–8.

MacDonald, R.A. (1956), A study of 356 carcinoids of the gastro-intestinal tract. *Am. J. Med.*, **21**, 867–76.

McGavran, M.H. *et al.* (1966), A glucagon-secreting alpha-cell carcinoma of the pancreas. *New Engl. J.*

Med., **274**, 1408–13.

Mallinson, C.N. *et al.* (1974), A glucagonoma syndrome. *Lancet*, **i**, 1–4.

Moldow, R.E. and Connelly, R.R. (1968), Epidemiology of pancreatic cancer in Connecticut. *Gastroenterology*, **55**, 677–86.

Moss, N.H. and Rhoades, J.E. (1960), Hyperinsulinism and islet cell tumors of the pancreas. In: *Surgical Diseases of the Pancreas*. (eds J.M. Howard and G.L. Jordan), J.B. Lippincott, Philadelphia.

Pearse, A.G.E. (1968), Common cytochemical and ultra-structural characteristics of cells producing polypeptide hormones (the APUD series) and their relevance to thyroid and ultimobronchial C cells and calcitonin. *Proc. Roy. Soc. London* (Biological Science), **170**, 71–80.

Percarpio, B. and Knowlton, A.H. (1976), Radiation therapy of adrenal cortical carcinoma. *Acta Radiol. Therapy Phys. Biol.*, **15**, 288–92.

Rapaport, E. *et al.* (1952), Mortality in surgically treated adreno-cortical tumors. *Postgrad. Med.*, **11**, 325–53.

Robins, S.L. (1967), The Pancreas. In: *Pathology*, W.B. Saunders, Philadelphia, p.963.

Schantz, A. and Castleman, B. (1973), Parathyroid carcinoma: A study of 70 cases. *Cancer*, **31**, 600–5.

Schein, P.S. *et al.* (1973), Islet cell tumours: current concepts and management. *Ann. Intern. Med.*, **79**, 239–59.

Schteingert, D.E., Cash, R. and Conn, J.W. (1966), Amino-glutethimide and metastatic adrenal cancer. *J. Am. Med. Assoc.*, **198**, 1007–10.

Service, F. *et al.* (1976), Insuloma. Clinical and diagnostic features of 60 consecutive cases. *Mayo Clinic Proc.*, **51**, 419–28.

Shons, A.R. and Gamble, W.G. (1974), Nonfunctioning carcinoma of the adrenal cortex. *Surgery Gynec. Obstet.*, **138**, 705–9.

Sipple, J.H. (1961), The association of phaeochromocytoma with carcinoma of the thyroid gland. *Am. J. Med.*, **31**, 163–6.

Stefanini, P. *et al.* (1974), Beta-islet cell tumours of the pancreas: Results of a study on 1067 cases. *Surgery*, **75**, 597–609.

Sworn, M.J., Reasbeck, P. and Buchanan, R. (1978), Intestinal ischaemia associated with ileal carcinoid tumour. *Br. J. Surg.*, **65**, 313–5.

Symington, T. (1969), In: *Functional Pathology of the Human Adrenal Gland*. Livingstone, London, pp. 219–324.

Szijj, T. *et al.* (1969), Carcinoma of thyroid associated with hypercorticism. *Cancer*, **24**, 167–73.

Turner, R.C. *et al.* (1978), Localisation of insulinomas. *Lancet*, **i**, 515–8.

Verner, J.V. Jr. and Morrison, A.B. (1958), Islet cell tumour and a syndrome of refractory watery diarrhoea and hypokalaemia. *Am. J. Med.*, **25**, 374–80.

Welbourn, R.B. *et al.* (1978), Apudomas of the Pancreas. In: *Gut Hormones* (ed. S.R. Bloom), Churchill Livingstone, Edinburgh, pp. 561–9.

Welch, J.P. and Malt, R.A. (1977), Management of carcinoid tumours of the gastrointestinal tract. *Surgery, Gynec. Obstet.*, **145**, 223–7.

Wells. S.A. Jr. *et al.* (1978), Medical adrenalectomy with aminoglutethimide: clinical studies in postmenopausal patients with metastatic breast carcinoma. *Ann. Surg.*, **187**, 475–84.

Wells, S.A. Leigh, G.S. and Ross, A.J. (1980), Primary hyperparathyroidism in *Current Problems in Surgery*, **17**, 435–64.

Wermer, P. (1954), Genetic aspects of adenomatosis of endocrine glands. *Am. J. Med.*, **16**, 363–71.

Wilson, C.B. and Dempsey, L.C. (1978), Transsphenoidal microsurgical removal of 250 pituitary ademonas. *J. Neurosurg.*, **48**, 13–22.

Zammit Maempel, F. and Modlin, I. (1978), Diagnosis and management of a gastric carcinoid tumour with hepatic metastases. *Br. J. Surg.*, **65**, 516–20.

Zollinger, R.M. and Ellison, E.H. (1955), Primary peptic ulcerations of the jejunum associated with islet cell tumours of the pancreas. *Ann. Surg.*, **142**, 709–28.

18 Thorax

T.J. Deeley and Ralph N. Sapsford, with a note on chemotherapy by Nicholas Thatcher

Part I: Lung

Incidence

There were few recorded cases of lung cancer in the medical literature until the beginning of this century. Since then there has been a steady increase due, firstly, to better diagnosis using radiographic and bronchoscopic techniques and more recently by sputum cytology and, secondly, a true increase in the number of patients presenting with the disease.

The incidence of the disease varies around the world (Table 18.1) and may vary tremendously within one country, industrial areas having a higher incidence and rural a lower. In large cities one part may have a higher incidence of cancer than another; in Great Britain this is the east side of a city.

It was predominantly a disease of men at one time; in more recent years we have seen more females affected and the male:female ratio is now about 6:1. This is a disease of older patients, some 90% occurring in patients over 50 years of age.

Aetiological factors

Smoking

The epidemiology of lung cancer reflects the pattern of smoking and it is now universally accepted that this disease is causally related to tobacco smoking.

We will briefly detail some of the factors involved:

1. There is a latent period between the cause and effect demonstrated by the lag between the rise in tobacco consumption and the increase in lung cancer (Fig. 18.1).
2. The incidence is related to the number of cigarettes smoked and to the duration of smoking (Fig. 18.2).

Table 18.1 Age standardized mortality per 100 000 from lung cancer in 24 countries, 1966–1967 (from Wynder and Hecht, 1976).

Country	Male	Female
Scotland	78.14	11.71
England and Wales	69.66	10.73
Finland	61.00	3.91
Netherlands	56.36	3.42
Austria	50.35	6.09
Belgium	50.09	4.36
USA (non-white)	44.83	7.14
Northern Ireland	43.29	7.14
Germany (Fed. Republic)	42.09	5.10
USA (white)	39.62	6.70
New Zealand	37.72	5.35
Australia	37.64	4.77
South Africa	37.63	6.93
Denmark	37.34	7.36
Switzerland	37.33	3.33
Canada	34.52	5.36
Ireland	33.54	7.88
Italy	30.23	4.53
France	27.71	3.74
Israel	22.51	7.62
Sweden	17.35	4.34
Chile	15.18	5.59
Norway	14.93	2.97
Japan	13.97	4.86
Portugal	10.91	2.74

3. There is an increasing risk of lung cancer going from non-smokers, to pipe smokers, to cigar smokers to cigarette smokers.
4. Discontinuing the habit reduces the risk of lung cancer. Doll and Peto (1976) found the age-adjusted death rates from cancer of the lung in male British doctors to be:

10/100 000 for non-smokers
83/100 000 for ex-smokers
104/100 000 for smokers.

5. There is some evidence to suggest that smokers who inhale have a higher incidence of lung cancer than non-inhalers; however, this is a complex problem and is bound up with other factors such as the length of cigarette smoked before it is dis-carded, the number of puffs, the use of filters and so on.

6. It is thought that the carcinogen is found in the tar and that the relative danger of a tobacco depends upon its tar yield.

7. Tobacco smoking is associated with squamous and, to a lesser extent, oat-cell tumours of the lung.

8. Among non-smokers, less than 1.0%, a few cancers will occur but of patients with proved lung cancer less than 1.0 per cent had never smoked.

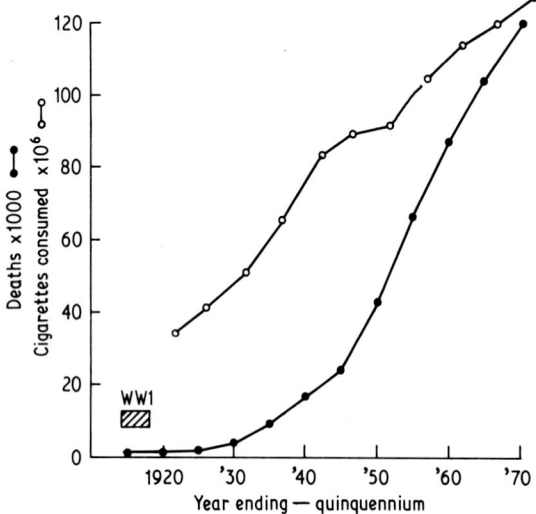

Fig. 18.1 Incidence of cancer of the lung and pleura in England and Wales, compared with number of cigarettes consumed. Cancer incidence from Division of Epidemiology, Institute of Cancer Research, London. Cigarette consumption, Wald (1976).

Other causes

Lung cancer has been associated with certain industries, such as gas and coke oven workers, the chrome and nickel ore industries and perhaps also arsenic, certain plastics and the asbestos industry. We must, of course, appreciate that the incidence may be greater in these workers if they also smoke.

Air pollution may account for some cases, especially in non-smokers; smoke from factories and homes may contain the same carcinogens as are found in tobacco and the increased incidence to the east of large urban areas may be due to the prevailing wind in this country being from the south-west. The motor car has increased the amount of pollution in the atmosphere from exhaust fumes, finely ground rubber particles and from asbestos used in brake linings; these substances may be responsible for some increased incidence of lung cancer especially in smokers.

Chronic infection in the lung may be a predisposing factor causing metaplasia, and chronic bronchitis is present in a large number of patients; cancer may develop also at the site of a tubercular scar.

Anatomy

The airway

The human airway within the chest consists of the trachea, the two major bronchi and the divisions of these bronchi to supply the lobes of the lungs. The trachea is held permanently patent by the presence of its 'C'-shaped cartilaginous rings. The rings are convex anteriorly. The posterior part of the trachea is unsupported and is known as the membranous part of the trachea. Cartilaginous rings also maintain the patency of the bronchi as far out as the commencement of the bronchioles. At the commencement of the main bronchi, they are also 'C'-shaped anteriorly but within a short distance come to surround the bronchi completely. The cartilaginous rings are supported and separated by smooth muscle which also forms the main constituent of the membranous part of the trachea. The airway is lined by a ciliated columnar epithelium

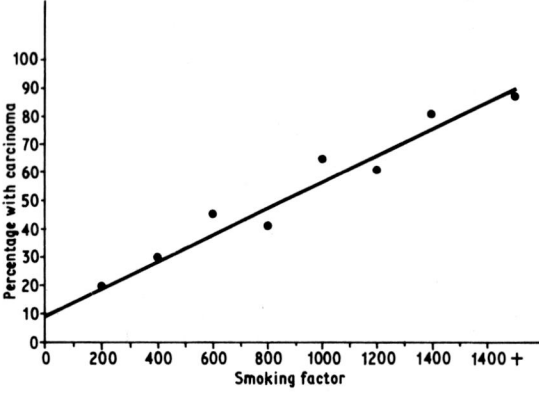

Fig. 18.2 The incidence of patients with carcinoma in people with the same smoking factors (cigarettes per day × number of years patient has smoked) (Deeley, 1974).

which extends out as far as the bronchioles. The respiratory bronchioles are a continuation of the bronchioles. The alveoli are minute sacular protrusions and are formed almost entirely by pavement epithelium lying on an exteriorly placed basement membrane. Outside this basement membrane the alveoli are separated by loose areolar tissue which contains the vessels of supply, the vessels of drainage and the lymphatics.

Special cells are to be found throughout the respiratory tree. There are mucus-secreting cells to be found amongst the ciliated epithelium of the trachea and bronchi. The respiratory bronchioles are lined by non-ciliated respiratory epithelium. The alveoli contain special cells responsible for the secretion of surfactant, called pneumocytes.

The lungs

The bronchi and all its divisions, together with the alveoli make up the two lungs. The right lung is a trilobed structure consisting of an upper, middle and lower lobe. The upper lobe has three segments namely the apical, the anterior and posterior segments. The middle lobe has two segments namely the medial and lateral segments. The lower lobe consists of five segments namely the apical, the anterior, posterior, lateral and the medial basal segments. A bronchoscopically identifiable tertiary bronchus supplies each of these segments.

The left lung is anatomically a bilobed structure consisting of an upper lobe and a lower lobe. The anatomical upper lobe consists of a true upper lobe and the lingular. The upper lobe has three segments but the apical and posterior segments come off a single tertiary bronchus and this is commonly known as the apicoposterior segment. The remaining segment is the anterior segment. The lingular bronchus arises from the upper lobe bronchus and divides into an upper and a lower segment. The lower lobe has four segments: the apical, the anterior, the posterior and the lateral base segment. Once again a bronchoscopically identifiable tertiary bronchus supplies each of these segments.

The pleura

Both lungs are covered and enclosed by a thin membrane of pavement epithelium called the visceral pleura. This structure is densely adherent to the surface of the lung. It reflects off the lung superiorly to, anteriorly to and posteriorly to the hilum and anteriorly and posteriorly to the inferior pulmonary ligament. The reflections contain the hilar structures above but are separated only by areolar tissue where they form the inferior pulmonary ligament. The pleura reflects away from the hilum and inferior pulmonary

ligament both superiorly, anteriorly and posteriorly to invest the mediastinum, where it is known as the mediastinal pleura. Finally it reaches the chest wall superiorly, anteriorly, posteriorly and the diaphragm inferiorly. It invests all these structures where it is now known as the parietal pleura. The pleura is bound loosely to the endothoracic fascia by areolar tissue. It is, however, firmly bound to the upper surface of the diaphragm. The two surfaces of the pleura are in close contact, separated only by a thin layer of fluid. The surface tension in this fluid maintains the contact between the two surfaces when placed under negative pressure during the respiratory cycle.

The blood supply

The lung has a dual blood supply, the main pulmonary artery divides into right and left branches which in turn subdivide progressively to become the lobar and segmental branches. The pulmonary artery branches accompany the bronchi, bronchioles and respiratory bronchioles and finally terminate as arterioles and capillaries in the areolar tissue which surrounds the alveoli.

Bronchial arteries arise from the descending thoracic aorta and enter the hilum of the lung. They ramify through the lung substance, again accompanying the bronchi and their branches. They terminate also as arterioles and capillaries in the areolar tissue surrounding the alveoli.

The two sources of arterial supply to the lung are drained by the pulmonary venous system. The pulmonary venous capillaries found in the areolar tissue surrounding the alveoli, return the blood through venules and then progressively larger channels which anatomically are situated in the planes between the lobules and segments. They terminate in four pulmonary veins, namely a superior and inferior pulmonary vein on each side which enters the left atrium.

Lymphatic drainage

The lungs have a very rich lymphatic drainage. Lymphatic drainage commences in the areolar tissue surrounding the alveoli and the lymphatic channels increasing steadily in size, and accompanying the pulmonary veins to the hilum of the lung. The lymphatics first drain into the interlobar nodes. These in turn drain into nodes surrounding the hilum of the lung. Notable amongst this group are the right and left superior tracheobronchial nodes and the nodes of the inferior pulmonary ligament. From these nodes further lymphatic drainage is into the mediastinal lymph nodes and these are to be found in groups in the following situations:

1. Along both sides of the trachea: these nodes are known as the paratracheal nodes and the lowest nodes in this chain are the superior tracheobronchial nodes. This group of nodes is continuous with the scalene nodes and the deep cervical nodes in the neck. On the left side the group of nodes, next above the tracheobronchial nodes, in this chain is known by surgeons as the sub-aortic group of nodes.
2. Inferior to the carina: these nodes, known as the subcarinal nodes are related directly to the oesophagus behind and the pericardium and the posterior wall of the left atrium in front.
3. In the anterior mediastinum.

From these groups of nodes drainage is finally into the blood stream. The lymphatic channels enter the thoracic duct, which in turn enters the left subclavian vein below which it is joined by the jugular vein to form the innominate vein.

In health, no lymphatics cross the pleural cavity. The left side of the chest wall is drained by lymphatics which enter the thoracic duct, as well as draining to the axillary lymph nodes. The entire diaphragm is drained by the thoracic duct. The right side of the chest wall is drained by the right lymphatic duct which enters the superior vena cava and also drains to the right axillary lymph nodes.

Pathology

Malignant change can occur from any tissues which constitute the human airway. Anatomically it can arise from the trachea, main bronchi, the lobar bronchi, the segmental bronchi or in the periphery of the lung having arisen from the bronchioles, respiratory bronchioles or alveoli. In addition malignant change can occur in the pleura. Very rarely malignant lesions of vascular origin are found in the lung.

Numerous classifications have been devised to cover all these lesions. The most widely accepted classification of malignant lung lesions today is that proposed by an expert committee of the World Health Organization (1960). This can be summarized as follows:

1. Squamous carcimona:
   (a) Keratinizing squamous carcinoma.
   (b) Dedifferentiated squamous cell carcinomas or polygonal cell carcinoma.
2. Anaplastic small cell carcinoma.
3. Adenocarcinoma:
   (a) Bronchiolar or bronchioloalveolar carcinoma.
4. Anaplastic large cell carcinoma.
5. Bronchial carcinoid.
6. Tumours of tracheobronchial mucous glands:

   (a) Adenoid cystic carcinoma (cylindroma).
   (b) Mucoepidermoid carcinoma.
   (c) Bronchial mucous gland adenocarcinoma.
7. Papilloma and papillary carcinoma.
8. Sarcoma:
   (a) Malignant lymphoma.
   (b) Leiomyosarcoma.
   (c) Others.
9. Teratomas, embryonal tumours and mixed tumours.
10. Pleural mesothelioma.
    (a) Epithelial or diffuse.
    (b) Fibrosarcomatous.
    (c) Other pleural sarcomas.

Four of these tumours constitute the great bulk of the carcinomas of the bronchus. They are the squamous carcinoma, the adenocarcinoma, the anaplastic small cell carcinoma and the anaplastic large cell carcinoma. Careful histological study of many of these tumours reveals more than one cell type in the same tumour. The clinical course of the patient is less predictable in these mixed cell types but usually follows the course of the least favourable type.

Squamous carcinoma

These lesions are the most common carcinomas of the bronchus. They comprise 40% of all lung cancers. They have a high correlation with smoking but do not as readily disseminate as other types of carcinoma. The degree of differentiation found in these lesions varies from the well differentiated keratinizing epidermoid carcinoma through all stages to the poorly differentiated or polygonal cell carcinoma. The degree of differentiation is related directly to the prognosis. Well differentiated tumours have a good prognosis whereas the poorly differentiated have a poor prognosis.

The doubling time of these tumours varies according to the degree of differentiation but it is approximately 103 days (Straus, 1974). Because they tend to metastasize late, they may reach a considerable size before they are detected. Direct spread through the lung and the involvement of adjacent structures may be extensive. Lymph node metastases are common; blood-borne metastases tend to occur late in the course of the disease.

Adenocarcinoma

These lesions comprise approximately 20% of all lung cancers. They are the most frequent type among non-smokers. They may arise from the surface epithelium of the bronchi or uncommonly from the bronchial glands. They can also arise from previous lung scarring. The doubling time of adenocarcinoma of the bronchus is approximately 187 days (Kreyberg, 1976). Characteristic acinar formation is found histologically. If the lesions are stained with mucicarmine they can be shown to produce mucin. Adenocarcinomas are usually more peripherally situated in the lung. The primary tumour has a lesser tendency to spread widely through the lung or to invade adjacent structures. They metastasize early to lymph nodes and extensive mediastinal lymph node involvement in this disease carries a grave prognosis (Kirsh *et al.*, 1972). Blood-borne metastases also can occur relatively early.

It is often difficult to be sure whether an adenocarcinoma of the bronchus is a primary lesion or a secondary from elsewhere. An extensive search for a primary outside the thorax is not justified normally unless the patient has symptoms or signs suggesting an extrathoracic primary.

Bronchiolar or bronchioloalveolar carcinomas are adenocarcinomas which arise from the most distal airway. They are nearly always peripheral in the lung. When they are localized entirely their prognosis is (somewhat) better than the prognosis for an adenocarcinoma. These tumours, however, have a tendency to be multicentric and the prognosis is poor in multicentric lesions.

Anaplastic small cell carcinoma

These lesions comprise approximately 35% of carcinomas of the bronchus. The majority arise in the larger central bronchi. They are the most malignant form of neoplasm encountered originating from the bronchi. They have a very characteristic and uniform histological appearance consisting either of small round oat-cell-shaped or spindle-shaped cells arranged in undifferentiated masses, ribbons, rosettes or ductules. The doubling time for this lesion is approximately 33 days (Straus, 1974). The primary lesion may be a small undetected lesion in a patient who is found to have widespread blood-borne metastases. Some patients present with a solitary small pulmonary lesion. Surgical excision of these lesions, which prove to be an oat-cell carcinoma, have yielded very good results. In a small series 36% of patients presenting in this way have survived five years (Higgins *et al.*, 1975). The majority of patients however, present with a large mass in the lung. Involvement of adjacent structures in this latter type is early. Lymph node metastases occur very early. They are often extensive and highly invasive. The most striking feature of this tumour is its tendency to spread via the blood stream at a very early stage. Between 50 and 70% of patients with oat-cell carcinoma of the bronchus have been found to have malignant cells in their bone marrow. This compares with 10% of patients with other carcinomas of the

bronchus, even when the disease is disseminated (Hansen *et al.*, 1971).

Oat-cell carcinoma is related to the bronchial carcinoids. Both are thought to arise from the Kultschitzy-cells (Bansch *et al.*, 1968). All grades from the completely benign bronchial carcinoid to the highly malignant oat-cell carcinoma have been found. They can produce the carcinoid syndrome which is caused only by tumours of the parocrine (APUD) systems of the cells (Bansch *et al.*, 1968; Hattori *et al.*, 1972). These lesions also have a high correlation with ectopic hormone production and with the production of other marker substances (see Chapter 17).

Anaplastic large cell carcinoma

It is difficult to give an incidence for this group of tumours as it is used to include the very poorly differentiated or anaplastic lesions of squamous or adenocarcinomatous origin. The cells which are clear or eosinophilic, form masses or nests within a fibrous stroma. The doubling time for these lesions is approximately 92 days (Straus, 1974). They usually present with a primary mass in the lung. Spread to the lymph nodes is early and extensive. Blood-borne metastases are common. They are quite frequently associated with paraneoplastic syndrome.

The other lesions listed in the World Health Organization classification are rare. Tumours of the tracheobronchial mucous glands are worthy of mention in that they tend to be confined to the trachea and the main bronchi where they are usually slow-growing and locally invasive and may present with serious airway obstruction problems.

Pleural mesotheliomas are not uncommon. They have a high correlation with exposure to asbestos. They are often well advanced at the time they are first detected. They are very resistant to all forms of treatment and have a bad prognosis.

Staging

Various characteristics of carcinoma of the bronchus have been correlated with prognosis. These have included the histological type, evidence of vascular invasion in the tumour, degree of spread and the extent of immunological activity. The most widely accepted classification for staging of carcinoma of the bronchus is that devised by the UICC. This staging system has been found to have a good predictive value for individual patients and also allows for reliable comparisons of results obtained from various surgical centres. The staging is based on the local extent of the tumour (T status), the extent of lymph node involvement (N status), and the presence of distant metastases (M status), Details of this staging are as follows:

T_{is} Carcinoma *in-situ*

T_0 No evidence of primary tumour

T_x Tumour proven by the presence of malignant cells in bronchio-pulmonary secretions but not visualized radiologically or bronchoscopically, or any tumour that cannot be assessed.

T_1 A tumour that is 3.0 cm or less in greatest diameter, surrounded by lung or visceral pleura and without evidence of invasion proximal to a lobar bronchus at bronchoscopy.

T_2 A tumour more than 3.0 cm in greatest diameter or a tumour of any size that either invades the visceral pleura or, with its associated atelactasis or obstructive pneumonitis, extends to the hilar region. At broncho-scopy the proximal extent of demonstrable tumour must be within the lobar bronchus or at least 2.0 cm distal to the carina. Any associated atelectasis or obstructive pneumonitis must involve less than an entire lung, and there must be no pleural effusion.

T_3 A tumour of any size with direct extension into an adjacent structure such as the parietal pleura or chest wall, the diaphragm or the mediastinum and its contents; or a tumour demonstrable bronchoscopically to involve a main bronchus less than 2.0 cm distal to the carina; or any tumour associated with atelectasis or obstructive pneumonitis of an entire lung or pleural effusion.

N_0 No demonstrable metastases to regional lymph nodes.

N_1 Metastases to lymph nodes in the peribronchial or the ipsi-lateral hilar region, or both (including direct extension).

N_2 Metastases to lymph nodes in the mediastinum (paratracheal, subcarinal or paraoesophageal).

M_0 No distant metastasis

M_1 Distant metastiasis such as in scalene, supraclavicular, cervical or contra-lateral hilar lymph nodes, brain, bones, liver or contralateral lung.

Occult carcinoma

$T_x\ N_0\ M_0$ An occult carcinoma with bronchopulmonary secretions containing malignant cells but without other evidence of the primary tumour or evidence of metastasis to the regional lymph nodes or distant metastasis.

Invasive carcinoma
Stage I

$T_1\ N_0\ M_0$
$T_1\ N_1\ M_0$
$T_2\ N_0\ M_0$
A tumour that can be classified T_1 without any metastasis or with metastasis to the lymph nodes in the ipsilateral hilar region only; or a tumour that can be classified T_2 without any metastasis to nodes or distant metastasis.

Stage II

$T_2\ N_1\ M_0$ A tumour classified at T_2 with metastasis to the lymph nodes in the ipsilateral hilar region only.

Stage III

T_3 with any N or M
N_2 with any T or M
M_1 with any T or N
Any tumour more extensive than T_2, or any tumour with metastasis to the lymph nodes in the mediastinum, or with distant metastasis.

After the investigations in a patient suspected of having a carcinoma of the bronchus have been completed the following information should be available:

1. The histological type of the lesion.
2. The presence or absence of extrathoracic lympha-tic metastases.
3. The presence or absence of distant blood-borne metastases.
4. The presence and extent of mediastinal lymph node involvement.
5. The site and size of the primary lesion.

This information will allow a preliminary staging to be carried out. This is essential because the form of treatment recommended for the patient will depend upon it. Patients who undergo surgical resection for their lesion can be staged finally at operation. It is important during the operation to record accurately all features of the local tumour and the lymph node spread so that the final staging can be used in prognostic fashion. Patients whose staging precludes surgery and who are treated by either radiography or chemotherapy or both, cannot have final staging carried out, particularly with reference to their interthoracic lymph nodes.

Metastases

The possibility of cure of a lung cancer is related to the presence, or not, of metastases; both surgery and radiotherapy are dependent on the disease being confined to the volume removed or ablated. Spread outside that volume means failure; cure now depends on the relative sensitivity of the tumour cells and normal cells to a chemotherapeutic agent or agents.

The function of the lung is to carry out gaseous interchange; thus it has an abundant blood supply of relatively small thin-walled vessels all contained in a loose tissue which can expand and contract with respiration. The inspired air may be infected so there is an abundant lymphatic supply. Thus tumour will spread rapidly by direct infiltration into the loose tissues, by the blood and the lymphatic system and indeed many patients have metastases on presentation.

The histology of the tumour determines the incidence of the metastases, well differentiated tumours, where the cells are in close apposition and, there is a high adhesion of cells, having a lower incidence of metastases than more rapidly growing tumours (Table 18.2).

In this series of patients only 9% were found to have no macroscopic evidence of metastases at necropsy. The site of metastases for the differing histological types is shown in Table 18.3.

The lymph node pattern of involvement seems to be radially away from the chest, thus the hilar nodes were involved in 83%, cervical nodes 16%, porta hepatitis 12%, axillary 4% and inguinal 1%.

The larger the organ the greater appeared to be the incidence of metastases but there was a disproportionate number of metastases in the adrenals and these were bilateral in 66% of cases. The commonest sites of

Table 18.2   Metastasis related to histology (from Line and Deeley, 1971).

Histological type	No. of patients	Lymphatic spread present (%)	Haematogenous spread present (%)
Squamous	255	54	60
Oat-cell	191	85	91
Anaplastic	179	76	79
Adenocarcinoma	56	75	82

Table 18.3   Sites of metastases related to histology (from Line and Deeley).

Site	Squamous (%)	Oat-cell (%)	Anaplastic (%)	Adeno-carcinoma (%)
Lymph nodes	54	85	76	75
Liver	23	64	38	47
Adrenals	21	44	39	30
Bones	23	39	30	41
Breast	17	42	24	39
Kidney	15	15	14	20
Pancreas	4	24	14	5
Lung	12	7	8	14
Pleura	7	11	5	5

bone involvement were vertebrae 25%, ribs 8%, sternum 3%, femur 2%, skull 1% and all other bones less than 1%.

Solitary metastases

The presence of solitary metastases in this lesion is important because it affects the measures taken in treatment; if a metastatic lesion is possibly solitary it dictates that a more radical approach should be taken than if it were part of a widespread dissemination. 'Solitary' implies that there are no other metastases present in the body. The possibility of a metastasis being solitary depends on the histological type of the tumour (Table 18.4).

The proportion of the metastases at certain sites of the body which were solitary is shown in Table 18.5.

Some of these lesions are amenable to treatment with a chance of ablation if the tumour is detected but detection may not be possible in some sites until the deposit reaches an advanced stage and at this time tertiary deposits may be present.

Presenting symptoms

The presenting symptoms may be:
1.   Chest symptoms present in 68% of patients; these are cough, dyspnoea, sputum, haemoptysis, chest pain and are not specific for cancer but may be found with other chest diseases.

Table 18.4   Solitary metastases related to histology (from Deeley and Line, 1969).

	Squamous	Oat-cell	Anaplastic	Adenocarcinoma	Total
Number of cases with metastases outside the chest	144	175	140	43	502
Number of solitary metastases	39	33	19	6	97
%	27	19	14	14	19

Table 18.5   Sites of solitary extrathoracic metastases (from Deeley and Line).

Site of metastases	Number with secondaries at that site	Number where metastasis was solitary	Solitary metastases (%)
Brain	109	22	20
Vertebrae	162	6	4
Other bones	94	6	7
Liver	265	24	9
Adrenals	214	14	7
Kidneys	100	8	8
Pancreas	79	2	3
Stomach	18	1	6
Eyes	2	1	50
Supra-clavicular nodes	87	10	11
Cervical nodes	78	3	4

Superior vena caval obstruction is strongly suggestive of a carcinoma of the bronchus but may be due to malignancy in mediastinal lymph nodes or occasionally to a benign condition, such as, constrictive pericarditis.

Chronic bronchitis, defined as a chronic cough of over three years' duration, was found in 40% of patients. Patients who already are diagnosed as having bronchitis may be at a disadvantage because fresh symptoms may be attributed to this disease and a diagnosis of cancer may be delayed.

2. General non-specific symptoms such as weight loss, anorexia, lassitude, without chest symptoms, may be found in 12% of patients.

3. Two per cent of patients present with paramalignant symptoms, either neurological, such as the neuropathies, myopathies and myasthenia; or endocrinal, such as gynaecomasia, hypercalcaemia, 'Cushing-like' syndrome, hyponatraemia, carcinoid, or thyrotoxicosis, or, cutaneous, such as acanthosis nigricans, erythema gyratum repens or hairy man.

4. A Pancoast tumour may give local pain, pain referred along an intercostal nerve or along a branch of the brachial plexus.

5. Five per cent of patients may have no symptoms at all and the mass may be found only on routine chest radiography.

Physical examination

Physical examination may reveal no detectable abnormality in some patients. The majority, however, do have physical signs which can lead one to be suspicious that the patient has a carcinoma of the bronchus. Mild clinical anaemia and weight loss are common. Careful examination of the finger nails often will reveal early, or in many cases, well developed clubbing. Tobacco staining of the patients' index and middle finger is all too common. A small percentage of patients will exhibit tender swollen wrists and ankles, suggesting hypertrophic pulmonary osteoarthropathy.

Superior vena caval obstruction is of serious prognostic significance in this disease and can be detected by the patients' facial appearance and distended veins in the neck, over the upper chest and in the arms. Occasionally this disease presents with features of Cushing's syndrome.

Careful examination of the skin might alert one to diagnosis by the presence of acanthosis nigricans, erythema gyratum repens or hairy man. The presence of migratory superficial thrombophlebitis is also very suggestive that the patient has a malignant process.

The chest

The presence of physical signs in the chest depends upon: 1. the degree of bronchial obstruction; 2. the size of the lesion; 3. the presence of atelectasis or infection beyond the lesion; 4. proximity to the chest wall; and 5. the presence of a pleural effusion.

As a consequence there may be no physical signs or very obvious physical signs in the more advanced patients. The common physical signs to which carcinoma of the bronchus can give rise, are diminished chest wall movement, dullness to percussion, diminished air entry, bronchial breath sounds, localized wheezing, crepitations and occasionally tenderness of the chest wall.

Metastases

An important part of the physical examination is to determine whether there is any evidence of spread beyond the chest. Cervical lymphadenopathy most commonly presents with palpable lymph nodes in the lower deep cervical chain. Axillary lymphadenopathy can result from retrograde spread from the deep cervical chain or may be due to the fact that the tumour has involved the chest wall. A careful examination of the abdomen, paying particular attention to palpation of the liver, may reveal the presence of metastases in this organ. Areas of skeletal pain should suggest the presence of skeletal metastases.

A careful neurological examination may reveal either the evidence to suggest cerebral metastases or the presence of a neuropathy or myopathy. Motor or sensory loss in one arm should suggest a brachial plexus lesion due to a Pancoast tumour.

The chest radiograph

The vast majority of carcinomas of the bronchus are evident on the chest radiograph. The lesions take on many different radiographic appearances, depending upon where they arise and to what extent they have advanced. Any of the following appearances should strongly suggest the diagnosis of carcinoma of the bronchus:

Hilar mass

This is a common presentation but the size and extent of the lesion is often difficult to determine because of the presence of dependent atelectasis or infection, or both. It is also often difficult to tell the central extent of the lesion because it overlaps with the other mediastinal structures.

Persistent segmental or lobar atelectasis
A small central lesion causing total obstruction to a segmental or lobar bronchus can often present simply with evidence of atelectasis in the dependent segment or lobe.

Discrete peripheral lesion
These lesions vary in density but usually can be identified as malignant because they do not possess a clear cut margin.

Diffuse cap-like apical lesion
This type of lesion, if it involves the brachial plexus, is known as a Pancoast tumour.

Any one of these forms of carcinoma may undergo central necrosis and present with a radiological appearance of a lung abscess. The clue to the malignant nature of a lung abscess lies in its thick and irregular wall.

The chest radiograph is also of value in suspecting or diagnosing spread of the tumour within the chest. Lymphatic spread to the mediastinum can be detected usually only if the spread is to the right and occasionally the left paratracheal nodes. Extensive metastases to the lymphatics draining the lung, result in a 'damming back' of malignant cells in the lymphatic channels, causing lymphangitis carcinomatosa. This can be diagnosed radiologically by its characteristic reticular pattern. Haematogenous spread to the same lung can usually be detected by the presence of discreet secondary lesions. A careful search of the other lung may well reveal contralateral spread.

Pleural effusions are not uncommon in patients with carcinoma of the bronchus. An effusion usually presents with the typical radiological appearances but if adhesions are present, it may well occur in the form of loculated effusions.

A phrenic nerve palsy can be suspected from a raised hemidiaphragm and confirmed by screening of the diaphragm. Careful attention to the ribs, particularly those adjacent to a carcinoma, is important to detect the presence of erosions. Occasionally distant ribs might show evidence of secondary spread.

The anatomical situation of a carcinoma of the bronchus is determined best by a good lateral radiograph of the same side. Accurate determination of the lobe segment and even bronchus from which the lesion arises usually can be made in this way.

Tomography

Anteroposterior and lateral tomograms of a lesion in the lung can often strengthen the diagnosis that the lesion is malignant. The solid central nature of the lesion can be shown. The thick ragged walls of a malignant lung abscess can be clearly shown. Tomography clearly shows the infiltrating periphery of a carcinoma. A tumour which has produced secondary atelectasis or infection can often be delineated from the secondary pathology by tomography. Mediastinal lymph node involvement can be more strongly suspected from the appropriate tomograms. Whole lung tomography is useful for detecting radiologically invisible blood-borne secondaries to the same lung and most important of all to the other lung.

Computerized axial tomography (CAT) is not available generally in this country at present. It is however, proving of great value in providing information about carcinoma of the bronchus and its endothoracic spread.

Sputum cytology

Sputum cytology is a valuable means of achieving a tissue diagnosis in patients with suspected carcinoma of the bronchus (Lukeman, 1973). A positive sputum cytology can nearly always be obtained from those patients with central lesions which have ulcerated the mucosa. These are commonly the patients who present with haemoptysis. The yield is not as high, but still high enough to make it a valuable investigation in patients with smaller non-ulcerating lesions or in patients with peripheral carcinomas. The difficult problem arises when a patient who has no detectable lesion radiologically is found to have positive sputum cytology. These cells arise either from an occult carcinoma or from a carcinoma in-situ. Ideally these patients should be submitted to an extensive bronchoscopic search using a fibreoptic bronchoscope under local anaesthetic through which multiple biopsies are taken from the entire bronchial tree, in order to localize the site.

In order to ensure the highest yield from sputum cytology, repeated early morning samples of sputum should be examined. Sputum cytology is also a useful adjunct during a bronchoscopic examination. Suckings can be obtained from the area under suspicion and these may help to provide a tissue diagnosis, particularly in those cases in whom there was nothing to biopsy.

Bronchoscopy

Three forms of bronchoscopy are now commonly practised. The older conventional bronchoscopy is carried out with a rigid bronchoscope. The second is a new method of carrying out bronchoscopy using a fibreoptic bronchoscope. The former today is almost always carried out under general anaesthesia, while the latter is commonly done transnasally under local anaesthesia. A third group of bronchoscopists combine the use of the rigid bronchoscope and the fibreoptic bronchoscope. This latter method seems preferable as it allows both the assessment of bronchial rigidity as well as the ability to see into parts of the bronchial tree which cannot be vizualized normally with the rigid bronchoscope.

Bronchoscopy is essential to establish a histological diagnosis in most patients, suspected of having a carcinoma of the bronchus, in whom the lesion is visible bronchoscopically. It is usually possible to obtain a biopsy from any lesion which is situated in the trachea, the main bronchi, the lobar bronchi and the tertiary segmental bronchi. With the use of the new biopsy forceps provided with the fibreoptic bronchoscope, it is often possible to obtain a histological diagnosis in a lesion situated in branches of the tertiary bronchi (Freda 1974). In patients with no visible lesion, bronchial brushings and suckings taken from an area under suspicion may yield positive cytological results. Bronchoscopy is also of great value in assessing the degree of endobronchial involvement in the malignant process. Examination of the carina might reveal this to be widened and rigid suggesting the presence of fixed carinal lymph nodes. Rigidity of a bronchus proximal to the visualized lesion suggests that the extrabronchial spread of the lesion has involved the surrounding bronchi. Indentation, narrowing or compression of adjacent bronchi also suggest that the extrabronchial spread of a carcinoma is extensive.

Other changes in the bronchial tree can be noted at the same time. Many of these patients are chronic bronchitics and the characteristic mucosal changes of this disease can be assessed.

Scalene node biopsy, mediastinoscopy and mediastinotomy

Palpable scalene nodes are normally routinely biopsied in the assessment of patients suspected of having carcinoma of the bronchus. The presence of malignant disease in these nodes precludes surgical treatment for the disease. Routine scalene node biopsy in patients with impalpable nodes however, has not proved to be very useful. Less than 5% of patients will be found to have histologically positive nodes in this group (Shields and Shocket, 1958).

Mediastinoscopy was first described in 1959 by Carlens. The procedure consists of making a skin crease incision just above the supra-sternal notch. The incision is deepened through the platysma and deep cervical fascia between the heads of the sternomastoid muscles. The strap muscles are separated longitudinally and the isthmus of the thyroid is exposed. This is retracted upwards to allow incision of the pre-tracheal fascia so as to establish the plane behind this fascia.

Digital and visual exploration of the entire pre-tracheal plane can now be undertaken. It is possible to palpate and obtain biopsies from the paratracheal nodes, the sub-aortic nodes, the superior tracheobronchial nodes and the sub-carinal nodes. Mediastinoscopy cannot be used for assessment of the involvement of the anterior mediastinal nodes or the nodes in the inferior pulmonary ligament. It is also of no value in assessing the involvement of the oesophagus, the pericardium or descending thoracic aorta.

Mediastinoscopy has greatly expanded the yield and value of the information which was previously sought by scalene node biopsy. It can produce the only histological diagnosis of carcinoma of the bronchus in 12–18% of patients. It is of value in assessing both the presence and extent of mediastinal lymph node involvement. It is particularly valuable in detecting those patients with contra-lateral mediastinal lymph node secondaries. Its value in the prognosis for the patient is now undisputed. It has been repeatedly shown that only 10–12% patients with mediastinal lymph node involvement can expect a 5-year survival rate; 40–45% patients with no mediastinal lymph nodes involved can expect a 5-year survival rate. Many chest physicians, oncologists and surgeons now feel that the presence of extensive mediastinal lymph node involvement is a contra-indication to surgical therapy for this disease.

Anterior mediastinotomy, as described by McNeill and Chamberlain (1966), can be used for exploration of the anterior mediastinal lymph nodes. It is normally carried out after excision of the second or third costal cartilage on the appropriate side. The anterior mediastinum is entered extra-pleurally through the opening so created. The area can be digitally and visually explored and lymph nodes palpated and biopsied. The thymus can also be explored and biopsied in this way.

Mediastinoscopy and anterior mediastinotomy have done much to reduce the number of thoracotomies for lesions which proved to be inoperable. Radinov (1962) reviewed 50 000 patients who were submitted to thoracotomy without mediastinoscopy. In 43% of these patients the lesion was not resectable. This figure was corroborated by a series of authors who found that from 16 to 40% were not resectable if mediastonoscopy was not used. When mediastinoscopy was used, this incidence dropped from 6 to 14%. The principle reason for non-resectability in this residual group was tumour involvement of those structures which could not be assessed by either of these methods. CAT scanning may well help in further reducing the number of unnecessary thoracotomies.

Drill biopsy

Material from lesions lying peripherally in the lung may be obtained by means of a needle or drill. Positive biopsies are reported in 81% of cases using a pneumatic drill. The contra-indication to such biopsies is the presence of superior vena caval obstruction. If the lesion is separated from the chest wall by a zone of normal lung there is a risk of pneumothorax especially if the lung is emphysematous; this occurs in about 3% of patients and is coped with in the usual way.

Biochemical and serological investigations

Biochemical investigation can be of considerable value in raising the suspicion of extrathoracic metastases. The most commonly used and valuable investigation is that of serum alkaline phosphatase. An elevated level can be due either to hepatic metastases or to bony metastases.

Patients presenting with a carcinoma of the bronchus causing the various endocrine syndromes require biochemical elucidation of the nature of this syndrome. Carcinoma of the bronchus has been described as capable of producing various hormone-like substances. These include adrenocorticotrophin, growth hormone, melanocyte-stimulating hormone, chorionic gonadotrophin, prolactin, placental lactogen, anti-diuretic hormone, parathormone, calcitonin, serotonin, oestrodyl, erythropoetin, insulin and glucogon. The hormonal deficiency states can be produced by metastatic involvement of the pituitary and the adrenals. Biochemical investigation will clarify the nature of these disorders.

Carcinomas of the bronchus are known to produce a variety of non-hormonal chemical products. The best investigated of these is the carcinoembryonic antigen (CEA). This substance has been used as a tumour marker and it has been found in pathological quantities in approximately 75% of patients with carcinoma of the bronchus (Lo Gerfo *et al.*, 1971). It tends to be higher in patients with more extensive disease and a very definite drop can be noted after successful surgical excision of the lesion (Vincent and Chu, 1973). It is relatively useful as an indicator of tumour recurrence but not perhaps as useful as it is in carcinoma of the colon.

Radioisotope scanning

Radioisotope scanning is essential and valuable in patients with suspected carcinoma of the bronchus who have neurological symptoms and or signs, hepatomegaly or hepatic tenderness, bone pain or tenderness or a raised alkaline phosphatase. Brain and bone scans are valuable in determining the presence of blood-borne metastases to these structures. A liver scan, however, is less specific and many surgeons require corroboration of a positive liver scan by liver biopsy before deciding that a patient is not suitable for resection of the primary lesion. These investigations are expensive and time-consuming and are probably not justified in patients who do not have symptoms or signs of distant metastases because the yield of useful information from these investigations is poor in this group of patients.

CAT is also proving valuable as an adjunct to radioisotope scanning. It is of particular value in confirming the presence of cerebral metastases and to a lesser extent of hepatic metastases.

Respiratory function studies

Respiratory function studies, although not contributing to the diagnosis of carcinoma of the bronchus, are nevertheless essential to assess the patient's respiratory status and reserve. This information is essential when treatment for the patient's condition is planned.

Treatment

Indications

The three methods of treatment currently available for cancer of the bronchus are surgery, radiotherapy and chemotherapy, either alone or in combination. Treatment is aimed at providing a cure or palliating troublesome symptoms. When a patient presents at the Outpatients' Department we have to choose between three treatment policies: radical treatment aimed at a cure; palliative treatment; or no treatment.

Radical treatment

Radical treatment aimed at producing a cure in a proportion of patients may cause some side-effects, sequelae or complications but provided the number of these is small it is justifiable to take some risk because the prognosis without treatment is hopeless. Although we normally assess the prognosis as five-year survival rates it is preferable to use 'normal life expectancy'; this is the time when the proportion of treated patients dying is approximately the same as that of a normal population of the same age and sex: in carcinoma of the bronchus this occurs at three years after treatment. The three-year survival rate is thus a satisfactory index of the success of treatment. For radical treatment to succeed when surgery or radiotherapy is used, the tumour must be contained within a volume which either can be removed totally or covered by fields of radiation which will raise the volume to a cancericidal dose. We have no records of three-year survival rates after chemotherapy and this mode of therapy, alone therefore, does not enter into discussions of radical treatment. When proposing radical treatment for a patient we need to assess the presence of other factors such as poor general health which may make it impossible to embark on such a region, other diseases which may limit the survival, and the age of the patient.

Palliative therapy

Palliative therapy is given when there is no chance of cure but the patient is distressed by his symptoms; this usually implies that the lesion has spread outside the chest. Any treatment given will be the minimum required to relieve; there is no justification for prolonging treatment, or risking sequelae.

No treatment

If a cure cannot be achieved and there are no distressing symptoms to palliate then any active treatment is contra-indicated; this is a clinical decision of equal importance to the other two.

It is possible to combine treatments; thus, radiotherapy may be given before radical surgery in the hope of attenuating any cells cast off into the blood stream so that they become incapable of division; radiotherapy and chemotherapy may be combined with the idea that radiation will kill the tumour in the chest, any microscopic occult metastases being ablated by cytotoxic agent.

Surgery

Surgery as the primary treatment for carcinoma of the bronchus should be confined to those patients who, after full investigation are found to have a lesion which is confined to one or other hemithorax. Controversy still surrounds the place of surgery in patients with known extensive mediastinal lymph node involvement. Patients with oat-cell carcinoma of the bronchus are not normally considered for surgical therapy. Occasionally surgical excision is used for small early oat-cell carcinomas, usually because no diagnosis had been reached before thoracotomy and resection.

The aim of surgical resection of a carcinoma of the bronchus is to achieve a monobloc resection of the lesion and all involved lymph nodes. The level of resection of the bronchus should be such that it is one or more centimeters proximal to the palpable tumour. The nature of the resection required will be determined by the site, the size, the extent of local spread through the lung, the extent of lymph node involvement and finally the involvement of adjacent structures.

Operation

Surgery for carcinoma of the bronchus is carried out under general anaesthesia. Most surgeons today request endobronchial anaesthesia as this allows the lung, being operated upon, to be collapsed and therefore improves access to the hilum. This form of intubation allows the operation to be carried out in the full lateral position which most surgeons prefer and prevents blood, mucus or pus from passing into the dependent lung as a result of handling of the diseased lung. A few surgeons still prefer to carry out the operation with a simple endotracheal tube and the patient in the face down position. This position precludes the risk of potentially septic material entering the good lung but does necessitate operating with an inflated lung on the diseased side.

A posterolateral thoracotomy is now virtually universally used irrespective of whether the patient is in the full lateral position or in the face down position. With few exceptions, the chest is entered through the bed of the unresected sixth rib. All pleural adhesions are divided so as to free the lung completely. If these adhesions are particularly dense or if they lie between a tumour which has reached or actually invaded the visceral pleural surface, this area of lung should be freed by extrapleural dissection. Occasionally the tumour will have invaded the pleural space and the chest wall. Under these circumstances excision of an area of chest wall is essential. Once the lung containing the carcinoma is entirely free, the lesion should be assessed digitally with care.

Particular attention is paid to the following points:

1. The size of the primary tumour.
2. The anatomical site of origin of the tumour. In many lesions it is often not possible to say more than that the tumour arises in one or other lobe. Smaller lesions however, can be more accurately defined in terms of the bronchus from which they arise or the segment in which they lie.
3. Encroachment through the lung substance across the major fissures. Sharp dissection is often necessary to provide the final information in this respect, as apparent tumour encroachment across a major fissure may simply be due to inflammatory adhesions set up by the tumour which initially give the appearance of tumour invasion of an adjacent lobe.
4. The presence of palpable nodules in apparently healthy lung tissue.
5. The central extension of tumour in the bronchial tree.
6. The central extension of the tumour along the pulmonary artery or the pulmonary veins.
7. The presence and extent of lymph node involvement.

8. Malignant involvement of adjacent structures such as the superior vena cava, the pericardium, the oesophagus, the aorta, diaphragm or the thoracic spine. This palpation, which should be gentle to avoid unnecessary blood-borne dissemination of the tumour before ligating the pulmonary veins, provides valuable information to help decide the extent of the pulmonary resection necessary to remove all macroscopic malignant tissue.

Sharp accurate dissection of the hilar structures is carried out now. The pulmonary artery and pulmonary veins should be dissected free of their adventitial coverings so as to assess whether it is possible to divide them between ligatures central to the tumour. If there is any doubt from the hilar dissection the pericardium should be opened behind the phrenic nerve and the structures assessed for length intrapericardially. The bronchial extension should likewise be assessed by sharp dissection. Tumour involvement of adjacent structures should always be diligently explored by sharp dissection as this involvement might be due to inflammatory adhesions, capable of division, rather than direct malignant invasion. A final decision can now be made as to the extent of the pulmonary resection which is necessary.

The best long-term results are obtained from resecting the least amount of lung tissue which is still consistent with an adequate monobloc dissection of the lesion. This can be accomplished by a variety of operations which vary from a wedge resection for a small peripheral carcinoma with no lymph node involvement; a lobectomy which, in the case of the upper lobes and occasionally the right middle lobe, may include a sleeve resection of the main bronchus; a bilobectomy on the right such as a combined upper and middle or a combined middle and lower lobe lobectomy, and finally a pneumonectomy. In order to achieve these resections the pulmonary veins draining the affected area are divided between ligatures. This step is carried out first to further cut down blood-borne dissemination as a result of handling the tumour. The pulmonary artery or its branches are then divided between ligatures. Finally, the bronchus is divided either between clamps, of open and closed with interrupted sutures.

Involved interlobar or hilar lymph nodes can normally be excised *en bloc* with the section of lung removed. The subcarinal nodes often can be excised together with the entire lung if a pneumonectomy is carried out. The sub-aortic and anterior mediastinal nodes invariably require to be excised separately.

Malignant involvement of adjacent structures may or may not preclude excision of the lesion. Wide excision around the tumour involving such structures as the pericardium, the fat of the anterior mediastinum, the upper surface of the diaphragm, is commonly carried out to free the lesion. Malignant involvement of vital structures such as the superior vena cava, aorta, oesophagus or the heart itself, are usually regarded as indications of inoperability. There are, however, reports of successful resections of tumour involving these structures together with reconstruction of the structure involved. If there is any doubt as to the efficacy of the clearance of malignant tissue from any part inside the chest, this area should be marked with silver clips to facilitate accurate irradiation later.

The thoracotomy is closed. Drainage always is used if a segmental resection or lobectomy has been carried out but most surgeons do not use drainage after a pneumonectomy.

Results of surgery for carcinoma of the bronchus

Surgical excision of carcinomas of the bronchus is currently the best form of treatment to offer the patient hope of a cure. The majority of patients are, however, too far advanced when first seen, even to be considered for surgical treatment. The principal reasons for this are extrathoracic spread of the tumour or a respiratory reserve which is inadequate to allow pulmonary resection.

About 40–70% of patients, depending on the thoroughness of the pre-operative assessment, will be found at operation to have resectable lesions. The outcome for patients with lesions which are resectable, is determined by the following factors: 1. the operative and perioperative mortality; 2. the stage grouping of the lesion; 3. the histological type of the lesion; 4. the presence of undetected distant metastases; 5. the respiratory reserve of the patient; 6. late local recurrence; 7. late recurrence of distant metastases; 8. the occurrence of new primary lesions in the remaining lung tissue.

1. Modern operative mortality for lung resections for carcinoma of the bronchus is of the order of 2–3%. Many of the patients are elderly and some have concomitant cardiac, hepatic or renal disease. Operative or perioperative deaths, as a consequence of inadequate respiratory reserve following the resection, should not occur today as modern respiratory function tests provide information sufficiently accurate to allow the exclusion of those patients who would not tolerate a lung resection. An important cause of perioperative mortality in surgery for this condition is post-operative infection in the remaining lung tissue. This is common because many of these patients have generalized lung disease, such as emphysema or chronic bronchitis, which makes them more prone to infection, particularly post-operatively and which may make the difference between someone with border-line pulmonary reserve surviving or dying as a result of the operation.

2. Stage grouping of the lesions has proved to be a valuable prognostic index. Patients with Stage 1 lesions, have been shown by numerous series to have a 40–45% five-year survival expectancy. This figure drops to 10–15% for patients with Stage 2 lesions. Patients with Stage 3 lesions, which are still surgically resectable, can expect a 5–10% five year survival rate (Mountain *et al.*, 1974).

3. The histological type of the lesion also influences the prognosis. There is a good correlation between the histological type and stage grouping. This is because the better differentiated lesions are often found earlier, they are slower growing and a greater percentage of them will be Stage 1 lesions. The poorly differentiated squamous carcinomata, the anaplastic small cell carcinomata and the anaplastic large cell carcinomata are likely to be much more advanced when first found and more of these will be Stage 2 and Stage 3 lesions. Adenocarcinomata as a result of their peripheral situation, are likely to be at an earlier stage, particularly the bronchiolar or bronchioalveolar lesion and they, as a consequence, carry a better prognosis. The tumours of tracheobronchial mucous gland origin, tend for the most part, to be slow-growing. They are often picked up early because of their bronchial obstructive effects and the prognosis from these lesions, as a consequence, is better. Sarcomata are rare but if they are still Stage 1 lesions, the prognosis is reasonable.

4. Matthews *et al.* (1973) found that 36% of 202 patients, who had undergone pulmonary resections for carcinoma and who died within 30 days of the operation, had undetected residual or local metastases and/or distant metastases. If these patients had survived the perioperative period, it is almost certain that these undetected metastases would have resulted in their death.

5. The patient's respiratory reserve after lung resection, although adequate to withstand the operation and the post-operative period, may prove to be inadequate later. This can be due to further deterioration as a result of an underlying generalized lung disease, such as chronic bronchitis or emphysema and these patients are particularly vulnerable to chest infections which may prove fatal. This is particularly so in patients who have undergone a pneumonectomy as opposed to a lobectomy.

6. Complete excision of the primary lesion, together with all its involved lymph nodes, often is not achieved. Histologically identifiable tumour at the level of section of the bronchus, can be found because the extent of proximal sub-mucosal spread was under-estimated at operation. In other patients poor respiratory reserve necessitates an inadequate operation leaving residual tumour at the level of bronchial section. Residual malignant lymph nodes may be left in the chest and these can later develop into invasive carcinomata. Involvement of the chest wall, pericardium, heart, the diaphragm or the great vessels may result in inadequate excision of the tumour. All residual tumour left in this fashion is likely to result in fatal tumour recurrence.

7. Excision of the primary tumour does not prevent the late occurrence of intrathoracic or distant metastases. This is a very important cause of death in patients with carcinoma of the bronchus. The tendency for these to occur falls off with the passage of time from the operation. The patients who have survived five years without recurrence of distant metastases are today regarded as cured.

8. Patients who have developed one carcinoma of the bronchus have a higher tendency to develop one or more additional primaries in their remaining lung tissues. This is most commonly seen in patients who have had previous well differentiated squamous carcinoma, adenocarcinomas of bronchiolar or bronchioalveolar lesions. It is seldom possible surgically to excise these lesions as they may well be in the contra-lateral lung and the patient's respiratory reserve precludes this.

Radiotherapy

The patients referred for radical radiotherapy have a tumour which is technically inoperable because of local extension, a respiratory reserve which is insufficient to allow lung resection; they are elderly, usually more than 70 years of age, in poor general condition, have another disease which reduces their expectation of life seriously or have refused operation. The results of operation in oat-cell and anaplastic tumours of the lung have been extremely disappointing and worse than those obtained by radiotherapy; as a result many surgeons now refer patients with these lesions for radiotherapy.

Radical treatment will only be given if clinical examination reveals that the tumour is confined to the chest and can be covered by fields of radiation of sufficient size to allow a full dose to be given. The frequency of metastatic spread suggests that a search should be made for occult metastases before starting a course of radical treatment. Kirkman *et al.* (1976) investigated radioactive isotopes in the detection of metastases within the body, their results showed that in a group clinically suitable for radical treatment only 36% had no detectable secondary deposits. Deposits were found in the brain in 5%, liver in 34% and bone in 33%.

In giving a radical course of radiotherapy aimed at a cure we must take into account the patient's general condition and also the late sequelae which may be expected. Tumour will kill tissues and radiation will also kill tissues; in both the damage will only be repaired by fibrosis. The patient will therefore need to have a fairly good initial respiratory reserve and to have no other illnesses which could kill him. Such desperate treatment techniques are only justified if there is a chance of producing a cure.

Selection of patients for radical radiotherapy
Patients receive a radical course of therapy if:

1. Their general condition is good.
2. The lesion is inoperable either on general grounds or technically and is a squamous or adenocarcinomatous lesion, or if operable is an oat-cell or anaplastic tumour. The following are not contra-indications: (a) age, because there are few untoward reactions with megavoltage therapy in the doses proposed; (b) chronic bronchitis, but it must be recognized that the late sequelae may be more severe in these patients. Acute exacerbations are always treated by a wide-spectrum antibiotic before starting treatment; (c) active tuberculosis; these patients are given appropriate anti-tubercular therapy at the same time.
3. There is superior vena caval obstruction and the disease is limited to the chest.
4. Chest aspiration reveals a straw coloured pleural effusion, but if blood is present this indicates potential involvement of the whole cavity and palliative treatment only is indicated.
5. Any metastases can be treated together with the tumour and if there is no evidence of other spread; widespread metastases are a contra-indication to radical treatment.

Preparation for treatment
Whilst every effort is made to improve the patient's health and general condition before therapy it is important that this is not unduly delayed because of the increased chances of dissemination. Anaemia, dehydration and dietary deficiencies are corrected and treatment instituted for infection. I prefer patients to be treated from their own homes because hospitalization increases the risk of cross-infection in patients with such low resistance.

Volume of isodose to be irradiated
The tumour opacity and a surrounding zone of at least 2.0 cm of apparently normal lung should be irradiated. The high incidence of mediastinal lymph node metastases demands that the mediastinum is included in the field of irradiation, the field thus includes the hilar region and the lower tracheal nodes and requires a vertical dimension of at least 15 cm and more should the paratracheal nodes be involved. The limits of the

tumour are determined from postero-anterior and lateral radiographs and transferred to the contour of the patient's chest.

Field arrangement
An adequate tumour volume can be irradiated using two fields with megavoltage therapy, arranged to avoid irradiating the spinal cord, thus one anterior and one oblique field are used. Wedged fields will help to produce a uniform dose over the whole volume (Fig. 18.3).

Tumour dose, fractionation and overall treatment time
For many years it was the intention to give the maximum dose of irradiation that could be tolerated but in more recent years we have tended to reduce this dose, because of the danger of producing radiation fibrosis which could proceed to right-sided heart failure and death. We need, therefore, to determine the optimum treatment conditions with the best balance between ablation of tumour, survival and radiation effects on normal tissue. In 1966, Deeley reported the results of controlled clinical trials comparing different doses of radiation. For squamous and adenocarcinomatous lesions the best results were obtained with 4000 rad given in 20 treatments in 28 days (4000/20/28) and in anaplastic and oat-cell tumours, with 3000/20/28. Patients receiving doses in excess of these were shown to have died from the effects of their radiation fibrosis; it must be remembered that the volume of irradiation needed in the lung is quite large. Since that time further controlled clinical trials have shown that a dose of 3200/8/28 is clinically equivalent to 4000/20/28 and 2400/8/28 is equivalent to 3000/20/28. There are obvious advantages to treating twice weekly; it is more convenient and less tiring to the patient, more adapt-

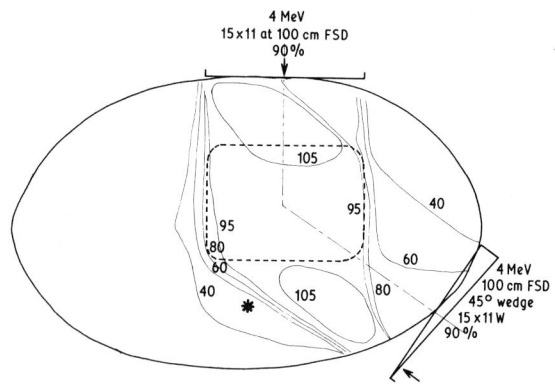

Fig. 18.3   Isodose distribution using anterior and wedged posterior oblique fields (– – – – = treatment volume, * = spinal cord).

able to out-patient treatment and is more convenient to the department. At the moment treatments are given on Tuesdays and Thursdays, a 3:4 spacing, but there are obvious alternatives, 2:5 and 1:6, to be investigated.

Dose distribution within the lung
The doses given have assumed unit-density of the whole of the irradiated fields, but this is not so; we have various tissues within the volume, bone, cartilage, muscle, solid growth, collapsed or consolidated alveoli and air containing alveoli. Exit dose measurements using lithium fluoride powder showed that the tumour dose could, in practice, be up to 60% greater than that calculated assuming unit tissue density (Svarcer *et al.*, 1965). If doses are measured daily it is found that there is often considerable variation throughout the treatment time; consolidated lung may be replaced by air if a secretion in the chest is coughed up; a bronchus blocked by growth may be re-aerated; the tissues may have increased vascularity because of the radiation; interstitial oedema may develop; fibrotic changes may collapse relatively small areas of the lung; a tumour may decrease in size and the surrounding lung be emphysematous and so on. This is an ever-changing condition. In practice we have three alternatives in calculating the doses:

1. To assume unit tissue density – knowing the limitations.
2. To calculate the correction factor at the beginning of the course and apply this throughout treatment – this is no more accurate than 1.
3. The only true method would be to measure the absorption factor by giving a test dose of radiation before each treatment and then correct – accurate but impractical considering the large number of patients involved and the necessary delay in giving each patient that day's treatment.

I prefer to adopt method 1. but this does mean that we do not really know the dose given, it could be up to 30% greater than that estimated; this must be taken into account when considering the doses I have given and also when comparing the higher doses given by some therapists, thus, an estimated dose of 6000 rad could be, in fact, nearer to 8000 rad within the tissues.

Results of radical treatment by radiotherapy
The results of treatment of carcinoma of the bronchus are distressingly poor, but a few patients can survive for many years after radical treatment. In a series of 513 patients who received radical radiotherapy for a carcinoma of the bronchus the yearly survival rates were 36, 15, 8, 7 and 6% (Deeley, 1974); other workers have produced similar results. For many years we have attempted to improve these results but we should

consider what we are trying to do and question whether this is possible.

We have already shown that a large proportion of patients with lung cancer had dissemination of the disease at necropsy; because of the rapid dissemination of this tumour and the poor survival time we can assume that the majority of these patients had small metastases at the time they presented for radical treatment; indeed this has been shown in our search for occult metastases and explains the poor survival in those with the best prognosis who are treated surgically. Probably only about 20% of patients are suitable for resection and of these the five-year survival rate is about 30% i.e. about 6 of 100 patients presenting. Of the remaining 80 patients radiotherapy may cure a further five, thus these two methods only satisfactorily treat about 11% of patients who present at hospital. However, considering that both surgery and radiotherapy are local methods of therapy and cannot control dissemination it is unlikely that these methods will control more of the presenting number than they do at present and it is not to such localized methods of treatment that we must look for control of the disease. Our only hope for improvement is to obtain some satisfactory method of treating the patients with disseminated tumour.

Factors affecting the prognosis after treatment by radiotherapy
There are certain factors which influence the prognosis:

1. Histology. Squamous lesion and adenocarcinoma have a better survival rate than anaplastic and oat-cell tumour: 10% three-year survival rate for squamous, 11% for adenocarcinomatous and 4% for both anaplastic and oat-cell tumours.
2. Site of primary tumour. In squamous tumours main bronchus lesions have a 13% three-year survival, upper and middle lobes 16% and lower lobes 2%; for anaplastic and oat-cell lesions, 3%, 7% and 0% respectively.
3. Mediastinal node involvement. In squamous tumours with no mediastinal node involvement there was a three-year survival rate of 11% but this dropped to 7% if nodes were involved; in anaplastic and oat-cell lesions the corresponding results were 5% and 2%.

It is also thought that the results are poorer in older patients; in women; in patients who appear to have a tumour with a rapid growth rate; where large masses are seen on radiography; where there is incomplete removal at thoracotomy; where there is associated chronic chest infection; and in patients with obvious weight loss, anaemia or cachexia.

Special cases

We must now consider some special circumstances where it is possible to give radical radiotherapy.

1. *Superior mediastinal obstruction.* Contrary to many reports in the literature the presence of superior mediastinal obstruction by itself does not denote a poor prognosis; this is because all such patients have been grouped together irrespective of whether the tumour is confined to the chest or disseminated. Obviously the latter group cannot be cured by localized radiotherapy; if we remove them we find that the survival rate for lesions localized to the chest after radical treatment is the same as for patients with no obstruction. For many years it was customary to start therapy with small daily doses building these up as treatment progressed; a cautious approach, but during this time the tumour continues to grow, to compress and possibly disseminate, and I now treat in the usual way.

2. *Solitary metastases.* If we know a patient has solitary metastases we can give radical treatment to both metastasis and primary, aiming for cure. We will consider three sites:

(a) The brain: if there is no clinical evidence of metastases elsewhere in the body, the brain and primary tumour are both treated. The brain is usually treated first, using two opposed fields to cover the whole brain and to give a total tumour dose of 800 rad in 2 treatments spaced 24 hours apart. Corticosteroids may be given to reduce the oedema. The survival rates after such treatment are 15% at one year, and 4% at three years.

(b) Supraclavicular and cervical lymph nodes: if these are involved, they are usually treated in continuity with the primary tumour and the mediastinum; survivals are 22% at one year, 7% at two years, 3% at three years and 1% at five years.

(c) Other sites: results at other sites have not been encouraging; in those treated, the one year survival was 6% but none survived for two years.

3. *Tuberculosis.* There is no evidence that radiation reactivates, accelerates or disseminates tuberculosis; patients with active disease should receive, however, appropriate antibiotic therapy.

4. *Endocrine and neurological disturbances.* The presence of these manifestations does not preclude radical treatment and in fact regression of the tumour is often associated with resolution of the disturbance.

5. *Post-operative irradiation.* A radical course of radiotherapy is given if the tumour is found to be inoperable at thoracotomy or cannot be completely removed. Survival rates reported are 12% at three years and 9% at five years. Radiation should be started when the skin sutures are removed.

Effects of radiation

The whole basis of radiotherapy is to kill malignant cells and we rely on a differential effect on normal and tumour cells; tumour cells being more rapidly dividing will be affected most but invariably some normal cells will also be damaged. Any permanent damage to tissues can only be repaired by fibrosis, but damage of normal tissues can occur from the tumour and from the irradiation and so the final effect will be a combination of both. Fibrosis in the tumour-bearing area therefore suggests resolution of the growth. Fibrosis of the normal tissues, especially if excessive, compels us to investigate the dose given and to determine whether the same effects on the tumour could be achieved if we reduced our radiation dose with less damage to normal tissue.

1. *Lung.* The effect of radiation on the lung resulting from the treatment of a carcinoma of the bronchus is described in two stages, the first merging into the second (Deeley, 1960).

Stage I   Reaction: this is the stage of reaction of normal tissues to an irritant, in this case radiation; the changes seen are exactly the same as those seen due to other irritants. The patient may have no symptoms, may have symptoms suggestive of acute chest infection or, in a few cases, symptoms may be very severe and occasionally may prove fatal. Radiography shows a diffuse opacity in the lung corresponding to the radiation fields. Histological section, at this time, shows the alveoli to be filled with exudate, necrotic cells, lymphocytes, foreign body giant cells and hyaline tissue, with an increased cellularity around the blood vessels. Recovery is possible but if the irradiation disrupts the elastic tissue around the alveoli, permanent damage will occur.

Stage II   Repair of damage: any permanent damage will be repaired by fibrosis. Radiographs taken over a period of time show at first fine bands of fibrosis extending throughout the consolidated area; these increase in density and coalesce and eventually cause movement of the mediastinal contents, the heart, trachea, and hilum of the lung, tenting of the diaphragm, retraction of the chest wall and eventually scoliosis. These effects are present in all patients by about thirteen months.

The severity of the complications depends on the site in the lung irradiated, the volume, the dose given and also on the presence of previous diseases in the lung especially those leading to fibrosis, such as bronchitis. In spite of the many attempts to reduce fibrosis there is no evidence that giving drugs such as corticosteroids or anti-coagulants has any effect on the progress. There is, of course, a marked individual variation to these effects of radiation.

The irradiated lung is prone to infection, the offending organism(s) cannot be isolated because of the fibrosis and wide-spectrum antibiotics should be prescribed; again, because of the fibrosis the blood supply is relatively poor and large concentrations of antibiotics may be needed. Yellow sputum is usually a good sign of infection and may or may not be associated with pyrexia and/or night sweats.

2. *Other tissues.* Oesophagus: this structure will inevitably be within the volume irradiated to a full dose; some patients develop dysphagia during treatment and all should be advised to take a light diet, with soft food, avoiding anything which will irritate the oesophagus, such as hard foods, acids, condiments, very hot or very cold foods and alcohol. In only about 2% of patients is it necessary to discontinue treatment for a few days.

Heart: the effects are somewhat non-specific; a reversal of the T-wave on ECG is possibly due to fibrosis of the pericardium.

Pleura: the pleura may show dense fibrosis.

Other structures: the ribs, vertebral body, skin and subcutaneous tissues may sometimes show radiation effects but less so than with orthovoltage therapy. Techniques now in use avoid the spinal cord but should this be included there is a possibility of radiation myelitis.

Palliation

Whilst the results of radical treatment are very disappointing we can obtain considerable symptomatic relief for many of our patients. We must emphasize that treatment must stop as soon as palliation is achieved and should take a few days only; much can be achieved by single treatments.

Bone pain due to metastases can often be relieved with one treatment which can be repeated if necessary. Haemoptysis is stopped in the majority of patients – 94% – and chest pain, cough and dyspnoea in about 70%. A collapsed lung, due to blockage by growth, can frequently be opened up with symptomatic improvement; constriction of the oesophagus may be relieved but invasion of the wall of the oesophagus may lead to a fistula if cancer cells are killed.

Cerebral metastases, even if part of a generalized dissemination, may be worth treating – two treatments giving 800 rad per tumour dose – because of the advantages to be gained in nursing, for the relatives, and patient; comatosed and paralysed patients often become more rational, co-operative and manageable.

Pleural effusion requiring repeated tappings may be treated by two large opposed fields of radiation which will cover the underlying malignant tissue.

Recurrent chest tumours

There is often a reluctance, on the part of radiotherapists, to retreat a tumour in the chest which has had previous irradiation; presumably this is because it is thought that further treatment increases the possibility of fibrosis. However, if a patient who has had a radical course of therapy subsequently develops a recurrence which causes distress I will treat palliatively; invariably he will not live long enough to develop late fibrosis.

Reasons for failure of treatment

Radical treatment for carcinoma of the lung frequently fails because we attempt to treat a tumour with local therapy when it has already disseminated; as yet we have no effective measures for these patients. However, if there is no evidence of metastases the patient should have the advantage of radical treatment, surgery being preferable to radiotherapy in most cases. It seems likely that the results of these two forms of therapy can be improved but little; successful management of the established lesion will only be achieved when we develop satisfactory methods of dealing with secondary deposits.

Future trends

Improvements in existing therapy are aimed at metastatic deposits, by means of chemotherapeutic or immunotherapeutic means. Radiotherapy or surgery may well be used to deal with the bulk of the primary tumour and chemotherapeutic agents given for metastases. Much work needs to be done to determine the optimal treatment conditions and this involves participation in controlled clinical trials.

Regrettably too many patients already have disseminated disease when they first attend hospital and we must develop methods of making an earlier diagnosis. Miniature mass radiography has little scope in malignant disease of the chest; routine sputum cytol-

Table 18.6   Response to single agent chemotherapy: influence of cell type* (modified from Selawry, 1974).

	Small cell (%)	Squamous cell (%)	Large cell (%)	Adenocarcinoma (%)
Cyclophosphamide	33	19	23	17
Methotrexate	34	25	17	32
Procarbazine	47	20	35	19
CCNU	17	30	17	23
Adriamycin	25	19	25	15
Hexamethylmelamine	32	12	18	15

* Number of patients studied of each histology $\geqslant 10$

Table 18.7   Actual relapse-free survival of 2 years or longer in limited stage small cell carcinoma (modified from Greco *et al.*, 1978).

Treatment*	Patient number	Complete response (%)	Number relapse-free 2 years or longer
CTX, VCR, RT	16	50	3
CTX, ADR, VCR, RT, CCNU, MTX, BCG	19	89	5
CTX, ADR, VCR, CCNU, MTX, RT	12	–	2
CTX, CCNU, MTX, VCR, RT	110	–	12
CTX, ADR, VCR, RT	10	100	4
CTX, VP-16, RT	12	40	4
ADR, VP-16, RT	9	33	1
CTX, ADR, VCR, MTX, RT	12	100	2
CTX, ADR, VCR, RT, HEXA, VP-16, MTX	16	94	2

* CTX, cyclophosphamide; MTX, methotrexate; ADR, adriamycin; RT, radiotherapy; HEXA, hexamethylmelamine; BCG, bacillus calmette guerin; VCR, vincristine; VP-16, epipodophyllotexein.

ogy, confined perhaps to those patients at high risk, involves considerable time, manpower and expense. Cancer information given to the general public may bring patients at an earlier stage. However, this is a preventable disease and the answer surely is to prevent the disease by removing the cause – tobacco.

Chemotherapy*

Chemotherapy is proving to be of increasing value in small cell bronchogenic carcinoma. The importance of histological tumour type in dictating response to chemotherapy has been reviewed by Selawry (1974); simplified in Table 18.6, small cell carcinoma being the cell type most sensitive to chemotherapy. Pooled data from reported studies of small cell carcinoma indicate

*A note by Nicholas Thatcher.

an increase over the years in complete response rate (mean 14%) with combination chemotherapy compared with the 2.5% mean complete response rate obtained with single agent treatment. The addition of radiotherapy to combination chemotherapy increased the mean complete response rate to 31% (Greco *et al.*, 1978). Obviously these results are difficult to interpret precisely due to the considerable heterogeneity of the patient populations. However, some increase in complete response rates has been achieved with the use of combination therapy (Selawry, 1974; Greco *et al.*, 1978; Weiss, 1978).

Improvement in chemotherapeutic response rates has quickened interest in the management of patients with small cell carcinoma of 'limited extent'. A situation previously viewed with great pessimism is now the subject of intense effort. The strategy of irradiation to the local-regional disease with chemotherapy to improve the local radiotherapy response and to remove undetected metastases is proving of value. The recent MRC study is an example of this type of management; a significant increase in response rate and survival was achieved when chemotherapy (using three agents) and irradiation were combined, 34% alive at one year compared with 18% alive when radiotherapy alone was used (MRC Lung Cancer Working Party, 1979).

True long term survival is uncertain at present, but a handful of reports with two years or more relapse-free survival are available (Table 18.7). Of the 216 patients treated with combined modalities, 35 (16%) remain in remission two years or more from the start of therapy (Greco *et al.*, 1978). A proportion of small cell carcinoma patients are therefore attaining long term survival and may be cured. There are still many deficiencies to be corrected, better evaluation of chemotherapeutic activity is emphasized by the detailed reviews of Selawry (1974) and Broder *et al.*, (1977); improvement in complete response rates and reduction of toxicity both for limited and extensive disease are clearly required. Various approaches to these problems, including prophylactic brain irradiation have been the subject of excellent recent reviews (Greco *et al.*, 1978; Weiss, 1978; Livingston, 1978).

The chemotherapy of non-small cell carcinoma is disappointing (Selawry, 1974; Hansen *et al.*, 1976). Difficulty in accurate evaluation of chemotherapy in this group of carcinomata is complicated by the wide range of reported response rates, the variation being a reflection of the lack of separation of prognostic features including disease stage, performance status etc. within the patient populations. The defects in study design do not allow any firm conclusions to be drawn concerning the value of chemotherapy used as an adjuvant to surgery or radiotherapy in limited disease. Response rates in ambulatory patients with limited disease are generally less than 50% with few complete responses, with little improvement in survival. The use of intensive combination regimes appears to be of little value for these patients and to be associated with unacceptable toxicity (Hansen *et al.*, 1976; Livingston *et al.*, 1975a, 1975b). Chemotherapy for non-small cell cancer should be restricted to carefully planned studies, perhaps with the addition of newer agents (e.g. platinum derivatives and more innovative regimes). The inclusion of immunotherapy would be one area of possible expansion and finds support from the positive result of McKneally using intrapleural BCG in early stage disease (McKneally *et al.*, 1976), though a random control trial has shown no clear effect on survival (Lowe *et al.*, 1980).

Although patients with non-small cell carcinoma do not appear to have benefited from the majority of reported chemotherapeutic regimes and more controlled studies are clearly required, the situation is much more optimistic with small cell carcinoma, a disease in which the possibility of cure can now be entertained.

Part II: Mediastinum

Oesophagus

Carcinoma of the oesophagus is a relatively uncommon disease accounting for about 3% of malignancies. It occurs in the 40–60 year age group, the male/female ratio being about 5:1, except in Scandinavia where there is a higher incidence among women. It is thought to be related to tobacco smoking and alcohol consumption, but may follow a benign lesion affecting the oesophagus, such as web, achalasia, or stricture.

Characteristic lesions may be found at three separate sites, the upper, middle and lower oesophagus, which correspond to the anatomical narrowings of this structure; the involvement of each site varies tremendously in the reported series, but is approximately 15%, 40% and 45% respectively.

The histology of the tumour depends on its site of origin. Upper and middle lesions are invariably squamous in origin and usually are moderately undifferentiated; adenocarcinomas may be found in the lower third but these could well be gastric in origin; sarcoma is very rare.

A lesion arising in the oesophageal mucosa can spread to the sub-mucosal tissues, the muscle is a definite barrier to further spread but spread is easy within the loose sub-mucosal tissues and will proceed fairly rapidly. Such spread may encircle the lumen producing a stricture and will then extend up and down the length of oesophagus. Penetration of the muscle layers occurs at a relatively late stage of the disease; the oesophagus has no serosal layer and once the muscle is penetrated spread can occur into the loose tissues of the mediastinum and involve such structures as the trachea, bronchus, large blood vessels, heart and the pleura.

Lymphatic spread from the upper third is to the deep cervical lymph nodes either directly or indirectly through the retropharyngeal or paratracheal nodes. Lower third lesions drain to the posterior mediastinum and also the abdominal lymph nodes. Middle third lesions have abdominal lymph node involvement in about one quarter of the cases.

It is estimated that at least 70% of patients have spread to lymph nodes on presentation and about 30% have blood-borne distant metastases; the oesophageal lesion is localized in only about one quarter of the patients. This dissemination is reflected in the poor prognosis obtained after treatment of this disease.

The commonest presenting symptom is dysphagia; initially intermittent it progresses to become persistent, first for solid food, then semi-solids then fluids. If sub-mucosal spread encircles the lumen entirely, symptoms may be produced quite early in the disease. More often though, spread occurs in all directions encircling and longitudinally and severe restriction of swallowing may not occur until later. In these patients there may be a feeling of 'something sticking', substernal pain, heartburn, increased salivation and regurgitation of food. Symptoms progress and the patient may lose considerable weight because of poor food intake and later become dehydrated when fluids are restricted.

The differential diagnosis is between an oesophageal web, Plummer-Vinson syndrome, found more frequently in women, for upper third lesions, mediastinal nodes for middle third lesions and achalasia and hiatus hernia for lower lesions.

Radiographs, using a fluid contrast media, will show persistent narrowing of the oesophagus and may give some indication of the extent of spread; tipping the patient's head allows some reflux and the lower limits of the lesion may then be seen. Occasionally fistulae may be seen into the trachea or main bronchus.

Oesophagoscopy will enable a biopsy to be taken, careful dilatation of a stricture, or the insertion of a tube to enable swallowing in inoperable patients; there is a risk of oesophageal perforation with mediastinitis and surgical emphysema.

The patient may need preparation before starting treatment. Dehydration may need rectifying as will any electrolyte balance which results. There may be chest infection from aspirated food and many of the patients are in poor general condition.

Treatment

Surgery is the treatment of choice in adenocarcinoma. It is suggested that because of the widespread infiltration of the squamous growths on presentation, radiotherapy is the treatment of choice.

The vast majority of patients are suitable for palliative treatment only; however, some can be treated radically aiming at cure and long-term survivors are reported.

Surgery

The first successful resection of a carcinoma of the oesophagus was carried out by Torek in 1913. He excised the entire oesophagus and left the patient with a cervical pharyngostomy and a gastrostomy. It was not until 1938 that Adams and Phemister recorded the first successful one-stage oesophagectomy and oesophagogastric anastomosis. Surgery for carcinoma of the oesophagus was viewed optimistically in the early days but subsequent experience has shown that this optimism was misplaced. Many factors have shown themselves to be responsible for this. The disease commonly occurs in elderly patients. The disease itself can cause marked malnutrition in the patients. Sub-mucosal spread is often extensive and is often underestimated at operation. The oesophagus does not possess a serosa which may result in invasion of important adjacent structures at an early stage. The oesophagus has a very rich lymphatic drainage and distant lymphatic involvement is common. This can be found both in the neck or below the diaphragm. The surgery of carcinoma of the oesophagus depends upon the site of the lesion.

Carcinoma of the upper third of the oesophagus

The surgery of these lesions poses many surgical problems. Today the most commonly used surgical approach is a three-stage operation.

The first stage consists of a laparotomy in which the stomach is mobilized. This mobilization consists of division of the left gastric and left gastroepiploic arteries together with the short gastric arteries. The right gastric and right gastroepiploic arteries are left as the blood supply to the mobilized stomach. All obviously involved lymph nodes around the stomach or around the coeliac axis are removed at the same time. The oesophagus is freed as it passes through the hiatus of the diaphragm. The right crus of the diaphragm is commonly divided to create more room. Finally a pyloroplasty is performed.

The second stage of the operation consists of placing the patient in position for a right posterolateral thoracotomy. The oesophagus and its lesion is explored and fully mobilized. This allows the previously mobilized stomach to be drawn through the hiatus in the diaphragm.

The third stage of the operation consists of exposing the oesophagus in the neck. The oesophagus is transected well above the lesion and the lesion, the oesophagus and the mobilized stomach are drawn up into the neck. The oesophagus is excised at the gastro-oesophageal junction which is oversewn. An anastomosis is carried out in the neck between the proximal oesophageal or pharyngeal stump and the fundus of the stomach to restore continuity of the alimentary tract.

Modifications of this approach have been described and consist either of bringing a Roux-en-Y loop up to the neck or using a length of transverse colon mobilized at the same time as the stomach to restore continuity of the gastrointestinal tract.

Carcinoma of the middle third of the oesophagus

Controversy still surrounds the best form of treatment for these lesions. Radiotherapy provides a good result and most oncologists believe there is little to choose between surgery and radiotherapy. If surgery is the treatment of choice for a particular patient this is most commonly carried out as a two-stage procedure. This operation was originally described by Lewis (1946).

The first stage is similar to that described for the three-stage operation. A laparotomy is performed and the stomach is mobilized to allow it to be drawn into the chest. The oesophagus is freed in the diaphragmatic hiatus.

The second stage consists of a right posterolateral thoracotomy through which the oesophagus containing the lesion is fully mobilized. The oesophagus is transected at least 2 cm above the lesion. The lower oesophagus containing the lesion, which is still attached to the mobilized stomach, is now drawn up through the hiatus in the diaphragm. The oesophagus is transected below at the level of the gastro-oesophageal junction. The defect so created is over-sewn. Direct oesophagogastric anastomosis is carried out to establish continuity of the gastrointestinal tract.

Carcinoma of the lower third of the oesophagus

These lesions may arise from the oesophagus. However many are of gastric origin arising at the cardia. Careful delineation of the site of origin of the lesion is important. Most oncologists believe that this lesion is best treated surgically unless it proves to be inoperable. Operation is normally performed as a one-stage procedure.

The lesion is either approached through a left lower posterolateral thoracotomy or through a thoracolaparotomy. The surgical method used will be determined by the level of origin of the tumour. The oesophagus is mobilized from the arch of the aorta downwards. If a thoracotomy alone is performed, a radial incision in the diaphragm is necessary in order to carry out that part of the operation below the diaphragm. If a thoracolaparotomy is performed, the thoracotomy is continued obliquely through the anterior abdominal wall and the diaphragm divided radially into the oesophageal hiatus. The stomach is mobilized so that it is supported only by the right gastric and right gastroepiploic arteries. All suspicious lymph nodes are excised during this mobilization. If the lesion arises in the lower third of the oesophagus, the oesophagus is transected a minimum of 2 cm above the lesion. The distal transection is usually carried out through the fundus of the stomach and includes the gastro-oesophageal junction. The level at which this is done is determined by how far down the tumour has encroached towards the cardia. The stomach is tubularized and brought up into the chest and a direct oesophagogastric anastomosis carried out. If the tumour arises at the cardia, when it is probably of gastric origin, it is necessary to excise a much greater amount of the stomach. This usually necessitates transecting the stomach at, or below, its mid-point. When this is done there is often not enough stomach to bring up into the chest to perform a direct oesophagogastric anastomosis. In this case either a Roux-en-Y or a colon interposition is used to reconstitute the gastrointestinal tract.

Palliative surgery

Many carcinomas of the oesophagus prove to be inoperable when first seen. These patients are commonly in very poor condition. Their dysphagia may well be complete. Their state of malnutrition is usually well advanced. Dysphagia for fluids if complete, rapidly results in gross dehydration. Surgical palliation in these patients with advanced disease is directed entirely to allowing the patients to swallow, certainly fluids, but if possible solids as well.

Various forms of intubation are available. The Souttars tube can be inserted through the lesion endoscopically. This tube is suitable for short circumferential tumours but as it has a poor flange it has a tendency to pass on through the tumour. The Mousseau-Barbin tube and the Celestin tube have larger flanges and are constructed with long leading bougies. It is necessary to perform a gastrostomy in order to pull these tubes down so as to lodge the flange above the lesion. These tubes also have a tendency to slip through the lesion, but less so than the Souttars tube. Patients with inoperable tumours who have developed tracheo-oesophageal or broncho-oesophageal fistulae can also be helped by palliative intubation. A well positioned tube can direct most of the patients saliva into the stomach, thus reducing the amount which enters the airway.

Some surgeons adopt a more aggressive approach to the palliation of the inoperable carcinoma of the oesophagus and a variety of bypass procedures have been described. Oesophagogastric anastomosis above the lesion, leaving the lesion *in situ*, has been described. Colon transplantation between the normal oesophagus above the lesion and the stomach below has also been used. Occasionally a Roux-en-Y anastomosis to the oesophagus above the stump has been used. Very few surgeons favour simple defunctioning of such a lesion by pharyngostomy and gastrostomy. Gastrostomy on its own should never be employed as the patient is quite unable to handle his or her saliva and also loses the ability to taste any food which in itself, has an adverse effect on the condition.

Results of surgery

The results of radical surgery for carcinoma of the oesophagus have proved universally disappointing. The operation carries a mortality which varies between 5 and 15% in nearly all described series (Gunnlaugsson *et al.*, 1970). A five-year survival for patients who have undergone resective surgery for carcinoma of the oesophagus approximately parallels the operative mortality. Very few authors have recorded a five-year survival in excess of 10%. In spite of these bad results the survivors are better off after their resection than before. The operation allows them to swallow. They are therefore able to maintain their state of hydration and their nutritional status often improves.

All forms of resections for carcinoma of the oesophagus are prone to anastomotic strictures. These may be cicatricial or due to malignant recurrence. The former can be dealt with by repeated dilatations. The latter may respond to irradiation, but they are a common cause of death. The other common cause of death is due to metastasis which may become widespread.

Radiotherapy

The patient's general health should be improved as much as possible before starting radical treatment but too long a delay only increases the chances of metastases. Intravenous fluids are necessary if there is complete obstruction. The patient may be distressed because he is unable to swallow saliva and the insertion of a Mousseau-Barbin or Celestin tube should be considered; gastrostomies are best avoided. In practice radical treatment is given to upper and middle third lesions but not often to lower third lesions.

Fields should extend at least 5 cm beyond the upper and lower limits of the tumour; in practice this means that fields smaller than 15 cm in length are to be considered inadequate to cover the growth.

The treatment of middle third tumours is relatively straight forward: a barium swallow, using a fluid contrast medium is taken with markers on the front and back of the chest to allow localization. Usually three fields are used, one anterior field and two posterior oblique fields, so that the spinal cord is spared a high dose. The fields must cover the tumour adequately and are usually 7–8 cm across, but involvement of the mediastinal nodes or tissues may require wider fields. A tumour dose of 5000 rad in 20 treatments over 4 weeks is usual, but there are many variations.

Lesions of the upper third pose specific problems because of the curvature of the upper oesophagus following that of the spine. The upper limit of the tumour in the oesophagus lies only a few centimetres from the anterior skin surface whilst the lower part is several

centimetres deep – at approximately the centre of the thorax. Techniques have been devised to counteract this and depend on using two anterior fields wedged in two directions, one in the horizontal plane and the other in the vertical plane (Deeley and Francois, 1958). In such lesions a dose of about 6000 rad is given in 30 treatments over 6 weeks.

This treatment will invariably cause some radiation oesophagitis; this is seldom serious and often settles down if a few days rest from treatment are given. Local anaesthetic agents help some patients. Foods which are likely to irritate the oesophagus should be avoided, for example rough foods, acids, spices, condiments, hot foods and alcohol. Radiation pneumonitis may develop but is usually limited to a relatively small part of the lung.

Growth may extend from the oesophagus to the trachea or bronchus and ablation of tumour may leave a fistula. It is possible that this may heal by scarring, food should be avoided by mouth and the patient should be placed on intravenous therapy. Chest and mediastinal infection needs to be treated with widespectrum antibiotics.

Treatment of an encircling growth may lead to fibrosis and subsequent dilatation of the fibrotic stricture may be needed.

The results of radiation treatment are not good and are usually about 5–7% five-year survival, but Pearson (1971) reported a 21% five-year survival in a series of 123 patients; these results are difficult to equal and there have been no others as good.

It has been suggested that pre-operative radiation may improve the surgical survivals but as yet there is no convincing proof of this.

Chemotherapy, at present, has no place in radical treatment at this site.

Palliative radiotherapy

Palliative radiotherapy can often relieve dysphagia for long periods of time. Radiation is limited to the immediate stricture, using shorter fields than in radical treatments. Even in the presence of widespread disease oesophageal patency may be achieved. Treatment is based on a day to day basis, giving about 200 rad daily or 400 rad twice weekly, and stops when the patient is able to swallow again; it may be repeated if stenosis recurs. Chemotherapy does not appear to be useful.

Treatment so often fails at this site because of the ease with which the tumour disseminates; many patients already have widespread disease on presentation. Major improvements in treatment will only be made if methods of early detection can be developed and there seems little hope of this.

Miscellaneous tumours

Tumours in the mediastinum are rare but include:

Anterior mediastinum

1. Retrosternal goitre; 2. thymic tumours and cysts; 3. teratomatous cysts and tumours; 4. dermoids; 5. lipoma; 6. spring water or clear water cysts.

Posterior mediastinum

1. Neurogenic cysts; 2. neurofibromas and ganglioneuromas; 3. paratracheal and parabronchial cysts; 4. cysts of gastric, oesophageal or enteric origin; 5. lymph nodes – these may be involved by the reticuloses or by secondary deposits; 6. seminoma from extragonadal germinal layers.

Treatment for benign lesions is surgical; this may also be the treatment of choice for well circumscribed malignant lesions. Other lesions including the reticuloses and secondary lymph nodes are treated by irradiation, in the former case to a radical treatment in the latter to relieve distressing symptoms.

Malignant thymomas

This is a very ill understood tissue; whilst present in childhood and adolescence it normally involutes in early adult age. A malignant tumour may be found in middle age presenting in the anterior superior mediastinum.

Histologically the tumour may have predominant cells, lymphocytes, epithelial cells, spindle cells or may have mixtures of these; a histological diagnosis of malignancy may be difficult. It is not certain whether Hodgkin's disease found at this site has originated in thymic remnants or in the loose mediastinal tissue.

Nearly half of the patients present with myasthenia gravis; the remainder may complain of discomfort in the chest or be picked up on routine chest radiography.

Treatment depends on the presence of myasthenia gravis. If this is not present surgical excision is performed. In inoperable tumours or incomplete excision, irradiation is given to the upper mediastinum, using either an anterior field or two oblique anterior fields, to cover the whole operation site, often needing 12–15 cm fields with a tumour dose of about 5000 rad in 20 treatments over four weeks.

The presence of myasthenia gravis increases the operation risk and it may be desirable to give pre-operative radiotherapy. It is usual to start treatment at a low dose rate of about 100 rad per day because of the risk of lightening-up the symptoms – a myasthenic crisis. Treatment of the myasthenia using parasympathetic stimulants requires close control. The symptoms may resolve and radical surgery can be carried out, giving post-operative radiotherapy if any spill has occurred or the tumour is incompletely excised.

The survival is reported to be in the region of 65% at five years and 50% at ten years irrespective of the presence of myasthenia and late recurrences have been reported.

Mesotheliomas

These lesions are usually associated with working in an asbestos environment. Patients complain of progressive dyspnoea and a dull ache in the chest. Severe dyspnoea may develop if a pleural effusion develops. Radiographs may reveal a pleural effusion only and the typical rounded pleural masses may only be visible when this fluid is removed. Differential diagnosis includes secondary deposits in the pleura. Diagnosis is made by needle or drill biopsy or by an open operation. Treatment is usually symptomatic. Radiation may, however, control the progress of the disease for a considerable time, two large opposed fields being used giving a tumour dose of 3000 rad in 20 treatments in two weeks; this covers the deep extension into the chest which may be missed by more sophisticated arcing methods aimed at treating a few centimetres of tissue below the skin surface.

References

Adams, W.E. and Phemister, D.B. (1938), Carcinoma of the lower thoracic oesophagus: report of a successful resection and oesophagogastrostomy. *J. Thorac. Surg.*, **7**, 621.

Bansch, K. *et al.* (1968), Oat cell carcinoma of the lung, its origin and relationship to bronchial carcinoma. *Cancer*, **22**, 1163.

Broder, L.E., Cohen, M.H. and Selawry, O.S. (1977), Treatment of bronchogenic carcinoma. II. Small cell cancer. *Cancer Treat. Rev.*, **4**, 219.

Carlens, E. (1959), Mediastinoscopy: A method for inspection and tissue biopsy in the superior mediastinum. *Dis. Chest*, **36**, 343.

Deeley, T.J. (1960), The effect of radiation on the lungs in the treatment of carcinoma of the bronchus. *Clin. Radiol.*, **11**, 33.

Deeley, T.J. (1966), A clinical trial to compare two different tumour dose levels in the treatment of advanced carcinoma of the bronchus. *Clin. Radiol.*, **17**, 299.

Deeley, T.J. (1974), National disease; basic concept. In: *A Guide to Oncological Nursing*, (eds T.J. Deeley, E.J. Fish and N.A. Gough), Churchill Livingstone, Edinburgh and London.

Deeley, T.J. (1974), Radiotherapy for carcinoma of the bronchus. *Cancer Treat. Rev.*, **1**, 39.

Deeley, T.J. and Line, D.H. (1969), Solitary metastases in carcinoma of the bronchus. *Br. J. Dis. Chest*, **63**, 150.

Deeley, T.J. and Francois, P.E. (1958), A technique for the irradiation of the upper oesophagus in megavoltage therapy. *Br. J. Radiol.*, **31**, 395.

Doll, R. and Peto, R. (1976), Mortality in relation to smoking: 20 years' observations in male British doctors. *Br. Med. J.*, **2**, 1525.

Freda, S. (1974), *Atlas of Flexible Bronchofiberoscopy*. University Park Press, Baltimore.

Greco, F.A. *et al.* (1978), Small cell lung cancer: Progress and prospectives. *Semin. Oncol.*, **5**, 323.

Gunnlaugsson, G.H. *et al.* (1970), Analysis of the records of 1,657 patients with carcinoma of the oesophagus and cardia of the stomach. *Surg. Gynec. Obstet.*, **130**, 997.

Hansen, H.H., Muggia, F.M. and Selawry, O.S. (1971), Bone marrow examination in 100 consecutive patients with bronchogenic carcinoma. *Lancet*, **2**, 443.

Hansen, H.H. *et al.* (1976), Combination chemotherapy of advanced lung cancer. A randomised trial. *Cancer*, **38**, 2201.

Hattori, S. *et al.* (1972), Oat cell carcinoma of the lung, clinical and morphological studies in relation to its histogenesis. *Cancer*, **30**, 1014.

Higgins, G.A., Shields, T.W. and Kechie, R.J. (1975), The solitary pulmonary nodule: ten-year follow-up of Veterans Administration – Armed Forces Cooperative Study. *Archs Surg.*, **110**, 570.

Kirkman, S. *et al.* (1976), Occult Metastases. In *South Wales Cancer Research Annual Report* (eds T.J. Deeley and W.H. Sutherland), Cancer Research Council, Cardiff Velindre Hospital.

Kirsh, M.M. *et al.* (1972), The effect of histological cell type on the prognosis of patients with bronchogenic carcinoma. *Ann. Thorac. Surg.*, **13**, 303.

Kreyberg, L. (1967), *Histological Typing of Lung Tumours*. WHO, Geneva.

Lewis, I. (1946), The surgical treatment of carcinoma of the oesophagus, with special reference to a new operation for growth of the middle third. *Br. J. Surg.*, **2**, 18.

Line, D.H. and Deeley, T.J. (1971), The necropsy findings in carcinoma of the bronchus. *Br. J. Dis. Chest*, **65**, 238-42.

Livingston, R.B. (1978), Treatment of small cell carcinoma: Evolution and future directions. *Semin.*

Oncol., **5**, 299.

Livingston, R.B. *et al.* (1975a), COMB (cyclophosphamide, Oncovin, methylCCNU and bleomycin). A four drug combination in solid tumours. *Cancer*, **36**, 327.

Livingstone, R.B. *et al*, (1975b), Combination chemotherapy with Bleomycin (NSC. 125066), Adriamycin (NSC. 123127), CCNU (NSC. 79037), Vincristine (NSC. 67574) and Mechlorethamine (NSC. 762) (BACON) in squamous cell lung cancer. Experience with 50 patients. *Cancer Chemother. Rep.*, Part 3, **6**, 361.

Lo Gerfo, P., Krupey, J. and Hausen, H.J. (1971), Demonstration of an antigen common to several varieties of neoplasia: assay using zirconyl phosphate gel. *New Engl. J. Med.*, **285**, 138.

Lowe, J. *et al.* (1980), Intrapleural BCG in operable lung cancer. *Lancet*, **i**, 11.

Lukeman, J.M. (1973), Reliability of cytologic diagnosis in cancer of the lung. *Cancer Chemother. Rep.*, **4**, 79.

McKneally, M.F., Maver, C. and Kausel, H.W. (1976), Regional immunotherapy of lung cancer with intrapleural BCG. *Lancet*, **i**, 377.

McNeill, T.M. and Chamberlain, J.M. (1966), Diagnostic anterior mediastinotomy. *Ann. Thorac. Surg.*, **2**, 532.

Matthews, M.J. *et al.* (1973), Frequency of residual and metastatic tumour in patients undergoing curative surgical resection for lung cancer. *Cancer Chemother. Res.*, **4**, 63.

Medical Research Council, Lung Cancer Working Party (1979), Radiotherapy alone or with chemotherapy in the treatment of small cell carcinoma of the lung. *Br. J. Cancer*, **40**, 1.

Mountain, C.F., Carr, D.T. and Anderson, W.A.D. (1974), A system for the clinical staging of lung cancer. *Am. J. Roentg.*, **120**, 130.

Pearson, J.G. (1971), The value of radiotherapy in the management of squamous oesophageal cancer. *Br. J. Surg.*, **58**, 794.

Selawry, O.S. (1974), The role of chemotherapy in the treatment of lung cancer. *Semin. Oncol.*, **1**, 259.

Shields, T.W. and Shocket, E. (1958), Preoperative evaluation of patients with clinically resectable bronchogenic carcinoma: role of biopsy of nonpalpable scalene nodes. *Archs Surg.*, **76**, 707.

Straus, M.J. (1974), The growth characteristics of lung cancer and its application to treatment design. *Semin. Oncol.*, **1**, 167.

Svarcer, V., Fowler, J.F. and Deeley, T.J. (1965), Exit doses for lung fields measured by lithium fluoride thermoluminescence. *Br. J. Radiol.*, **38**, 785.

Torek, F. (1913), First successful resection of the oesophagus. *J. Am. Med. Assoc.*, **60**, 1533.

Vincent, R.G. and Chu, T.M. (1973), Carcino-embryonic antigen in patients with carcinoma of the lung. *J. Thorac. Cardiovasc. Surg.*, **66**, 320.

Wald, N.J. (1976), *Lancet*, **i**, 136.

Weiss, R.B. (1978), Small cell carcinoma of the lung: Therapeutic management. *Ann. Int. Medicine*, **88**, 522.

World Health Organization (1960, *Epidemiology of cancer of the lung*. Technical Report No. 192, Geneva.

Wynder, E.L. and Hecht, S. (eds) (1976), *Lung Cancer* International Union Against Cancer, Geneva.

19 Gastrointestinal tract

Kenneth C. Calman

Gastrointestinal cancer has a very high incidence in western countries and remains one of the main causes of death. Results of treatment have not improved greatly during recent years. Fresh approaches are very much needed. Most tumours have been treated by surgery alone and it is only now that combined treatment strategies, investigating the integration with surgery of better and more sophisticated radiotherapy, chemotherapy and perhaps immunotherapy are being performed. This chapter outlines the present position for cancer of stomach, small and large bowel, and rectum.

Cancer of the stomach

Gastric carcinoma, for long known as one of the 'Captains of the men of death' continues to remain a problem in spite of its falling incidence. Survival rates remain poor unless the disease is diagnosed at an early stage. Systemic therapy, for example with chemotherapy has, as yet, made little impact on the disease.

Incidence

One of the most striking features of gastric carcinoma is the marked geographical variation in its incidence. Thus in Europe and North America the incidence is low, while in Japan the incidence is extremely high (Table 19.1). In the United Kingdom gastric carcinoma is the third leading cause of death from cancer while in Japan it is first. A further interesting feature has been the fall in the incidence and mortality from the disease over the last 30 years. This fall has occurred consistently over the Western Hemisphere and is not simply due to changes in diagnostic procedures. It represents a real decrease in incidence of the disease.

Aetiology

The geographical variation and falling incidence have suggested that an environmental factor (or factors) is associated with the cause of gastric carcinoma. Dietary factors in particular have been implicated but, in spite of careful searching, no specific factors have been positively identified. At the present time nitrates in water or food seem to be the most likely factors. These compounds may be converted into nitrites or nitrosamines by bacterial action.

Genetic factors do, however, seem to be of some importance in that it is known that persons with blood group A have a higher incidence of gastric cancer. Several diseases seem to predispose to gastric cancer. These include pernicious anaemia, atrophic gastritis and gastric polyps. The arguments continue concerning the relationship between benign and malignant gastric ulcer. One of the most interesting relationships, and perhaps the most controversial, is the relationship between peptic ulceration, its treatment, and the subsequent development of gastric cancer. Several series have now been reported which suggest that gastric cancer can develop following gastric resection or even vagotomy and drainage. It has been suggested that achlorhydria with biliary reflux and bacterial contamination of the stomach act together resulting in the development of cancer (Ellis et al., 1979).

One factor which seems to be universally accepted is that of socioeconomic status; the lower the status the higher the incidence of gastric cancer.

Anatomy

The stomach is an intraperitoneal organ, communicating with the thoracic cavity via the oesophagus. The importance of anatomical considerations relate to the mechanisms of spread of gastric cancer. The neoplasm spreads locally to the serosa and then to the local and regional lymph nodes. These nodes occur along the inferior and superior surfaces and spread to the coeliac nodes. Nodes along the bed of the splenic vessels may also be involved. There is a small group of nodes in the cardiac region which may be of considerable importance in proximal lesions. The supra-clavicular nodes

Table 19.1   Standardized international death rates per 100 000 population showing ranking, for cancer of the stomach, large intestine and rectum, 1971 (Standardizing Population, Scotland 1971), (From *World Health Statistics Annual*, 1971 (1974)).

Country	Stomach (ICD 151) Standard-ized rate	Rank	Large intestine (ICD 153) Standard-ized rate	Rank	Rectum (ICD 154) Standard-ized rate	Rank
Canada	16.5	26	23.6	5	7.9	17
Austria	42.4	4	18.5	12	12.0	3
Belgium	27.6	13	22.2	6	10.3	7
Czechoslovakia	41.7	5	12.3	20	13.4	1
Denmark	19.8	22	19.6	8	13.1	2
Finland	34.5	9	9.6	22	8.3	15
France	19.4	23	18.3	13	7.7	18
Germany (Federal Republic)	36.5	7	19.5	10	11.8	4
Greece	16.4	25	7.9	23	0.8	27
Hungary	46.5	2	16.3	16	10.2	9
Ireland	29.0	12	24.4	4	9.5	10
Italy	34.8	8	15.1	17	7.5	21
Netherlands	26.7	14	19.2	11	8.4	14
Norway	23.9	19	14.6	18	9.3	12
Poland	40.6	6	6.7	24	6.4	23
Portugal	43.6	3	13.6	19	7.7	19
Roumania	32.8	10	5.4	26	4.5	26
Spain	32.2	11	10.8	21	4.8	25
Sweden	21.2	21	17.1	15	8.1	16
Switzerland	26.2	15	18.3	14	8.8	13
England and Wales	23.5	20	19.5	9	11.0	5
Northern Ireland	25.5	18	24.4	3	9.4	11
Scotland	26.1	16	25.4	1	10.8	6
Yugoslavia	25.7	17	5.0	27	5.4	24
Australia	16.5	24	21.4	7	7.6	20
New Zealand	15.2	27	24.6	2	10.3	8
Japan	68.8	1	6.3	25	7.0	22

are not infrequently involved (Virchow's node). Spread, however, also occurs across the peritoneum resulting in multiple deposits on the serosal surfaces with associated ascites. When spread to the ovaries occurs the patient may present with an ovarian tumour (Krukenberg tumour). Pelvic metastases may result in a rectal shelf which can be palpated by digital examination.

Spread by vascular routes also occurs and liver metastases occur in around 30% of patients. Lung, skin and bone metastases also occur but are less frequent.

Pathology

Adenocarcinomas are by far the most common his-

tological type though lymphomas and sarcomas do occur. The tumour may be described macroscopically as polypoid, ulcerated, invasive or infiltrating. The infiltrative types may occur as superficial spreading lesions or as linitus plastica where the stomach becomes thickened, shortened and infiltrated with neoplastic cells. More commonly, however, the tumour is diffusely infiltrating and extends microscopically beyond the limits which can be defined macroscopically.

Histologically the adenocarcinomas may be more or less mucinous in nature. When mucin is a major feature, 'signet ring' cells may be noted. Occasionally squamous metaplasia occurs. While this may be difficult to quantify, the more anaplastic the tumour, the more aggressively it behaves.

Symptoms and presentation

One of the major problems with gastric carcinoma is that the symptoms associated with it may be vague and non-specific, hence the late presentation of the disease in many instances. Amongst the most common presenting features are upper gastrointestinal symptoms, weight loss, non-specific anaemia and depression. In more advanced disease ascites, abdominal masses, hepatomegaly or enlarged lymph nodes may be found. Occasionally the disease may be recognized during investigation for dyspepsia or at operation as an incidental finding. Gastric carcinoma can occur in the young and should not be forgotten during investigation (Stock, 1963).

Diagnosis

Because of the difficulty in recognizing the problem at an early stage when symptoms alone are considered, the argument for early diagnosis in asymptomatic patients is a strong one. Upper gastrointestinal radiology and endoscopy are the cornerstones of diagnosis. Using double contrast barium meals and endoscopy, lesions as small as 1 mm can be visualized, and biopsied. While the bulk of the investigative work has been done in Japan, there is good evidence that similar early diagnostic pick-up rates can be achieved elsewhere (Evans *et al.*, 1978).

Other methods of diagnosis include gastric cytology either from brushings taken at the time of endoscopy or from examination of gastric fluid following aspiration. This latter method has also been used to study biochemical features of gastric juice but in spite of assessing a variety of tests such as β-glucuronidase, lactic dehydrogenase, total DNA content etc., no single test has found clinical acceptance. Measurement of serum and gastric fluid carcinoembryonic antigen (CEA) levels has also been used but has been found to be unhelpful for diagnosis.

In high risk populations, aggressive screening programmes with radiology and endoscopy would seem to be able to pick up small, and hence potentially curable, gastric cancers. It has been argued, however, that the cost of such screening and the expertise required would not justify its widespread use. If improvements cannot be made in the treatment of the disease, however, this statement must be challenged.

Investigations

In most instances the diagnosis is established by radiology and biopsy. Subsequent investigations are aimed at assessing the disease spread and would include isotopic liver scan, ultrasonic examination of the abdomen and chest X-ray. Clinical examination may well define spread outside the stomach. Measurement of CEA levels in serum may be useful for follow-up purposes.

On the basis of such investigations the lesion may be deemed 'operable' or 'non-operable'. However in most instances a laparotomy (or laparoscopy) is performed to confirm the diagnosis, assess extent of spread and to remove or by-pass the tumour.

Staging

The TNM classification of gastric cancer is shown in Table 19.2. This is a clinical classification and is often difficult to implement. At laparotomy the lesion may be classified as resectable, or non-resectable, and the extent of spread be defined. It should be remembered that the aim of staging is to define such spread and to allow comparability of reporting of results.

Treatment

In most instances the diagnosis will have been established prior to treatment though in some cases the diagnosis will only be made at the time of surgery. An attempt should be made, pre-operatively, to assess operability and to define the treatment procedure to be adopted.

Before a programme of management is instituted careful consideration should be given to the location of the tumour, the symptoms associated with it, prognostic factors and the extent of spread. Where possible these should be assessed pre-treatment. Thus symptoms of outlet obstruction or dysphagia may dictate the treatment policy. In an elderly patient with minimal symptoms but evidence of disease spread the plan of management may be quite different.

The treatment of gastric carcinoma is predominantly surgical, this being the most effective way of dealing with tumour bulk and preventing recurrence. The use of radiotherapy and chemotherapy will be discussed later and these two modalities are usually used following surgery. There is increasing use of combined modality therapy, with chemotherapy or radiotherapy being used before surgery, or after surgery, in integration.

Pre-treatment support may be essential in some patients. Anaemia should be corrected and nutritional support given by intravenous or oral routes. Vitamin supplementation may also be used. Where gastric obstruction has been a problem nasogastric suction and intravenous fluids may be required to correct metabolic abnormalities. In a small group of patients where bleeding is a problem, blood will be required and this should be readily available during the opera-

Table 19.2 TNM classification for gastric cancer.

ANATOMICAL REGIONS

1. Upper third
2. Middle third
3. Lower third

In order to delimit these regions the lesser and greater curvatures are divided at three equidistant points and these are joined

Upper third includes the cardiac area and fundus
Middle third includes the bulk of the corpus
Lower third includes the antral area

The tumour is assigned to the region in which the bulk of it is situated

REGIONAL LYMPH NODES

The Regional Lymph Nodes are the perigastric nodes; the nodes located along the left gastric, coeliac and splenic arteries; the nodes along the hepatoduodenal ligament; the para-aortic and other intra-abdominal nodes

TNM TREATMENT CLINICAL CLASSIFICATION

T – *Primary tumour*

T_{is} Pre-invasive carcinoma (carcinoma in situ)

T_0 No evidence of primary tumour

T_1*   Tumour limited to the mucosa *or* mucosa and sub-mucosa regardless of its extent or location

T_2 Tumour with deep infiltration occupying not more than one half of one region

T_3 Tumour with deep infiltration occupying more than one half but not more than one region

T_4 Tumour with deep infiltration occupying more than one region *or* extending to neighbouring structures

T_x The minimum requirements to assess the primary tumour cannot be met

N – *Regional lymph nodes*

N_0 No evidence of regional lymph node involvement

N_1 Evidence of lymph node involvement within 3 cm of the primary tumour along the lesser or greater curvatures

N_2 Evidence of lymph node involvement more than 3 cm from the primary tumour including those along the left gastric, splenic, coeliac, and common hepatic arteries

N_3 Evidence of involvement of the para-aortic and hepatoduodenal lymph nodes *and/or* other intra-abdominal lymph nodes

N_x The minimum requirements to assess the regional lymph nodes cannot be met

M – *Distant metastases*

M_0 No evidence of distant metastases

M_1 Evidence of distant metastases

M_x The minimum requirements to assess the presence of distant metastases cannot be met

---

tion. Adequate blood should be cross-matched.

The modalities of therapy will be described individually, then the possibilities of combined therapy will be discussed.

Surgery

As with many surgical procedures there have been fashions in treatment. The operation performed depends not only on the location of the tumour and extent of spread but on the aggressiveness and experience of the surgeon.

The definition of operability, or inoperability, also depends on the experience of the surgeon. In most large series 75% of patients will be deemed operable before the surgical procedure and approximately 50% will have a definite resection. One of the first decisions to be made is the site of the incision. For distal lesions a midline or paramedian incision may be used. For proximal lesions a thoracoabdominal incision may be employed.

Following the opening of the abdomen, exploration is first carried out. The extent of the local lesion is defined and a careful search made for intraperitoneal and liver metastases. The lesser sac is opened and the region of the coeliac axis and splenic bed is examined. If at this stage the lesion is considered to be inoperable, it is essential that clips are placed on the lesion, any enlarged or involved nodes or areas of secondary spread. Biopsy should be taken from all relevant sites. If surgery is to be undertaken the following procedures may be used:

1. *Sub-total gastrectomy*. In this procedure two thirds of the stomach is removed. For adequate resection of nodes almost all of the lesser curvature of the stomach should be included. The duodenum is transected to allow at least 5 cm of tissue clear of the tumour. In almost all instances the spleen is also removed. The subsequent anastomosis depends on the tumour site and the mobility of the stomach remnant. It is usual to use a proximal jejunal loop, and a valve-type closure may be employed.

2. *Total gastrectomy*. The entire stomach is resected together with a cuff of oesophagus. A thoracoabdominal approach is usually required to give adequate exposure. Once again several forms of anastomosis may be used to restore continuity. These include the use of a jejunal loop (with end-to-side anastomosis) a Roux-en-Y procedure and the use of an interposed colonic segment. The type of anastomosis may well affect the short and long-term side-effects of the procedure.

* The clinical evidence for T_1 is the recognition of:
(a) a malignant pedunculated polyp, (b) a malignant sessile polypoid lesion, (c) a cancerous erosion, or (d) an area of cancerous erosion on the margin of, or surrounding a peptic ulcer.

3. *Extended total gastrectomy*. In addition to removing the entire stomach and spleen, the body and tail of the pancreas are resected. The morbidity and mortality from this procedure are naturally higher.

4. *Resection of adjacent organs*. Where the tumour has invaded locally then it is occasionally justifiable to resect the adjacent involved organs. These would include colon and small bowel. Where the greater omentum is involved then this may also be resected. The reasons for carrying out such extensive procedures are to remove as much tumour bulk as possible (debulking) and also to prevent, or diminish, the subsequent effect of local recurrence.

5. *Palliative procedures*. Where it is not possible to resect the tumour *en bloc*, there may still be merit in removing the bulk of the neoplasm. In these circumstances it is essential that remaining sites of the tumour are marked using radio-opaque clips. Where the cancer is quite inoperable then a bypass procedure may allow relief of symptoms and permit the use of additional modalities of therapy. Once again delineation of the lesion and metastases should be performed.

6. *Second look operations*. This procedure may be considered in the patient who is clinically and radiologically free of disease. This may be used for restaging or to reach a decision regarding the continuation, or termination, of other modalities of therapy.

7. *Recurrent disease*. If the patient develops locally recurrent disease demonstrable radiologically or at endoscopy, consideration should be given to further surgical procedures. A second resection may be possible and the extent of disease can be assessed at the same time.

8. *Emergency procedures*. If the patient develops a surgical emergency, such as an obstructive lesion or upper gastrointestinal bleeding, the surgeon faces a difficult and complex clinical decision. Each individual case has to be judged on its merits, and considerable surgical expertise may be required.

Post-operative management. Standard surgical textbooks should be consulted regarding the detailed problems involved. From the point of view of the clinical oncologist the important features relate to the subsequent integration of other therapeutic modalities. Thus the healing of the wound, the presence of infection or fistulae and the nutritional state of the patient may delay or modify subsequent therapy.

Complications. In the short-term these relate to the factors mentioned above. In the long-term, the patient may develop anaemia (iron deficiency and megaloblastic), dumping syndrome, weight loss and nutritional deficiencies. These are not only serious in themselves but may present a difficult diagnostic problem when tumour recurrence is suspected. The morbidity associated with such operative procedures should be assessed before the institution of other therapies (e.g. chemotherapy) as this may accentuate some of these problems.

Radiotherapy
The role of radiotherapy in the treatment of gastric carcinoma still remains to be defined. It has however been used in several ways, some of which are still under investigation.

Gastric cancer is not a particularly radiosensitive tumour. Palliative doses of radiotherapy using 2000–4000 rad given as a wide field have been most frequently used. If the extent of the tumour has been defined at operation and radio-opaque clips used, treatment planning is facilitated. Kidney shielding may be required and in the post-operative patient the treatment is usually started two to three weeks after the operation. A major problem with large gastric cancers is that large areas may be hypoxic, minimizing the effect of the radiation. This may be overcome by the use of large fractions, radiosensitizers or the use of neutron therapy.

Primary treatment with radiotherapy. This procedure has normally been reserved for inoperable lesions, or in patients who are 'unfit' for surgical procedures. This, in itself, may make the results difficult to interpret. The use of super voltage technique has met with little success, though more recently the use of neutron therapy has been encouraging. In patients treated with neutrons there is good evidence that the primary tumour was well controlled but the overall survival rate did not appear to be altered (Kingsley *et al.*, 1976).

Pre-operative radiotherapy. Several clinical trials have been reported using pre-operative radiotherapy. The subsequent surgical morbidity has not been increased and the treatment, in general, has been well tolerated. However, little long-term benefit has been achieved.

Post-operative radiotherapy. In most instances this has been used to treat sites of disease not removed at operation. Little evidence of long-term benefit is available.

Treatment of complications, or recurrent disease. Under some circumstances, radiotherapy may be used to relieve an obstructive lesion and to stop haemorrhage.

Chemotherapy
In contrast to other tumours where cytotoxic agents now have a clearly defined place, the use of

chemotherapy in gastric cancer still requires elucidation. Because of the difficulty in evaluating the results of treatment only a limited number of studies are available for evaluation (Comis and Carter, 1974).

The drug which has been most extensively used is 5-flourouracil (5-FU). This may be given in several dose schedules. These include the use of a loading dose followed by weekly injections, oral use or as infusions. In general the results obtained do not show specific benefit from any one technique. The weekly intravenous dose is said to be less toxic and easier to administer. More recently the use of high dose infusions of 5-FU with allopurinol has been described (Fox *et al.*, 1979). An increased response rate has been reported with this technique, though results must await confirmation. The use of oral preparations is of some interest though the absorption is variable. The overall response rate with 5-fluorouracil is between 20 and 25%, responses lasting between 4 and 6 months.

Mitomycin C is another single agent which has been extensively investigated. It is commonly given on an intermittent basis using between 0.05 and 1 mg/kg i.v. At the high dose level, however, the toxicity was considerable. Response rates of 30% have been reported with this drug with a short duration of effectiveness.

Other drugs which have been used include anamycin, cytosine arabinoside, cyclophosphamide, methotrexate and the nitrosoureas. Variable results have been reported with these drugs and they are often used in combination. In gastric cancer there is a striking lack of information on the use of many of the commonly used drugs. Many more single agent studies are required.

Combination chemotherapy. While important advances have been made in the use of combination chemotherapy in several types of solid tumour, the same cannot be said at this time of gastric cancer. One of the first combinations to be used was that of 5-FU and the nitrosoureas. Initial results showed promise but these have not been confirmed. 5-FU and mitomycin C, with or without adriamycin, has also been assessed. Initial results seem promising.

Combined modality therapy

The combination of radiotherapy and 5-FU has been explored (Moertel *et al.*, 1969) in locally unresectable gastric cancer treated with 900–1200 rad/week to a total tumour dose of 4000 rad. There was a significant benefit in the use of both modalities with an increase in the survival time. This has not however been adequately followed up.

Several studies have been carried out in which chemotherapy was given after operation as an adjuvant to surgery. Many of these have suffered from being poorly planned and the results have been difficult to evaluate. Several drugs have been used including thiotepa, 5-FU, mitomycin C and a variety of combinations. The majority of these studies have given equivocal or negative results. A very few however have indicated that the thesis may be correct though these require urgent confirmation.

Results of treatment

Over the last twenty years the overall five year survival rate of all patients has remained stable at between 10 and 15%. Thus in spite of the introduction of new modalities of therapy and the more frequent use of combined modality therapy, no significant improvements have occurred. Gastric cancer remains an area for research and development.

Cancer of the small bowel

Malignant tumours of the small bowel are not common, accounting for only 2% of all malignant neoplasms of the gastrointestinal tract. Yet the small bowel covers 75% of the length of the alimentary tract. When all neoplasms of small bowel are considered, benign and malignant, 50% are found to be carcinomas, lymphomas, carcinoid tumours and sarcomas. The remainder are benign. The relative rarity of small bowel tumours compared to stomach and colon cancer has been commented on many times and several explanations put forward. These include rapid transit time preventing contact with an intraluminal carcinogen; rapid cell turnover eliminating neoplastic cells; immunological mechanisms because of the large amount of lymphoid tissue in small bowel (Calman, 1974). Whatever the cause, for every small bowel tumour there are 14 stomach cancers and 46 colon cancers. There is a variation in the incidence of malignant disease along the length of the small bowel, most tumours being twice as frequent in the ileum (Southam, 1974).

Pathology

Apart from secondary tumours of small bowel (which again are rare) malignant lesions can be divided into four broad groups – adenocarcinomas, lymphomas, carcinoid tumours and sarcomas. Both lymphomas and sarcomas are covered fully elsewhere in this volume and will not be considered further. Carcinoid tumours (see Chapter 17) arise from the argéntaffin cells of the small bowel mucosa and are classified as Apud cells (amine precursor uptake and decarboxylation). These apudomas may secrete a variety of hormones including insulin, gastrin, glucagon, 5-hydroxytryptamine and many others.

Carcinoid tumours may be benign or malignant. In those which are malignant there is infiltration locally, and spread to involve the liver and other organs. When liver metastases occur the clinical symptoms of the carcinoid syndrome become apparent. Normally the release of 5-hydroxytryptamine in the portal venous system is metabolized with no systemic effects. When liver metastases are present, however, this does not occur. The symptoms of carcinoid syndrome, diarrhoea, abdominal discomfort, facial flushing, bronchoconstriction and valvular lesions are not simply due to the release of 5-hydroxytryptamine, but also related to the release of other agents including kinins and possibly the prostaglandins.

Symptoms and presentation

Tumours of the small bowel may present with symptoms, or as an incidental finding at laparotomy. In most instances the patient complains of abdominal distension, obstructive symptoms or of malabsorption. Anorexia, weight loss and pain are common. Nausea and vomiting may occur and the patient may present with gastrointestinal bleeding. A factor of considerable importance in relation to treatment is that the patient may present as an abdominal emergency, with perforation, obstruction, intussusception or bleeding. At the time of surgery the diagnosis may not be suspected and, either for this reason or for surgical problems, a definitive operative procedure may not be performed.

Diagnosis

The diagnosis may be suspected from the history and the physical findings. It may be confirmed by radiological studies, using a variety of methods for visualizing the small bowel. It is however crucial to establish the diagnosis histologically. This may be done at laparotomy or occasionally at laparoscopy. The diagnosis may also be confirmed retrospectively following an emergency procedure and biopsy should be taken of representative areas. The importance of establishing the diagnosis histologically is related to the number of other conditions which may mimic neoplasia. These include the chronic infections, such as tuberculosis, Crohn's disease, benign neoplastic diseases and other causes of malabsorption.

Treatment

The treatment of cancer of the small bowel is primarily surgical, hence the importance of the primary procedure. At the initial operation, either because of perfo-ration or other complications, it may not be possible to carry out an adequate resection. Under these circumstances it is essential that, at the earliest time convenient to the patient, a second laparotomy is performed and a definitive resection completed. In all instances, radio-opaque markers should be placed at the site of the tumour and where metastases have been located. For resection to be adequate, 5–10 cm of macroscopically normal bowel on the side of the lesion should be excised, together with the mesentery and involved nodes. For proximal lesions pancreaticoduodenectomy may be required.

Because of the relative rarity of adenocarcinomas of the small bowel, there is little data on the effects of the radiotherapy or of chemotherapy on such tumours. In general, they behave like adenocarcinomas of the colon and the management of these is discussed later. The treatment of lymphomas and sarcomas will not be discussed further here (see Chapters 31 and 36).

The treatment of neoplasms of the appendix is of some interest. The majority of these (90%) are carcinoid tumours and most of these will be discovered at laparotomy for acute appendicitis. In the majority of instances no further action will be required. The remainder of appendicial tumours are mucoceles. As with mucus-producing neoplasms of the gastrointestinal tract, rupture into the peritoneal cavity may occur producing the clinical picture of pseudomyxoma peritonei. This is typically related to a slow-growing adenocarcinoma of the colon, normally well differentiated histologically.

The treatment of malignant carcinoid tumours is covered in Chapter 17. Symptomatic control may be achieved using methysergide, cyproheptidine or phenoxybenzamine. As vitamin usage may be altered because of tumour requirements for niacin, vitamin supplements may be required. A number of chemotherapeutic agents have been used in the treatment of malignant carcinoid tumours. The most commonly used, however, are 5-FU and streptozotocin. Approximately 25% of patients will respond to such agents.

Cancer of the large bowel

Incidence

The death rate of large bowel cancer varies widely throughout the world. It ranges from being high (15/100 000) in Western Europe and the United States, to low in Africa and Japan (4/100 000) (Table 19.1). These differences have suggested that environmental factors, notable in the diet, are responsible for the aetiology of this disease. However, not only does the incidence of the disease vary from country to country, so does the site of the lesion. In high incidence areas cancer occurs most frequently on the left side of the colon. In low incidence areas it is more frequent on the right. While it is often difficult to separate rectal and rectosigmoid lesions anatomically, the epidemiology of these two sites is different. The incidence of rectal cancer does not show marked variations around the world and this tumour affects predominantly males (1.4:1, male:female).

Aetiology

From the epidemiological studies detailed above, it was considered that environmental factors might be the most important in the causation of colorectal cancer. It has been suggested that the intraluminal contents of the large bowel contain a carcinogen which acts directly on the bowel mucosa. The most likely environmental association is with the diet and numerous epidemiological studies have been carried out to elucidate this problem. High fat, low fibre and high beef content of the diet are the major contenders and it should be noted that these factors are not mutually exclusive. Some of the most fruitful sources of research have been migrant populations, particularly native born Japanese who have moved to the United States. After this movement the incidence of colon cancer rises sharply to approach that of the United States (Wynder and Reddy, 1973).

A search has been made in the faeces for compounds which would be putative carcinogens. Several such compounds have been identified both directly and indirectly. Initial studies centred on the role of faecal bile acids and bacteria in the aetiology of colorectal cancer. These studies in metabolic epidemiology suggested faecal bile acids might indeed be carcinogens or cocarcinogens (Hill et al., 1975). Other compounds, especially nitroso compounds have also been isolated. The importance of this aspect of aetiology is that once the carcinogen has been identified, attempts can be made to eliminate this compound or to render it non-carcinogenic. This is currently being investigated in animals and man.

Colon cancer can now be induced in a variety of animals by carcinogenic compounds such as 1,2-dimethylhydrazine. These experimental models have been useful in the understanding of the mechanisms of carcinogenesis and in the way in which diet, bacteria and the continuity of the gastrointestinal tract can influence tumour development.

Predisposing factors

In carcinoma of the colon, as in many other forms of cancer, it is useful to identify those patients who are at high risk of developing malignant disease. With carcinoma of the colon there are a number of such pre-malignant conditions which have been identified and allow screening of this population to be carried out regularly.

Chronic inflammatory disease

Ulcerative colitis is now well recognized to be associated with an increased risk of developing colon cancer. This risk is estimated to be 8–10 times that of the normal population, and will occur in 5–12% of the population at risk. When ulcerative colitis has been present for over ten years and has been active during this time the question of panproctocolectomy should be raised. There is some debate as to whether a colostomy or an ileorectal anastomosis should be performed. In Crohn's disease affecting the colon there is a small but definite increased risk of developing colon cancer. Other chronic inflammatory processes such as radiation proctocolitis, schistosomiasis and post-ureterosigmoidostomy have been shown to be associated with an increased incidence of colon cancer.

Dysplastic polypoid lesions

These include solitary tubular and villous adenomas together with multiple colonic polyps. Familial polyposis and Gardner's syndrome (intestinal polyposis, soft tissue abnormalities, bone abnormalities) are the most common of these multiple polyp syndromes. The cancer family syndrome (colon, breast and female genital tract) can also be included in this group.

Of general importance is the mechanism by which such adenomas or polyps become malignant and the biological model of carcinogenesis presented by such a clinical problem is a fascinating one. It has been suggested (Hill et al., 1978) that normal colonic epithelial cells are transformed by a carcinogen into a small adenoma. This event only occurs when the carcinogen is present and when the epithelial cell is genetically capable of this change. A small proportion of these small adenomas will develop into malignant lesions under the influence of a second carcinogen. In the majority of instances the small adenoma develops into a large adenoma and it is at this stage that the malignant transformation occurs. There is circumstantial and epidemiological evidence to support such a hypothesis. Thus the regular removal of rectosigmoid polyps reduces the subsequent incidence of the development of cancer and the greater the size of the adenoma the greater would appear to be its malignant potential. Not all evidence, however, is in favour of the hypothesis and it must be concluded that, at present, there is the potential for such a progression but that the exact mechanism remains to be established.

Hamartomatous polypoid lesions

These include juvenile polyposis coli and the Peutz-Jeghers syndrome. In both instances there is a small chance of development of carcinoma of the colon.

Pathology

In Western countries 70% of all cancers of the colon occur in the rectosigmoid region. This implies that over 30% can be reached by the examining finger and 60% by the sigmoidoscope. In gross terms the lesion may be polypoid, obstructive, ulcerating or nodular. Microscopically the lesion may be well or poorly differentiated and this can be correlated with prognosis. Pathologically invasion into surrounding tissues and lymph nodes may be noted. Of considerable prognostic importance is venous invasion which requires to be looked for with special care. The degree of mucin production varies from tumour to tumour. The pathological examination of the operative specimen is relevant to staging and this will be discussed later.

Symptoms and presentation

Patients with colorectal cancer may present in a variety of ways, depending on the site of the lesion and the extent of its spread. Right-sided colonic lesions tend to present with weight loss, anaemia and the presence of an abdominal mass. Left-sided lesions may present with rectal bleeding, colicky abdominal pains, obstructive symptoms or evidence of altered bowel habits or a mass.

Patients may also present for the first time as abdominal emergencies with bowel obstruction, perforation or bleeding. Unfortunately many patients still present late in spite of symptoms being present for some time. There is certainly scope for patient education in this regard. Altered bowel habit and rectal bleeding are important warning signs and should not be taken lightly by the patient or his doctor.

Diagnosis

Physical examination, including digital rectal examination and sigmoidoscopy, together with the history of the presenting complaints will usually suggest the diagnosis. It will however be necessary to confirm this histologically either by colonoscopy (if it is not accessible to the sigmoidoscope) or at laparotomy. A barium enema examination should be carried out as a routine procedure even when the lesion can be palpated and biopsied directly, because of the dangers of missing a second lesion.

Early diagnosis

Because of the high incidence of this disease, its late presentation and its treatability when discovered early, a great deal of effort has been put into diagnosing the cancer early. The methods employed include the use of faecal occult blood tests, colonoscopy, double contrast barium enemas and cytology. As these latter techniques are time-consuming and expensive, it is useful if a preliminary screening procedure can be used thus narrowing down the number of patients screened by defining high risk populations (Gillespie *et al.*, 1979).

Of the faecal occult blood tests, the most promising at present is the 'Haemoccult' test. This test is easy to use but is still being evaluated. It is hoped that this test will allow widespread screening for the disease and select patients for further investigations.

Several years ago the use of oncofetal proteins in the diagnosis of colon cancer came into prominence. A glycoprotein, carcinoembryonic antigen (CEA) was described. This biological marker was found in foetal colon and initially it was said to be present specifically in the blood of patients with colon cancer. It was therefore considered that this would be an ideal screening test for colon cancer. Unfortunately, however, as time has passed it would appear that CEA is not specific for colon cancer, nor indeed for malignant disease. It is therefore of little value in screening but, if elevated may be of great value in the follow up of patients, as the level of CEA can be used to monitor the effects of therapy (Holyoke *et al.*, 1975).

Cytology of colonic washings has also been used for early diagnosis of colon cancer. The technique, however, is time consuming and requires special expertise in the assessment of the washings.

Investigations

Following clinical examination and sigmoidoscopy, several other investigations may be performed aimed at defining the extent of spread of the disease. These would include barium enema, isotope scan and/or ultrasonic examination of liver, biochemical tests of liver function, baseline CEA and chest X-ray. Colon cancer may metastasize to bone more frequently than is usually recognized and an isotope bone scan may be useful. Unless the tumour is considered to be inoperable, laparotomy is one of the most useful investigations, in that it will allow full examination of the abdominal cavity, biopsy of lesions and marking of metastatic deposits.

Staging

Many methods have been devised for the staging of colorectal cancer. The earliest of these was the Duke's classification which initially applied only to rectum but was extended to colon. The A, B, C (and subsequently D) stages were established by pathological examination of the resected specimen and the stage was shown to correlate with prognosis thus:

Dukes A – Tumour into muscle coat but not through it (95% 5-year survival rate)
Dukes B – Tumour through serosa but nodes not involved (77% 5-year survival rate)
Dukes C – Draining nodes involved (32% 5-year survival rate)
Dukes D – Distant metastases (12% 5-year survival rate)

More recently the UICC have developed the TNM staging for colorectal cancer and this is shown in Tables 19.3 and 19.4. It cannot be emphasized too strongly that accurate pathological staging requires a great deal of work by the pathologist but that this does have important prognostic implications.

Table 19.3   TNM Staging for colonic carcinoma.

TNM PRE-TREATMENT CLINICAL CLASSIFICATION

T – *Primary tumour*

T_{is} Pre-invasive carcinoma (carcinoma *in situ*)

T_0 No evidence of primary tumour

T_1 Tumour limited to the mucosa *or* mucosa and sub-mucosa

T_2 Tumour with extension to muscle *or* muscle and serosa

T_3 Tumour with extension beyond colon to immediately contiguous structure

T_{3a} Tumour without fistula formation
T_{3b} Tumour with fistula formation

T_4 Tumour extending beyond the immediately adjacent organs or tissues

T_x The minimum requirements to assess the primary tumour cannot be met

N – *Regional and juxtaregional lymph nodes*

N_0 No evidence of regional lymph node involvement

N_1 Evidence of involvement of regional lymph nodes

Note: The categories N_2 and N_3 are not applicable

N_4 Evidence of involvement of juxtaregional lymph nodes

N_x The minimum requirements to assess the regional *and/or* juxtaregional lymph nodes cannot be met

M – *Distant metastases*

M_0 No evidence of distant metastases

M_1 Evidence of distant metastases

M_x The minimum requirements to assess the presence of distant metastases cannot be met

p.TNM POST-SURGICAL HISTOPATHOLOGICAL CLASSIFICATION

pT – *Primary tumour*

The pT categories correspond to the T categories

G – *Histopathological grading*

G_1 High degree of differentiation

G_2 Medium degree of differentiation

G_3 Low degree of differentation *or* undifferentiated

G_x Grade cannot be assessed

pN – *Regional and juxtaregional lymph nodes*

The pN categories correspond to the N categories

pM – *Distant metastases*

The pM categories correspond to the M categories

STAGE GROUPING

Stage Ia	T_1	N_0	M_0
Stage Ib	T_2	N_0	M_0
Stage II	T_3, T_4	N_0	M_0
Stage III	Any T	N_1	M_0
Stage IV	Any T	N_4	M_0
	Any T	Any N	M_1

SUMMARY

Colon

T_1/pT_1	Mucosa or sub-mucosa only
T_2/pT_2	Muscle or serosa
T_{3a}/pT_{3a}	Extension to contiguous structures No fistula
T_{3b}/pT_{3b}	With fistula
T_4/pT_4	Extension beyond contiguous structures
N_1	Regional
N_4	Juxtaregional

Treatment

At the present time the most effective method of treatment is the surgical removal of the lesion. Other modalities do have parts to play and these will be defined later. Each method of treatment will be described in turn, followed by a discussion of the integration of these methods of treatment.

Surgery

Surgical treatment has been the mainstay of management for the patient with colorectal carcinoma. Since 1908 when Miles first described the abdominoperineal resection a variety of operative procedures have been used, and the principles behind such operations defined.

1. *Selection of patients*. With improved surgical and anaesthetic techniques most patients can now have a laparotomy to define the extent of the tumour spread. Clearly, however, those patients who present with very

Table 19.4   TNM classification for rectal carcinoma.

TNM PRE-TREATMENT CLINICAL CLASSIFICATION

T –	*Primary tumour*
T_{is}	Pre-invasive carcinoma (carcinoma *in situ*)
T_0	No evidence of primary tumour
T_1	Tumour limited to the mucosa *or* mucosa and sub-mucosa
T_2	Tumour with extension to muscle *or* muscle and serosa
T_3	Tumour with extension beyond colon to immediately contiguous structure

T_{3a} Tumour without fistula formation
T_{3b} Tumour with fistula formation

T_4	Tumour extending beyond the immediately adjacent organs or tissues
T_x	The minimum requirements to assess the primary tumour cannot be met
N –	*Regional and juxtaregional lymph nodes*
N_0	No evidence of regional lymph node involvement
N_1	Evidence of involvement of regional lymph nodes

Note: The categories N_2 and N_3 are not applicable

N_4	Evidence of involvement of juxtaregional lymph nodes

N_x	The minimum requirements to assess the regional *and/or* juxtaregional lymph nodes cannot be met
M –	*Distant metastases*
M_0	No evidence of distant metastases
M_1	Evidence of distant metastases
M_x	The minimum requirements to assess the presence of distant metastases cannot be met

p.TNM POST-SURGICAL HISTOPATHOLOGICAL CLASSIFICATION

pT –	*Primary tumour*
	The pT categories correspond to the T categories
G –	*Histopathological grading*
G_1	High degree of differentiation
G_2	Medium degree of differentiation
G_3	Low degree of differentation *or* undifferentiated
G_x	Grade cannot be assessed
pN –	*Regional and juxtaregional lymph nodes*
	The pN categories correspond to the N categories
pM –	*Distant metastases*
	The pM categories correspond to the M categories

STAGE GROUPING

Stage Ia	T_1	N_0	M_0
Stage Ib	T_2	N_0	M_0
Stage II	T_3, T_4	N_0	M_0
Stage III	Any T	N_1	M_0
Stage IV	Any T	N_4	M_0
	Any T	Any N	M_1

SUMMARY

Rectum

T_1/pT_1	Mucosa or sub-mucosa only
T_2/pT_2	Muscle or serosa
T_{3a}/pT_{3a}	Extension to contiguous structures No fistula
T_{3b}/pT_{3b}	With fistula
T_4/pT_4	Extension beyond contiguous structures
N_1	Regional
N_4	Juxtaregional

advanced disease may not require a major procedure. Age itself is no barrier to operation.

2. *Pre-operative preparation*. The nutritional status of the patient should be evaluated and pre-operative nutritional support, blood and intravenous fluids given as required. Adequate bowel preparation is essential and many methods are available to accomplish this.

3. *The extent of the resection*. Depending on the site of the lesion a wide margin of normal bowel with adjacent lymph nodes taken to the root of the mesentery is excised. In most large series recurrence at the site of the primary tumour occurs and can be reduced by adequate primary excision. With rectal lesions the site of the lesion will be the most important factor in dictating the operative procedure performed. With low-lying lesion an abdominoperineal resection is preferred.

4. *Sphincter-sparing operations*. For low rectal lesions a rectal anastomasis may be performed, without excision of the anal sphincter. This procedure is open to the objection that insufficient tissue on either side of the lesion has been removed. Small rectal lesions may be approached via the perineum and removed without interfering with the sphincter.

5. *Ligation of colonic vessels*. Considerable attention has been focused on the value (or otherwise) of early ligation of colonic vessels. Initial reports (Turnbull *et al.*, 1967) suggested that this was associated with an improved survival rate. Such a technique was based on the assumption that handling the tumour would result in an increase of blood-borne cells with a consequent increase in metastases. Griffiths *et al.* (1967) did indeed show that there was an increase in cells in the venous blood following resection but that there was no increase in metastases. The work of Turnbull has been challenged and may be explained on the basis of extended tumour resection (Block and Enker, 1978).

6. *Colostomy*. Where continuity of the gastrointestinal tract cannot be restored, even on a temporary basis, a colostomy will be required. A wide variety of surgical procedures have been used and the reader is referred to standard surgical texts for details of the techniques involved. The presence of a colostomy, however, has important physical and psychological effect. Attention to the construction and siting of the colostomy has improved the quality of life of patients. Newer appliances have made rehabilitation much easier and faster. The development of stoma therapists and patient organizations has done a great deal to improve the lot of the patient. The psychological effects, however, are still underestimated. Impotence, for example, (related to the operation or to the colostomy) is a serious problem. These effects can only be overcome by a sympathetic understanding of the patient, his home and his family.

Indications for surgical procedures

1. *Primary surgical treatment*. The techniques and philosophy of treatment have been described above. *En bloc* resection of the tumour and adjacent lymph nodes is the treatment of choice.

2. *Emergency surgical treatment*. A percentage of patients will present primarily to the surgeon as an emergency. The operative procedure carried out will depend not only on the site of the lesion, but the condition of the patient, the extent of contamination of the operative field or degree of obstruction, and the experience of the surgeon. Thus with a small lesion with only local perforation involving a mobile area of the sigmoid colon a one-stage resection may be performed in experienced hands. Where the patient is unwell and the procedure potentially very hazardous, a defunctioning colostomy may be performed and resection delayed until the patient is improved.

3. *Treatment of recurrence*. Where a local recurrence has been demonstrated or suspected, laparotomy may be useful in that the lesion may be resectable. Where a solitary liver metastasis has been demonstrated, partial hepatectomy may be indicated. Surgical techniques may also be required for the insertion of a catheter into the hepatic artery or umbilical vein prior to infusion.

4. *Second look operation*. This procedure is carried out where the patient is suspected of being free from the disease. It is used to assess the effects of therapy, and to restage the patient. The 'second look' operation may be of great value in a selected group of patients.

Post-operative problems. Wound healing and infection are the major early post-operative problems. They are important in that they may delay the use of other modalities of therapy. The long-term problems are similar to those of other major abdominal operations. The presence of a colostomy has, however, other long-term implications for the patient some of which have been discussed above.

Radiotherapy

In the early years of the century radiotherapy was widely used in the treatment of rectal cancer. However, because the techniques available were poor and associated with significant morbidity the use of radiotherapy fell into disrepute. Coincidentally, the operative procedures improved and there seemed to be little use for radiotherapy in rectal cancer.

In the last few years there has been an important reappraisal of the role of radiotherapy in the treatment of rectal cancer with the development of newer techniques. It would be fair to say now that radiotherapy has an important part to play in the management of rectal cancer and that lack of awareness of its value has been its major stumbling block (Priestman, 1977).

Pre-operative radiotherapy. Initially this was used to convert an inoperable lesion into an operable one. While this may still be an important objective, the scope has widened and radiotherapy has been used as an adjunct to surgery in operable lesions. The initial studies were performed in the United States and a large series (Stearns *et al.*, 1959) indicated that both the 5- and 10-year survival rates could be improved. On the basis of these results, several prospective studies were initiated. The Veteran Administration Study (Roswit *et al.*, 1973) showed a decrease in lymph node involvement after surgery, and a significant improvement in the 5-year survival rate (40.4% vs 27.5%) in the treated group over the controls in those patients having abdominoperineal resection. Several other studies are now under way in an attempt to confirm these findings.

Post-operative radiotherapy. Because of the delay in healing following abdominoperineal resections (often taking over two months), post-operative radiotherapy has been found to be of little use in the immediate post-operative period.

Intracavitary radiation. This technique, which has been popularized on the Continent of Europe, is of considerable interest in the management of rectal cancer. Initially the technique was used in the treatment of inoperable lesions or in patients who were unfit for surgery. More recently it has been used in the treatment of well localized tumours (Papillon, 1975). Using a 50 kV machine which gives a circular radiation beam with limited penetration, 78% 5-year survival rates have been reported. It is recommended that following this, an iridium wire implant is inserted following contact therapy. There are obvious advantages of this technique over abdominoperineal resection and the risk of infection, perforation and haemorrhage are small.

Palliative radiotherapy. Radiotherapy may be particularly helpful in the management of local problems following surgery. The pain associated with perineal recurrence can often be very well controlled, as can haemorrhage and rectal discharge. Bone pain associated with spread may also respond well to radiotherapy. The use of radiosensitizers and neutron therapy may well improve these results.

When hepatic metastases are a problem because of pain, good palliation may be achieved by treating the whole liver to a dose of 4500 rad in 4.5 weeks by supervoltage therapy (Stearns and Leaming, 1975). This may be considered to be an excessive dose, and half this dose in 2 weeks may be sufficient for symptom relief.

Chemotherapy

Extensive studies have been conducted on the use of single drugs in the treatment of large bowel cancer. Most of the currently available cytotoxic drugs have been assessed, though not all of these have been used at optimal doses or schedules.

As with gastric cancer the most commonly used drug is 5-FU. This has been used in many dose schedules and routes (Table 19.5). On average a 20% response rate has been achieved. Toxicity is mild and mainly gastrointestinal. The response rate varies according to the site of the metastases, abdominal secondaries responding reasonably well while lung metastases respond poorly (Gerard, 1975).

Mitomycin C has been reasonably well evaluated though it does not appear to be as useful as 5-FU. A number of other drugs including cyclophosphamide, methotrexate, the nitrosoureas, hexamethylmelamine and DTIC (dacarbazone) have all been used with variable degrees of success. Most other agents appear to have little value though some require re-evaluation in the light of more recent pharmacological information.

The use of intra-arterial perfusion of the liver in patients with colon cancer has been assessed on many occasions (Taylor, 1978). While drugs levels are undoubtedly higher, there seems to be no real advantage in this route of administration in patients with advanced disease. The technique has also been used after surgery and initial results are of some interest though they require confirmation (Taylor *et al.*, 1977).

Of the drugs more recently available Iphosphamide may have some activity, though cis-platinum, in initial studies, seems to be an inactive agent.

Combination chemotherapy. A very large number of two and three drug combinations has been assessed (Carter and Friedman, 1974). Most of these have involved the use of 5-FU with other drugs. A combina-

Table 19.5 The use of 5-fluorouracil in the treatment of large bowel cancers (Carter and Friedman, 1974).

	Response rate (%)
Intravenous, standard loading dose	19
Intravenous, standard loading dose then weekly maintenance	39
Intravenous, weekly	21
Modified standard loading dose	30
8–24 infusions	17
Oral	19
Overall	21

tion which appeared more active than single agents was 5-FU, methyl-CCNU and vincristine. In subsequent studies, however, this combination was found to be ineffective; and had greater toxicity. It must be stated therefore that considerable efforts are still required to develop an active combination of drugs for colorectal cancer.

Adjuvant chemotherapy
Once again a large number of studies employing single agents and combinations of drugs in the treatment of colorectal cancer following surgery have been performed. In general the results have been disappointing with no real benefit in terms of survival or extension of disease-free interval. A more recent study (Taylor *et al.*, 1977) using immediate post-operative intra-arterial perfusion of the liver, has shown some benefit, though these results require confirmation. At the present time, therefore, adjuvant chemotherapy in the treatment of carcinoma of the colon must still be considered as a trial procedure and much more information is required regarding its value.

There are theoretical advantages in the use of 5-FU as a radiosensitizer, together with radiotherapy in the management of this disease. Although several studies have been performed (Moertel *et al.*, 1969; Henderson *et al.*, 1968), there has been no real benefit. One retrospective study (Vongtama *et al.*, 1975) did show some benefit, though this remains to be confirmed.

Immunotherapy
Several studies using BCG, *Corynebacterium parvum* or levamisole either alone or in combination with chemotherapy have been made (Calman, 1975). In some of these (Mavligit *et al.*, 1976) initial benefit was shown though this has not been fully substantiated. Until further trials are available, this must also remain an experimental procedure.

Results of treatment
In the treatment of colorectal cancer the results of treatment depend most on the stage of the lesion and on the extent of the surgical procedure. Radiotherapy has a great deal to offer in the management of rectal cancer, both in early disease and for palliation. The role of chemotherapy still remains to be defined.

Further Reading

Carter, S.K. and Comis, R.L. (1977), Gastric cancer: Current status of treatment. *J. Natn. Cancer Inst.*, **58**, 567-78.
En, W.E. (ed.) (1978), Cancer of the Colon and Rectum. Year Book Medical Publishers.
Everson, T.C. and Cole, W.H. (1969), Cancer of the

gastrointestinal tract. Butterworths, London.
Gerard, A. (ed.) (1978), *Gastrointestinal Tumours*. A Clinical and Experimental Approach. Pergamon Press.
Lipkin, M. and Good, R.A. (eds) (1978), *Gastrointestinal Tract Cancer*. Plenum Medical Book Co.
McConnell, R.B. (1978), Epidemiology of gastrointestinal tumours: a review. *J. R. Soc. Med.*, **71**, 278-81.
Morson, B.C. (ed.) (1978), The Pathogenesis of Colorectal Cancer. W.B. Saunders.

References

Block, G.E. and Enker, W.E. (1978), Controversies in large bowel cancer. In: *Carcinoma of the Colon and Rectum*. (ed. W.E. Enker) Year Book Medical Publishers.
Calman, K.C. (1974), Why are small bowel tumours rare? *Gut*, **15**, 552-4.
Calman, K.C. (1975), Tumour immunology and the gut. *Gut*, **16**, 490-9.
Carter, S.K. and Friedman, M. (1974), Integration of chemotherapy into combined modality therapy of solid tumours. II. Large bowel carcinoma. *Cancer Treat. Rev.*, **1**, 111-30.
Comis, R.L. and Carter, S.K. (1974), Gastric cancer. *Cancer Treat. Rev.*, **1**, 221-8.
Ellis, D.J. *et al.* (1979), Gastric carcinoma and previous peptic ulceration. *Br. J. Surg.*, **66**, 117-9.
Evans, D.M.D. *et al.* (1978), Comparison of 'early gastric cancer' in Britain and Japan. *Gut*, **19**, 1-9.
Fox, R.M. *et al.* (1979), Allopurinol modulation of high dose fluorouracil toxity. *Lancet*, **i**, 677.
Gerard, A. (1975), Carcinoma of the colon and rectum: Prognostic facors and criteria of response. In: *Cancer Therapy. Prognostic Factors and Criteria of Response*. (ed. M. Staquet), Raven Press, New York., pp. 199-227.
Gillespie, P.E. *et al.* (1979), Colonic adenomas and colonoscopic survey. *Gut*, 240-5.
Griffiths, J.D. (1973), Carcinoma of the colon and rectum: Circulating malignant cells and five-year survival. *Cancer*, **31**, 226-310.
Henderson, I.W.D., Lipowska, B. and Lougheed, M.N. (1968), Clinical evaluation of combined radiation and chemotherapy, in gastrointestinal malignancies. *Am. J. Roentg.*, **102**, 545-57.
Hill, M.J. *et al.* (1975), Faecal bile acids and clostridia in patients with cancer of the large bowel. *Lancet*, **i**, 535-9.
Hill, M.J., Morson, B.C. and Bussey, H.J. (1978), Aetiology of adenoma – carcinoma sequence in large bowel cancer. *Lancet*, **i**, 245-7.
Holyoke, E.D., Chu, T.M. and Murphy, C.P. (1975),

CEA as a monitor of gastrointestinal malignancy. *Cancer*, **35**, 830-6.

Kingsley, D., Gad, A. and Catterall, M. (1976), Adenocarcinoma of the stomach: radiological and pathological correlation of effects of treatment with fast neutrons. *Gut*, **17**, 624-32.

Mavligit, G.M. *et al.* (1976), Prolongation of post-operative disease free interval and survival in human colorectal cancer by BCG or BCG plus 5-fluorouracil. *Lancet*, **i**, 871-6.

Moertel, C.G. *et al.* (1969), Combined 5-fluorouracil and supervoltage radiation therapy of locally unresectable gastrointestinal cancer. *Lancet*, **ii**, 865-7.

Papillon, J. (1975), Intracavity irradiation of early rectal cancer for cure. *Cancer*, **36**, 696-701.

Priestman, T.J. (1977), The place of radiotherapy in the management of rectal adenocarcinoma. *Cancer Treat. Rev.*, **4**, 1-12.

Roswit, B. *et al.* (1973), Preoperative irradiation of operable adenocarcinoma of the rectum and rectosigmoid : Report of a randomised study. *Radiology*, **108**, 389-95.

Southam, J.A. (1974), Primary tumours of the small intestine. *Ann. Coll. Surg.*, **55**, 129-33.

Stearns, M.W. and Leaming, R.H. (1975), Radiation in in-operable cancer. *J. Am. Med. Assoc.*, **231**, 1388.

Stearns, M.W., Deddish, M.R. and Quan, S.H.Q. (1959), Pre-operative roentgen therapy for cancer of the rectum. *Surg. Gynec. Obstet.*, **109**, 225-31.

Stock, F.E. (1963), Carcinoma of the stomach in young patients. *Lancet*, **i**, 805-6.

Taylor, I. (1978), Cytotoxic perfusion for colorectal liver metastases. *Br. J. Surg.*, **65**, 109-14.

Taylor, I., Brooman, P. and Rowling, J.T. (1977), Adjuvant liver perfusion in colorectal cancer : Initial results of a clinical trial. *Br. Med. J.*, **2**, 1320-1.

Turnbull, R.B. *et al.* (1967), Cancer of the colon : influence of no-touch technique on survival rates. *Ann. Surg.*, **166**, 420-5.

Vongtama, V. *et al.* (1975), End results of radiation therapy, alone and combination with 5-fluorouracil in colorectal cancer. *Cancer*, **36**, 2020-5.

World Health Statistics Annual, 1971 (1974), WHO, Geneva.

Wynder, E. and Reddy, D. (1973), Studies of large bowel cancer human leads to experimental application. *J. Natl. Cancer Inst.*, **50**, 1099-1106.

20 Exocrine pancreas and biliary tract

Christopher Mallinson
and John Hermon-Taylor

Incidence and epidemiology

Pancreatic exocrine adenocarcinoma kills 6000 people a year in the UK and 20 000 in the USA where it is the fourth commonest cause of cancer death after cancers of the bronchus, colon and breast. The disease has increased in frequency throughout the century in industrialized countries and shows a marked urban distribution (Krain, 1970). In 1976 in England and Wales, 17.6% more men and 27.5% more women died of the disease than in 1964; in 1969 in the US and 1975 in the UK a plateau appeared for men but not for women among whom the incidence throughout the world has begun to catch up that for men. The frequency increases with age and cohort analysis suggests the presence of environmental aetiological factors (Bernarde and Weiss, 1977) of which the only ones identified so far are cigarette smoking and working in the rubber industry. Within countries the incidence may show geographical variation but parallel differences between men and women: for example in central and southern Britain the male incidence is 104 per million per year and in southern Scotland 128. The highest global incidence is seen in male Hawaiians (314 per million), in Maoris (266) and Detroit blacks (250). The disease is least common in Spain, Bombay and Thailand (Waterhouse et al., 1976).

Cancer of the bile ducts is also increasing but gall bladder cancer is decreasing. In the USA where the two are distinguished in the mortality statistics, gall bladder cancer is twice as common in females as males and, in the different ethnic groups runs parallel but of course not equal to the incidence of gallstones. Biliary tract cancer is slightly commoner among men and appears related to exposure to benzidine, infestation with *Clonorchis sinensis* and is ten times more common in patients with ulcerative colitis.

Anatomy

The anatomy of the pancreas and biliary tract is well known and only a few points need emphasizing in the context of pancreatic cancer.

The pancreas from head to tail is closely related to most of the structures in the upper abdomen. The kidneys and the hollow viscera are highly radiosensitive and limit the dose of radiotherapy which can be administered. The relationship of the body of the pancreas to the coeliac axis and the neck of the gland to the portal and superior mesenteric veins are important determinants in the resectability of pancreatic tumours. The variable arterial blood supply to the pancreas may be an indication for selection angiography prior to pancreatic surgery.

The rich supply of intralobular lymphatics communicating freely with the peripancreatic channels leading to the five groups of local lymph nodes (Fig. 20.1) are an important consideration in the spread of pancreatic cancer. A useful surgical point is that the middle colic vein usually enters the front of the superior mesenteric vein; thereafter the left and anterior surfaces of the portal vein are free of tributaries.

Pathology

The site of origin of exocrine pancreatic cancers is shown in Table 20.1. The distinction between periampullary cancer, cancer of the head and cancer of the body of the pancreas has great bearing on the treatment and its outcome. As shown in Table 20.2 the majority of pancreatic exocrine cancers arise from duct cells. They show a differentiation into glandular structures and the cells contain mucin. In ampullary lesions in particular, papillary structures are frequent. Fibrous reaction is often intense. Pancreatitis around the tumour may increase its apparent volume; it is due to duct obstruction as well as trypsinogen activation by tumour cell proteases (Grant et al., 1978). Tumour proteases which act on the blood coagulation system may also contribute to the local or disseminated venous throm-

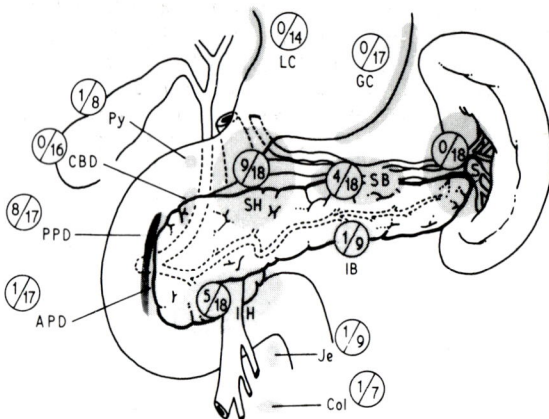

Fig. 20.1 Distribution of lymph nodes draining the pancreas. SH = superior head; SB = superior body; IH = inferior head; IB = inferior body; APD = anterior pancreaticoduodenal; PPD = posterior pancreaticoduodenal; CBD = common bile duct; Py = pyloric; LC = lesser curve; GC = greater curve; S = tail of pancreas and splenic; Je = jejunal; Col = mid colic. Numerator of the fraction on each group represents the number of patients with metastases in the group. Denominator indicates the number of groups examined in 18 regional resection specimens (from Cubilla *et al.*, 1978).

Table 20.2   Histological classification of 406 primary non-endocrine tumours of the pancreas (Cubilla and Fitzgerald, 1975).

	%
Duct cell adenocarcinoma	76
giant cell carcinoma	5
microadenocarcinoma	4
adenosquamous carcinoma	4
mucinous adenocarcinoma	2
anaplastic carcinoma	2
Acinar cell carcinoma	1
Cystadenocarcinoma	1
Carcinoma in childhood	<1
Unclassified	7

bosis which is found in a third of cases.

Two thirds of patients fall into the two higher grades of malignancy in Broders' classification of cell differentiation (Carter and Comis, 1975). In these grades the primary tumour is commonly larger than in the lower grades and is associated with more widespread metastases and venous thrombosis. Cubilla and Fitzgerald (1975) found that in half of their surgically resected specimens marked atypia or carcinoma in-situ of the duct epithelium was present at a distance from the primary tumour. Such changes were not found at autopsy in age and sex matched controls dying of non-pancreatic cancer. Metastatic permeation along perineural lymphatics is particularly characteristic and is associated with a circumferential fibrotic response.

Rare sub-types of pancreatic cancer are those arising from digestive enzyme-synthesizing acinar cells, which liberate secretory enzymes into the circulation, and cystadenocarcinoma which may grow to a large size, are usually well differentiated, and carry a relatively good prognosis.

Hermreck et al. (1974) have proposed the following

Table 20.1   Site of origin of non-endocrine tumours of the pancreas in three large series.

Author	Number of cases	Ampulla	% Head region Terminal CBD	Pancreas	% Body and tail
Hertzberg, 1974 (Norway)	303	7.6	3.4	64	25
Webster, 1975 (Wales)	100	4.0	4.0	75	17
Nakase *et al.*, 1977 (Japan)	3206*	14.3	9.7	57	19

* Carcinoma of the duodenum and of the entire pancreas excluded.

staging scheme:

I   Local disease.
II Invasion of surrounding tissues.
III Local lymph node metastases.
IV Widespread metastases, mainly to liver, peritoneum and lungs.

Lymphatic spread is almost invariably found in resected specimens from pancreatic cancer and the frequency with which different groups are involved with tumours at different sites is described in detail by Cubilla *et al.* (1978).

The common form of bile duct cancer is a scirrhous adenocarcinoma spreading intramurally and obstructing the lumen; it may be difficult to distinguish from sclerosing cholangitis. Polypoid forms occur and may be associated with haemobilia, probably aggravated by the hypoprothrombinaemia secondary to obstructive jaundice. Lymphatic spread occurs later than biliary obstruction which, together with secondary liver failure, is the common cause of death from tumours which cannot be bypassed. Cancer of the gall bladder is most commonly diagnosed by accident in specimens resected for gallstones when it is usually well localized: tumours presenting otherwise have usually undergone widespread metastasis.

Clinical presentation and course

The earliest symptoms of cancer of the exocrine pancreas in any site are abdominal pain, weight loss and nausea. Constipation and mental changes are found in one to two thirds of patients and jaundice is the first symptom in only one fifth of patients with carcinoma of the head of the gland. During the two to four months which elapse before investigation the picture changes to one of obstructive jaundice with a dilated biliary tree and gall bladder in patients with cancers in the head of the pancreas or progressive pain with a malignant hepatomegaly, an abdominal mass and often an arterial bruit over the gland in patients with carcinoma of the body. Bile duct cancers present almost invariably with obstructive jaundice which may be fluctuant at first. The majority of gall bladder cancers are discovered accidentally at cholecystectomy for gallstones, the remainder present with pain, a mass or malignant hepatomegaly.

The median survival of pancreatic and biliary tract cancers associated with certain prognostic variables is shown in Table 20.3. Data for pancreatic cancer is abbreviated from that cited by Carter and Comis (1975) and since it was acquired retrospectively in a non-randomized fashion it may be misleading. No attempt has yet been made to assess the comparative weight of these variables when found in combination.

Table 20.3 Prognostic factors in pancreatic adeno-carcinoma (modified from Carter and Comis, 1975).

Prognostic variable	Median survival (months)
Site of primary tumour	
Head	4.0
Body	3.0
Tail	2.5
Grade of malignancy (Broders)	
I and II	5.5
III and IV	3.0
Extent	
Regional	6.0
Distant (within abdomen)	3.0
Hepatic	2.5
Extra-abdominal	2.0
Surgical treatment	
None	2.0
Bypass	4.5
Radical resection	15
Chemotherapy	
South East England Regime (SEER)	11
Streptozotocin/Mitomycin-C/5-FU (SMF) (responders)	8
Chemotherapy and radiotherapy	
Dobelbower *et al.* (1978)	13
Moertel *et al.* (1976b)	8

Two reports of the influence of age and sex on survival have produced contradictory conclusions. The course of pancreatic cancer depends upon whether an adequate radical resection can be performed, in which patients the five-year survival is 10%, while survival in bile duct cancer depends upon whether the obstruction can be bypassed or cannulated (Welton *et al.*, 1969). With gall bladder cancer the length of survival depends on whether the tumour was found by accident at cholecystectomy or not (Nevin *et al.*, 1976).

Diagnosis

A complete pre-operative anatomical and histological diagnosis can now be made in the majority of patients within two days. Even this improvement in expertise cannot be expected to raise the overall five-year survival of 1% to more than 2%. Quicker referral of patients complaining of the earlier symptoms would help, but a great improvement in survival figures awaits the development of a satisfactory screening method for asymptomatic patients. Such a programme is not yet feasible since high risk groups have not been identified

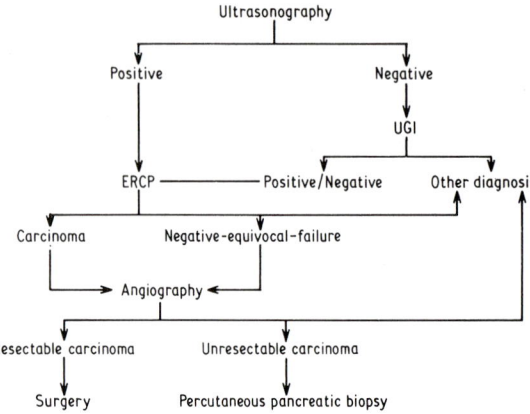

Fig. 20.2 Scheme for investigation of a patient suspected of pancreatic disease in a unit where ERCP is preferred over transhepatic cholangiography. In many units the latter would be carried out before ERCP in jaundiced patients (Freeny and Ball, 1978).

in the public at large (outside Hawaii, New Zealand, Detroit and the rubber industry) and no reliable screening test has yet appeared. Several candidate tests have been explored among symptomatic patients but the most promising markers of pancreatic oncofoetal antigen, carcinoembryonic antigen and ribonuclease, have not proved either sufficiently specific or reliable (Gelder *et al.*, 1978; Mackie *et al.*, 1979).

The symptomatic patient

A systematic approach to diagnosis suggested by Freeny and Ball (1978) is outlined in Fig. 20.2. Ultrasound (U/S) or computerized axial tomography (CAT-scan) are both useful in detecting and localizing mass lesions: they discriminate accurately between medical and surgical jaundice and between malignant and benign surgical jaundice (Lees *et al.*, 1979). Endoscopic retrograde cholangiopancreatography (ERCP) is preferred over percutaneous transhepatic cholangiography (PTC) or transjugular cholangiography (TJC) as the second step in diagnosis for the U/S-positive patient since it can demonstrate lesions in the pancreatic ducts as well as the bile ducts. However, in the jaundiced patient PTC or TJC are highly informative and are generally more widely available than ERCP. Laparoscopy has been found to be a useful adjunct to diagnosis in several units.

Percutaneous fine-needle biopsy can be carried out at laparoscopy or under guidance of U/S or CAT-scan shown in Fig. 20.3. This is safe and, in experienced hands, gives 80–95% diagnostic accuracy (Smith *et al.*, 1975). The place of angiography is usually in detecting the involvement of major blood vessels and in the demonstration of the vascular anatomy prior to surgery (Tylen and Arnesjo, 1973). To be able to confirm the histology of a pancreatic tumour without laparotomy in elderly and unfit patients can be extremely useful: in the unjaundiced patient the decision for or against palliative treatment can be taken without further intervention. In selected patients with obstructive jaundice both pruritis and jaundice can be relieved without a laparotomy by inserting an endoprosthesis through the obstruction at PTC as shown in Fig. 20.4.

Duodenal intubation is useful in a number of centres but the accuracy much depends on the extent of local skills. Isotope scanning is of very limited value in relation to other diagnostic methods.

Operative diagnosis

In spite of diagnostic advances patients still come to laparotomy undiagnosed. The problem is then the histological nature of a solitary mass in the head of the gland; it should be biopsied by fine-needle aspiration and submitted to frozen section (Shorey, 1975). However, a clinical decision may still have to be made as to whether to resect a lesion which is not confirmed as malignant. A useful clinical sign of malignancy in such patients is the finding of a widely dilated, thin walled common bile duct.

Treatment

Pancreatic cancer is the most difficult of all the common solid abdominal malignancies to treat. Optimal

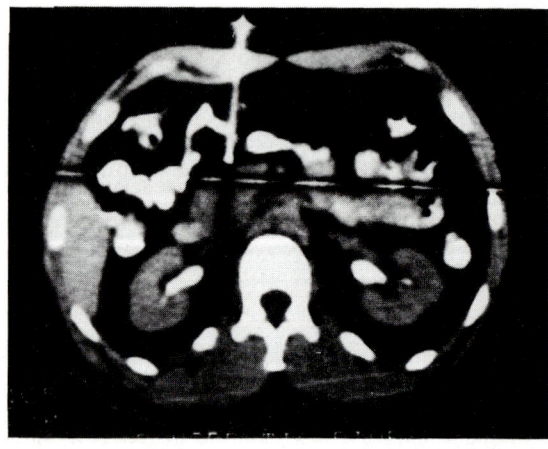

Fig. 20.3 Percutaneous needle biopsy of a pancreatic tumour under CAT-scan control (by kind permission of Dr Afsel Riaz).

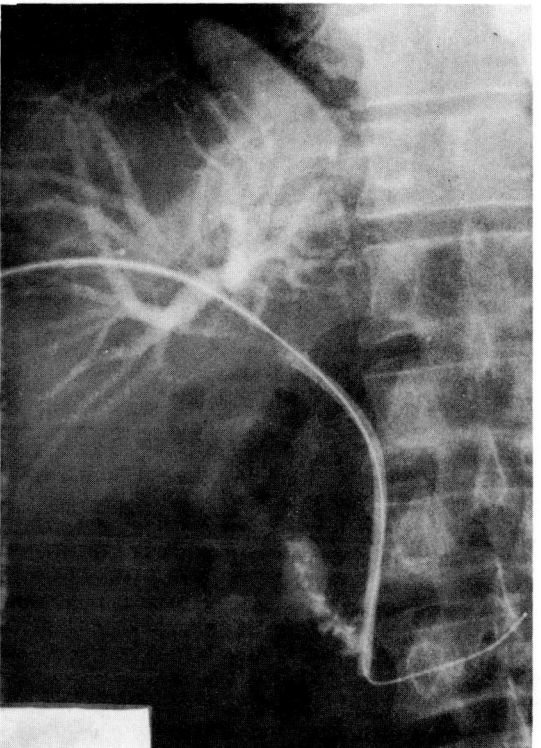

Fig. 20.4 An endoprosthesis has been installed in the lower end of the common bile duct through an obstructing carcinoma. The prosthesis was pushed over the guide wire which is still in position. The latter is removed leaving the prosthesis to drain into the duodenum. Contrast medium is seen passing from the dilated intrahepatic bile ducts into the duodenum (by kind permission of Dr Duncan Irving).

Table 20.4 Outlines of surgical procedures discussed in text.

Proximal pancreaticoduodenectomy
Removal of the distal 2/3 of the stomach, duodenum and upper few cm of jejunum together with the uncinate process head and neck of the pancreas, pancreatic, retroduodenal and part of supra-duodenal common bile duct and including the superior and inferior head and anterior and posterior lymph nodes with adjacent soft tissue. The pancreas is divided to the left of the portal vein.

Distal pancreatectomy
Removal of the spleen, tail and body of the pancreas which is divided to the right of the portal vein. Includes the splenic, superior and inferior body lymph nodes and associated connective tissue and if necessary includes the left adrenal, kidney capsule, left mesocolon and a segment of transverse colon or hepatic flexure.

Regional (total) pancreatectomy
Removal of the distal 2/3 of the stomach, duodenum and upper few cm of jejunum together with the whole pancreas and spleen, common bile duct and gall bladder and all associated lymph nodes. Includes the transverse meso-colon and middle colic vessels, the blood supply to the transverse colon coming from the anastomotic arcade between the ileo-colic and inferior mesenteric. Portal vein is also resected if this is involved, with end-to-end anastomosis of superior mesenteric and portal veins.

Bypass
Palliative operation to relieve obstruction of the common bile duct by anastomosis of the proximal dilated biliary tree to the small intestine. Best performed as gall bladder or hepatic duct, to Roux loop of jejunum brought up through transverse mesocolon, but may be gall bladder to duodenum. Prophylactic gastroenterostomy because of the frequency of subsequent duodenal obstruction by infiltrating tumour.

management involves the combined and collaborative application of resection with multiple chemotherapy and radiotherapy. To date, there is all too little experience with such combined regimes largely due to high operative mortality and low surgical resection rate.

Palliative chemotherapy and radiotherapy have had some success in improving pain and, more recently, in prolonging useful life.

Surgical aspects of the treatment of non-endocrine pancreatic and peri-ampullary cancers (Table 20.4)

There are several alternative surgical policies: laparotomy and biopsy alone, bypass of biliary and duodenal obstructions, drainage of an obstructed pancreatic duct, partial pancreatectomy or total and regional pancreatectomy. The essence of the debate about which to choose for an individual patient, is the necessity of balancing the chance of premature loss of life due to operative mortality, with the low cure rate so far achieved with pancreatic ductal cancers after apparently successful resection. At present the information available about survival after various surgical procedures is largely that which follows resection as the only form of treatment. This section sets out a surgical policy which recognizes the desirability and necessity of combining resection with effective chemotherapy and radiotherapy as a means of extending survival and improving its quality. It also recognizes that research

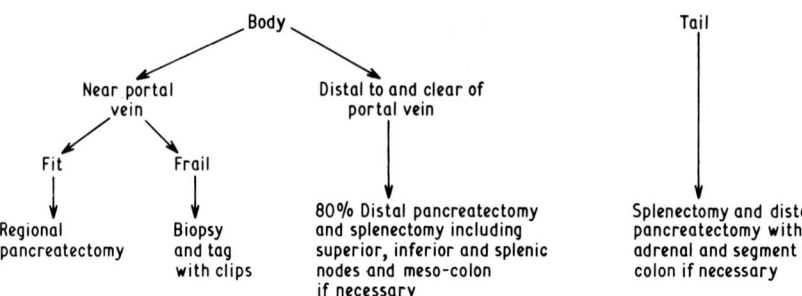

Fig. 20.5 Guidelines for the surgical treatment of non-endocrine tumours of the body and tail of the pancreas.

into the causes and prevention of surgical death after these operations together with increased specialization in the field are likely to be followed by a continued reduction in operative mortality.

Pancreatic exocrine cancers should be resected whenever possible, in a single procedure. There are three types of operation according to whether the pancreatic tissue removed is the head and neck, the body and tail, or the whole organ. The operations are called proximal pancreaticoduodenectomy (Whipple's procedure), distal pancreatectomy and regional pancreatectomy, respectively. The latter includes total pancreatectomy and is documented principally by Pliam and ReMine (1975), Ihse *et al.* (1977) and Fortner *et al.* (1977). Details of these procedures are given in Table 20.4 and guidelines to surgical policy shown diagrammatically in Figs. 20.5 and 20.6.

Tumours of the body and tail
Lesions of the tail should be removed by distal pancreatectomy (Fig. 20.5). After division of the gastrocolic omentum, the peritoneum is incised lateral to the spleen and the spleen and pancreas mobilized to the right; adjacent lymph nodes with or without the mesocolon are taken and the pancreas is divided at the portal vein. If the adrenal is involved this is removed; if the left transverse colon is infiltrated a segment is excised. The operation is straightforward and should have a mortality of under 3%.

Surgical management of cancers of the body depends upon the size of the tumour, its relation to the portal vein and the age and condition of the patient. Too often cancers of the body are not removed because the surgeon feels that it is fixed and infiltrating the aorta. In fact this is rarely the case and it is usually feasible to separate even large lesions from the aorta. The removal of a substantial tumour mass in this way is often followed by dramatic relief of severe pain and provides chemotherapy and radiotherapy with a better

chance of success. If there is sufficient macroscopically uninvolved pancreatic tissue between the tumour and the portal vein (2–3 cm) then distal pancreatectomy should be carried out, removing adjacent soft tissue as described above but dividing the pancreas as far to the right of the portal vein as possible. This ignores the probability that in approximately 18% of cases there will be multifocal carcinoma in-situ in the major duct system of the remaining pancreas as well as the possibility of tumour cells at the resection line. However, it avoids the greater mortality of total or regional pancreatectomy which is the only other practical alternative to leaving the tumour in place. If the tumour mass is close to the portal vein and the patient is reasonably fit a regional pancreatectomy should be performed, taking a segment of portal vein if necessary. If the general condition of the patient is poor, a biopsy and insertion of markers for post-operative radiotherapy should be carried out.

Tumours in the region of the head
The more controversial subject of the management of non-endocrine tumours in the region of the head of the pancreas is outlined in Fig. 20.6. It is important to remember the exceptions to Courvoisier's law and also that periampullary lesions and gallstones can coexist.

In the case of ampullary tumours the decision is simple: carcinomas of the papilla of Vater should be diagnosed pre-operatively by endoscopic biopsy and percutaneous cholangiography, and treated by elective proximal pancreaticoduodenectomy. This should be done wherever possible, since operative mortality is less than 5% in practised hands and the five-year survival is 30–40% after resection alone. If the patient is very frail, bypass should be carried out. Local excision is not an alternative since tumour resection is likely to be inadequate and the mortality of the procedure is about the same as a pancreaticoduodenectomy.

Now we come to the heart of the matter; the tumours

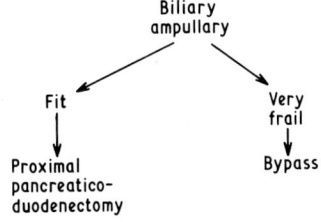

Fig. 20.6 Guidelines for the surgical treatment of non-endocrine tumours of the head of the pancreas, papilla of Vater and pancreatic common bile duct. (CBD = common bile duct; PD = pancreatic duct.)

of the head of the pancreas itself. Whether to bypass them and accept the inevitable early death of most of the patients with the occasional pleasant surprise a year or two later when, because of the inaccuracies of establishing a tissue diagnosis, the continued survival of one of them suggests that the original lesion was probably not cancer at all but pancreatitis; or whether to try to take them all out, and apparently have to accept the erosive immediacy of a high operative mortality, and poor ultimate survival after resection alone. The accumulated information from which an optimum solution to this dilemma can logically be resolved is available in the following publications; it shows a clear overall advantage for resection in practised hands (Crile, 1970; Feduska *et al.*, 1971; Smith, 1973; Gilsdorf and Spanos, 1973; Aston and Longmire, 1973; Hermreck *et al.*, 1974; Hertzberg, 1974; Warren *et al.*, 1975; Webster, 1975; Pliam and ReMine, 1975; Shapiro, 1975; Tepper *et al.*, 1976; Brooks and Culebras, 1976; Wise *et al.*, 1976; Sato *et al.*, 1977; Nakase *et al.*, 1977; Ihse *et al.*, 1977; Fortner *et al.*, 1977).

The 30-day operative mortality for resection of carcinomas of the lower common bile duct is in the range 8–17%; the five-year survival after resection alone is in the range 16–30%. The operative mortality associated with resection of pancreatic duct carcinomas arising in the head of the gland is in the range 8–25%; the five-year survival after resection alone may be 0% (Hertzberg, 1974) or between 3 and 15%. It is usually not possible to distinguish carcinomas of the lower end of the bile duct and pancreatic duct cancers at the time of operation. The operative mortality of bypass procedures is 7–33% and, except for mistaken diagnosis and the occasional tumour with a very benign course, nobody survives five years. With the exception of Crile (1970) and a statistical study by Shapiro (1975) the weight of evidence shows that resection is associated with better palliation and longer survival than bypass and this is supported by our own experience. In fit

patients therefore, carcinoma of the lower end of the common bile duct and head of the pancreas should be resected whenever possible (Fig. 20.6). If the surgeon is not sufficiently practised, biliary decompression should be performed and the patient referred to a centre specializing in this field (see below).

We must now examine the type of resection to perform. The main resources for considering regional (total) pancreatectomy for lesions of the head of the pancreas are: that there should be a lower operative mortality by avoiding jejunopancreatic anastomosis, and that it should improve survival and reduce the incidence of local recurrences (which may be as high as 50%) by a better clearance of regional lymph nodes and by removing foci of carcinoma in-situ elsewhere in the duct system of the pancreas which may be present in 16–18% of cases (Cubilla and Fitzgerald, 1976; Ihse *et al.*, 1977). Haemorrhage and anastomotic leakage, however, still occur after total pancreatectomy and the mortality is about the same as after proximal pancreaticoduodenectomy. The operation causes a brittle, insulin-dependent diabetes mellitus which has itself been the cause of death from hypoglycaemia, which is difficult to manage in a quarter of patients, and which almost certainly impairs the quality of life in the remainder (Pliam and ReMine, 1975; Ihse *et al.*, 1977). So far there is insufficient evidence of any improvement in survival to justify the use of this procedure for all carcinomas in the head of the pancreas (Fortner *et al.*, 1977). It is better to accept that microscopic tumour persists at the level of pancreatic division in about 13% of cases, and rely on post-operative chemotherapy and radiotherapy. For the smaller pancreatic ductal cancers in the head of the gland and those of the lower end of the common bile duct, proximal pancreaticoduodenectomy should be performed. If the lesion is Stage II or III, regional pancreatectomy for fit younger patients, and bypass for older and unfit patients are the operations of choice (Fig. 20.6).

Reduction in operative mortality

We must look to developments in chemotherapy for improvements in ultimate survival after resection, but an increase in the proportion of cancers which can be successfully resected with a lower operative mortality as part of a combined treatment plan is well within contemporary organizational and technological capability.

Surgical specialization

A major pancreatic operation involves the resection and anastomosis of all the major producers of the gastrointestinal digestive secretions. The dissection must proceed in a complex anatomical field close to large fragile and essential blood vessels. Add to this the uncertainties even of operative diagnosis, the difficulties of assessing accurately the extent of blood vessel involvement and the necessity on occasion of making an irreversible operative commitment on the basis of inadequate information, and it becomes clear why these are unquestionably the most difficult operations in general surgery. Selection of the most appropriate operation is a decision which has to be made at the time, and in order to be able to choose the best procedure for an individual patient, the surgeon must be practised in doing them all. The number of cases which present to a general surgical service not specializing in this field is likely to be too small to develop the necessary experience in these particular procedures, as well as in the all important collaborative system of perioperative care. The essential requirement of specific training in pancreatic surgery and of centres specializing in the field, is self-evident and supported by the published experience of others (Aston and Longmire, 1973; Gilsdorf and Spanos, 1973; Pliam and ReMine, 1975; Warren *et al.*, 1975; Tepper *et al.*, 1976 and Ihse *et al.*, 1977).

Analysis and reduction of principle complications

The principle causes of operative death after pancreatic resection are haemorrhage and breakdown of the pancreaticojejunal anastomosis. The average incidence of haemorrhage after proximal pancreaticoduodenectomy is 13% with a 50% mortality; the incidence appears to be about the same after total pancreatectomy but in this case the mortality from this complication seems to be a little lower. There are two types of bleeding; the more frequent is a diffuse haemorrhage from the mucosa of the gastric remnant, suture line or upper jejunum but bleeding from an acute penetrating gastric ulcer can also occur. Both the incidence and severity of this type of haemorrhage are reduced by adequate gastric resection with or without vagotomy; cimetidine in doses sufficient to achieve maximum reduction in gastric acid secretion should be given just before, and during the operation, and maintained for at least three weeks afterwards since haemorrhage may be triggered by feeding. The second type of haemorrhage can come from the pancreaticojejunal anastomosis and diffusely from the abdominal cavity and the wound. It is suggested that this is due to the anastomotic or intra-abdominal effects of activated pancreatic proteases on exposed tissue planes.

The pancreaticojejunal anastomosis breaks down on average after 11% of pancreaticoduodenectomies with a 40% mortality. The frequency of this complication is not affected by putting little tubes in the pancreatic duct (Braasch and Gray, 1977). The real reason is much more likely to be the immediate activation of the pancreatic juice flowing out of the divided duct by high enterokinase containing upper jejunal mucosa which is now adjacent to the unprotected cut surface of the gland. Maximum enterokinase secretion by the small intestinal mucosa in man ends geographically 10–20 cm distal to the duodenojejunal flexure (Hermon-Taylor *et al.*, 1977). Although low levels of enterokinase activity are found beyond this limit it is suggested that until non-toxic specific inhibitors become available, dividing the intestine at least 20 cm distal to the duodenojejunal flexure will bring about a reduction in the complication rate from this anastomosis without much additional nutritional impairment after proximal pancreaticoduodenectomy.

Surgical relief of pain

Surgical resection of coeliac ganglia and nerves, or their injection with phenol or 50% alcohol has long been advocated. Similar procedures can be carried out percutaneously after operation; results are variable but with careful technique pain reduction may occur in some patients (Flanigan and Kraft, 1978).

Biliary tract and gall bladder

Unresectable tumours of the gall bladder may lead the surgeon to carry out a right hemihepatectomy. This formidable operation seldom saves the patient since distant metastases are usually present: the role of chemotherapy and radiotherapy are being investigated (Davis *et al.*, 1978). A lesion high in the common bile duct or at the junction of the hepatic ducts is also seldom resectable. Where possible the obstruction should be cannulated either percutaneously or at operation. An alternative is Longmire's operation in which a loop of jejunum is brought up and anastomosed, mucosa to mucosa, to a dilated intrahepatic bile duct in the right lobe of the liver. All these procedures may improve survival for patients who would otherwise die of liver failure with unrelievable pruritus. The mitotic activity of these tumours is often low, and survival after relief of anatomical obstruction alone may be surprisingly long. Chemotherapy and radiotherapy are likely to improve this further (Davis *et al.*, 1978).

Chemotherapy and radiotherapy

Chemotherapy with or without radiotherapy should be offered to all patients with pancreatic cancer who are fit enough to tolerate the side-effects. Neither can be expected to be effective in the treatment of large tumour masses which contain a high proportion of hypoxic central cells which are radioresistant and less accessible to blood-borne chemotherapeutic agents. There is some clinical evidence to support the concept that chemotherapy is more effective against smaller metastatic lesions than large primary tumours (Wiggans *et al.*, 1978). It remains to be seen whether radiotherapy is more effective than chemotherapy in the control of primary tumours and their local lymph glands. Both modalities have been tested separately, chemotherapy more widely than radiotherapy, and combinations of the two appear to show greater promise than either used alone. However chemotherapy has been far more extensively investigated than radiotherapy, and the best results so far have been achieved without radiotherapy using combinations of chemotherapy only.

Chemotherapy

The most consistently prescribed medications in pancreatic cancer are analgesics. It is our experience that analgesics are seldom given frequently enough or in sufficient dose to forestall and control pain in terminal pancreatic cancer.

Anti-tumour chemotherapy has had a consistent modest success in pancreatic cancer. 5-Fluorouracil (5-FU) and mitomycin-C (MTC) are the two most effective single agents and appear to have additive effects when used in combination. Less potent single agents are methotrexate, adriamycin and streptozotocin. Chlorambucil, ifosfamide, ICRF 159 and ftorafur appear to have some effect but are, so far, unproven.

5-FU

This is the most commonly prescribed cytotoxic drug for all gastrointestinal cancers and is a constant ingredient in all combination regimes. Combination regimes have shown such promise that it is probably unjustified to use 5-FU as a single agent. If this is done, the original regime described by Curreri in 1958 is still as effective as any and has been described elsewhere (Carter and Comis, 1975).

5-FU causes regression of pancreatic cancers as judged by a reduction in measured palpable diameter (Wiggans *et al.*, 1978) in 20–30% of patients. This may

be an optimistic estimate, and regression is seldom complete; the effect on survival is still unknown after tens of thousands of patients have received treatment. A promising new derivative of 5-FU, is FT207 (ftorafur) which has been found effective in other gastrointestinal tumours in Japan but has so far not been evaluated satisfactorily in pancreatic cancer.

Mitomycin-C (MTC)

This drug is reported to produce tumour regression in 20–30% of patients with pancreatic cancer and is the second most widely used agent for this tumour both singly and in combination. While it is most effective when given by daily injection the incidence of haematological and renal toxicity with this regime is unacceptably high and it is now almost invariably used, in the West at least, as intermittent treatment in combination with other drugs.

Streptozotocin (STZ) and other nitrosoureas (BCNU, CCNU and methyl-CCNU)

STZ is a nitrosourea which is widely effective on pancreatic endocrine tumours as described in Chapter 17. The first, over optimistic, reports of this drug in pancreatic exocrine cancer suggested a 50% tumour regression rate. In combination with 5-FU or cyclophosphamide STZ causes regression in 12% of patients only. Although a high percentage of these were complete regressions, the median survival of the patients treated was only 2.5 months (Moertel *et al.*, 1977). The promising results of a combination of STZ, 5-FU and MTC, described below, may in fact owe little to the STZ.

BCNU, CCNU and methyl-CCNU have all been extensively tested in pancreatic cancer and appear to have no worthwhile effect, with a response rate of 6% when maximum doses of methyl-CCNU were combined with 5-FU (Moertel *et al.*, 1976a).

Methotrexate

In one abstract (Djerassi *et al.*, 1974) methotrexate was reported to be surprisingly effective in five patients with Stage IV pancreatic cancer. All survived eight months and three for over a year. Intermittent, moderately high doses of 50 mg/kg were given intravenously every three weeks followed by citrovorum factor 'rescue'. This regime appears more promising than the use of 10 mg/kg weekly which gave a response rate of 10% (Schein *et al.*, 1978). MTX is part of the initiation regime used by Mallinson *et al.* (1976).

Alkylating agents

Apart from MTC only occasional reports of alkylating agents exist. Chlorambucil in a dose of 0.2 mg/day for 42 days produced tumour regression in four out of six patients (Carter and Comis, 1975). Cyclophosphamide has proved ineffective singly and in combination with STZ (Moertel *et al.*, 1977) but a new analogue, ifosfamide, given in a large, fractionated dose has produced a response in 85% of 13 patients in a preliminary report (Hoeffer-Janker and Scheef, 1977).

Combination chemotherapy

Three regimes of combined chemotherapy, which included in each case 5-FU and MTC, have shown significant prolongation of survival in patients with advanced pancreatic cancer. In the two studies in which it was measured, tumour regression was better than 40%.

Earlier combinations of 5-FU with nitrosoureas, cyclophosphamide and testolactone have failed to show any consistent effect on tumour regression or patient survival, probably because the effective drug, 5-FU, was combined with agents which have little or no activity when used singly. The surprising effect of testolactone reported in 1975 by Waddell has not been confirmed (Schein, personal communication).

SEER

The first chemotherapy regime to show a convincing lengthening of survival in pancreatic cancer was reported by Mallinson *et al.* (1976) using a combination which is referred to as SEER (South East England Regime). The regime which relies heavily on 5-FU in the initiation course and the combination of 5-FU and MTC in the follow-up treatment is shown in Table 20.5. It was given intravenously by sequential bolus injection. Toxicity was low, the most common side-effect being nausea with occasional vomiting, moderate hair loss, requiring a wig in only exceptional

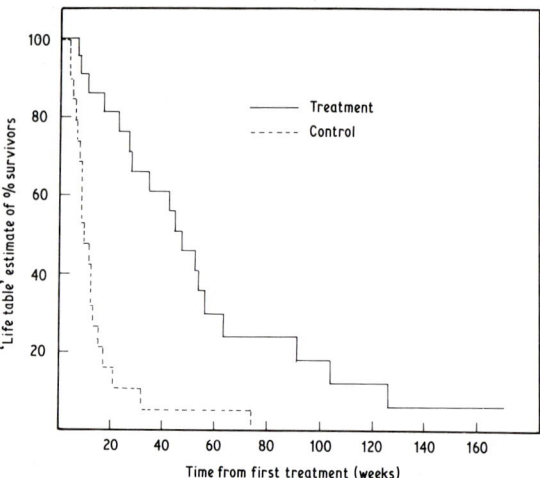

Fig. 20.7   Actuarial survival curves for the SEER regime (Mallinson *et al.*, 1976). Median survival of control group is 2.5 months and that of treated group 11 months (P = 0.0006).

patients, and modest haematological toxicity. No course of treatment had to be interrupted because of toxicity. The study was a controlled, prospective, randomized comparison of chemotherapy versus no treatment. It was interesting that patients receiving no chemotherapy had almost as high a prevalence of the symptoms and laboratory changes usually attributed to drug toxicity as treated patients. Treated patients had a median survival of 11 months compared with 3 months in the controls as shown in Fig. 20.7. Tumour size was not evaluated in these patients, and since most patients did not have a marker lesion which could be measured, the patients in this study are not directly comparable

Table 20.5   Drug regime used for the initiation and follow-up course in SEER. Figures in brackets indicate dose if patient's weight falls outside 60–80 kg.

Day	Cyclophosphamide	5-Fluorouracil	Vincristine	Methotrexate
1	300 mg	500 mg	–	20 mg
2	–	500 mg	1 mg	–
3	–	500 mg	–	–
4	–	500 mg	–	20 mg
5	300 mg	500 mg	1 mg	–
	(4.5 mg/kg)	(7.5 mg/kg)	(0.02 mg/kg)	(0.3 mg/kg)

Maintenance courses (at 5 week intervals):
5-Fluorouracil   10 mg/kg ⎫
Mitomycin-C   100 μg/kg ⎬ Daily for 5 days

with those in the two below who all had such lesions and probably therefore had more advanced cancer (Moertel *et al.*, 1974). Nevertheless, the control and treated groups were highly comparable and the improved survival in the treated group appears to be attributable to the chemotherapy rather than patient selection.

Streptozotocin, mitomycin-C and 5-FU (SMF)
Wiggans *et al.* (1978) reported the use of streptozotocin 1 g/m^2 and 5-FU 600 mg/m^2 given on days 1, 8, 29 and 36 of a 56-day cycle with MTC 10 mg/m^2 given on day 1. Doses were modified according to toxicity as shown in Table 20.6. Nausea and vomiting were experienced by most patients as would be expected in a combination containing STZ and 5-FU, but this caused interruption of the regime in only 1/23 patients. Marrow depression was moderate and neither cumulative nor related to response. Nephrotoxicity was seen in 30% of cases but blood urea levels were not markedly raised and did not rise further when STZ was withdrawn, in spite of continued MTC treatment. The survival figures in Fig. 20.8 show the advantage of separating data on responders, patients with stable disease, and non-responders. Ten of 23 patients responded (43%) with one complete response lasting for 7 months. The median survival was 7.5 months in responders, 9 months in patients with stable disease and 3 months in non-responders. Thus it seems that a regime which only stops pancreatic cancer increasing in size, can be advantageous. Tumour regression was commoner in patients in whom a large liver was the marker lesion than those with an abdominal mass, suggesting that chemotherapy is more effective against multiple secondary lesions which are usually smaller than a palpable primary tumour.

A variation of the SMF regime (Abderhalden *et al.*, 1977) also showed a comparable response of 31% using 5-FU 500 mg/m^2 and STZ 300 mg/m^2 on five days every four weeks, with MTC 10 mg/m^2 every eight weeks. Used in this way STZ does not produce a high proportion of complete responses, and among many experienced workers even at comparatively low doses it is regarded as a notoriously nauseating drug.

5-Fluorouracil, adriamycin and mitomycin-C (FAM)
Haller *et al.*, (1978) reported in abstract the results of using 5-FU and MTC as described in the SMF regime but substituting adriamycin 30 mg/m^2 on days 1 and 29 in place of the STZ. This regime has been described in detail in the chapter on stomach cancer (Chapter 19) for which this combination is particularly effective. Six of 14 patients with advanced pancreatic cancer (43%) showed a partial response for a mean duration of 5 months. The median survival of responders was 6.5 months which was significantly longer than 3 months in non-responders. Marrow toxicity, which was to be expected with this combination, was moderate and controllable. The patients did not survive long enough to get near to the cardiotoxic dose of adriamycin. More recent reports (Bitran *et al.*, 1979; Smith *et al.*, 1979 and 1980) confirm this impression.

Radiotherapy

Radiotherapy alone
External beam irradiation of pancreatic cancer in conventional doses of 3500–4000 rad has shown no beneficial effect on symptoms or survival. However, 5000–6500 rad given in doses of 200 rad daily on six days a week produces useful relief of pain and improvement in performance status in two thirds of the patients with tolerable toxicity but no significant improvement in survival.

Implantation of radioactive beads directly into pancreatic cancers has been the subject of intermittent research, and is a technique showing some promise clinically and theoretically since a permanent afterloading implantation with radioactive gold grains is feasible producing a total dose of 7000–10 000 rad (Carter and Comis, 1975). It may also be possible to transfix primary and larger secondary tumours using thread impregnated with radioactive isotope or bearing radioactive seeds.

Table 20.6 Modification of doses of drugs in relation to toxicity in the SMF regime.

WBC	Platelets	Dose reduction
Early (2–3 weeks) <2000		↓ 5-FU by 25%
Late (4–5 weeks) 1500–2500		↓ MMC by 25%
<1500		↓ MMC by 50%
	50–75 000	↓ MMC by 25%
	<50 000	↓ MMC by 50%

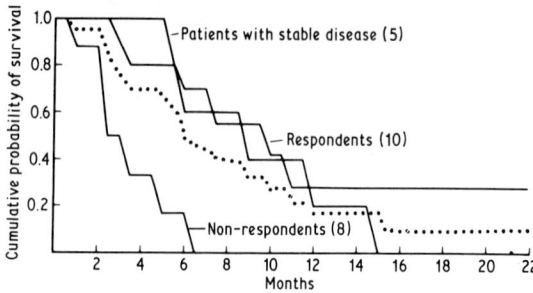

Fig. 20.8 Actuarial survival curves for patients on SMF (Wiggans *et al*., 1978). The dotted line represents the overall survival of the group, the continuous lines the survival of patients according to tumour response.

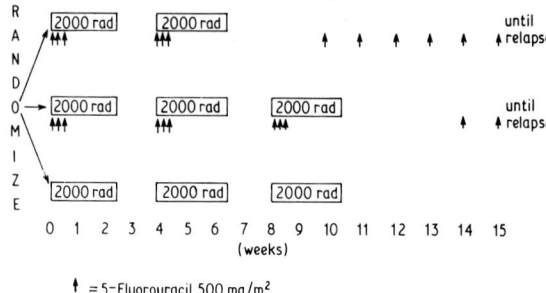

Fig. 20.9 The protocol of fractionated radiotherapy with and without 5-FU reported by the GITSG (Moertel *et al*., 1976*b*).

The topic of radiotherapy in pancreatic cancer has been reviewed by Carter and Comis (1975) and Macdonald *et al*. (1977), and interstitial implantation by Hilaris (1978). Several problems concern the radiotherapist in this disease: the tumours are not particularly radiosensitive and are surrounded by more radiosensitive structures such as the stomach, liver, small intestine and the kidneys. The central core of the tumours consist of particularly radioresistant hypoxic cells which may however be made more treatable by the use of radiosensitizers, at present the object of intensive research (Courtenay, 1978). The problem of acute or chronic damage to the tissue surrounding the pancreas has been approached by administering the dose in fractions separated by intervals without treatment to allow recovery of normal tissue as described below. A more adventurous technique still is the use of sophisticated external beam equipment to deliver a high dose of irradiation directly onto the tumour at operation while radiosensitive tissues are held aside and shielded.

It is in fact impossible to evaluate the results of the two earlier reports of fractionated external beam irradiation because many of the patients included were also treated with a variety of chemotherapeutic agents. Indeed the results of the two prospective, randomized studies of radiotherapy with and without chemotherapy favour the combined modality approach (Moertel *et al*., 1969 and 1976*b*).

Split course radiotherapy
Haslam *et al*. (1975) described a method which is still that used in the majority of current studies in the USA. Tumours are localized at laparotomy by clips, or afterwards by ultrasound or CAT-scan. The tumour is treated to a midplane dose of up to 6000 rad in 10 weeks using approximately 2000 rad over 2 weeks separated by 2-week intervals as illustrated in Fig. 20.9. Irradia-

tion is administered by a cobalt unit using a double split-course technique via anteroposterior opposed fields. The tumour to be treated must be confined to a field 20 cm × 20 cm or 400 cm³. The initial report of this method demonstrated a 34% 12-month survival in 23 patients with a median survival of 7.5 months; 70% of patients experienced good to fair palliation but 10% developed acute morbidity during treatment requiring unplanned interruption or cancellation of it. A number of these patients received chemotherapy, usually with 5-FU, but with other agents as well, singly or combined with the 5-FU. It was apparent that the impact on survival and palliation was greater than in previous reports of conventionally fractionated radiotherapy.

In 1978 Dobelbower *et al*. reported a modification of this technique using the Betatron. The tumour was localized as above with care to localize the kidneys by CAT-scan or an IVP with a cross-table lateral view in the nephogram phase. External beam irradiation was administered by 45 MeV betatron to an area encompassing the demonstrated tumour volume with a 1–2 cm margin. In patients where the posterior margin of the target was 12 cm or less from the anterior abdominal wall a 3-field technique was used as shown in Fig. 20.10. (Opposed lateral 45 MeV-photon fields and one anterior fixed beam of 45 MeV-photons and 50% 15–35 MeV electrons). The proportion of electron energy was based on the posterior extent of the target volume: where the posterior surface of the target was more distant than 10 cm from the anterior abdominal wall a 4-field box or a 3-field box with the anterior beam entirely of photons was used. The minimum dose to the target was in the range of 6300–6700 rad and encompassed by the 90–95% isodose curve. This was delivered in doses of 180 rad fractions split between 5 days a week over 7–9 weeks (mean 7.5 weeks). The mean target volume was 1000 cm³ or less; the dose to the spinal cord was well within tolerance but one eighth to

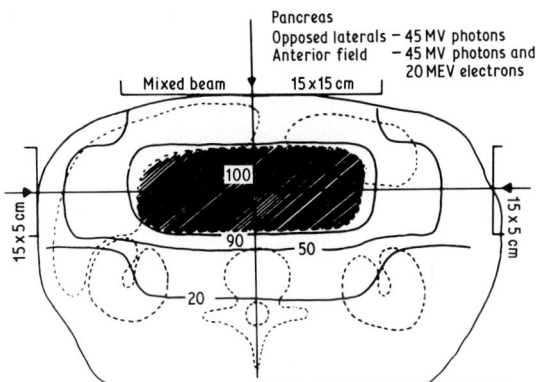

Fig. 20.10 Technique for treating regional pancreatic carcinoma with a three-field anterior mixed beam (Dobelbower *et al.*, 1978).

one half of the renal parenchyma was within relatively high dose volume. Eighteen patients were treated thus: in two, treatment was interrupted on account of severe sepsis. Side-effects of mild nausea or diarrhoea were readily controlled; weight loss was rare and slight, and improvement in appetite and relief of pain occurred in 10 of 13 patients. Long-term side-effects have not been adequately evaluated in this small group followed up for a short time, but there has been no case of radiation-induced myelitis or significant hepatic or renal damage, though mild exocrine and endocrine pancreatic damage has been indicated.

The actuarial survival rate in this series is 59% at 12 months. Seven of the patients alive at one year were clinically free of disease, and the median length of survival was 11.8 months. However, 7 patients received adjuvant chemotherapy with a median survival of 13 months compared to 7.5 months for the 11 patients who received radiation alone. The patients treated had locally unresectable disease only, without metastases, and are therefore not strictly comparable with the majority of patients in chemotherapy trials with Stage III and IV disease but appear to have survived longer than historical controls of comparable staging and to have done so without detectable disease.

Combined modality treatment

The combination of surgical resection with either chemotherapy, radiotherapy or immunotherapy has not been satisfactorily tested, and in the centres which have started such studies difficulty is being experienced in recruiting patients. In patients with unresectable cancer only two prospective, randomized studies of radiotherapy with and without chemotherapy have been published. Moertel *et al.* (1969) compared super

voltage radiation treatment of locally unresectable pancreatic cancers using an unfractionated technique with and without 5-FU. The mean survival of patients on combined treatment was 10 months, significantly longer than that in patients on radiotherapy alone. More recently the Gastrointestinal Tumour Study Group (Moertel *et al.*, 1976) has published the results of their prospective, randomized, well-stratified study. Three arms of treatment were compared:

6000 rad alone.
6000 rad plus 5-FU, 250 mg/m² given on the first 3 days of each fraction or radiotherapy and then at weekly intervals starting 6 weeks after the end of radiotherapy as shown in Fig. 20.9.
4000 rad plus 5-FU as above.

The two combined modality arms proved preferable to radiotherapy alone and 4000 rad with 5-FU was as effective as 6000 (Moertel *et al.*, 1976). A similar schedule of irradiation with a combined chemotherapy of 5-FU, methyl-CCNU and testolactone showed no advantage over the simpler GITSG regime. This is unsurprising since neither methyl-CCNU nor testolactone have shown single-agent effect. This does not mean that other combinations of effective single agents in conjunction with fractionated radiotherapy will not improve on the GITSG results: these showed a median survival of approximately 8–9 months in each arm, and no significant difference between each but consistently longer survival in the 4000 rad plus 5-FU arm.

By British standards the field used in these studies is large, and may contribute to morbidity and indeed mortality. Most radiotherapists in Britain would use a smaller field in spite of the lack of side-effects mentioned by both Haslam and Dobelbower.

Carcinoma of the biliary tract and gall bladder

There are few reports of chemotherapy and none of radiotherapy or immunotherapy for these rather rare tumours. The earliest reports on 5-FU from the Mayo Clinic suggested that carcinoma of the gall bladder responded in 50% of patients. Since then occasional reports of different drugs used on isolated cases have appeared with a consistent pattern of rather high response rates. Stratification is particularly important in prospective, randomized trials of cancer of the gall bladder as mentioned above (Nevin *et al.*, 1976). Two studies are in progress, both by the Eastern Co-operative Oncology Group: in one, 5-FU 600 mg/m²/day on 5 days at monthly intervals is compared with the same regime plus streptozotocin 500 mg/m²/day on the same days and again with 5-FU 500 mg/m²/day × 5, days 1–5 and 36–40, given by mouth plus methyl-

CCNU 150 mg/m² on day 1 also by mouth. In the other trial, a comparison is being made of radiotherapy to a dose of 4000 rad with radiotherapy of the same dose plus 5-FU 600 mg/m² intravenously on the first 3 days of radiotherapy then weekly as in the GITSG study in Fig. 20.9

Future progress

At present the overall results of the treatment of most pancreatic cancers is so bad that it can only get better. Improvements must come from progress in two fields; research and specialized collaborative clinical management. In research the priorities are the identification of environmental causes by widely applied epidemiological studies exploiting the regional, geographic, occupational, and migratory differences in incidence. Legislative and educational measures to reduce the impact of risk factors must be introduced and extended. The second main priority is laboratory research, the rate-limiting step in which is now lack of research *money* not lack of knowledge or research opportunity. Improvements in specific early diagnosis are unlikely to come from the detection of oncofoetal macromolecules since they are not iso-immunogenic. What is needed is a detailed biochemical and immunological characterization of pancreatic exocrine cancer cells themselves, directed particularly at the post translational modification of polypeptides and the nature of the cell surface. These studies will be facilitated by exploiting contemporary advances in *in vitro* and *in vivo* culture and by encouraging the close collaboration between career scientists and informed clinicians. Such collaboration is also most likely to result in the development of effective laboratory methods for testing new chemotherapeutic agents.

On the clinical side the priorities are firstly an increase in the proportion of pancreatic cancers that are successfully resected. Such an increase will only come about by recognition of the need for special training in pancreatic surgery, by the application of research development to reduce operative mortality, and by the establishment and referral of patients to centres specializing in the collaborative perioperative management of these cases. Secondly it must be recognized that resection is only part of management and that chemotherapy with or without radiotherapy is essential. Progress in these fields will come from the identification through properly designed multicentre clinical trials, of optimal combinations of drugs and treatment schedules, together with the application of chemo- and radiosensitizers. 'Heavy particle' radiotherapy may well show special benefit for pancreatic cancer (see Chapter 4). Another approach which shows promise already is the development of radiosensitizers which are possibly chemosensitizers as well.

References

Abderhalden, R.T. *et al.* (1977), Streptozotocin (STZ), 5-fluorouracil (5-FU) with and without mitomycin-C (Mito) in the treatment of pancreatic adenocarcinoma. *Proc. Am. Soc. Oncol.*, **18**, 301.

Aston, S.J. and Longmire, W.P. (1973), Pancreaticoduodenal resection: twenty years' experience. *Archs. Surg.*, **106**, 813–7.

Bernarde, M.A. and Weiss, W. (1977), A cohort analysis of pancreatic cancer. *Cancer*, **39**, 1260–3.

Bitran, J.D. *et al.* (1979), Treatment of metastatic pancreatic and gastric adenocarcinoma with 5 F.U., adriamycin and mitomycin (FAM). *Cancer Treat. Rep.*, **63**, 2049–51.

Braasch, J.W. and Gray, B.N. (1977), Considerations that lower pancreatoduodenectomy mortality. *Am. J. Surg.*, **133**, 480–4.

Brooks, J.R. and Culebras, J.M. (1976), Cancer of the pancreas. Palliative operation, Whipple's procedure or total pancreatectomy. *Am. J. Surg.*, **131**, 516–20.

Carter, S.K. and Comis, R.L. (1975), The integration of chemotherapy into a combined modality approach for cancer treatment. VI. Pancreatic adenocarcinoma. *Cancer Treat. Rev.*, **2**, 193–214.

Courtenay, V.D. (1978), The effect of misonidazole on the radiation response of clonogenic human pancreatic carcinoma cells. *Br. J. Cancer.* (Supplement), **37** (3), 225–7.

Crile, G. (1970), The advantages of bypass operations over radical pancreatoduodenectomy in the treatment of pancreatic carcinoma. *Surg. Gynec. Obstet.*, **130**, 1049–53.

Cubilla, A.L. and Fitzgerald, P.J. (1975), Morphological patterns of primary non-endocrine human pancreas carcinoma *Cancer Res.*, **35**, 2234–48.

Cubilla, A. and Fitzgerald, P.J. (1976), Morphological lesions associated with human primary invasive non-endocrine pancreas cancer. *Cancer Res.*, **36**, 2690–8.

Cubilla, A.L., Fortner, J. and Fitzgerald P.J. (1978), Lymph node involvement in carcinoma of the head of the pancreas area. *Cancer*, **41**, 880–7

Davis, H.L. et al. (1978), Gastrointestinal cancer. In: *Randomised Trials in Cancer: A Critical Review by Sites.* (ed. M.J. Staquet), Raven Press, New York, pp. 147–230.

Djerassi, I., Kim, J.S. and Suvansri, V. (1974), 'Pulse' methotrexate and citrovorum factor 'rescue' in common solid tumours (including lung and pancreas) of the adult. *Proc. Am. Ass. Cancer Res. Am. Soc. Clin. Oncol.*, **15**, 78.

Dobelbower, R.R. *et al.* (1978), Pancreatic carcinoma treated with high dose, small-volume irradiation. *Cancer*, **41**, 1087–92.

Flanigan, D.P. and Kraft, R.O. (1978), Continuing experience with palliative chemical splanchnicectomy. *Arch. Surg.*, **113**, 509–11.

Feduska, N.J., Dent, T.L. and Lindenauer, S.M. (1971), Results of palliative operations for carcinoma of the pancreas. *Archs Surg.*, **103**, 330–4.

Fortner, J.G. *et al.* (1977), Regional pancreatectomy: en bloc pancreatic, portal vein and lymph node resection. *Ann. Surg.*, **186**, 42–50.

Freeny, P.C. and Ball. T.J. (1978), Rapid diagnosis of pancreatic carcinoma. *Radiology*,**127**, 627–33.

Gelder, F.B. *et al.* (1978), Purification, partial characterization and clinical evaluation of a pancreatic oncofetal antigen. *Cancer Res.*, **38**, 313–24.

Gilsdorf, R.B. and Spanos, P. (1973), Factors influencing morbidity and mortality in pancreaticoduodenectomy. *Ann. Surg.*, **177**, 332–7.

Grant, A., McGlashan, D. and Hermon-Taylor, J. (1978), A study of pancreatic secretory and intracellular enzymes in pancreatic cancer tissue, other gastrointestinal cancers, normal pancreas and serum. *Clin. Chim. Acta*, **90**, 75–82.

Haller, D. *et al.* (1978), Fluorouracil (F), Adriamycin (A) and Mitomycin-C (M), FAM, for advanced colorectal and pancreatic cancer. *Proc. Am. Ass. Cancer Res. Am. Soc. Clin. Oncol.*, **19**, 342.

Haslam, J.B., Cavenaugh, P.J. and Stroup, S.L. (1973), Radiation therapy in the treatment of irresectable adenocarcinoma of the pancreas. *Cancer*, **32**, 1341–5.

Hermon-Taylor, J. *et al.* (1977), Immunofluorescent localisation of enterokinase in human small intestine. *Gut*, **18**, 259–65.

Hermreck, A.S., Thomas, C.Y. and Friesen, S.R. (1974), Importance of pathologic staging in the surgical management of adenocarcinoma of the exocrine pancreas. *Am. J. Surg.*, **127**, 653–7.

Hertzberg, J. (1974), Pancreaticoduodenal resection and bypass operation in patients with carcinoma of the head of the pancreas ampulla and distal end of the common duct. *Acta Chirurg. Scand.*, **140**, 523–7.

Hilaris, B.S. (1978), Interstitial implantation of pancreatic cancer. In: *Renaissance of Interstitial Brachytherapy.* (eds J.M. Vaeth *et al.*) Karger, Basel.

Hoeffer-Janker, W. and Scheef, W. (1977), Clinical experience with Holoxan. In: *Proceedings of International Holoxan Symposium.* Asta, Dusseldorf, pp.99–103.

Ihse, I. *et al.* (1977), Total pancreatectomy for cancer: an appraisal of 65 cases. *Ann. Surg.*, **186**, 675–80.

Krain, L.S. (1970), The rising incidence of carcinoma of the pancreas: an epidemiologic appraisal.*J. Surg. Oncol.*, **2**, 115–24.

Lees, W.R. *et al.* (1979), Prospective study of ultrasonography in chronic pancreatic disease. *Br. Med. J.*, **1**, 162–4.

Macdonald, J.S., Widerlite, L. and Schein, P.S. (1977), Biology, diagnosis and chemotherapeutic management of pancreatic malignancy. *Adv. Pharmac. Ther.*, **14**, 107–42.

Mackie, C.R. *et al.* (1979), Prospective evaluation of some candidate tumour markers in the diagnosis of pancreatic cancer. (In preparation).

Mallinson, C.N. *et al.* (1976), Chemotherapy for pancreatic cancer. *Gut*, **17**, 826–7.

Mallinson, C.N. *et al.* (1980), Chemotherapy for pancreatic cancer results of a prospective randomised controlled trial. *Brit. Med. J.*, **281**, 1589–91.

Moertel, C.G. *et al.* (1969), Combined 5-fluorouracil and supervoltage radiation therapy of locally unresectable gastrointestinal cancer. *Lancet*, **ii**, 865–7.

Moertel, C.G. *et al.* (1974), Effects of patient selection on results of Phase II chemotherapy trials in gastrointestinal cancer. *Cancer Chemother. Rep.*, **59**, 257.

Moertel, C.G. *et al.* (1976*a*), Phase II study of methyl-CCNU in the treatment of advanced pancreatic carcinoma. *Cancer Treat. Rep.*, **60**, 1659–61.

Moertel, C.G. *et al.* (1976*b*), An evaluation of high dose radiation and combined radiation and 5-fluorouracil (5-FU) therapy for locally unresectable pancreatic carcinoma. *Proc. Am. Ass. Cancer Res.*, **17**, 244.

Moertel, C.G. *et al.* (1977), Treatment of advanced adenocarcinoma of the pancreas with combinations of streptozotocin plus 5-fluorouracil and streptozotocin plus cyclophosphamide. *Cancer*, **40**, 605–8.

Nakase, A., Matsumoto, Y. and Uchidak, Honjo I. (1977), Surgical treatment of cancer of the pancreas and peri-ampullary region. *Ann. Surg.*, **185**, 52–7.

Nevin, J.E. *et al.* (1976), Carcinoma of the gall bladder. Staging, treatment and prognosis. *Cancer*, **37**, 141–8.

Pliam, M.B. and ReMine, W.H. (1975), Further evaluation of total pancreatectomy. *Archs. Surg.*, **110**, 506–12.

Sato, T. *et al.* (1977), Follow-up studies of radical resection for pancreaticoduodenal cancer. *Ann. Surg.*, **186**, 581–8.

Schein, P.S. *et al.* (1978), Randomised Phase II clinical trial of adriamycin, methotrexate and actinomycin-D in advanced measurable pancreatic carcinoma: a Gastrointestinal Tumour Study Group Report. *Cancer*, **42**, 19–22.

Shapiro, T.M. (1975), Adenocarcinoma of the pancreas : a statistical analysis of biliary by-pass v's Whipple resection in good risk patients. *Ann. Surg.*, **182**, 715–21.

Shorey, B.A. (1975), Apsiration biopsy of carcinoma of the pancreas. *Gut*, **16**, 645–7.

Smith, R. (1973), Progress in the surgical treatment of pancreatic disease. *Am. J. Surg.*, **125**, 143–53.

Smith, E.H. *et al.* (1975), Percutaneous aspiration biopsy of the pancreas under ultrasonic guidance. *New Engl. J. Med.*, **292**, 825–8.

Smith, F.P. *et al.* (1979), Phase II evaluation of FAM, 5-Fluorouracil, adriamycin, and mitomycin-C in advanced pancreatic cancer. *Proc. Am. Soc. Clin. Oncol.* (abstract), **20**, 415.

Smith, F.P. *et al.* (1980), 5-Fluorouracil, adriamycin and Mitromycin-C (FAM) chemotherapy for advanced adenocarcinoma of the pancreas. *Cancer*, **46**, 2014–18.

Tepper, J., Nardi, G. and Smit, H. (1976), Carcinoma of the pancreas : review of MGH experience from 1963 to 1973. Analysis of surgical failure and implications for radiation therapy. *Cancer*, **37**, 1519–24.

Tylen, U. and Arnesjo, B. (1973), Resectability and prognosis of carcinoma of the pancreas evaluated by angiography. *Scand. J. Gastroenterol.*, **8.**, 600–10.

Waddell, W.R. (1973), Chemotherapy for cancer of the pancreas. *Surgery*, **74**, 420–9.

Warren, K.W. *et al.* (1975), Results of radical resection for peri-ampillary cancer. *Ann. Surg.*, **181**, 534–40.

Waterhouse, J. *et al.* (eds) (1976), *Cancer Incidence in Five Continents*. Vol. III. IACR Scientific Publications No. 15, Lyon, pp. 500–3.

Webster, D.J.T. (1975), Carcinoma of the pancreas and peri-ampullary region: a clinical study in a district general hospital. *Br. J. Surg.*, **62**, 130–4.

Welton, M.J. *et al.* (1969), Carcinoma of the junction of the main hepatic ducts. *Qu. J. Med.*, **38**, 211–30.

Wiggans, R.G. *et al.* (1978), Phase II Trial of streptozotocin, mitomycin-C and 5-fluorouracil (SMF) in the treatment of advanced pancreatic cancer. *Cancer*, **41**, 387–91.

Wise, L., Pizzimbono, C. and Dehner, L.P. (1976), Periampullary cancer. A clinicopathologic study of sixty-two patients. *Am. J. Surg.*, **131**, 141–8.

21 Liver

Walter M. Melia
and Roger Williams

The term 'primary liver cancer' is used to describe hepatocellular carcinoma or hepatoma and cholangiocarcinoma as well as the rarer tumours – haemoangioendothelioma, haemangiosarcoma, and Kupffer cell sarcoma. Little information is available with respect to the response of the rarer variants to treatment and the particularly small group of hepatoblastomas in infants and children have also not been considered. Hepatocellular carcinoma is far commoner (75–80% of cases in most series) than cholangiocarcinoma (15–20%). In some series a small proportion (about 5%) of 'mixed' tumours is described with elements of cholangiocarcinoma occurring in hepatocellular carcinoma, or *vice versa*. The clinical course of such tumours is usually not significantly different from that of their major histologic component.

Possible modes of therapy have been grouped into surgery, cytotoxic agents, and radiotherapy. Within each section hepatocellular carcinoma (HCC) will be considered first, then cholangiocarcinoma where procedure or results of therapy differ significantly, and finally metastatic liver cancer. Since management of hepatic metastases from primary carcinoid tumours poses additional problems because of the associated carcinoid syndrome, the possible therapeutic approaches will be discussed separately.

Survival with untreated tumour

Hepatocellular carcinoma is one of the most rapidly growing of the solid organ tumours. Most untreated patients die within six months of diagnosis, with mean survival periods of less than three months. In the African, the tumour is known to behave especially aggressively and Geddes and Falkson (1970) report a mean duration of symptoms of 1.5 months in South African Bantu miners.

It is more useful to consider the prognosis of HCC in relation to grading. Cochrane *et al.* (1977) have analysed age, length of history, levels of serum bilirubin and AST, the presence of cirrhosis and/or ascites and weight loss in relation to duration of survival. Probability figures for each of these were combined to yield a total patient 'score' (Table 21.1). All patients with scores of more then 35 survived over 3.5 months (Fig. 21.1). Primack *et al.* (1975) has divided patients into three prognostic grades on the basis of presence or absence of ascites, portal hypertension, marked weight loss and hyperbilirubinaemia but found age and underlying cirrhosis of little significance.

Deterioration after detection of hepatic metastases is usually rapid, average survival being between 2.5 and 4.5 months, although where the primary tumour is colorectal, life expectancy is better (Foster, 1970). Patients with some of these may live 12–36 months or even longer without treatment.

Initial assessment

Hepatic arteriography is a most useful investigation in the decision as to whether treatment of HCC should be surgical and, if so, whether lobar resection is feasible or

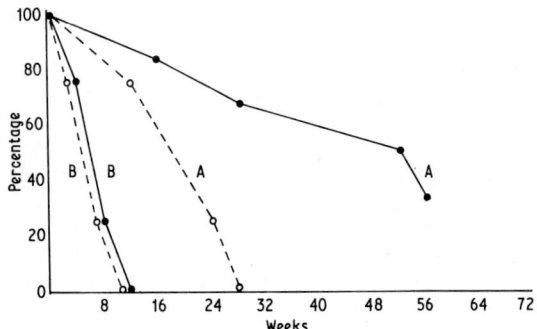

Fig. 21.1 Patient survival (weeks) from onset of treatment: for patients treated by chemotherapy (solid line) and radiotherapy followed by chemotherapy (broken line) for Grade A and Grade B cases.

Table 21.1   Scoring system used in the Cochrane method of grading hepatocellular carcinoma. Patients with scores of less than 35 have Grade B: severe disease; while those with scores of over 35 have Grade A: less severe disease.

		Score		*Score*
Age (years)	< 50	10.0	> 50	2.5
Symptoms present	> 3/12	5.8	< 3/12	3.3
Weight loss (% of body)	< 15%	6.7	> 15%	3.3
Ascites	Absent	7.3	Present	1.4
Cirrhosis	Absent	10.0	Present	2.5
Aspartate transaminase (IU/l)	$< \times 2$	6.3	$\geqslant \times 2$	4.0
Bilirubin (μmol/l)	$< \times 2$	6.0	$\geqslant \times 2$	0.0

whether a more limited approach such as partial resection for carcinoid metastases or hepatic artery devascularization, could be considered. For lobar resection the tumour should be limited to one lobe in an otherwise normal liver. More extensive tumours could be treated by trisegmentectomy where only the lateral segment of the left lobe remains. These procedures are not usually possible in patients with underlying cirrhosis. Delineation of the tumour within the liver is also obtained with [99m]technetium sulphur colloid scanning. The demonstration of selective uptake of [75]selenomethionine within the filling defects is seen with HCC but not with cholangiocarcinoma or other primary liver tumours. Both ultrasound examination and computerized axial tomography (CAT-scan) of liver can give information on the extent and nature of the tumour (particularly in the distinction from cyst or abscess), but comparative information as to their respective values and also their use in relation to scanning procedures and arteriography is not yet available.

Detailed investigation for metastatic spread, which occurs mainly to lymph nodes, lung and skeleton, is vital in the initial assessment because it will determine broad separation between surgical and medical forms of therapy as well as being of major importance in prognosis. Small metastases are particularly difficult to detect in the lymph nodes of the porta hepatis and para-aortic areas. Detection may be aided by inferior vena cavography and abdominal lymphangiography, although CAT-scan could replace these procedures. It is essential to include whole lung tomography in screening for pulmonary metastases and in the examination for skeletal metastases bone scintiscanning should be carried out in addition to the conventional skeletal X-ray survey.

Metabolic assessment should not be overlooked as HCC can be associated with various endocrine systemic manifestations; hypercalcaemia, due to release of a parathyroid hormone-like protein from tumour cells, is the commonest. Hypoglycaemia, due to secretion of metabolites with insulin-like activity, and polycythaemia due to the release of an erythropoietin-like substance from the tumour are rare in Great Britain and USA although found in many cases in the Far East. Primary liver tumour may present as hypercalcaemic crisis, and measurement of serum calcium level is imperative in a patient with encephalopathy since this may otherwise be attributed to liver failure. Similarly low blood sugar levels in a patient with HCC will explain a history of recurrent fainting. Proof that hypercalcaemia is HCC-associated requires the demonstration by radioimmunoassay of an elevated serum parathormone. The hypercalcaemia usually responds to oral corticosteroid therapy.

Response to therapy can be assessed clinically, serologically and radiologically. Improvement in patients' well-being, loss of abdominal pain and weight gain are useful subjective clinical indicators, while a palpably smaller liver, loss of jaundice and/or ascites are objective signs of response. We use the Karnovsky scale (Karnovsky, 1961) to assess changes in the patients' activity. Changes in α-fetoprotein are of the greatest significance and assay should be carried out at least every four weeks. Serial isotopic liver scanning can be particularly helpful in patients being treated by surgery to assess the degree of regeneration or appearance of new deposits in remaining liver. Where tumour has apparently regressed, according to these various markers, hepatic arteriography is repeated. Complete disappearance of malignant vascularity may be observed.

Treatment

Hepatic resection

In some patients reasonable pallation has been obtained with resection. Some survivors after resection have lived between 10 and 21 years, but it can only be used in the few patients in whom the tumour is restricted to one lobe and where there is no evidence of extrahepatic spread. In one series, a 33% operative mortality rate has been quoted despite the employment of prior hilar dissection (Brasfield *et al.*, 1972) and individual ligation of the lobar branches of portal vein and hepatic artery. However, Fortner *et al.* (1974), using the technique of lobectomy by complete vascular isolation initially, thus reducing blood loss, and cold perfusion, describe only two operative deaths from 33 resections from liver cancer.

In a review of the world literature, Foster (1970) analysed results obtained from over 300 resections published in 25 reports of adult HCC; 24% died in the perioperative period and of 227 adequately followed up, 33% survived two years. Survival was significantly better in non-Asians than in Asians, a 59% two-year survival and 36% five-year survival compared with 23% and 6% respectively. As 8% of the non-Asians had cirrhosis compared with 74% of the Asians, survival figures may relate to a higher mortality of hepatic resections in cirrhosis. Indeed, except in HCC seen in the Far East, clinical experience would indicate that resection is contra-indicated in cirrhosis. In children, results appeared better: 80·4% of 46 primary liver tumours resected in Foster's unit, all without cirrhosis, survived operation and 43% of survivors lived for two years and 18% for five years. Other series worthy of note include that of Adson and Sheedy (1974) who report a favourable outcome to a series of 30 resections in adult patients, all but two non-cirrhotic. Of those with adequate follow-up, 84% survived for three years and 46% five years; 53% had either died or developed recurrent tumour, but 3 of 4 patients treated over ten years before were still alive. Among 23 cases of primary liver cancer in Japanese patients resected by Honjo and Mizumoto (1974) between 1951 and 1973, overall operative mortality was 9%, and 22% survived for three years and 13% for five years. Unfortunately, separate survival figures for the cirrhotic group were not included but one cirrhotic patient lived for 17·4 years after the resection, only to die in a road traffic accident. Interestingly, 16 of the 19 adults described by Foster who survived five years following resection had either left lobectomy or left lateral segmentectomy, suggesting that tumour confined to the left lobe may behave less aggressively. Most recently Starzl *et al.* (1975) described the technique of 'hepatic trisegmentectomy' which is an extended right lobectomy leaving only the lateral segment of the left lobe. This involves resecting over 85% of the liver. Most of their cases were HCC patients deemed unresectable by standard right lobectomy who had been referred for transplantation, but whether such radical methods of resection

for right lobe lesions improve survival remains unproven.

Cholangiocarcinoma
Intraheptic cholangiocarcinoma might be expected to present with localized resectable disease. Reviewing almost 200 cases, McBride (1976) reported a 26% incidence of cholangiocarcinoma and noted that all with unresectable disease died within eight months, while one patient resected survived five years.

Metastatic liver disease
Foster (1970) in a review of 166 resections for metastatic liver cancer, including 51 of his own cases, noted a 17% operative mortality. Two-year survival was 48% and five-year survival 21%, and survival was similar in the sub-group with primary colorectal tumours. Three of 6 patients whose primary tumour was a Wilm's tumour survived two, four and a half and five and a half years. There were no survivors at five years following resection when the primary tumour was in the stomach (30% initial survivors). Where resection was carried out for spread of adjacent tumour from gastric or colonic cancer (*en bloc* resection), Foster noted that 2 of 14 patients lived for nine years and one for six years. Eleven of 14 with extension from primary gall-bladder cancer died within two years, the three survivors living for three, three and a half and five years.

Survival was improved if the interval between surgery of the primary tumour and detection/resection of hepatic metastases was long. When this was greater than two years, mean survival was 35 months, as compared with 23 months when both resections coincided. Five-year survival rates were 31% and 12·5% respectively. Good results are reported by Adson and Van Heerden (1980).

Devascularization techniques

Hepatic artery ligation
Hepatic neoplasms, both primary and metastatic, derive the bulk of their blood supply from the hepatic artery, although a significant portal vein supply to metastatic lesions may sometimes exist (Breedis and Young, 1954). Hepatic artery ligation has been found to have significant palliative effect in both HCC and metastases especially in combating pain. In the early years, operative mortality rate approached 60% but now this figure is significantly less. Kim *et al.* (1973), using hepatic artery ligation from 1951 to 1971, noted a 6·8% operative mortality and, although Foster (1970) reported four deaths following hepatic artery ligation in 23 patients with unresectable liver cancer, none of the deaths could be attributed to the ligation.

Pre-operative hepatic arteriography is essential to

delineate the exact arterial supply of the tumour. Collateral tumour supply from other branches of the coeliac axis may also be discovered. The aim must be to ligate close to the liver so as to ensure complete devascularization but this may be very difficult technically with marked enlargement of the liver. The gall-bladder should be removed as there is a significant risk of necrosis from infarction. In addition, penicillin needs to be administered because of the risk of clostridia and similar organisms invading necrotic areas. A patent portal vein is also a pre-requisite. Ultrasound examination of the upper abdomen may also be used pre-operatively to detect portal vein patency and the portal vein should also be palpated at the time of surgery before ligation is carried out. Although ligation is dangerous if the portal trunk is obstructed, there have been patients with HCC in whom hepatic dearterialization was safely and successfully performed although one portal vein branch was occluded by tumour invasion or thrombus. An underlying cirrhosis and/or marked hepatocellular dysfunction associated with the tumour are also contra-indications to hepatic artery ligation.

Xenon injections studies have shown that after hepatic artery ligation blood flow through tumour is almost totally stopped. Revascularization occurs within days from capsular vessels and along the major blood vessels at the hilum. Arteriography at 4–6 weeks has delineated collateral supply from the phrenic, intercostal, coeliac and superior mesenteric artery. Although tumour necrosis of varying degree is induced, some viable tumour usually persists, especially in sub-capsular areas. Metastases may be affected even more than HCC, particularly when cytotoxic drugs are infused into the portal vein following the procedure. This was done in a series of patients with hepatic metastases from primary colonic tumours (Murray-Lyon *et al.*, 1970). Elevated liver enzymes were noted in the blood in all cases following the procedure, the tumour necrosis was demonstrable in four follow-up liver biopsies. Most gained weight and defervescence occurred in 7 of 8 cases where pyrexia was attributable to the presence of liver metastases. A mean survival of 10·7 months was achieved and two patients survived over two years.

Some idea of the benefits of ligation can be obtained from the history of one of our patients (Johnson *et al.*, 1978). A 29-year old garage mechanic was referred to hospital for investigation of non-specific complaints of faintness and sweating with right-sided abdominal pain occurring two or four times a day. Liver scan showed a filling defect in the left lobe and hepatic arteriography demonstrated a corresponding area of increased malignant-type vascularity. Both HB_sAg and α-fetoprotein were detectable in serum. At laparotomy in October 1975, a tongue of tumour mass extended posteriorly into the right lobe, precluding left lobectomy. Instead, two hepatic artery branches to the left lobe were ligated and the patient returned home to await transplantation which was performed three months later. Pathological examination of the removed liver revealed that there was massive necrosis of the tumour with only a rim of viable hepatocellular carcinoma cell remaining. Recovery was relatively uncomplicated and he has returned to work on standard immunosuppressive therapy and remains well 2·75 years later, and is still HB_sAg-negative. Nevertheless, despite the usefulness of ligation, it has largely been replaced by recent techniques for embolization of the hepatic artery by which similar results can be achieved without the need for surgery.

Embolization of the hepatic artery

This is achieved by injecting emboli under fluoroscopic control at the time of diagnostic hepatic arteriography, until blood flow ceases. The procedure has been widely used in the management of primary tumours at other sites (head, neck, colon), either pre-operatively to reduce both blood loss and risk of disseminating viable cells while handling the tumour at operation, or as a palliative procedure in unresectable cases. As with hepatic artery ligation, it can greatly relieve the pain of hepatic tumours, whether primary or secondary, by reducing tumour bulk. Embolization is preferable to surgical ligation not only because anaesthesia and laparotomy are avoided but subsequent growth of collateral circulation is less likely or at least delayed, as occlusion is induced at the periphery. A variety of embolizing agents have been used such as blood clot, sub-cutaneous fat, muscle fragments, oxycel, wool, cotton, steel balls, lead shot, plastic or glass beads, radioactive particles, wire springs, tantalum powder, silicone compounds, instantly setting polymers, isobutyl-2-cyano-acrylate, balloon catheters and 'Lyodura' (lyophilized dura mater). The ideal agent should be sterile, should be easily injected, should not precipitate sensitivity reactions and, while dispersible, should maintain occlusion of the vessel. Gelatin foam, thrombin, or 'Lyodura' are currently most favoured. Side-effects from the procedure include pain over the liver for the first 24–48 hours, inadvertent embolization of other tissue, passage of emboli to lung via large arteriovenous shunts, adherence of the catheter tip to the vessel wall if instant-setting polymers are used, and sensitivity reactions to the embolizing agents injected. Systemic or local infection of the necrotic area with abscess formation may occur, retrograde propagation of thrombus and release of active humoral agents from infarcted tumour masses, especially in the carcinoid syndrome are other complications. We have treated two patients with histologically-proven HCC employing gelatin foam and thrombin for embolization (Wheeler *et al.*, 1978). In both, α-fetoprotein levels fell precipitously. Subsequently, adriamycin therapy was initiated when the levels had plateaued at a low level. Both remain well and symptom-free, four and six months later (Fig. 21.2).

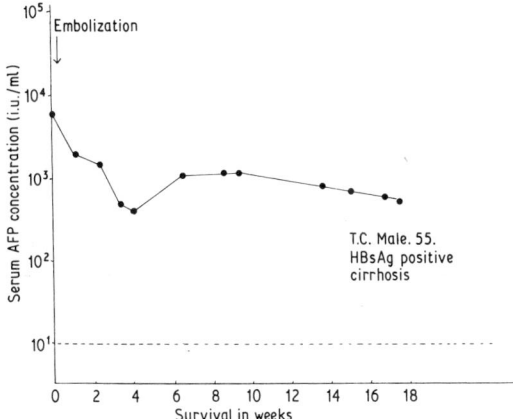

Fig. 21.2 Changes in α-fetoprotein (AFP) concentration after hepatic artery embolization followed by intravenous adriamycin therapy in T.C., a 55-year old West Indian with hepatoma secondary to HbsAg positive chronic active hepatitis.

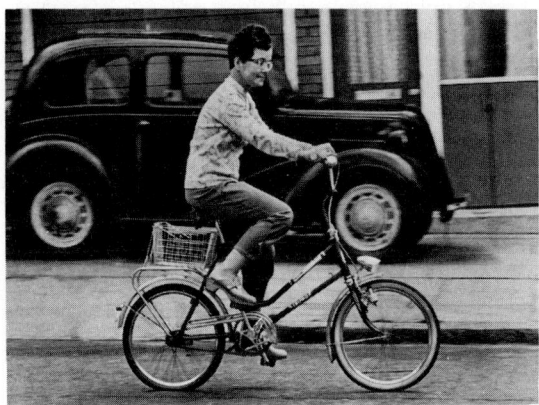

Fig. 21.3 In 1971, when she was 31 years old, R.W. underwent a hemihepatectomy for a primary hepatocellular carcinoma apparently confined to the left lobe of the liver. She remained well until early 1974 when evidence of tumour recurrence in the remaining lobe was detected. Transplantation was carried out shortly afterwards and during the 4·5 years since transplantation she has led an active life. The biliary tract anastomosis had to be reconstructed in June 1975 because of calculi within the biliary tract.

Liver transplantation

In both the Cambridge/King's College Hospital (McDougall and Williams, 1978) and Denver groups (Putnam *et al.*, 1977) improved results have been achieved in recent years, attributable to better methods of biliary drainage and recipient selection. To date, 30 HCC patients have received a transplant in the Cambridge/KCH series. Twenty-eight of these have died, 7 during operation or in the early post-operative period, and 21 at a later stage. Three of the 7 who died perioperatively had residual tumour at autopsy and 13 of the 21 late deaths had tumour at autopsy, either residual or recurrent, giving a 43% recurrence rate. Both patients who are still alive are tumour-free and well. There have been six survivors of over one year (20% one-year survival rate) and two of these are still alive and have reached 2·75 and 4·5 years (Fig. 21.3). In addition, 7 achieved good palliation in that they were discharged from hospital and resumed normal activity, surviving up to 11 months. Our longest survivor (5·5 years) died from cholangitis and septicaemia and had no evidence of tumour recurrence at autopsy. In our experience, one of the major problems in selecting HCC patients for transplantation is in the exclusion of small metastases, particularly at the porta hepatis and in the lung.

A review of the Denver experience (Putnam *et al.*, 1977) showed that of 117 transplants, 12 patients with primary hepatoma were treated. In addition, 2 children selected for transplantation for intrahepatic biliary atresia were found to have small hepatoma in the removed liver. One of these is still alive and well eight years later, the only survivor. Of those operated on for HCC, 7 patients died soon after transplantation from complications unrelated to their malignancy. The other 5 developed tumour recurrence and died 87 to 432 days after transplantation.

One of the dramatic results of transplantation is the prompt disappearance of endocrine manifestations associated with the tumour. In one of our patients whose hypercalcaemia was demonstrably related to secretion by the tumour of a metabolite immunologically similar to parathyroid hormone (PTH), abnormal serum calcium and PTH levels returned to normal within 36 hours of transplantation (Fig. 21.4). In another with massive hepatic metastases and severe hypoglycaemia, normoglycaemia was demonstrated from the time of anastomosis.

One problem that appears to have been satisfactorily overcome is the prevention of hepatitis B reinfection of the donor liver in the HBsAg-positive recipient. Three patients in the Cambridge/King's group have been successfully treated with anti-HBs immunoglobulin immediately following removal of the infected liver,

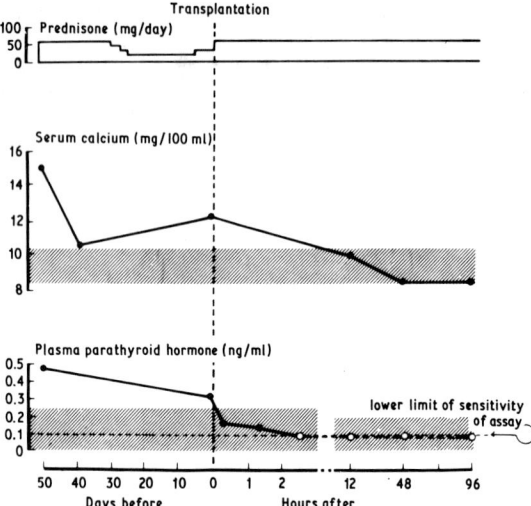

Fig. 21.4   Serum calcium and plasma parathyroid hormone levels in a patient with hepatoma-associated hypercalcaemia before and after treatment by hepatic transplantation (from Knill-Jones *et al.*, 1970).

including the patient already referred to with the familial HCC. Following this, HBsAg titres fell to low levels in serum and eventually cleared completely.

In the few patients treated by transplantation for metastatic liver disease tumour recurrence occurred rapidly and this applies also to cholangiocarcinoma. From 1963 to 1975 in all centres combined, 23 cases of cholangiocarcinoma have had liver transplants and of 5 then alive, survival ranged from 3 to 23 months. Of those who had died, only 4 survived more than 3 months and two of these died from tumour recurrence at 8 months. Our group has treated 4 cases of intrahepatic cholangiocarcinoma and 8 cases of extrahepatic high duct carcinoma (Klatskin tumour). Only 2 patients survived one year and, with most of the early deaths there was recurrence also.

Radiotherapy

There are diverse reports on the value of radiotherapy. No intrahepatic tumour can be considered truly radiosensitive. In a small group of African patients with histologically proven HCC, Geddes and Falkson (1970) found significant prolongation of survival – six months from commencement of therapy compared with two months for symptomatically treated patients. In contrast, when combined with chemotherapy (procarbazine or hydroxyurea), radiotherapy failed to aid survival in another small group.

Since we had treated some patients with apparent

improvement we carried out a controlled clinical trial in which radiotherapy followed by chemotherapy was compared with similar chemotherapy (Cochrane *et al.*, 1977). Radiotherapy was applied using ^{60}Co γ-rays to three fields – right anterior, posterior oblique, and left anterior oblique, giving a total tumour dose of 3000 rad in three to four weeks. Mean survival in the radiotherapy group was three months and only 2 survived to enter the chemotherapy phase, 1 of whom developed extensive pulmonary metastases and died within three months and the other died of massive ascites after four courses of chemotherapy. Whereas 60% of those, initially given chemotherapy were alive at three months, only 37% given radiotherapy survived to three months and none were alive at seven months. Forty per cent of those treated with chemotherapy were still alive at seven months (Fig. 21.1). Dose-related radiation hepatitis is a complication seen with dosage exceeding 3000 rad and its detection is difficult when liver function is already deranged either as a result of tumour or the presence of underlying cirrhosis. Although prolonged remission may be achieved in the occasional patient, overall the results in this trial can only be considered as disappointing and the use of radiotherapy for unresectable HCC has for the present been superseded by developments in cytotoxic drug therapy (see later). Delay in beginning radiotherapy may also be the reason for poor results and radiotherapy may still be of value *after* initial chemotherapy.

Cytotoxic drug therapy

5-Fluorouracil (5-FU)
This has some effect in patients with HCC and in those with metastatic liver disease but most series reported contain only small numbers of patients. Response has been seen in 40% of 28 patients with HCC (Carter and Livingstone, 1970). Three of 8 patients with biopsy-proven HCC treated by Moertel (1974) with once weekly intravenous 5-FU achieved measurable response. In contrast, Link *et al.* (1977) found that 5-FU (15 mg/kg body weight) given intravenously once weekly to a mean total dose of about 6g over a mean of 1·5 months had no significant effect in 10 patients with HCC. Absorption of 5-FU after oral therapy has been demonstrated to be variable and unsatisfactory. However, Kennedy *et al.* (1977) treated 12 patients with unresectable HCC with 15 mg oral 5-FU/kg body weight once weekly in a controlled trial. Fifty per cent responded with over 30% decrease in liver size and one patient was cured of recurrent hypoglycaemia. Survival was significantly improved in these patients – a mean of eleven months compared with one month in untreated patients. In contrast, Link

et al. (1977), comparing oral with i.v. 5-FU, found no objective or symptomatic response in 10 patients using 15 mg/kg weekly as an oral dose.

Metastatic liver tumour

Lahiri *et al.* (1971) have reported an uncontrolled trial of oral 5-FU (15 mg/kg body weight once weekly after an initial six day induction course) in hepatic metastases of colorectal primary tumours. Eight of 14 patients had evidence of partial tumour regression while 3 went into complete remission with complete disappearance of hepatic metastases on scanning, this being maintained in one patient for over a year. Therapy was less effective in treating pulmonary or skeletal metastases. Hahn *et al.* (1975) found, in a double-blind controlled trial, that oral 5-FU was equivalent to i.v. 5-FU for hepatic metastases using a 5-day course 5 times weekly on the basis of response at 2·5 months although blood levels after oral 5-FU therapy were erratic. Moertel (1974) similarly found that response rates for oral and i.v. 5-FU were similar.

Intra-arterial infusion of cytotoxic drugs

Some success has been reported for infusion of cytotoxic agents directly into the tumour mass via the hepatic artery whether at open celiotomy or by retrograde transfemoral closed catheterization. Hepatic and superior mesenteric arteriography is initially performed to determine which artery supplies the tumour. Complications of the technique are common, especially thrombosis of the common hepatic artery. Goldman *et al.* (1975) describe some degree of thrombosis in 34%, completely occluding the artery in 10%. Systemic heparinization has not been found to reduce the incidence of thrombotic complications. Catheter displacement occurs occasionally and there have been case reports of peritonitis following this. The largest and, so far, most favourable report is that of Cady and Oberfield (1974) who review a 14-year experience with 5-fluorodeoxyuridine (5-FDU) by arterial infusion. Intra-arterial 5-FDU was continued as long as arterial and catheter patency was arteriographically demonstrable, i.e. for a mean of 8·5 weeks. Five patients (28%) died from complications of the technique, but 4 of those deaths occurred in the early part of the series. Symptomatic improvement, largely pain relief, was seen in 61% and substantial improvement was achieved in 44%, with overall mean survival periods improving to 16.5 months for males and 8 months for females. Misra *et al.* (1977) in an uncontrolled trial in Indian patients report a median survival of 8·2 months (range 3–16 months) using a combination of 5-FU and mitomycin. Median survival for the responders was 7·2 months and for 21 with histologically proven hepatic metastases similarly treated was

9·4 months. Fifty per cent had failed to respond to systemic chemotherapy with the same agents. Of 13 patients with primary cancer of the gall-bladder and liver secondaries, 70% achieved objective response with a decrease in liver size and sustained fall in serum AST and alkaline phosphatase levels. McIntyre *et al.* (1976) report prolonged survival (mean 7 months) and diminishing α-fetoprotein levels in 5 of 8 patients with HCC given intra-arterial methotrexate, although none had clinical or radiological evidence of tumour regression. Geddes and Falkson (1970) found significant prolongation of survival using intra-arterial methotrexate in a group of Bantu patients with HCC (mean survival of 9·75 months compared with 2 months in controls). El Domeiri and Mojab (1978) compare their experience infusing 5-FDU alone with a combination of initial chemotherapy and intermittent hepatic artery occlusion achieved by twice daily inflation of a balloon catheter over a three-week period. They believe this to be superior to hepatic artery ligation, as a limited period of warm ischaemia is more likely to destroy tumour cells than damage normal liver. There was no major difference in survival between the two groups, 50% of all patients living 18–30 months and some showing clinical and radiographic evidence of partial tumour regression. Most recently, in a controlled trial, Bern *et al.* (1978) have shown a similar response duration following either intra-arterial or intravenous adriamycin. Intra-arterial infusion did not protect against the most important systemic side-effects.

Combination chemotherapy

Geddes and Falkson (1970) have reviewed results of various chemotherapeutic agents given either orally or intravenously to 127 Ugandan patients with biopsy-proven HCC. The sub-groups unfortunately contained only small numbers of patients (less than 10). Single courses of cyclophosphamide, hydroxyurea, mitomycin-C, actinomycin-D etc. were ineffective and various combinations, including quadruple chemotherapy (methotrexate, 5-mercaptopurine, procarbazine and vincristine) likewise. In the controlled trial carried out on this unit already referred to, combination chemotherapy (5-FU 500 mg, cyclophosphamide 500 mg, methotrexate 50 mg and vincristine 2 mg) was given intravenously as a single bolus once every three weeks. Dosage was adjusted if there was evidence of myelosuppression or if body weight fell below 50 kg. Patients were randomly allocated to receive either combination chemotherapy alone or radiotherapy for two months initially, followed two months later by similar chemotherapy. Patients with severe disease (Grade B) did poorly with mean survival of 1·25 months for chemotherapy alone and 2 months for radiotherapy and chemotherapy combined.

However, in patients with less severe disease (Grade A category) median survival was 13·5 months after chemotherapy alone but only six months after chemotherapy and radiotherapy. One of these patients survived 18 months, while none of the patients given radiotherapy was still alive, 40% of the chemotherapy group were surviving.

Adriamycin

Of all the cytotoxic agents used singly or in combination for HCC, the most encouraging and consistently reported success has been with intravenous adriamycin (doxorubicin).

The first reported use of adriamycin in hepatoma was that of Tormey *et al.* (1973) who achieved significant results using it in combination with bleomycin. In 1975 Olweny *et al.* reviewed their experience in an uncontrolled trial of 14 African subjects employing a regimen of 75 mg/m² intravenously every three weeks. All 11 patients adequately completing the course, showed evidence of at least partial remission, with at least 50% reduction in bulk of measurable tumour. In three patients apparently complete regression occurred and α-fetoprotein became undetectable, remission lasting 3, 6 and 7 months, and the patients surviving 8, 9 and 13 months respectively. At this dosage, three patients developed severe myelosuppression and one died from gram-negative septicaemia. In 1977 Vogel *et al.* reported a joint study of 19 Bantu patients and 29 patients living in the USA with HCC, employing a regime of 20–75 mg/m² intravenous adriamycin three weekly, the dose being varied according to serum bilirubin level, and degree of myelosuppression observed. Only 3 of 18 patients given 20 or 35 mg/m² responded, but 4 of 7 Zambians with advanced disease in whom dosage was increased to 60 mg/m² achieved definite response, as did 4 of 16 given 75 mg/m². Disease 'stabilization' was noted in 4 others, with disappearance of tumour-related polycythaemia in 1. Myelosuppression was more severe and frequent at a regimen of 75 mg/m² with one death from gram-negative septicaemia.

We have treated 44 patients with HCC between January 1976 and October 1977, at a dosage of 60 mg/m² three weekly to a total dose of 550 mg/m² (Johnson *et al.*, 1978). If serum bilirubin was raised above normal, only 50% of the standard dose was used and if the serum bilirubin was over twice normal, only 25% was given. Similarly, if total leucocyte count fell below 2000/μl or platelet count below 100 000/μl dosage was halved and if leucocyte count fell below 1000/μl or platelets below 50 000/μl dosage was reduced to 25% of the standard dose. Thirty-two per cent showed an objective response with loss of pain, weight gain and decrease in liver size. Twelve of the 14

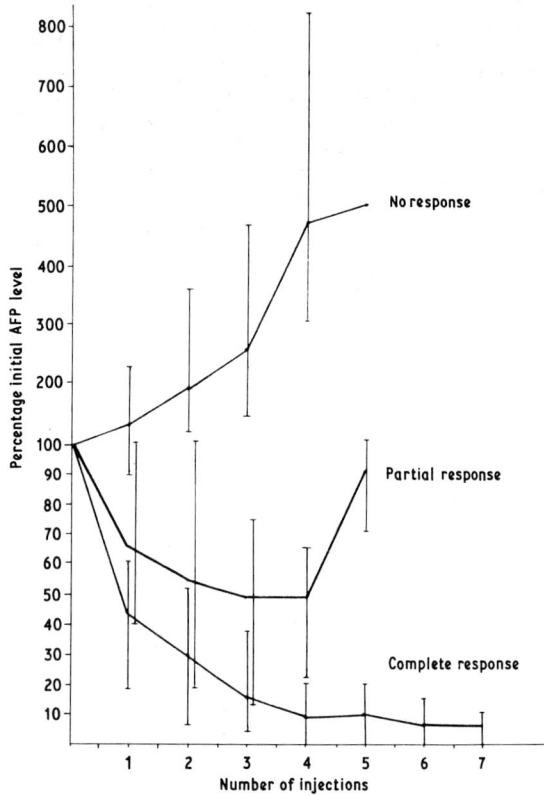

Fig. 21.5 Mean and range of α-fetoprotein levels expressed in percentage of level at presentation in patient showing complete, partial and no response.

responders were α-fetoprotein positive. Levels fell within 3 weeks of the first infusion in 11 and following the second injection in the other. The extent of the fall in AFP levels was also related to the completeness of the response (Fig. 21.5). In the 4 AFP-positive patients who achieved a complete clinical response, levels fell by more than 80% (Fig. 21.6). Five of 14 patients responding to chemotherapy were considered to have achieved a complete clinical remission, having lose all clinical indicators of HCC, surviving 12, 12, 16, 20 and 24 months, still alive today. Falkson *et al.* (1978) report encouraging results.

VP 16-23

Encouraging results have recently been published by Cavalli *et al.* (1977) employing a podophyllotoxin derivative, VP 16-23. Twelve Swiss patients were treated in all, 6 with oral VP 16-23 100 mg/m² for 3 consecutive days weekly, and 6 with concurrent 5-FU intravenously. Five of 11 with measurable tumour

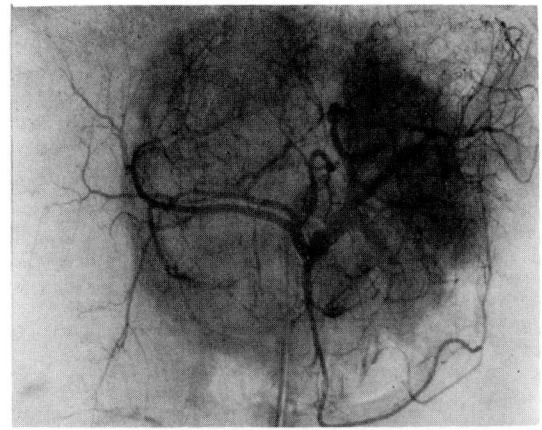

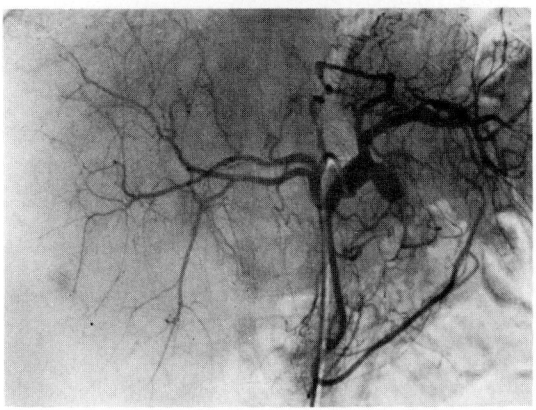

Fig. 21.6 Hepatic arteriograms before (upper) and after (lower) a complete course of adriamycin (550 mg/m²) in a patients with hepatoma superimposed on alcoholic cirrhosis, who remains well at 30 months after presentation.

criteria responded with objective weight gain, diminution in liver size and changes in α-fetoprotein levels. Responders showed a median survival of 7·2 months compared with 1·5 months in those not showing response. Myelosuppression was not seen.

Therapy of hepatic carcinoid

As the pharmacological mediators of the symptoms of the carcinoid syndrome, 5-HT, histamine, kallikrein and prostaglandins are normally metabolized by the liver, the occurrence of carcinoid syndrome where the primary tumour is intestinal, is synonymous with the presence of hepatic metastases. The presence of hepatic carcinoid does not imply poor life expectancy and about 25% survive five years. Symptoms usually benefit from the use of adrenergic blockade (for flush-

ing) and anti-serotonin agents (methysergide, parachlorphenylalanine, cyproheptadine) for diarrhoea but, where still troublesome, other treatment has to be considered. Most of the modes of therapy previously described for primary liver tumour have been tried in therapy of liver carcinoid metastases.

Hepatic resection has yielded remissions of up to two years in small numbers of cases reported. As the carcinoid is usually multilobar in distribution, complete removal by lobectomy is rarely possible and the aim is to resect as much as possible to give relief from the major effects of the carcinoid syndrome. Murray-Lyon *et al.* (1970) have reported on the results of hepatic artery ligation and intraportal cytotoxic infusion in three cases of the malignant carcinoid syndrome. Symptom remission was achieved for 2, 5, 5 and 5 months with survivals of 2, 5, 12 and 16 months respectively (Fig. 21.7). The first patient developed a carcinoid crisis in the immediate post-operative period and prior intra-arterial chemotherapy combined with methysergide and flufenamic acid, a kinin inhibitor, is essential in patients with severe symptoms to ensure a more controlled release of pharmacologic mediators from tumours. Bengmarck *et al.* (1974) describes a technique of intermittent temporary dearterialization aimed to give controlled ischaemia, avoiding carcinoid crisis. Reports of successful hepatic artery embolization for liver carcinoid have recently appeared.

Most of the reported cytotoxic experience is with systemic 5-FU and periods of objective remission have in general been short. Some response has also been achieved with streptozotocin, singly or in combination, although Moertel (1975) found this incomplete. There is one report of rapid regression of extensive metastatic

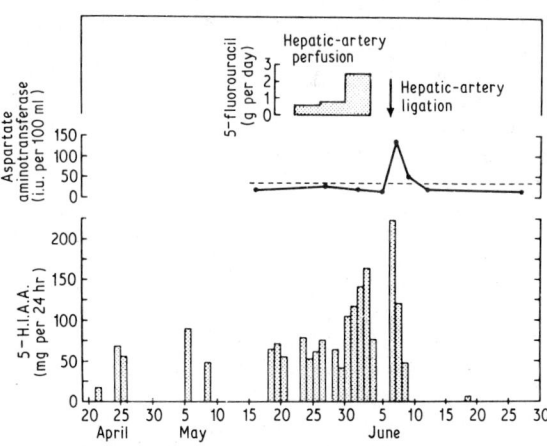

Fig. 21.7 Serial measurement of 24-hour urinary 5-HIAA levels before and after hepatic artery infusion of 5-FU followed by hepatic artery ligation.

liver carcinoid on three separate occasions using a combination of adriamycin, cyclophosphamide and methotrexate. Moertel has found no response to actinomycin-D, phenylalanine mustard, fluoromethalone, mitomycin-C and a combination of 5-FU and BCNU. Both surgery and chemotherapy may precipitate an intractable, potentially fatal carcinoid crisis, usually heralded by constant intense flushing, rapidly rising urinary 5-HIAA levels with rapid evolution of coma, failing to respond to serotonin antagonists. Caution is needed therefore when giving initial chemotherapy.

Further reading

Bagshawe, A.F. (1975), Hepatocellular carcinoma. In: *Modern Trends in Gastroenterology*, Butterworths, Burough Green, pp. 115-34.
Foster, H. and Berman, Martin M. (1977), *Solid Liver Tumours*, Vol. XXII of Major Problems in Clinical Surgery, W.B. Saunders Co., Philadelphia, London and Toronto.
Kahan, B.D. (1981), Cosmos and Damian in the 20th century. *New Eng. J. Med.*, **305**, 280-1.
Okuda, K. and Peters, R.L. (1976), *Hepatocellular Carcinoma*, John Wiley and Sons Inc.

References

Adson, M.A. and Sheedy, P.F. (1974), Resection of primary hepatic malignant lesions, *Archs Surg.*, **108**, 599-604.
Adson, M.A. and Van Heerden, J.A. (1980), Major hepatic resections for metastatic colorectal cancer. *Ann. Surg.*, **191**, 576-83.
Bengmarck, S. (1974), Hepatic arterial ligation, *Prog. Surg.*, **13**, 141.
Bern, M.M. *et al.* (1978), Intra-arterial hepatic infusion and intravenous adriamycin for treatment of hepatocellular carcinoma. *Cancer*, **42**, 399-405.
Bloom, K.R. *et al.* (1978), Echocardiography in adriamycin toxicity. *Cancer*, **41**, 1265-9.
Brasfield, R.D., Bowden, L. and McPeak, C.J. (1972), Major hepatic resection for malignant neoplasms of the liver. *Ann. Surg.*, **176**, 171-7.
Breedis, C. and Young, G. (1954), The blood supply of neoplasms in the liver. *Am. J. Path.*, **30**, 969-85.
Cady, B. and Oberfield, R.A. (1974), Arterial infusion chemotherapy of hepatoma. *Surgery, Gynec. Obstet.*, **138**, 381-4.
Carter, S.K. and Livingstone, R. (1970), *Single Agents in Cancer Chemotherapy*. Plenum Publishing Corporation, New York, pp. 217-8.
Cavalli, F. *et al.* (1977), Therapie resultate mit VP 16-213 allein oder kombiniert mit 5-FU beim

leberzellkarzinoma. *Schweiz. Med. Wschr.*, **107**, 1960-4.
Cochrane, A.M.G. *et al.* (1977), Quadruple chemotherapy versus radiotherapy in treatment of primary hepatocellular carcinoma. *Cancer*, **40**, 609-13.
El Domeiri, A. and Mojab, K. (1978), Intermittent occlusion of hepatic artery and infusion chemotherapy for carcinoma of liver. *Am. J. Surg.*, **135**, 771-81.
Falkson, G. *et al.* (1978), Chemotherapy studies in primary liver cancer. *Cancer*, **42**, 2149-56.
Fortner, J.G., Shiu, M.H. and Kinne, D.W. (1974), Major hepatic resection using vascular isolation and hypothermic perfusion. *Ann. Surg.*, **180**, 644-52.
Foster, J.H. (1970), Survival after liver resection for cancer. *Cancer*, **26**, 493-502.
Geddes, E.W and Falkson, G. (1970), Malignant hepatoma in the Bantu. *Cancer*, **25**, 1271-8.
Goldman, M.L. *et al.* (1975), Complications of indwelling chemotherapy catheters. *Cancer*, **36**, 1983-90.
Hahn, R.G., Moertel, C.G. and Schutt, A.J. (1975), A double blind comparison of intensive course of 5-FU by oral versus intravenous route in the treatment of colorectal carcinoma. *Cancer*, **35**, 1031-5.
Honjo, I. and Mizumoto, R. (1974), Primary carcinoma of the liver. *Am. J. Surg.*, **128**, 31-6.
Johnson, P.J. *et al.* (1978), Induction of remission in hepatocellular carcinoma with Adriamycin. *Lancet*, **i**, 1006-9.
Johnson, P.J. *et al.* (1978), Familial HbsAg-positive hepatoma: treatment by orthoptic liver transplantation and specific immunoglobulin. *Br. Med. J.*, **1**, 6107-10.
Karnovsky, D.A. (1961), Meaningful clinical classification of therapeutic responses to anti-cancer drugs. *Clin. Pharmacol. Ther.*, **2**, 2709-21.
Kennedy, P.S., Lehane, D. and Smith, F.E. (1977), Oral fluorouracil therapy of hepatoma. *Cancer*, **39**, 1930-5.
Kim, D.K., Kinne, D.W. and Fortner, J.G. (1973), Occlusion of the hepatic artery in man. *Surgery, Gynec. Obstet.*, **136**, 966-8.
Knill-Jones, R. *et al.* (1970), Hypercalcaemia and increased parathyroid hormone activity in a primary hepatoma: studies before and after transplantation. *New Engl. J. Med.*, **ii**, 704-8.
Lahiri, S.R., Boileau, G. and Hall, J.C. (1971), Treatment of metastatic colorectal carcinoma with 5-fluorouracil by mouth. *Cancer*, **28**, 902-6.
Link, J.S. *et al.* (1977), 5-Fluorouracil in hepatocellular carcinoma: 21 cases. *Cancer*, **39**, 1936-9.
McBride, C.M. (1976), Primary carcinoma of the liver. *Surgery*, **80**, 322-7.
McDougall, B.R.D. and Williams, R. (1978), The

indications for orthotopic liver transplantation. *Proc. Int. Cong. Transplant. Soc.*, **9**, 247-51.

McIntyre, K.R., Vogel, C.L. and Primack, A. (1976), Effect of surgical and chemotherapeutic therapy on alpha fetoprotein levels in patients with hepatocellular carcinoma. *Cancer*, **37**, 677-83.

Misra, N.C. *et al*. (1977), Intrahepatic arterial infusion of a combination of mitomycin-C and 5-flourouracil in treatment of primary and metastatic liver carcinoma. *Cancer*, **39**, 1425-9.

Moertel, C.G. (1974), Letter. *J. Am. Med. Assoc.*, **229**, 1109.

Moertel, C.G. (1975), Clinical management of advanced gastrointestinal cancer. *Cancer*, **36**, 675-82.

Murray-Lyon, I.M. *et al*. (1970), Treatment of secondary hepatic tumours by ligation of hepatic artery and infusion of cytotoxic drugs. *Lancet*, **ii**, 172-5.

Olweny, C.L.M. *et al*. (1975), Treatment of hepatocellular carcinoma with Adriamycin: preliminary communication. *Cancer*, **36**, 1250-7.

Primack, A. *et al*. (1975), A staging system for hepatocellular carcinoma: prognostic factors in Ugandan patients. *Cancer*, **35**, 1357-64.

Putnam, C.W. *et al*. (1977), Progress on liver transplantation. *Wld. J. Surg.*, **1**, 165-75.

Starzl, T.E. *et al*. (1975), Hepatic trisegmentectomy or extended right lobectomy: relation to other liver resections. *Surgery, Gynec. Obstet.*, **141**, 429-37.

Tormey, D.C. *et al*. (1973), Preliminary trials with a combination of Adriamycin (NSC 123127) and Bleomycin (NSC 125066) in adult malignancies. *Cancer Chemother. Rep.*, Part I, **57**, 413-8.

Vogel, C.L., Bayley, A.C. and Brooker, R.J. (1977), A phase II study of Adriamycin (NSC 123127) in patients with hepatocellular carcinoma. *Cancer*, **39**, 1923-30.

Wheeler, P.G. *et al*. (1978), Tumour devascularisation by embolisation in conjunction with doxorubicin for induction of remission in hepatocellular carcinoma. *Brit. Med. J.*, **2**, 242-5.

22 Kidney

Brigit van der Werf-Messing
and Fritz H. Schroeder

Incidence

The incidence of renal cell carcinoma varies from country to country: it is highest in Denmark (incidence per 100 000: 7.7 males, 6.3 females) and lowest in Japan (ratio of incidence male : female = 1.5 : 0.6). There is no reported increase during the last decades (Doll *et al.*, 1970). It constitutes about 2% of all malignancies (Everson and Cole, 1966), and occurs usually in the age group above 50 years, the average age being about 55 years. Up to 1972 renal cell carcinoma has been reported in 60 children.

Aetiology

An association between contact with cadmium and the incidence of renal cell carcinoma has been reported by Kolonel (1976). A relationship has been suggested between smoking and this malignancy. The low incidence amongst Jews and Japanese has been associated with diet (Wynder, 1974).

Anatomy

This short description will only include surgically and oncologically important parts of the renal anatomy. Both kidneys are positioned retroperitoneally; the left kidney stands higher than the right one. The upper pole superimposes the twelth rib. The kidneys are enveloped by a double fascial system: the fascia renalis or renal capsule which surrounds the kidney tightly but can be separated from the parenchyma, and the fascia retrorenalis (Gerota, Zuckerkandl). The retrorenal fascia unites ventrally into the peritoneum, and can dorsally be separated from the psoas fascia. It includes the adrenal glands and is cranially suspended at the diaphragm. The perirenal fat is ventrally interpositioned inbetween the renal capsule and the peritoneum, dorsally inbetween the renal capsule and the retrorenal fascia.

Adjacent organs on the right side are the adrenal, the vena cava, the liver, the duodenum, the colon ascendens and the diaphragm. On the left side the adrenal gland, the aorta, the spleen and its pedicle, the tail of the pancreas, the colon descendens and the diaphragm are located closely to the kidney and may be involved by tumour.

The renal hilus is situated medially and contains three groups with usually a total of twelve calyces, the renal pelvis, the renal artery(ies) and vein (veins) with their branches, lymph vessels and nerves. Normally vein, artery and renal pelvis are found in this sequence in anterior-posterior direction.

The vascular supply differs between the right and left side. On the right the renal artery originates from the aorta, is long and runs dorsally to the vena cava. The right renal vein reaches the vena cava inferior without having any major accessories. The right renal vein is short. On the left side the renal artery originating out of the aorta is short. The vein has major accessory vessels: the left spermatic (ovarium vein), the adrenal vein, and the first lumbar vein. It crosses the aorta ventrally and connects to the vena cava. Vascular abnormalities are frequent (Fig. 22.1).

Lymphatic drainage

The first lymph node station, i.e. the regional lymph nodes, consists of the para-aortic (high infrarenal and suprarenal) nodes, the para-aortic low nodes, for the right kidney of the lateral caval nodes and for the left kidney of the renal vein nodes. The second station, the juxtaregional nodes, comprises the common iliac nodes, the external iliac nodes, the mediastinal and the supraclavicular (usually left) nodes. The routes of preference for tumours in the lower part of the kidney are the anterior renal pathways, for the middle and the superior part of the kidney respectively the middle and posterior renal routes (Fig. 22.2).

Table 23.4   Prognosis after external megavoltage irradiation.

Author	Type of external irradiation	5-year survival by T-category		
Sagerman *et al.* (1965)	4 Field technique or rotation technique including bladder and regional lymph nodes (in deeply invading ca.): 6000 rad to pelvis + 1000 rad booster to bladder/6–8 wk, 200 rad/day	$B_1 + B_2$	(76)	32%
		C	(46)	25%
		D_1	(54)	3%
Rider and Evans (1976)	3500 rad/16 f/3 wk to pelvis × lymph nodes incl. L2 + bladder 1500 rad/5 f/5 days	T_1	(142)	58%
		T_2	(120)	50%
		T_3	(162)	17%
		T_4	(74)	26%
Scanlon and Furlow (1970)	5000–5500 rad in 2 equally divided courses (3–4 wk rest) (2 or 3 fields, 10 × 10 cm or 8 × 8 cm)	T_4	(47)	19%
Finney (1971)	Fractionation 200 rad ⎫ 250 rad ⎬ 300 rad ⎭	T_2	(28) 18% (25) 20% (24) 29%	
Edsmyr *et al.* (1971)	Treated by ^{60}Co unit 6 Mev acc. between 1957–1964	T_2	(86)	34%
		T_3	(125)	25%
		T_4	(89)	7%
Morrison (1975)	4 portals, 20 daily fractions, all portals treated daily T_1 T_2: ⎧ 6250 rad fields covering bladder only Trial ⎨ 5500 rad ⎩ T_3: ⎧ 4250 rad fields covering whole pelvic cavity Trial ⎨ 5000 rad ⎩	$T_1 + T_2$ $T_1 + T_2$ T_3 T_3	2-year survival (44) 80% (46) 61% (45) 38% (40) 55%	
Goffinet *et al.* (1975)	5000 rad/5 wk via 4 portals to pelvis + 2000 rad/2 wk small field rotation to bladder or 7000 rad/7 wk rotation to bladder (less invasive cancer)	A	(33)	35%
		B_1	(68)	42%
		B_2	(123)	35%
		C	(95)	20%
		D_1	(65)	8%
Van der Werf (1978)	Palliative and curative treatment unsuitable for interstitial radium implant, because of tumour or bad condition 6000 rad/6 wk or 6500 rad/6½ wk, 200 rad/day	T_1	(86)	20%
		T_2	(119)	15%
		T_3	(290)	10%
		T_4	(396)	5%
		M_1	(124)	0%

Number of patients treated within brackets.

nal irradiation can be given either by multiple fields or rotation technique (Figs. 23.2*a*, *b*; 23.3.) A dose of at least 6000–7000 rad (or its biological equivalent) in about 7 weeks should be planned. As T_1 growths are only moderately radiosensitive and the dose of ionizing radiation which can be given to the tumour by external irradiation – without permanent damage to the healthy intrapelvic structures – is biologically much lower than the dose given by interstitial implant, cure rates, as present in the larger series, do not exceed 50%. However, in case of failure a cystectomy still can be performed, though with increased risk of morbidity due to the radiation changes in pelvic tissues.

Attempts to cure multiple or extensive T_1 growths by intracavitary application of solid or liquid sources of radioactive material have yielded promising results, but have not become widely accepted. If the general condition of the patient allows and if the patient does not object to mutilation, for multiple or large T_1 growths simple or radical cystectomy is the alternative therapeutic approach.

In spite of positive selection for surgery and negative selection for radiotherapy, treatment results after cystectomy and after radiotherapy do not differ significantly.

T_2

A category T_2 cancer, infiltrating into but not beyond the superficial muscle can occasionally be controlled by transurethral resection. However, most clinicians

Table 23.5 Prognosis after pre-operative irradiation followed by cystectomy (comparison with cystectomy only and with external irradiation only).

Author	Type of treatment	Type of growth T-Category		5-year survival	
Scott *et al.* (1973)	Non-randomized study:				
	1. 5000 rad/4–6 wk, field	O, A, B_1		(13)	69%
	size 7 × 7 cm 4–6 wk later	B_2, C		(11)	27%
	cystectomy				
	2. Cystectomy only	O, A, B_1		(19)	53%
		B_2, C		(7)	0%
Whitmore	1. 4000 rad/4–6 wk to true	O, A, B_1		(44)	36%
(1963, 1968, 1977)	pelvis;	B_2, C		(65)	30%
	1–3 m later cystectomy				
	2. Cystectomy only	O, A, B_1		(51)	43%
	(historical control group)	B_2, C		(89)	20%
	3. 2000 rad/1 wk;	T_3		(52)	39%
	after 1 wk radical cystectomy				
Prout *et al.* (1973)	Cooperative prospective randomized study:				
	1. 4500 rad/28–32 days,	B_2, C	tumour in cytological specimen	(39)	±29%
	varying technique,		no tumour in cytological specimen	(19)	51%
	4–8 wk later cystectomy	B_1, B_2, C		(99)	40%
	2. Cystectomy	B_2, C		(72)	25%
		B_1, B_2, C		(129)	27%
Van der Werf	4000 rad/4 wk, portal:	All cases T_3		(141)	50%
(1978)	until 1972: true pelvis	$T_3 \longrightarrow P_3$		(43)	20%
	after 1972: including juxta-	$T_3 \longrightarrow P_0\ P_1\ P_2$		(96)	60%
	regional nodes level L5				
	± immediately followed by	$T_3 \longrightarrow P_2$		(30)	45%
	cystectomy	$T_3 \longrightarrow P_1, P_{is}$		(24)	75%
		$T_3 \longrightarrow P_0$		(42)	60%
		$T_3 \longrightarrow Px$		(2)	
Miller (1977)	5000 rad/5 wk	T_3		±(69)	30%
	after 6 wk simple cystectomy				
	7000 rad/7 wk	T_3		(137)	±20%
	Randomized study				
	5000 rad/5 wk + simple	T_3		(35)	46%
	cystectomy				
	7000 rad/7 wk	T_3		(32)	16%
Wallace and Bloom	Prospective cooperative randomized study:				
(1976)	1. 4000 rad/4 wks followed by	All T_3		(98)	33%
	cystectomy after 4 wk	<60 years		(43)	±40%
	(including juxtaregional nodes				
	level L5)	P_0, P_{is}, P_1, P_2		(36)	±50%
		P_3, P_4		(41)	±25%
	2. External irradiations only	All T_3		(91)	21%
	4000 + 2000 rad/5 weekly	<60 years		(34)	±25%
	fractions of 200 rad				
Reid *et al.* (1976)	2000 rad/4 days +	P_3, P_4		(92)	35%
	radical cystectomy after 1 day	(pathological staging only)			

Number of treated patients within brackets.

Table 23.6 Effect of adjuvant systematic chemotherapy.

Author	Type of chemotherapy	Results
Prout *et al.* (1970)	Pre-operative radiation + cystectomy + randomized adjuvant 5-FU	*18-months' survival* (170) 5-FU 55% no 5-FU 66%
Yagoda *et al.* (1977)	Adriamycin	*Significant response*: (35) 14%
Murphy (1977)	5-FU (15 authors) Adriamycin (4 authors) Adriamycin + cyclophosphamide (Rosw. Mem.)	*'Response'* 26/74 30/87 8/15
Kenny *et al.* (1972)	Limited irradiation (2000–4500 rad) combined with 5-FU (150 cases) or hydroxyurea (20 cases)	*5-year survival by T-Category* T_3/T_4 (± 30?) 138% T_4/M_1 (± 140?) 2.2%

Number of treated patients within brackets

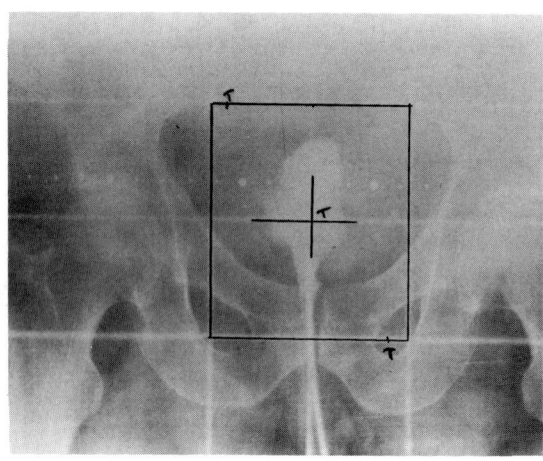

(a)   (b)

Fig. 23.2 Rotation irradiation of the urinary bladder. (*a*) X-ray showing the anterior view of the irradiation field. The bladder is partially filled with contrast. The outlines drawn on the film indicate the superior, inferior and lateral borders of the fields. (*b*) Lateral view of the irradiation field. The ventral border and the dorsal border of the field are drawn on the film.

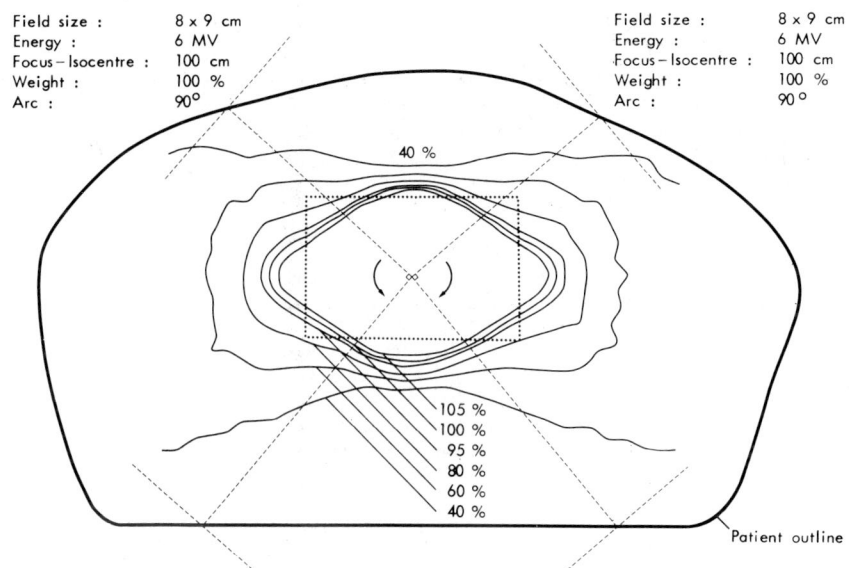

Field size :	8 x 9 cm
Energy :	6 MV
Focus – Isocentre :	100 cm
Weight :	100 %
Arc :	90°

40 %

105 %
100 %
95 %
80 %
60 %
40 %

Patient outline

Fig. 23.3 Technical data of rotation therapy planning of the urinary bladder. Patient outline and the target area (surrounded by a dotted line) are based on the X-rays presented in Figs. 23.2 (*a*) and (*b*). The isodose curves presenting isodose lines varying from 105% to 40% of the intended dose have been calculated by computer.

prefer a more radical approach with a higher chance of cure. Segmental resection can be indicated for a small cancer in the mobile part of the bladder. The most elegant and effective treatment is probably interstitial application of radioactive material for a solitary growth, not exceeding about 5 cm in diameter (Fig. 23.4). Since in the T_2 category the incidence of lymph node involvement is negligible, a local approach is the application of a very high dose of ionizing irradiation to the moderately radiosensitive primary, and irradiation with a low dose to the remainder of the bladder to destroy possible tentacular spread and pre-carcinoma, without significantly affecting the adjacent bladder structures. Interstitial treatment by implant of radioactive material will achieve this approach. The results of this non-mutilating procedure surpass those of cystectomy and of external irradiation. Addition of a short course (3 × 350 rad) pre-implantation external irradiation will reduce the incidence of iatrogenic metastases and abolish scar implants (van der Werf, 1969, 1978). If the general condition of the patient does not permit interstitial therapy or if the T_2 growth is too extended or multiple, a full course of external megavoltage irradiation can be considered. Various techniques (Figs. 23.5 *a*, *b*; 23.6) covering the bladder with a high dose and by some clinicians the adjacent external iliac and hypogastric nodes with a lower irradiation dose

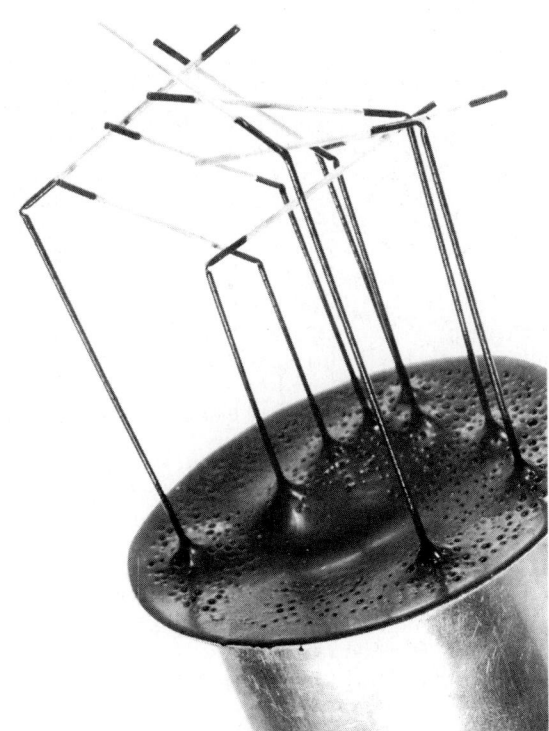

Fig. 23.4 Three-dimensional reconstruction of a one-plant implant in a bladder cancer, category T_2. In this reconstruction the radium needles are fixed on vertical metal bars. The reconstruction corresponds exactly to the situation in the bladder of the patient.

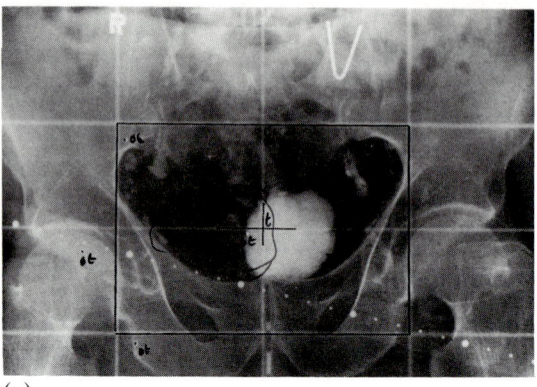

(a)

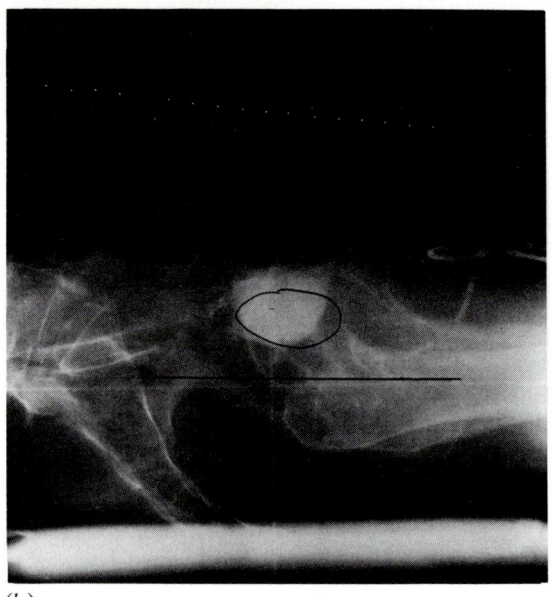

(b)

Fig. 23.5   Three-field irradiation technique for a bladder carcinoma category T₂. (a) Anterior view of the irradiation field. The bladder is partially filled with contrast. The assumed tumour site, the cranial, caudal and lateral borders of the field are drawn on the film. (b) Lateral view of the irradiation field. The ventral and dorsal border of the irradiated area and presumed tumour are drawn on the film.

will result in moderately satisfactory survival rates. If the general condition of the patient permits radical or simple cystectomy, this type of treatment should be considered as an alternative to a full course of external irradiation. The beneficial influence of pre-cystectomy irradiation in the T₂ category has not been proven. Many studies are underway and an answer to this problem can be expected within the next decade.

Cure rates after cystectomy or after a full course of external irradiation do not differ significantly, in spite of the patient selection.

T₃

A category T₃ cancer infiltrates into the deep muscle or the perivesical fat. Solitary small T₃ growths can be treated by interstitial implant similar to corresponding T₂ growths; however, these implants only cover the primary growth with a small margin, hence adjacent involved lymph nodes have only a minimal chance of being sterilized. Since the percentage of involved lymph nodes in T₃ growths approaches about 30%, cure rates exceeding 50% can hardly be expected by interstitial methods.

A full course of external megavoltage irradiation with doses comparable to 6000–7000 rad in 6–7 weeks to the bladder and the adjacent tissues (Figs. 23.5 a, b; 23.6) with or without lower doses to regional and juxtaregional lymph nodes, depending on the policy of the centre and on the selection of the patients, results in cure rates in nearly all large series varying between 20% and 30%. Radical cystectomy only has proven to

be most disappointing. The combination of pre-operative external irradiation followed by cystectomy is based on the following hypotheses.

The pre-operative irradiation might reduce the depth of infiltration of the growth, hence facilitating the complete removal of the primary; it might have a sterilizing effect on involved lymph nodes: the lymph node involvement is usually less massive than the carcinomatous bladder involvement and hence the cancer cells are less hypoxic and more radiosensitive; spill and iatrogenic lymphogenous and haematogenous dissemination might not result in metastases as theoretically the cancer cells have to some extent been 'devitalized' by the external irradiation. Various authors have demonstrated the beneficial influence of pre-operative irradiation: 4000 rad, in 200 rad daily fractions, given to the midline of the true pelvis by two opposing daily fields (Fig. 23.7) followed by cystectomy as soon as possible, or pre-operative irradiation of 2000 rad in 1 week seem to yield comparable results (Whitmore, 1977). As the results of pre-operative irradiation followed by simple cystectomy (van der Werf, 1971 a, b, 1973, 1975 and 1979; Miller, 1977), are at least as good as those of pre-operative irradiation followed by radical cystectomy (with lymphadenectomy), it is debatable whether lymphadenectomy is indicated at all. The beneficial influence of pre-cystectomy external irradiation is made clear by the fact that in those growths where the previous T₃ carcinoma has been reduced to a lower P-category, as seen microscopically in the cystectomy specimen, prognosis is considerably

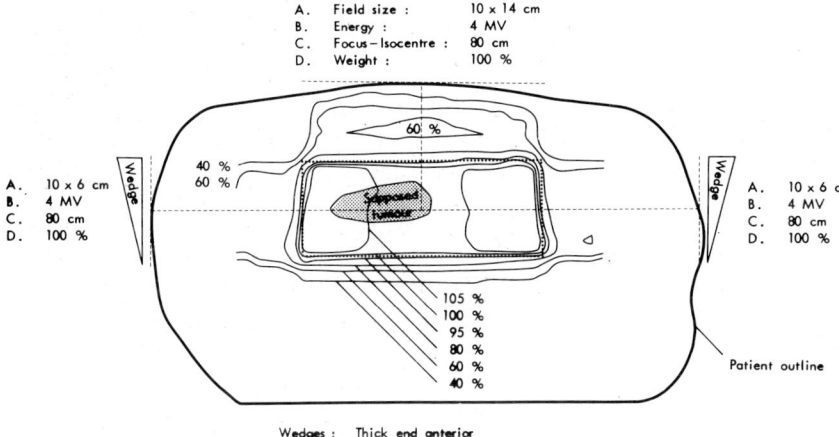

A. Field size : 10 x 14 cm
B. Energy : 4 MV
C. Focus – Isocentre : 80 cm
D. Weight : 100 %

A. 10 x 6 cm
B. 4 MV
C. 80 cm
D. 100 %

A. 10 x 6 cm
B. 4 MV
C. 80 cm
D. 100 %

Patient outline

Wedges : Thick end anterior
Nominal angle of isodose curve of wedged fields : 45°

Fig. 23.6 Technical data of a three-fields irradiation plan for a bladder cancer category T_2. One anterior and two lateral (wedge) fields are employed. The supposed tumour area has been drawn on the film; target area (surrounded by a dotted line) and patient outline are derived from X-rays (Figs. 23.5 *a* and *b*). The 105–40% isodose curves of the intended dose have been calculated by computer.

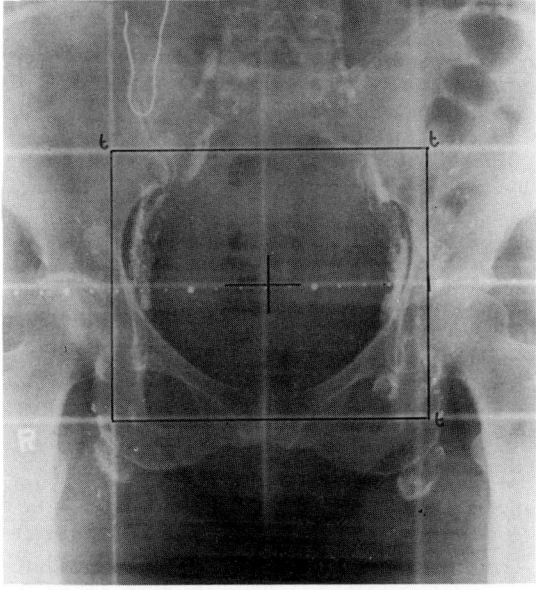

Fig. 23.7 Preoperative irradiation followed by cystectomy for bladder cancer category T_3: X-ray, showing the irradiation field. The lateral, cranial and caudal borders of the portal are drawn on the film. The dose, given by two opposing anterior and posterior fields, is calculated in the midplane of the patient.

better than in case of no such 'T-reduction' (van der Werf, 1971, 1973, 1975, 1979; de Weerd and Colby 1973; Prout *et al*., 1973; Wallace and Bloom, 1976).

The relationship of this 'T-reduction' to effects on possibly involved lymph nodes is confirmed by the fact that in the case of T-reduction (T_3 corresponds to P_0, P_{IS}, P_1, P_2) those who die during the follow-up period have a significantly lower incidence of clinical lymph node involvement than those patients who die without T-reduction ($T_3 = P_3$) (7% and 40% respectively) (van der Werf, 1975, 1978). Moreover, Wallace and Bloom (1976) found in a historical series of cystectomies about 30% lymph node involvement whereas after 4000 rad pre-operative irradiation this incidence had been reduced to 23% in the total group and to only 8% in the sub-group with T-reduction. This again supports the concept, that T-reduction indicates a beneficial influence of irradiation on involved lymph nodes.

Since prognosis with no 'T-reduction' is identical to that after a full course of external irradiation, it would be useful to find a criterion to identify after irradiation but before cystectomy, those patients in whom T-reduction has not occurred, in order to avoid mutilating cystectomy. Unfortunately so far attempts to do this have not been satisfactory (van der Werf, 1975, 1979).

Transabdominal lymph node cytology (Wallace *et al*., 1977) or lymph node biopsy (with frozen section microscopy) just cranial to the irradiation field, could, if yielding cancer cells, prevent mutilating unnecessary cystectomy since the prognosis is then nearly hopeless. Though additional chemotherapy might theoretically improve prognosis, by killing sub-clinical minimal metastases beyond the pre-operative irradiation field, a prospective clinical trial with adjuvant 5-FU has shown no such effect (Prout *et al*., 1968).

With increasing experience it is hoped that the complication and mortality rate will decrease. However, apparently, patients older than about 65 years, should not be submitted to this vigorous treatment (Wallace and Bloom 1976; van der Werf, 1978).

T₄

Category T₄ cancers are fixed to pelvis and/or infiltrate into other organs. In this category, external irradiation is the only justifiable curative treatment since radical surgery usually can not be complete. Moreover, the risk of lymph node involvement beyond the pelvis is considerable. In cases with good general condition a full course of external irradiation covering the whole bladder including the adjacent lymph nodes, using either two opposing fields or multiple fields, will result in a cure rate of about 5%. In highly selected patients with a T₄ growth, Rider and Evans (1976) achieved a cure rate of about 26% by including the regional and juxtaregional lymph nodes up to lumbar two in the irradiation field.

Radiotherapy combined with systemic chemotherapy – 5-FU and hydroxyurea – in a selected group of patients might improve prognosis (Kenny *et al*., 1972). If distant metastases (M₁) are present, local treatment of the bladder is still indicated, if the primary is causing symptoms. Transurethral resection or palliative irradiation (10 × 300 rad) might be sufficient to suppress bleeding and other local symptoms until death follows from metastases.

In women, intravaginal radium application can suppress symptoms for a long period – sometimes even permanently – from the primary in the bladder. Intravesical hyperbaric therapy, developed by Helmstein (1972), can effectively control bleeding and prolong life (England, 1973; Hirose *et al*., 1977; Hammonds *et al*., 1974).

Metastasis itself, such as painful bone lesions, can successfully be irradiated palliatively, alleviating pain and preventing fractures. A pulmonary metastasis approaching the size of 10 cm, the critical size for the onset of distressing bleeding, can be irradiated to prevent this.

Chemotherapy*

Chemotherapy for carcinoma of the urinary bladder has been in use since the earlier part of the twentieth century (Table 23.7).

Table 23.7   Uses of chemotherapy in bladder cancer.

Topical/intravesical therapy
Adjunctive to surgery/radiation therapy
Single agent therapy
Combination chemotherapy
Adjuvant chemotherapy
Radiosensitization
Intra-arterial perfusion

* Contributed by Haydn Bush

Topical installation of several agents has been used for non-invasive bladder cancer typical results being reported by Riddle (1973).

5-Fluorouracil was used adjunctive to surgery and radiation therapy in the early 1960s. Two prospective randomized studies suggested that there was no added survival but that the incidence of distant metastases could be reduced (Bush *et al*., 1979).

Arterial perfusion chemotherapy has been used by few authors and although palliative benefits have been claimed (Nevin *et al*., 1973; Burn, 1966; Ogata *et al*., 1973) for 5-fluorouracil, methotrexate and mitomycin-C used in this way, considerable technical skill is required; there is no good evidence that arterial perfusion is superior to systemic therapy.

Many single agents have been used in the therapy of advanced bladder cancer (Table 23.8). Strict criteria of response have seldom been used and Yagoda has attempted to identify these agents which consistently produce objective responses. So far three agents appear to fulfil these criteria – adriamycin, methotrexate and cis-platinum (Yagoda, personal communication).

Recent results suggest that cis-platinum may be one of the more active agents in bladder cancer (Table 23.9).

The place of combination chemotherapy in the management of bladder cancer is not yet established. In a continuing series of studies Yagoda (Table 23.10) has evaluated a number of single agents and combinations in 211 patients with measurable disease (lymph nodes, lung metastases, liver, skin and subcutaneous metastases). Only 2/211 patients had complete responses and cyclophosphamide appeared to confer no advantage over cis-platinum alone. These early results suggest that the combination of adriamycin and cis-platinum may produce a higher rate of objective responses. Einhorn, using the combination of cis-platinum, adriamycin and 5-fluorouracil has produced 14 objective responses in 27 patients with advanced bladder cancer (52%). In this small series the overall duration of response was 6.6 months, the median survival of the overall group was 9.0 months whilst responders survived somewhat longer, 11.5 months.

More recent approaches to the management of invasive bladder cancer have involved the use of methotrexate for primary disease (i.e. prior to irradiation or surgery) with interesting preliminary findings (Oliver, personal communication). Table 23.11 shows the early results of the primary use of methotrexate and cis-platinum; 24% of the whole series achieved complete remissions as assessed cystoscopically and pathologically, and this opens up an exciting avenue for further study in the management of locally advanced primary bladder cancer.

Table 23.8 Response rates to single agents in bladder cancer (collected series) (from Bush *et al.*, 1979).

Drug	No. of patients	Average objective response (%)	Range
Methotrexate	88	24	17–36
Adriamycin	235	23	0–37
5-Fluorouracil	56	39	0–75
Cyclophosphamide	41	41	0–53
Mitomycin-C	50	20	16–33
Cis-platinum	24	35	–
Neocarcinostatin	15	66	–
Vincristine	20	30	–
Epipodophlyotoxin (VM26)	24	25	–

Table 23.9 Cis-Platinum as a single agent in bladder cancer.

Number of patients	Objective responses (number)	(%)	Author
17	8	47	Soloway
14	8	57	Merrin
33	11	33	Yagoda
Totals 64	27	42	

Five-year survival rates of only 30–40% in patients with T$_3$ bladder cancer, achieved with radiotherapy alone or with a combination of radiation and surgery, suggest that there is potential for adjuvant chemotherapy. Several such studies are now in progress (EORTC Urologic Study Group).

Summary

Progress in the management of advanced metastatic bladder cancer by chemotherapy is slow, but newer agents are now showing promise of producing consistent objective responses.

Areas of current major interest include the treatment of primary bladder cancer with chemotherapeutic agents, the use of adjuvant chemotherapy and the use of radiation-sensitizing agents.

Follow-up

After each treatment, regular cystoscopy follow-up has to be performed. Early recurrence can, according to the stage and extent of the recurrence and to the general condition of the patient, still be treated either with curative or with palliative intent. 'New' lesions might be discovered early and treated curatively. In case of a recurrence after transurethral resection only, or after radium implant, a full course of external irradiation or a cystectomy can still be performed, depending on the stage of the growth and on the condition of the patient. If routine follow-up cystoscopy is too great a burden for the patient, routine urine cytology with only occasional cystoscopy can be the alternative. Routine urine cytology can also lead to the early diagnosis of a ureteral or renal pelvis cancer even though there is completely normal cystoscopic appearance of the bladder. Though theoretically each follow-up examination should include bimanual palpation under general anaesthesia, it is debatable whether these older patients should be submitted to frequent anaesthesia. However, this is mandatory if there are suspicious findings on cystoscopy or palpation.

Table 24.8 Results of radical prostatectomy for prostatic carcinoma category T_3.

Author	Treatment		Survival in % 5 years	10 years	15 years
Flocks (1973)	Total perineal prostatectomy + interstitial irradiation + lymphadenectomy N_0 (–)	(68)	74.0	66.7	27.5
Scott and Boyd (1969)	Oestrogen pre-treatment + total perineal prostatectomy	(39)	74.4	60.6	29.0
Schroeder and Belt (1975)	Total perineal prostatectomy	(213)	64.0	35.9	20.3

(Number of patients treated within brackets)

Survival figures of T_1, T_2 patients are identical with the expected survival. The enthusiasm for these results must be limited because it is unknown whether the same could not be achieved with less effort and damage to the patient. An extremely low rate of local recurrences of 6.8% in Stage B and a low overall cancer mortality (11.5%) indicate the high efficiency of the operation in controlling the disease in this stage (Schroeder and Belt, 1975).

It can be seen from data in Table 24.8 that prostatic carcinoma in the T_3 category (Stage C) has a significantly worse prognosis than T_1, T_2. The results of surgical treatment of this tumour are superior to all forms of conservative management. However, patients eligible for radical surgery, are more highly selected than in the reference groups. The data of Flocks (1973) show that survival of T_3 (Stage C) patients can be further improved in those who have negative lymph nodes at the time of surgery. The combination with interstitial irradiation has produced the lowest rate of local recurrence ever reported.

The role of lymphadenectomy has already been discussed and it will be seen in the future whether this procedure has therapeutic importance.

The preliminary results of TUR alone and cryosurgery alone will not be discussed.

Radiation therapy
Many reports of external megavoltage treatment of prostatic cancer, are now available but comparison of results is hazardous in view of the differences in classification, selection and the details of radiotherapy technique. The 5-year survival rate in the category T_1M_0 and T_2M_0 (comparable to Stage B) varies between 70% and 90%. In the category T_3, T_4M_0 (Stage C), 5-year survival rates vary between 50% and 70% (Table 24.9). All authors confirm that in each T-category (or stage) poorly and undifferentiated growth has a significantly worse prognosis than dif-

ferentiated: differentiation improves prognosis by about 20%.

Variations in dose between 6000 and 7000 rad do not demonstrably influence prognosis. Additional hormone therapy has also not led to better survival. Systematic irradiation of all regional nodes has not convincingly resulted in better prognosis than irradiating the prostate with only adjacent periprostatic regional nodes.

After interstitial therapy, 5-year survival rates reached 100% in category T_1 and T_2 and dropped to 90% in selected T_3 and T_4 growths. (Table 24.10).

Conservative treatment
Results have been previously discussed and Table 24.11 summarizes some results of conservative management.

The results of chemotherapy are limited to 'partial objective responses' of short duration. Results of the most promising forms of treatment, with Estramustine phospate and cis-platinum, have been discussed in the chemotherapy section.

Reasons for failure of treatment

Surgery
Obviously, the most common reason for failure of attempts of radical removal of prostatic carcinoma is understaging. Locally, incomplete removal results in local recurrence at the level of the anastomosis of bladder-neck and urethra or behind the bladder. Local recurrence has been observed in the cited series to occur in 2–15% of the patients and is an ominous sign. In Belt's series (Schroeder and Belt, 1975) local recurrence was found in Stage B and C in 6.8 and 12.7% of the patients. Interstitial irradiation apparently controls residual tumour quite efficiently (Flocks, 1973). Transurethral resection is an effective means of palliative treatment of obstruction from local

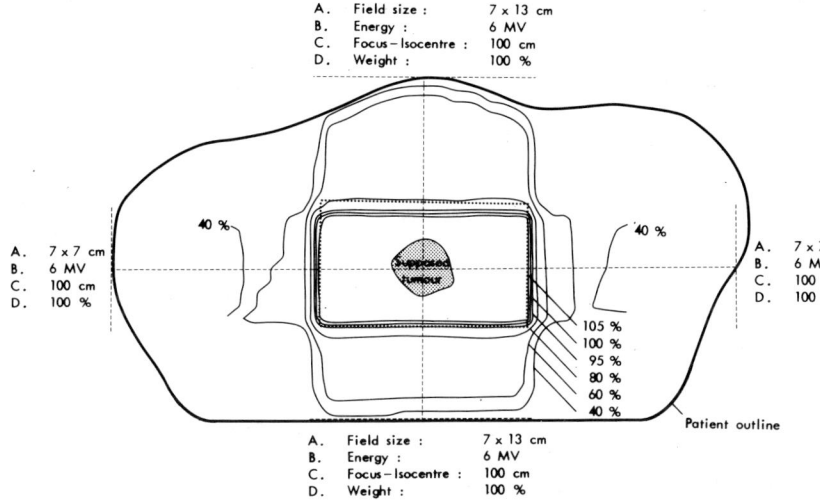

A. Field size : 7 x 13 cm
B. Energy : 6 MV
C. Focus – Isocentre : 100 cm
D. Weight : 100 %

A. 7 x 7 cm
B. 6 MV
C. 100 cm
D. 100 %

40 %

40 %

A. 7 x 7 cm
B. 6 MV
C. 100 cm
D. 100 %

105 %
100 %
95 %
80 %
60 %
40 %

Patient outline

A. Field size : 7 x 13 cm
B. Energy : 6 MV
C. Focus – Isocentre : 100 cm
D. Weight : 100 %

Fig. 24.5 Technical data of a 4-field irradiation planning of the prostate (2 lateral fields, 1 anterior and 1 posterior field). The data concerning patient outline and location of the tumour and the target area are based on the films presented in Figs. 24.4 (*a*) and (*b*). Isodose curves from 105–40% of the intended dose have been calculated by computer.

recurrence but carries a high risk of urinary incontinence.

Development of distant metastases after total prostatectomy usually leads to death within 1–2 years. All techniques of conservative management should be used. The presence of occult metastases at the time of treatment must be considered to be the reason for failure. The incidence of distant metastases and death from carcinoma should decrease after exclusion of patients with lymph node metastases identified through surgical staging. Table 24.1 illustrates the inherent treatment failure for T_1, T_2 and T_3 tumours if lymphadenectomy is not done. In addition, lymphadenectomy may have a therapeutic effect; the limits of curability of prostatic carcinoma are not clear at present.

Radiation therapy
The main reason for failure after external radiation therapy and after interstitial therapy is the clinical appearance of distant metastases. These might have come from a persistent primary growth (10% to 20%) or they might develop from sub-clinical metastases present at the time of first treatment. The latter reason applies mainly to undifferentiated and poorly differentiated growths. After interstitial therapy, Hilaris (1975) demonstrated that metastases will develop within 3 years in 60% of cases with lymph node involvement at more than one level, and in only 20% of those with less lymph node involvement, in spite of radical lymphadenectomy or additional regional lymph node irradiation.

The prognostic significance of positive prostate biopsy or transrectal prostate cytology after radiation therapy is still controversial. Kurth *et al.* (1977) found no metastasis in 66 patients in cases of negative prostate biopsy, whereas 12 out of 30 patients with biopsy proved residual growth developed metastases within 1–4 years. However, van der Werf-Messing (1978) and Cox and Stoffel (1977) could not establish a correlation between positive prostatic cytology or biopsy and the development of metastasis. There is no clear correlation between the clinical findings on palpation and the transrectal cytology results since fibrosis can mimic malignancy and normal findings might still coincide with positive cytology. The long local persistence of malignant cells might only reflect the long period which is required to remove killed cells of this slowly growing tumour. In case of local failure and/or distant metastases, hormone treatment is still applicable, hence radiation therapy offers the patient at least a postponement of hormone treatment up to several years; in a high percentage hormone treatment will never be necessary (relapse-free survival rates, Table 24.9).

Hormonal treatment
Failure of hormonal treatment is thought to be due to loss of hormone responsiveness of the carcinoma. The precise mechanisms are unknown, and parameters to determine the hormone dependence of individual tumours are unfortunately not yet available. Steroid receptor studies applied to prostatic carcinoma tissue have not yet shown a good correlation with prognosis. It has been thought that poorly differentiated carcinoma does not respond to androgen withdrawal but daily clinical experience demonstrates the contrary.

Table 24.9 Results after treatment of prostate cancer with external megavoltage irradiation with or without hormone or surgical treatment.

Author	Type of treatment and selection	Type of growth		Prognosis
Cantril (1974)	Megavolt photons 60% of patients: 7000–7500 rad/7–7.5 wks ± 40 patients: $^{60}Co/4$ MeV 4 fields/rotation to prostate + periprostatic tissue	$T_{3,4}M_0$ well differentiated poorly differentiated	(166) (71)	*5-year survival* 60% 30%
Edsmyr et al. (1974)	Megavolt photons 500 rad/5–7 wks 2 anterior wedge fields, 1 posterior field + Hormones Stilboestrol and/or Estradurin (all patients received antibiotics)	$T_{3,4}M_0$ poorly differentiated	(20)	3-year survival: 55% (2 patients interc.)

| | | | | *Survival* | |
				5-year	*10-year*
Bagshaw et al. (1975)	Megavolt photons 7000–7600 rad/7–7½ wks to prostate and periprostatic tissue (rotation or R + L lateral arc therapy)	Limited to prostate $(T_{1,2}M_0)$	(230)	72%	44%
		Extracapsular $(T_{3,4}M_0)$	(200)	51%	38%

| | | | | *5-y. survival with NED* | | *10-y. survival with NED* | |
				dissemination		*dissemination*	
Ray et al. (1975)	Megavolt photons Small field to prostate + periprostatic tissue ± 7000–7500 rad/7–7½ wks	Limited to prostate	(81)	72%	2% (28)	46%	4%
		Extracapsular extension	(82)	42%	6% (23)	26%	5%

| | | | | *Follow-up period 1–50 m (median: 22 m)* | |
				Disease-free	
Bagshaw et al. (1977)	Patients ≤ 70 years of age lymph node biopsy at laparotomy A. Nodes negative – randomized:	Stage A, B, C $(T_{1,2,3,4}M_0)$			
Megavolt photons	a. 7000 rad/7 wks to prostate b. a + pelvic nodes radiation 4000 rad/7 wks c. a + b + para-aortic radiation		(17) (18) (2) (37)	15 16 1 32	87%
	B. Pelvic nodes positive. – randomized: b. c.		(9) (5) (14)	7 3 10	72%
	C. Para-aortic nodes positive c.		(10)	3	30%
		Total	(61)	45	74%

| | | | | *5-year survival* | | |
				NED	*alive with tumour*	*dead with tumour*
Perez et al. (1977)	22 MeV photons	Stage C $(T_{3,4}M_0)$				
	total 7000 rad to prostate		(97)	42%	0	22
I (47)	total 6000 rad to true pelvis total 5000 rad to pelvis incl. L5					
II (50)	Idem + Hormone therapy (orchiectomy + oestrogens)		No difference between I and II			

Table 24.9 (continued)

Author	Type of treatment and selection	Type of growth	Prognosis
			5-year Survival
Taylor et al. (1977)	10 MeV photons	Stage C ($T_{3,4}M_0$)	(221) 58%
	whole pelvic fields + booster to prostate		Additional hormone therapy had no bearing on prognosis
Neglia et al. (1977)	22 MeV Photons	Stage $B_1C_1C_2$	Mean follow-up: 4 yr 7 m.
	I. 4 fields (10 × 10 cm to 12 × 15 cm)	(T_2M_0 : 4	5-year survival
	Trial 5000 rad/± 5 wks	T_4M_0 : 97	(79) 74.7% after radiation
	Prostate booster 1000–2000 rad	T_4M_0 : 53)	only
	via anterior + posterior field		(75) 61.3% after radiation
	additional hormones		+ hormones
	Randomized ⟨ DES 5 mg/day		No difference between 7000 rad
	no hormones		± 6000–6500 rad.
	II. Previous series (no trial): 6000–7000 rad/6–7 wks to true pelvis with or without hormones		No difference between 'small' and 'large' radiation-fields
			5-year survival NED
McGowan (1977)	Patients ≤ 75 years	A ($T_1N_0M_0$)	(21) 88% 84%
	Only patients with negative	B_1 ($T_2N_0M_0$)	(43) 90% 61%
	lymphography are included in	B_2 ($T_3N_0M_0$)	(30) 66% 43%
	study	C ($T_4N_0M_0$)	(13) 39% 37%
	^{60}Cobalt 6000 rad/6 wks, 5 fields daily		
van der Werf-Messing (1976)	Trial:	Stage C ($T_{3,4}M_0$)	5-year survival
	A. 1 mg Lynoral daily		(26) 65%
	B. 1 mg Lynoral daily + Megavolt photons 7000/7 wks by 2 opposing fields covering prostate and surroundings		(30) 55%

			Actual uncorrected survival			
			3-year NED		5-year NED	
van der Werf-Messing (1978)	Megavolt photons	T_3M_0 differentiated (40)	80%	65%	80%	65%
	4000 rad + 2 wks split + 3000 rad	T_3M_0 undifferentiated (15)	55%	35%	follow-up too short	
	4 portals to prostate and	T_4M_0 differentiated (22)	65%	65%	65%	63%
	surrounding tissue	T_4M_0 undifferentiated (7)	50%	25%	follow-up too short	

(Number treated within brackets)
(NED = no evidence of disease)

Future trends

The effectiveness and limitations of surgical treatment are well established. Progress can be made from prospective trials including an arm having no treatment, identifying patients who may not require any treatment and those who should be treated aggressively. The role of lymphadenectomy should be better defined by randomized trials.

Further research on new combinations and new dosage schemes might improve prognosis especially when there are metastases with low differentiation not responding to hormones. Combinations of chemotherapy with hormones and immunotherapy might be of value. When clinically demonstrable metastases are absent (M_0), elective adjuvant chemotherapy and immunotherapy might improve prognosis in high risk cases after radiation therapy and/or surgery. High risk groups are considered to be those with an undifferentiated growth or with regional lymph node involvement beyond the adjacent periprostatic region. This kind of vigorous elective com-

Table 24.10   Results of treatment of prostate cancer by interstitial radiotherapy.

Author	Type of treatment	Type of growth		Prognosis	
Flocks (1973)	Radical surgery + interstitial therapy (100 mCi ^{198}Au, 2 cc diluent)	$T_3, T_4 \, M_0$	(147)	*5-year survival* 60%	
Chan and Gutierrez (1976)	Gold grain implant (± 4000 rad) + external megavoltage to a total dose of ± 8000 rad	Stage C		*3-year survival*	*NED*
		normal acid phosph.	(13)	13	8
		abnormal acid phosph.	(3)	0	0
		Total Stage C	(16)	13/16	8/16
				All controlled locally	
Hilaris *et al.* (1977)	Retropubic bilateral lymphadenectomy + prostate implant with ^{125}I (16000 rad/1 year = 2030 rets)			*crude 5-year survival*	
		$T_1 \, M_0$	(65)	100%	
		$T_2 \, M_0$	(40)	100%	
	'limited'	$T_3 \, M_0$	(23)	77%	
		$T_4 \, M_0$	(80)	87%	
				actual 5-year survival	
		Lymph-nodes negative	(102)	92%	
		Lymph-nodes positive	(84)	46%	

(Number of patients treated within brackets)
(NED = no evidence of disease)

Table 24.11   Results of endocrine management of prostatic carcinoma.

Author	Tumour category	5-Year survival in %				Remarks
		No treatment or placebo	Oestrogens	Orchiectomy	Orchiectomy + oestrogens	
Barnes and Ninan (1972)	A/B (78)	–	60.6 5-year 36.0 10-year	–	–	+ TUR
Hanash *et al.* (1972)	B (129)	19.0 5-year 40.0 10-year 5.0 15-year	–	–	–	only TUR
VACURG (1967)	C (1362)	57.0	50.0	55.0	43.0	prospective, randomized
Nesbit and Baum (1950)	C/D (578)	10.2	29.0	31.2	43.6	retrospective, multicentric

(Number of patients treated within brackets)

bined modality treatment might well be worthwhile for patients in good general condition.

Radiation therapy might yield better results by different fractionation, by combination with radiosensitizers, and with hyperthermia. A mixture of all these approaches also has to be evaluated. Irradiation with neutrons and pi-mesons is theroetically promising in view of the supposed high percentage of anoxic cells in prostatic cancers. Pi-mesons have the additional advantage of sparing most surrounding tissues (Shipley *et al.*, 1979; Batata *et al.*, 1980).

CT-scan assessment of the extent of the primary, supported and supplemented by ultrasound data will be helpful in identifying cases most suitable for treatment. Immunochemical methods might contribute by sparing patients from too vigorous local therapy by early indication of sub-clinical metastases, and providing an opportunity for initial adequate systemic therapy (Chu 1978).

Organized screening procedures will contribute to detecting many early cases (category T_1 and T_2M_0). By randomizing those patients in a prospective trial comparing treatment (radiation therapy or surgery) with no treatment, knowledge would accrue of the need to treat these early cases; criteria might be assessed to help identify those early cases who benefit from treatment and distinguish them from those who have an excellent prognosis without any treatment.

Elective total body irradiation of high risk patients, who have a high risk of sub-clinical metastases, might postpone or even prevent the development of clinical metastases and thus postpone or preclude further hormone treatment or chemotherapy.

Further reading

Bagshaw, M.A. *et al*. (1975), External beam radiation therapy of primary carcinoma of the prostate. *Cancer*, **36**, 723-8.

Scott, W.W. and Schirmer, H.K.A. (1970), Carcinoma of the prostate. In: *Urology*, **2**, (eds M.F. Campbell and J. Hartwell Harrison), W.B. Saunders Co., Philadelphia, p. 1143.

References

Akazaki, K. and Stemmerman, G.N. (1973), Comparative study of latent carcinoma of the prostate among Japanese in Japan and Hawaii. *J. Nat. Cancer Inst.*, **50**, 1137-44.

Alsheik, H.I. *et al*. (1977), The effect of transurethral resection of the prostate on lymphocyte response in patients with prostatic cancer. *J. Urol.*, **118**, 1022-3.

Arduino, L.J. and Glucksman, M.A. (1962), Lymphnode metastases in early carcinoma of the prostate. *J. Urol.*, **88**, 91-3.

Bagshaw, M.A. *et al*. (1975), Extended-field radiation therapy for carcinoma of the prostate: a progress report. *Cancer Chemother. Rep.*, **59**, 165-73.

Bagshaw, M.A. *et al*. (1977), Evaluation of extended-field radiotherapy for prostatic neoplasm: 1976 progress report. *Cancer Treat. Rep.*, **61**, 297-306.

Barnes, R.W. and Ninan, C.A. (1972), Carcinoma of the prostate – biopsy and conservative therapy. *J. Urol.*, **108**, 897-900.

Barzell, W. *et al*. (1977), Prostatic adenocarcinoma: relationship of grade and local extent to the pattern of metastases. *J. Urol.*, **188**, 278-82.

Batata, M.A. *et al*. (1980), Radiation therapy in adenocarcinoma of the prostate with pelvic lymph node involvement on lymphadenectomy. *Int. J. Radiat. Oncol. Biol. Phys.*, **6**, 149-153.

Belt, E. and Schroeder, F.H. (1971), Oestrogenbehandlung des Prostatacarcinoms nach totaler Prostatektomie: Ueberlebensraten und Cardiovasculäre Komplikationen in den Serien von MELLINGER und BELT. *Urologe*, **A 10**, 56-8.

Belt, E. and Schroeder, F.H. (1972), Total perineal prostatectomy for carcinoma of the prostate. *J. Urol.*, **107**, 91-6.

Berlin, B.B. *et al*. (1968), Radical perineal prostatectomy for carcinoma of the prostate – survival in 143 cases treated from 1935 to 1958. *J. Urol.*, **99**, 97-101.

Bisson, J., Vickers, M. Jr. and Fagan, W.T. Jr. (1974), Bone scan: in clinical perspective. *J. Urol.*, **111**, 665-9.

Broders, A.C. (1926), Grading and practical application. *Arch. Pathol.*, **2**, 376-81.

Bush, R.B. and Bush, I.M. (1977), Early developments in the history of prostatic disorders. In: *Urologic Pathology: The prostate*, (ed. M. Tannenbaum), Lea and Febinger, Philadelphia, pp. 7-22.

Byar, D.P. (1977), VACURG studies on prostatic cancer and its treatment. In: *Urologic Pathology: The Prostate*, (ed. M. Tannebaum), Lea and Febinger, Philadelphia, pp. 241-67.

Byar, D.P. and Mostofi, F.K. (1972), Carcinoma of the prostate: prognostic evaluation of certain pathological features in 208 radical prostatectomies. *Cancer*, **30**, 5-13.

Cantril, S.T. *et al*. (1974), Radiation therapy for localized carcinoma of the prostate: correlation with histopathological grading. *Front. Radiat. Ther. Onc.*, **9**, 274-94.

Castellino, R.A. *et al*. (1973), Lymphangiography in prostatic carcinoma: Preliminary observations. *J. Am. Med. Assoc.*, **233**, 877-81.

Catalona, W.J. and Scott, W.W. (1978), Carcinoma of the prostate: A review. *J. Urol.*, **119**, 1-8.

Chan, R.C. and Gutierrez, A.E. (1976), Carcinoma of the prostate. Its treatment by a combination of radioactive gold-grain implant and external irradiation. *Cancer*, **37**, 2749-54.

Chisholm, D.G., O'Donoghue, E.P.N. and Kennedy, C.L. (1977), The treatment of estrogen-escaped carcinoma of the prostate with Estramustine phosphate. *Br. J. Urol.*, **49**, 717-20.

Chu, T.M. *et al*. (1978), Immunochemical detection of serum prostatic acid phosphatase: Methodology and clinical evaluation. *Invest. Urol.*, **15**, 319-23.

Cook, G.B. and Watson, F.R. (1968), Twenty single nodules of prostatic cancer not treated by total prostatectomy. *J. Urol.*, **100**, 672-4.

Cooper, J.F. *et al*. (1978), A solid phase radioim-munassay for prostatic acid phosphatase. *J. Urol.*, **19**, 388-91.

Cox, J.D. and Stoffel, T.J. (1977), The significance of needle biopsy after irradiation for stage C adenocarcinoma of the prostate. *Cancer*, **40**, 156.

Culp, O.S. and Meyer, J.J. (1973), Radical prostatec-tomy in the treatment of prostatic cancer. *Cancer*, **32**, 1113-8.

Dhom, G. and Hautumm, B. (1975), Die Morphologie des klinischen Stadiums O des Prostatacarcinoms (incidental carcinoma). *Urologe*, **A 14**, 105-11.

Edsmyr, F. *et al*. (1974), Carcinoma of the prostate; the place of radiotherapy. In: *Radiology*, Proc. 13th Int. Cong. Radiol., **2**, Madrid, 15-20 October 1973, (eds J. Gomez Lopez and J. Bonmati), Excerpta Medica, Amsterdam, pp. 63-6.

Einhorn, J. and Franzen, S. (1962), Thin needle biopsy in the diagnosis of thyroid disease. *Acta Radiol.*, **58**, 321-36.

Esposti, P.L, (1966), Cytologic diagnosis of prostatic tumours with the aid of transrectal aspiration biopsy. *Acta Cytol.*, **10**, 182-6.

Farnsworth, W.E. (1969), A direct effect of estrogens on prostatic metabolism of testosterone. *Invest. Urol.*, **6**, 423-7.

Faul, P., Klosterhalfen, H. and Schmiedt, E. (1971), Erfahrungen mit der Feinnadelbiopsie der Pros-tata. *Urologe*, **A 10**, 120–6.

Fergusson, J.D. and Hendry, W.F. (1971), Pituitary irradiation in advanced carcinoma of the prostate: analysis of 100 cases. *Brt. J. Urol.*, **43**, 514-9.

Flocks, R.H., Culp, D. and Porto, R. (1959), Lympha-tic spread from prostatic cancer. *J. Urol.*, **81**, 194-6.

Flocks, R.H. (1973), The treatment of stage C prosta-tic cancer with special reference to combined surgi-cal and radiation therapy. *J. Urol.*, **109**, 461-3.

Foti, A.G. *et al*. (1977), Detection of prostatic cancer by solid phase radioimmunassay of serum prostatic acid phosphatase. *New Engl. J. Med.*, **297**, 1357-61.

Franks, L.M. (1977), Etiology and epidemiology of human prostatic disorders. In: *Urologic Pathology: The Prostate* (ed. M. Tannenbaum), Lea and Febinger, Philadelphia, P. 23.

Franks, L.M. and Durh, M.B. (1956), Latency and progression in tumours. The natural history of pros-tatic cancer. *Lancet*, **ii**, 1037-9.

Gleason, D.F. (1966), Classification of prostatic car-cinoma. *Cancer Chemother. Rep.*, **50**, 125-8.

Gleason, D.F. (1977), Histologic grading and clinical staging of prostatic carcinoma. In: *Urologic Pathol-ogy: The Prostate* (ed. M. Tannenbaum) Lea and Febinger, Philadelphia, pp. 171-97.

Gleason, D.F., Mellinger, G.T. and the VACURG (1974), Prediction of prognosis for prostatic adenocarcinoma by combined histological grading and clinical staging. *J. Urol.*, **111**, 58-64.

Glenn, J.F. and Boyce W.H. (1969), *Urologic Surgery*. Hoeber, Harper and Row, New York.

Golimbu, M. *et al*. (1978), Presentation at the Ameri-can Urological Association Meeting, Washington, D.C. (submitted for publication to the *J. Urol.*).

Goodwin, W.E. (1953), Carcinoma of the prostate gland. *Calif. Med.*, **78**, 440-3.

Grayhack, J.T. (1963), Pituitary factors influencing growth of the prostate. *Nat. Cancer Inst. Monogr.*, **12**, 189-9.

Hanash, K.A. *et al*. (1972), Carcinoma of the prostate – A 15-year follow-up. *J. Urol.*, **107**, 450-3.

Harada, M. *et al*. (1977), Preliminary studies of histo-logic prognosis in cancer of the prostate. *Cancer Treat. Rep.*, **61**, 223-5.

Higgins, I.T.T. (1975), The epidemiology of the pros-tate. *J. Chron. Dis.*, **28**, 343-48.

Hilaris, B.S. (1975), *Handbook of Interstitial Brachytherapy*. Publ. Sci. Group, Acton.

Hilaris, B.S. *et al*. (1977), Behavioural patterns of prostatic adenocarcinoma following an iodine 125 implant and pelvic node dissection. *Clin. Bull.*, **7**, 168-9.

Huggins, C. and Hodges, C.V. (1941), I. The effect of castration, of oestrogen and of androgen injection on serum phosphatases in metastatic carcinoma of the prostate. *Cancer Res.*, **1**, 293.

Jacobi, G.H. *et al*. (1978), Bromocriptine and prostatic carcinoma: plasma, kinetics, production and tissue uptake of ^{3}H testosterone in vivo. *J. Urol.*, **119**, 240-3.

Jewett, H.J. (1956), Significance of the palpable pros-tatic nodule. *J. Am. Med. Assoc.*, **160**, 838-41.

Jewett, H.J. (1970), The case for radical prostatec-tomy. *J. Urol.*, **103**, 195-9.

Jewett, H.J. (1975), The present status of radical pros-tatectomy for stages A and B prostatic cancer. *Urol. Clin. N. Am.*, **2** (1), 105-24.

Jewett, H.J. *et al*. (1968), The palpable nodule of pros-tatic cancer. *J. Am. Med. Assoc.*, **203**, 403-6.

Jewett, H.J., Eggleston, J.C. and Yawn, D.H. (1972), Radical prostatectomy in the management of car-cinoma of the prostate: probable causes of some therapeutic failures. *J. Urol.*, **107**, 1034-7.

Khan, R. *et al*. (1977), Bone marrow acid phosphatase: another look. *J. Urol.*, **117**, 79-80.

Kimborough, J.C. (1956), Carcinoma of the prostate – five-year follow-up of patients treated by radical surgery. *J. Urol.*, **76**, 287-91.

Kipling, M.D. and Waterhouse, J.A.H. (1967), Cad-mium and prostata + carcinoma. *Lancet*, **i**, 730-1.

Kopecky, A.A., Laskowski, T.Z. and Scott, R. (1970), Radical retropubic prostatectomy in the treatment of prostatic carcinoma. *J. Urol.*, **103**, 641-4.

Kurth, K.H. *et al.* (1977), Follow-up of irradiated prostatic carcinoma by aspiration biopsy. *J. Urol.*, **117**, 615-17.

McGowan, D.G. (1977), Radiation therapy in the management of localized carcinoma of the prostate. A preliminary report. *Cancer*, **39**, 98-103.

McNeal, J.E. (1968), Regional morphology and pathology of the prostate. *Am. J. Clin. Pathol.*, **49**, 347–57.

Mayer, E.J. (1975), Orales Estracyt^R – Behandlung beim Prostatakarzinom. *Therap. Umsch.*, **32**, 114-19.

Merrin, C. (1978), Treatment of advanced carcinoma of the prostate (stage D) with infusion of CIS-diammine dichloroplatinum (II NSC 119875): A pilot study. *J. Urol.*, **119**, 522-4.

Mostofi, F.K. (1975), Grading of prostatic carcinoma. *Cancer Chemother. Rep.*, **1**, 111-7.

Murphy, G.P. (1977), Chemotherapy of advanced prostatic cancer. *Rev. Surg.*, **34**, 75-87.

Nagel, R. und Koelln, C.P. (1976), Behandlung des fortgeschrittenen Prostatakarzinoms mit Estracyt$_R$. *Med. Klin.*, **71**, 3-15.

Neglia, W.J., Hussey, D.H. and Johnson, D.E. (1977), Megavoltage radiation therapy for carcinoma of the prostate. *Int. J. Radiat. Oncol. Biol. Phys.*, **2**, 873-82.

Nesbit, R.M. and Baum, W.C. (1950), Endocrine control of prostatic carcinoma. Clinical and statistical survey of 1818 cases. *J. Am. Med. Assoc.*, **143**, 1317-20.

Perez, C.A. *et al.* (1974), Radiation therapy in the treatment of localized carcinoma of the prostate. Preliminary report using 22 MeV-photons. *Cancer*, **34**, 1059-68.

Perez, C.A. *et al.* (1977), Radiation therapy in the definitive treatment of localized carcinoma of the prostate. *Cancer*, **40**, 1425-33.

Pontes, J.E. *et al.* (1977), Indirect immunoflourescence for identification of prostatic epithelial cells. *J. Urol.*, **117**, 459-63.

Potts, C.L. (1965), Occupational exposure to cadmium and prostate carcinoma. *Ann. Occup. Hyg.*, **8**, 55-61.

Ray, G.R., Cassady, J.R. and Bagshaw, M.A. (1975), External-beam megavoltage radiation therapy in the treatment of post-radical prostatectomy residual or recurrent tumour; preliminary results. *J. Urol.*, **114**, 98-101.

Robinson, M.R.G. and Thomas, B.S. (1971), Effect of hormonal therapy on plasma testosterone levels in prostatic carcinoma. *Br. Med. J.*, **4**, 391-4.

Schroeder, F.H. and Belt, E. (1975), Carcinoma of the prostate: A study of 213 patients with stage C tumours treated by total perineal prostatectomy. *J. Urol.*, **114**, 257-60.

Schroeder, F.H., Belt, E. and Mostofi, F.K. (1978), Prostatic carcinoma; late results on 484 patients treated by total perineal prostatectomy. Unpublished data.

Scott, W.W. and Boyd, H.L. (1969), Combined hormone control therapy and radical prostatectomy in the treatment of selected cases of advanced carcinoma of the prostate: a retrospective study based upon 25 years of experience. *J. Urol.*, **101**, 86-91.

Shearer, R.J. *et al.* (1973), Plasma testosterone: An accurate monitor of hormone treatment in prostatic cancer. *Br. J. Urol.*, **45**, 668-77.

Shipley, W.U. *et al.* (1979), Proton radiation as boost therapy for localized prostatic carcinoma. *J. Am. Med. Assoc.*, **241**, 1912-15.

Silverberg, E. and Holleb, A.I. (1974), Cancer statistics, 1974 – worldwide epidemiology. *Cancer*, **24**, 2-21.

Tannenbaum, M. (1977), *Urologic Pathology: The prostate*, Lea and Febinger, Philadelphia.

Taylor, W.J., Richardson, R.G. and Hafermann, M.D. (1977), Radiation therapy of prostate cancer. *Int. J. Radiat. Oncol.*, **2**, Suppl. 2, abstr. 12 + 13.

Veenema, R.J., Lattimer, J.K. and Gursel, E. (1973), Prostate cancer treated by retropubic prostatovesiculectomy. *XVI$_e$ Congr. Soc. Int. Urol.*, Rapports 1, 103-8.

Veenema, R.J. *et al.* (1977), Bone marrow acid phosphatase; prognostic value in patients undergoing radical prostatectomy. *J. Urol.*, **117**, 81-2.

Veterans Administration Urological Research Group (VACURG) (1967), Treatment and survival of patients with cancer of the prostate. *Surgery, Gynec. Obstet.*, **124**, 1011-7.

Van der Werf-Messing, B., Sourek-Zikova, V. and Blonk, D.I. (1976), Localized advanced carcinoma of the prostate: radiation therapy versus hormonal therapy. *Int. J. Radiat. Oncol. Biol. Phys.*, **1**, 1043-8.

Van der Werf-Messing, B. (1978), Prostatic cancer treated at the Rotterdam Radiotherapy Institute. *Strahlentherapie*, **154**, 537-41.

Whitmore, W.F. and Mackenzie, A.R. (1959), Experiences with various operative procedures for the total excision of prostatic cancer. *Cancer*, **12**, 396-405.

Whitmore, W.F., Hilaris, B. and Grabstalt, H. (1972), Retropubic implantation of Iodine-125 in the treatment of prostatic cancer. *J. Urol*, **108**, 918-20.

Whitmore, W.F. Jr. (1973), The natural history of prostatic cancer. *Cancer*, **32**, 1104-12.

Wynder, E.L., Mabuchi, K. and Whitmore, W.F. Jr. (1971), Epidemiology of cancer of the prostate. *Cancer*, **28**, 344-60.

25 Urethra

Fritz H. Schroeder and Brigit van der Werf-Messing

Incidence

In 1834, Thiaudierre described the first urethral cancer (Hotchkiss and Amelar, 1954). This malignancy is extremely rare, no reliable incidence data are available. It is more frequent in female than in male (ratio varies between 4 to 1 and 10 to 1).

Aetiology

Cancer of the urethra has causally been related to strictures due to gonorrhoea and due to previous instrumentation. Iatrogenic implant after transurethral resection of papillary bladder cancers has also been suggested (Hendry, 1974; Richie and Skinner, 1978).

Primaries in the posterior part of the urethra (transitional cell carcinomas) have probably the same aetiology as bladder cancers.

Anatomy

In males about 75% of the urethral cancers are located in the prostatic and bulbomembraneous part of the urethra (posterior part) and about 25% in the penile and meatus region (anterior or pendulous part).

In females no exact data about the location are available in literature.

Lymphatic drainage

The regional lymph nodes of the anterior part of the urethra are the inguinal and the external iliac nodes. The posterior part of the urethra drains to the deep iliac and hypogastric nodes. The glans penis drains to the deep and superficial inguinal nodes (see Fig. 24.3).

Metastasis and natural history

In males, the primary urethral cancer, originating from the urethra epithelium, will infiltrate into the surrounding tissues. If located in the posterior part of the male urethra it will infiltrate into the prostate and into the bladder; if located in the anterior part spread by continuity will occur into the corpora cavernosa, the tunica and the skin.

In females, the labia, the anterior vagina and the parametria can be involved by continuity. Lymphatic spread to the regional lymph nodes usually occurs before the evidence of haematogenous metastases.

Haematogenous metastases are rare and occur late. Spontaneous regression has not been reported. Untreated urethral cancer will lead to death by local extension associated with infection; by uraemia due to lymph node involvement; by general cancer cachexia due to distant lymphatic and haematogenous spread.

If treated, the prognosis is usually better with anterior location of the malignancy, because of earlier diagnosis and greater accessibility for treatment (general prognosis after treatment for anterior cancers: 50% cure; for posterior cancers: 16% to 19% cure).

Pathology and histological classification

The urethra is covered by columnar epithelium. Foci of squamous cell metaplasia might lead to the development of squamous cell cancer, 88% of the cancers are squamous cell carcinomas with various degrees of differentiation. The remainder are transitional cell carcinomas in the posterior part of the urethra, with the same microscopic characteristics as bladder cancers. Adenocarcinoma is rare and usually originates from periurethral glands.

Symptoms and presentation

The main symptoms are bleeding (more than 50% of the cases), dysuria, discharge, dyspareunia, incontinence, urinary obstruction, a mass, fistula formation, and in the male haemospermia.

Diagnosis

By external palpation or rectal/vaginal palpation a mass can be diagnosed. Urethroscopy and urethrography can lead to the clinical diagnosis, transurethral biopsy, urine cytology and swab cytology from the urethra will confirm the clinical diagnosis.

Careful palpation of the inguinal nodes provides reliable information of carcinomatous involvement in case of anterior location of the primary (Grabstald, 1973), simply and correctly confirmed by biopsy or needle aspiration. To assess regional lymph nodes, in case of posterior location, lymphography can be useful.

Clinical classification and staging

There is no staging proposed by the International Union against Cancer or by the American Joint Committee.

Most clinicians propose a classification according to localization (anterior part and posterior part) and according to the depth of infiltration (Grabstald, 1973; Bracken et al., 1976; Chau and Green, 1965; Ray et al., 1977).

Treatment

Indications and treatment policies

An untreated urethral cancer will inevitably lead to death. Spontaneous regression has never been reported. In localized tumours curative treatments should be attempted. Both surgical and radiotherapeutical approach can be worthwhile if the growth is not deeply infiltrating and limited to the anterior part of the urethra. Elective treatment of the regional lymph nodes has not led to increased cure rates in these cases.

Palliative surgical or radiotherapeutic treatment in case of gross local involvement with or without clinical evidence of lymph node invasion is usually indicated in order to prevent pain, bleeding, infection and extreme discomfort due to the local mass.

Surgical treatment

Surgery is the oldest treatment for urethral cancer; transurethral resection or local excision is usually incomplete, especially in the posterior part of the male urethra. Partial or complete amputation cures about 50% of males with a not too deeply infiltrating growth in the anterior part. In females wide local excision of superficial growths and vulvectomy for deeper infiltrating malignancies may result in cure. However, quite often on microscopic examination of the operation specimen, surgery turns out not to have been complete.

Radiotherapy

Radiotherapy is mainly applied in females. Urethra cancer is only moderately radiosensitive. Its destruction requires a high dose of ionizing irradiation, whereas the surrounding tissues of the urethra are vulnerable to irradiation. Therefore interstitial radiotherapy, which gives a high dose to the growth and spares largely the surrounding tissues, is the method of choice, especially in growths limited to the anterior third of the urethra and not infiltrating too deeply (Fig. 25.1).

External irradiation by electrons or photons, depending on the location and the depth of the growth,

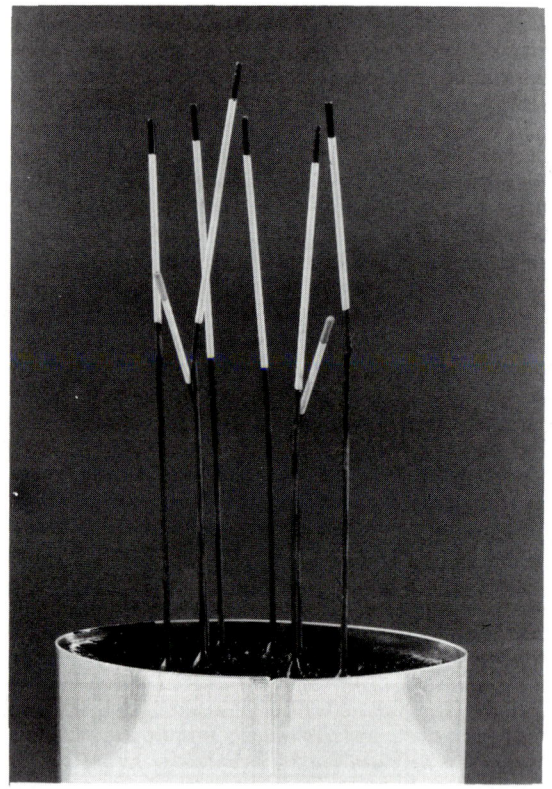

Fig. 25.1   Three-dimensional reconstruction of a radium implant in a carcinoma of the urethra of a female. The eight radium needles are fixed by a metal bar.

delivering doses of about 6000 rad in 5 to 6 weeks via 2 opposing fields, occasionally with an additional perineal field, adapted to the site and characteristics of the growth, may result in cure.

A combination of primary excision followed by interstitial therapy in small lesions is a well accepted procedure. The combined approach for larger lesions consists usually of pre-operative irradiation delivering a dose of 4000 to 5000 rad in 4 to 5 weeks followed by radical excision. In case of demonstratable lymph node involvement either a lymphadenectomy of the inguinal nodes or irradiation of this area can be done. The result is usually only palliative.

Demonstratable involvement of pelvic nodes usually requires irradiation, again with mainly palliative results.

The results after surgery and radiotherapy, by characteristics of the therapy and by type of growth are presented in Tables 25.1 and 25.2.

Chemotherapy

There are no reports in literature presenting data on the effect of systemic chemotherapy in urethral cancer, neither on the local growth nor on its metastases.

Ueda and Omoto (1976) observed a palliative effect of mitomycin-C instillations into the urethra.

Complications

Pointon and Poole-Wilson (1968) report an operative mortality of 4 out of 20 surgically treated patients. Lymph node dissection can result in severe oedema of the legs and the pubic region. No systematic accounts of complication incidence after surgery are presented in the literature. After radiotherapy, Chu (1973) reports four complications in 22 patients: ulceration, urethra dilatation, pelvic abscess. After interstitial irradiation, with or without external irradiation, Taggart *et al.* (1972) had four complications in 37 patients: urethra-vaginal fistula, radiation ileitis, recto-vaginal fistula, necrosis of distal urethra.

Future possibilities

Failure to cure is usually due to local recurrence and lymphatic spread. A more sophisticated combined modality approach consisting of surgery, radiotherapy and more effective chemotherapeutic agents might improve prognosis, especially in deeply infiltrating growths, located in the posterior urethra. In view of the extremely low incidence of this growth randomized trials to assess the value of various therapeutic approaches are really not feasible.

Improved diagnostic procedures to assess pelvic lymph node involvement (CT-scan, transabdominal lymph node cytology after lymphography) might exclude these patients from mutilating and time-consuming therapy when the chance of cure is nearly zero.

Further reading

Grabstald, H. *et al.* (1966), Cancer of the Female Urethra *J. Am. Med. Assoc.*, **197**, 835–42.

Table 25.1 Prognosis after surgery.

Author	Type of growth	Type of treatment	Results at 5-year survival
	Surgery for Males		
Ray *et al.* (1977)	Pars pendulans	Amputation and inguinal node dissection	6/9 cured
	Pars bulbomembraneous + prostatic	Radical surgery (excision, cystectomy, penectomy, emasculation, pelvic node dissection, ileal conduit)	3/14
Marshall (1957)	'All types'	Deep excision	4/8
	Surgery for Females		
Pointon and Poole-Wilson (1968)	'All types' (11 after failure of previous irradiation)	All types of surgery	8/20
Grabstald (1973)	'Entire' urethra involved	All types of surgery	3/14 cured
	Anterior part involved	Excision with wide margin, vulvectomy	7/9 (living 5–240 mth.)

Table 25.2 Prognosis after radiotherapy in females.

Author	Type of growth	Type of treatment	Results
			Cured
Hilaris and Batata (1975)	< 5 cm Ø }	Radium needle implant 5000–6000 rad/5–7 days irradiation	{ 5/5 3/6
	> 5 cm Ø		
Chu (1973)	All types of growth	Interstitial + external irradiation } Total dose 6000–8000 rad	*Cured*
		< 3500 rad	4/13
		> 3500 rad	1/3 } 7/22 32%
		External irradiation only	6/
		Radium only	2/2
	Distal urethra (anterior)	All types of irradiation	7/11 64%
			3-year crude survival
Pointon and Poole-Wilson (1968)	Small lesions	Permant Au implant	(26) 77%
	Large lesions	Radium implant 5500 rad/7 days	(40) 40%
	Too large for implant	Radical external irradiations (5500 rad/3 weeks)	(12) 42% } 52%
		Intracavitary irradiation	(3) 33%
			5-year survival
Bracken *et al.* (1976)	All types of growth	Interstitial irradiation (gold grains, radium, iridium)	(25) 45%
		Interstitial irradiation + External irradiation } 5500–7000 rad individualized	(21) 37%
		External irradiation only (anterior-posterior opposing fields ± perineal field	(16) 12%
	< 2 cm	All types of irradiation	(10) ±60%
	2–4 cm	All types of irradiation	(22) ±46%
	≥ 5 cm	All types of irradiation	(31) ±13%
	Stage A (submucosal)	All types of irradiation	(11) ±45%
	Stage B (muscular)	All types of irradiation	(19) ±40%
	Stage C (periurethral)	All types of irradiation	(28) ±25%
	Stage D (metastases, lymph node and distant)	All types of irradiation	(16) ±20%
Taggart *et al.* (1972)	All types of tumour	Radium needles 7000 rad/7 days (or equivalent)	*2-year NED*
		External irradiation (22 MeV photons) + interstitial irradiations 4000–6000 rad/4–6 wk + 3000–4000 rad radium/3–4 days	(37) 32%
	Anterior urethra	Radium or radium + external irradiation	(11) 16%
Prempree and Wizenberg (1977)	No metastases, limited infiltration	Interstitial irradiation only or interstitial irradiation + external irradiation	(10) 80% cure rate
	100% failure in case of involvement of inguinal nodes, abdominal nodes, parametrium, bladder-neck		

Within brackets: number of treated patients
NED: no evidence of disease

References

Bracken, R.B. *et al.* (1976), Primary carcinoma of the female urethra. *J. Urol.*, **116**, 188–92.

Chau, P.M. and Green, A.E. (1965), Radiotherapeutic management of malignant tumors of vagina. In: *Progress in Clinical Cancer.* **I**, (ed. I.M. Ariel), Grune and Stratton, Inc., New York, p. 728.

Chu, A.M. (1973), Female urethral carcinoma. *Radiology,* **107**, 627–30.

Grabstald, H. (1973), Tumors of the urethra in men and women. *Cancer*, **32**, 1236–55.

Hendry, W.F. (1974), Surgical treatment of urethral tumors associated with bladder cancer. *Proc. R. Soc. Med.*, **64**, 304–7.

Hilaris, B.S. and Batata, M.A. (1975), Cancer of the female urethra. In: *Handbook of Interstitial Brachytherapy* (ed. B.S. Hilaris), Publishing Sciences Group, Inc., Acton, Massachusetts, p.235.

Hotchkiss, R.S. and Amelar, R.D. (1954), Primary carcinoma of the male urethra. *J. Urol.*, **72**, 1181–91.

Marshall, V.F. (1957), The choice of surgical therapy for epithelial neoplasms of the urinary bladder. *Br. J. Urol.*, **29**, 228–31.

Pointon, R.C.S. and Poole-Wilson, D.S. (1968), Primary carcinoma of the urethra. *Br. J. Urol.*, **40**, 682–93.

Prempree, T. and Wizenberg, M.J. (1977), Treatment planning in radiation management of primary carcinoma of the female urethra. *Int. J. Radiat. Oncol. Biol. Phys.*, **2**, 833–41.

Ray, B., Canto, A.R. and Whitmore, Jr., W.F. (1977), Experience with primary carcinoma of the male urethra. *J. Urol.*, **117**, 591–4.

Richie, J.P. and Skinner, D.G. (1978), Carcinoma in situ of the urethra associated with bladder carcinoma: the role of urethrectomy. *J. Urol.*, **119**, 80–1.

Taggart, C. G., Castro, J.R. and Rutledge, F.N. (1972), Carcinoma of the female urethra. *Am. J. Roentg.*, **11**, 145–51.

Ueda, T. and Omoto, T. (1976), Tumorrezidive in der Harnröhre nach totaler Zystektomie bei Blasenkarzinomen. *Acta Chir. Austriaca*, **4**, 81–3.

26 Testis and epidydimis

M.J. Peckham, T.J. McElwain
and W.F. Hendry

Testicular tumours may occur in childhood and early or late adult life. However, they commonly present between the ages of 20 and 40 years and in this age group constitute the fourth most common cause of death from malignant disease. This chapter is concerned with the discussion of seminoma and teratoma testis and the rarer categories of testicular malignancy will not be discussed. The classification of testicular tumours described by the British Testicular Tumour Panel is set out in Table 26.1 (Pugh, 1976).

Age distribution and prevalence

Fig. 26.1 shows the age distribution of testicular tumour patients in England and Wales and Fig. 26.2 (*a, b, c*) the age distribution according to pathological

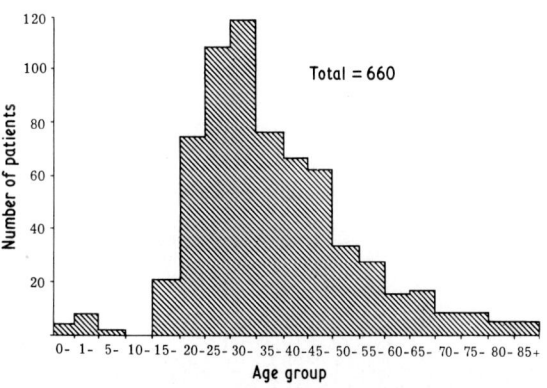

Fig. 26.1 Age distribution of testicular tumour patients (England and Wales, patients registered, 1970) Registrar General's Review (1975).

subtype. It is seen that seminomas tend to present a decade later than malignant teratomas, with combined tumours occupying an intermediate position. The prevalence of teratomas and seminomas varies from country to country and evidence of an increased incidence has been reported from several countries over the last few decades. Fig. 26.3 summarizes data from the Testicular Tumour Panel illustrating the apparent increase in incidence of testicular tumours which has occurred over the past 20 years.

Aetiology and predisposing factors

The aetiology of testicular tumours is unknown; trauma, mumps, orchitis and tight clothing fashions have been suggested as possible aetiological factors, but remain purely speculative. Testicular maldescent, on the other hand, is known to predispose to the development of testicular malignancy, increasing the chance of tumour formation by a factor of 35 to 40 times. It is of interest that approximately one in four

Table 26.1 Classification of testicular tumours.

Classification		Relative frequency* (%)†
Seminoma		39.5
Teratoma	(i) Teratoma differentiated (TD)	
	(ii) Malignant teratoma intermediate (MTI)	
	(iii) Malignant teratoma undifferentiated (MTU)	31.7
	(iv) Malignant teratoma trophoblastic (MTT)	
Combined seminoma/teratoma		13.5
Yolk sac tumour		1.9
Sertoli cell tumour		1.2
Interstitial cell tumour		1.6
Malignant lymphoma		6.7

* From a total of 2793 patients reported by the Testicular Tumour Panel (Pugh, 1976)
† A further 3.0% includes miscellaneous tumours, metastases and tumours of uncertain histogenesis

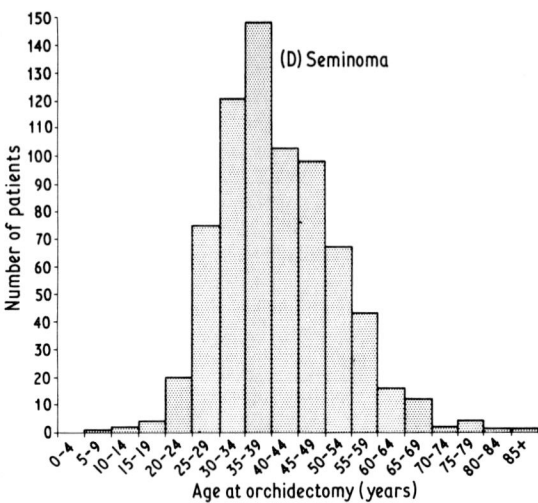

Fig. 26.2a   Seminoma testis: age distribution (from Pugh, 1976).

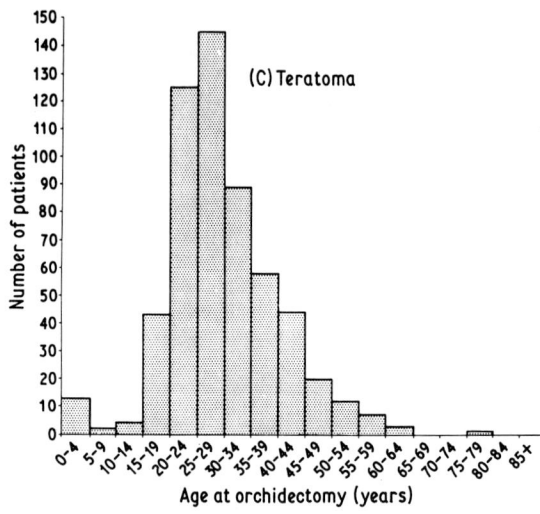

Fig. 26.2b   Testicular teratoma: age distribution (from Pugh, 1976).

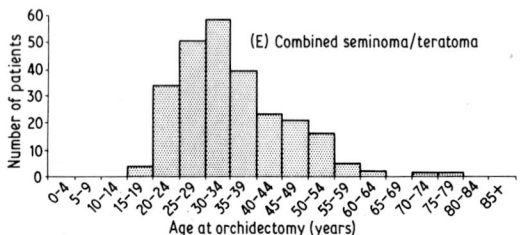

Fig. 26.2c   Combined seminoma/teratoma of the testis: age distribution (from Pugh, 1976).

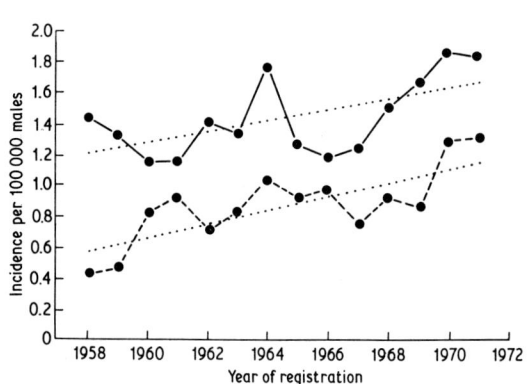

Fig. 26.3   Age-standardized incidence rates of seminoma (solid line) and teratoma (broken line) per 100 000 males, South Metropolitan Region of England (1958–1971). Regression of incidence rate on year of registration is shown by a dotted line (from Pugh, 1976) (reprinted with permission of Dr. Roger Pugh).

tumours developing in men with a history of maldescent occur in the normally descended testis. Patients with bilateral maldescent are particularly at risk, not only of developing one testicular tumour but of developing a malignancy in the contra-lateral testis. In most series approximately 7% of patients with testicular tumours give a history of maldescent. There is no clear evidence that orchidopexy carried out before the age of 10 years materially influences the susceptibility of the testis to subsequent neoplastic evolution. The fact that tumours can arise in the normally descended testis in patients with maldescent suggests that the maldescent *per se* is not responsible for tumorigenesis but the factors underlying failure of the testis to migrate from its site of embryological origin into the scrotal sac, may predispose to malignant change.

Bilateral testicular tumours

The man who has had one testicular tumour is more at risk than the general male population of developing a tumour of the remaining testis. In our own series, 2.8% of patients have developed second testicular malignancies (Sokal *et al.*, 1979). The second tumour may occur at time intervals ranging up to 15 years following the diagnosis of the first tumour, both tumours may present synchronously. In 9/21 patients developing second tumours, the second malignancy was diagnosed within two years of the first.

History and clinical examination

Although classically the tumour-bearing testis is described as being hard and deficient in sensation, pain and tenderness, usually misdiagnosed initially as epididymo-orchitis, are equally common presenting features. Some patients give a history of progressive shrinkage in testicular volume preceding the detection of a lump and in a minority of patients who present with symptoms relating to the presence of metastases, the testis may feel perfectly normal with a history of transient swelling and tenderness having occurred some time previously. As noted above, a history of testicular maldescent and orchidopexy will be elicited in 5% to 10% of testicular tumour patients and patients with a history of bilateral maldescent are at risk of developing a tumour in the contra-lateral testis and need to be followed closely after primary treatment. In most instances the primary tumour is clinically obvious as a hard irregular swelling. Occasionally, a patient is referred with upper abdominal tumour thought to have arisen in the retroperitoneal area, but who, on careful examination, proves to have a small primary testicular tumour. In exceptional cases where metastatic spread has occurred and been verified histologically, the testes feel normal. If a history of transient swelling of one testis is obtained, removal of this testis may reveal a micro primary tumour or a scar suggesting spontaneous regression (Azzopardi *et al.*, 1961). Small hydroceles may occur; larger fluid collections are uncommon. Occasionally the testis is exquisitely tender and may be mistaken for an inflammatory condition or torsion. The presence of metastases in a patient with a normal testis and in whom there is a history of absence since childhood of the contra-lateral testis should alert the clinician to the possibility of a tumour-bearing intra-abdominal testis, since the risk of malignant change in testes in this situation is approximately 1 in 20.

A history of breast enlargement and tenderness in a testicular tumour patient usually, but not invariably, indicates the presence of a tumour producing human chorionic gonadotrophin (HCG). The commonest symptom referable to metastases is diffuse lumbar backache due to the presence of enlarged retroperitoneal lymph nodes. In patients with more extensive disease, breathlessness may occur if there are multiple metastases; haemoptysis is uncommon and may be due to parenchymal metastases or, rarely, endobronchial deposits. Weight loss and anorexia accompany liver involvement and, in such patients, there is almost invariably evidence of metastatic spread to other extralymphatic sites, particularly the lungs. Symptoms referable to intracranial (and rarely extradural) metastases may occur but spread to these sites is more usually a late event.

Staging

In most instances the patient will already have undergone orchidectomy before referral to the treatment centre. It is important to ascertain whether the tumour-bearing testis was removed via an inguinal incision with high cord ligation, since trans-scrotal orchidectomy may increase the chance of scrotal recurrence. It is important, also, to note whether the testis was replaced in the scrotal sac following biopsy or whether trans-scrotal needle biopsy was attempted. Both procedures predispose to tumour recurrence in the scrotum.

In a minority of patients widespread tumour dissemination renders intensive staging inessential and pre-treatment investigation can be limited to an assessment of renal and hepatic function, chest radiograph and full blood count. Wherever possible, however, it is our policy to stage patients as precisely as possible using non-invasive investigative methods. The staging protocol employed is outlined below and several aspects then considered in more detail. Staging procedures are summarized in Fig. 26.4.

The objective of detailed patient investigation is the detection of extent and sites of tumour spread. Furthermore, since the volume of metastases exerts an influence on therapeutic response, this parameter is also incorporated into the clinical staging system.

The investigative procedures selected depend upon an appreciation of the pattern of spread of the tumour. In the absence of inappropriate surgery, spread of tumour to the scrotum and inguinal nodes is uncommon. Spread via the lymphatic pathways is common and the nodes predominantly involved are in the para-aortic region. Lymphography, ultrasonography and computerized tomography (CT) scanning are employed to evaluate the retroperitoneal area. Involved lymph nodes may be present above L_1, at which level

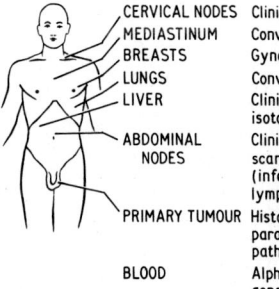

Fig. 26.4 Schema for patient assessment in testicular teratoma. Procedures not usually performed at The Royal Marsden are shown in parenthesis.

the thoracic duct commonly forms to pass through the posterior thorax to the left neck. Thus, extension to the left supraclavicular region is not infrequent and when it has occurred the probability of extra lymphatic dissemination is extremely high. The commonest extranodal site to be involved is the lung, which can be assessed in considerable detail with the advent of CT.

The following sequence of investigations is routinely carried out:

1. Histology review. If possible, the entire operative specimen is obtained for detailed examination, pathological staging and identification of β-human chorionic gonadotrophin (β-HCG) and α-feto protein (AFP) using immunoperoxidase staining. This aspect is discussed in more detail later. If the histological material is inadequate, further biopsy from, for example, cervical nodes may be feasible.
2. Whole lung tomography is performed in patients with a negative chest radiograph or less than three visible metastases.
3. Lymphography and intravenous urography.
4. Liver isotopic scan.
5. Liver and retroperitoneal ultrasonography.
6. CT scans of the lungs, unless multiple lung metastases are identified using routine radiographic methods.
7. CT scans of the liver and retroperitoneal area.
8. Full blood count, liver function tests, serum calcium, urea and electrolytes.
9. Blood for tumour markers (β-HCG and AFP).
10. Assessment of renal function (ethylene diamine tetra-acetic acid clearance; EDTA).
11. Sequential pulmonary function tests are performed in patients receiving high dose bleomycin.
12. During the past year it has been our policy to bank semen samples from patients likely to be sterilized by treatment.

Histology

Malignant teratoma

The classification proposed by the British Testicular Tumour Panel (Pugh, 1976) differs in terminology but not radically in concept from the system in use in the United States. In the British system the following categories are recognized:

Malignant teratoma intermediate (MTI)
This tumour type contains incompletely differentiated tissue and elements having the histological characteristics of malignancy as well as fully mature adult tissues. This category corresponds to the Dixon and Moore (1952) category of teratocarcinoma.

Malignant teratoma undifferentiated (MTU)
This is a malignant teratoma without mature or organoid elements varying from solid sheets to an adenocarcinomatous appearance. MTU corresponds to embryonal carcinoma.

Malignant teratoma trophoblastic (MTT)
This tumour is characterized by the presence of true trophoblastic elements, that is a syncytial cell mass and malignant cytotrophoblast. MTT corresponds to the Dixon and Moore (1952) category of chorioncarcinoma.

Yolk sac tumour
Although this term is restricted to the distinctive adenocarcinoma of childhood, yolk sac elements are recognized in a proportion of adult malignant teratoma. The recognition of such elements does not modify the histological classification at the present time.

Combined tumour
This is a malignant testicular tumour in which one or more of the above elements are present in combination with seminoma.

Seminoma

In contrast to the cystic and often haemorrhagic appearance of the cut surface of malignant teratoma, seminomas tend to be uniform in appearance, often lobulated from the presence of fibrous intersections. The tumour tends to be pale in colour and in most cases the entire testis is replaced by seminoma. The characteristic histological feature, in contrast to teratoma, is the uniform appearance of the seminoma cell population. In classical seminoma – the most common variant – the cells are rounded with finely granular cytoplasm and a well defined chromatin network. In addition to classical seminoma, several variants are recognized: spermatocytic seminoma, anaplastic seminoma and what Friedman and Pearlman (1970) have described as 'seminoma with trophocarcinoma'. Seminomas may be combined with malignant teratoma in the same testis; such combined tumours constitute 14% of the total testicular tumour population.

Spermatocytic seminoma
The characteristic feature is the presence of a small and large cell population, the former resembling spermatogonia and the latter spermatocytes. This subtype constitutes less than 5% of seminomas, tends to occur in an older age group and is associated with an excellent prognosis.

Anaplastic seminoma

This variant, which shows marked nuclear pleomorphism and a higher mitotic rate than classical seminoma, constitutes approximately 3% of seminomas and is associated with a more aggressive evolution and a worse prognosis.

Seminoma with trophocarcinoma

This subtype, described by Friedman and Pearlman (1970) is composed predominantly of anaplastic seminoma with occasional foci of syncytial cells and/or cytotrophoblast. In their series 7.5% of seminomas showed this appearance and the clinical course was aggressive.

Functional pathology

It has become abundantly clear that the above classification defines an arbitrary series of groupings, whereas, in reality many tumours are composed of a range of elements in which undifferentiated tissue, yolk sac tumour, mature adult somatic tissue and malignant trophoblast may be identified. The use of immunoperoxidase staining methods in which the presence of β-HCG or AFP is detected in tissue sections using antisera linked to horseradish peroxidase (Heyderman and Neville, 1978) has demonstrated that even when trophoblast and yolk sac tumour elements are not recognized histologically, either or both tumour markers may be identified. The value of more complex sub-divisions of histological classification remains to be evaluated and at the present time the simpler system summarized above should be retained since it has been shown to have prognostic significance.

Pathological staging of the primary tumour

It has been shown that the probability of dissemination and hence prognosis, is influenced by the local extent of the primary tumour (Pugh, 1976). Thus, in the British Testicular Tumour Panel's series of patients, the survival figures at three years for P_1 (tumour confined to testis), P_2 (tumour involving epididymis and lower cord), and P_3 (tumour cells present in the upper cord), were for MTI, 65%, 44% and 11% and for MTU 61%, 35% and 21% respectively. No information is available on the prognostic significance of pathological staging in patients undergoing intensive clinical staging as described above.

Lymphography

Lower limb lymphangiography opacifies the inguinal, external iliac and para-aortic nodes to the origin of the thoracic duct, usually at the level of L_1–L_2. The lymph drainage of the testis is to the para-aortic nodes and there is a relatively constant lymphatic which discharges into the upper external iliac node on the same side. Nodes in the hilum of either kidney may (rarely) be involved by metastases and these nodes are not opacified by pedal lymphography (Macdonald and Paxton, 1976). The rich plexus of vessels leads to cross over which is more likely from right to left (56%) than left to right (32%). The appearance of metastatic involvement in nodes is variable. In 10% of positive lymphograms the appearance resembles lymphoma. However, the most usual manifestation of involvement is the presence of filling defects. In cases with gross involvement there may be virtual nodal replacement with tumour and little or no opacification at lymphography. Displacement of one or both ureters and in some cases an obstructive uropathy may result. Table 26.2 summarizes the positive lymphogram rate in the Royal Marsden Hospital series. The accuracy of lymphography may best be assessed by correlation of nodal histology and radiological diagnosis. Unfortunately, since nodal dissection as primary treatment is not performed in our institution, the diagnostic accuracy of lymphography employing our criteria for radiological interpretation cannot be assessed directly.

Table 26.2   Positive lymphogram rate in testicular tumours (from Wilkinson and Macdonald, 1975).

Classification	Total patients	Positive	%
Seminoma	116	30	26
Teratoma	96	40	42
Combined tumours	38	20	53
Total	250	90	36

Table 26.3 summarizes details from the literature of 316 patients reported as having negative lymphograms. Of this group 25% had histological evidence of lymph node metastases at surgery.

Opacification of left supraclavicular nodes is usually observed but if mediastinal nodes are visualized, this is to be regarded as a possible indication of involvement by tumour.

Role of CT-scanning in the management of malignant teratoma

Approximately 20% of Stage I patients relapse in the lungs following treatment by orchidectomy and radiation therapy. These metastases may be presumed to have been present at the time of orchidectomy and

Table 26.3 Occult metastases from testicular teratoma in negative lymphogram patients.

Author(s)	Number patients with negative lymphograms	Postitive histology
Fein and Taber (1969)	30	10
Wallace and Jing (1970)	49	8
Hussey *et al.* (1977)	73	13
Maier and Schamber (1972)	24	6
Hultén *et al.* (1973)	16	4
Jonsson *et al.* (1973)	10	2
Safer *et al.* (1975)	21	3
Durant and Barrat (1977)	14	6
Kademian and Wirtanen (1977)	16	4
Lasser *et al.* (1977)	11	4
Cook *et al.* (1965)	12	4
Seitzman and Halaby (1964)	12	6
Storm *et al.* (1977)	28	10
Total	316	80 (24.7%)

CT-scanning of the lungs may be a method of detecting at least some of this group and identifying them *ab initio* as Stage IV patients in need of systemic treatment. This is currently being explored. CT-scanning may also be useful in the investigation of the mediastinum and is already of proven value in the abdomen, particularly for delineating nodal masses for staging purposes, radiation therapy planning, monitoring of chemotherapeutic response and choice of surgical approach (Husband *et al.*, 1979).

Staging classification

The staging classification employed at the Royal Marsden Hospital includes a statement of tumour extent, site(s) of metastases and tumour volume. The four stages and their sub-divisions are shown in Fig. 26.5 (*a–d*).

Pattern of spread in seminoma and malignant teratoma

Malignant teratomas of the testis are rapidly growing tumours with a propensity for early spread via the lymphatic system and by the blood stream to extralymphatic sites, particularly the lungs and liver. Seminomas, on the other hand, tend to be more indolent, although rapid growth may be encountered occasionally.

The stage-distribution at presentation of patients with malignant teratomas is unknown since each centre is referred a selected patient population. A recent study from the Leeds Regional Centre suggests that approximately 25% of patients have advanced disease at diagnosis (Corbett, P.J: personal communication). Experience at our own centre suggests that although spread beyond the lymphatic system may have occurred by the time the primary tumour is diagnosed, this is initially confined to the lungs and often pulmonary metastases are small in volume. Liver involvement at presentation is relatively uncommon. The cure rates obtained by nodal dissection or radiation therapy in patients with abdominal lymph node metastases confirms that tumour spread may be limited to the retroperitoneal lymph nodes, although the probability of extralymphatic spread when the cervical nodes are involved, or when abdominal metastases are bulky, is high.

Conversely, the large majority of seminoma patients are Stage I. Tumour spread when it occurs tends to be less predictable than is the case with teratoma, with more frequent involvement of soft tissues (for example sub-cutaneous, mesentery, prostate). Pulmonary metastases may be ill defined and fluffy in appearance compared with the characteristic cannon ball metastases of teratoma.

Treatment of malignant teratoma

Historically, the management of Stage I and II malignant teratomas has been by orchidectomy and radiation therapy in Great Britain and orchidectomy and radical node dissection in the United States. Both forms of treatment produce essentially similar results (Peckham, 1976). It is clear that the advent of more effective chemotherapy necessitates a reconsideration of the roles of both radiation therapy and surgery. In the section which follows it will be argued that orchidectomy and radiation should be employed for a precisely defined group of early stage patients, reserving chemotherapy for relapse, and that treatment should be initiated with chemotherapy in all other stage groupings. The extent to which chemotherapy needs to be supplemented with radiation therapy and-/or surgery is not known and needs evaluation in a controlled clinical study. Experience indicates that relapse in bulky tumour may occur following chemotherapy. The preliminary results of sequential treatment with drugs, radiation and surgery will be discussed.

Cure by orchidectomy alone

It is evident from early experience that a proportion of

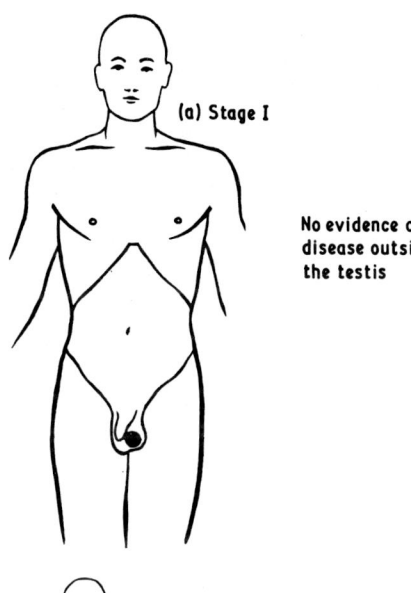

(a) Stage I

No evidence of
disease outside
the testis

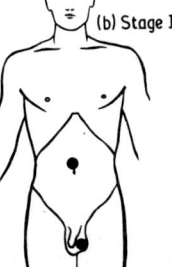

(b) Stage II. Infradiaphragmatic node involvement

This is subdivided according to the maximum
diameter of metastases into the following
substage categories:

IIA maximum diameter of metastases < 2 cm
IIB maximum diameter of metastases 2–5 cm
IIC maximum diameter of metastases > 5 cm

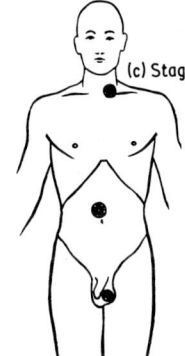

(c) Stage III. Supra- and infradiaphragmatic node
involvement

This is subdivided as follows:

Abdominal nodes: A, B and C as for stage II
Mediastinal node involvement: M +
Neck nodes: C +

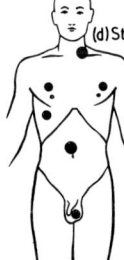

(d) Stage IV. Extension of tumour to extralymphatic sites

The following suffixes define the extent and
volume of metastatic spread:
(i) Abdominal nodes: O = negative lymphogram
                    A, B, C as for stages II and III
(ii) Mediastinal and neck nodes as for stage III
(iii) Lungs: L_1 < 3 metastases
             L_2 multiple metastases < 2 cm max diameter
             L_3 multiple metastases > 2 cm max diameter
(iv) Liver involvement is denoted as H +
(v) Other sites e.g. bone and brain, are specified

Fig. 26.5 *(a–d)* Staging classification for testicular teratoma
(Royal Marsden Hospital).

testicular teratoma patients are cured by removal of
the primary tumour. Thus, in a historical series of 79
patients quoted by Whitmore (1968), 27 (34%) were
alive at five years following only orchidectomy. Since
approximately one third of this group of patients would
be expected to have a positive lymphogram, it is possible that as many as 50% of patients who would now be
classified as Stage I, might be cured by orchidectomy.
It is possible that the combined used of improved clinical staging procedures and a better understanding of
the signficance of elevated tumour markers, might
eventually allow those patients cured by orchidectomy
to be identified. It is likely that future clinical studies
will investigate the role of radiation therapy in the
clinical Stage I patient by comparing elective nodal
irradiation with careful observation and no immediate
treatment after orchidectomy.

Post-orchidectomy treatment

Following the completion of the staging procedures
outlined above, it is our policy to treat patients according to the protocols summarized below.

Stage I: Radiotherapy

The para-aortic and ipsilateral pelvic nodes are irradiated by anterior and posterior fields using 6–8 MeV
photons from a linear accelerator and delivering a
midplane tissue dose of 4000 rad in four weeks. The
field extends from the upper border of D_{10} to the
obturator foramen. The contra-lateral testis is protected by 1-cm thick lead cups and the scrotal sac and
groin nodes not irradiated unless there has been an
orchidopexy, scrotal interference or penetration of the
tunica by tumour. Using this approach the radiation

dose to the testis is of the order of 50–70 rad and fertility in many men is preserved (Smithers *et al.*, 1973; Thomas *et al.*, 1976). Van der Werf Messing (1976) reported that 21 men in her series of patients fathered children after successful radiation therapy and Orecklin *et al.* (1973) described 16 men primarily irradiated for testicular malignancy who subsequently produced a family. At the Royal Marsden Hospital, Smithers *et al.* (1973) reported a total of 52 children born to 34 men who had had pelvic and para-aortic node irradiation. Sandeman (1966) and Thomas *et al.* (1976) have reported post-irradiation oligospermia with recovery of sperm count at between one and two years.

Stage IIA
In a retrospective analysis of the Royal Marsden Hospital series it was demonstrated that abdominal node metastases ≤ 2 cm in maximum diameter could be satisfactorily controlled with radiation therapy (Tyrrell and Peckham, 1976). It is our policy in this group to treat as for Stage I with a supplementary dose of 500–1000 rad using small fields to treat the involved node(s). Previously it was our policy to treat the mediastinum and neck but this has now been omitted since the probability of supra-diaphragmatic node involvement is probably low (*vide supra*), and when supra-diaphragmatic node involvement is present, the probability of extranodal extension is high rendering localized therapy inappropriate. Furthermore, the irradiation of large volumes of bone marrow compromises subsequent chemotherapy should this become necessary. In practice the Stage IIA category is uncommon.

Stage IIB, IIC and III
In this group of patients results with radiotherapy alone are poor (*vide infra*) and treatment should be initiated with chemotherapy. Details of chemotherapy are given later in the chapter. Initially, vinblastine and bleomycin (VB) (Samuels *et al.*, 1976) was used but currently we are employing the combination of cis-diaminedichloroplatinum (II), vinblastine and bleomycin (PVB) (Einhorn and Donohue, 1977a; Einhorn and Donohue, 1977b). After four cycles the patient is reassessed (Figs. 26.6 and 26.7). If there is a complete tumour marker remission and no evidence of tumour volume enlargement, the patient proceeds to irradiation. If there is progressive marker reduction, but a persistently elevated titre, chemotherapy is continued to six courses. In Stage II patients, four weeks to six weeks after completion of chemotherapy the para-aortic and pelvic nodes are irradiated to a dose of 4000 rad and initially (or persistently) enlarged nodes irradiated using multiple smaller fields to a total dose of 4500

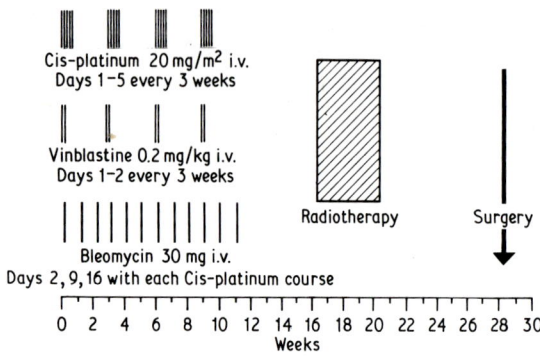

Fig. 26.6 Royal Marsden Hospital protocol for combined chemotherapy-radiotherapy and surgery in the management of advanced testicular teratoma.

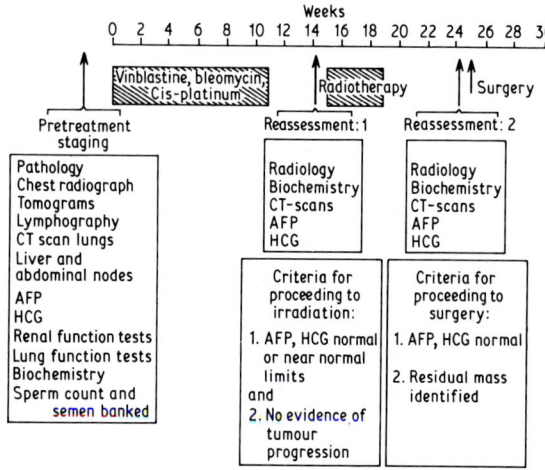

Fig. 26.7 Schema showing Royal Marsden Hospital investigative and reassessment protocols in advanced testicular teratoma.

to 5000 rad. In Stage III patients the mediastinum and left supra-clavicular fossa receive 4000 rad and initially involved nodes boosted as for the abdomen, if this is technically feasible. Four to six weeks after completion of irradiation Stage IIB/C patients undergo laparotomy with exploration and excision of residual masses if these are identified. This is also undertaken in Stage III patients if small volume supra-diaphragmatic tumour is associated with large volume abdominal disease.

Stage IV L₁
These patients receive four–six courses of chemotherapy followed by irradiation to the abdominal nodes and sites of lung metastases followed by

surgery if bulky abdominal nodes (B or C) are present initially.

Stage IV L₂

These patients receive chemotherapy alone unless bulky abdominal nodes (B or C) are present when they are managed as for Stage IV L₁ patients.

Stage IV L₃ and IV H+

These patients receive chemotherapy alone.

Role of radiotherapy in testicular teratoma

The role of radiotherapy can be considered under three headings:

1. An assessment of the response of non-seminoma germ cell tumour metastases to radiation.
2. Deployment of radiation therapy in overall treatment strategy. This aspect involves consideration of the results of treatment, the pattern of treatment failure and the morbidity of orchidectomy and nodal irradiation.
3. Patient tolerance to surgery and chemotherapy before and after radiation therapy.

Response of metastases to irradiation

As shown in Table 26.3 approximately one in four patients with negative lymphograms harbour occult tumour deposits. Following irradiation to the para-aortic and pelvic nodes local recurrence is an exceptionally rare event (Peckham *et al.*, 1977). From these observations we may conclude that small volume metastases are readily eradicated by doses of the order of 4000 rad. Furthermore, even when small metastases are visible on the lymphogram, so long as their size does not exceed 2 cm in diameter the probability of control is high (Tyrrell and Peckham, 1976). Further evidence supporting these observations comes from observations made in patients undergoing nodal resec-

tion after pre-operative irradiation. Thus, Klein and Maier (1977) have reported that the incidence of positive nodes was reduced in patients receiving 2500–3000 rad before surgery (Table 26.4).

Deployment of radiation therapy in overall treatment strategy

In order to discuss this aspect it is necessary to consider the rationale of employing a local treatment method and to discuss the relative merits and demerits of radical node dissection as opposed to radiotherapy. The evidence of the results presented below points to the effectiveness of orchidectomy and radiation therapy in early stage disease and more recent experience indicates that chemotherapy for early relapse is practicable and effective. If, with further experience, a cure rate approaching 100% is confirmed adopting this policy, then eight of every 10 men treated will never have had chemotherapy or major surgery, thus preserving potency and, in many cases, fertility.

Radical retroperitoneal lymphadenectomy was developed during the period before effective systemic therapy and together with radiation therapy provided the only hope of cure for patients with spread to the abdominal nodes. With present techniques a reasonably thorough clearance of nodes can be achieved bilaterally up to the renal vessels. Clearance can be extended above the renal vessels by using a thoracoabdominal approach or by complete mobilization and elevation of the pancreas (Donohue *et al.*, 1977). The procedure is a major undertaking associated with significant morbidity. The overall complication rate in two large series has been reported as 11% (Lindsey and Glenn, 1976) and 12% (Staubitz *et al.*, 1974). Ejaculatory impotence is common after bilateral lymphadenectomy. The results obtained by radical node dissection are summarized for several large series in Table 26.5. The results for negative nodes (83%) and positive nodes (49%) are similar to those obtained by radiotherapy in clinical Stage I and II patients respec-

Table 26.4 Results of node dissection ± pre-operative irradiation (from Klein and Maier, 1977).

Clinical stage	Pre-operative radiation therapy	Incidence of histologically positive nodes at dissection	
		M.D. Anderson	*Walter Reed*
I	−	18/106 (17%)	6/24 (25%)
	+	0/5 (0%)	1/30 (3%)
II	−	20/22 (91%)	32/35 (91%)
	+	15/28 (54%)	11/21 (52%)

Table 26.5 Survival (minimum 3 years) in testicular teratoma patients after retroperitonal node dissection.

	Histology	
	Negative nodes	Positive nodes
Whitmore (1968)	43/49	9/16
Bradfield et al. (1973)*	28/40	11/34
Culp et al. (1973)*	13/15	6/10
Skinner and Leadbetter (1971)*	27/30	15/27
Castro (1969)*	31/37	11/22
Maier et al. (1969)*	80/109	44/97
Walsh et al. (1971)	24/25	3/4
Staubitz et al. (1974)	42/45	15/20
Lindsey and Glenn (1976)*	20/23	13/27
Total	308/373	127/257
	82.6%	49.4%

* Some had supplementary radiotherapy

tively (van der Werf-Messing, 1976; Hussey *et al.*, 1977; Peckham *et al.*, 1979). An important decision for the future must relate to a reappraisal of the contribution of this major surgical intervention in non-seminomatous tumours. Donohue *et al.* (1978) have recently advocated the continuance of a thorough and complete node dissection in spite of the fact that all their patients have ejaculatory impotence and that 52% had histologically negative nodes. Their argument is based upon the results of treating 58 patients between 1965 and 1975. These are summarized in Table 26.6

It is impossible to equate pathologically staged with clinically staged patients but as indicated below our recent experience with a policy of post-orchidectomy irradiation in early stage disease (which can be approx-

imately equated with Stages A and B₁ above) followed by intensive chemotherapy on relapse has been encouraging since all 28 patients are alive and free from disease. Similarly our preliminary experience with bulky Stage II disease using a sequence of chemotherapy and radiotherapy shows this approach to be a practicable alternative to chemotherapy and major surgery.

In recent years it has been suggested that radical nodal dissection may be justifiable as a staging procedure. Given the demonstration that the non-surgical management of early stage patients carefully investigated with non-invasive procedures should rarely, if ever, result in death from testicular cancer, it is difficult to justify the role of radical node dissection solely on the basis of the staging information provided. These points are summarized in Table 26.7

Patient tolerance to surgery and chemotherapy before and after radiation therapy

This important question is discussed below. Toxicity of treatment is of critical importance since it is probable that more than one treatment approach may produce identical results. In such a situation therapeutic choice must hinge on a consideration of relative toxicities.

Chemotherapy of testicular teratoma

It has been appreciated for many years that testicular teratomas are chemosensitive tumours. Thus, actinomycin D which was used widely as a single agent before the introduction of effective combinations occasionally effected a cure and in most series of patients treated in the 1960's between 5% and 10% of Stage IV patients are long term disease-free survivors. Smithers (1972) reviewed the chemotherapy literature and found 31 cases of complete remission with single agents including mithramycin, nitrofurazone, methotrexate and hydroxyurea. In more recent years

Table 26.6 Non-seminomatous germ cell tumours of the testis: node dissection as initial treatment (from Donohue *et al.*, 1978).

Stage		Total patients	Relapsing as stage C	Surviving NED†
A	(negative nodes)	30	3 (10%)	30 (100%)
B₁	(positive nodes, minimal disease)	14	4 (28.5%)	13 (92%)
B₂	(gross nodal enlargement)	11	7 (63.7%)	7 (63.7%)
B₂	(bulky disease)	3*	0	3 (100%)

* Two received post-operative irradiation + actinomycin D and one patient actinomycin D
† No evidence of disease

Table 26.7 Relative merits and disadvantages of radical node dissection and nodal irradiation in early testicular cancer.

		Radical node dissection	Radiation therapy (Royal Marsden Hospital data)
Performance as a curative procedure (% cure rate)	−ve nodes*	82.6%†	82.4%
	+ve nodes	49.4%	51.1%
Complication rate		11%‡	< 2%
Mortality		1%‡	0%
Interference with sexual function		Retrograde ejaculation	None, fertility often preserved
Compromising effect on subsequent chemotherapy		None	Immediate chemotherapy: gut toxicity. Effective chemotherapy possible after abdominal node irradiation for early stage disease
Clinical vs pathological staging		Pathalogical staging data obtained. Major operative procedure required to obtain it.	25% false negative lymphogram rate: irrelevant since radiation therapy and deferred chemotherapy give a high disease-free survival rate.

* Histology −ve or +ve for radical node dissection
  Lymphography −ve or +ve for radiation therapy
† Collected data as shown in Table 23.5
‡ Data from Williams (1977)

experience with newer agents such as cis-diammine-dichloroplatinum (II) (cis-DDP), adriamycin and the epipodophyllotoxin VP 16–213 has underlined the chemoresponsive nature of testicular teratoma.

Between 1960 and 1970 combinations of drugs were investigated but although responses could be readily achieved, long-term responses were obtained only in a minority of patients. In an early study Li *et al.* (1960) reported a series of 23 patients treated with chlorambucil, actinomycin D and methotrexate, 12 of whom showed objective responses with one patient disease-free at 18 months

Vinblastine and bleomycin
Although a variety of combinations was explored in the ensuing years it was not until the introduction by Samuels *et al.* (1976) of the combination of vinblastine and bleomycin at high dosage that durable complete regressions were achived. In an initial study eight patients were treated and all eight responded. In more recent reports (Samuels *et al.*, 1975a; Samuels *et al.*, 1975b; Samuels *et al.*, 1976) results obtained with two different combinations are described. In the VB₁ regime vinblastine 0.4 mg/kg is given in two divided fractions intravenously on days 1 and 2 with bleomycin 30 mg intramuscularly twice weekly (Samuels *et al.*, 1975a).

Courses are repeated at four to six week intervals depending on toxicity. VB₃ is vinblastine in the same dosage on days 1 and 2 followed by bleomycin 30 mg/day for five days by continuous intravenous infusion. Both regimes were extremely toxic and patients needed to be in hospital.

In MTU complete response rates were seven of 26 patients (26%) with VB₁ and 21 of 36 patients (58%) with VB₃. In MTI the rates were 10 of 24 patients (44%) with VB₁ and seven of 21 patients (33%) with VB₃.

There were nine patients with MTT treated with vinblastine-bleomycin regimes. There were only two complete remissions. Only one of these remained alive and disease-free.

The success of Samuels' (1975; 1976) vinblastine-bleomycin combination led us to study this regime beginning at the end of 1975. A small group of patients were treated with vinblastine 9 mg/m² on days 1 and 2 followed by bleomycin 30 mg intramuscularly twice weekly for five weeks. The increased complete remission rate described with the VB₃ regime led to the adoption of a slight modification of this regime in early 1976. Vinblastine 9 mg/m² was given by intravenous injection on days 1 and 2 and bleomycin, 30 mg per day by continuous infusion over 24 hours was started after

Table 26.8 Malignant teratoma, Royal Marsden Hospital, 1976–1977 vinblastine/ continuous bleomycin chemotherapy.

Histology	No. of patients	CR		PR		Overall response	
MTU ± seminoma	31	15	(48%)	12	(39%)	27	(87%)
MTI ± seminoma	10	1	(10%)	2	(20%)	3	(30%)
MTT ± seminoma	6	1	(17%)	1	(17%)	2	(34%)
Other teratomas (mediastinal, retroperitoneal, differentiated)	4	–		3		3	
Overall	51	17	(33%)	18	(35%)	35	(68%)

CR = Complete remission
PR = Partial remission

Table 26.9 Malignant teratoma, Royal Marsden Hospital, 1976–1977 VB₃ chemotherapy. Response of metastases according to site.

Site	No. of patients	CR		PR		Overall response	
Lung	41	21	(51%)	10	(25%)	31	(76%)
Abdominal nodes	27	6	(22%)	11	(41%)	17	(63%)
Supra-clavicular and mediastinal nodes	8	3	(37%)	5	(63%)	8	(100%)
Liver	5	1		2		3	

CR = Complete remission
PR = Partial remission

the first injection of vinblastine and continued for five days, to a total dose of 150 mg per course. Courses were repeated at four to five week intervals depending on haematological toxicity.

Initially, no patients received more than two courses of vinblastine and bleomycin because the overall treatment plan included whole lung irradiation as a later treatment option. Subsequently patients received up to a maximum of six courses of vinblastine and bleomycin.

Table 26.8 sets out the response rates in 51 evaluable patients subdivided according to histology. The majority of responses occurred in patients with undifferentiated teratoma. The response rates in intermediate and trophoblastic teratoma were low, although patient numbers were small.

Table 26.9 shows the results according to the site of metastases. A definite difference was observed in complete response rate between pulmonary metastases and abdominal nodal metastases. Much of this can probably be explained by the large number of patients with bulky abdominal metastases.

Analysis of this group of patients made it clear that the volume of metastases was an important predictor of response (Table 26.10). Tyrrell and Peckham (1976) have shown this to be true for abdominal disease treated by radiotherapy alone and Samuels *et al.* (1976) have described similar findings with chemotherapy. The results of his accumulated chemotherapy experience have led Samuels to alter his approach to staging. Similarly, the differing responses according to bulk and site have led to a change in the detailed staging system used at this hospital which is summarized above.

Toxicity of the VB regime. The vinblastine/continuous

Table 26.10 Response of teratoma testis metastases to VB chemotherapy: influence of tumour volume.

Site of metastases	Substage	Total patients	Complete (CR) and partial (PR) remission	
			CR	PR
Lung metastases	L₁, L₂	21	16 (76.2%)	1 (5%)
	L₃	20	5 (25%)	9 (45%)
Abdominal metastases	A	3	3 (100%)	0

bleomycin regime is extremely toxic. There have been three treatment related deaths in the VB series, all associated with septicaemia. Infectious complications remain the major danger of treatment and may require therapy with granulocyte transfusions as well as appropriate systemic antibiotics. Neutropenia reaches its nadir, usually below 600 WBC/mm³, on days 8–10 with recovery evident by day 14. Thrombocytopenia occurs on days two to four, often below 30 000/mm³ with recovery proceeding through the period of leukopenia. Haemorrhage has occurred in only one patient, with duodenal invasion by massive abdominal disease. He had a haematemesis while responding well during his first course of VB₃. Subsequent courses were not associated with bleeding.

Less significant but almost universal side-effects are alopecia, stomatitis and constipation; the latter two require vigorous local treatment. The haemoglobin falls by one to 3 gm% with each course but recovers between courses and transfusion is rarely required. Bleomycin skin rashes and pigmentation are common and bleomycin also produces febrile reactions and symptoms rather like severe influenza. No bleomycin pneumonitis has been seen, other than in patients who have had previous lung irradiation. Patients usually lose from 5 to 10 kg with each course, but most recover to near their pre-treatment weight between courses.

All aspects of toxicity tend to become more severe with continuing treatment. One patient had chemotherapy terminated after the fifth course with severe neuropathy, gastrointestinal upset and inability to regain weight.

The toxicity is such that this regime should only be used by those experienced in the management of neutropenic patients in a hospital with adequate facilities.

Cis-diamminedichloroplatinum (II) (cis-DDP)
The reports by Higby *et al.* (1974*a*, *b*) of the effect of cis-DDP in testicular tumours and the more recent reports (Cvitkovic *et al.*, 1977; Hayes *et al.*, 1977) demonstrating that nephrotoxicity could be largely prevented by forced diuresis led us to study the drug as a single agent in doses of 50–130 mg/m² by intravenous infusion over 20 to 30 minutes. Mannitol was used with normal saline, 6l/24 hours, and intravenous frusemide as required to ensure a high urine flow. Infusions were repeated at three-week intervals depending on haematological and biochemical toxicity. Nephrotoxicity was monitored carefully using EDTA clearances.

Twenty-five patients received one to four infusions of cis-DDP. Twenty-three can be fully assessed. Three of the assessable patients received low doses (50 mg/m²) of cis-DDP. Two showed no response. The other, who had haemoptysis without evidence of a mass lesion, responded. The remaining 20 patients received cis-DDP in doses of 100–130 mg/m². Results are summarized in Table 26.11

Toxicity was not a major problem with cis-DDP. There was a transient fall in haemoglobin by 1–2 gm% which always recovered by three weeks. White cell count did not fall below 3000 or platelets below 100 000 except in a small group of patients who had had extensive prior chemotherapy and/or radiotherapy. Only three of four patients admitted to tinnitus, which has been described as a side-effect by Gottlieb and Drewinko (1975), although audiograms were not performed. Fig. 26.8 shows serial EDTA clearance in a patient having two infusions of cis-DDP.

It is clear that cis-DDP shows high activity in testicular teratoma and is of obvious interest to combine with vinblastine and bleomycin. Its toxicity is qualitatively different from both vinblastine and bleomycin and there is experimental evidence that it may have a specific effect on tissues arising from the urogenital anlage in that it produces testicular atrophy in monkeys (Higby *et al.*, 1974*a*).

Platinum: effect on EDTA clearance

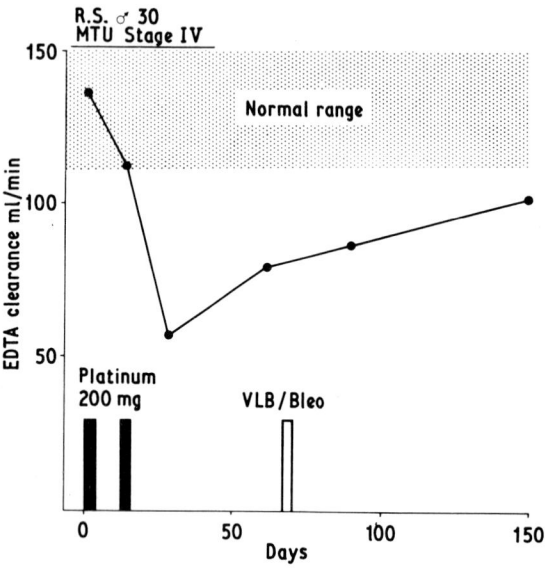

Fig. 26.8   Effect of cis-DDP on EDTA clearance (VLB = Vinblastine; Bleo = Bleomycin).

Cis-diamminedichloroplatinum, vinblastine and bleomycin (PVB) combination chemotherapy
This regime has been extensively explored by Einhorn and his colleagues (Einhorn and Donohue, 1977 *a, b*). Between August 1974 and September 1976, 50 patients with disseminated testicular teratoma were

treated. Three patients died within the first two weeks after presentation and were excluded from the analysis. Of the remaining 47 evaluable patients, 33 (70%) achieved complete remission and a further five patients were rendered disease-free by resection of residual tumour. Of the whole group 27 (57.4%) remain disease-free at 21 to 45 months (Einhorn and Williams, 1979).

It is clear that the PVB regime constitutes a major advance in the management of testicular teratoma and since relapses tend to occur within the first year following treatment the majority in this initial series are probably cured of their disease.

Drug dosage. Cis-DDP was given in a dosage of 20 mg/m² as a 15-minute infusion for five consecutive days every three weeks initially for three courses and more recently for four. Vinblastine was given initially at a dose of 0.4 mg/kg body weight in divided doses on days 1 and 2. More recently the vinblastine dose has been reduced to 0.3 mg/kg without loss of effectiveness but with reduction in toxicity (Einhorn and Williams, 1979). Bleomycin (30 mg iv) was given on days 2, 9 and 16 of each platinum course. Maintenance chemotherapy was employed in the form of vinblastine (0.3 mg/kg) every four weeks for a total of two years' duration.

Toxicity. The toxicity of cis-platinum includes nausea and vomiting, nephrotoxicity and tinnitus. Bleomycin is associated with fever, chills, cutaneous striae, alopecia and pneumonitis. Vinblastine produces myalgia, myelosuppression and gastrointestinal disturbance including pain and constipation. In the series of patients reported by Einhorn and Donohue (1977*b*), 18 required admission to hospital because of

Table 26.11   Malignant teratoma, Royal Marsden Hospital, 1976–1977 cis-DDP chemotherapy.

Histology	No. of patients	CR		PR		Overall response	
MTU ± seminoma	14	4	(29%)	4	(29%)	8	(57%)
MTI ± seminoma	4	–		2		2	(50%)
MTT ± seminoma	2	–		–		–	
Mediastinal teratoma	1	–		–		–	
Orchioblastoma	1	1		–		1	
MTD/yolk sac	–	–		–		–	
Overall	23	5	(22%)	6	(26%)	11	(48%)

CR = Complete remission
PR = Partial remission

Table 26.12 Influence of volume of metastases on response to
PVB (from Einhorn and Donohue, 1977*b*).

Extent of disease	Number of patients	Complete remission
Elevated HCG only	3	3 (100%)
Minimal lung	10	9 (90%)
Minimal abdomen + lung	9	8 (88%)
Total small volume disease	22	20 (91%)
Advanced lung	9	6 (67%)
Advanced abdomen	16	9 (56%)
Total large volume disease	25	15 (60%)

granulocytopenia and fever. Seven patients had proven septicaemia and one died.

Tumour volume and PVB response. Table 26.12 summarizes the relationship between volume of tumour and chemotherapy response for the PVB regime (Einhorn and Donohue, 1977*b*).

Results of treatment in testicular teratoma

Patients treated 1962—1975
The results obtained at the Royal Marsden Hospital between 1962 and 1975 are summarized below.

Stage I — Between 1962 and the end of 1975, 111 Stage I patients were treated by orchidectomy and radiation therapy. Of these 90 (81%) remain alive and disease-free.

Stage IIA — During the same period 21 Stage IIA patients were treated and 17 (80.9%) are alive and disease-free.

Stage IIB/C — In these patients with bulky abdominal disease, of 24 only six (25.0%) are alive and disease-free.

Stage III — Stage III is a less common stage category and only 16 patients were treated between 1962 and 1975. Of these five (31.2%) have survived.

Stage IV — A total of 112 Stage IV patients were treated up to December 1975 with a variety of single agent or combination regimes. Of these, only 11 (9.8%) survive.

Pattern of relapse in stage I and IIA. The time to initial relapse is short with 80% occurring during the first post-treatment year (Peckham *et al.*, 1977). Extension is predominantly to the supra-diaphragmatic nodes

and lungs. The time to and sites of relapse are summarized in Figs 26.9 and 26.10.

Significance of histology in the early stage patients. Fig. 26.11 shows the survival of Stage I and IIA patients treated between 1962 and 1975 according to histologic subtype. The difference between MTU and MTI is significant (p <0.05).

Follow-up, early detection of relapse and results of treatment for first relapse. The timing to first relapse, site(s) of relapse and the identification of MTU as the highest risk group in Stage I are relevant to patient follow-up. It is our practice to see MTU Stage I and IIA patients at monthly intervals for the first year. At each visit a chest radiograph is performed and blood taken for β-HCG and AFP measurement. CT-lung scans are performed at three and six months. Relapses are detected early and promptly treated with four to six courses of chemotherapy with or without further radiation therapy depending on restaging.

Patients treated 1976—1977
Patients treated after December 1975 were managed according to the protocols outlined above. Initially the chemotherapy regime was VB and, subsequently, PVB. Stage I and IIA patients were managed by orchidectomy and nodal irradiation, chemotherapy being deferred until relapse was established either by rising serum AFP and/or β(HCG, or by clinical detection of tumour. Stage IIB, C, III and IV patients received chemotherapy initially, as indicated above. The results obtained in patients treated between January 1976 and March 1978 are summarized in Tables 26.13 and 26.14 and the survival curves shown in Fig. 26.12. During this period only the VB regime was employed.

Early stage categories (Stage I and IIA, Table 26.13).

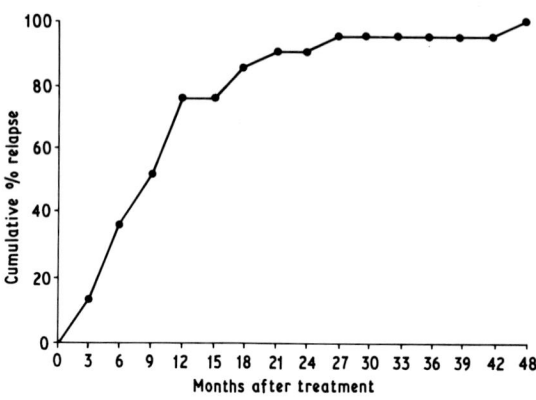

Fig. 26.9 Time to relapse in 32 patients treated for Stage 1 and IIA testicular teratoma (Royal Marsden Hospital 1962–1975).

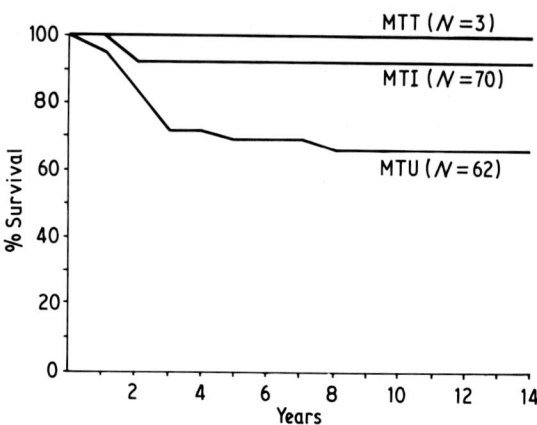

Fig. 26.11 Survival of Stage I and IIA testicular teratoma according to histology (Royal Marsden Hospital 1962–1975).

Sites of relapse in Stage I and IIA testicular teratoma patients treated by orchidectomy and nodal irradiation

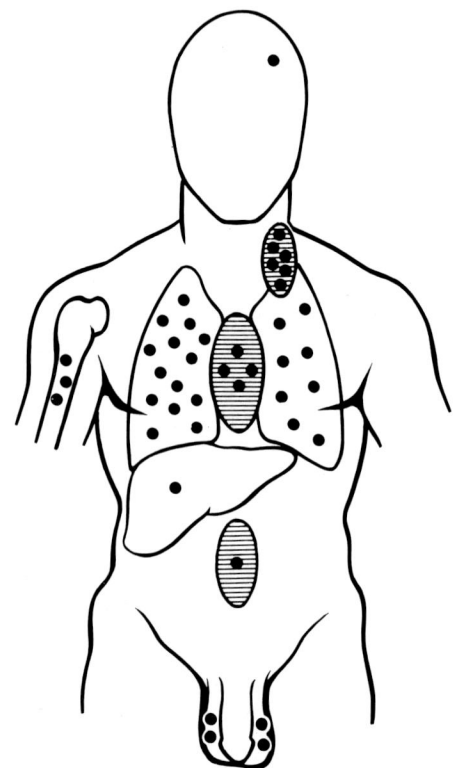

Fig. 26.10 Spread pattern in early stage testicular teratoma (Royal Marsden Hospital 1962–1975).

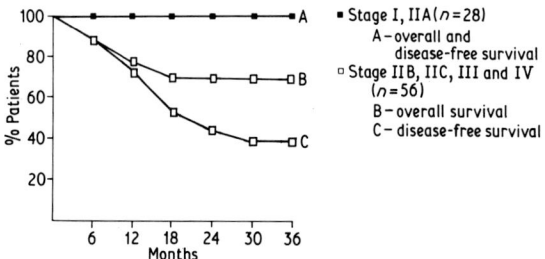

Fig. 26.12 Results of treatment in testicular teratoma (Royal Marsden Hospital Jan. 1976–March 1978).

All 28 patients treated remain alive and disease-free with follow-up times of 13 to 37 months (median 23) (Fig. 23.12). Of this group, three patients (11%) relapsed after radiation therapy and were treated for small-volume metastases with VB. They remain in complete remission at 12, 27 and 28 months.

Advanced stage categories. Table 26.14 summarizes the disease-free survival figures by clinical stage and previous treatment. Patients are subdivided into two broad groups; those considered suitable for multimodality therapy, as indicated above, and those with bulky multiple lung metastases and/or hepatic involvement (IV, L_3, IV, H_+) receiving chemotherapy alone. Fig. 26.12 shows the survival curve for the whole group of patients and Fig. 26.13 survival of the advanced presentation broken into the two broad subgroups as described above. The difference in disease-free survival between these two groups is highly significant (p <0.001). Of the first group, 17/21 (80.9%) of previously untreated patients are disease-free compared

Table 26.13 Testicular teratoma: results of treatment of stage I and IIA patients (Royal Marsden Hospital, 1976–1977).

Total patients	Number relapsing	Number alive and disease-free
28	3* (10.7%)	28 (100%)

* Alive and disease-free at 12, 24 and 32 months

Table 26.14 Advanced testicular teratoma: disease-free survival by stage (Royal Marsden Hospital, January 1976–March 1978).

Stage		Previously untreated patients	*Previously irradiated patients
II		2/3	1/2
III		3/4	0/1
IV O/A L_1	Group	6/6	1/2
IV B/C L_1	I	2/2	0/1
IV O/A L_2		2/2	3/4
IV B/C L_2		2/4	1/2
Total		17/21 (80.9%)	6/12 (50%)
IV O/A L_3	Group	3/7	1/2
IV B/C L_3	II	0/7	0/2
IV H+		0/4	0/1
Total		3/18 (16.7%)	1/5 (20%)
Grand total		20/39 (51.3%)	7/17 (41.2%)

* Staging refers to clinical stage on referral *after* relapse

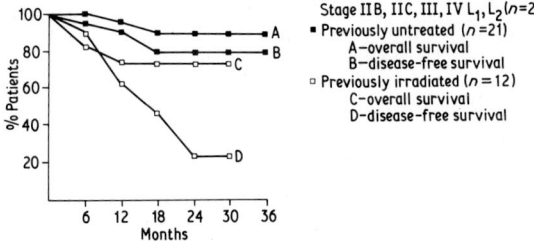

Fig. 26.13 Results of treatment in advanced testicular teratoma (Group I) by previous treatment status (Royal Marsden Hospital Jan. 1976–March 1978).

with 3/18 (16.7%) of the IV L_3 and IV H+ group. Overall, 51.3% of previously untreated patients are currently alive and disease-free compared with 41.2% of the patients referred following relapse after radiation therapy (Fig. 26.14).

Of 56 patients treated for advanced disease 33 (58.9%) had MTU, 16 (28.6%) MTI and seven (12.5%) MTT. MTI patients fared less well than MTU (57.6% vs 31.3% disease-free survival rates respectively); the difference did not reach significance.

Tumour markers in testicular tumours

Alphafoeto protein

AFP is produced by the vitelline cells of the yolk sac origin and its production by the tumour represents a derepression of the original response for the production of the protein. AFP is a major plasma protein of early foetal life and its content in the serum rapidly falls after birth. Its physiological function is unknown although it probably functions as foetal albumen. Its value as a marker in testicular tumours was proposed by Abelev *et al.* (1967) and is now clearly established. AFP is produced by yolk sac components of the tumour and its synthesis has been demonstrated in yolk sac tumour growth *in vitro* and *in vivo* as xenografts in nude mice. In patients without metastases and in whom

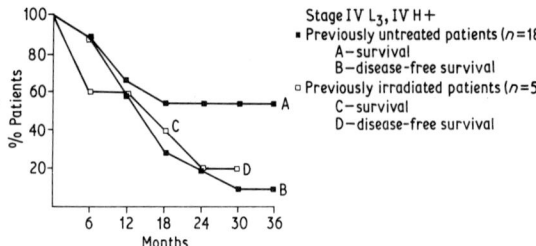

Fig. 26.14 Advanced testicular teratoma (Group II): results of treatment by previous treatment status (Royal Marsden Hospital Jan. 1976–March 1978).

elevated serum AFP levels can be entirely attributed to production by the primary testicular neoplasms the serum half life following orchidectomy is 3.5–5.0 days.

Human Chorionic Gonadotrophin

HCG is a glycoprotein normally secreted by specialized cells of the placenta. HCG, follicular stimulating hormone (FSH) and luteinizing hormone (LH) each consist of two polypeptide chains, alpha and beta. All three hormones are structurally, biochemically and in part antigenically similar. The β chain of HCG is immunologically distinct and can be accurately measured by the sensitive radioimmunoassay developed by Vaitukaitis and Ross (1973). The plasma clearance of HCG is approximately 16 h.

As noted above elevated serum levels of β-HCG and AFP detected post-orchidectomy may reflect production of marker by the primary tumour. It is thus important, if possible, to obtain a pre-orchidectomy sample

and at least two sequential samples post-orchidectomy before treatment is initiated. The prognostic significance, if any, of marker production by the primary tumour *per se* is not yet clear but should be elucidated in the near future. Persistence of elevated levels after orchidectomy indicate the presence of metastases, but the prognostic significance of elevated marker levels over and above the significance of tumour stage is not yet clear. Both β-HCG and AFP are valuable monitors of therapeutic progress and post-treatment marker elevation is a clear indication of relapse. Conversely, falling β-HCG and AFP levels do not necessarily indicate continued tumour regression, since progression of non-marker producing tumour elements may occur.

Tumour marker levels in Stage I patients

Pre-orchidectomy sampling may show elevated serum levels of β-HCG or AFP due to marker production by the primary tumour with, in some patients, an associated contribution from metastatic tumour. In the absence of metastases the markers will be cleared from the blood and fall to undetectable levels. If either AFP or β-HCG is produced by metastases the levels may remain elevated after initial incomplete reduction in the serum. Pre-therapeutic marker levels may be of prognostic significance in several different ways.

1. Pre-orchidectomy marker production by the primary tumour may be in itself of prognostic significance.
2. Persisting levels after clearance following orchidectomy of marker produced by the primary tumour will indicate metastases and hence are

Table 26.15   Treatment outcome and tumour markers (AFP and HCG) in Stage I testicular teratoma (Royal Marsden Hospital, 1973–1978).

AFP	β-HCG	Total patients	Number continuously disease-free	Observation time (months) Range	Median	NED†	Relapsed patients On treatment	Dead
	−	36	31	9–77	28	2	2	1
−	ND‡	9	6	46–72	60	2	−	1
	+	3	2	13–26	−	−	−	1
	−	15	11	10–66	29	1	−	3
+	ND	1	−	−	−	−	−	1
	+	2	1	62	−	1	−	−
Total patients		66	51			6	2	7

59/66 Alive   = 89.4%
51/66 cdf*   = 77.3%
7/66 Dead   = 10.6%

* continuous disease-free survival
† no evidence of disease
‡ not done

likely to be prognostically significant.

3. The absolute levels of persisting post-orchidectomy marker are likely to be a measure of the volume of metastatic tumour.

Although it is not yet possible to analyse these events in detail (due to paucity of information on pre-orchidectomy AFP and β-HCG levels), a preliminary assessment of the role of AFP and β-HCG in early stage patients can be made. Table 26.15 summarizes marker details on 66 Stage I patients seen between 1973 and 1978. Of 36 patients in whom both AFP and β-HCG were measured and found to be normal (following orchidectomy and before radiation therapy) only five (13.9%) relapsed subsequently. In 21 patients showing elevation of either AFP or β-HCG, seven (33%) relapsed.

These results suggest that pre-treatment marker elevation in Stage I is associated with abdominal node metastases in 2/3 of patients and with extralymphatic spread in 1/3. In marker negative patients the probability of cure with orchidectomy and radiation therapy is high. This may reflect the presence of small tumour aggregates confined to the abdominal nodes (readily controlled by irradiation but inadequate to produce detectable levels of AFP and β-HCG or alternatively patients who have been cured by orchidectomy and who have no metastatic tumour.

Future studies are likely to test the value of elective radiotherapy in the marker negative Stage I patient and of chemotherapy as initial therapy in the patient in whom elevated AFP and β-HCG levels fails to return to normal after orchidectomy.

AFP and β-HCG in advanced presentations

As shown in Fig. 26.15 the proportion of patients with elevated serum marker levels increases with more advanced disease and particularly with bulky tumour masses. The most important determinant of patient outcome is complete or incomplete reversal of marker levels to normal on chemotherapy. As shown in Table 26.16 no patient who failed to achieve marker remission has survived free from disease.

Combined modality treatment in testicular teratoma

Surgery, radiation and chemotherapy are each capable of curing a proportion of patients when employed as the sole method of treatment. With the introduction of effective chemotherapy the role of radiation and surgery needs reappraisal. The following points can be made. Effective chemotherapy for testicular teratoma is toxic and hence should be avoided if its use is not

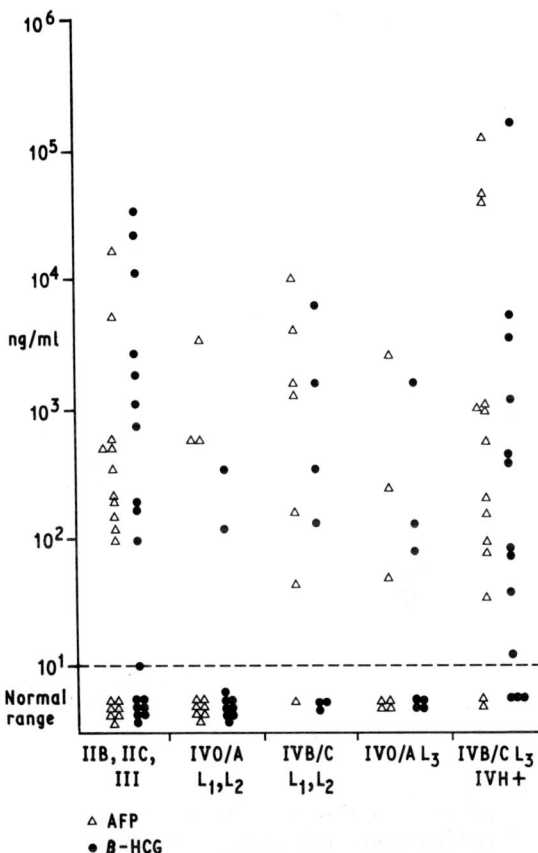

Fig. 26.15 Advanced testicular teratoma: tumour markers by sub-stage (Royal Marsden Hospital 1976–1978).

essential. Thus, in early stage patients where 80% of men are cured by orchidectomy and radiation therapy, chemotherapy should not be employed unless relapse is proven. As discussed in the management of the Stage I patient, if there are *persistently* high marker levels after orchidectomy the probability of relapse following irradiation is high and chemotherapy should be the initial form of therapy. In the marker negative Stage I patient it may be possible to omit any form of treatment following orchidectomy and institute a policy of careful follow-up.

It seems not to substantiate any case for node dissection as a primary treatment method and surgery is more effectively deployed following chemotherapy to excise residual tumour masses. Whether its role is diagnostic or therapeutic is unclear but if further chemotherapy can be given in situations where the histology of excised material is positive then the role of surgery

Table 26.16 Advanced testicular teratoma: results of treatment by serum AFP and β-HCG response to chemotherapy, Royal Marsden Hospital (January 1976–March 1978).

	Total patients	Initial marker levels		Marker response to chemotherapy		NED
		Normal	Elevated	CR	NR/PR	
(A) Previously untreated patients	39	10				6
			29*	19		14
					9	0
(B) Previously irradiated patients	17	5†				3
			12‡	8		4
					3	0

* One patient died with first course of chemotherapy
† One patient died from treatment in complete remission
‡ One patient died from treatment following one course of chemotherapy

KEY: CR = Complete remission
NR = No response
PR = Partial response
NED = No evidence of disease

may well be both diagnostic and therapeutic.

So far as radiation therapy is concerned it is clear that small volumes of teratoma are highly responsive to irradiation. With this observation and the development of a chemotherapeutic combination comparable or even superior to MOPP in Hodgkin's disease, it is important to consider whether chemotherapy followed by irradiation of sites of initial bulky disease might not be a highly effective method of management.

The influence of tumour volume on drug response is clear (Table 26.17) and provides a sound rationale for such an approach to management. Preliminary experience with combined treatment at the Royal Marsen Hospital has been summarized above.

Radiation therapy following chemotherapy

Whereas chemotherapy (VB) given soon after nodal irradiation may produce severe acute toxicity, particularly in the gastrointestinal tract, our experience to date has been that following chemotherapy, radiotherapy is tolerated satisfactorily and not associated with unexpected immediate or subsequent toxicity. In testicular tumours, as in other clinical situations, it would appear logical to deploy systemic therapy initially. The bone marrow reserve is uncompromised, small-volume tumour is eradicated and bulky tumour masses reduced in volume, thus facilitating subsequent irradiation and/or resection.

Table 26.18 summarizes our early experience with combined therapy.

For the moment, we are continuing to employ surgery following chemotherapy and radiotherapy but it may eventually be possible to identify patients in whom a combination of chemotherapy and carefully individualized radiation therapy to bulky tumour sites, may be a suitable form of management. It is intended to test the combination of chemotherapy and surgery against chemotherapy and radiotherapy in a randomized study.

Treatment of testicular seminoma

Seminomas are characterized by their prompt and marked responsiveness to radiation. Information on the chemosensitivity of advanced seminoma is scanty, although it is generally assumed that their radiosensitivity is paralleled by sensitivity to a range of cytotoxic drugs including alkylating agents. The overall cure rate in seminoma exceeds 90% and this is, in large part, a reflection of the early stage presentation of the majority of patients.

Age at presentation

The large experience of the Testicular Tumour Panel (Pugh, 1976), is summarized in Fig. 26.2*a*, showing a peak age incidence at 35 years. Most seminomas in men over 70 are of the spermatocytic type (*vide infra*).

Stage presentation

As shown in Table 26.19 more than 70% of seminoma patients present with Stage I disease. In our own series

Table 26.17 Influence of tumour volume on chemotherapy response in testicular teratoma.

Author	Small volume			Large volume		
	Total	CR	%	Total	CR	%
*Samuels *et al.* (1976)	26	23	88.5	63	24	38.1
†Juttner and McElwain (1979)	24	19	79.2	44	8	18.2
Total (VB)	50	42	(84)	107	32	(29.9)
‡Einhorn and Donohue (1977*b*)	22	20	91	25	15	(60)
§Stoter *et al.* (1979)	3	3	100	36	20	(55.5)
Total (PVB)	25	23	92	61	35	(57.4)

* Small volume includes: 3A supra-clavicular metastases only
                                 3B gynaecomastia only
                                 $3B_2$ minimal pulmonary disease
  Large volume includes: $3B_3$ advanced pulmonary disease
                                   $3B_4$ advanced abdominal disease
                                   $3B_5$ visceral metastases (excluding lung)
† Small volume includes Stages IVA and IV L_1 L_2
  Large volume includes Stages IVB, C and IV L_3
‡ Small volume includes: raised HCG only
                                 minimal lung disease
                                 minimal abdomen + lung
  Large volume includes: advanced lung disease
                                 advanced abdominal disease
§ As above raised HCG only category excluded
CR = Complete remission

Table 26.18 Combined management of previously untreated patients with advanced testicular teratoma, Royal Marsden Hospital (January 1976–March 1978).

Stage	Total patients	Total receiving combined treatment	C—R—S‡	C–R	C–S–R	C–S	Total
II	3	3	1/1	–	1/1	–	2/2
III	4	3	2/2	1/1	–	–	3/3
IV L_1	8	8*	2/2	6/6			8/8
IV L_2	6	3	–	1/2†	–	1/1	2/3
Total	21	16	5/5	8/9	1/1	1/1	15/16 (93.8%)

* One patient had lung irradiation for residual disease
† One patient currently being assessed for possible surgery
‡ C = Chemotherapy; R = Radiotherapy; S = Surgery
   Order of letters denotes time-sequence of therapy

of patients (Table 26.20) 54/190 (28%) had positive lymphograms but no evidence of metastases elsewhere (Stage II). Stage III and IV disease presentations are uncommon. Thus, there were only 8/190 Stage III patients (4.2%) and seven Stage IV presentations (3.6%).

Investigation and clinical staging procedures

The approach to patient investigation is essentially similar to that described for malignant teratoma. Since the majority of patients present with early stage disease and have an excellent prognosis, staging is generally limited to chest radiography, intravenous pyelography, lymphography, routine biochemistry and examination of the blood for tumour markers (AFP and β-HCG).

If there is evidence of abdominal node involvement it is important to determine the extent of disease accurately, since failure to include metastatic tumour within the radiation field has led to treatment failure in the past. For this reason, in patients with bulky disease, we have advocated laparotomy with accurate surgical delineation of the extent of the tumour. With the advent of CT-scanning it is possible to avoid a surgical intervention since adequate information on the disposition of retroperitoneal tumour can be obtained in most cases.

In patients suspected of harbouring distant metastases [67] Gallium scanning is a useful tumour localizing method in seminoma, although not in malignant teratoma (Paterson *et al.*, 1976).

Table 26.19 Seminoma testis: incidence of Stage I disease.

	Total seminomas	Stage I
Ytredal and Bradford (1972)	80	71
Saxena (1973)	77	75
Castro and Gonzalez (1971)	96	58
Van der Werf-Messing (1976)	257	153*
Maier *et al.* (1968)	80	78
Kademian *et al.* (1976)	52	36
Calman *et al.* (1979)	191	121
Total	833	592 (72.7%)

* This includes 95 patients designated Nx in the absence of lymphography

Table 26.20 The results of treatment by stage of 190 previously untreated patients with seminoma testis (The Royal Marsden Hospital, 1963–1975).

	Total patients	Lost to follow-up	Relapsed	Died of intercurrent disease	Died seminoma	Died teratoma	Developed second tumour
Stage I	121	13	4	4	1 (second tumour)	0	7
Stage IIA	38	1 (42 months)	6	4	6	0	0
Stage IIB	16	0	4	1	3		0
Stage III	8	1 (67 months)	1/ 1 NC	0	2	2	2 (both died teratoma)
Stage IV	7	1 (9 months)	0/ 4 NC	0	4	1	1 (died teratoma)

NC = never controlled by therapy

AFP and HCG in seminoma testis

It is important to examine the serum levels of AFP and β-HCG even if the histological appearance of the primary tumour is that of pure seminoma. In some combined tumours where both seminoma and non-seminoma elements are both present in the primary tumour, the malignant teratoma element may be small and thus overlooked if the entire tumour is unavailable for detailed histological examination. Moreover, even in apparently pure seminoma tissue, β-HCG-containing cells can be demonstrated in some cases using immunocytochemical staining methods. The presence of raised serum markers should be taken as evidence of a teratomatous component and this should influence treatment choice. The presence of small foci of trophoblast in a minority of seminoma cases raises the interesting possibility that seminoma and teratoma may represent different points along the histogenetic pathway of germ cell tumours and that, at least in some instances, seminoma may evolve into malignant teratoma.

History before presentation

Some patients with seminoma give a long history of testicular swelling before a diagnosis of malignancy is finally made. Length of history has been examined in relation to the extent of abdominal lymph node disease in our own series of patients and the results summarized in Fig. 26.16. It is seen that the length of history may extend to 10 years with 11 patients giving a history of testicular swelling for more than two years. It is of interest that the median length of history (six months and 11 months) are significantly different ($p < 0.05$) for patients with small volume and large volume abdominal node metastases respectively.

Treatment policy in seminoma testis

This is summarized as follows:

Stage I

Disease is treated by radiation therapy of the para-aortic and ipsilateral pelvic lymph nodes from $D_{10/11}$ to the lower border of the obturator foramen. The scrotal sac and inguinal nodes are only irradiated if there has been a trans-scrotal needle aspirate, scrotal orchidectomy, or previous orchidopexy. A dose of 3000 rad in three weeks is delivered to the nodes, using a 6–8 MeV linear accelerator.

Stage II

As pointed out above, if bulky disease is present, the extent and position of tumour is determined accurately to minimize the risk of a geographic miss with radiation therapy. If large volume disease is present it is now our

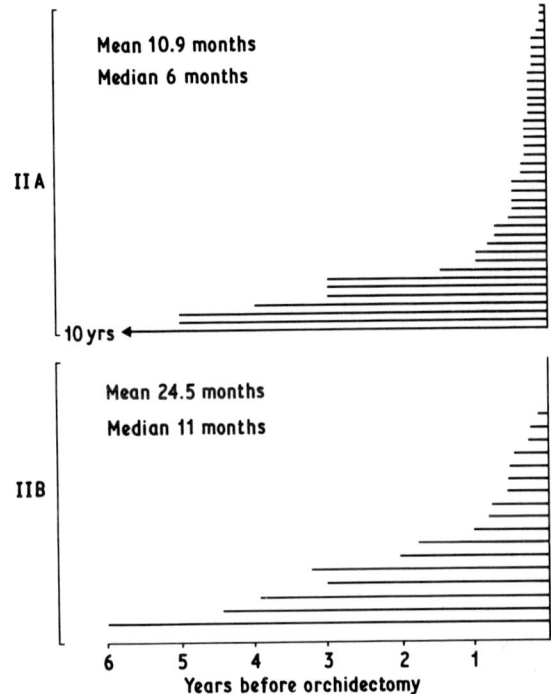

Fig. 26.16 Seminoma of testis (Royal Marsden Hospital 1963–1975): length of history in relation to volume of abdominal node metastases.

policy to shrink the tumour with prior chemotherapy before embarking on irradiation. Initially, we employed high dose cyclophosphamide (5 g with forced diuresis) but currently we are exploring the PVB combination, as employed in the treatment of the non-seminoma germ cell tumours. Para-aortic and pelvic node irradiation is given as for Stage I patients except that the contra-lateral pelvic nodes are irradiated if there is low para-aortic disease. A minimum tumour dose of 3500 rad in three and a half to four weeks is given with a supplementary boost to residual abdominal nodes. After an interval of one month the mediastinal and supra-clavicular nodes are irradiated (3000 rad in three weeks). This is omitted if the patient has had prior chemotherapy.

Stage III

Here the approach is essentially similar to that described for the Stage II patient. Supplementary radiation doses are given by reduced fields to supra-diaphragmatic tumour following delivery of 3000 rad in three weeks to the mediastinal and supra-clavicular nodes.

accounts for between 1% and 1.5% of all gynaecological cancer. Because of its rarity few clinicians gain wide experience in its treatment. The number of deaths in England and Wales is about 130 per year. Most primary cancers of the vagina occur between the ages of 50 and 80 years with the late fifties as the predominant age. Parity appears to have no bearing on the incidence of the disease, neither does previous irradiation for other gynaecological cancers. Trauma and ulceration following prolonged wearing of a supportive vaginal pessary is an aetiological factor.

In recent years there have been reports in the USA of clear cell adenocarcinoma of the vagina occurring in adolescent girls and young women who were born of mothers treated with stilboestrol during the early stages of pregnancy, to prevent recurrent abortion. The aetiological relationship between maternal stilboestrol therapy in the 1940s and the development of this disease in female children in the late 1960s was quickly recognized. This therapy was rarely used in the United Kingdom.

The common primary lesion is a squamous cell carcinoma and the most frequent site of origin is in the upper vagina on the posterior wall, although any segment may be involved. Carcinoma in-situ occurs in the vagina, most commonly in the upper vagina, but may occur throughout its whole length and is often multicentric in origin. It may be found in association with carcinoma in-situ of the cervix and if it is first demonstrated by cytology following hysterectomy for a cervical in-situ lesion, the presumption must be that it had pre-existed when the cervical lesion was diagnosed.

Secondary carcinoma of the vagina is very uncommon and such lesions are usually secondary to endometrial carcinoma; typically they present just inside the introitus on the anterior wall immediately behind the urethra and may be due to retrograde lymphatic spread. Lesions may occur due to direct invasion from cancer of the cervix; there may be secondary invasion by extensive cancer of the rectum or bladder. Very rarely ovarian cancer may erode through the pouch of Douglas.

Spread of disease

Carcinoma of the vagina spreads principally by direct extension either laterally into the parametrial tissue and to the pelvic walls, anteriorly into the bladder, or posteriorly into the rectum; the main mode of spread is lymphatic. The vaginal mucosa and muscularis contain an anastomotic meshwork of lymphatics which combine laterally into larger drainage trunks. The lymphatics from the upper portion of the vagina communicate with branches from the cervix and drain to the internal and external iliac lymph nodes. The lower half of the vagina drains to the pelvic and to the inguinal and femoral nodes. The anterior vaginal wall drains to the nodes on the lateral pelvic wall, especially the internal iliacs, and the posterior vaginal wall tends to drain to the deep pelvic lymph nodes such as the inferior gluteal, the sacral and the rectal nodes. Occasionally metastases may be found in bones, lungs and liver. Patients tend to die from locally uncontrolled disease leading to pressure on the ureters and to uraemia or, more rarely, from the effects of distant metastases in the liver or lungs. Sepsis and toxic absorption is an important cause of death.

Pathology

Primary vaginal carcinoma is nearly always a squamous cell carcinoma of a fairly well differentiated variety. Adenocarcinomas are very rare, as are mixed mesodermal tumours and also sarcomas. Very occasionally, a melanoma of the urethra may present as a mass in the vagina.

Symptoms and presentation

Vaginal bleeding and blood-stained discharge are the commonest symptoms of this disease. Post-coital bleeding is a possible presenting feature in young patients with adenocarcinoma, but post-menopausal bleeding is encountered more frequently because of the older age of these patients. Pain is associated only with very extensive disease. Urinary symptoms or rectal bleeding may also be presenting symptoms and these again are associated with extensive disease. Once a bleeding tumour is established secondary infection and purulent discharge is inevitable.

Diagnosis

Carcinoma in-situ of the vagina may be picked up on cytological smear, and an alert cytologist may comment that malignant cells were present on the vaginal but not on the cervical smear. A cone biopsy performed because of a suspicious smear may be reported negative and subsequent cytological smears remain positive; in such circumstances carcinoma in-situ of the vagina must be considered. All patients presenting with vaginal bleeding and discharge must be fully examined. The examination must include careful manipulation of the vaginal speculum so as to ensure that the whole of the vaginal mucosa is visualized. Special investigations include chest X-ray, blood count and blood chemistry, an intravenous pyelogram and lymphography if this is available. The diagnosis rests upon an examination under anaesthesia including a cystoscopy, dilatation and curettage, cervical biopsy, bimanual examination and sigmoidoscopy. A biopsy is taken of any and every abnormal lesion seen on the vaginal mucosa. The colposcope now allows well directed biopsy.

Staging of carcinoma of the vagina

Very few published series have been staged according to the UICC system of TNM and it is impossible to reassess reports and restage them. Also it is very difficult to assess the pelvic lymph nodes by either vaginal or rectal examination even under anaesthesia. Even lymphography is of doubtful value in central pelvic lymph node involvement. The FIGO staging is therefore preferable for this particular tumour.

It should be noted that primary adenocarcinoma of the vagina should not be diagnosed unless endometrial carcinoma has been positively excluded.

A diagnosis of primary carcinoma of the vagina must not be made if the cervix is involved unless it can be demonstrated conclusively that such cervical involvement was definitely secondary.

Treatment

The results of treatment of carcinoma of the vagina are poor. To improve them it is essential that clinicians must realize that limited or conservative management is unlikely to be successful. Radiotherapy is the treatment of choice because surgery if used at all must be very extensive. Only for Stage I lesions is surgery even feasible and here total hysterectomy, total vaginectomy and pelvic lymphadenectomy is the minimum procedure which can be classified as potentially curative. Not only does the operation carry substantial risk of damage to bladder function but the removal of the

Table 27.1 FIGO Staging of carcinoma of the vagina (from Perez *et al.*, 1973).

	Stage	Carcinoma
Pre-invasive	0	Carcinoma in-situ (intra-epithelial)
Invasive	I	Carcinoma limited to the vaginal mucosa
	II	Sub-mucosal infiltration and into parametrium but not extending out to the pelvic wall
	III	Tumour extends to pelvic wall
	IV	Tumour extends to bladder or rectum or metastases outside true pelvis (a bullous oedema of the bladder mucosa does not necessarily indicate involvement or permit allotment of the case to Stage IV)

vagina is psychologically distressing and successful split-skin vaginoplasty is doubtfully compatible with radical excision. For Stage I lesions in the lower third of the vagina, total hysterectomy, vaginectomy, vulvectomy and inguinal node dissection would be obligatory. Surgery may be indicated in patients with total procidentia when total hysterectomy and total vaginectomy can be combined with pelvic irradiation. Surgical salvage can be employed in some patients where radiation has failed and the persistent disease is not too extensive. It is an adjunctive to irradiation in special cases such as rectovaginal or vesicovaginal fistula when preliminary colostomy or ileal loop bladder formation must precede definitive treatment.

Carcinoma in-situ

Carcinoma in-situ of the vagina may be multicentric and in view of this, it is important to treat the whole of the vaginal mucosa. This is best done with a delrin or nylon applicator which extends from the vaginal vault to the introitus in the centre of which are placed the radioactive sources, the number of sources depending upon the length of applicator in the vagina (Fig. 27.2). The size of the applicator is variable, usually between 2.5 to 3 cm in diameter. The aim is to give 6500 to 7000 rad to the mucosal surface. Care must be taken to avoid overdosage as this can lead to severe mucosal reaction and vaginal stenosis. Within two weeks of treatment, the patient should be encouraged to perform daily vaginal douching as this helps prevent vaginal stenosis, and she should be encouraged to resume intercourse as soon as she is no longer sore.

Invasive carcinoma of vagina

In virtually all cases of invasive carcinoma of the vagina, there is a place for external beam therapy associated with some form of intracavitary or interstitial treatment. The latter may be individualized according to the position of the lesion in the vagina and to its extent.

Stage I

If the lesion is small and in the posterior vaginal vault it may be treated similarly to carcinoma of the cervix with three intracavitary insertions of caesium utilizing a uterine tube and vaginal sources to a total of 9000 rad to Point A, three insertions of 22 hours each at 2 and 1 week intervals. This is followed by external irradiation to the whole pelvis by a parallel opposed pair of fields on a Linear Accelerator or Cobalt Unit with central shielding so that the dose to parametria and pelvic walls will be 4800 rad. If, however, the lesion extends further down the vaginal wall, or is at the introitus, then the patient should be treated by external irradia-

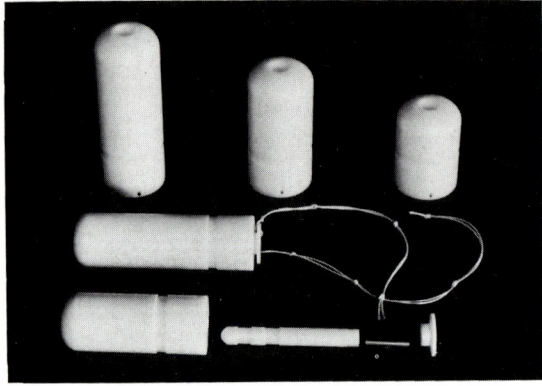

Fig. 27.2   After-loading Dobbie applicators.

tion to the whole pelvis, preferably by one anterior and two posterior oblique fields covering the pelvis from the top of the fifth lumbar vertebra down to the lower border of the obturator foramen and extending laterally to cover the pelvic side walls, giving a dose of 4000 to 4500 rad in 4 to 5 weeks followed either by a vaginal cylinder giving a surface dose of 8000 rad in two insertions separated by 2 weeks, or by an interstitial implant with either caesium needles or after-loading iridium wires. The implant may either be a single plane implant or a double plane implant, depending on the thickness of the lesion, planning to give a dose of 4000 to 5000 rad in 3 to 5 days. To obtain a good parallel application it is important when inserting the needles to place them with their tips converging slightly because when the patient is taken down from lithotomy, the proximal ends of the needles splay outwards.

Stage II

In Stage II disease the patient should have external irradiation to the whole pelvis as described for Stage I, with one anterior and two posterior oblique fields, to a dose of 4500 to 4800 rad in 5 weeks, care being taken to keep the lower rectal dose as low as possible. This is followed by the insertion of an intracavitary cylinder carrying radioactive sources in tandem to fill the entire length of the vagina, and left *in situ* for a time calculated to bring the total minimal dose to the tumour of 7000 to 8000 rad. If the tumour is near the introitus, then the possibility of inguinal node involvement is high, and these should be treated with external beam therapy with a Linear Accelerator preferably with careful fractionation and with care to prevent any overlap from the previous anterior pelvic fields to a dose of 5000 to 6000 rad in 5 to 6 weeks. In doubtful cases, node biopsy is indicated. Bilateral superficial lymphadenectomy may obviate the need for external irradiation.

Stage III

Stage III carcinoma of the vagina, where the tumour extends to the pelvic wall, is best treated entirely by external irradiation, whether the lesion has arisen in the upper or the lower part of the vagina. The whole pelvis should be treated, preferably with supervoltage on a Linear Accelerator or Cobalt Unit, with an anterior and posterior pair of fields extending from the introitus up to the middle of the body of L5 and laterally to encompass the pelvic walls, the posterior field having a central lead block 4 cm in width extending the whole length of the field for rectal protection, and two posterior oblique fields which may or may not be wedged depending on the configuration of the patient's buttocks (Fig. 27.3). The highest dose in the region of the parametrium is taken to 4800 rad in 5 weeks. The patient is then replanned with smaller fields to encompass the whole of the vagina, usually four oblique fields of about 10×8 cm size extending from the introitus upwards to cover the top of the vagina including the cervix, this volume being taken to a total of 6000 rad (Fig. 27.4).

Stage IV

Here treatment is purely palliative and as the tumour has already invaded either the bladder or the rectum, the dangers of irradiation producing a rectovaginal fistula or a vesicovaginal fistula are high, as the tumour regresses in the rectovaginal septum or in the vesicovaginal septum. Dosage should therefore be designed solely to relieve symptoms. Treatment should be by irradiation with an external beam from a Linear Accelerator or Cobalt Unit to the whole pelvis to a dose of 4000 rad in 4.5 weeks.

Complications of treatment and follow-up

It is essential that careful follow-up is carried out so that recurrence may be detected early and treated surgically. If the primary tumour is well controlled but the patient has developed inguinal node metastases, node dissection may render her clear of tumour again. During and immediately after irradiation, patients may be troubled by diarrhoea and tenesmus but this can usually be controlled with the use of codeine phosphate tablets 30 mg t.i.d. and Lomotil tablets 1 t.i.d. or a mixture of kaolin and morphia. Vaginal fibrosis can be avoided by the judicious use of vaginal douching. Proctitis may develop at a later stage and this may be alleviated by the use of intrarectal steroid preparations. Radiation cystitis may also occur during treatment and it is important to make cetain that the urine is clear of infection at all times during radiotherapy. Rectal or urethral stricture may occur as late complications but

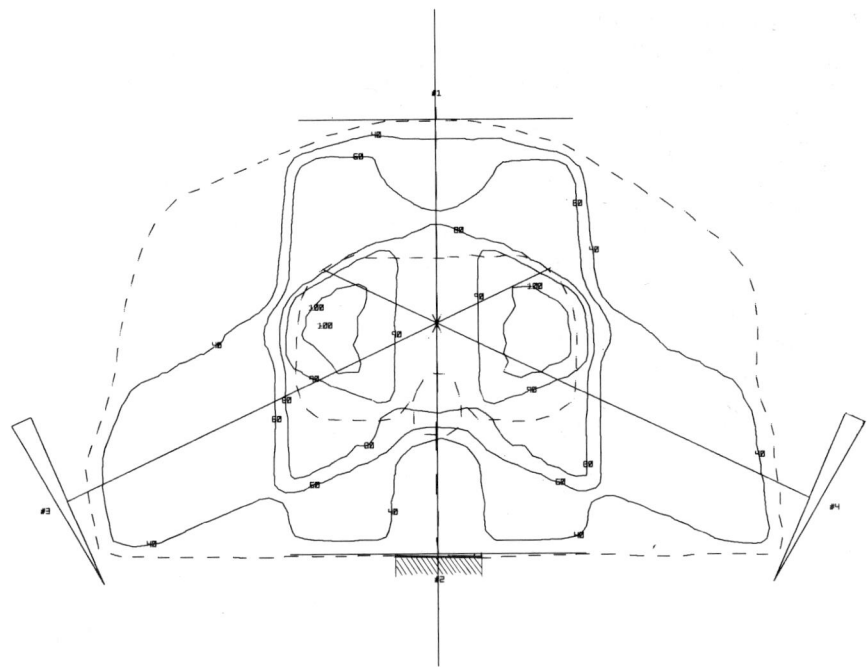

Fig. 27.3   8 MeV Linear Accelerator: 4-field treatment plan for carcinoma of the vagina.
Beam   1   14.0 × 13.0, Weight 47%
Beam   2   14.1 × 14.1, Weight 23%
Beam   3 and   4   15.0 × 8.5, Wedge No.1, Weight 46%

these generally follow excessive dosage. Rectovaginal or vesicovaginal fistula, the former being more common, may occur but this is usually due to tumour regression within the rectovaginal septum or the vesicovaginal septum. Alleviation by colostomy or ileal loop conduit may be needed.

Results

The absolute 5-year survival results are in the range of:

Stage 0	In-situ	83%
Stage I		70–80%
Stage II		26–68%
Stage III		27–30%
Stage IV		0–9%

Patients die either from uraemia due to uncontrolled local disease or from distant metastases because of failure to control local disease. It is highly likely that the failure to control local disease is due to an hypoxic sub-population of cells within the tumour volume. Squamous cell carcinomata have a fair prognosis but melanomata and sarcomata bear a very poor prognosis indeed. The earlier the patient is seen and the earlier the stage of the disease, the better the outlook.

Future trends

One would hope that radiosensitizers with the use of misonidazole or other similar drugs might improve the results of the radiotherapy treatment of carcinoma of the vagina. The place of the laser beam and of cryosurgery have yet to be established.

Part III: Ovaries

Cancer of the ovary is a common disease and in recent years, the annual incidence of primary ovarian malignancies has shown a steady rise and is now responsible for about twice as many deaths as either cervical or uterine carcinoma. There are approximately 4000 deaths a year from ovarian cancer in England, and the incidence of new registrations per 100 000 women per year is about 16.

Aetiology

Hembold (1961) analysed 14 different patient populations, comprising a total of 1300 cases of ovarian tumour. He found the frequency of ovarian carcinoma

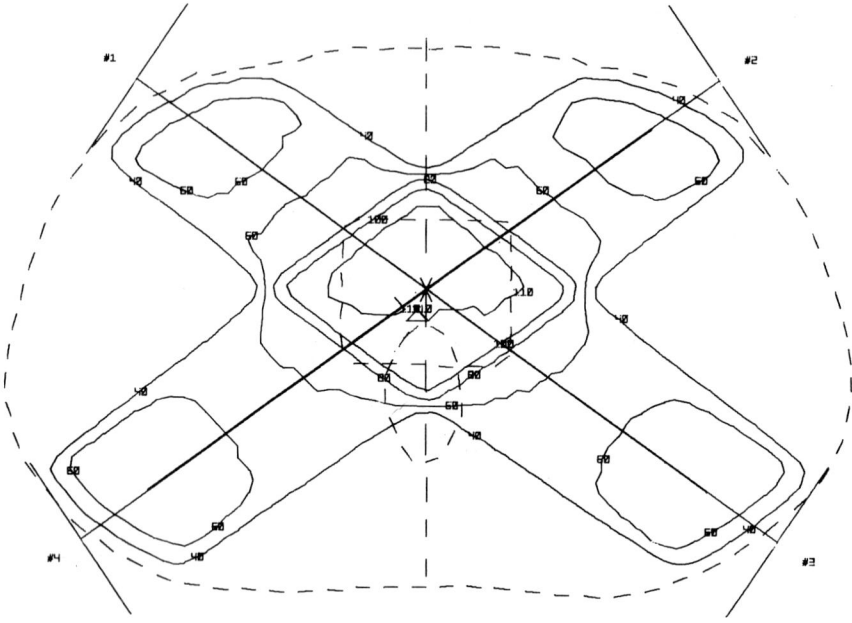

Fig. 27.4 8 MeV Linear Accelerator: 4-field plan treatment
of carcinoma of the vagina.
All Beams   8.0 × 6.5, Weight 38%

to be 1.165 : 1 in women with blood group A, relative
to those in blood group O. This difference was significant at a level of $P = 0.018$ Osborne and de George
(1963), in a group of 713 women, confirmed this
association with blood group A. The group analysed by
Fox and Langley (1976), found that both benign and
malignant mucinous ovarian tumours occurred signfic-
antly more frequently in women of blood group A, but
women with benign teratomata did not show this
association. It would seem that these findings need
closer study. No definitive environmental factors have
been isolated so far, but Japanese women, living in
their homeland, have a relatively low incidence of
ovarian carcinoma; if, however, they move to the
United States, their incidence of ovarian carcinoma
reaches that of American women. In the USA, the
mortality rate for ovarian carcinoma is higher for single
women than for married, widowed or divorced women
in all age groups.

Tumours of the ovary traditionally tend to be large,
often develop very rapidly and do not produce symptoms until late. Benign or malignant tumours may grow
to a very large size before a patient consults her doctor.
Malignant tumours are often bilateral, due either to
spread or to multicentric origin. The frequency with

which these malignancies occur as a secondary change
in a formerly benign ovarian cyst is difficult to ascertain, but it may be high. Symptomless metastases in the
ovaries are found fairly frequently at autopsy in
patients who have suffered with carcinoma of other
organs.

Ovarian tumours tend to spread transperitoneally
and may then pass through the diaphragm and involve
the pleura and mediastinum. Multiple peritoneal
deposits may cause ascites. Implantation growth may
also be found in the fallopian tubes, uterus, vagina and
rarely even vulva. They frequently produce multiple
implants on other abdominal organs by this trans-
peritoneal spread. The omentum is particularly likely
to be involved. Lymphatic spread is to the upper group
of the para-aortic nodes at the level of the renal
arteries. If the thoracic duct is invaded, the axillary,
supra-clavicular or other cervical nodes may be
involved. Distant spread via the blood stream may
occur to involve the lungs, the liver, or the bones.

Unfortunately, more than 70% of all cases of ovarian
carcinoma have spread beyond the ovary by the time
the diagnosis is made. Symptomatology associated
with carcinoma of the ovary occurs late and is indefi-
nite in character so it does not take the patient to the

doctor at an early stage. Patients may complain of gastrointestinal disturbances, some increase in abdominal girth which they put down to 'middle-age spread', vague abdominal pain, dysuria, diarrhoea and, only occasionally, of abnormal vaginal bleeding.

If improvement in treatment is to be made, earlier diagnosis is essential and every doctor performing a smear on a patient should also do a full pelvic examination. A palpable ovary in a post-menopausal woman should be immediately suspect and the patient referred for surgery. Ovarian cancer is rare below the age of 35 years, but, unfortunately, it does occur and ovarian enlargement below this age must never be assumed to be due to a simple cyst or benign teratomata. If an ovarian swelling is palpated in a young woman, the patient should aways be submitted to laparoscopy and possibly laparotomy. The majority of ovarian cancers occur in peri- and post-menopausal women, who on clinical examination may be found to have a single mass arising out of the pelvis, or several masses which may be irregular, semi-solid with cystic areas. They are usually fixed and, more commonly, the condition is bilateral. If the disease has spread beyond the ovary, there may be an irregular mass felt in the pouch of Douglas, or there may be other masses palpable in the abdomen. Ascites is frequently present by the time the woman first presents and is demonstrable in about 30% of cases. Any ovarian enlargement found in a peri- or post-menopausal woman calls for immediate laparotomy. The differential diagnosis includes pelvic inflammatory disease, endometriosis, diverticulitis-/osis, pedunculated fibroids, Meigs' syndrome, retroperitoneal tumours, such as lymphomas, colonic tumours, pelvic, kidney, hydatid cysts and indeed any cause of ascites.

Pelvic inflammatory disease is usually differentiated by the history, the presence of vaginal discharge, the absence of nodularity in the pouch of Douglas and marked excitory pain on moving the cervix. Diverticular disease is confined to the left side of the pelvis associated with bowel symptomatology on careful history taking; barium enema is an important but not utterly reliable diagnostic aid. Endometriosis is commonly encountered at an earlier age; here thickening of the uterosacral ligaments is classical and the relationship of pain to menstruation enables the diagnosis to be made in most cases. When in doubt, laparoscopy is particularly effective. The common simple benign ovarian cyst is unilateral, cystic with smooth wall and completely free of attachment, but the existence of early malignant change within the cyst cannot be excluded except by histology, so such a tumour should always be removed immediately.

Histology

Tumours of surface epithelium (common epithelial tumours)

Serous cystadenoma
Pseudomucinous cystadenoma
Brenner tumour
Serous cystadenocarcinoma
Pseudomucinous cystadenocarcinoma
Endometrioid carcinoma
Clear Cell ('Mesonephric') carcinoma
Malignant Brenner tumour
Adenocarcinoma unclassified
Carcinoma undifferentiated

Tumours of mullerian mesoderm

Mixed mesodermal tumour 'Carcinosarcoma'

Sex cord-mesenchyme tumours (gonadal stromal tumours)

Granulosa cell tumour
Theca cell tumour
Stromal luteoma
Luteoma, luteoma of pregnancy
'Sertoli cell', 'Sertoli-Leydig cell' and 'Leydig cell' tumours (arrhenoblastoma)
Hilus cell tumours

Germ cell tumours

Dysgerminoma
Teratoma, differentiated (dermoid cyst)
Malignant teratoma, intermediate
Malignant teratoma, undifferentiated
Malignant teratoma, trophoblastic (choriocarcinoma)
'Yolk sac carcinoma' ('endodermal sinus tumour')
Combined tumour (teratoma + dysgerminoma)

Tumours of dysgenetic gonad

Gonadoblastoma

Lymphoreticular tumours

Malignant lymphoma

Miscellaneous tumours

Lipid cell tumours of indeterminate type
Adrenal rest tumours
Others

Classification

The prognosis of a tumour depends to some extent on its nature and also on the degree of differentiation but the spread of the tumour is of major prognostic importance and methods of classifying the extent have been devised by a number of workers. In 1964 the International Federation of Gynaecologists and Obstetricians adopted the following scheme.

FIGO staging of ovarian carcinoma

Stage	Description
I	Growth limited to the ovaries (26%).
Ia	Growth limited to one ovary; no ascites.
	(i) no tumour on the external surface; capsule intact.
	(ii) tumour present on the external surface or capsule ruptured (or both).
Ib	Growth limited to both ovaries: no ascites.
	(i) no tumour on the external surface: capsule intact.
	(ii) tumour present on the external surface or capsule(s) ruptured (or both).
Ic	Tumour either Stage 1a or Stage 1b, but with ascites present or positive peritoneal washings.
II	Growth involving one or both ovaries with pelvic extension (21%).
IIa	Extension or metastases to the uterus or tubes.
IIb	Extension to other pelvic tissues.
IIc	Tumour either Stage IIa or Stage IIb, but with ascites present or positive peritoneal washings.
III	Growth involving one or both ovaries with intraperitoneal metastases outside the pelvis or positive retroperitoneal nodes; tumour limited to true pelvis, with histologically proved malignant extension to small bowel or omentum (37%).
IV	Growth involving one or both ovaries with distant metastases; if pleural effusion is present there must be positive cytology to allot a case to Stage IV; parenchymal liver metastases equals Stage IV (16%).

Special category

Unexplored cases thought to be ovarian carcinoma.

UICC TNM classification of ovarian cancer

There must be histological verification of the disease to permit division of cases by histological type.

The extent of disease is assessed on clinical examination and the findings at operation, but before definitive treatment. It is recognized that some cases will remain unclassified and therefore the total number seen must be recorded.

The regional lymph nodes are the abdominal para-aortic nodes including those situated in the renal pedicles.

Histopathological findings must not determine or alter the T category. The histological type of tumour has to be determined and for some types, e.g. cystadenomas, grading is also indicated.

T	– *Primary Tumour*
T_{is}	– Pre-invasive carcinoma (carcinoma in-situ).
T_x	– Tumour cannot be assessed (laparotomy not done).
T_1	– Tumour limited to one ovary.
T_2	– Tumour limited to both ovaries.
T_3	– Tumour extending into the uterus and/or Fallopian tubes.
T_4	– Tumour extending directly to other surrounding anatomical structures.

Note: No regard is paid to the presence of ascites.

N	– *Regional Lymph Nodes*
N_x	– When it is not possible to assess the regional lymph nodes, the symbol Nx will be used permitting eventual addition of histological information, thus: N_x- or N_x+.
N_0	– No abnormal regional lymph nodes demonstrated.
N_1	– Abnormal regional lymph nodes demonstrated.

M	– *Distant Metastases*
M_0	– No evidence of distant metastases.
M_1	– Implantation or other metastases present.
	M_{1a} In the true pelvis only
	M_{1b} Within the abdomen
	M_{1c} Beyond the abdomen and pelvis

G	– *Histopathological Grading*
G_1	– Tumour of low potential malignancy.
G_2	– Tumour obviously malignant.

Stage Grouping

Stage IA:	T_1	N_0	M_0	
Stage IB:	T_2	N_0	M_0	
Stage IIA:	T_3	N_0	M_0	
Stage IIB:	T_4	N_0	M_0 ————Any M_{1a}
Stage III:	Any N_1 ————————Any M_{1b}
Stage IV:	————————————Any M_{1c}

The International Union Against Cancer has developed a system (TNM) which takes account of the extent of the primary tumour, the presence or absence of lymph node involvement and the site of secondary implantation or metastases. However, as the majority of the world's literature reports the FIGO staging, in order to make comparison of results possible, it is suggested this be retained.

Treatment

The role of surgery in the treatment of carcinoma of the ovary

Surgery is the keystone in the treatment of ovarian neoplasms and, as a rule, it should be the initial method of therapy. It can have three distinct roles, namely prophylactic, diagnostic and therapeutic. The prophylactic role consists primarily in the removal of both ovaries at the time of hysterectomy for some other indication. Since the vast majority of hysterectomies are performed because of menstrual disorders, often associated with fibroids, conservation of the ovaries is commonly practised in younger women and the argument that they should be removed rests solely on the possibility that malignant change may take place subsequently. It has been established that hysterectomy alone has no effect (Terz *et al.*, 1967) upon the likelihood of the development of carcinoma of the ovary, but conversely the operation confers no protection and Kaplan (1977) reporting on a series of 142 cases of carcinoma of the ovary noted that 15 had undergone previous hysterectomy and that in 11, hysterectomy had been performed when the woman was aged 45 or more; he suggested therefore that in peri- and post-menopausal women both ovaries should be removed if hysterectomy is necessary. Recent developments in hormone replacement therapy allow safe and effective treatment of any resultant menopausal symptoms and strengthen the case for such a course. McLeish (1977) has suggested that if a benign epithelial cystoma is removed from a young woman, there is an increased liability of a similar change in the surviving ovary in later life, and that a malignant change may take place unnoticed, thus constituting an indication for prophylactic hysterectomy and oophorectomy when such a woman reaches the menopause.

The final diagnosis of carcinoma of the ovary depends upon surgery; the staging of the disease and the planning of treatment is based upon the laparotomy findings. It cannot be stressed too strongly that the surgeon who first opens the abdomen and finds ovarian carcinoma has the obligation to carry out a very full exploration of the entire abdominal cavity with particular reference to the undersurface of the diaphragm, and to the lymphatic drainage site of the ovaries, namely the para-aortic nodes in the region of the renal arteries. If ascites is present a sample should be sent to the cytologist for examination for malignant cells and many advocate the routine instillation of normal saline into the pelvis from which it is then reaspirated and sent for cytological examination. The routine removal of the whole of the omentum whenever ovarian cancer is suspected may well reveal that the disease has microscopically disseminated at the time of operation. Any enlarged lymph nodes either in the pelvis or para-aortic region should be biopsied as an integral part of the staging process. Even when one ovary only is clinically involved the other must always be removed, because in primary ovarian malignancy, microscopic lesions may be found in the contra-lateral ovary in up to 43% of cases (Buka and McFarland 1964). The uterine serosa may be involved microscopically in Stage I disease and hysterectomy is indicated on these grounds; it is also advisable in young women whenever bilateral oophorectomy is performed, since the absence of the uterus makes subsequent hormone replacement therapy easier and safer.

In the young women with Stage IA disease at laparotomy, conservative surgery aimed at preserving hormonal and reproductive function has been advocated. Munnell (1968) showed that the 5-year survival rate was less with such treatment particularly when the tumour was mucinous. Other workers (Parker *et al.*, 1970) found no difference between simple oophorectomy and total hysterectomy with bilateral salpingo-oophorectomy, but their studies did not include assessment of the lymph nodes at laparotomy nor by subsequent lymphography. With such an aggressive malignancy as ovarian carcinoma conservative surgery has no place.

Laparotomy for ovarian carcinoma presents several special problems. Full visualization and exploration of the pelvis is clearly essential, but in addition, the undersurface of the diaphragm is a common site for secondary tumour deposits and must be inspected with possible excision biopsy of any nodules found and their sites marked with clips. Thus the chosen incision must be capable of allowing both facilities, and a paramedian incision should normally be selected.

A malignant cystic tumour is liable to rupture and an exfoliative friable solid tumour may be broken so that in either case, intraperitoneal tumour dissemination may occur. Intraperitoneal spread is extremely common in ovarian carcinoma and thus accidental rupture can greatly increase the chance of metastases. Great care should always be taken to avoid this accident most particularly when clinically the woman has Stage I disease. On the other hand, microscopic spread may have already occurred in any case, so the proposed treatment plan should not be altered merely because rupture occurs. The accident must be recorded and the prognosis may be adversely affected, but after careful removal of any 'spilt' tissue, the original planned regime should be implemented.

Even in Stage I disease, surgical treatment alone has not yielded a satisfactory cure rate and the mortality is such as to call for total effort of eradication in as early a stage as possible. Aggressive surgery followed by routine chemotherapy or intracavitary colloidal radio-phosphorus in Stage I disease seems promising. Currently 5-year survival rates of 80–90% (Langley, 1976; Piver *et al.*, 1975) seem to be obtainable.

Stage II ovarian carcinoma is undoubtedly the most difficult to assess (the more careful the assessment the more frequently it will be transferred to Stage III) and to treat. Total hysterectomy and bilateral salpingo-oophorectomy with omentectomy and gland dissection wherever feasible should be done. Sites of malignant adhesions to pelvic wall or gland biopsy sites should be marked with clips. Subsequent management can then be planned on the basis of this accurate localization.

The diagnosis of Stage III and Stage IV disease may be clinically obvious and can be confirmed by paracen-tesis with cytological examination of the aspirated effusion. Nevertheless laparotomy should always be done as it will provide accurate histological diagnosis and also the exact sites of fixed tumour masses can be identified, thereby allowing more accurate future planning. In addition it is often possible for a great bulk of the tumour to be removed at the same time and this is helpful in reducing the future formation of ascites. It has been demonstrated that if more than 80% of tumour can be removed and residual masses are less than about 2 cm in diameter, survival with combined further therapy is very significantly improved.

Brunschwig and others have shown that excision of isolated secondary tumours in bowel with end to end anastomosis can be followed by prolonged survival. Ileo-enterectomy, whereby a loop of ileum (or other small bowel) is isolated and then opened and inverted to leave the mucosa exposed within the peritoneal cavity whilst retaining the blood supply intact has been used to reabsorb ascitic fluid but with limited success. Appropriate radiotherapy, chemotherapy and radioactive colloidal gold or phosphorus have been found to be more effective and the operation is no longer recommended. The modern technique of tumour bulk reduction decreases the incidence of severe recurrent ascites.

Intestinal obstruction following therapy for advanced ovarian cancer is not infrequent and will often respond to a regime of 'drip and suction' with careful electrolyte balance. A repeat laparotomy may enable the obstruction to be freed with or without a need for bowel resection. Occasionally the presence of carcinomatosis with massive pelvic recurrence will necessitate a permanent colostomy or a small to large bowel bypass anastomosis. Chemotherapy and radiotherapy can be continued with much worthwhile palliation.

If any malignant tissue has to be left *in situ*, it can be 'marked' with metal clips so that subsequent radiotherapy can be accurately directed. Lymphogra-phy is a valuable diagnostic tool and should be per-formed post-operatively on all patients with carcinoma of the ovary; it gives information regarding the state of the para-aortic lymph nodes at the time when it is performed and subsequent changes can be monitored by check X-rays whilst the dye persists in the nodes.

Combined therapy

Surgery, radiotherapy and chemotherapy all form part of the treatment of the different stages of carcinoma of the ovary and on reviewing the world's literature, there is an overwhelming multiplicity of treatments with sur-prisingly similar survival results when analysed at five years. In Stage I the results vary from 60% to 90%; in Stage II from 35% to 50% and in Stage III from 0 to 20%. The overall 5-year survival rate including all stages runs at approximately 20% (Bush *et al.*, 1977; Tobias and Griffiths, 1976; Kolstad *et al.*, 1975; Delclos and Quinlan 1969).

The evaluation of different treatment techniques is exceedingly difficult because the numbers included in each group are small. This arises from the fact that only relatively small numbers of patients are seen at any one centre and because of the many sub-groups which arise from the staging and from the histological differences. Kottmeier (1976) says it is difficult to draw conclusions from statistics as to the best methods of therapy. It is even questionable whether it is possible to estimate the value of different therapeutic methods on the basis of consecutive series of cases treated at one and the same institution. Kolstad *et al.* (1977), reporting a series of 2175 cases treated between 1967 and 1975 states that, even with this number of cases, it is clearly difficult to reach definite conclusions as to which mode of treat-ment is to be preferred in malignant ovarian neoplasia because it takes such a long time to collect a uniform and sufficiently large quantity of material. Further-more, the follow-up period must be long enough to enable definite conclusions to be made.

In analysing past treatment with a view to recom-mending therapy appropriate to each stage, the various sub-groups in the stage must be taken into account.

Stage I

In a large series from the Mayo clinic, 111 patients with Stage I intracystic tumours had a 5-year survival rate of 98% (Webb *et al.*, 1973). With extracapsular excrescences the survival rate fell to 68%. With intraoperative rupture, the survival rate was 56% and with adherence of the tumour to surrounding structures, the 5-year survival rate was 51%. In view of these findings there would seem no place for any form of adjuvant therapy in patients with Stage IA(i) disease where there is no tumour on the external surface of the ovary and the capsule is totally intact and histologically there is no penetration. However, in IA(ii) disease where perhaps the capsule has ruptured or there is tumour present on the external surface of the ovary, in IB and IC disease where there has been rupture of the capsules or there is already ascitic fluid or positive peritoneal washings, it has been shown by Clark *et al.* (1976) that the results of instilling radioactive ^{32}P chromic phosphate in a colloidal suspension improved the 5-year survival from 65% to 90%. The instillation of radioactive colloidal gold has been used in the past, but has been shown by Muller, Kettle and Kolstad to have a significant morbidity. ^{32}Phosphorus only emits β-particles with a maximum range of 3.8 mm and it has been used in a wide series of cases (Alderman *et al.*, 1977) without undue morbidity. The colloidal radioactive chromic phosphorus forms a physical bond with the peritoneal surface and so the patient does not require isolation and there are no special precautions which have to be taken in her nursing care. This procedure is best carried out within the first 48–72 hours after laparotomy during which nylon tubes with multiple side holes should have been placed in the peritoneal gutters for afterloading with colloidal chromic ^{32}P, purse string sutures having been placed around the abdominal stab wounds, where the tubes are extruding; 250 ml of normal saline from a 550 ml bottle are introduced into the peritoneal cavity by hydrostatic pressure and a tracer dose of 0.5 mCi of technetium^{99} pertechnetate are injected into the peritoneal ccavity via the nylon tubes. The patient is then positioned from the supine to the sitting position and then to lying on the right and left sides and prone, and is placed under a gamma camera. If scanning shows a homogeneous distribution of the tracer isotope, a dose of from 10–15 mCi of colloidal radioactive phosphorus, suspended in 30% of glucose, is introduced as a bolus, using an additional 50–100 ml of normal saline. The nylon tubes are removed and the purse string sutures are tied to ensure a watertight seal. Any materials contaminated by the radioactive isotopes are retained in the Department of Nuclear Medicine and stored until decay has taken place. During the next 24 hours the patient is encouraged to move and to turn frequently, so that she spends time lying on her sides, her abdomen and also on her back, sitting up and lying down, so that the colloid is spread over the entire peritoneal surface.

This method of treatment ensures that the whole of the peritoneal cavity is treated. It carries less morbidity than the use of radioactive colloidal gold. It is preferable to the use of alkylating agent chemotherapy in these early cases because although such drugs carry a good long term prognosis of 90% survival for five years, they can induce leukaemia in patients who survive for a long period of time. This leukaemia risk (Reimer *et al.*, 1977) is acceptable for women with advanced carcinoma of the ovary where survival rate is not very favourable but would seem an unnecessary risk for patients with early disease.

Stage II

In Stage II carcinoma of the ovary where there is pelvic extension of the tumour involving one or both ovaries, external radiotherapy to the pelvis and the whole abdomen should be given because in about 30% of these patients, there will already have been occult extraplevic spread. Whole abdominal irradiation with a boosting dose to the pelvis is therefore the main line of treatment. It may be given either by a fixed field technique of parallel opposed pair of fields or by a moving strip technique using either a Linear Accelerator or Cobalt Unit. The latter method is perhaps less taxing to the patient and delivers a sufficiently high dose in a short period of time to be effective. It is more difficult to set up accurately if the patient happens to be obese. The anterior and posterior aspects of the abdomen from the xiphisternum to the lower border of the obturator foramen are divided into transverse strips 2.5 cm wide. Alternating daily between the anterior and posterior positions, the strips are irradiated, beginning at the obturator foramen with the first 2.5 cm strip. A daily dose of 350–450 rad skin dose is given. Each day the next superior strip is added to the port until four strips have been irradiated. Each day thereafter one new strip is added superiorly, and the most inferior strip, which by then has been treated four times, is omitted. If a Linear Accelerator is used in order to avoid cold spots, the strips are staggered so that the posterior surface lines project to the centre of the anterior opposed strip. An additional exposure is given to the lowest and uppermost strips. To avoid any possibility of radiation nephritis occurring, kidney shields with lead blocks are used after proper localization so that the kidneys do not receive more than 1500 rad throughout treatment. An additional 2000–3000 rad are then delivered to the pelvis through a parallel opposed pair of fields. If a fixed field technique is used then a Linear Accelerator has to be employed in order to achieve a large enough field to cover the patient's whole abdomen, extending from above the poles of the diaphragm to the lower border of the obturator foramen and laterally to take in the whole of the abdominal cavity (Fig. 27.5). A parallel opposed pair of fields is used and a dose of 2500–3000 rad is given to this volume at a mid-point dose rate of 750 rad per week; both fields are treated daily. Kidney shields are employed when the whole volume has received 1500 rad. Radiation induced hepatitis has not occurred within doses of 2500–3000 rad but may occur at doses above this level. When 2500–3000 rad have been reached, the abdominal irradiation is stopped and a pelvic boost is given with one anterior field and two posterior obliques to take the total dose to the pelvis to 4500–4800 rad (Fig. 27.6). If a lymphogram has been performed and this has shown that the para-aortic nodes are involved with tumour, then a para-aortic strip field is treated so that the total dose to the para-aortic lymph nodes is 4000 rad; this is inclusive of the whole abdominal irradiation already given. Total abdominal irradiation carries some morbidity.

During treatment patients are troubled by quite severe nausea, sometimes vomiting and also diarrhoea. These symptoms can be alleviated by the use of anti-emetics such as Fentazin 4 mg t.i.d. or Maxolon 10 mg t.i.d. by mouth. Diarrhoea may be controlled by the use of Lomotil tablets 1 t.i.d. or codeine phosphate 30 mg t.i.d. Very occasionally, if the symptoms are particularly bad, two or three days' rest from treatment enables the patient to continue the irradiation without further problems provided they continue regular medication. It is important that a good nutritional intake is obtained by these patients, and it is a wise precaution to warn them that excessive intake of green vegetables and fruit is likely to exacerbate diarrhoea. Providing the dose rate is kept at 750 rad per week while the whole abdomen is being treated and only increased to between 850 and 900 rad per week when the pelvis alone is under treatment, few patients develop severe side-effects. Survival of patients with Stage II disease is markedly improved when there has been surgical removal of gross tumour mass before irradiation. It has been shown by Long *et al.* (1967), Delclos and Quinlan (1969), and Rubin *et al* (1962) that the 5-year survival rate in patients with Stage II disease is improved by the addition of post-operative radiotherapy.

Stage III and IV

Because carcinoma of the ovary is such an insidious disease, many women have already reached Stage III or Stage IV by the time they are first seen and undergo laparotomy. Despite improvements in chemotherapy and in irradiation, the prognosis for such women remains poor. Less than 10% of Stage III ovarian carcinoma patients treated either by single agent chemotherapy or by irradiation alone will survive for five years. There are numerous studies of varied treatment regimes involving whole abdominal irradiation, single-agent chemotherapy and multiple-agent chemotherapy in all combinations published in the United States of America, United Kingdom, Scandinavia and Europe but evaluation is difficult because response criteria vary from series to series and such criteria are often imprecisely stated. Even from large institutions, the number of cases is small and the follow-up time is usually too short.

Chemotherapy

In the past chemotherapy has tended to be used only for patients with advanced stages of ovarian cancer who have failed to respond to or have been considered unsuitable for radiotherapy. Logically it would seem

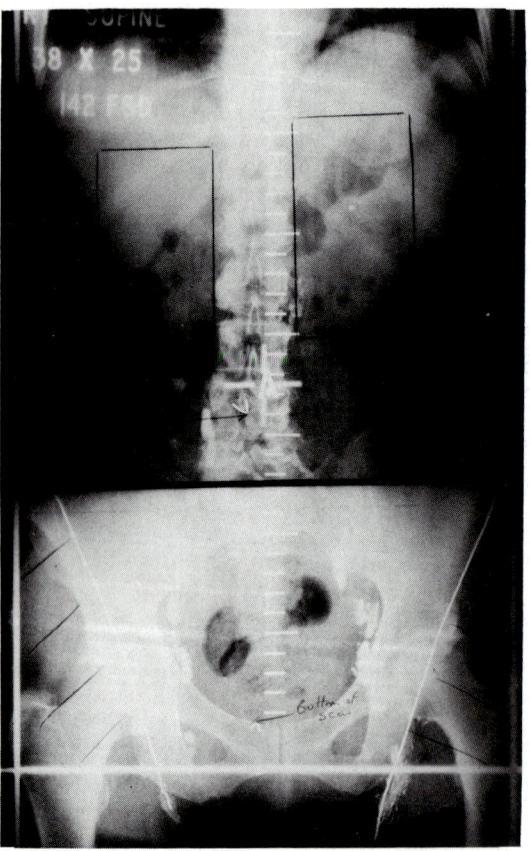

Fig. 27.5 Photograph to show simulator planning film for whole abdominal irradiation. Kidney shield marked.

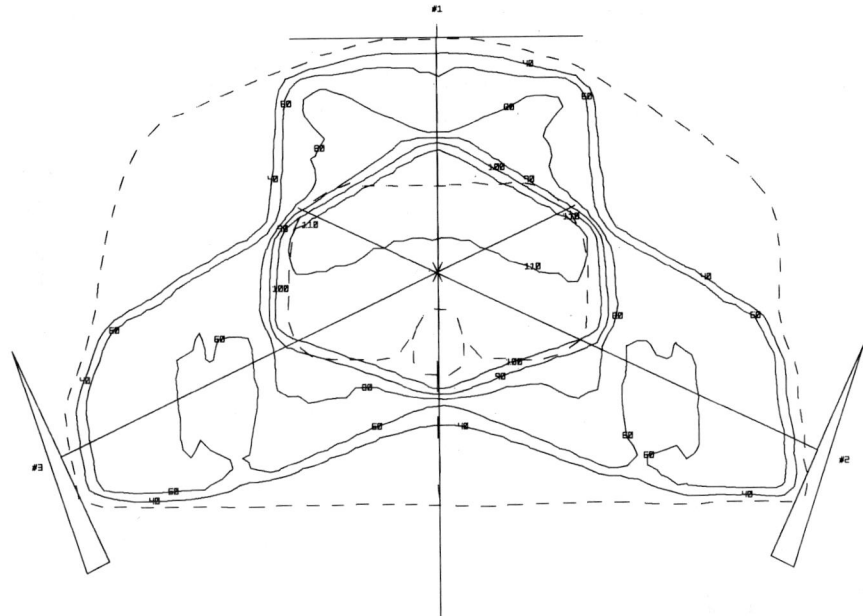

Fig. 27.6   8 MeV Linear Accelerator: 3-field plan for treatment of the pelvis.
Beam   1   14.0 × 13.0, Weight 60%
Beam   2 and 3   15.0 × 10.0, Wedge No. 1, Weight 60%

preferable as a primary treatment for patients with widespread abdominal disease where it is unlikely that an effective dose of irradiation can be safely delivered to large tumour masses.

To date, the most commonly used form of chemotherapy for ovarian cancer has been the alkylating agents. Chlorambucil, cyclophosphamide, melphalan and triethylene thiophosphoramide have all produced very similar initial objective response rates of between 35% and 65% (Bagley *et al.*, 1972). The median survival of patients who respond to chemotherapy is 17 to 20 months and for those who fail to respond is 6 to 13 months. Treatment regimes using oral loading doses, oral maintenance (daily) doses or intermittent intravenous doses appear to be equally effective. Also the response to treatment is poorly correlated with cell type though remissions are less frequent and of shorter duration with undifferentiated tumours compared to those of higher histological grade.

Because the alkylating agents have generally been considered as first choice, there is less reliable data on the alternative forms of chemotherapy. The antimetabolites methotrexate and 5-fluorouracil have produced a response rate of approximately 32% but this is only in a small series of patients. More recently

objective responses have been shown to other antitumour agents. Adriamycin, an antitumour antibiotic, has shown an overall reported response rate of approximately 33%. Cis-dichlorodiammineplatinum (II) has also been used with a reported objective response rate of 26.5% with a 6 month median duration of response. As further experience with cis-platinum is obtained, it looks more encouraging as a single agent therapy but the follow-up time is still too short for true evaluation at present. Both adriamycin and cis-platinum have been shown to be non-cross-resistant drugs (Wiltshaw and Carr, 1974; Wiltshaw and Kroner, 1976).

In a large series of patients treated with melphalan alone, Smith *et al.* (1972) reported a mean duration of complete clinical response for mucinous carcinoma as 46 months, for serous cystadenocarcinoma 28 months, and for undifferentiated carcinoma 22 months. The mean duration for those showing partial response was less than 12 months. This is not significantly better than the survival of non-responding or even untreated patients. De Palo *et al.* (1977) randomized 30 previously untreated patients between adriamycin and melphalan. Tumour regression was obtained with both agents and when treatment began to fail, cross-over was performed and further responses were obtained. Following this a further randomized study was made between adriamycin and adriamycin-plus-melphalan. Tumour regression occurred in 7 out of 12 patients receiving adriamycin and in 10 out of 14 patients on combined adriamycin and melphalan. This study therefore failed to provide evidence for a synergistic effect between the two compounds. Possibly the failure of the combination to be more effective than either agent alone was because when given together, the dosage of each had to be markedly reduced in order to avoid myelosuppression. It must also be remembered that prolonged administration of adriamycin carries a high risk of cardiac toxicity – a cumulative dose of 550–600 mg/m² should not be exceeded (Bonadonna *et al.*, 1975).

Buchler *et al.* (1977) studied the use of multiple drugs against single agents and could find no significant difference. This study did show that those patients who had a pelvic mass of less than 8 cm diameter or who had nodules in the upper abdomen of less than 2 cm diameter had a better response to all drugs than those who had more massive tumours. The trial also demonstrated that patients with a significant amount of residual disease after laparotomy benefited more from chemotherapy than from irradiation.

The treatment of Stage III carcinoma of the ovary remains in a state of flux and there has been little gain following the use of combined as against single agents. The recent marginal improvement in prognosis is likely to be due to more aggressive surgery rather than to the chemotherapeutic agents employed. There is no doubt that extensive surgery, removing as much tumour bulk as possible, provides a better chance of a good response to adjuvant therapy. Thus when laparotomy reveals Stage III disease, meticulous dissection with removal of all possible tumour is worthwhile and, specifically, any pelvic mass greater than 8 cm diameter or upper abdominal mass greater than 2 cm diameter must be removed if possible.

Single alkylating agents are probably the chemotherapeutic agents of choice and these can be either melphalan, chlorambucil, cyclophosphamide or thio-tepa. Melphalan is one of the better tolerated drugs and can be given in doses of 4 mg/m² for 5 days repeated at 6-week intervals providing the blood count is satisfactory with a white cell count of 3000/mm³ and a platelet count of 150 000/mm³. If the count is below these levels then the chemotherapy must be delayed until the levels are satisfactory again; 45% of patients treated in this manner will show partial or complete response for anything from 6 to 20 months.

In the event of a relapse, other single-agents such as adriamycin in a dose of 40–60 mg/m² intravenously repeated at 21-day intervals can be given. No benefits have yet been demonstrated from the use of combination regimes using different chemotherapeutic agents and such techniques carry considerable toxicity with liability to myelosuppression particularly when following previous chemotherapy. Individual reports have been interesting and synergistic combinations may yet be discovered. Tobias and Griffiths (1976) showed

encouraging results from a combination of cyclophosphamide 500 mg/m² with adriamycin 40 mg/m² intravenously in a 3-week schedule. The regime can cause severe myelosuppression and they have used autogenous bone marrow support. Further evaluation is needed.

Table 27.2 Summary of treatment by staging.

Stage 1a (ii), b and c
Total hysterectomy, bilateral salpingo-oophorectomy, omentectomy with careful assessment of lymph nodes and of under-surface of diaphragm. Intraperitoneal radioactive colloidal ³²P.

Stage IIa, b and c
Hysterectomy, bilateral salpingo-oophorectomy, omentectomy. Careful assessment of diaphragm, liver and lymph nodes. Whole abdominal irradiation with pelvic boosting dose.

Stage III and IV
Hysterectomy, bilateral salpingo-oophorectomy, omentectomy and removal of all bulk tumour, patient's general condition permitting. Chemotherapy.

Second look laparotomy (Tepper *et al.*, 1977)

Laparotomy and subsequent radiotherapy or chemotherapy must be followed by careful and systematic observation of the patient. Where chemotherapy is being used continuously or sequentially, it is important to know if and when such treatment can be safely discontinued. So long as a palpable mass or definite tumour exists, there is no place for laparoscopy though there may well be an indication for a 'second-look' laparotomy. Sometimes at a second laparotomy, it is possible to remove previously inoperable masses and to offer the chance of a curative procedure which had previously been considered impossible. When the patient is well and the disease appears to be in remission, there is a strong case for laparoscopy which is a relatively minor procedure. If residual tumour is not seen at laparoscopy, then laparotomy with multiple peritoneal biopsy must be done so that residual tumour will not be missed and chemotherapy prematurely stopped (Gary Smith *et al.*, 1977). Laparoscopy is not an alternative to 'second-look' laparotomy but is a useful adjunct for determining the presence of resectable, unresectable or diffuse disease after chemotherapy; it can only detect macroscopic lesions and these only within its limited field of view, thus it must never be used as proof of freedom from disease.

In experienced hands abdominal ultrasound can give valuable information about abdominal masses, but it should not replace laparoscopy or laparotomy.

Dysgerminoma

Dysgerminoma is the female equivalent of the male seminoma but among the germ cell tumours it is the most common. It occurs in the young age group and spreads by the lymphatics to the retroperitoneal lymph nodes, to the nodes in the mediastinum and the supraclavicular fossa. Treatment is by a combination of surgery and radiotherapy. The patient should have a hysterectomy and bilateral salpingo-oophorectomy with para-aortic lymph node biopsy. This should be followed by lymphography. If the para-aortic lymph nodes are involved then the whole pelvis and the para-aortic lymph nodes should be treated, the whole pelvis by an anterior and two posterior oblique fields and the para-aortic lymph nodes by a parallel opposed pair to a dose of 2500 rad in three weeks as these tumours are very radiosensitive. If the lymphogram is positive in the para-aortic region or if these nodes have been found to be positive, on histological examination, then 6 weeks later the mediastinum and left supraclavicular fossa should be treated with a further 2500 rad in 3 weeks. The 5-year survival rates from this disease range from 68% to 78% but as the disease is rare, it is difficult to get a clear cut statement of survival rates related to treatment.

Granulosa cell tumour

Granulosa cell tumours are also very rare. These are hormone-producing neoplasms and have a potential degree of malignancy. They tend to recur ten or twenty years after surgical removal. They can occur at any age group but if the patient is post-menopausal then it is probably wise to give post-operative irradiation to the pelvis.

Embryonal carcinomas, teratomas and the rare sarcomas of the ovary are probably best treated by combination chemotherapy but they all carry a very poor prognosis. Irradiation has no part to play in their treatment.

Future trends

Even with the advent of new chemotherapeutic agents, the results of treatment of ovarian cancer are still extremely disappointing. Improved management and resultant improved survival may be achieved by discovering what is the optimal existing therapy for each histological type and stage of the disease (Fisher and Young, 1977). We need carefully controlled prospective randomized clinical trials with careful staging and meticulously thorough surgery, and universally established criteria for response rate and a 5-year follow-up period.

Table 27.3 Results of treatment for carcinoma of ovary.

Stage Ia	(i)	93%
Ia	(ii)	
b		} 60%–90%
c		
Stage IIa		
b		} 35%–50%
c		
Stage III and IV		0%–20%

Immunological studies may have an important role to play, and some encouraging results have been reported by Alberts (1977) in Arizona on the use of adjuvant immunotherapy with BCG in combination with chemotherapy. *Corynebacterium parvum* has also been used in a similar manner but with slightly less encouraging results (Knapp and Berkowitz, 1977). These studies are in a very early stage at present and need full evaluation over a long period of time; if they are then statistically significant, they may provide an important new approach to the treatment of patients with Stage III and IV disease.

If xenografting can be perfected, then new drugs and present drugs may be tried against the patient's disease *in vitro* and this may give useful information for *in vivo* treatment.

Part IV: Fallopian tube

This is a rare form of malignancy. Kinzel writing in 1976 could trace less than 1000 recorded cases. No single series is large enough to yield statistically reliable data but the 41 cases seen in the Gynaecologic Oncology Centre, British Columbia from 1946 to 1976 varied in age from 33 years to 80 years with a median age of 54. In common with many other series, parity was below average suggesting that relative infertility and carcinoma of the Fallopian tube may have a common aetiological factor such as salpingitis in earlier life.

Symptoms are minimal and late. The most common presenting symptom is abnormal vaginal bleeding or discharge but the classical picture of profuse watery orange-coloured discharge is rarely seen. Abdominal pain occurs in about half of all cases but is non-specific in character. Cytological smears are rarely abnormal. The difficulty in making a correct diagnosis is emphasized by the fact that in the Canadian series 22 women presented with abnormal bleeding or discharge and were subjected to dilatation and curettage, but in 9 cases this failed to reveal a malignancy and one women underwent the procedure 3 times and still her carcinoma was not discovered.

Staging of this disease is as for carcinoma of the ovary. Actual involvement of the tube secondary to ovarian cancer is far more common than primary Fallopian tube carcinoma but the differentiation is not difficult. The histological picture is of a papillary adenocarcinoma. Anaplastic undifferentiated tumours are exceedingly rare.

Treatment is exactly as for primary ovarian cancer. Early cases require thorough laparotomy and staging with total hysterectomy, bilateral salpingo-oophorectomy and omentectomy. Tumour and metastases are sensitive to radiotherapy and response to chemotherapy is similar to that of ovarian carcinoma. The common embryological origin of tube and endometrium suggests that progestogens may have a therapeutic role but this has not yet been established.

In the Canadian series the overall 5-year survival rate was under 35% although for patients with early disease, the prognosis was more than twice as good. The single most important factor affecting survival was the extent of the disease at diagnosis and it is therefore clear that an increased willingness to resort to laparotomy or laparoscopy in suspicious cases could be a most significant advance in treatment.

Further reading

Fletcher, G.H. (1973), *Textbook of Radiotherapy*. Lea and Febiger, Philadelphia.

Fox, H. and Langley, F.A. (1976), *Tumours of the Ovary*. Heinemann, London.

Langley, F.A. (ed.) (1976), *Clinics in Obstetrics and Gynaecology*, 3 (2), W.B. Saunders Co. Ltd., London, Philadelphia, Toronto.

Moss, W.T. (1973), *Radiation Oncology*, Kempton.

Tobias, J.S. and Griffiths, C.T. (1976), Management of ovarian carcinoma – current concepts and future prospects. *New Eng. J. Med.*, **294**, 818–23; 877–882.

Way, S. and Hennigan, M. (1966), The late results of extended radical vulvectomy for carcinoma of the vulva. *J. Obstet. Gynec. B. Commun.*, **73**, 594.

References

Alberts, D.S. (1977), Adjuvant immunotherapy with BCG of advanced ovarian cancer: A preliminary report. In: *Adjuvant Therapy in Cancer* (eds S.E. Sa, and S.E. Jones), North Holland, Amsterdam, pp. 327–34.

Alderman, S.J. *et al.* (1977), Postoperative use of radioactive phosphorus in stage I ovarian carcinoma. *Obstet. Gynaec.*, **49**(6), 659–62.

Bagley, C.M. *et al.* (1972), Treatment of ovarian carcinoma – possibilities for progress. *New Engl. J. Med.*, **287**, 856–62.

Bonadonna, G. *et al.* (1975), Adriamycin (NSC-123127) studies at the Instituto Nazionale Tumori, Milan. *Cancer Chemother. Rep.*, Part 3, 6(2), 231–45.

Brunschwig, D.D. Intestinal surgery of advanced carcinoma of the ovary. In: *Ovarian Cancer*, (UICC Monograph Series), **III**, 165–71.

Buchler, D.A. *et al.* (1977), Stage III ovarian carcinoma: treatment and results. *Therap. Radiol.*, **122**, 469–72.

Buka, N.J. and MacFarland, K.T. (1964), Malignant tumours of the ovary. *Am. J. Obstet.*, **90**, 383–7.

Bush, R.S. *et al.* (1977), Treatment of epithelial carcinoma of ovary: operation, irradiation and chemotherapy. *Am. J. Obstet. Gynec.*, **127**, 692–703.

Clark, D.G. *et al.* (1976), Treatment of cancer of the ovary. *Clin. Obstet. Gynaec.*, **3**, 159–79.

Delclos, L. and Quinlan, E.J. (1969), Malignant tumours of the ovary managed with post-operative megavoltage irradiation. *Radiology*, **93**, 659–63.

De Palo, G.M., De Lena, M. and Bonadonna, G. (1977), Adriamycin versus Adriamycin plus Melphalan in advanced ovarian carcinoma. *Cancer Treat. Rep.*, **61**, 355–7.

Dewhurst, C.J. (1976), *Integrated Obstetrics and Gynaecology*, 2 edn., Blackwell Scientific Publications Oxford, p.679.

Fisher, R.I. and Young, R.C. (1977), Advances in the staging and treatment of ovarian cancer. *Cancer*, **39**, 967–72.

Gary Smith, W., Day, T.G. and Smith, J.P. (1977), The use of laparoscopy to determine the results of chemotherapy for ovarian cancer. *J. Reprod. Med.*, **18**,(5), 257–60.

Helmbold, von W. (1961), Sammelstatistik zur Prufung auf Korrelationen Zwischen dem weiblichen genital carcinom und dem ABO und rhesus system. *Acta Genet.* (Basel), **11**, 29–51.

Kaplan, E. (1977), Cancer of the ovary. *S. Afr. Med. J.*, **52**, 1123.

Kinzel, G.E. (1976), *Am.J.Obstet. Gynec.*, **125/b**, 816–820.

Knapp, R.C. and Berkowitz, R.S. (1977), Corynebacterium parvum as an immunotherapeutic agent in an ovarian cancer model. *Am. J. Obstet. Gynec.*, **128**, 782–6.

Kolstad, P. (1977), Report of cases treated between 1967 and 1975. *Am. J. Obstet. Gynec.*, **128**.

Kolstad, P., Davy, M. and Hoeg, K. (1977), Individualized treatment of ovarian cancer. *Am. J. Obstet. Gynec.*, **128**.

Kolstad, P., Davy, M. and Scheinert, H. (1975), Individualized treatment of ovarian neoplasia. In: *Diagnosis and treatment of ovarian neoplastic alterations*, (eds H. de Watteville *et al*.) Excerpta Medica, Amsterdam pp.166–71 (ICS No. 364, 1974).

Kottmeier, H.L. (1976), Presentation of therapeutic results in carcinoma of the female pelvis: experience of the annual report on the results of treatment in carcinoma of the uterus, vagina and ovary. *Gynaec. Oncol.*, **4**, 13–9.

Long, R.T.L., Johnson, R.E. and Sala, J.M. (1967), Variations in survival among patients with carcinoma of the ovary. Analysis of 253 cases according to histologic type, anatomical shape and method of treatment. *Cancer*, **20**, 1195–202.

McLeish, G.R. (1977), The surgical management of ovarian carcinoma. *Australas. Radiol.*, **21**(1), 81.

Morris, J.M. (1977), A formula for selective lymphadenectomy – its application to cancer of vulva. *Obstetrics and Gynaecology*, **50**, 2, 152–8.

Muller, J.H. (1963), Curative aim and results of routine intraperitoneal radiocolloid administration in the treatment of ovarian cancer. *Am. J. Roentgenol. Radium Therap. Nucl. Med.*, **89**, 533–40.

Munnell, E.W. (1968), The changing prognosis and treatment in cancer of the ovary: a report of 235 patients with primary ovarian carcinoma 1952–1961. *Am. J. Obstet. Gynec.*, **100**, 790–805.

Osborne, R.H. and de George, F.U. (1963), The ABO blood groups in neoplastic disease of the ovary. *Am. J. Human. Genet.*, **15**, 380–8.

Parker, R.T., Parker, C.H. and Willbanks, G.D. (1970), Cancer of the ovary: survival studies based upon operative therapy, chemotherapy, and radiotherapy. *Am. J. Obstet. Gynec.*, **108**, 878–88.

Parry-Jones, E. (1976), Management of vulval malignant and pre-malignant conditions. *Clin. Obstet. Gynec.*, **2**(2), 222.

Perez *et al.* (1973), Treatment of carcinoma of vagina. *Cancer*, **31**, 36–44.

Piver, M.S. *et al.* (1975), Sequential therapy for advanced ovarian adenocarcinoma: operation, chemotherapy, second-look laparotomy, and radiation therapy. *Am. J. Obstet. Gynec.*, **122**, 355–7.

Reimer, R.R. *et al.* (1977), Acute leukaemia after alkylating-agent therapy of ovarian cancer. *New Engl. J. Med.*, **297**(4), 177–80.

Rubin, P., Grise, J.W. and Terry, R. (1962), Has postoperative irradiation proved itself? *Am. J. Roentgenol. Radium Therap. Nucl. Med.*, **88**, 849–66.

Rutledge, F., Smith, J.P. and Franklin, E.W. (1970), Carcinoma of the vulva. *J. Am. Obstet. Gynec.*, **106**, 1117–30.

Smith, J.P. and Rutledge, F. (1970), Chemotherapy in the treatment of cancer of the ovary. *Am. J. Obstet. Gynec.*, **107**, 691–703.

Smith, J.P., Rutledge, F. and Wharton, J.T. (1972), Chemotherapy of ovarian cancer: new approaches to treatment. *Cancer*, **30**, 1565–71.

Staging and treatment of ovarian carcinoma (1975). *Seminars in Oncology*, **II**(3).

Tepper, E. *et al.* (1977), Second look surgery after radiation therapy for advanced stages of cancer of the ovary. *J. Roentg.: Radium Ther. Nucl. Med.*, **112**(4), 755–9.

Terz, J.J., Barber, H.R.K. and Brunschwig, A. (1967), Incidence of carcinoma in the retained ovary. *Am. J. Surg.*, **113**, 511.

Tobias, J.S. and Griffiths, C.T. (1976), Management of ovarian carcinoma – current concepts and future prospects. *New Engl. J. Med.*, **294**, 818–23; 877–882.

Way, S. (1951), *Malignant Disease of the Female Genital Tract*, Churchill, London.

Way, S. (1954), Results of a planned attack on carcinoma of the vulva. *Br. Med. J..*, **ii**, 780–2.

Way, S. (1964), Microinvasive carcinoma of the cervix. *Acta Cytol.* (Philadelphia), **8**, 14.

Way, S. and Hennigan, M. (1966), The late results of radical vulvectomy for carcinoma of the vulva, *J. Obstet. Gynec. Br. Commonwealth*, **75**, 594–8.

Webb, M.J. *et al.* (1973), Factors influencing survival in Stage I ovarian cancer. *Am. J. Obstet. Gynec.*, **116**, 222–8.

Wiltshaw, E. and Carr, B. (1974), Cis-Platinum (II) diamminedichloride: clinical experience of the Royal Marsden Hospital and Institute of Cancer Research, London. *Recent Results Cancer Res.*, **48**, 178–82.

Wiltshaw, E. and Kroner, T. (1976), Phase II study of Cis-dichlorodiammine platinum (II) (NSC-119875) in advanced adenocarcinoma of ovary. *Cancer Treat. Rep.*, **60**, 55–60.

28 Uterus

Charles A.F. Joslin
and K.R. Peel

Cancer of the uterus constitutes about 20% of all cancers in woman. It can be separated into cancer of the cervix uteri and of the corpus uteri. The pathogenesis is different in the two situations which in turn affects the problems of management.

Irrespective of the type of management, the best results of treatment occur with early disease. As a result, the classification by clinical staging and histopathological grading play a vital part when comparing results of treatment for the various modalities.

Aetiology and epidemiology

Cervix cancer

A number of pre-disposing factors have been identified but, as yet non-confirmed as being the primary cause of cervix cancer. The more important of these factors are listed in Table 28.1 which indicates that among the causes some may be interlinked. In particular, the work of Reid and Coppleson suggests the disease as being venereally transmitted which, for predisposed subjects leads to a transformation from a metaplastic state in the cervix epithelium through a series of biochemical changes to a malignant state. A review on this subject is provided by Reid and Coppleson (1976).

Endometrial cancer

Endometrial cancer differs from cervix cancer in a number of ways. It occurs more frequently in the nulliparous woman, is less aggressive than cervix cancer and most patients present with early symptoms.

These patients have a pre-disposition to obesity, diabetes and heart disease and thus often constitute a poor surgical risk.

It has long been suspected that women developing endometrial cancer have either an inborn irregularity of endocrine function or fail to receive the 'protective' endocrine changes associated with pregnancy. The former view supported by Chamlian and Taylor (1970)

indicates how transition from a typical hyperplasia to endometrial carcinoma can occur. This should not be confused with 'benign' cystic hyperplasia although this has been reported in association with adenocarcinoma in women aged over 50 years (Ritzman, 1978). A review on the subject is covered by Brush and Taylor (1975).

Incidence

The reported incidence rates for cervix and endometrial cancer vary for different parts of the world (Table 28.2) in different proportions for both cervix and endometrial cancer from one country to another, suggesting entirely unrelated aetiologies for the two.

The age-specific rates for endometrial cancer compared with cervix cancer show that an older age group of women are more commonly affected and that 95% of cervix cancer occurs in women over the age of 30 years and 95% of endometrial cancer in women over 40 years (Fig. 28.1).

Anatomy of the uterus

The uterus is a pear-shaped thick walled muscular hollow organ made up of corpus, isthmus and cervix. It normally measures about 9–10 cm in length, 6 cm in its widest part and 4 cm in overall thickness. The walls are 1–2 cm thick providing a cavity of 7–8 cm.

It is supported by the levator ani muscle and overlying fascia, thickened to form ligaments. It is anteverted and inclined forwards at angle of 90° to the axis of the vagina (Fig. 28.2). In 10–15% of women it may be either retroverted, retroflexed or occasionally both. Anteversion is maintained by the weight of the uterus, the round and the uterosacral ligaments pulling the supra-vaginal cervix backwards, being supported laterally by the broad ligaments. The body accounts for two thirds and the cervix one third of the organ which is covered with peritoneum and lined by endometrium.

The relations of the uterus are important. The blad-

Table 28.1   Associated risk factors for developing cervix cancer.

Associated factor	Increased risk	Reference
Marriage at an early age	2:1 for a woman marrying before 20 years	Lombard and Potter (1950)
Divorced, separated or widowed women	3:1 compared with matched controls	Lombard and Potter (1950); Priden and Lilienfield (1971)
Prostitution	4:1 compared with normal population	Levin *et al.* (1942) Røjel (1953)
Ethnic groups	5:1 Non-Jewish to Jewish depending on geography of domicile	Weiner *et al.* (1951) Rotkin (1973)
Occupation of consort	3:1 Manual workers compared with professional groups	Wakefield *et al.* (1973)
Herpes type 2 virus	Cervix cancer patients have a high titre	Adams *et al.* (1974)
High risk males	3.5:1 increased incidence in second and third wives	Singer (1973)
Biochemical morphological and genetic differences in male ejaculate	Correlation still required	Reid and Coppleson (1978)

der base is anterior to its lower half and in the upper half small intestine may lie in approximation. Posteriorly the pouch of Douglas, which may contain loops of small bowel, forms the posterior vaginal fornix.

Laterally, the broad ligaments with the fallopian tubes above, carry blood vessels and nerves. The ureter passes through the broad ligament and 1 cm from the supra-vaginal cervix lies below the uterine artery. On the posterior surface of each broad ligament is an ovary attached to the uterus by the ovarian ligament.

The uterus derives its blood supply primarily from the uterine branches of the internal iliac arteries and branches of the ovarian arteries which are themselves branches of the aorta. Venous drainage is via plexuses

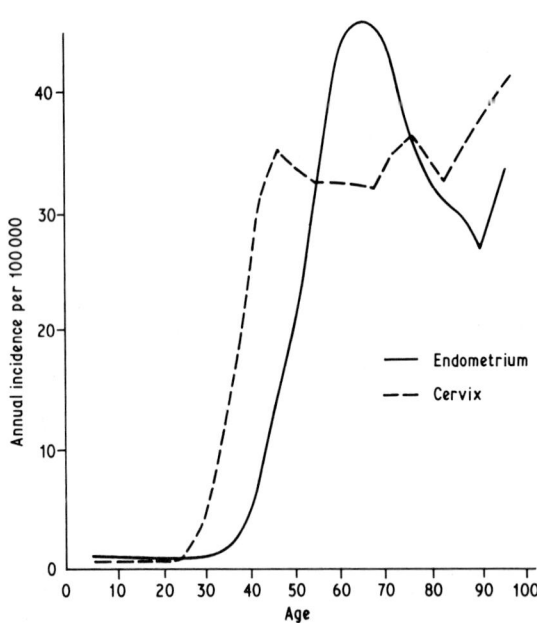

Fig. 28.1   Age specific rates for cervix and endometrial cancer (from data reported by Waterhouse, 1974).

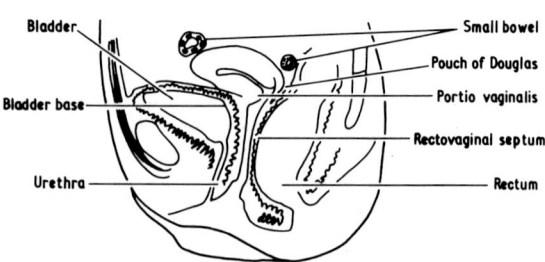

Fig. 28.2   The anatomical relations of the uterus to other pelvic structures.

Table 28.2 Age-standardized incidence rates for cervix and corpus cancer (from Segi, 1977).

Place of Assessment	Age-standardized rate/100 000*		Ratio† $\dfrac{CX}{CP}$
	Cervix (CX)	Corpus (CP)	
El Paso (Spanish)	80.9	9.5	8.5
Recife (Brazil)	58.1	2.2	26.4
Denmark	31.6	11.4	2.8
Mar. Prov. (Canada)	22.6	12.3	1.8
Norway	18.1	9.8	1.9
Osaka (Japan)	16.2	0.9	18.0
UK South West	12.7	11.3	1.1
New York State	10.8	12.7	0.85
Israel (All Jews)	4.5	10.8	0.42

* Annual age-standardized rate against a truncated world population/100 000
† Different ratios appear affected more by geographical location than anything else.

in the broad ligament to the uterine and ovarian veins as well as vaginal and vertebral venous plexuses.

Lymphatic drainage

Lymphatic vessels drain the cervix through the broad and utero-sacral ligaments. Lymph nodes exist alongside the cervix and in groups described according to the adjacent arteries, that is the obturator, sacral, internal iliac and external iliac groups. They ultimately drain into the para-aortic chain. The lower corpus has the same lymphatic system but from its upper part drains to the inguinal nodes via the inguinal canal and with the ovarian vessels to the pre- and para-aortic node groups.

Hartgill (1971) and Kolbenstedvt and Kolstad (1973) describe the lymphatic pathways, and the use of lymphangiography both as an aid to pre-operative diagnosis and to the surgeon at operation.

Histological classification

Cervix

Sufficient histopathological data now exist to demonstrate the natural history of cervix cancer from an early pre-invasive stage to clinically invasive disease. This has come about by cytological studies and from controlled biopsies obtained using colposcopic techniques. These show that the majority of cancers develop from an *in-situ* or atypical phase; the time taken varies but all such lesions should be considered potentially invasive. Stromal invasion may be a forerunner of invasive cancer and the reader is referred to Langley (1976) for further information.

Histologically, approximately 95% of cervix cancer can be classified as squamous and most of the remaining 5% as adenocarcinoma.

Squamous cell carcinoma

These are graded according to the degree of differentiation. Grade I shows distinct keratinization with the production of epithelial pearls. Grade II reveals stratification as less clear with the possible appearance of spindle cells. Grade III is either dedifferentiated or anaplastic with no stratification.

As pointed out by Willis (1960) the structural pecularities are legion and often diverse in any one tumour and several biopsies are advisable. The reported variations include 'clear' and spindle cell carcinomas.

Adenocarcinoma of cervix

The precise origin of these lesions is still debated. However, there is little doubt that they do exist as a distinct entity arising from the glandular epithelium, some of which are mucus secreting. The two primary sites are the endocervical canal and external os. Mixed adenosquamous lesions sometimes occur which behave more like cervical squamous than endometrial lesions and should be managed accordingly.

Body of the uterus

Cancer of the endometrium may occur as a single polypoid growth or less often be multifocal. The commonest site is the uterine fundus and the majority are adenocarcinomas. Some contain both adeno and squamous elements, the so called adenoacanthomas which arise in areas of metaplasia. Adenocarcinomas appear to develop from atypical proliferative endometrial hyperplasia and in some cases the differential diagnosis is difficult with both conditions coexisting.

In practice, histological grading is only of value to patients with Stage I disease. Grading is done according to the worst area seen on microscopy. Grade 1 is highly differentiated adenomatous carcinoma. Grade 2 is differentiated adenomatous carcinoma with partly solid areas. Grade 3 is predominantly solid and entirely undifferentiated carcinoma. Most tumours are classified as Grade 1. Such tumours have a reduced tendency to penetrate the myometrium which, in turn, is associated with a reduced chance of lymph node involvement and consequently an improved prognosis. The poorly differentiated lesions tend to invade locally and spread to pelvic lymph nodes and beyond.

Less common tumours of the corpus
Sarcomas occur both within the endometrium and in pre-existing fibromyomas. However, they also occur in the myometrium with a tendency to spread both locally and to metastasize outside the pelvis.

The commonest cause of secondary deposits occurring within the uterus are those originating from the ovary. Management of these tumours is best determined by the amount of spread revealed at the time of the initial investigation.

Metastases and natural history

Cervix cancer

The morphological development of cancer of the cervix can be considered under three headings:

1. Endophytic or infiltrative.
2. Excavating or ulcerative.
3. Exophytic or cauliflower growth.

Endophytic lesions
These invade the tissues underlying the cervical epithelium without ulcerating the surface until a late stage. As such they can have lateral extension and/or uterine spread before symptoms occur. These lesions are occasionally missed initially and difficult to biopsy. One particular variant is the so-called 'barrel' carcinoma. These are of endocervical origin, histologically adenocarcinomas and cause expansion of the lower uterine segment.

Excavating lesions
These lesions cause extensive ulceration of the cervix as the normal tissues are destroyed. They invariably have a shaggy base with superimposed infection and

may give rise to a serosanguinous offensive discharge. They bleed easily which results in many of them presenting with post-coital or intermenstrual bleeding.

Exophytic lesions
These originate from a definitive base from which they expand into the vagina to produce an extremely soft and friable cauliflower-type growth. The surface of the tumour has a papillary appearance, is often infected and bleeds easily.

Spread of disease
Most commonly spread occurs to the adjacent structures through the interstitial spaces of the parametrial tissues and along the epithelial surface of the uterus. Occasionally, the disease invades the bladder base anteriorly or rectum posteriorly. An important structure which can be affected by compression or local infiltration is the lower ureter which comes within 2–3 cm of the endocervical canal.

The chance of lymphatic spread varies with local infiltration and grade of tumour. Lymph node metastases are reported in 15–20% of stage Ib lesions rising to about 60% for stage IIIb disease. The chance of lymph node metastases tends to follow the same general rules as for squamous carcinoma at other sites with the proximal lymph nodes being affected first.

Blood-borne metastases occur more commonly in the late stages of disease affecting bone, liver, lungs and skin. As the cure rate for advanced disease increases the number of cases returning with blood-borne metastases seems also to increase. However, the commonest association of distant metastases is with recurrent or residual pelvic disease. Death from cervical cancer is often due to uraemia as a result of ureteric compression by growth within the pelvis, otherwise the end result can be extremely unpleasant with prolonged cachexia and the unpleasant sequelae of vesicovaginal or rectovaginal fistula.

Endometrial cancer
Fortunately, because of post-menopausal bleeding, endometrial cancer commonly presents at an early stage with disease confined to the endometrium although the myometrium may be invaded. It has been shown that the depth of myometrial invasion is related to histological grading (Joslin *et al.*, 1977), and in turn to lymph node involvement and prognosis. Where disease is limited to the endometrium the chance of pelvic lymph node involvement is some 7% rising to about 50% when disease reaches the serosa.

The chance of distant spread is small; Joslin (1978) reported only 5 of 41 cases with poorly differentiated tumours and 4 of 210 with well differentiated tumours showing distant spread at up to five years from treatment. The tissues most commonly affected are lung, liver, bone and adrenals.

Local spread may involve the fallopian tubes or ovaries by seeding. This can extend to produce pelvic peritoneal deposits. Spread can also occur down the vagina with a predilection for the sub-urethal area.

Death occurs less often from uraemia than in cervix cancer and is principally due to the invasion of other organs.

Symptoms and presentation

Carcinoma of the cervix

This commonly presents in pre-menopausal woman as intermenstrual bleeding, usually precipitated by intercourse, or after the menopause as post-menopausal bleeding. Bleeding can mimic prolonged or heavy menstruation and the loss can be profuse. If the tumour outgrows its blood supply then surface ulceration with secondary infection can occur with the patient noticing an offensive vaginal discharge.

Bladder involvement can lead to frequency or urgency of micturition with or without haematuria and if the rectum is involved, with tenesmus or diarrhoea. With extensive disease, urinary or faecal incontinence may be the presenting symptoms. Less often pain is a presenting symptom as a result of visceral or lateral pelvic wall involvement, invasion of the sacroiliac plexus or acute compression of the ureters within the parametria. Occasionally, presentation may be due to distant metastases.

Carcinoma of endometrium

Carcinoma of the endometrium invariably causes irregular or, more commonly post-menopausal bleeding. However, any woman over 35 years of age who complains of prolonged or heavy menstruation or intermenstrual bleeding should be fully investigated. Occasionally, a watery or purulent vaginal discharge due to pyometria may indicate a carcinoma. Nearly always symptoms due to local disease will precede those due to metastatic spread.

Diagnosis

A full general and pelvic examination including a diagnostic curettage and biopsy is necessary. A speculum examination should precede any digital examination in order to initially see and assess the size and extent of any vaginal disease. Care is necessary to prevent bleeding and a good technique is to slowly advance a long narrow speculum of the sims type along the posterior vaginal wall with the patient in the left lateral position.

A cervical smear for cytological examination should be taken. A bimanual examination will reveal the size, shape, consistency and mobility of the uterus or any adnexal mass. If an obvious cervical lesion is present a punch biopsy can easily be obtained during the examination. The clinical examination should include a search for involved lymph nodes in the supra-clavicular fossae and groins and of the abdomen for a palpable liver, kidney or abdominopelvic mass.

A rectal examination is done in all cases to determine the extent of possible parametric spread and to search for pathology in the pouch of Douglas.

Cervical cytology is a technique with proven value in the diagnosis of cervical malignancy which during recent years has been supplemented by colposcopic examination of the cervix.

Various methods of obtaining endometrial cells are in use, most of which are unsatisfactory for diagnosing endometrial carcinoma but especially aspirates from the post-vaginal fornix.

Examination under anaesthesia is the next most important step. It reveals the nature and extent of the lesion and allows biopsies for histological confirmation. Before this is done, however, a full blood count, blood urea, serum electrolytes, liver function tests and a chest X-ray are necessary as part of the general routine preceding a general anaesthetic.

With the patient in the lithotomy position, a speculum is inserted to expose the vagina and cervix after which the pelvic organs are bimanually palpated to establish the size and mobility of the uterus and any possible spread of disease. A uterine sound is passed and the cavity measurement recorded since this is of prognostic significance in carcinoma of the corpus. Dilatation of the cervix followed by fractional curettage is then done. Curettings are first taken from the endocervix and subsequently from the endometrial cavity. If obvious cervical cancer exists a punch biopsy is taken.

Staging is done according to the FIGO recommendations discussed in the next section. Finally, it is essential again to carry out a rectal examination in all patients. Additional procedures such as cystoscopy and sigmoidoscopy are done where indicated although it is sometimes suggested that a cystoscopy should always be done for cervix cancer.

Once the histological diagnosis is available an intravenous pylogram should be performed in all patients to complete the disease staging process. Lymphography referred to earlier, can be helpful in cervix cancer to assess (it is suggested that the diagnostic accuracy is up to 85%) any possible nodal metastases and to help the surgeon achieve a total clearance of the relevant lymph nodes. It can also aid the radiotherapist in treatment planning.

Clinical classification and staging

The classification used by the authors is that of the International Federation of Gynaecology and Obstetrics. It is permissible to make the examination under anaesthesia and to take into account the findings at cystoscopy and radiological evidence resulting from an intravenous pylogram. Any special radiographic investigations such as lymphography, venography and arteriography may provide valuable pre-operative information, but should not be taken into account in the staging process. Once staging is done it must stand regardless of any subsequent operative findings and, also, histological grading is important.

International classification of cervix cancer

Stage 0	Carcinoma in-situ, intraepithelial carcinoma.
Stage Ia	Microinvasive carcinoma (early stromal invasion).
Stage Ib	Carcinoma strictly confined to the cervix. (i) Occult carcinoma should be marked 'Occ'. (ii) Extension to the corpus should be disregarded.
Stage IIa	The tumour involves the upper two-thirds of the vagina but has not reached the lower third and there is no obvious parametrial involvement.
Stage IIb	The carcinoma extends into the parametrium on one or both sides but has not extended on to the pelvic wall.
Stage IIIa	The tumour involves the lower third of the vagina but has not extended to reach the pelvic wall.
Stage IIIb	The carcinoma has extended to the pelvic wall on one or both sides and/ or hydronephrosis or a non-functioning kidney is present.
Stage IV	The carcinoma has extended beyond the true pelvis or has clinically involved the mucosa of the bladder or the rectum. (A bullous oedema of the bladder base, as such, does not permit a case to be allocated to Stage IV).

Note 1. Microinvasive carcinoma is diagnosed from the histological findings in a biopsy specimen. Occult carcinoma is an invasive cancer that cannot be diagnosed by routine clinical examination and thus again the diagnosis will have been the result of histological findings.

Note 2. When parametrial fixation to the pelvic wall is smooth it may be cancerous or merely inflammatory. The patient should only be staged as IIIb if the parametrium is nodular or the cervix is pulled towards the pelvic wall.

International classification of corpus cancer

Stage 0	Pre-invasive carcinoma.
Stage I	Carcinoma confined to the corpus. Stage 1a Uterine cavity measures 8 cm or less. Stage 1b Uterine cavity measures more than 8 cm.
Stage II	The carcinoma also involves the cervix.
Stage III	The carcinoma has extended outside the uterus both not outside the true pelvis. This may include spread to the vagina.
Stage IV	The carcinoma has extended outside the true pelvis and has involved the mucosa of the bladder or rectum (bullous oedema of the bladder base is not sufficient evidence).

Treatment policies for cervix cancer

Cancer of the cervix can be treated by either surgery, radiotherapy or a combination of both. Kottmeier (1976) reported 5-year survival rate of more than 90% for Stage I carcinoma following treatment by either radiotherapy alone or combined with surgery.

A distinction between Stage II disease which has spread either to the vagina (Stage IIa) or parametrium (Stage IIb) is important for treatment and prognosis. For Stage IIa the patient can be treated as for Stage Ib, with similar results but Stage IIb cases are usually best dealt with by radiotherapy alone.

Radiotherapy is used for all Stage III cases, but occasionally surgery may be necessary to relieve a uraemic patient by bilateral ureterostomies before commencing radiotherapy. Patients with Stage IV disease may require treatment by radiotherapy, chemotherapy or surgery depending upon the affected organs. However, there are a few patients in this group who are better left untreated.

The place for surgical treatment in carcinoma of the cervix

Carcinoma in-situ

A cone biopsy is normally used for diagnosis and almost always is adequate for definitive treatment. In some centres colposcopically controlled laser beam therapy is being used, particularly in young women, so as to reduce the degree of surgical intervention and conserve reproductive function. Only rarely is a total hysterectomy and partial vaginectomy required.

The importance of cytological follow-up for life, so as to detect recurrence cannot be overemphasized no matter what method of treatment is chosen.

Microinvasive cancer

Lymph node involvement occurs in no more than 1% of microinvasive cancer. However, where invasion is more than 1 mm deep from the surface of the lesion more radical surgery is advisable (Nelson *et al.*, 1975).

The current FIGO staging separates microinvasive (Ia) from occult invasive cancer (previously Ia, now Ib occult). Boronow (1977) reports that this subdivision results in no involved nodes with microinvasion compared with over 20% for occult lesions. The value of this substaging should, therefore, become clear as more reports are made.

Invasive cancer

Primary surgical treatment (Peel, 1978) needs considering for the young patient with restricted disease (Stages Ib occult, Ib and IIa). It should also be considered when the pelvis has been the site of previous inflammatory disease or when benign pathology prevents the proper application of intracavitary radiation sources. Radical hysterectomy should include removal of the uterus, tubes, parametria and upper-third of the vagina coupled with pelvic node lymphadenectomy. Ovaries are rarely the site of metastases from cervical carcinoma in its early stages and can, therefore, be conserved to provide hormone production in the young women. However, where post-operative histological examination confirms node involvement, post-operative external irradiation is recommended. It should be unnecessary to remove more than the upper third of the vagina but in those cases where it is removed then Symmonds and Pratt (1961) have described a technique in which the peritoneum on the front of the rectum and the bladder can be used to extend the vagina.

Pre-treatment laparotomy is practised in a number of centres in the USA although its value remains unproven. In one series Averette *et al.* (1972) reported an error of 38.6% due to mis-staging, principally from involved para-aortic nodes, undetected by clinical examination. Less than 50% of patients had positive findings on lymphography. When para-aortic nodes are involved surgery is abandoned and para-aortic irradiation added to the usual radiotherapeutic regime. (The experience of the Author is that radiotherapy cures only a small number of these patients.) The frequency of node involvement has been reported as 8% for Stage I, 16% for Stage II and 26% for Stage III by Chism *et al.* (1975). It should be emphasized that para-aortic node biopsy is not without complication and all authors emphasize the experimental nature of their work.

Surgical complications

Surgical treatment has an operative mortality approaching 1% and for those who do not regularly do this operation the complications are greater. Post-operative bladder morbidity is not uncommon, the patient experiencing difficulty initiating micturition or having intermittent urinary incontinence. Damage to the ureter during dissection may pass unnoticed. For surgery in combination with radiotherapy a urinary fistula rate of about 0.5% is usual but is significantly less for surgery alone. The elderly and obese patient also presents special surgical problems and is best dealt with by radiotherapy. Although pre-operative lymphography has made the surgeon's task of removing nodes much easier, it is still almost impossible to guarantee complete dissection.

Pre-operative radiotherapy

Pre-operative local radiotherapy is combined with surgery in the belief that it destroys viable tumour cells around the cervix which may implant in the vaginal wall during operation. It will also shrink the primary tumour making surgery easier and reduce bleeding. Normally, intracavitary ^{226}Ra or ^{137}Cs is used to deliver a dose of 4000 rad at the Manchester point A in 70 hours continuous treatment, with surgical treatment 3–4 weeks later. It should be explained that it is unlikely that these doses, often referred to as 'half' doses will eradicate any but the most superficial lesions.

It is usually suggested that endocervical adenocarcinoma should be treated by a combined approach because of poor response to radiotherapy but this is not the experience of the author who normally treats these by radical radiotherapy. However, should a biopsy confirm residual disease two months later, a total hysterectomy is advisable although some morbidity must be expected.

Other indications for surgical treatment

Surgical treatment may prove necessary if patients treated primarily with radiotherapy later have histological proven residual disease. Before starting any surgical procedure, metastatic deposits outside the pelvis should first be excluded. Even so, the first step in any subsequent surgical procedure is to confirm the pre-operative findings under anaesthesia and take biopsies from para-aortic lymph nodes and lateral pelvic wall tissues for frozen section examination. Radical excision of the uterus, tubes and ovaries not only runs the risk of incomplete tumour removal but is associated with a high incidence of post-operative fistula. It is for this reason that pelvic exenteration has been recommended. Brunschwig did his first exenteration in 1946 and since then Way (1976), Rutledge and Burns (1965) and Symmonds *et al.* (1975) have all reported on the procedure. This latter series report a mortality rate of 3% in 102 patients operated on since 1963.

Primary pelvic exenteration also needs consideration for the Stage IV disease involving either the bladder or rectum and especially if a fistula exists. Even so exenteration should only be done if the disease is restricted to the pelvis.

The place of radiotherapy in carcinoma of the cervix

Carcinoma in-situ

There is little place for treating carcinoma in-situ by radiotherapy except for patients considered unfit for surgery because of obesity, age or infirmity. Under these circumstances local intracavitary irradiation is sufficient. In the older patient, considered unfit for radical surgery, the same follow-up considerations apply as have been discussed previously. Where there is likely to be an underlying invasive lesion it is reasonable to treat with intracavitary radiotherapy.

Microinvasive cancer

The treatment of choice is surgery for the fit patient but otherwise radical intracavitary radiation is recommended.

Invasive cancer

Radiotherapy should be given on a regional basis for all stages using a combination of external beam and intracavitary therapy.

Essentially, intracavitary treatment is concerned with controlling the primary tumour and its local ramifications, whereas external beam therapy is concerned with the bulky primary tumour and spread to other pelvic structures including the lymphatic system. Thus, for early disease the major contribution is provided by the intracavitary therapy and for advanced disease by external beam therapy, thereby providing highly individualized treatment.

General principles of radiotherapy for treating carcinoma of the cervix

Intracavitary treatment for cervix cancer was introduced in the early part of this century as the mainstay of management. The position changed when attempts to improve cure rates, by using supervoltage X-ray therapy for advanced disease appeared to be successful. More recent developments have paid particular attention to protecting staff from radiation exposure as well as improving the standards of dose distribution in the pelvis.

With the introduction of these new treatment modalities to protect staff the major problems have been to at least maintain established cure rates and at the same time reduce morbidity and inconvenience to the patient.

Intracavitary treatment

Intracavitary treatment is firmly established as a practical method for treating cervix cancer because:

1. the cervical canal and vaginal vault form a suitable vehicle to carry radioactive sources,
2. the normal tissues of the uterus and the vaginal vault are relatively radioresistant and tolerate high doses of radiation in comparison to squamous carcinoma and
3. the intensity of radiation falls off rapidly at quite short distances from the cervical region therapy protecting vital normal structures such as bladder and rectum.

The combination of these three facts has made it possible to deliver extremely high doses of radiation to the primary tumour and to its immediate surroundings.

Dose distribution

Although intracavitary therapy alone is fully capable of controlling local disease its ability to deliver a cancericidal dose to tumour extension becomes progressively less as the distance from the radiation source increases. This problem can be reduced to some extent by placing radioactive sources within each of the lateral fornices of the vagina. This will effectively provide a high dose of radiation in the direction of tumour spread, whereas attempting to increase the dose to any lateral tumour extension by increasing the central dose alone provides a high risk of radiation necrosis.

Fig. 28.3 illustrates the dose distribution obtained from a number of radioactive sources, arranged to encompass the primary tumour. Since any dose distribution will have a three-dimensional configuration, the magnitude of dose in any one plane can be increased by altering either the relative positions of the

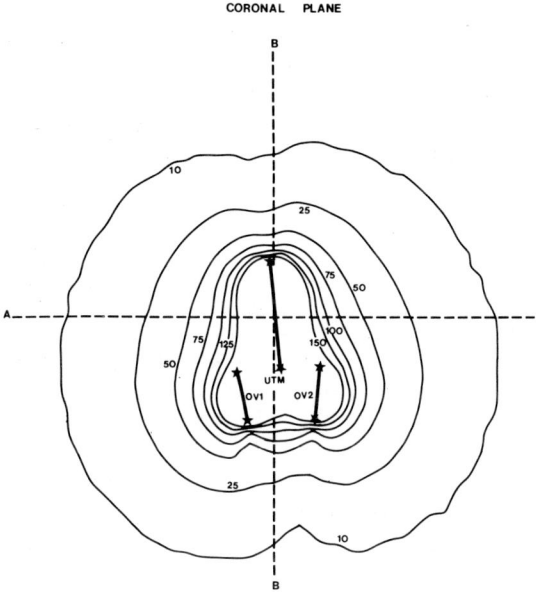

CORONAL PLANE

Fig. 28.3 Dose distribution from a three source system for treating cervix cancer. The isodose curves are expressed as a percentage of the Manchester point 'A' dose.

sources, the individual loading of each source or the time each source is left in position. In practice the position taken up by the sources is determined by the size and shape of the tumour. Any effect this has on dose distribution can be compensated for in some modern systems which allow independent control of the time each source is left in position.

Prescribed dose

In principle, the concept of a treated volume irradiated to a specified absorbed dose and a specified time dose pattern follows the same general principles as for external beam therapy. However, due to the steep dose-rate gradient occurring within the treated volume the point at which the prescribed dose is specified must be related to the expectation of cure and acceptable morbidity. An alternate system which still has many advocates is to prescribe, for a particular source arrangement, the product of the source strength in milligrammes of radium or milligrammes equivalent of radium and the treatment time in hours. Within fairly close limits this simple system is practical but can be dangerous. It has, in the author's opinion little place in current radiotherapy practice since the radiobiological damage produced is not a constant relationship to dose rate and as a result it is important to state both parameters when reporting results and if possible the dose rate at different points.

A disadvantage of defining the absorbed dose at one or more points is that the points in question usually relate to the normal anatomical structures and not to the tumour, except by approximation. The concept of a treatment volume contoured by a specified isodose containing the tumour and local extension leads to a better understanding of the treatment, especially when external therapy is added.

Intracavitary techniques

Despite the many different intracavitary techniques for treating cervical cancer there are only two basic methods:

The Stockholm method

The Stockholm method was first described by Forsell in 1917. Briefly it utilizes the uterus and vagina as vehicles for carrying a combination of intrauterine and vaginal radium, selected individually for each patient. The intrauterine sources are placed in tandem and adjusted according to the length of the uterine canal, containing up to 74 mg of radium. The vaginal applicator(s) take the form of boxes or a tapered collar to cover the vaginal component of the tumour containing up to 100 mg of radium. The applicators are retained during treatment by gauze packing to avoid the rectal or bladder tissues coming into contact with the radium applicators. In order to minimize the normal tissue reactions and achieve maximum tumour control, treatment is divided into two fractions each lasting between 20 and 24 hours, separated by an interval of 3 weeks. The total treatment provides between 7000 to 8000 mg hours but is reduced when external beam therapy is added. The most fundamental and important principle which Heyman (1947) stressed was individualized treatment and dedicated expertise and Heyman's classical paper should be studied.

The Paris method

The Paris method originally developed by Regaud (1926) is similar to the Stockholm method in using uterine and vaginal sources. However, the intravaginal sources are placed in a colpostat comprising two impermeable cork cylinders, one in each vaginal fornix, banded by a metal spring. A central source overlying the cervix is also used in selected cases. The quantities of radium used are less than in the Stockholm method, corresponding to units of 6.66 mg each. The number of units and loading factors are selected according to the lengths of uterine canal but never exceed 40 mg. The vaginal loading is usually 30 mg and treatment is continued for 5 days. This provides for a total treatment of 7000 to 8000 mg hours. Any reader interested in the original description should refer to Regaud (1934).

The important principle of the Paris method was the protracted low dose rate used as opposed to the Stockholm method which used a higher dose rate but fractionated treatment.

Both methods prescribed treatment in milligramme hours as previously discussed.

The Manchester technique

The most well-known development of the Paris method was the Manchester technique originated by Tod and Meredith (1938), later modified. Hard rubber ovoids replaced the colpostats, being held apart by a washer or a spacer. These ovoids were shaped to produce a radiation dose uniform to within 10%, over the surface of the ovoids.

A selection of three sizes for both the intrauterine tubes and vaginal ovoids, with different source loading, are available to meet the problems of differing sizes of uterus and vagina. Treatment is separated into two fractions of 70 hours each in a total time of 10 days to deliver 8000 Roentgens to the Manchester point A which is discussed later.

One important principle of the Manchester system is to prescribe treatment in terms of a dose of radiation to defined points of interest within the paracervical tissues and to the pelvic wall. Accurate source positioning in relation to the normal anatomical structures is strongly stressed and check X-rays following insertion of the sources should always be carried out.

As a working proposition the source loadings were designed to deliver a standard radiation dose rate to a defined point, the Manchester point A, irrespective of the combination of ovoid or uterine source used (Table 28.3).

The Manchester point A came into use as a prescribing point because of the importance of limiting the dose of radiation within the paracervical tissues, where the uterine artery and ureter are closely related and where the least variation in dose occurs. Todd (1941)

extended this work to show the effect of localized high doses of radiation to the anterior rectal wall tissues, the so-called intrinsic rectal reaction, and the generalized pelvic fibrosis which can occur following full pelvic irradiation, the so-called extrinsic reaction.

The Manchester point A is defined as that point 2 cm lateral to the central uterine canal and 2 cm up from the vaginal skin of the lateral fornix in the plane of the uterus. A second point, point B, lying in the same plane and 5 cm from the patient's midline (originally 3 cm lateral to point A) is also used and this gives an indication of the dose to the pelvic nodes and of the slope of the dose rate curve. The reader is referred to Easson (1973) for a review of the Manchester method.

These basic methods and techniques are fundamental to all our present day concepts on management by intracavitary radiation for cervix cancer. There are now numerous modifications and an abundance of techniques available, but the fundamental principles remain unaltered.

Afterloading

One recent technical development has been introduced to reduce or eliminate the radiation exposure to staff and has also increased the versatility of treatment. This development involves the loading of source carriers only after they are satisfactorily inserted within the patient. The empty source carriers are connected to hollow tubes, either flexible or rigid of plastic or metal which project from within the vagina to the patient's exterior (Fig. 28.4). The techniques for insertion are very similar to those for pre-loaded carriers but with the advantage that there is no radiation exposure to the theatre staff. This provides more time for the therapist to place the source carriers in position and to provide some measure of controlling dose distribution by having independent source control. Loading is achieved by inserting the radioactive sources, carried on semi-flexible cables either manually or by some semi- or fully automated device. At the completion of

Table 28.3 Dose rates for the standard Manchester system.

Source of radiation	Radium loading	Type of applicator	Dose rate at point 'A'*
Intrauterine tube	10, 10, 15 mg	Long	35.4 rad/h
	10, 15 mg	Medium	35.2 rad/h
Vaginal ovoids	22.5 mg	Large	18.9 rad/h
	20.0 mg	Medium	19.4 rad/h
	17.5 mg	Small	19.6 rad/h

* Dose rates from the intrauterine and vaginal sources are such that whatever the combination of sources used, the total approximate dose to point A is 54.4 rad/h.

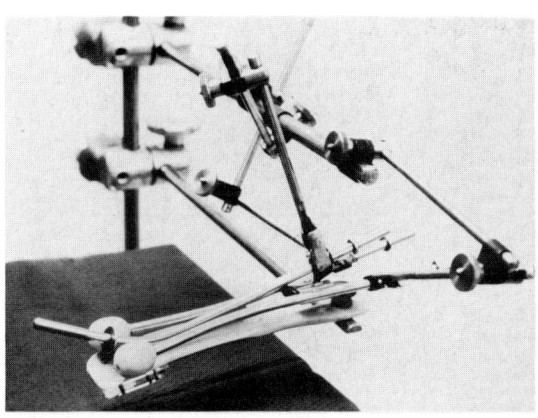

Fig. 28.4 This illustrates an afterloaded system suitable for treating cervix cancer.

treatment sources are as easily removed. Such techniques either eliminate or greatly reduce the exposure from radiation to the various theatre and ward staff.

Among the manual after-loading systems which have been described are those of Henschke (1960) and Suit *et al.* (1963) and for automated after-loading of low activity sources that of Walstram (1965) and of high-activity sources Joslin (1971).

Alternate treatment sources
Recent developments involve the replacement of radium with ^{60}Co or ^{137}Cs (Table 28.4). The advantages include the reduced danger of radiation leakage and reduced protection problems. Because of its high specific activity ^{60}Co, physically no larger than a radium tube yet of several Curies' strength can be used. This permits treatment to be given in minutes rather than hours or days. However, as already indicated, the use of high activity sources necessitates a fractionated treatment programme.

High activity source loading
Intracavitary treatment utilizing high activity sources,

of several Curies, necessitates isolation of the patient during treatment. The essential requirements are: a source storage container, a source carrier system from the storage container to the patient, a suitably protected room to house the patient and a suitable control panel outside the treatment room.

The principal advantage to be gained from remote after-loading is the total elimination of radiation exposure to all staff.

The same dosimetry problems face the therapist when using high as opposed to low activity sources. The aim is to project the dose laterally with limitation in the direction of the bladder and rectum. As for low activity source applicators the size and shape of the tumour will affect the source position. However, since treatments are normally separated by several days, shrinkage of the tumour should occur between treatments and provide for an improved source(s) position.

One suitable device, which has been in use for over ten years, is the 'Cathetron' first described by O'Connell *et al.* (1967). It consists basically of a storage safe containing several separate ^{60}Co sources (Fig. 28.5). By means of connecting cables and a control unit, up to three ^{60}Co sources may be independently driven into each of three stainless steel catheters. These sources terminate in two Manchester style ovoids and an intrauterine tube. The position and setting of the catheters is maintained by means of clamps suspended from a horizontal bar supported by a vertical pillar attached to the treatment couch. The technique has been discussed in detail elsewhere (Joslin, 1971).

The dose prescribed, the number of fractions and the overall treatment time will depend upon whether external beam therapy is also used. Suitable dose regimes will be discussed later but for intracavitary treatment alone, indicated in Stage Ib (occult) cases, a total of 4250 rad in 5 fractions of 850 rad at weekly intervals to the Manchester point A is prescribed.

When using treatment combined with surgery O'Connell (1973) advised 5 or 6 fractions of 600 rad each to point A on a daily basis with a Wertheim hysterectomy 3 to 4 weeks later.

Table 28.4 Properties of radionuclides suitable for intracavitary techniques.

Radionuclide	^{60}Co	^{226}Ra	^{137}Cs
% Transmission through 2 cm Pb	39%	30%	12%
Average photon energy	1.17 MeV + 1.33 MeV	1.0 MeV	0.66 MeV
Half-life	5.26 yr	1604 yr	30.0 yr

Rectal dose measurement

Irrespective of the intracavitary technique used it is essential to avoid rectal reaction; rectal dose measurements are thus made at each insertion. It is also essential to insert the measuring probe in such a way that it provides a good indication of the dose of radiation to the anterior rectal wall so that this can be related to clinical experience. In general, provided the maximum rectal dose does not exceed 60% of the prescribed point A dose, complications are unlikely to occur.

Combined intracavitary and external beam therapy

The chance of lymph node involvement will increase with the stage of disease, therefore unless the chance of cure is to be denied to some women with Stage Ib or later disease, a regional approach to management is necessary. This can only be done by combining both external beam and intracavitary treatment.

Where there is a large central tumour mass or spread to the lateral pelvic wall, intracavitary treatment alone will only deliver an effective dose to the central tumour. Therefore it is essential initially to treat such cases by external beam therapy in order both to shrink the primary tumour mass and at the same time treat the pelvic lymph nodes. Although a mid-pelvic dose of 4500 rad in 20 fractions over 28 days will normally produce an initial regression without further treatment many of these cases will later recur centrally. Where good regression has occurred further treatment to the residual tumour mass by intracavitary therapy is logical since this will result in a high dose to a small treatment volume containing a proportion of hypoxic tumour cells.

Although some tumours shrink quickly the majority only show partial regression by the time external therapy finishes. Therefore further assessment should be delayed by two to three weeks and this will also give an opportunity for the normal tissue reactions to settle.

When a satisfactory response has been obtained the patient should be taken to theatre for an examination under anaesthesia. If examination confirms the previous clinical findings routine dilatation of the cervical canal and a biopsy should be done. Intracavitary treatments can be either:

1. A single intracavitary low activity source technique. One such system is to use the Manchester method to deliver approximately 2500 rad at the Manchester point A in about 45 hours.
2. Two, high activity, after-loaded treatments spaced a week apart each delivering 800 or 850 rad to the Manchester Point A.

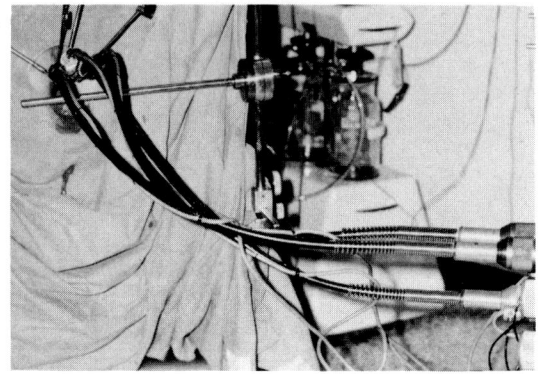

Fig. 28.5 Afterloading is affected by a series of hollow flexible tubes connecting the treatment source carrier to a suitable storage safe.

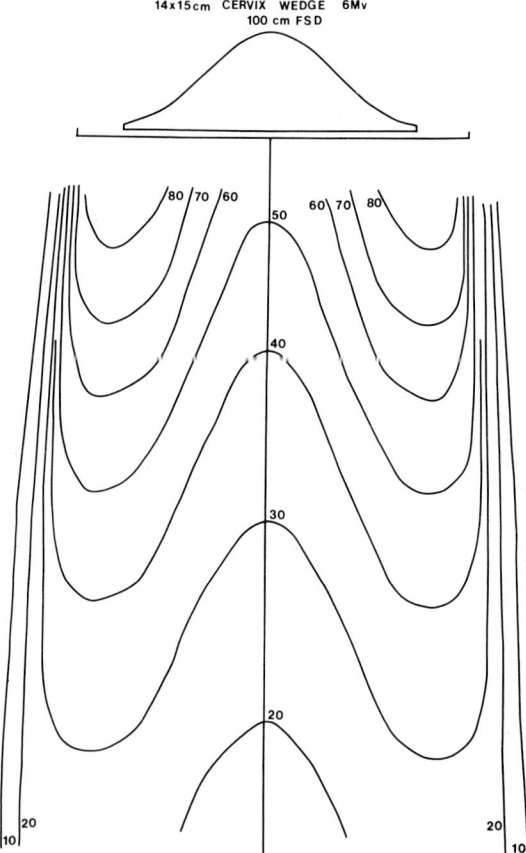

Fig. 28.6 Depth dose curves using a central wedge with 6 MeV photons.

One possible complication following external beam treatment is that of vaginal stenosis making it difficult to place the vaginal ovoids in anything but a tandem position or to use only one. With the 'Cathetron' it is sometimes possible to place an ovoid in one lateral fornix, to treat one side and then the other. However, this does mean that a high local dose is delivered to the vaginal vault tissues and it is not advisable to repeat this on the second occasion when a central tube only should be used, to deliver 500 rad to point A.

For the less advanced case (Stage Ib and early IIb) the problem of combining external and intracavitary treatment differs since the cervical tumour is likely to be controlled by the intracavitary treatment alone. As a result central structures such as the bladder and rectum can be protected from the effects of external therapy by a central shield which allows a higher dose to be given to the pelvic lymph node groups. Various techniques for shielding the central structures have been described ranging from a simple lead block 4 cm wide, centred in the mid-pelvis and extending the length of the field, to compensatory wedges which are designed to allow for the fall-off in dose from the intracavitary sources either laterally (Fig. 28.6) or laterally and vertically. The dose contribution for one such system is illustrated in Table 28.5.

Special situations

Barrel lesions

These tumours, usually adenocarcinomas, are said to originate in the endocervical canal. Shrinkage of the primary mass should first be attempted by using external beam therapy. We use 200 rad daily for 5 treatments followed by routine Cathetron therapy and wedged external beam therapy.

Prediction of radiocurability

It is well recognized that some patients with cervical cancer respond badly to radiotherapy. A major difficulty is to determine which patients fall into this category before radiotherapy is completed in order that surgery can be substituted. Some reports suggest that radiation sensitivity is affected by the histology, an example being the large adenomatous barrel lesion. Our experience suggests that adenocarcinoma is radiocurable even though less sensitive.

One attempt to establish tumour radiosensitivity was developed by Glucksmann and Spear (1945). By taking serial biopsies during treatment they showed a correlation between prognostically favourable tumours and cellular differentiation. The assessment included counting the numbers of resting, mitotic and degenerating cells. Walter *et al.* (1971) reported improved results for the radioresistant cases by recourse to surgery. This produced a 10-year survival rate of 35% for Stage I and 29% for Stage II as compared with 12% and 7% when radiotherapy alone was used.

Walter *et al.* (1964) stressed the value of histological grading, showing that anaplastic cases fared worse than well differentiated ones. However, we suggest that prognosis is more closely related to the clinical stage of disease. More recently Atkin (1971) has shown the importance of chromosomal variability in cervix cancer cells as having prognostic value independent of histological grading. Dixon and Stead (1977) have shown that sequential biopsies during treatment permit a qualitiative assessment of the proliferative state of the tumour which can be directly related to radiocurability.

Complications of radiotherapy

Failure to eradicate cancer of the cervix at the first attempt is invariably followed by the disease destroying the patient. The price of cure is something which the therapist must decide but the patient has to suffer. The decision can be difficult, for as treatment is

Table 28.5 Pelvic doses for cervical carcinoma by combined high activity after-loading and external beam therapy.

Treatment modality	Manchester point A dose*	Dose 3 cm lateral to point A	Rectal dose†
Cathetron 5 fractions	5 × 850 = 4250 rad	5 × 235 = 1175 rad	5 × 510 = 2550 rad
External 16 fractions	(16 × 150) = 2400 rad	(16 × 210) = 3360 rad	(16 × 125) = 2000 rad
Total dose	6650 rad	4535 rad	4550 rad

* The prescribed dose is the point A dose. † The rectal dose from the Cathetron treatments is expressed as a maximal dose, which should not be exceeded

increased in dose or volume to bring about improved tumour control the morbidity also increases.

With the advent of high energy machines many of the complications which were previously commonplace have largely disappeared only to be replaced by others. For example, with the virtual elimination of skin reactions because of the higher energies now used it is easy to become complacent about what may be happening to the underlying tissues. As a result careful attention must be given to any symptoms occurring during treatment.

Reactions during treatment

These will vary with the tissue and radiation parameters. Radiation reactions may be assessed symptomatically by clinical observation or by laboratory measurement. Criteria for an acceptable reaction and whether it heralds immediate or long term morbidity are the result of experience.

One symptom which commonly occurs during the second half of treatment is proctitis. Various conservative measures are available, the commonest being a mixture of kaolin amd morphine. Patients aged over sixty years are best rested for a few days as they tend to be less tolerant to radiation and take longer to recover. In severe cases Predsol enemas may provide considerable relief.

Patients developing cramp-like abdominal pain or colic with or without diarrhoea should be suspected of having a small bowel reaction and rested until symptoms subside. In patients who have had previous pelvic inflammatory disease or surgery a loop of small bowel and particularly terminal ilium may be adherent within the pelvis. Reactions occurring shortly after the start of radiotherapy should be taken as an indication to consider surgery.

External beam therapy may cause reduced absorption of vitamin B12 and neutral fats from the terminal ileum during the second half of treatment (Tankel *et al.*, 1965).

Urinary symptoms may occur including urgency, frequency of micturition and dysuria. It is important to exclude infection and urinary culture should always be done. A liberal intake of fluids can help and analgesics may be indicated.

Other complications include vaginal haemorrhage which may usually be controlled by vaginal packing but occasionally an immediate hysterectomy is indicated. Where hysterectomy is not technically possible ligation of the internal iliac arteries may be necessary but the prognosis in such cases is invariably poor.

Patients with a pyometra at the time of insertion of low activity radioactive sources are best rested from treatment and given antibiotics. When high activity sources are used the treatment time is short and therapy need not be delayed but culture and sensitivity tests with treatment by appropriate antibiotics are still necessary.

Where a tumour has penetrated the rectum or bladder a fistula may occur during radiotherapy. For all these cases it is worth considering a defunctioning colostomy or urinary diversion before radiotherapy commences.

Reactions following treatment

Reactions following treatment can be classified as those which produce mild complications and little inconvenience to the patient and those which produce severe complications of which some are remedial. After meticulous treatment, as already described, the incidence of serious complications should be very low, as after surgery, but it is all the more important to manage those that do occur correctly.

Vaginal complications
The commonest complication is recurrent vaginal adhesions which may be followed by vaginal stenosis or occlusion. The latter will produce dyspareunia which, for some patients, can be classified as a severe complication. Stenosis and occlusion invariably occur where previous malignant infiltration of the vaginal tissues has occurred. One advantage claimed for the short treatment times of high activity intracavitary sources is that the resultant vaginal scarring is less than that seen from protracted treatment, possibly as a result of free drainage and lack of prolonged vaginal packing.

Sub-dermal complications
Sub-dermal fibrosis and fat necrosis are commonly seen after using parallel opposed fields in obese patients treated with ^{60}Co radiation at less than 100 cm SSD (source to skin distance). Such patients are best treated by either a box technique or at an energy of not less than 8 MeV photons at 100 cm FSD (tube focus to skin distance). Affected patients present with a hard plaque in the anterior abdominal wall and buttocks. It can be unsightly and produce discomfort; unfortunately little can be done for it.

Rectal complications
In the early days of intracavitary treatment rectal complications occurred in as many as 20% of patients. Tod and Meredith (1938) showed the importance of limiting the dose directly to the anterior rectal wall, to avoid any intrinsic reaction. It was then realized that rectal dose must be limited and that confirmatory rectal dose measurements must be made at the beginning of treatment. This form of injury is therefore now uncommon.

Unfortunately, rectal bleeding and pain often progress to a rectovaginal fistula. Healing of a rectal ulcer may follow a defunctioning colostomy but almost invariably the colostomy has to be permanent. Transvaginal closure of a fistula following colostomy has been reported but the chance of a successful outcome is small.

Sigmoid colon complications
The reported incidence of these is low, but they do produce recurrent sigmoiditis, stricture or ulceration with perforation and occasionally a fistula. They occur particularly following a high localized dose, due to either a retroverted uterus or in the case of a rigid after-loading system the uterus being pushed too far posteriorly.

The presenting symptom is usually bleeding, occasionally as an acute haemorrhage and is best treated by a transverse defunctioning colostomy. In some cases after a few months rest bowel continuity may be restored but occasionally a hemicolectomy is required. Fistulae to other portions of bowel have been reported but the numbers are small.

In all cases of this nature, careful assessment is needed by gynaecologist, gastrointestinal surgeon and radiotherapist.

Small bowel complications
Small gut is extremely sensitive to irradiation and doses of more than 4000 rad in 20 fractions over 4 weeks can cause small bowel complications. Since this order of dose is at the lower limit of that normally prescribed some risks have to be taken.

Malabsorption may occur in the terminal ileum leading to malnutrition and occasionally a stricture leading to obstruction or perforation and peritonitis. Presenting symptoms include a history of repeated attacks of colic followed by vomiting, steatorrhea and progressive weight loss. Occasionally patients present with peritonitis from a perforated ulcer.

Where malabsorption occurs replacement therapy should be started. However, to delay further investigation and laparatomy in any patient with sub-acute obstructive symptoms is subjecting the patient to the serious risk of total obstruction or perforation. Such cases are best managed by surgeons who appreciate the problems of vascular damage from irradiation since experience has shown that a bypass of the affected gut rather than an end-to-end anastomosis produces the best chance of a successful outcome (Smith *et al.*, 1969).

Bladder complications
The most common symptom is haematuria. Cystoscopy will often reveal ruptured capillaries in the bladder base within an area of telangectasia and not recurrent cancer. This usually settles quite quickly and interference by fulgarization or biopsy can lead to frank ulceration or fistula.

Increasing urgency of micturition and frequency with no confirmatory evidence of infection may be due to a contracted bladder at least, or early onset of an ulcer later followed by a vesicovaginal fistula. Occasionally a fistula may appear without warning. For a contracted bladder or a fistula the only alternative to a life of misery for the patient is some form of urinary diversion such as an ileal conduit since attempts at closing a fistula usually fail (Burns and Upton, 1969).

Cancer of the cervical stump

Cancer of the cervical stump following a sub-total hysterectomy is less frequent now that this operation is performed less often. However, when it does occur one particular problem is the loss of the uterine cavity to hold the intracavitary sources. A further problem is that of disease spread onto the pelvic floor. Because of this, treatment should start with external beam therapy to the whole pelvis to deliver 4500 rad in 20 fractions over 28 days, followed by a modified intracavitary insertion one week later. However, with a canal of less than 2 cm length difficulty may be experienced in retaining the intracavitary source in position, although it may be possible to apply a retaining suture. For low activity sources 2500 to 3000 rad are delivered to the Manchester point A in 48 hours. Alternatively, using high activity sources a dose of 850 rad to the Manchester point A on two occasions spaced a week apart is usually sufficient.

Cervix cancer in pregnancy

Cervical cancer is usually discovered at the first antenatal visit when a cervical smear is taken for cytology. When reported as abnormal a colposcopically directed punch biopsy should be done for histology and if doubt still exists a cone biopsy performed.

The treatment of carcinoma in-situ can be deferred until after delivery provided regular colposcopic examination is undertaken throughout pregnancy.

Patients with microinvasion must be dealt with on an individual basis with due consideration of the age and parity of the patient and the likelihood of cure resulting from a cone biopsy.

Cancer in the first trimester
Treatment can be carried out as for a non-pregnant woman. Radiotherapy is inevitably followed by abortion and it is preferable to carry out evacuation first. In

general we prefer surgery for patients with early disease as a rapid solution for a possibly disturbed patient. Where positive nodes are found, post-operative radiotherapy is indicated. For advanced lesions radiotherapy is the treatment of choice.

Cancer in the second trimester

This group of patients pose a most difficult problem and generally we prefer a radical hysterectomy with lymphadectomy followed by post-operative radiotherapy in those cases with positive nodes.

For the advanced case external radiotherapy alone may be necessary in the first instance. This should cause a spontaneous abortion but in general it is preferable to carry out a hysterotomy followed by radiotherapy.

Cancer in the third trimester

From the 28th week the foetus can be delivered by a classical section before definitive treatment but not without risk to the foetus. The patient's personal wishes need considering during assessment. Treatment delay will increase the chance of a live baby but also the risk to the patient. Weekly assessment will indicate the tumour growth rate and whether it remains local. On balance, the risk to the patient by delaying treatment for four weeks, is not great and should be taken, provided intensive neonatal care is available for the baby.

Once a decision to effect delivery has been taken a classical Caesarian operation should be done and radiotherapy started within a few days.

Treatment of recurrent disease

Recurrence can occur within or outside the previous treated volume as an isolated lesion or as generalized disease. Following radical radiotherapy a series of 290 cases followed for two years or more, shows how central, pelvic, or distant metastases occur, the majority appearing within one year (Table 28.6).

Pelvic recurrence following surgery

This can occur:
1. Where microinvasive cancer, treated radically, later produces positive vaginal vault smears for invasive cancer. This indicates possible multifocal disease which if confirmed by biopsy is best treated by radical radiotherapy. Even though the chance of lymph node involvement is low, full pelvic irradiation to 3500 rad in 15 fractions over 21 days followed by three daily fractions of 500 rad at 0.5 cm from the surface of a 2.5 or 3.0 cm diameter vaginal obturator using high activity after-loaded sources is indicated.
2. Where clinically invasive disease has been previously treated by radical surgery, sometimes after preoperative intracavitary radiation. Despite the fact that most of the previously irradiated tissues have been removed, the effects of radiation may still exist in the anterior rectal wall. A further problem is that of adherent small bowel in the pelvis. It is advisable to treat these patients with external beam therapy at a rate of 200 rad per day 5 times weekly to a total dose of 4500–5000 rad. After one week's rest a decision must be made whether to reduce the treatment volume to encompass the recurrent lesion and treat to a further 1000 rad but much will depend on how well the patient has tolerated treatment this far and the tissues involved.

Recurrence outside the treated volume

Among the sites for recurrence outside the primary irradiated volume are the para-aortic nodes and when excluded from external beam therapy by central screening, the sub-urethral area.

Para-aortic nodes

Unfortunately, early symptoms are unusual and when clinically palpable the nodes are considerably enlarged. Radiotherapy is the only radical treatment available and the chance of cure is low. A dose of 4500 rad in 20 fractions over 28 days should be aimed for or

Table 28.6 Sites of recurrence for each state of disease in a total of 290 cases followed for two years or more.

| Stage | No. | Recurrence site | | | Total no. failing radiotherapy |
		Local	Regional	Distant	
IB	83	3	2	3	4
IIA and B	120	11	21	12	23
IIIA and B	87	18	23	13	26

(Many cases recurred both on the pelvic wall and centrally).

alternatively 5000 rad at 200 rad on a daily basis.

A 2-cm gap between the lower edge of the treatment field and the upper edge of any original pelvic field is necessary to avoid possible complications.

In planning treatment an intravenous urogram is necessary with computerized tomography if possible. A laparotomy may be indicated at least for difficult cases.

Sub-urethral deposits

Treatment is preferably by an interstitial volume implant for the larger lesions and a single curved plane implant for the smaller ones using radium or ^{137}Cs needles. A dose of 5500 rad in 7 days is usually sufficient to provide local control. For a single implant the needles should be in the plane of the anterior vaginal wall and insertion started well below the lesion and retained in position by suturing. It is unusual for the urethra itself to be involved but in advanced cases disease may extend towards the bladder neck. Where this occurs the chance of urinary control is reduced and reconstructive surgery may require consideration.

Distant metastases

The primary consideration is to assess the need for relieving symptoms. Where immediate palliation is indicated this takes precedence and further investigations can be done later. Where asymptomatic disease is discovered at routine clinical examination it is best to determine any further spread before embarking on treatment.

Where disease appears to be localized, palliation is best achieved by a radical approach since these patients may live for some time without further trouble.

If evidence indicates that more than one site is involved chemotherapy should be considered and this is discussed later.

Bone metastases

Although uncommon these do occur, particularly in the spine. Palliative radiotherapy should be considered first but where symptoms indicate spinal cord compression the first priority is a neurosurgical opinion for possible decompression followed by radiotherapy. Where surgery is refused or contra-indicated radiotherapy should be given but the chance of successfully reversing paraplegia is small. A given dose of 2500 rad in 5 days to the involved site using high energy radiation may relieve symptoms.

Cytotoxic chemotherapy for cervix cancer

The use of chemotherapy in cervix cancer has remained restricted because of the superior results of surgery and radiotherapy. However, for pelvic recurrence following radiotherapy or when widespread systemic disease is present, cytotoxic agents are worth consideration but it is important to assess each case carefully, particularly in relation to renal function.

Adjuvant treatment

As an adjunct to surgery or radiotherapy, with the intention of obtaining an improved degree of local control within the pelvis and to reduce the incidence of metastatic disease, particularly for Stage III cancer, the value of cytotoxic agents for cervix cancer remains debatable. As a result an interest in controlled clinical studies has developed; in particular the Cancer Treatment Evaluation Programme of the Division of Cancer Treatment of the American National Institute has initiated several studies of combined systemic chemotherapy and local radiotherapy against radiotherapy alone.

Therapeutic indications

Where widespread disease is suspected or known to exist and particularly if symptoms are produced in an otherwise fairly active patient systemic treatment by chemotherapy should be considered. The possibilities include either single or multiple agents each of which has its advocates.

Single agents

The use of single agents has been poorly assessed but remains the commonest method of treating either local or widespread recurrent disease. Most reported studies have been small but objective remissions of about 20% can be obtained.

One such agent is methotrexate which is convenient since it produces little toxicity if given intravenously every two weeks. The dose used on the first two occasions can be 50 mg which is then reduced to 25 mg. However, it is important that patients have normal renal function and both blood urea and urinary creatinine clearance should be checked before starting treatment. The only morbidity which we have encountered is ulceration of the mouth in a few cases in whom the plasma folate levels were probably low.

Multiple agents

Response to multiple chemotherapy regimes is reported as being superior to single agents. However, the numbers reported as having complete remission, apart from those of Miyamoto *et al.* (1978) and Guthrie and Way (1978), remain small and disappointing (Table 28.7). The overall survival is also poor and does

Table 28.7   Multiple agent chemotherapy for cervix cancer.

Author	Agents	No. of cases	% Response	Comments
Miyamoto *et al.* (1978)	Bleomycin + mitomycin	15	80%	Complete remission 3/12
Baker *et al.* (1976)	Vincristine + bleomycin + mitomycin	27	48%	Greater than 50% reduction in measured tumour volume
Conroy *et al.* (1976)	Methotrexate + bleomycin	20	60%	
De Palo *et al.* (1976)	Adriamycin + bleomycin versus cyclophosphamide + vincristine	15 / 19	20% / 10%	Complete + partial remission
Bond *et al.* (1976)	Adriamycin + vincristine + methotrexate versus the above + bleomycin	21 / 20	48% / 35%	Partial + complete remission
Guthrie and Way (1978)	Adriamycin + methotrexate	12	17% / 50%	Complete remission Partial remission

not greatly exceed that for single agents or indeed for untreated cases (De Palo *et al.*, 1976).

Treatment policies for carcinoma of the body of the uterus

When compared with carcinoma of the cervix the treatment of endometrial carcinoma is relatively non-controversial. Fortunately, most cases present as Stage I disease and the most common practice is to perform an abdominal total hysterectomy and bilateral salpingo-oophorectomy. Unfortunately, not every patient is fit enough for surgery due either to obesity or cardiovascular problems and in such patients radical radiotherapy is preferred.

The cure rates for surgery alone are reported at around 70%, failure being due to pelvic lymph node metastases, vaginal vault recurrence and sub-urethral deposits. To reduce the problem of node involvement more radical operations have been advocated (Lewis *et al.*, 1970) but the general view is that the incidence of pelvic node involvement, and the ability of surgery to control it, is not so high as to justify a Wertheims hysterectomy as a primary form of treatment. Pre-operative intrauterine irradiation has been successfully used to reduce the incidence of vaginal vault recurrence and shrink the primary tumour (Rutledge *et al.*, 1958). An alternative is to follow surgery with post-operative radiotherapy depending on the extent of myometrial invasion and proximity of growth to the cervix.

The place for surgical treatment in endometrial cancer

The primary task is to remove the uterus together with the adnexa and upper vagina. This will be sufficient to cure a large proportion of cases with disease limited to the superficial tissues. However, the chance of lymph node involvement increases with the depth of myometrial invasion. Since the latter has been shown to be related to histological grading, Lees and Bar-Am (1978) advocate that tumour grading should be done first in order to plan a more radical approach in the poorly differentiated case.

A similar argument can be made for carrying out a fractional curettage, because where disease reaches the isthmus or approaches the endocervical region the chance of hypogastric node involvement increases and as a result a Wertheim hysterectomy may be advocated.

Although we support a Wertheim hysterectomy for the obvious Stage II cases, for Stage I we prefer a simple total hysterectomy and bilateral oophorectomy with the removal of the upper vagina followed by post-operative radiotherapy.

Surgical complications

Surgical treatment may cause complications analagous to cervix patients but where limited surgery is used the technical complications are less. However, generally these patients are older and medically less fit than cervix patients resulting in an increased risk of secondary complications.

Pre-operative radiotherapy

The major advantage claimed for pre-operative intracavitary irradiation is reduction in tumour bulk to simplify surgery and in incidence of vaginal vault recurrence. However, there are those who feel it delays the patient's definitive treatment and should not be carried out routinely. Disadvantages are that it makes any post-operative assessment of possible myometrial invasion difficult and that it does not provide treatment to the pelvic lymph nodes.

Various techniques exist but in general treatment is about one half of that normally given for radical treatment. For a Manchester system this corresponds to approximately 4000 rad being delivered at a distance of 2 cm from a central tube.

When a greatly enlarged uterus is present, 4000 rad external irradiation to the whole pelvis in 20 fractions over 4 weeks is worth considering, followed by surgery 3–4 weeks later.

The place of radiotherapy in carcinoma of the endometrium

The results of treating corpus cancer by radiotherapy alone can equal those for surgery but the general inconvenience to the patient and the care needed usually outweigh the disadvantages that surgery may have. The few exceptions to this include the obese patient, the medically unfit patient and advanced disease. Intracavitary treatment alone only treats the uterus and upper vagina, it offers no greater chance of controlling lymph node metastases than does total hysterectomy.

Intracavitary treatment

The application of intracavitary irradiation for endometrial cancer follows the same general rules as for cervix cancer. However, the major difference facing the radiotherapist is that the isodose envelope needs to be much wider at the fundus than at the isthmus. Since the fall-off in dose from a single line source is such that a cancericidal effect becomes virtually impossible at distances greater than about 2 cm from the source and since the tumour itself may well exceed 2 cm in thickness this method is not ideal as radical treatment. However, various techniques have been described to overcome this problem, the most successful being the Heyman technique.

Manchester technique

This single line source technique follows similar principles to that for cervix cancer with a central tube and two ovoids. However, the central tube is differentially loaded with a 25 mg radium source at the fundal end (Fig. 28.7*a*) and below this a series of 10 mg tubes are inserted in tandem, the number depending upon the length of the uterine canal. The vaginal ovoids are usually small and loaded with only 10 mg of radium. The insertion is for 72 hours repeated after 4–7 days to deliver a total dose of 8000 rad at 2 cm from the central tube.

Heyman technique

This technique was first introduced in Stockholm in 1936 by Heyman and published from 1941. The method involves packing the uterine cavity with radium tubes finally leaving a single tube in the endocervical canal. By packing the uterine cavity tightly with applicators the walls of the uterus will

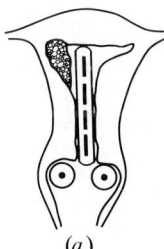 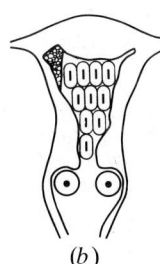 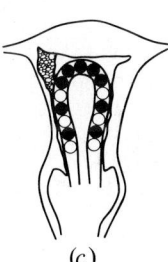

(*a*)   (*b*)   (*c*)

Fig. 28.7 (*a*) Manchester system. Single line source technique. The major problem is obtaining a satisfactory dose at depth within the myometrium.
(*b*) Heyman system. Packing the uterus with encapsulated individual sources provides a means of obtaining a fairly even dose distribution.
(*c*) Strickland system. This technique provides a high fundal dose which is also projected laterally.

stretch allowing a greater depth dose to be achieved within the uterine wall (Fig. 28.7*b*). Where tumour has infiltrated the myometrium the amount of stretching may be greater, thereby increasing the depth of radiation where it is most needed. At the same time if a considerable bulk of tumour is present it may equally prevent an effective dose at the tumour base. Repeating treatment three weeks after the initial insertion will reduce this problem although fewer sources will normally be used on this occasion due to shrinkage of the uterus following the first treatment. Vaginal vault radium is inserted to reduce the chance of vaginal metastases, on one or both occasions. A total dose of 7000 rad to the vaginal vault surface should be given.

It is important to insert each capsule in sequence with numbered tags on the connecting threads. This permits the sources to be removed in the reverse order and prevents tangling of the threads and obstruction of the sources. The sources are retained for 30–50 hours to deliver 3000 rad 1.5 cm from the endometrial surface, repeated 3 weeks later.

A particular problem encountered occasionally is perforation of the uterus although it is not reported as producing dangerous problems (Kottmeir, 1959).

The cure rate for radiotherapy alone has been reported as 55–60% which is similar to that for surgery alone. With suitable adjustment of the treatment time external beam therapy can be added to provide treatment to the pelvic lymph nodes. This requires particular consideration in those cases with disease approaching the isthmus or with a poorly differentiated tumour. Full pelvic irradiation to deliver 4000 rad in 20 fractions over 28 days followed by one intracavitary insertion to deliver a combined total dose of 6000 rad at 1.5 cm from the endometrial surface is one method.

After-loading techniques

One of the major problems with the Heyman technique is the high exposure dose received by staff during insertion and removal of the sources. Efforts at overcoming this have been made and such systems will become more important with the present trends to reduce staff exposure. The substitution of ^{137}Cs or ^{60}Co beads for radium has become the practice in many centres now but despite this the amount of radiation received by the radiotherapist or gynaecologist can still exceed 50 millirems per patient.

After-loading involves no more than a direct connection from the intrauterine source(s) to the patient's exterior. This applies to sources of low or high activity. However, the problem of dose distribution in the uterine cornua still remains although some after-loading techniques have been developed to overcome this.

Manual after-loading

One technique which has been in use for a number of years is that described by Strickland (1971). This takes the form of a helix of stainless steel wire in the form of a loop which is inserted in the uterine cavity terminating in a stainless steel plug which, in turn, is 'keyed' into an endocervical cannula. The device (Fig. 28.7*c*) is afterloaded with ^{60}Co sources each of 6.5 mCi to provide a total loading of 60–75 mCi. The device offers the advantage of an improved dose distribution with a reduced exposure of about 25 millirems to the operator for each loading. Treatment is aimed at delivering 6000 rad at 1.5 cm from the spring in 2 fractions, each of approximately 15 hours separated by one week. A 5-year disease-free rate of 60% is claimed in a series exceeding 200 patients.

After-loading of Heyman system.

A method of after-loading Heyman-type capsules has been developed (Simon and Silverstone, 1972) which retains the advantages of the Heyman system without the problems of exposure. It consists of hollow plastic tubes with a bulbous end identical in shape and size to the Heyman capsule. Insertion is extremely straightforward following which each applicator is loaded with ^{137}Cs (25 mCi), equivalent to 10 mg of radium. Each source is carried on a stainless steel wire to facilitate loading into the hollow capsules.

The technique provides for a much greater degree of flexibility in management since the capsules are not loaded until the therapist is satisfied that the insertion is satisfactory and the patient returned to her room. Exposure is reduced to only 1–2 millirems which is an obvious advantage.

Remote after-loading

The principles are the same as for cervix treatment. We use a high activity source loading system combined with external beam therapy. Initially we irradiate the whole pelvis to a dose of 4500 rad in 20 fractions over 28 days. Two weeks later, after the uterus has shrunk, further treatment is given on a 'Cathetron' after-loader to deliver 850 rad at 2 cm from the uterine tube which is differentially loaded. This is repeated 1 week later.

Radiation following surgery

While many reports claim superiority for pre-operative radiotherapy, post-operative intravaginal treatment offers the same degree of control of vaginal vault recurrence and does not delay surgery (Table 28.8). Unfortunately neither procedure will treat lymph node disease and we prefer a combination of post-operative intravaginal and external beam therapy.

Table 28.8 Survival following post-operative radiotherapy for endometrial cancer.

Category	Intravaginal therapy only		Combined external beam therapy + intravaginal therapy		Probability of difference at 6 years
	No. of cases	% Survival at 6 years	No. of cases	% Survival at 6 years	
Superficial	56	84	11	100	p < 0.04
Less than half myometrial penetration	25	76	57	100	p < 0.03
More than half myometrial	7	40	100	80	p < 0.09

Intravaginal treatment

One of the most satisfactory techniques that has been described is that by Dobbie (1953). This takes the form of a vaginal obturator which is divided into sections of diameter 2 cm, 2.5. cm or 3 cm, which can be screwed into each other in tandem. Each section can be individually loaded with a radium tube of either 15 or 10 mg. When joined in tandem it provides treatment from the vault to the introitus to deliver a dose at 0.5 cm from the surface of the obturator of 6000 rad in 96 hours.

This technique will effectively reduce vaginal vault recurrences to less than 1% but rectal complications do occur and this disadvantage must be faced. It is important to reduce the prescribed dose at 0.5 cm when an obturator of 2 cm diameter is used otherwise a very high surface dose will result.

A simple modification enables the obturator to be used for high activity after-loading (Joslin, 1971). The obturator is made of perspex and carries a central stainless steel catheter throughout its length. This is attached to an after-loading device containing high activity ^{60}Co sources to deliver treatment by 5 daily fractions each of 600–700 rad at 0.5 cm from the surface of the obturator depending upon the diameter of obturator used and age of patient. Using this technique alone we have reported (Joslin, 1978) a 5-year vaginal vault recurrent rate of about 1% (Fig. 28.8).

Combined external and intravaginal treatment

Patients with poorly differentiated tumours or myometrial invasion have an increased chance of node involvement. Since a total hysterectomy will not control lymphatic spread external beam therapy is indicated. As long ago as 1950, Czech reported an improved 5-year survival figure for patients given post-operative radiation (72.5%) against those not having radiation (54%).

Since much of the node involvement will involve small deposits a radiation dose which is at the low end of the radical dose range should be sufficient. This in turn will minimize the chance of producing gut morbidity. At the same time to take advantage of the radiation tolerance of the vaginal vault tissues, supplementary intravaginal therapy can be given to further reduce the chance of vaginal recurrence.

Since 1967 we have used a technique of giving 3500 rad in 15 fractions over 21 days (3000 rad in women over 55 years) followed by 4 daily fractions of intravaginal treatment prescribed to 500 rad at 0.5 cm from the surface of a 2.5-cm obturator. The later treatment is given with a high activity after-loading system.

Table 28.8 gives the results of treatment for a series of 256 cases over six years. These show that seven cases

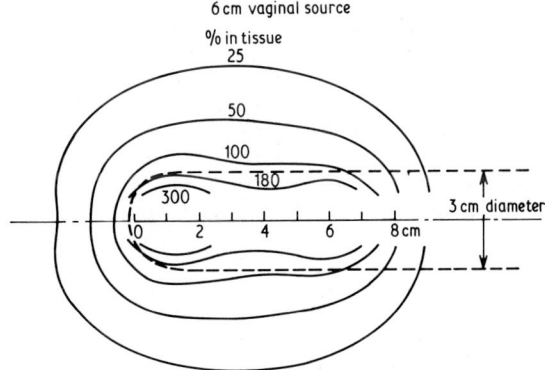

Fig. 28.8 This illustrates the isodose distribution from a vaginal obturator used for treating the full length of vagina followed hysterectomy for corpus cancer. The prescribed dose is given at a depth of 0.5 cm from the surface of the obturator.

with deep myometrial invasion not having external beam therapy did badly. For this reason external beam therapy was then introduced for cases with myometrial involvement. The overall survival of this group of cases was 78% at five years which is appreciably better than anything achieved previously (67%), when external therapy was not used (p<0.01%).

Treatment of advanced disease

Fortunately late disease (Stage III and IV) is not commonly seen. Initially the aim is to achieve bulk reduction of the primary tumour by external beam therapy. A total dose of 4500 rad in 20 fractions over 4 weeks is given with assessment of response 2–3 weeks later. On this occasion a decision is made regarding operability or intracavitary treatment. Where little or no response is seen further treatment is invariably of little use and consideration should be given to hormone therapy.

Where stage IV disease is present with spread outside the pelvis radiotherapy is best used to control local symptoms and systemic treatment with hormones started.

Recurrent disease

Recurrent disease in Stage I corpus does not often occur. In a series of 256 cases Joslin (1977) reports recurrence within the vagina in three, within the pelvis in thirteen and in only seven cases had distant metastases occurred without pelvic involvement. In the 168 patients who had pelvic irradiation only eleven developed some form of recurrence, three of whom had no apparent pelvic disease.

Radiotherapy has little part to play in managing recurrent disease in previously irradiated patients except on a strictly localized palliative basis. However, in cases not previously having radiotherapy, or at most pre- or post-operative intracavitary treatment, full pelvic radiation to 4500–5000 rad can be given accepting the fact that in the previously irradiated cases rectal or bladder morbidity may be high. Such treatment should not be attempted on a radical basis until spread to other sites particularly lungs, liver and bone, has been excluded.

Hormone therapy for endometrial cancer

Progestogens may suppress growth of both malignant and hyperplastic endometrial tissues. The mode of action is not fully understood but the biological effect appears to be directly upon the endometrial tissues (Hustin and Kremers, 1975). However, even before this progestogens were used for treating recurrent endometrial cancer (Kelley and Baker, 1961), using 17-hydroxyprogesterone caproate, leading to an objective response in 30% of cases. Since then many other progestogens have been tried but that which has found greatest favour has been medroxyprogesterone acetate.

It has been reported that pulmonary and skeletal lesions respond better than visceral ones. However, the time taken to show a response can be considerable. In one of our cases it was nine months from the start of treatment before pulmonary metastases finally disappeared. It has been suggested that a large loading dose of progestogens will shorten this period (Kistner and Griffiths, 1968).

We normally give 100 mg of medroxyprogesterone acetate three times daily without a loading dose. The well differentiated tumours tend to respond more often than the poorly differentiated ones and in particular tumours with a long cancer-free interval respond more readily than aggressive tumours which recur rapidly following primary treatment (Kennedy, 1963). The length of remission varies and may last as long as 4–5 years.

The major virtue of giving progestogens to patients is that they do not produce any unpleasant side-effects. In fact patients report an increased sense of well-being, although patients prone to fluid retention should be carefully observed.

Prophylactic use

It is difficult to argue the case for treating patients routinely with progestogens following surgery. The case for their use is to provide an increased cancer-free interval for those cases who have not been cured (about 20% of Stage I cases) and the fact that progestogens do not upset the patient. However, until the results of existing clinical trials are completed the case will continue to be debated if only on the grounds of unnecessary expense and inconvenience to the 80% who have already been cured.

Cytotoxic therapy for endometrial cancer

The results of treatment have been disappointing with no clear indication for cytotoxic therapy. The only single agents reported as producing more than a 10% response are 5-fluorouracil and adriamycin. The latter is reported as having a 36% response rate (Slavik, 1975).

Combination cytotoxic therapy

Only limited experience is available and among the regimes reported is one using adriamycin and cyclophosphamide (Lloyd *et al.*, 1976). It is clear that further studies are necessary but the fact that no one centre has large numbers of cases points to the need for multicentre trials.

The future prospects for uterine cancer

Perhaps for more than any other organ there is already very good evidence that treatment of early disease by conventional therapy cures a large proportion of patients. However, advanced and recurrent disease still pose a considerable problem and better methods of systemic control are required. More Phase II chemotherapy studies and properly conducted multicentre clinical trials are necessary. For advanced local disease the future possibilities include combined modality treatment with radiotherapy and chemotherapy, the use of radiosensitizers and the place for high energy neutrons. The fact that such studies will require a multidisciplinary approach using all the available expertise, both clinical and scientific, should not need emphasizing.

Further reading

Brush, M.G., King, R.J.B. and Taylor, R.W. (eds) (1978), *Endometrial Cancer*. Ballière Tindall, London.

Deeley, T.J. (ed.) (1971), *Modern Radiotherapy: Gynaecological Cancer*. Butterworths, London.

Jordan, J. and Singer, A. (eds) (1968), *The Cervix*. Saunders, London.

References

Adams, E. *et al.* (1974), Sero-epidemiologic studies of herpes virus type 2 and carcinoma of the cervix IV. *Am. J. Epidemiol.*, **98**, 77–87.

Atkin, N.B. (1971), Cytogenic factors influencing the prognosis of uterine cancer. In: *Modern Radiotherapy: Gynaecological Cancer*, (ed. T.J. Deeley). Butterworths, London, pp. 138–54.

Averette, H.E., Dudan, R.C. and Ford, J.H. Jr. (1972), Exploratory celiotomy for surgical staging of cervical cancer. *Am. J. Obstet. Gynec.*, **113**, 1090–6.

Baker, L.H., Opipari, M.E. and Izbiki, R.M. (1976), Phase II study of mitomycin-C, vinstristine and bleomycin in advanced squamous cell carcinoma of the uterine cervix. *Cancer*, **38**, 2222–4.

Bond, W.H. *et al.* (1976), Combination chemotherapy in the treatment of advanced squamous cell carcinoma of the cervix. *Clin. Oncol.*, **2**, 173–8.

Boronow, R.C. (1977), Stage I cervix cancer and pelvic node metastasis. *Am. J. Obstet. Gynec.*, **127**, 135–7

Brunschwig, A. (1948), Complete excision of the pelvic viscera for advanced carcinoma. *Cancer*, **1**, 177–83.

Brush, M.G. and Taylor, R.W. (eds) (1975), *Gynaecological Malignancy: Clinical and Experimental Studies*. Baillière Tindall, London.

Burns, B.C. and Upton, R.T. (1969), Management of urinary tract complications of treatment for carcinoma of the uterine cervix. In: *Cancer of the Uterus and Ovary*. 11th Annual Clinical Conference on Cancer, 1966. M.D. Anderson Hospital, Houston, Texas. Year Book Medical Publishers, Chicago pp. 257–68.

Chamlian, I.L. and Taylor (1970), Endometrial hyperplasia in young women. *Obstet. Gynaec.*, **36**, 659.

Chism, S.F., Park, R.C. and Keys, H.M. (1975), Prospects for para-aortic irradiation in treatment of cancer of the cervix. *Cancer*, **35**, 1505–9.

Conroy, J.F. *et al.* (1976), Low dose bleomycin and methotrexate in cervical cancer. *Cancer*, **37**, 660–4

Czech, H., Kepp, R.K. and Wolthaus, G. (1950), Ergebnisse der Behandlung der bosartigen Genital-tumoren an der Universitats – Frauenklinik Gottingen in den Jahren 1937–1944. *Strahlentherapie*, **82**, 321–54.

De Palo, G.M. *et al.* (1976), Adriamycin plus bleomycin versus cyclophosphamide plus vincristine in advanced carcinoma of the uterine cervix. *Tumori*, **62**, 113–22.

Dixon, B. and Stead, R.H. (1977). Feulgen microdensitometry and analysis of S-phase cells in cervical tumour biopsies. *J. Clin. Path.*, **30**, 907–13.

Dobbie, B.M.W. (1953), Vaginal recurrences in carcinoma of the body of the uterus and their prevention by radium therapy. *J. Obstet. Gynaec. Br. Commonw.*, **60**, 702–5.

Easson, E.C. (1973), *Cancer of the Uterine Cervix*. (ed. E.C. Easson) Saunders, London.

Forsell, G. (1917). Uebersicht uber due Resultate die Kreksbehandlung am Radiumhemmet. Stockholm 1910–1915. Fortschr. a.d. *Geb.d. Rontgenstrohlen*, **25**, 142–9.

Glucksmann, A. and Spear, F.G. (1945), The qualitative and quantitative histological examination of biopsy material from patients treated by radiation for carcinoma of the cervix uteri. *Br. J. Radiol.*, **18**, 313–22.

Guthrie, D. and Way, S. (1978), The use of adriamycin and methotrexate in carcinoma of the cervix. *Obstet. Gynaec.*, **52**, 349–54.

Hartgill, J.C. (1971), Lymphogram control during pelvic lymphadenectomy. *Proc. R. Soc. Med.*, **64**, 401–3.

Henschke, U.K. (1960), Afterloading application for

radiation therapy of carcinoma of the uterus. *Radiology*, **74**, 834.

Heyman, J. (1947), Improvement of results in the treatment of uterine cancer. *J. Am.Med. Assoc.*,**135**, 412–16.

Hustin, J. and Kremers, P. (1975), Steroid 17-hydroxylase activity in normal and cancerous endometria. *J.Clin. Endo. Metab.*, **41**, (Pt. II), 419–421 [quoted in *Br. J. Obstet. Gynaec.*, **82**, 493].

Joslin, C.A. (1971), Radical and post operative treatment of uterine carcinoma by intracavitary after-loaded high intensity ⁶⁰Co sources. In: *Modern Radiology: Gynaecological Cancer*. (ed. T.J. Deeley) Butterworths, London, pp. 71–92.

Joslin, C.A. (1978), The indications for post operative radiotherapy In: *Endometrial Cancer*, (eds Brush, King and Taylor) Baillière Tindall, London, pp.158–62.

Joslin, C.A., Vaishampayan, G.V. and Mallik, A. (1977), The treatment of early cancer of the corpus uteri. *Br. J. Radiol.*, **50**, 38–45.

Kelley, R.M. and Baker, W.H. (1961), Progestational agents in the treatment of carcinoma of the endometrium. *New Engl. J. Med.*, **264**, 216–22.

Kennedy, B.J. (1963), A progestogen for treatment of advanced endometrial cancer.*J. Am. Med. Assoc.*, **184**, 758–61.

Kistner, R.W. and Griffiths, C.T. (1968), Use of progestational agents in the management of metastatic carcinoma of the endometrium. *Clin. Obstet. Gynecol.*, **11**, 439–56.

Kolbenstedvt, A. and Kolstad, P. (1973), Pelvic lymph node dissection under pre-operative lymphogram control. *Gynaec. Oncol.*, **2**, 39–59.

Kottmeier, H.L. (1959), Carcinoma of the corpus uteri. *Am. J. Obstet. Gynec.*, **78**, 1127–40.

Kottmeier, H.L. (1976), *Annual Report of the Results of Treatment for Carcinoma of the Uterus, Vagina and Ovary*. **16**, (ed. H.L. Kottmeier), Cancer Committee of the International Federation of Gynaecology and Obstetrics, Stockholm.

Langley, F.A. (1976), The pathology of cervical neoplasia. In: *The Cervix*, (eds J. Jordan and A. Singer) Saunders, London, pp.345–63.

Lees, D.H. and Bar-Am, A. (1978), A rational approach to the surgical treatment of endometrial carcinoma. In: *Endometrial Cancer*. (eds Brush, King and Taylor) Baillière Tindall, London, pp.139–48.

Levin, M.L., Kress, L.C. and Goldstein, H. (1942), Syphilis and cancer; Reported syphilis prevelance among 7761 cancer patients. *N.Y. St. J. Med.*, **42**, 1737–45.

Lewis, B.V. *et al.* (1970), Primary adenocarcinoma of the cervix. *J. Obstet. Gynaec. Br. Commonw.*, **77**, 277–9.

Lloyd, R.E. *et al.* (1976), Combination chemotherapy with adriamycin (NSC-123127) and cyclophosphamide (NSC-262271) for solid tumours:- a phase II trial. *Cancer Treat. Rep.*, **60**, 77–83.

Lombard, H. and Potter, E. (1950), Epidemiological aspects of cancer of the cervix II heriditary and environmental factors. *Cancer*, **3**, 960–8.

Miyamoto, I. *et al.* (1978), Effectiveness of a sequential combination of bleomycin and mitomycin-C on an advanced cervical cancer. *Cancer*, **41**, 403–14.

Nelson, J.H., Averette, P. and Richard, R.M. (1975), *Dysplasia and Early Cervical Cancer*. American Cancer Society, Professional Education Publications, New York.

O'Connell, D. (1973), A technique of afterloading: high dose-rates. *Proc. R. Soc. Med.*, **66**, 938–9.

O'Connell, D. *et al.* (1967), The treatment of uterine carcinoma using the cathetron Part I – Technique. *Br. J. Radiol.*, **40**, 882–7.

O'Connell, R.B. (1978), Epidemiology of gastrointestinal tumours a review.*J. R. Soc. Med.*, **71**, 278–81.

Peel, K.R. (1978), The surgery of cervical carcinoma. *Clinics Obstet. Gynec.*, **5**, 659–73.

Priden, H. and Lilienfield, A.M. (1971), Carcinoma of the cervix in Jewish women in Israel 1960–1967. *Israel. J. Med. Sci.*, **7**, 1465–70.

Regaud, C. (1926), Traitment des cancers du col de l'uterus par les radiations: idée sommaire des methodes et des resultats; indications therapeutiques. *Rapp. VIIe Cong. Soc. Int. Chirurg.*, **1**, 35.

Regaud, Cl. (1934), Considerations sur la radiotherapie des cancers cervico uterus d'apres l'expérience et les resultats acquis a L'Institut du Radium de Paris. *Radiophys. Radiother.*, **3**, 155–70.

Reid, B.L. and Coppleson, M. (1976), Natural history: recent advances. In: *The Cervix*. (eds J. Jordan and A. Singer) Saunders, London, pp.317–31.

Ritzman, H. (1978), Types of endometrial hyperplasia and their relationship to carcinoma of the endometrium. In: *Endometrial Cancer*. (eds Brush, King and Taylor) Baillière Tindall, London, pp.118–23.

Røjel, J. (1953), Interrelation between uterine cancer and syphilis. *Acta Path. Microbiol. Scand.*, Suppl. **97**, 1–82.

Rotkin, I.D. (1973), A comparison review of key epidemiological studies in cervical cancer related to current searches for transmissible agents *Cancer Res.*, **33**, 1353–67.

Rutledge, F.N., Tan, S.K. and Fletcher, G.H. (1958), Vaginal metastases from adenocarcinoma of the corpus uteri. *Am. J. Obstet. Gynec.*, **75**, 167–74.

Rutledge, F.N. and Burns, B.C. (1965), Pelvic exenteration. *Am. J. Obstet. Gynec.*, **91**, 692–708.

Segi, Mitsuo. (1977), *Graphic representation of cancer*

incidence by site and by area and population. Segi Inst. Cancer Epidemiology, Nagoya, Japan, p.25.

Simon, N. and Silverstone, S.M. (1972), Intracavitary radiotherapy of endometrial cancer by afterloading. *Gynaec. Oncol.*, **1**, 13–16.

Singer, A. (1973), The male factor in the aetiology of cervical cancer. *Oxford Med. Sch. Gaz.*, **25**, 18–21.

Slavik, M. (1975), Adriamycin (NSC-123127) activity in genitourinary and gynaecologic malignancies. *Cancer Chemother. Rep.*, **6**, 297–303.

Smith, J.P., Golder, P.E. and Rutledge, F. (1969), The surgical management of intestinal injuries following irradiation for carcinoma of the cervic. In: *Cancer of the Cervic and Ovary.* University of Texas M.D. Anderson Hospital, Year Book Medical Publishers, Chicago, pp.241–56.

Strickland, P. (1971), The treatment of carcinoma of the body of the uterus. In: *Modern Radiotherapy: Gynaecological Cancer.* (ed. T.J. Deeley) Butterworths, London, pp.167–85.

Symmonds, R.E. and Pratt, J.H. (1961), Prevention of fistulas and lymphocysts in radical hysterectomy. *Obstet. Gynec.*, **17**, 57–64.

Symmonds, R.E., Pratt, J.H. and Webb, M.J. (1975), Exenterative operations: experience with 198 patients. *Am. J. Obstet. Gynec.*, **121**, 907–18.

Suit, H.D. *et al.* (1963), Modification of the Fletcher ovoid system for afterloading, using standard sized radium tubes. *Radiology*, **81**, 126–31.

Tankel, H.I., Clark, D.H. and Lee, F.D. (1965), Radiation enteritis with malabsorption. *Gut*, **6**, 560–9.

Tod, M.C. and Meredith, W.J. (1938), A dosage system for use in the treatment of cancer of the uterine cervix. *Br. J. Radiol.*, **11**, 809–24.

Todd, T.F. (1941), Urological complications of carcinoma of the cervix uteri. *J. Obstet. Gynaec. Br. Empire.*, **43**, 334.

Wakefield, J. *et al.* (1973), Relation of abnormal cytological smears and carcinoma of the cervix uteri to husband's occupations. *Br. Med. J.*, **ii**, 142–3.

Walstram, R. (1965), Remotely-controlled afterloading radiotherapy apparatus. *Phys. Med. Biol.*, **7**, 225–8.

Walter, L.H., Cherry, C.P. and Glucksman, A. (1971), Serial biopsies. In: *Modern Radiotherapy: Gynaecological Cancer.* (ed. T.J. Deeley) Butterworths, London, pp.101–19.

Walter, L. *et al.* (1964), Assessment of response of cervical cancers to irradiation by routine histological methods. *Br. Med. J.*, **i** (5399), 1673–5.

Waterhouse, J.A.H. (1974), *Cancer Handbook of Epidemiology and Prognosis,* Churchill Livingstone, Edinburgh and London.

Way, S. (1976), The surgical management of advanced cervical carcinoma-pelvic exenteration. In *The Cervix.* (eds J. Jordan and A. Singer) Saunders, London, pp.507–16.

Weiner, I., Burke, L. and Goldberger, M.A. (1951), Carcinoma of the cervix in Jewish women. *Am. J. Obstet. Gynec.*, **61**, 418–22.

Willis, R.A. (1960), *Pathology of Tumours.* 3rd edn, Butterworths, London.

29 Trophoblastic tumours

K.D. Bagshawe

The treatment of gestational choriocarcinoma may be considered in the context of a spectrum of neoplastic processes arising from the trophoblastic epithelium of the placenta (Park, 1971; Ober *et al.*, 1971). Choriocarcinoma may occur after any form of pregnancy and the total number of cases arising after hydatidiform mole equals or exceeds that arising from all other pregnancies going to term or aborting without recognized molar change at an earlier stage. Since hydatidiform mole occurs in Western populations with a frequency of 1 in 1000 to 1 in 3000 pregnancies, it is clear that the risk after mole is of the order of 1000 times greater than after non-mole pregnancy. Even so the risk of true choriocarcinoma arising from hydatidiform mole probably does not greatly exceed 3% but the picture is complicated by the occurrence of invasive mole (Bagshawe, 1969).

The distinction between choriocarcinoma and invasive mole lies in their morphological appearances and in their natural history. In contrast to gestational choriocarcinoma, invasive mole probably arises only from a placenta that has undergone some hydatidiform change. The essential morphological distinction lies in the absence from choriocarcinomatous lesions of villous structures containing stroma. The trophoblast tends to be pleomorphic, there are multiple nucleoli, the mitotic figures may be abundant. Foci of necrosis and haemorrhage are surrounded by cytotrophoblast and syncytial elements are normally present. Invasive mole may also show extensive areas of trophoblastic proliferation but these are associated at least in some areas with persisting villous structures. The distinction between the two lesions may be difficult or impossible when the only material for examination is obtained for instance by curettage after hydatidiform mole. It is not uncommon in such curettings to see extensive areas of trophoblastic proliferation without villi but a subsequent curettage or hysterectomy specimen reveals persisting villi. The problem is almost restricted to the patient who has recently had a hydatidiform mole removed since any persistence of trophoblastic elements after the removal of a non-mole abortion or after a normal pregnancy for more than five to six weeks has to be regarded as choriocarcinoma until proved otherwise.

However, since choriocarcinoma can arise from the normal placenta and since the placenta contains numerous villous structures it is evident that at some stage choriocarcinoma is associated with villi. Tumour specimens from the uterus which are otherwise characteristic of choriocarcinoma may reveal an occasional villus usually at an advanced stage of degeneration. In these cases the great bulk of the trophoblast is not associated with villi and the other morphologic features of choriocarcinoma are present.

Evidence from the measurement of trophoblastic products following the evacuation of hydatidiform mole indicates that even when the uterine cavity has been carefully emptied, trophoblastic activity persists in 75% or more of these patients for periods ranging from a few weeks to several months (Bagshawe *et al.*, 1973). It seems highly probable that these patients have invasive mole but that the lesion resolves spontaneously in the great majority of patients.

It is recognized that some invasive moles become large and occasionally metastasize, particularly to the lungs and vagina. Yet invasive mole is a threat to life principally through its capacity to cause severe haemorrhage into the uterine cavity and to perforate the serosal surface and cause intraperitoneal haemorrhage. Invasive mole clearly has powerful invasive properties and may metastasize but it does not, in our experience, produce progressive metastatic disease unless it undergoes transformation to choriocarcinoma and this does not appear to be a common occurrence. In the pre-chemotherapeutic era invasive mole most often killed as a result of its local invasive properties. Although it carried a mortality rate of about 20% it was, for the most part, adequately treated by hysterectomy. Except in the multiparous or menopausal woman it is now better treated by chemotherapy and in the present series which includes more than 200 invasive moles there have been no fatalities.

The problem of defining when an invasive mole requires therapeutic intervention is one that will be considered in relation to the follow-up of patients after evacuation of hydatidiform mole. The arbitrariness of the criteria for therapeutic intervention has, however, had an important influence on the comparability of data from different series. Clearly if less than 10% of the patients who had hydatidiform mole are selected for treatment with cytotoxic agents, as is the practice in the UK, then roughly one in three of these patients can be expected to have choriocarcinoma, whereas the methods of selection used in North America where 20–30% of patients are treated after hydatidiform mole means that possibly only one in ten of these patients has choriocarcinoma and that two-thirds of them receive cytotoxic agents for lesions which would undergo spontaneous regression without therapy.

Ideally one would only use chemotherapy either for histologically proven choriocarcinoma or for a situation where invasive mole is known to exist and is likely to cause serious morbidity if left untreated. However, the fact that in the majority of instances evidence for the presence of a gestational trophoblastic lesion can be compelling if not completely unequivocal in the absence of morphological evidence, presents a different situation from that which usually obtains in cancer practice. Thus clinical, radiological and hormonal evidence for a trophoblastic neoplasm are often so strong and the difficulty of obtaining adequate material for histological examination sufficiently disadvantageous to merit a clinical diagnosis being acceptable. Indeed with the exception of the patient who has had hydatidiform mole evidence of a progressive trophoblastic lesion has to be regarded as equivalent to morphological proof of choriocarcinoma if the patient is not to be at a disadvantage. Moreover where the lesion follows hydatidiform mole the distinction between invasive mole and choriocarcinoma can sometimes be made on the basis of the length of time which has lapsed since the mole was removed. It is very uncommon for invasive mole to persist more than six to eight months after primary evacuation of the mole without causing uterine haemorrhage or perforation. Also, extensive metastatic disease at any time after evacuation of mole is likely to be choriocarcinoma.

The disadvantages of trying to establish a morphological diagnosis by hysterectomy when the clinical picture of choriocarcinoma is evident lies in multiple factors. First, hysterectomy for a large, highly vascular tumour carries a mortality. It will, in any case, delay the introduction of chemotherapy for at least 10 to 14 days and during this time metastases may be established in the brain. Handling the uterus may result in dissemination. In 10–15% of cases there is no lesion to be found in the uterus despite evidence of metastatic disease although this can be determined with moderate reliability by ultrasound and arteriography. Finally, the patient may be deprived of child-bearing function unnecessarily.

In the absence of morphological evidence the diagnosis of a trophoblastic tumour rests in part on the history of a pregnancy, generally in the preceding twelve months, but intervals of up to 17 years have been recorded before recurrent disease has been found. The metastatic disease pattern is that of haematogenous spread from the uterus. There has been no case in the author's series with an active trophoblastic neoplastic process that was radiologically or clinically detectable that was not associated with elevated values of human chorionic gonadotrophin (HCG). Elevated HCG values are of course inadequate evidence by themselves since it is essential to exclude pregnancy, a matter which is still not entirely without difficulty in the first eight to ten weeks. It is also necessary to exclude the possibility that the tumour is teratomatous in origin or a tumour producing HCG as an ectopic product. Tumours producing HCG as an ectopic product usually, but not always, produce relatively small amounts of the hormone. This is not true of course with malignant teratoma and here the distinction may be aided by the presence of elevated serum alpha-fetoprotein (AFP) which is not found in patients with choriocarcinoma unless there is extensive hepatic dysfunction. Malignant teratoma or dysgerminoma arising after a pregnancy can present most difficulty but these cases have usually presented with abdominal pain, and required laparotomy on that account, so that the diagnosis has been established on the basis of the site of the lesion and also histological examination. In principle therefore the diagnosis of choriocarcinoma can usually be established without recourse to hysterectomy or other major surgery, provided the diagnosis is suspected and the appropriate investigations performed.

Human chorionic gonadotrophin

A patient with large tumours which are suspected of being a trophoblastic tumour will almost invariably have a positive 'pregnancy test'. But with the exception of the primary diagnosis of such patients pregnancy tests have little application. Quantitative estimates by radioimmunoassay or enzyme immunoassay should be used and these should be capable of detecting $<1\mu g$ HCG/1 of serum or urine (<5 international units/1).

In general, the serum assay using antibody to the HCG-β-subunit is the most satisfactory system (Kardana and Bagshawe, 1976), although valuable information was obtained for many years with a less specific assay which detected both HCG and pituitary luteinizing hormone (LH) and which still has a place (Wilde *et al.*, 1967). The β-subunit assay is however, effectively 10 to 30 times more sensitive than the HCG/LH assay by virtue of its improved specificity. The problem is that it is difficult to produce antisera which clearly discriminates between HCG and luteinizing hormone. It is essential also that the results of these assays should be available without undue delay since the choice of therapeutic regimen often depends on them and time considerations in treatment are of great importance. Assays with incubation times as short as 2 to 3 hours can be used although overnight incubation giving a result the day after the sample is taken is probably adequate. During the treatment of a patient 'with a trophoblastic tumour by chemotherapy twice weekly assays are desirable.

The serum concentration of HCG and the urinary excretion rate show a quantitative relationship with the amount of viable trophoblast in the patient. This relationship holds both in the first two months of normal pregnancy and in patients with an established invasive mole or choriocarcinoma. Although there is much biological variation between the tumours of different individuals this variation is comparatively small when set against the scale of cell numbers involved. The patient with a body burden of $10^{11}-10^{12}$ tumour cells out of a total body population of approximately 5×10^{13} is likely to have a serum HCG in excess of 10^6 IU/l of serum and a somewhat higher value in the 24-hour urine sample. Studies on excised tumour and on choriocarcinoma cells grown *in vitro* suggest that one cell produces something of the order of $10^{-4}-10^{-5}$ IU HCG per day.

Since the limit of sensitivity is approximately 2 IU HCG/l of serum, it follows that the tumour becomes detectable when the viable cell mass has reached the order of 10^5 cells. Similarly when the tumour is undergoing destruction the assay becomes negative when the population of cells has been reduced to below this level. The implications of this for the duration of chemotherapy are important. If treatment is discontinued as soon as a negative HCG is obtained from the patient with choriocarcinoma, tumour growth is invariably renewed. Renewed growth does not invariably occur if the lesion is hydatidiform or invasive mole. In the case of choriocarcinoma the duration of continued chemotherapy after negative values have been obtained is best adjusted according to a consideration of a number of factors (Bagshawe, 1969). In general these are the prognostic factors which will be considered

below and the rate of fall of HCG during treatment. Thus if a tumour has responded only slowly to treatment it is likely that the residual cells will take longer to eradicate than where the rate of fall of HCG values has been made more rapid.

Following the completion of treatment the patient should be followed up with regular HCG assays and at least for the first year it is desirable to have HCG assays on serum. Later it may be more convenient to revert to the urinary HCG/LH assay. The frequency of performing assays can again be adjusted to the likelihood that the patient will relapse so that for some patients it is more important that assays should be performed than it is for others. The rate of increase of HCG in relapse tends to be rapid in early relapse and slower in late relapses but there are exceptions to this generalization.

In the majority of patients with choriocarcinoma elevated HCG values persist after radiological and clinical resolution of the tumour masses has occurred. However, in some patients the situation is reversed and whereas the HCG assays suggest that the tumour has been eradicated radiological opacities remain in the lungs. Thoracotomy for such metastases sometimes proved that the lesions were sterile and therefore in other cases it has been found possible to wait for their progressive resolution, which has taken one to two years to complete. Clearly when radiological opacities persist it is essential that regular radiological follow-up be maintained as well as the usual follow-up with HCG assays.

Detection and monitoring of intracranial metastases

One of the hazards of choriocarcinoma is metastatic disease within the central nervous system (CNS). Such lesions may be present at the time of presentation and about 10% of patients with choriocarcinoma have intracranial metastases as the presenting symptom. The introduction of radionuclear scanning and computerized axial tomography have greatly improved the radiological capability of detecting intracranial metastatic disease. The blood/brain barrier, however, facilitates still earlier diagnosis by its effect on HCG values in the serum and cerebrospinal fluid (Bagshawe and Harland, 1976). In the absence of CNS metastases the concentration of HCG in the cerebrospinal fluid (CSF) is low and the serum/CSF ratio is greater than 60. When HCG is produced within the central nervous system the concentration of HCG increases and the serum/CSF ratio falls below 60 and the CSF concentration may exceed that in the serum. The lead-in time between HCG detection and scanning or clinical detection of metastatic tumours to the CNS has been several weeks in some cases.

Patients with pulmonary metastases are at high risk to develop CNS metastases so long as there are viable tumour cells in the lungs. The measurement of serum/CSF ratios during treatment provides information which is generally commensurate with the trauma entailed by repeated lumbar puncture. Follow-up determinations of CSF HCG are indicated in patients who have been treated successfully for CNS metastases for about six months. In three instances in this series, intracranial or spinal cord metastases have been detected or have been clinically apparent in patients who have not had pulmonary metastases. There is therefore a case for submitting all patients requiring chemotherapy to a single determination of the CSF/HCG ratio even when pulmonary metastases are not present.

Follow-up of patients with hydatidiform mole

HCG values in serum and urine fall to undetectable levels within 11 to 17 days of a normal term delivery. This is also the case after most non-mole abortions although a few of these take longer to reach normal and these are generally associated with persisting products of conception in the uterine cavity.

In contrast, HCG excretion tends to persist for a longer period after evacuation of hydatidiform mole. The fact that HCG concentration tends to be higher at the time a hydatidiform mole is evacuated accounts for part of this but the principal cause is persisting trophoblast which has penetrated deep into the myometrium. Sometimes repeated curettage is useful in cases where mole tissue recurs in the uterine cavity but in most cases repeat curettage yield little tissue and has little or no effect on HCG values. At two months post-evacuation approximately 40% of patients still have detectable levels of HCG. However, the process of progressive resolution of mole tissue may continue for up to six months following evacuation and the process can be followed by serial estimations of HCG in serum or urine. To avoid frequent venepuncture, radioimmunoassay by HCG/LH assay on urine is adequate at least until HCG values have fallen to the normal range. It is then appropriate to do serum HCG assays until these are also giving negative results.

It is exceptional for recrudescence of trophoblastic growth to occur after HCG has fallen spontaneously to normal values. In 0.3% of the mole patients followed up by this Unit recurrent growth has however occurred and generally in the second year of follow-up.

The traditional duration of follow-up after mole has been two years and it would seem advisable to persist with this rule whenever practicable. On the other hand, where HCG values have fallen rapidly and the patient is anxious to proceed with a further pregnancy the risk of doing so more than six months after HCG has ceased to be detectable, is very small and may be acceptable.

The follow-up system for patients with hydatidiform mole adopted in the United Kingdom has been based on three central laboratories. The patient collects 12-hour urine specimens, measures and records the volume and posts a 5-ml aliquot in a special pack directly to the central laboratory, which in turn reports the results to her gynaecologist. The first assay is performed three weeks after primary evacuation and subsequent assays are performed every two weeks until normal results are obtained, then monthly for one year post-evacuation, then three monthly during the second year of follow-up. Patients are also advised to have a radioimmunoassay for HCG three weeks after the end of any pregnancy subsequent to mole. In the present series 3% of cases gave a history of mole in a pregnancy preceding that directly antecedent to choriocarcinoma.

Indications for treatment following hydatidiform mole

Although marked proliferation of the trophoblast of a hydatidiform mole is associated with a slightly increased risk of malignant sequelae this in no way forms a guide to the need for follow-up management. The use of radioimmunoassays as described above has provided a means for detecting those patients where trophoblast persists for several months. It has also become evident that the interval between the end of an antecedent pregnancy and the time at which chemotherapy is started has a critical effect on the ability to eradicate that tumour. Were this not so it would perhaps be reasonable to wait for say nine to twelve months after evacuation of mole before instituting chemotherapy. Unfortunately some patients have proved resistant in the past even though chemotherapy was started as early as six to seven month's post-mole. Patients with persisting trophoblastic activity five months after evacuation of the mole, are therefore treated with chemotherapy even in the absence of evidence of metastatic disease, provided that at the time they are admitted to hospital their HCG values are not showing a progressive fall. Other indications for treatment include:

1. Histological evidence of choriocarcinoma.
2. Opacities on chest radiograph unless associated with falling HCG values.
3. Recurrent or persistent uterine haemorrhage, or haemorrhage from vaginal metastases.
4. Evidence of metastases at any non-vaginal or non-pulmonary site.
5. Very high HCG values, e.g. 40 000 IU/l, more

than four weeks post-evacuation.

6. Progressively increasing HCG values at any time; these high values even early after evacuation of the mole generally reflect a highly active invasive lesion which is liable to cause uterine perforation.

Factors affecting the risk of requiring chemotherapy after mole

In a series of 611 cases of hydatidiform mole, to which the above criteria for treatment were applied, it was found that hysterectomy or hysterotomy, or evacuation with the aid of oxytocin or prostaglandins was associated with twice the risk of requiring chemotherapy as evacuation by vacuum or curettage or spontaneously (Stone and Bagshawe, 1979).

Another analysis (Stone *et al.*, 1976) showed that where oral contraceptives were taken while HCG was still detectable, the rate of decline of HCG values was slowed and the risk of requiring treatment was increased above two-fold. There was no statistically significant effect where oral contraception was started after HCG had become undetectable. Three patients who developed choriocarcinoma after HCG had become undetectable and then reappeared had been on oral contraception. It would seem advisable to avoid oral contraceptives until radioimmunoassay for HCG has been normal for two months or more.

Alternative methods for management of patients after hydatidiform mole

In some centres, notably in North America, it has been the practice to treat all patients still excreting HCG six to eight weeks after hydatidiform mole and on this basis 20–30% of all mole patients receive cytotoxic chemotherapy (Curry *et al.*, 1975). The proportion of patients for whom treatment is indicated on this basis would tend to increase with improved sensitivity to the assay method. At other centres, particularly in southeast Asia, the use of chemotherapy at the time the mole is evacuated, so-called 'prophylactic chemotherapy' has been used. It is evident that since only 2–3% of moles are followed by choriocarcinoma and a slightly larger percentage by persisting invasive mole, this policy results in giving chemotherapy to ten women or more for every one that requires it. If chemotherapy could be proven to be harmless and effective, such a policy might be justified. The potential teratogenic action of these agents administered during unsuspected early pregnancy is a considerable hazard. However, the main deficiency of prophylactic chemotherapy is its dubious effectiveness. In some series where so-called prophylactic chemotherapy has been reported, the incidence of chemotherapy for subsequent lesions has been higher than in the series in the UK where prophylactic chemotherapy was not employed (Curry *et al.*, 1975). Methotrexate alone does not appear to be adequate to eradicate all the tumours which can arise after mole and the toxicity and depilatory effect of actinomycin-D and other agents are a deterrent to prophylactic use.

Indication for treatment after term delivery or non-mole abortion

When there is no history of hydatidiform mole and the previous pregnancy was a term delivery or non-mole abortion, evidence of persisting trophoblastic activity must be assumed to be due to choriocarcinoma until proved otherwise. All such patients require full investigation and treatment.

Investigatory procedures in patients with trophoblastic tumours

In addition to frequent and regular measurements of HCG concentration in serum or urine it is appropriate to carry out the usual tumour localization procedures. Choriocarcinoma produces identifiable metastases in lymph nodes in less than 1% of all cases and bone marrow metastases have not been identified at all in this series. Spread is essentially by haematogenous route and chest radiograph is the principal means of detecting metastatic spread. Pulmonary tomography and CT-scan will however reveal metastases not evident on plain chest X-ray but are not an essential routine. Pelvic arteriography can be used to reveal the dramatic vascular changes which occur in the pelvis of these patients and to demonstrate the remarkable arterial venous connections between the main tumour mass and vaginal metastases when these are present. However, in the absence of vaginal metastases arteriography provides little in the way of clinical information above that provided by HCG and general clinical examination. Arteriographic examination of the kidneys and liver is appropriate when metastases are present in these organs and again the highly vascular nature of the lesions is shown. Arteriographic examination of the brain and suspected brain metastases may reveal lesions but is less reliable for this purpose than CT-scan and serum CSF values for HCG. Unexplained anaemia calls for investigation of the gastrointestinal tract as a source of blood loss. Barium and arteriographic studies, however, have not proved useful in our experience since the lesions are generally small but tend to be multiple and unsuitable for surgical resection.

Staging and prognostic factors

The purpose of staging patients with malignant disease is to provide criteria for comparability between different patients and to provide a basis for the matching of therapeutic methods to the patient's requirements. In the case of gestational trophoblastic tumours the TNM classification provides inadequate information in comparison with alternative methods. The alternative method here is to apply a scoring system which is based on factors known to influence prognosis. The prognostic factors which have been found most useful in this respect are listed in Table 29.1 and the evidence for this prognostic scoring system has been presented elsewhere (Bagshawe, 1976). In brief, the overall prognosis of patients was better if the antecedent pregnancy were mole rather than term birth or non-mole abortion. It was better if HCG values were low, indicating a small total body burden of cells and was better if the tumours were young rather than old as measured by the interval between the end of the antecedent pregnancy and the start of chemotherapy. It was better for patients whose husbands were group B or AB and worse for patients whose own blood group was B or AB. The prognosis was also affected to some extent by a marked mononuclear cell infiltrate where histological examination was performed and small masses were more amenable to treatment than large masses. Metas-

tatic site also plays a part and metastases in the brain or liver tend to be unfavourable.

These prognostic factors appear to operate collectively. Thus it has proved possible to get a good guide to the overall prognosis by simple arithmetic summation of numerical values given to each of the prognostic factors.

Prognosis in this context in effect means the risk or potential to develop drug resistance. The difficulty of overcoming resistance to methotrexate and actinomycin-D with other agents has been described (Lewis, 1976). The story of the treatment of gestational choriocarcinoma is therefore one of attempting to avoid or overcome the development of drug resistance.

Historical development of chemotherapy for trophoblastic tumours

The early studies in the mid 1960s showed that many trophoblastic tumours were highly sensitive to methotrexate but it became clear, even at that time, that resistance to methotrexate frequently occurred. To overcome or avoid the development of such resistance drug combinations were used in this series from an early stage and the combination used between 1957 and 1964 was methotrexate with 6-mercaptopurine (Bagshawe and McDonald, 1960). This reduced the

Table 29.1 Prognostic score in choriocarcinoma.

	0	10	20	40
Age (years)	< 39	> 39		
Parity	1, 2, > 4	3 or 4		
Antecedent pregnancy	Mole	Abortion	Term	
Interval (AP-chemotherapy in months)	< 4	4–7	7–12	> 12
HGC (plasma mIU/ml or urine IU/day)	10^3–10^4	< 10^3	10^4–10^5	> 10^5
ABO *female* × *male*	A × A × B × AB	O × O A × O	B × AB ×	
No. of metastases	Nil	1–4	4–8	> 8
Site of metastases	Not detected Lungs Vagina	Spleen Kidney	GI tract Liver	Brain
Largest tumour mass	< 3 cm	3–5	> 5 cm	
Lymphocytic infiltration	Marked	Moderate Unknown	Slight	
Immune status	Reactive		Unreactive	
Previous chemotherapy	Nil		Yes	

Total score   Low < 55   Medium 55–60   High > 100

incidence of drug resistance but was relatively toxic and the safety margin was low. By 1962 it was evident that it was appropriate to use chemotherapy for some early post-mole cases and it seemed inappropriate that they should be submitted to the severe toxicity incurred with the chemotherapeutic methods then in use. For this reason methotrexate/folinic acid combinations were introduced, at first using intra-arterial infusion (Bagshawe and Wilde, 1964) or intravenous infusion and later combinations of intramuscular methotrexate with oral or intramuscular folinic acid (Bagshawe, 1969). These relatively non-toxic regimens proved highly satisfactory for the majority of early post-mole cases and a marked cytoreductive effect was obtained even in most cases of metastatic choriocarcinoma.

The general pattern in the 1960s therefore was to treat all patients with a non-toxic drug regimen and provided they went into remission no further treatment was required. Actinomycin-D was found to be an effective agent (Hertz, 1967) and those who showed resistance then went on to other drugs or drug combinations including actinomycin-D, vincristine, cyclophosphamide and other agents. It was also found at this time that 6-azauridine used in conjunction with methotrexate and folinic acid had an augmentation effect but occasional cerebral complications have led to its eventual withdrawal. By 1970 the pattern of prognosis and risk was beginning to emerge clearly and it appeared advantageous to distinguish between low and high risk patients and later it became advantageous to distinguish between low, medium and high risk patients. It had also become apparent that it was disadvantageous to allow drug resistance to develop and that where the probability of drug resistance to single agents could be predicted then it might be better to institute multidrug therapy from the outset.

Stratification

On the basis of the scoring system described above, patients in this series are defined as in the low risk, middle risk and high risk categories according to whether their prognostic scores are below 55, between 55 and 100 and in excess of 100 respectively. Up to 1973 there had been no deaths in the group with scores less than 55 on admission and there had been no survivors in the group with scores in excess of 180. By recognizing the different risk categories, however, and identifying the very high risk patients at the outset, some patients with very bad prognostic factors with scores in excess of 220 have gone into remission and the remission has so far been sustained.

Thus the 'low risk' patients are treated with the relatively non-toxic regimen (Regimen 1, Table 29.2), which causes little or no stomatitis, no significant hair loss and no detectable nephrotoxicity. 'Middle risk' patients cycle through a series of courses (Regimen, 2, 3, 4 and 5) and these patients suffer various degrees of toxicity which generally includes moderate to severe alopecia. Patients in the 'high risk' category are treated with a complex multidrug regimen (Regimen 6) from the outset and these patients suffer mild to moderate toxicity and alopecia but even so are generally able to return home between courses of therapy. Regimen 6 may be alternated with Regimen 5. Multidrug combinations may succeed where the middle-risk regimen has failed (Fig. 29.1). The chamoca regimen used in this case has now been largely replaced by the less toxic MECA regimen (Regimen 6).

Resistance to a drug regimen is judged to have occurred when the HCG value, at the time of haematological recovery, is not lower than it was at the start of the preceding treatment and partial resistance when the net fall in HCG during this period is less than half. If drug resistance develops in a patient receiving treatment in the 'low risk' category she is then treated with the regimen used in the 'middle risk' group. Similarly, a patient in the middle risk group who develops resistance receives the regimen otherwise used in only the 'high risk' category. The overall objective, however, is to try to select out those patients in whom the risk of resistance is high and to avoid the situation where resistance is seen to emerge. Although toxicity is frequently incurred there is nothing to suggest from the study of choriocarcinoma that toxicity is essential to achieve a cure or that toxicity is in any way proof of effectiveness of a regimen.

Timing of courses

In much cancer chemotherapy where palliation is the objective it is accepted that a single course of treatment at an interval of 3 to 4 weeks is close to the limits of acceptability. In the case of choriocarcinoma intervals of this duration often allow the tumour to recover to its pre-treatment size. It is therefore imperative that the interval between successive courses of treatment be kept to a minimum consistent with safety. With the low risk methotrexate/folinic acid regimen the interval between successive courses can be safely kept to 7 days provided there is no intercurrent infection.

With the middle risk regimen the treatment-free interval has to be adjusted according to haemopoietic and mucosal recovery but is generally of the order of 7 to 9 days. With the MECA regimen used in the high risk protocols the interval between successive courses is generally 7 days.

Table 29.2   Treatment schedules

Regimen 1   (MTX/FA)

MTX 1.0 mg/kg every 48 hours × 4 i.m. or 50 mg
every 48 hours × 4
FA 6 mg 30 hours after each injection of MTX i.m. or
p.o.

Regimen 2   (HU[a], MTX/FA 6-MP[a])

Days 1 and 2
   HU 0.5 g every 12 hours p.o. × 4
Days 3–10
   12 hours after last dose of HU start Regimen 1 as
   above and give 6-MP 1 mg/kg × 3 daily on FA
   days only.

Regimen 3   (VC[a] CY[a])

VC 1 mg/m² on Days 1 and 3 CY 400 mg/m² i.v. on
Days 1 and 3. The regimen can be repeated on Day 5
but myelosuppression is more marked.

Regimen 4   (AD)

AD 0.5 mg (or 10 μg/kg) i.v. daily for 5 days.

Regimen 5   (VP16-213)

VP16-213 100 mg/m², by i.v. infusion in 200 ml N
saline during 30 min, daily for 5 days.

Regimen 6   'MECA'

Day 1	VP 16213 100 mg/m² in 200 ml N. saline by 30 min i.v. infusion.
	AD 0.5 mg i.v. stat.
	MTX 100 mg/m² i.v. stat.
	MTX 200 mg/m² by 12 hour i.v. infusion.
Day 2	VP 16213 100 mg/m² as Day 1.
	AD 0.5 mg i.v. stat.
	FA 15 mg every 12 hours, × 4 starting 24 hours after start of MTX.
Day 8	VC 1 mg/m² i.v. start.
	CY 600 mg/m² by 30 min. i.v. infusion.
Day 15	Repeat cycle as from Day 1.

Regimen 7   (VC, MTX/FA, Cis-plat.)

Day 1	VC 1 mg/m² i.v. starting 5 hours later MTX 300 mg/m² is given by i.v. infusion in 500 ml N saline during 12 hours.
Day 2	FA 18 mg i.m. or p.o. 24, 48 and 72 hours after start of MTX infusion.
Day 3	1 l N saline + 1 l 5% dextrose overnight.
Day 4	Cis-plat. (NSC–119875) 120 mg/m² i.v. with mannitol 12.5 g i.v. then mannitol 10 g hourly × 6, with hourly infusions of 1 l N saline (× 1 g KCl), alternating with 5% dextrose (× 1 g KCl). Fluid and weight monitored.

Regimen 8   High dose MTX-FA.

---

* Check that WBC > 2 × 10⁹/l and platelets > 80 × 10⁹/l before
giving. It may also be justifiable to proceed with lower counts in some
circumstances.

Abbreviations: Cis-plat, Cis-dichlorodiammine platinum;
HU, hydroxyurea; 6-MP, 6-mercaptopurine; VC, vincristine;
CY, cyclophosphamide; MTX, methotrexate; FA, folinic acid;
AD, actinomycin D;
VP16-213, epipodophyllotoxin; N, normal; KCl, potassium chloride;
WBC, white blood cells; i.m., intramuscular; i.v., intravenous; p.o., oral

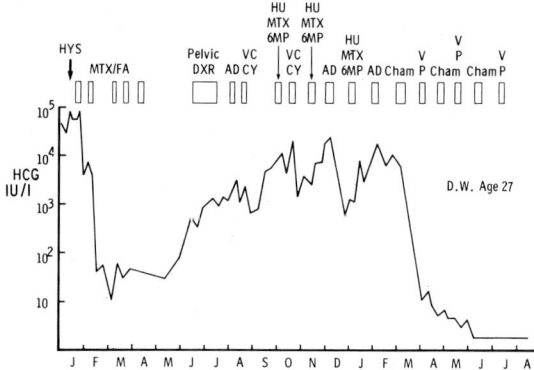

Fig. 29.1   The HGC values for this patient illustrate a
number of important points. This 'high-risk' patient was treated elsewhere initially with the 'low-risk' methotrexate/
folinic acid regimen. There was a good response during the
months Jan. to Feb. but later resistance was apparent.
Radiotherapy (DXR) to the pelvis failed to affect the rising
HCG levels and reduced haemopoietic reserves. Subsequent
treatment with hydroxyurea (HU), methotrexate (MTX),
6-mercaptopurine (6-MP), actinomycin-D (AD), vincristine
(VC) and cyclophosphamide (CY) also failed to control the
tumour. On admission to Charing Cross Hospital she had
multiple pulmonary metastases. The same agents used in the
multiple-drug regimen CHAMOCA were however effective
one year after the start of chemotherapy (HYS = hysterectomy, VP = VP16213).

Treatment is continued after HCG values have become undetectable for varying periods of time, depending on the patient's prognostic score and on the rate of response to treatment. In general patients in the low risk category have two to three courses of treatment after HCG values have become undetectable. Patients in the middle risk category need to continue treatment for approximately eight to ten weeks after HCG values have become undetectable. Patients in the high risk category need to continue treatment, whenever possible, for at least three months after values have become undetectable. Even so occasional relapses will occur but should not amount to more than 5% of the total number of cases treated and reinduction of remission can be expected but reinduction must then be associated with still more prolonged treatment.

Patients with pulmonary metastases should also receive treatment directed at preventing the occurrence of brain metastases. The methotrexate component of Regimen 6 incorporates a moderately high dose but this probably does not result in effective concentrations of methotrexate throughout the central nervous system. However, it has been found that by combining this with intrathecal methotrexate 12.5 mg, given with each course of treatment, brain metastases appear to be effectively prevented from development. As an alternative to this, high dose methotrexate 1–3 g/m² has recently been introduced for evaluation in this department but it is not yet clear whether it is advantageous in comparison with the standard high dose regimen plus intrathecal methotrexate. It is a question of balancing the risk and trauma of intrathecal methotrexate with that of the renal risks of high dose methotrexate. High dose methotrexate is also very expensive and by itself was not found to be an effective method of overcoming drug resistance in systemic choriocarcinoma.

Two new useful drugs have been introduced in recent years. These are VP 16–213, an epipodophyllin derivative (Regimen 5) and given either by itself or in combination with other has proved to be a useful addition, overcoming resistance in some cases. The second agent is cisdiamminoplatinum and although this has not proved highly effective in resistant choriocarcinoma by itself, in conjunction with vincristine and methotrexate useful effects have been obtained in a small number of patients who had proved resistant to all other drug combinations used (Regimen 7).

Patients with brain metastases

In general patients with brain metastases come into the high risk category and are treated with the MECA regimen, which incorporates a moderately high dose of methotrexate. As indicated above for the prevention of brain metastases in patients with pulmonary lesions, it is necessary to combine this regimen whenever possible with intrathecal methotrexate. This, however, is not possible in the case of patients who have raised intracranial pressure, at least not in the early stage of treatment. In these situations it is therefore necessary to obtain effective concentrations of methotrexate in the central nervous system by using a high dose of methotrexate followed by folinic acid.

Patients with brain metastases present on admission have responded well to treatment. That is to say the lesions have not only regressed completely but there has been remarkable recovery of even extensive neurological deficits in the majority of cases. A few patients have however been left with homonymous field defects and residual pareses. Brain metastases from choriocarcinoma must therefore be regarded as lesions which are potentially reversible through haemorrhage into them remains a serious initial hazard.

Patients who have no evidence of brain metastases on admission but who develop brain metastases during the course of treatment have however, fared badly. It is for this reason that prophylactic anti-CNS therapy has been introduced. In contrast with the situation of acute lymphoblastic leukaemia the risk of developing brain metastases remains until complete eradication of systemic disease has been achieved. It does not appear to be possible to prevent the development of intra-CNS choriocarcinoma for instance by giving a single course of radiotherapy. Moreover radiotherapy has not in our hands added significantly to the results obtained by chemotherapy. In general the prevention of development of CNS metastases during the course of chemotherapy for systemic disease is one of the most important developments in the management of this tumour in recent years.

Further reading

Bagshawe, K.D. (1969), *Choriocarcinoma: The Clinical Biology of the Trophoblast and its Tumours*. Edward Arnold, London.

Holland, J.F. and Hreschchshyn, M.M. (eds) (1967), *Choriocarcinoma: Transactions of a Conference of the International Union against cancer*. Springer-Verlag, Berlin.

Park, W.W. (1971), *Choriocarcinoma: a study of its Pathology*. Heinemann, London.

References

Bagshawe, K.D. and McDonald, Janetta M. (1960), Treatment of choriocarcinoma with a combination of cytotoxic drugs. *Br. Med. J.*, **ii**, 426–31.

Bagshawe, K.D. and Wilde, C.E. (1964), Infusion therapy for pelvic trophoblastic tumours. *J. Obstet. Gynaec. Br. Commonw.*, **LXXI**, 565–70.

Bagshawe, K.D. (1969), *Choriocarcinoma: The Clinical Biology of the Trophoblast and its Tumours*. Edward Arnold, London.

Bagshawe, K.D. *et al.* (1973), Follow-up after hydatidiform mole: studies using radioimmunoassay for urinary human chorionic gonadotrophins. *J. Obstet. Gynaec. Br. Commonw.*, **80**, 461–8.

Bagshawe, K.D. (1976), Risk and prognostic factors in trophoblastic neoplasia. *Cancer*, **38**, 1373–85.

Bagshawe, K.D. and Harland, S. (1976), Immunodiagnosis and monitoring of gonadotrophin producing metastases in the central nervous system. *Cancer*, **38**, 112–8.

Curry, S.L. *et al.* (1975), Hydatidiform mole: diagnosis, management and long-term follow-up of 347 patients. *Obstet. Gynec.*, **45**, 1–8.

Hertz, R. (1967), Eight years experience with the chemotherapy of choriocarcinoma and related trophoblastic tumours in women. In: *Choriocarcinoma: Transactions of a Conference of the International Union Against Cancer*. (eds J.F. Holland and M.M. Hreschchshyn) Springer-Verlag, Berlin,

Kardana, A. and Bagshawe, K.D. (1976), A rapid, sensitive and specific radioimmunoassay for human chorionic gonadotrophin. *J. Immunol. Meth.*, **9**, 297–307.

Lewis, J.L. (1976), Current status of treatment of gestational trophoblastic disease. *Cancer*, **38**, 620–6.

Ober, W.B., Edgcomb, J.H. and Price, E.B. (1971), The pathology of choriocarcinoma. *Ann. N.Y. Acad. Sci.*, **172**, 299–426.

Park, W.W. (1971), *Choriocarcinoma: a Study of its Pathology*. Heinemann, London.

Stone, M. and Bagshawe, K.D. (1979), An analysis of the influence of maternal age, gestational age, contraceptive method, and the mode of primary treatment of patients with hydatidiform moles on the incidence of subsequent chemotherapy. *Br. J. Obstet. Gynaec.*, **86**, 782–92.

Wilde, C.E., Orr, A.H. and Bagshawe, K.D. (1967), A sensitive radioimmunoassay for human chorionic gonadotrophin and luteinising hormone. *J. Endocr.*, **27**, 23–35.

30 Skin (including anus and penis)

Margaret F. Spittle
and R.C.G. Russell

Skin cancer is frequently dismissed as an unimportant topic, yet the highest incidence of cancer involving any site occurs in the skin. Collectively, the tumours of the skin are unique in that some are very easy to treat while others are among the most complicated to diagnose, treat and otherwise manage. Although cancers of the skin generally are more amenable to therapeutic measures, accurate differential diagnosis presents many problems, making cooperation with a pathologist, preferably a dermatopathologist, more necessary than is the case for most other types of cancer. Education of the public in the early signs of skin cancer has a greater potential for cure, than for any other cancer.

Aetiology

In the majority of patients who develop skin cancer in Great Britain an aetiological factor can be implicated in the development of that cancer; in many instances the aetiology is multifactorial. Such cancers develop more commonly in the Scottish, Irish and Welsh peoples – those of Celtic extraction – rather than in Anglo-Saxons. It is considered that this is due to a relative lack of pigmentation and thus increased sensitivity to the carcinogenic effects of ultraviolet light. There is an increased incidence of skin cancer in patients who were fair-haired or auburn in their youth. Nevertheless lesions are seen even in people of Mediterranean extraction. The Albino has a high incidence of both basal cell epitheliomas and squamous carcinomas in exposed skin sites. Long-term sun exposure is therefore an important aetiological factor. It is considered that the most potent wavelengths of ultraviolet light are those found in the mid-range (approximately 290–320 nm), and their potency for carcinogenesis is proportional to their potency for erythema production. Thus, many of those who suffer with skin cancer have a history of war service in a hot climate, or are outdoor workers such as farmers. Because of the slow growth of these tumours there is invariably a long latent period.

Since the late 19th century the importance of carcinogens in the development of skin tumours has been recognized. Coal tar, creosote, mineral oils and crude paraffin are skin carcinogens, the lesions being manifest after a long latent period. Chronic arsenical poisoning may also result in the development of skin tumours. Arsenic was commonly given for diseases such as petit mal and psoriasis; such patients, and others exposed to arsenicals, may present many years later with multiple hyperkeratoses, with the subsequent development of skin tumours. These tumours may develop not only in the sun-exposed areas of the body but also on the trunk, between the toes and at other uncommon sites. There is a high incidence of coexistent carcinomas; thus arsenic-exposed patients should be fully investigated in order to exclude tumours of internal organs.

X-rays have been known to be carcinogenic since shortly after they were discovered, and an interesting group of patients are those who present with basal cell epitheliomas on the face and scalp, having in the past had epilation for ringworm infection (*micro-sporum ouadini*, (Epstein *et al.*, 1969). This endothrix fungus infection affects the hair follicles and was resistant to all forms of treatment prior to the manufacture of griseofulvin. The Kienbock-Adamson technique of epilation, which was used for some years prior to 1956, aimed to give the whole hair-bearing scalp a single dose of approximately 500 rad at 50–70 kV. A five-field technique was used with the result that there were occasional areas of high dose due to overlapping fields or erroneous calibration. In general, the technique was successful, causing total alopecia with cure of the ringworm infection and complete hair regrowth in most subjects. After a long latent period of thirty to sixty years some subjects present with basal cell epitheliomas within the hair-bearing scalp. In addition, there is also an increased incidence in these patients of basal cell epitheliomas on the face as in many instances shielding from scattered irradiation was inadequate. Occasionally, there is evidence of late radiation sequelae on these patients' scalps, with the hair sparser and finer than would be expected. Where there are areas of frank radiation damage, with permanent alopecia, tethering of the skin to the scalp, telangiectasia or pigmentation, basal cell epitheliomas are rare but in the adjacent zones which received a lower dose of irradiation, epitheliomas can be frequently found (Albert and Omran, 1968). The particular interest of these radiation-induced tumours lies in the fact that they have the longest latent period for carcinogenesis, and may occur in the total absence of any stigma of radiation damage. When these tumours arise in apparently normal skin with no evidence of late radiation change, they can be treated by radiation without unusual reactions. Other tumours have been described to occur in the scalp of these patients (Fig. 30.1), and some series have shown an increased incidence of carcinomas and sarcomas at other sites, particularly in the head and neck region (Modan *et al.*, 1974).

Anatomy

The epidermis is an avascular cellular structure that varies in thickness from 0.66 mm to 0.8 mm. The border between the epidermis and the dermis is irregular due to the indentation of the epidermis by cone-shaped dermal papillae. The ridges of epidermis between the papillae are known as the rete pegs. The epidermis is divided into four layers of cells: 1. the basal cells; 2. prickle layer or stratum malpighii; 3. granular layer or stratum granulosum and 4. the horny layer of keratin or stratum corneum. The cells in the various layers represent different stages in the gradual evolution and maturation of the basal cells. In the basal layer, there are basal cells and melanocytes. It is from this layer that basal cell cancer develops. Melanocytes are of neural origin and are wedged between the basal cells. Squamous cell carcinoma arises from the prickle layer. Under normal conditions, it takes approximately 26–28 days for an epithelial cell to migrate from the basal layer to the surface. Mitoses occur in the basal and prickle layers. The mitotic index, the number of dividing cells per 1000 cells, varies from two to eight or higher, depending upon the number of desquamated cells, since the thickness of the epidermis remains quite constant. Mitotic activity is greatest during rest and sleep; it is reduced during activity, in a cool environment, and during stress and starvation. Methotrexate

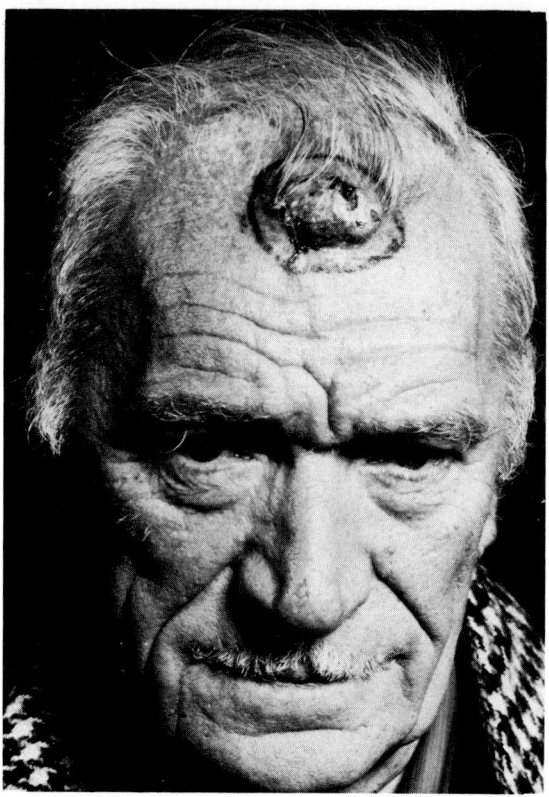

Fig. 30.1   Basal cell carcinoma arising on the hair-bearing scalp of a man irradiated 45 years previously for ringworm.

and other anti-cancer drugs depress division of cells in the skin.

The dermis constitutes the bulk of the skin; it is composed of three types of fibre: collagen, elastic and reticulum; blood vessels, lymphatics and nerves are present. Few cancers arise in the dermis, but their variety is great.

Pathology and histological classification

The approach to the classification of skin tumours must be essentially histological, but relevant clinical information is utilized to categorize further certain entities. Part of this problem arises from the fact that it is difficult to decide whether a skin lesion is a true neoplasm or a pseudotumour (Sanderson, 1972). Included in this category are the hamartomas and processes in which there is a more or less exuberant growth of tissue. Some tumours, such as basal cell carcinomas, are relatively benign and terms other than carcinoma have been introduced to express their relative benign course. Contrariwise, dermatofibrosarcoma protuberans is not as malignant as the name implies, but because of a disposition to recurrence it is regarded as a malignant tumour. The classification listed below follows closely the classification published by the World Health Organization.

I. *Epithelial tumours and tumour-like lesions*

A   Basal cell carcinoma
     1. Variants of basal cell carcinoma
       (a) superficial multicentric type
       (b) morphoea type
       (c) fibroepithelial type
       (d) naevoid basal cell carcinoma syndrome
B   Squamous cell carcinoma
     1. Variants of squamous cell carcinoma
       (a) adenoid squamous cell carcinoma
       (b) spindle cell squamous carcinoma
C   Metatypical carcinoma
D   Adnexal carcinoma
E   Tumours and related lesions of sweat gland
     1. Benign, for example papillary syringadenoma, papillary hidradenoma etc.
     2. Malignant (sweat gland carcinoma)
F   Tumours and tumour-like lesions of sebaceous gland
     1. Benign
       (a) sebaceous adenoma
     2. Malignant
       (a) carcinoma of sebaceous glands
     3. Tumour-like lesions
       (a) naevus sebaceus of Jadassohn
       (b) adenoma sebaceum (Pringle)
       (c) steatocystoma multiplex
       (d) hyperplasia of sebaceous glands
       (e) rhinophyma
G   Tumours and tumour-like lesions of hair follicle
     1. Trichoepithelioma
     2. Trichofolliculoma
     3. Trichilemmoma
     4. Pilomatrixoma (calcifying epithelioma of Malherbe)
     5. Inverted follicular keratosis
H   Undifferentiated carcinoma
I   Cysts
     For example, keratinous cysts, dermoid cysts and bronchogenic cysts
J   Tumour-like lesions
     1. Keratoacanthoma
     2. Seborrhoeic keratosis
     3. Benign squamous keratosis (keratotic papilloma)
     4. Virus lesions

     5. Hamartomas
     6. Others
K   Unclassified

II. *Pre-cancerous lesions and conditions*

A.   Actinic keratosis (solar, senile keratosis)
B.   Radiation dermatosis
C.   Bowen's disease
D.   Erythroplasia of Queyrat
E.   Intraepidermal epithelioma of Jadassohn
F.   Arsenical dermatosis
G.   Paget's disease
     1. Mammary
     2. Extramammary
H.   Xeroderma pigmentosum
I.   Others

III. *Tumours and lesions of the melanogenic system*

A.   Benign (naevus)
     1. Junctional naevus
     2. Compound naevus
     3. Intradermal naevus.
     4. Epithelioid and/or spindle cell naevus (juvenile melanoma)
     5. Balloon cell naevus
     6. Halo naevus
     7. Giant pigmented naevus
     8. Fibrous papule of nose (involuting naevus)
     9. Blue naevus
     10. Cellular blue naevus
B.   Pre-cancerous
C.   Malignant
D.   Non-tumourous pigmented lesions

IV. *Tumours and tumour-like lesions of soft tissue*

A.   Tumours of fibrous tissue
     1. Benign
       (a) fibroma
       (b) dermatofibroma (histiocytoma, sclerosing haemangioma)
       (c) recurring digital fibroma
       (d) fibrous hamartoma of infancy
       (e) connective tissue naevus
     2. Malignant
       (a) dermatofibrosarcoma protuberans
       (b) fibrosarcoma
     3. Tumour-like lesions
       (a) cutaneous fibrous polyp (skin tag, acrochordon)
       (b) hyperplastic scar

(c) keloid
(d) nodular fasciitis
(e) fibromatosis
B.   Tumours of fat tissue
C.   Tumours of muscle
D.   Tumours of blood vessels
  1. Benign
  2. Malignant
E.   Tumours of lymph vessels
  1. Benign
    (a) lymphangioma
      (i) capillary lymphagioma
      (ii) cavernous lymphangioma
      (iii) cystic lymphangioma (hygroma)
  2. Malignant
    (a) lymphangiosarcoma (malignant lymphangioendothelioma)
    (b) postmastectomy lymphangiosarcoma
F.   Tumours of peripheral nerves
  1. Benign, e.g. neurofibroma
  2. Malignant, e.g. malignant schwannoma
  3. Tumour-like lesions, e.g. traumatic neuroma
G.   Tumour-like xanthomatous lesions
H.   Miscellaneous tumours
    e.g. Granular cell tumour

V. Tumours and tumour-like conditions of the haematopoietic and lymphoid tissues

A.   Mycosis fungoides
B.   Sezary disease
C.   Hodgkin's disease
D.   Lymphomas
E.   Leukaemias
F.   Reactive lymphoid hyperplasia
G.   Benign lymphocytoma cutis
H.   Benign lymphocytic infiltrate of Jessner
I.   Lymphomatoid papulosis
J.   Pathogenic granuloma (Wegener's granuloma)
K.   Histiocytosis X
L.   Urticaria pigmentosa (Mastocytoma)

VI. Metastatic tumours

VII. Unclassified tumours

Clinical recognition

Skin neoplasms do not have a standard appearance, and the variation in presentation is such that biopsy is the only accurate diagnostic method – even then difficulties can and do arise. It is now standard practice to submit all skin tumours to biopsy before a planned approach to treatment is considered, unless the lesion is so small that simple excision biopsy will satisfactorily treat and at the same time provide a diagnosis. Of great importance in the management of skin tumours is the state of the surrounding skin, and evidence of actinic or radiation damage should be sought as well as other factors which may predispose to cancer.

Selected pre-cancerous skin and mucocutaneous lesions

Some skin and mucocutaneous disorders exhibit a natural history for the development of carcinoma often enough to be classified as pre-cancerous disease. These conditions frequently occur in patients with skin cancer, and thus merit consideration in their own right. These diseases initially show microscopic features of carcinoma in-situ (Freitaig and Culmane, 1976).

Solar keratosis
Senile or actinic keratosis is the most common precancerous cutaneous disease; the lesions develop in sun-exposed areas of aging skin, which is dry, wrinkled, atrophic and sometimes pigmented. The lesions are round to irregular in shape, scaly, keratotic, usually flat and vary from grey to brown in colour. Without treatment, 12% of patients with solar keratosis develop a squamous cell carcinoma, but metastases are rare. The invasive lesions appear as keratotic papules, nodules or plaques with crusting, ulceration and elevated pearly margins. There is disruption of the dermoepidermal basement membrane and atypical squamous keratinocytes extend into the corium with squamous pearl formation. The prognosis is excellent, the neoplasm being non-aggressive and should be classified as a separate entity, distinct from malignant squamous cell skin and mucocutaneous tumours which do metastasize. Solar keratosis with acantholysis represents the precursor lesion of adenoid squamous cell carcinoma, and this type of skin cancer also deserves separate classification because 3% of patients with nodules 2 cm or greater in size exhibit evidence of metastases.

Bowen's disease
This condition involves predominantly Caucasians living in sun-exposed areas, and occurs in both sexes. Chronic arsenical administration is a well documented predisposing factor. The lesions occur equally on exposed and covered areas. Typical lesions appear as plaques which are round to irregular, lenticular, polycyclic, erythematous, pigmented, scaly, keratotic, fissured, crusty, nodular and eroded. The plaques are free of hair, and usually appear sharply demarcated from the surrounding skin. Treatment of Bowen's disease is necessary because at least 5% of patients with this disease show clinical and microscopic evidence of

an invasive carcinoma occurring in larger lesions. In 2% of all patients with Bowen's disease, there is evidence of metastases to internal structures, but this occurs only after *in-situ* atypical epithelial cells disrupt the dermoepidermal basement membrane and invade the underlying stroma as a carcinoma. Once invasive carcinoma develops, at least one third of patients with this type of disease develop metastases unless early and adequate treatment is given. Between five and ten years after the onset of Bowen's disease, at least 40% of patients develop other skin and mucocutaneous pre-malignant and malignant lesions. Early adequate treatment of Bowen's lesions has no preventative effect on the subsequent development of systemic pre-malignant and malignant lesions. At least 5% of patients with Bowen's disease have occult internal cancer.

Extramammary Paget's disease

This disease occurs in both sexes, but is more common in the female; it affects the anogenital area, axillae, umbilicus, external ear canal and orbital skin. At least 20% of patients show multiple lesions. The lesions appear erythematous to whitish grey, elevated, crusted, eczematoid, eroded and occasionally papillary. More than 50% of patients complain of itching and some experience pain and/or bleeding. In at least 40% of patients, a cutaneous adnexal carcinoma arising from apocrine structures is present immediately subjacent to the Paget's lesion. Approximately 40% of patients with extramammary Paget's disease have their lesions in the perianal skin, and three quarters of these show an associated subjacent adnexal carcinoma, breast carcinoma or adenocarcinoma of the rectum. In patients with extramammary Paget's disease of other areas, only 40% show an associated carcinoma. The prognosis of the condition is related to the presence or absence of a subjacent carcinoma and its stage. Before or at the time of death, 95% of the patients with extramammary Paget's disease have some type of cancer.

Intraepidermal epithelioma of Jadassohn

This lesion occurs as a single grey to brown, keratotic, scaly, flat and irregularly shaped plaque, sharply demarcated from normal skin. Occasionally, the lesions appear papillary and show areas of erosion and ulceration. The lesions occur on all parts of the body except the palms and the soles, with a predilection for the lower extremity. It is seen predominantly in Caucasians, and is seen more often in men than in women. Eight per cent of patients show clinical and microscopic evidence of invasive carcinoma in their primary lesions, while 5% of these patients with invasive carcinoma show evidence of metastases. Of

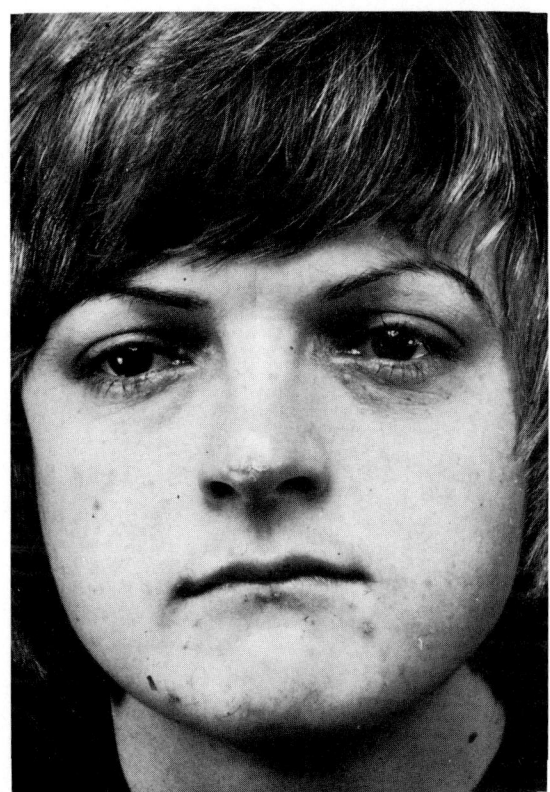

Fig. 30.2   Gorlin's syndrome. Note basal cell epithelioma on tip of nose.

patients with follow-up to their death, only one death was directly related to intraepidermal epithelioma of Jadassohn with carcinoma and metastases.

Related conditions

Gorlin's syndrome (multiple naevoid basal cell carcinoma syndrome)

This rare syndrome (Fig. 30.2) is a predominantly inherited disease with many manifestations. The diagnostic triad consists of multiple basal cell lesions on the face, squamous lined cysts in the mandible, and other bony abnormalities, the commonest of which is bifid ribs (Fig. 30.3). Other features of the syndrome which occur less consistently are frontal bossing, hypertelorism, abnormal dentition, bridged pituitary fossa, falx calcification, palmar pits and ovarian tumours (Fig. 30.4). There is a high incidence of medulloblastoma in these patients or their offspring. The cutaneous manifestations of this disease are variable, ranging from

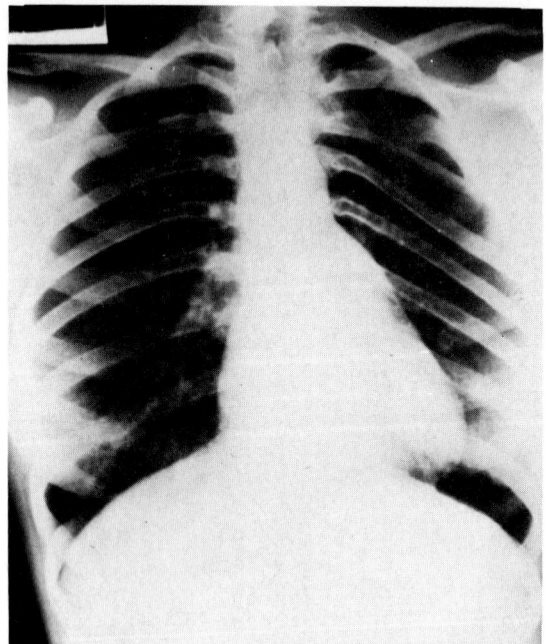

Fig. 30.3   Gorlin's syndrome – note bifid ribs.

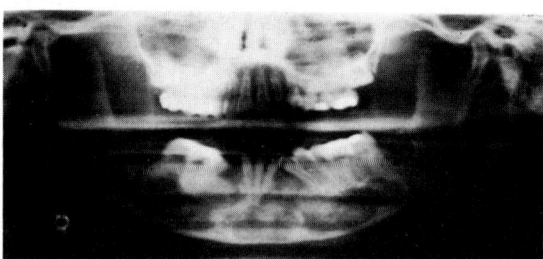

Fig. 30.4   Mandible of the same patient – note cysts and abnormal dentition.

multiple small lesions on the face, which may be regularly treated and kept under control, to widespread infiltrating nodular lesions, particularly on the face, down the centre of the back, and the perineum. Great care in detecting and treating early lesions in patients with Gorlin's syndrome may prevent the disfiguring and disastrous sequelae of widespread uncontrolled disease. Some patients with Gorlin's syndrome have an euphoric affect and attend poorly for follow-up.

Xeroderma pigmentosa
This is a rare genodermatosis with an increased sensitivity to sunlight causing multiple squamous and

basal cell carcinomas to develop in exposed areas (Cleaver, 1968). These lesions manifest themselves in the patient while in childhood. The basic defect is an inability to remove ultraviolet induced thymine dimers from DNA. Several distinct defects have been described, and these have been demonstrated in epidermal cells, fibroblasts, and circulating lymphocytes of patients with xeroderma pigmentosa. Like Gorlin's syndrome, these patients present a difficult treatment problem.

Other diseases in which a higher incidence of basal cell carcinomas can be found are epidermolysis bullosa and porphyria cutanea tarda.

Clinical classification

The UICC classification applies to histologically verified tumours of the skin, excluding malignant melanoma for which there is no standard classification. The classification is based on division into six regions. In defining the regional lymph nodes the body is divided horizontally at the level of the umbilicus. The regions and regional nodes are as follows:

Regions
(a) Eyelid, ear and nose
(b) Face, excluding (a),
    scalp and neck
(c) Upper limb
(d) Trunk above the umbilicus
(e) Trunk below the umbilicus
(f) Lower limb

Regional nodes
Cervical (bilateral)
Cervical (bilateral)
Axillary and epitrochlear
(unilateral)
Axillary (bilateral)
Inguinal (bilateral)
Inguinal and popliteal
(unilateral)

Multiple tumours

In the case of multiple simultaneous tumours, the tumour with the highest T category will be identified and the number of separate tumours will be indicated in parenthesis: e.g. (5) T_2. Successive tumours should be classified independently.

T – *Primary Tumour*
Tis   Pre-invasive carcinoma (carcinoma in-situ).
To   No evidence of primary tumour.

T_1 Tumour 2 cm or less in its largest dimension, strictly superficial or exophytic.

T_2 Tumour more than 2 cm but not more than 5 cm in its largest dimension or with minimal infiltration of the dermis, irrespective of size.

T_3 Tumour more than 5 cm in its largest dimension or with deep infiltration of the dermis, irrespective of size.

T_4 Tumour involving other structures such as cartilage, muscle or bone.

N – *Regional Lymph Nodes*
N_0 No palpable nodes
N_1 Movable homolateral nodes
N_{1a} Nodes not considered to contain growth
N_{1b} Nodes considered to contain growth
N_2 Movable contra-lateral or bilateral nodes
     N_{2a} Nodes not considered to contain growth
     N_{2b} Nodes considered to contain growth
N_3 Fixed nodes

M – *Distant Metastases*
M_0 No evidence of distant metastases
M_1 Distant metastases present including lymph nodes beyond the region in which the primary tumour is situated, or satellite nodules more than 5 cm from the border of the primary tumour.

Treatment for pre-cancerous skin lesions

The methods available for the management of these lesions include: 1. simple excision; 2. electrosurgery and curettage; 3. cryosurgery; 4. topical chemotherapy – the use of caustics such as trichloroacetic acid or cytotoxic agents (5-fluorouracil); 5. dermabrasion; 6. radiotherapy – the use of superficial X-rays and 7. immunotherapy – the use of delayed hypersensitivity reactions against epidermal tumours.

Actinic keratosis

Multiple methods of treatment may be utilized for eradicating these lesions. A single superficial lesion may be cured by cautery and curettage, cryotherapy or the application of trichloroacetic acid. If the lesion is nodular or infiltrated and carcinoma is suspected, surgical excision is preferable. For numerous superficial actinic keratoses, topical 5-fluorouracil (5-FU) is useful; a 5% concentration of 5-FU is applied for 2–3 weeks for lesions on the face while a longer period (4–6 weeks) is required for the hands or forearms. Dermabrasion although effective offers no distinct advantage.

Bowen's disease

Excision or cautery and curettage are standard methods of treatment, although simple excision is preferable as a better specimen for histology is obtained. Cryosurgery has been found to be effective, as has topical 5-FU in concentrations of 5% with and without occlusion; the 5-FU cream should be applied for 3 weeks. A steroid cream may reduce the inflammatory response. Superficial X-ray therapy has been used giving 500 rad twice weekly for 5 weeks. X-ray treatment is worthy of consideration when the disease is on the lower eyelid, the finger, the hand, or large lesions which would require extensive surgery, and for patients who are not fit for surgical treatment. Bowen's disease occurs occasionally on the lower leg which tolerates poorly both surgery and radiotherapy. The latter should be avoided particularly in the elderly.

Intraepidermal epithelioma of Jadassohn

This lesion should be excised in order to obtain an adequate histological examination; alternatively curettage and cautery can be used after biopsy (Mehregan and Pinkus, 1964). If the lesion is very extensive low voltage irradiation can be used.

Treatment of early squamous cell and basal cell carcinoma

Tumours in this category are those primary lesions without local or distant metastases, which are limited to the skin and sub-cutaneous tissues, and which may on occasion superficially infiltrate underlying muscle or cartilage. Many methods of treatment are used, but the three common methods are excision, radiation and curettage. It is important that experts in all modalities should be available for joint discussion of the appropriate treatment. Curettage with local application of various chemicals such as podophyllin, trichloroacetic acid or Millon's reagent (acid nitrate of mercury) have been used, but the chemical agents cause pain and inflammatory response. Mohs' chemosurgery has proved effective but the technique is too cumbersome and time consuming for routine use; however, its prime indication is the advanced cancer which has recurred after other methods have failed.

Topical 5-FU has produced cures but only in patients with very superficial disease. Tubercidin (7 DEAZA-adenosine 7) is said to be more effective. Probably, the only indication for topical chemotherapy is the presence of a large number of small tumours.

Based on limited studies, dermatocryosurgery has become established using either the cryoprobe or the more popular cryojet system (Braun *et al.*, 1976). A multiple freeze-thaw cycle is monitored by thermocouples placed deep in the tumour. Cryosurgery seems to be the method of choice for young people (in whom ionizing radiation is contra-indicated because of the long latent period available for possible carcinogenesis) who develop cancers in certain anatomic sites which are difficult to treat by excision or curettage.

For the vast majority of tumours the choice of treatment lies between excision, curettage and radiotherapy. To a large extent the decision rests on the doctor's preference, but the following factors should be considered. If the patient is young, the cancer arises in excessively sun-damaged skin or previously irradiated skin, the lesion is not localized on the head and neck, or there is evidence of chondritis, then radiotherapy should be avoided. However, radiotherapy is specifically indicated in patients who are unfit for surgery, or whose lesions are large, or the site of the lesion is such as would require complex reconstructive surgery, or for lesions extending into areas such as the paranasal fold, auriculotemporal sulcus, or around the readily protected eye, and for those lesions which have been inadequately excised (Moss *et al.*, 1973). For tumours not included in these strictures, cosmetic considerations and the convenience of the patient become of paramount importance.

Radiotherapy

Skin tumours have a very long doubling time relative to other tumours. Although there is a high rate of cell loss, and the labelling index is high, the normal skin also has a high mitotic index, and hence there is no radiobiological necessity for rapid fractionation. With increased fractionation better cosmetic results will be obtained, yet many patients will not attend regularly for what is to them a minor lesion, and thus a balance must be struck between the ideal and the practical. However, considerable flexibility in the treatment regimens can be chosen varying from a single dose technique in the elderly with a small lesion, to a multiple dose regimen in the younger patient with an obvious facial lesion. In planning the treatment schedule it should be borne in mind that, although 90% of lesions are cured by the first course of treatment, of those which do recur 50% will recur yet again. Recurrence is associated with particular histological patterns, and certain sites such as the nasolabial fold where a wider treatment margin is indicated. Thus all malignant skin tumours should have a full histological assessment before the treatment is planned.

The size of the tumour should be considered, larger lesions requiring a more fractionated treatment.

Moulds and afterloading techniques have been used for these large lesions, especially if overlying bone or cartilage. The electron beam has made treatment of these lesions safer and cosmetically more acceptable (Grosch and Lambert, 1979). Large lesions on the nose and ear which overlie cartilage may be readily treated with the electron beam without fear of necrosis because the radiation is not disproportionately absorbed in bone or cartilage (Tapley, 1975). When treating the nose a rim of normal nostril should, if possible, be left untreated, as this will prevent contraction and deformity. The result of electron beam treatment of the pinna may well be cosmetically superior to wedge resection.

For a small lesion typical dosage schedules of superficial X-rays are as follows: for the single dose in the elderly patient 2000–2250 rad at 50 kV–90 kV is appropriate; for the face a fractionated dose at 80–100 kV is suitable, while more superficial lesions may be treated with 60 kV, and exophytic or infiltrative disease will require 120 kV. Appropriate regimens for a 2 cm treatment volume are:

750 rad × 5 in 7 days
600 rad × 9 in 19 days
500 rad × 10 in 12 days

In an attempt to blur the edges of the radiotherapy field, the lesion may be treated by a different shaped cut-out daily. An applicator with a crenated edge or circle, square or diamond applicator may be alternated daily, thus avoiding the punched out areas seen after radiation. The usual fractionations all cause permanent hair loss, and it is important to warn patients of this sequela. Infection may supervene in the treated area, and to prevent this complication, topical antibiotic cream may be used while the radiation reaction subsides. The occasional use of a corticosteroid cream is also recommended.

Gorlin's syndrome

Treatment should always be directed towards discovering the lesions early and using the least invasive form of therapy. The basal cell carcinomas are frequently nodular and invasive when they occur and excision with histological clearance is the most appropriate form of therapy. Radiation should be avoided where possible in these patients except when the lesions are extensive or in sites difficult for surgery, such as on the nose or periorbital regions. The widespread nature of the disease means that new lesions will occur close to previously treated ones and this may make treatment by irradiation hazardous. Due to the nodular nature of the basal cell epitheliomas in these patients treatment such as topical 5-FU is rarely satisfactory. Intravenous cytotoxic chemotherapy, using regimens including bleomycin, which is said to normalize squamous epithelium, have been used, but with minimal success. The tumours are not sensitive to chemotherapy and seem to be in the more radioresistant spectrum of basal cell epitheliomas. It has been suggested that there is an increased tendency to scarring and these patients are therefore prone to disfiguring radiation reactions. However, this may be due to the fact that patients with Gorlin's syndrome have often had much radiation, occasionally with sub-optimal fractionation schedules.

Xeroderma pigmentosa

In this condition the main pillar of management is prevention of developing skin cancers by avoiding exposure to sunlight, and the extensive use of barrier creams and ultraviolet protective screens. Sunglasses and protective clothing should always be worn. Considerable time counselling these patients is well spent. The most conservative forms of treatment are also the most effective if the disease can be caught early, and radiation should only be used when the lesions have become extensive or involve sites not amenable to surgery. Chemotherapy, either topical or intravenous has been of little value in these patients.

Treatment of advanced carcinoma

Extensive carcinoma develops either due to delay in treatment or following previously unsuccessful treatment. It is in this area that cooperation between excisional surgeon, reconstructive surgeon and radiotherapist must be of primary consideration before treatment is started. Treatment for advanced lesions is wide surgical excision, with or without planned postoperative radiotherapy. The trend towards early surgical excision has arisen because of the problems of skin coverage which follow other forms of therapy. The vast majority of these extensive lesions occur in the head and neck, and it is proper that references should be made to units dealing with these rare problems. The surgical approach must be vigorous, persistent and should now allow reconstructive considerations to prevent a complete removal of affected tissues. Involvement of regional lymphatics makes a block dissection of lymphatic tissue mandatory. The surgical margin of the resected specimen should be examined by intraoperative frozen section in an attempt to ensure adequate removal. However, it should not be forgotten that tumour spreads beneath the skin in planes of muscle or of scar tissue, thus a wide margin of excision is necessary (2 cm on the face and 5 cm elsewhere). Reconstruction is initiated at the time of the ablative procedure. When the patient is elderly or unfit for

complex surgical procedures, supervoltage radiotherapy techniques give good palliation, and occasionally a cure. The treatment of this group of patients must be individualized, and in management the whole patient, including his psychological make-up, must be taken into account. The treatment plan must be flexible so that it can be altered according to the response of the tumour or the patient.

Malignant melanoma

Aetiology

Melanoma is increasing in its incidence in white races, not only in areas where melanoma is common, such as Queensland, Australia, but also in Norway, Britain, the United States and Canada. In Queensland it is estimated that the incidence of melanoma has quadrupled in the last 30 years and for the other countries it has probably doubled in the same period. Factors in the aetiology of melanoma include the relationship of the disease to skin naevi, to racial factors, to sunlight, to familial factors and to hormones.

Relationship to naevi
Nearly two thirds of patients state that their melanoma arose from a pre-existing pigmented lesion, in which there had been a recent change. Associated intradermal naevi can be demonstrated histologically in about one quarter of all melanomas. It is probable that a further third arise in junctional naevi, and the remainder arise *de novo*. It is estimated that one per 100 000 pigmented naevi become malignant, and the average person has between 10 and 16 naevi. However, the giant congenital naevi frequently become malignant.

Relationship to race
It is said that there is a higher incidence of melanoma in the fair skinned Celt. In Sweden and Norway the occurence of melanoma is more frequent than in England and Wales, where the incidence for the years 1962–1965 was 1.4 per 100 000 for men and 2.4 for women. Pigment protects, the incidence being lower in dark skinned races. However, the site incidences in dark skinned races are different, melanoma on the sole of the foot and mucosae being more common.

Relationship to sunlight
The mortality of melanoma increases with proximity to the equator. It is probable that sunlight has a general as well as local effect because melanoma even in those parts of the body not exposed to the sun is more common nearer the equator.

Familial relationship
There are certain families in which melanoma has

occurred more frequently than can be attributed to chance and in these families there is a greater incidence of multiple primaries. The mode of inheritance is not clear.

Hormonal aspects

In many published series there is a higher incidence of melanoma in women than in men, due to the larger number of lesions on the lower leg of women, but paradoxically the mortality rate is higher in men than in women; these differences continue past the menopause. It is now accepted that pregnancy does not induce melanoma and does not have an adverse effect on the survival of patients who have had a melanoma in the past.

Classification

In 1972 at the time of the UICC Cancer Congress in Sydney a number of pathologists devised the following classification (McGovern *et al.*, 1973):

1. Invasive malignant melanoma with an adjacent intraepidermal component of Hutchinson's melanotic freckle type.
2. Invasive malignant melanoma with an adjacent intraepidermal component of the superficial spreading type.
3. Invasive malignant melanoma with an adjacent intraepidermal component of unclassifiable type.
4. Invasive malignant melanoma without an adjacent intraepidermal component.

Histological appearance

Hutchinson's melanotic freckle

This lesion occurs most commonly in the malar region and often involves the lower eyelid. It is an irregular macular lesion varying in colour between brown and black. It often has paler areas which represent spontaneous regression. The lesion is impalpable. After 10–15 years and sometimes much longer one or more nodules, which may be amelanotic, of an invasive melanoma appear. Microscopically the melanocytes are large and round with irregular nuclei, and these atypical melanocytes extend down the outer root sheath of the hair follicle. Eventually small clusters form, and at this stage there is usually invasion of the dermis. It is very unusual for a melanoma arising in Hutchinson's freckle to give rise to metastases in women.

Melanoma with an adjacent intraepidermal component of superficial spreading type

This type of melanoma commences as a flat macular lesion and sooner or later a recognizable nodule appears representing invasion of the dermis. The lesions are black or dark brown in colour, with palpable and clearly defined margins. These lesions are up to 2 cm in size, although on rare occasions they may be more extensive. Melanoma of this type can occur on any part of the body, and is rarely surrounded by skin showing the changes of solar degeneration. Microscopically this lesion is characterized by invasion of the epidermis as well as the dermis. The term superficial spreading means that there is a wave of malignancy spreading out from the centre and transforming the melanocytes in the basal region, which thereupon invade both the epidermis and the dermis.

Melanoma without an adjacent intraepidermal component

This type appears as a nodule, a so-called nodular melanoma. There is no surrounding pigmented macule; the lesion may be polypoid and ulcerated with a faster growing rate than other types of melanoma. This tumour has minimal involvement of the adjacent epidermis, and involvement of no more than three rete ridges. These lesions are more active than the other lesions with more mitoses, and as a result have a poorer prognosis.

Mitotic activity

It has been shown that survival rate can be correlated with the degree of mitotic activity. The tumour can be graded according to its mitotic activity as follows:

1. Fewer than one mitosis per five high power fields.
2. Between one mitosis per five high power fields and one in each high power field .
3. One mitosis per high power field and over.

These figures are obtained using a 300 times magnification.

Levels of invasion

The levels of invasion have been divided into five groups and the name Clark (Clark *et al.*, 1969) is usually associated with this classification: 1. intraepidermal; 2. papillary dermal; 3. papillary-reticular dermal interface; 4. reticulo-dermal and 5. subcutaneous fat.

The level of invasion can be correlated with prognosis; however, one of the difficulties in the histological staging is that the papillary zone varies in thickness. A melanoma may fill the papillary layer depressing the reticular zone downwards instead of invading it. In this way a tumour at level 3 may be twice the depth of a tumour which has penetrated to level 4, the reticular zone. Thus an alternative classification based on the depth of a tumour, as measured with an occular micrometer, has been introduced and found to correlate with survival. Thus tumours up to 0.75 mm in thickness have a good prognosis, while those measuring from 0.76 to 1.50 mm had an unpredictable prognosis with 70% survival rate whether or not the lymph nodes were resected. Tumours more than 1.50 mm in depth had only a 30% survival rate but lymph node resection increased the survival rate in this group.

Diagnosis

The patient presents with a pigmented lesion which has grown, changed colour, itches or bleeds. The lesion may not have a typical appearance, and can easily be confused with a freckle, junctional naevus, compound naevus, halo naevus, blue naevus, seborrhoeic naevus, localized pigmentation due to blood, or a sclerosing haemangioma. Even experienced dermatologists may be no more than 66% accurate in their clinical diagnosis. For this reason a biopsy is the mainstay of diagnosis. Partial excision of a suspected melanoma is unwise because malignant degeneration of a benign lesion is not homogeneous. Also the treatment of the tumour is influenced by the maximum depth of penetration. Thus excision biopsy is the procedure of choice unless it is impracticable.

Treatment

Appropriate treatment is determined by pre-operative diagnosis. Extensive pre-operative staging by use of liver scans, bone scans or brain scans is unlikely to alter the initial management, because local control of the disease is important in the symptomatic as well as curative approach to the condition. Primary treatment is surgical excision. The extent of the excision is open to debate. There is reasonable evidence that excision of a tumour, which is less than 0.5 mm in depth or histological level I or II with a margin of 2 cm is adequate; these wounds can be closed by primary suture. Deeper lesions or those extending beyond level II require a wide excision; the extent of excision is open to debate, but a 5 cm lateral and distal margin with a 10 cm margin in the line of the draining lymphatics is adequate. Many suggest that carrying the dissection below the deep fascia is not necessary; on the other hand, excising the deep fascia ensures that the excision is well clear of the affected tissue, especially the area disturbed by the excision biopsy. A 5-cm margin is impracticable in the face, and probably a 2-cm margin is adequate. In order to cover the defect left by the wide excision, a split skin graft is applied, the graft having been taken before the excision is started from

an area which is not conceivably in the line of lymphatic drainage from the tumour. The size of the defect can be decreased by undercutting the edges of the excised area and suturing them down to the muscle with a sub-cuticular absorbable suture.

A point of controversy is the management of the regional lymph nodes; however, with the more accurate staging of the disease a rational policy can be advocated. Tumours, whose thickness is more than 1.75 mm, have a bad prognosis, and thus, prophylactic block dissection is appropriate in this group if they have a single lymphatic drainage area such as the groin for a leg melanoma. For those tumours between 1.5 mm and 1.75 mm, block dissection is performed if the tumour is near the draining lymph nodes, has a high mitotic index, occurs in a middle aged man or is on the trunk. These decision levels are arbitrary, and American writers suggest that 1 mm is the level at which block dissection should be performed. For the patient who presents with lymph node involvement, a full assessment, including lymphangiogram or CAT-scanning, should be undertaken before proceeding with radical local treatment. If disseminate disease is present a debulking procedure should be carried out, as a prelude to treatment by chemotherapy, immunotherapy or radiotherapy.

Radiotherapy
Radiotherapy plays no significant role in the primary treatment of cutaneous melanoma; however, it is of considerable value as an adjunct to chemotherapy or immunotherapy, for the treatment of the local mass of melanoma which cannot easily be excised, for the management of pain caused by metastases, and probably most valuable as a palliative management of brain metastases. The whole brain is irradiated with a midline dose of 3000 rad in 10 fractions over 12 days. Dexamethasone is given during the irradiation to reduce local oedema. Prolonged survival has been achieved with this regimen.

Chemotherapy
Despite extensive experience in the management of this disease with different chemotherapeutic regimens, none has shown evidence of significant benefit to more than a small minority of the patients treated. The mainstay in the chemotherapy of melanoma is DTIC (dimethyl-triazeno-imidazole carboxamide), a drug with a response rate of approximately 20% with a median duration of about three months. The dosage schedule is 250 mg/m^2 i.v. daily for 5 days, repeated every 4 weeks. The primary toxicity is gastrointestinal, with severe nausea and vomiting, usually occurring on the first day of chemotherapy. Tolerance appears to develop, and after the second or third course the side-

effects become less marked. Myelosuppression is rarely severe, and DTIC appears to be relatively free of immunosuppressive toxicity. There is no evidence that increasing doses affect the response rate. The only other agents with significant activity against melanoma are the nitrosoureas with a response rate between 13 and 18%. Actinomycin D, adriamycin and vindesine have been reported to be of value, but their role has not yet been fully evaluated.

Immunotherapy

There is a growing body of evidence, suggesting that melanoma tumour cells express tumour-associated antigen on their surfaces. Thus, activation of the host immune response against tumour cells containing foreign antigen appears to be a logical therapeutic approach. Of importance in this approach is the fact that tumour cells appear in regional lymphatics prior to haematogenous dissemination in more than 75% of patients. It is therefore reasonable to expect that activation of the immune system within the regional lymphatic system might enable the host to retard further tumour growth or prevent distant spread of the tumour.

The group of patients who are ideally suited to immunotherapy are those with locally recurrent disease, and no evidence of distant metastatic spread. Removal of as much tumour as possible by surgical excision or even radiotherapy may well aid the control of this disease.

A standard immunotherapeutic regimen has not been established; the background to this approach is discussed in Chapter 7. Commonly, high numbers of viable units of lyophilized BCG are given by intradermal injection or scarification every week for three months, and then at monthly intervals. For patients with disseminated disease, combination of immunotherapy with chemotherapy can be given. It is doubtful if this method of treatment should be undertaken outside a clinical trial, or by a clinician without specific knowledge of immunotherapy as the results have yet to be fully evaluated to be certain that actual harm is not done to some patients.

Tumours and tumour-like conditions of the haematopoietic and lymphoid tissues

Tumours of these tissues have specific dermatological manifestations. Although infiltration of the skin is relatively rare in Hodgkin's disease, except in the terminal stages, it is more common in the leukaemias and is frequently seen in the other reticuloses. Specific eruptions may be papular, nodular, tumorous or ulcerative. Mycosis fungoides is a lymphoma predominantly affecting the skin, and the extracutaneous manifesta-

tions of this disease are relatively rare. The non-specific dermatological expressions of lymphomas and leukaemias include purpura, pigmentation, pruritus, prurigo, atrophy, alopecia, exfoliative dermatitis and herpes zoster. With the exception of mycosis fungoides, cutaneous manifestations of the leukaemias and systemic lymphomas rarely need specific treatment and respond to chemotherapy regimes with the other manifestations of the disease.

Mycosis fungoides

This disease (Fig. 30.5) was described by Alibert in 1832; it is a reticulosis affecting the skin for most of the duration of the disease, and only in some instances progressing to lymph nodes and visceral involvement. The cause is unknown, as are any aetiological factors. Histological features of the disease are difficult to interpret and in the early stages may be entirely non-specific. It is said to progress through a superficial prodromal phase, to an infiltrative phase and finally the phase of tumour formation. However, all these phases may be present at the same time, and it is important when seeking confirmation of the diagnosis to biopsy the most advanced lesion. Microscopically, there is an upper dermal infiltration of mononuclear cells and histiocytes, some of which are atypical cells with hyperchromatic nuclei. The mycosis cell, which is said to be the same as the sezary cell, has a large nucleus with minimal cytoplasm, and is characterized as a T-cell. The mycosis cell can be found in lymph nodes draining the affected area of skin, but the commoner cause for lymph node enlargement is due to dermatopathic lymphadenopathy. However, this non-specific lymph node change is important because prognosis is worse in those patients with dermatopathic lymphadenopathy (Fuks *et al.*, 1973).

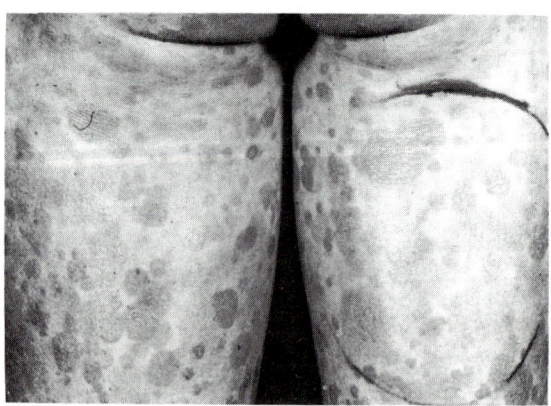

Fig. 30.5 Mycosis fungoides. Classical Alibert form.

The clinical manifestations of mycosis fungoides are varied (Samman, 1976). The classical Alibert form may show early non-specific eczematous lesions with patches of varying size and colour, common sites of occurence are the breasts and buttocks. The erythrodermic variety of mycosis fungoides is a rare variant and total skin redness with occasional patches of normal skin may be found. The *tumeur d'emblee* form shows rapid progression to advanced tumour lesions in one area with minimal background patterning over the rest of the skin.

There is a 2:1 male predominance, and, although disease has been described in young children, it is commonly an affliction of middle life. In the classical Alibert variety, progression to the tumour stage takes up to 40 years.

Poikloderma atrophicans vasculare

This may be associated with the development of mycosis fungoides. The areas of poikloderma found in these patients show atrophy, depigmentation and telangiectasia, mimicking late radiation changes. The association with the Alibert form of mycosis fungoides is usually indicative of a good prognosis.

Woringer Kolopp variant

This recently described condition is mycosis fungoides in-situ, the infiltrate being confined to the epidermis (Fig. 30.6). The patient presents with a solitary patch of superficial scaling eruption, most usually on the limbs. Some cases eventually disseminate, manifesting the classical Alibert form of mycosis fungoides.

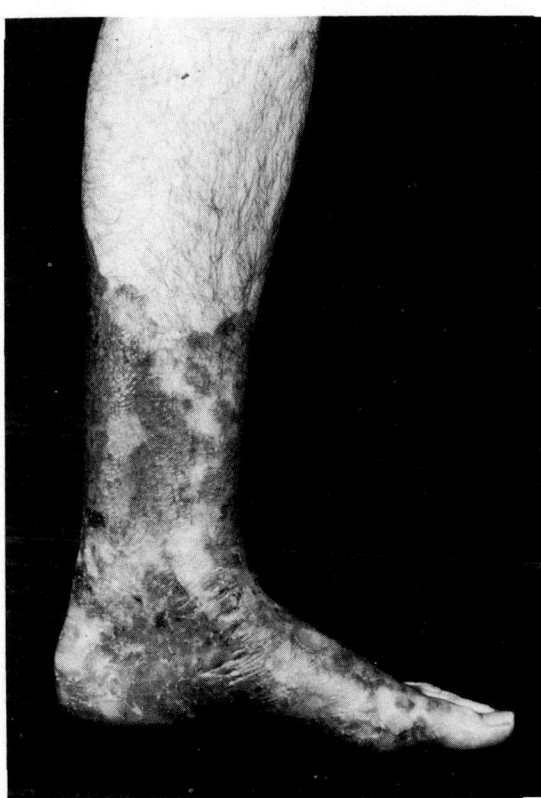

Fig. 30.6 Woringer Kolopp variant of mycosis fungoides. Note abrupt border with normal skin.

Treatment

The philosophy of treatment in this condition stems from the poor response to chemotherapy and the excellent local response to X-ray therapy. As the natural history of the disease may be up to 40 years in evolution, symptomatic measures will form a large part of the management of these patients; thus local topical steroids, antihistamines and emulsifying creams are important. Where superficial involvement is the main manifestation of the disease especially in the breast and buttock areas, ultraviolet light in erythema doses may produce long-term control. Eventually, as more skin becomes involved and infiltration increases, therapy with psoralens and ultraviolet light (PUVA therapy) may be considered (Gilchrist *et al.*, 1976). Therapy has to be continued and pigmentation may occur; nevertheless, there is good control of the superficial disease which helps greatly with the morale of the patient, a factor of great importance in this chronic condition. The long-term disadvantages of this chronic ultraviolet exposure have not yet been evaluated.

In advanced infiltrated disease or where other therapies have failed, whole skin electron beam therapy can completely clear the skin for periods from months to many years.

Electron beam therapy of mycosis fungoides (Fig. 30.7) was initially described in 1939 but later developed by Trump and Bagshaw in America (Fuks *et al.*, 1973) and by Szur and Bewley in England (Spittle, 1975). It is difficult to attain homogeneity of dose over the whole skin. Several methods have been devised to do this. At the Hammersmith Hospital the patient stands 6 m from the horizontal electron beams of a linear accelerator; at Cambridge a strontium-90 strip traverses the length of the prone or supine patient and in other centres multiple field techniques or moving couches have been used (Spittle, 1979). The production of low voltage electrons is often unreliable and a higher energy may be more efficiently produced and decelerated by a material of low atomic number. The beam may also need scattering to achieve the appropriate field size. X-ray contamination must be minimal – less than 1%.

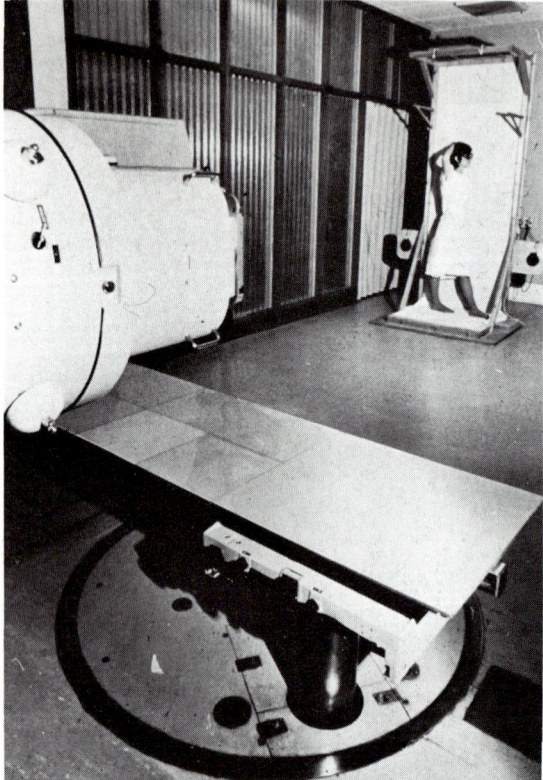

Fig. 30.7 Electron beam therapy of mycosis fungoides.

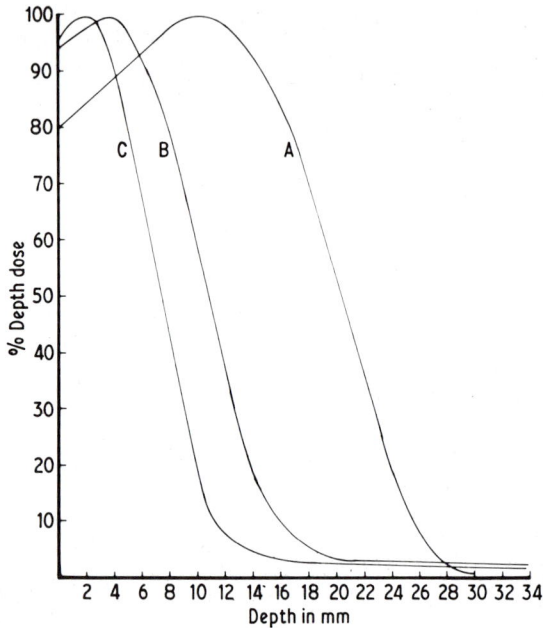

Fig. 30.8 Depth-dose curves for electron beams of differing energies in the 6 Mev linear accelerator A. Full electron energy; B. 4 mm carbon decelerator; C. 7 mm carbon decelerator.

Electron energies of 2.5, 3 or 3.5 MeV are produced giving an 80% isodose distribution at between 6 and 12 mm depending on the depth of infiltration of the disease (Fig. 30.8). Approximately 400 rad can be given twice weekly to all body surfaces for 6–10 treatments. There is some suggestion that higher doses may give a longer disease-free survival and possibly cure. However, the long natural history of the disease makes this difficult to assess and higher doses may result in later complications such as telangiectasia and subcutaneous fibrosis.

As mycosis fungoides frequently affects the head, the patient's face and scalp are treated and the eyes shielded by lead goggles – alopecia is temporary. The testicles are also shielded. Few systemic effects of whole skin electron beam treatment are noted – temporary peripheral oedema, male gynaecomastia and loss of finger and toe nails may occur.

Clearance of the disease occurs in most patients treated with whole skin electron beam therapy (Fig. 30.9) but recurrence may occur. If advanced cases are chosen most will have recurred by eighteen months.

New studies attempting to maintain the remission initiated by electron beam therapy with PUVA or topical nitrogen mustard (Van Scott and Kalmanson, 1973) on a long-term basis show encouraging results.

Local radiotherapy to tumour stage disease is effective whether the condition has been previously treated or has recurred following electron beam therapy. A dose of 900 rad in 3 treatments over a period of 1 week to the local lesions may cause long-term suppression of the disease. Topping up doses in the groins, between the natal clefts, around the scrotum, in the axilla and to the plantar surfaces of the feet following whole skin electron beam therapy are advantageous as these are the common sites of recurrence after electron beam therapy due to treatment inhomogeneity.

There is no consistent response to chemotherapy in mycosis fungoides. For this reason much care has been given to perfecting whole skin irradiation. Procarbazine, cyclophosphamide and intravenous nitrogen mustard given as single agents have some reputation in this disease. Regimens useful for systemic lymphomas such as CHOP and MOPP have had only moderate success with mycosis fungoides. Topical nitrogen mustard has proved useful in superficial disease; 10 cm³ mustine is diluted to 50 cm³ in tap water and this is

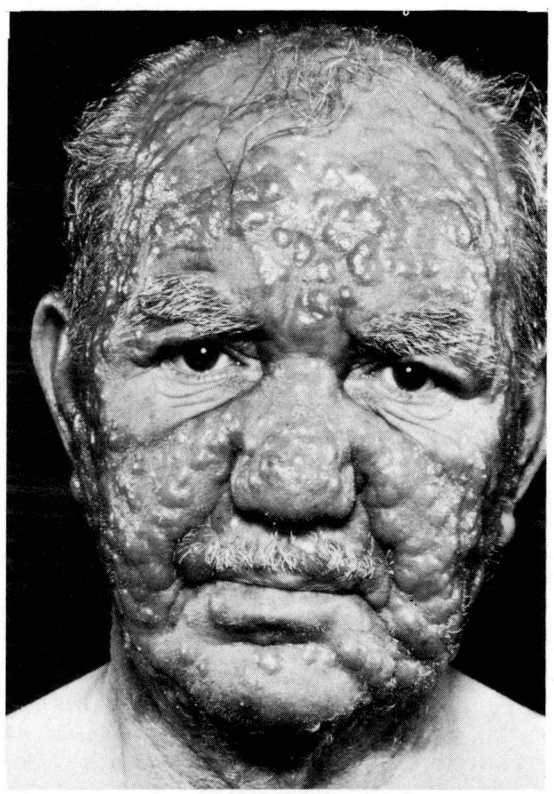

(a)

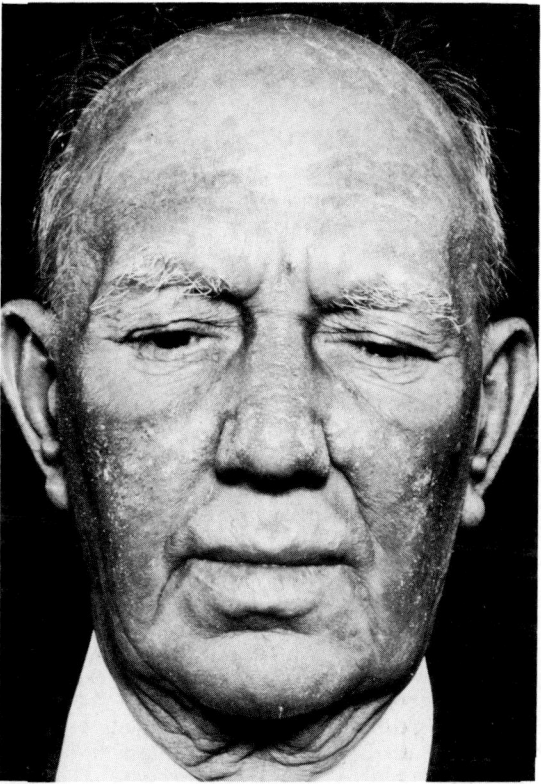

(b)

Fig. 30.9 Non-Hodgkin's lymphoma predominantly affecting the face skin: (a) before electron beam therapy (b) after electron beam therapy.

rubbed over the whole skin daily by the patient wearing plastic gloves. Treatment must be continued and sensitization may occur. Regimens for desensitization have been elaborated so that therapy may continue if useful. Results of systemic steroid therapy are variable and they may be used to control intractable pruritus.

Sézary syndrome

This syndrome possibly represents the leukaemic phase of mycosis fungoides. It presents as a generalized erythroderma, with facial oedema, pruritus, pigmentation, lymphadenopathy, hyperkeratosis of the palms and soles and ectropion due to infiltration of the lower eyelids. The histological feature of the condition is the Sézary cell which is found in increased numbers in the peripheral blood. It is a large T-lymphocyte with pale cytoplasm and a large crenated nucleus; however, the cell is not specific to this syndrome, being also found in

mycosis fungoides and other reticuloses. The bone marrow is normal.

Treatment is unsatisfactory, since the response to chemotherapy is poor. The electron beam is useful for intractable pruritus and skin oedema. Immunotherapy and leucophoresis have been used with minimal success. As the symptoms become progressively severe, the only therapeutic approach remaining is aggressive chemotherapy which frequently is the immediate cause of death. Steroid therapy may alleviate intractable pruritus.

Benign lymphocytoma cutis

This condition is characterized by single or multiple papules or nodules occurring round the face, neck and scalp, particularly in the female. The disease may be circumscribed or disseminated. Diagnosis is made by biopsy of the lesion. Treatment is by radiation to which the lesions are extremely sensitive. A dose of 1000–1500 rad is given in 5 treatments over 7 days at 80–100 kV. The size of the field is arbitrary, but adjacent skin is often involved, and thus a wider field is preferable. Permanent regression of the local lesion is to be expected.

Benign lymphocytic infiltration of Jessner

This condition is a variable of benign lymphocytoma cutis. Flat pink papules on the face may remit and relapse. There is gross lymphocytic infiltration of the dermis which characteristically sleeves blood vessels. Radiotherapy (300 rad × 5 at 80–100 kV) is indicated and effective for the management of the local disease.

Other lymphomas

Both lymphocytic and histiocytic lymphomas may arise in the skin, particularly on the trunk and, although appearing histologically aggressive, may be cured by local superficial radiotherapy, 3000 rad being given over a 2-week period at 80–100 kV. The limits of the disease may be difficult to determine and recurrence due to a geographical miss may occur.

The penis

Neoplastic disease of the penis is rare, and with better hygiene is becoming less common in Westernized society. The commonest neoplasm is that of a carcinoma, but there are certain pre-malignant conditions whose importance lies in their correct diagnosis to prevent their natural history progressing to a life-threatening disorder.

Pre-malignant lesions

Erythroplasia of Queyrat

This lesion is a hyperplastic epithelial condition of the glans, usually the dorsum, which practically never occurs in the circumcised. Chronicity and periods of partial regression and recurrence are common. The lesions are often painful. The condition presents as an area of intense erythema or velvety red plaques with ill-defined margins. Microscopy shows the stratum corneum and stratum germinativum to be hyperplastic with prominent interpapillary acanthosis. The dermal inflammatory reaction is usually intense and mitotic figures are prominent in the epithelium.

Evolution of these lesions to carcinoma in-situ and frank malignancy is well documented (Goette, 1974). Treatment is primarily surgical, excision biopsy of the lesion with circumcision to enable easier observation of the glans being sufficient. If the lesion is extensive, partial amputation of the penis is necessary. Recurrence following surgical excision is unusual, provided excision is complete, and there is no evidence of carcinoma. Other treatments such as radiotherapy and

topical 5-fluorouracil have been tried but the need for an excision biopsy to exclude carcinoma rules out these modes of therapy, except if the patient refuses surgical treatment.

Leukoplakia

This lesion is probably related to lack of hygiene; it rarely occurs as an isolated abnormality, and is most often found adjacent to areas of frank squamous carcinoma. The areas of leukoplakia should be completely excised, and a careful histological examination made of the whole specimen for invasive carcinoma. A circumcision should be performed to aid hygiene, and the patient followed on a long-term basis to exclude recurrence.

Bowen's disease

On the penis, intraepithelial carcinoma is similar to disease in other areas. The lesions must be completely excised with a margin of 2 mm clear of disease on microscopy, as local recurrence is common. If excision will distort the penis, the topical application of 5-fluorouracil is effective. The risk of metastases is extremely small, and probably never occurs.

Buschke-Lowenstein tumour

The giant penile condyloma, although histologically benign, grows to a large size, having a malignant appearance, and will eventually destroy the penile tissue. With the lesion, there may be foci of carcinoma, thus an excision biopsy is essential. Because of the large size of the lesion a distal amputation is frequently the only way to obtain an excision biopsy. If invasion is present subsequent treatment should be the same as that for a penile carcinoma.

Malignant penile lesions

Epidermoid carcinoma

Carcinoma is the most common malignant neoplasm of the penis, yet accounts for less than 1% of deaths from malignant disease in the United Kingdom. In Burma, and in China the incidence may be as high as 18% of tumours in males. The highest reported incidence in Africa is in Uganda, where 12% of male cancers are in the penis.

The aetiology is unknown, but the distribution suggests that circumcision and poor hygiene are major pre-disposing causes. Further evidence to implicate the carcinogenic role of smegma is found in the fact that many patients present with a long history of phimosis, but no single carcinogen has been identified. Venereal disease, inflammatory disease and trauma have been incriminated in the past, but the rise in venereal disease in the United Kingdom has been followed by a fall, rather than a rise in penile carcinoma.

Penile cancer spreads to the regional lymph nodes – the prepuce and the skin of the penis drain to the superficial inguinal nodes, whereas the glans and the corpora drain to the deep inguinal nodes (De Kermon and Persky, 1978). Invasion of the corpora cavernosa will lead to blood-borne dissemination, which involves primarily lung and bone, although this is unusual.

Any exophytic or diffuse lesion in the penis should be considered to be a penile carcinoma until proved otherwise by biopsy, which should include adjacent normal tissue. The differential diagnosis includes lymphogranuloma venereum, condyloma acuminatum, chancroid, traumatic ulceration and the pre-malignant lesions. In addition to biopsy, a chest X-ray and possibly a bone scan is indicated. Lymphangiography probably contributes little to staging, since enlarged groin nodes are readily palpated and the frequently coexistent infection cannot thus be differentiated from metastatic spread. However, if block dissection is considered then a lymphangiogram or CAT-scan of the iliac or aortic nodes should be performed to exclude metastases beyond the limits of dissection.

Clinical classification and staging

The TNM classification is less commonly used than the staging system recommended by Jackson. In the former classification T_1 is a tumour 2 cm or less in its largest dimension, strictly superficial or exophytic; T_2 is a tumour between 2 and 5 cm in maximum diameter with minimal infiltration; T_3 is a lesion larger than 5 cm in diameter or a tumour infiltrating deeply, while a T_4 lesion is one which infiltrates neighbouring structures. The staging system defines Stage I tumours as those limited to the glans penis or prepuce; Stage II lesions involve invasion into the shaft of the penis or corpora without nodal or distant metastases; Stage III tumours are those confined to the shaft with proven node metastases, and Stage IV lesions are those in which there is local invasion from the shaft of the penis, inoperable regional node metastases or distant metastases. Staging penile carcinoma is particularly difficult because between 35 and 50% of patients will have palpable inguinal adenopathy when first seen, because of associated infection.

Treatment

Surgical treatment has been most widely employed, but the desire to preserve the penis, especially in younger patients, has prompted a less aggressive approach. Thus, tumours of the prepuce can be treated effectively by circumcision; however, tumours involving the glans penis which spread rapidly to the deep iliac nodes through the profuse glandular lymphatics require amputation of the penis. The extent of penile amputation is determined by taking the incision 2 cm proximal to the tumour margin, thus shaft tumours will require a total amputation. The major complication of treatment of the primary tumour is local recurrence, which occurs in approximately 10%.

Radiation therapy has been proposed as a method of treating the primary tumour with preservation of the penis. When the lesion is superficial with no invasion of the corpus cavernosum, radiotherapy can be used. Low voltage X-rays have the disadvantage that the penile skin seems unusually prone to radionecrosis at doses tolerated by other organs. Electron beam therapy, using build-up to reduce the slight skin-sparing effect of low voltage electrons, is good treatment of superficial lesions (Mantell and Morgan, 1969): 400 rad given daily for 10–11 treatments in 12–17 days gives a good functional result when care is taken to avoid infection and trauma after therapy. Where the squamous penile carcinoma is more infiltrating and invades the corpus cavernosum attempts have been made to irradiate with supervoltage therapy enclosing the penis in a wax block to improve dose homogenity. This treatment is usually unsuccessful as the penis tolerates radical radiotherapy poorly and the disease is commonly extremely extensive and gross infection is present. However if recurrence does occur after 6000 rad given in 30 treatments over 40 days nothing is lost as surgical amputation obviously removes the irradiated area. Control and cure can be achieved in a small proportion of patients and this is useful for the elderly patient who is unfit for operation or for those patients refusing surgery. Using the electron beam, local control in 65% can be obtained. Unfortunately, stricture of the urethra can occur in up to 12% of patients. Occasionally, severe ulceration and necrosis of the penis can occur, and this necessitates total removal of the penis. External beam irradiation will control a small tumour in 85% of patients.

Management of regional lymph nodes

Because 35–50% of patients have node enlargement at the time of presentation, and only half of these will have tumour in the nodes, it is difficult to evolve a policy for the routine management of inguinal lymph nodes. In Stage II disease the incidence of lymph node metastases is well above 50%, and thus all those with persistently palpable lymph nodes should have a block dissection of the inguinal nodes on the affected side. In those without palpable nodes there appears to be no advantage in undertaking a prophylactic node dissection. In Stage III disease, block dissection of the groin is undertaken on the affected side. There are no data to suggest that bilateral block dissection is of advantage to the patient. External beam radiation therapy has been advocated for the treatment of inguinal nodes, but few cures have been achieved by patients treated in this manner. High dose fractionated irradiation would be necessary. Treatment of the inguinal or external iliac and inguinal nodes in palliative cases can be given using supervoltage irradiation: 4500 rad given in 15 treatments over 21 days can result in palliation but as advanced inguinal nodes affected by squamous carcinoma of the penis are often infected and ulcerate, oedema of the lower leg, venous stasis and thrombosis, local induration and terminal haemorrhage may occur. Surgical treatment is not indicated for Stage IV cases although the course of the disease may be distressing and long. Bleomycin initially had a good reputation as the cytotoxic for choice in penile carcinoma but has not yet justified the initial enthusiasm. Nonetheless combinations of cytotoxics, including bleomycin and methotrexate give the best hope of palliation.

Prognosis

Stage I tumours should be cured by treatment in all cases, while Stage II and III are associated with 40–70% cure rate. It is rare for a patient with Stage IV disease to live five years.

The anus

Tumours of the anus and the perianal skin are rare. Malignant epithelial growths in the anal region may be subdivided into five types: adenocarcinoma of the rectum descending into the anal canal; squamous cell carcinoma; basal cell carcinoma; malignant melanoma and primary adenocarcinoma of the anal canal and perianal tissues. The commonest of these lesions is the squamous cell carcinoma yet only 1–3% of all anorectal growths are anal squamous carcinomas. Basal cell carcinomas are even less common, having an incidence of only 0.25% of all anorectal growths.

Squamous cell carcinoma

Histologically this tumour varies from well differentiated tumours to almost completely undifferentiated growths. The carcinomas in men, in whom growths are more common, tend to be well differentiated and of low malignancy, whilst squamous carcinoma of the anal canal, which is generally poorly differentiated and much more malignant in character occurs more frequently in the female. Intermediate types of growth may occur in the anal canal, such as basisquamous, mucoepidermoid and transitional cell tumours.

The lesion usually presents as an ulcer or a raised warty growth. Digital examination determines its extent, and a biopsy determines its nature. In the female a vaginal examination is performed to exclude involvement. The inguinal lymph nodes should be examined carefully, and the size of the enlarged nodes noted. Spread of the tumour is by way of the lymph nodes, blood spread being late. Assessment of spread by lymphangiography or CAT-scan is necessary unless block dissection of the nodes is being considered.

Treatment

There has been a divergence of opinion as to the relative merits of some form of irradiation and surgical treatment in the management of squamous cell carcinoma of the anus. Because of the rarity of the condition series tend to be small and not comparable. For growths which extend up to the rectal mucosa, lymphatic spread to the mesenteric nodes occurs in 43% of cases, hence radical excision of the rectum and anus by an abdominoperineal excision is indicated (Golden and Horsley, 1976). On the other hand, for growths below the pectinate line a wide local excision with sacrifice of some of the lower part of the anal sphincters is appropriate.

Approximately 40% of anal carcinomas have inguinal metastases. However, treatment of these glands is usually postponed until the management of the primary lesion has been completed. This allows a period of observation of the glands to ensure that they are not inflammatory. Block dissection of both groins should be undertaken when there are easily palpable hard nodes present two months after the primary treatment. If the inguinal glands do not appear clinically implicated, an expectant policy appears appropriate, as in the management of all squamous cell carcinomas.

If the inguinal lymph nodes are fixed, or the primary tumour is inoperable, radiotherapy will be of value in palliation of the not inconsiderable discomfort associated with persistent anal disease. External beam irradiation has had only limited success in anal carcinoma. Supervoltage radiation using a planned approach of posterior angled wedged fields or a rotation technique reaching 6000 rad in 30 treatments over 40 days may cure occasional early cases but will achieve palliation in patients with advanced disease. Good results have been reported in early cases of anal carcinoma using interstitial irradiation with iridium wire (Papillon, 1974). The obvious advantage in successful irradiation treatment is preservation of the normal anatomy and anal continence (Dalby and Pounton, 1961).

Multimodality treatment has been reviewed by Bruckner *et al.*, (1979) and some encouraging trends towards reduction of treatment morbidity and increasing survival using concomitant intravenous chemo-therapy with 5-fluorouracil and mitomycin-C are described.

Prognosis
Prognosis for cancer of the anus is usually considered to be poorer than that for cancer of the colon, but collected experience suggests that the condition has an acceptable prognosis with an absolute 5-year survival rate of 40% and a 10-year survival rate of 20%.

Basal cell carcinoma

These lesions represent as a pile, an ulcer or a small sore spot in the anal region. It is rarely larger than 1 cm in size, and never spreads. Excision biopsy is the method of diagnosis and treatment, although radiotherapy is equally effective. The prognosis is excellent provided that the initial treatment has been adequate.

Further reading

Braun Falio, O., Lukacs, S. and Goldschmidt, H. (1976), *Dermatologic Radiotherapy*. Springer Verlag, New York.
Freitag, S.B. and Culmane, D.L. (1976), *Neoplasms of the Skin and Malignant Melanoma*. Year Book Medical Publishers, Chicago.
Milton, G.W. (1977), *Malignant Melanoma of the Skin and Mucus Membranes*. Churchill Livingstone, Edinburgh.

References

Albert, R.E. and Omran, A.L. (1968), Follow up study of patients treated by X-ray epilation for tinea capitis. 1. Population characteristics, post treatment illnesses and mortality experiences. *Archs Environ. Hlth*, **17**, 899.
Braun, Falco O., Lukacs, Sr. and Goldschmidt, H. (1976), *Dermatologic Radiotherapy*. Springer Verlag, New York.
Bruckner, H.W. *et al.* (1979), Carcinoma of the anus treated with a combination of radiotherapy and chemotherapy. *Cancer Treat. Rep.*, **63**(3), 395–8.
Clark, W.H. Jr. *et al.* (1969), The histogenesis and biologic behaviour of primary human malignant melanomas of the skin. *Cancer Res.*, **29**, 705–27.
Cleaver, J.E. (1968), Defective repair replication of DNA in xeroderma pigmentosa. *Nature*, **218**, 652–6.
Dalby, J.E. and Pointon, R.S. (1961), The treatment of anal carcinoma by interstitial irradiation. *Am. J. Roentg.*, **85**, 515–20.

De Kermon, J.B. and Persky, L. (1978), Neoplastic lesions of the penis. In: *Genito-Urinary Cancer*. (eds D.G. Skinner and J.B. De Kermon) Saunders, Philadelphia, pp.494–508.
Epstein, J.H., Fukerjama, K. and Dobson, R.L. (1969), Ultra-violet light carcinogenesis. In: *The Biologic Effects of U.V. Radiation*, Pergamon Press, New York, pp.551–68.
Freitaig, S.B. and Culmane, D.C. (1976), *Neoplasms of the skin and malignant melanoma*. Year Book Medical Publishers, Chicago.
Fuks, Z.Y., Bagshaw, M.A. and Farber, E.M. (1973), Prognostic signs and the management of mycosis fungoides. *Cancer*, **32**, 1385–95.
Gilchrist, B.A. *et al.* (1976), Oral Melthoxsalen photo-chemotherapy of mycosis fungoides. *Cancer*, **38**, 683–9.
Goette, D.K. (1974), Erythroplasia of Querat. Treatment with topically administered 5-fluorouracil. *Arch. Derm.*, **110**, 271.
Golden, G.T. and Horsley, J.S. III (1976), Surgical management of epidermoid carcinoma of the anus. *Am. J. Surg.*, **131**, 275–80.
Grosch, E. and Lambert, H.E. (1979), The treatment of difficult cutaneous basal and squamous cell carcinomata with electrons. *Br. J. Radiol.*, **52**, 422–78.
Mantell, B.S. and Morgan, W.Y. (1969), Querats erythroplasia of the penis treated by beta particles of irradiation. *Br. J. Radiol.*, **42**, 855–7.
McGovern, V.J. *et al.* (1973), The classification of malignant melanoma and its histologic reporting. *Cancer*, **32**, 1446–57.
Mehregan, A.H. and Pinkus, H. (1964), Intra-epidermal epithelioma: a critical study. *Cancer*, **17**, 609–36.
Modan, B. *et al.* (1974), Radiation induced head and neck tumours. *Lancet*, **1**, 277.
Moss, W.T., Brand, W.N. and Battiflora, H. (1973), *Therapeutic Radiology*, 4th edn, C.V. Mosby, Saint Louis.
Papillon, J. (1974), Radiation therapy in the management of epidermal carcinoma of the anal region. *Dis. Colon Rectum*, **17**, 181–7.
Samman, P.D. (1976), Mycosis fungoides and other cutaneous reticuloses. *Clin. Exp. Derm.*, **1**, 197.
Sanderson, K.V. (1972), Tumours of the skin. In: *Textbook of Dermatology*, 2nd edn, (eds A. Rook, D.S. Wilkinson and F.J.G. Eblin) Blackwells, Oxford pp.1911–2007.
Spittle, M.F. (1975), The treatment of mycosis fungoides. *Trans. St. John's Hosp. Derm. Soc.* (London), **61**, 31–4.
Spittle, M.F. (1979), Electron beam therapy in England. *Cancer Treat. Rep.*, **63**, 639–41.
Tapley, N. du V. (1975), Skin and lips. In: *Clinical*

Applications of the Electron Beam. (ed. N. du V. Tapley), John Wiley and Sons, Ashington, pp.93–123.

Van Scott, E.J. and Kalmanson, J.D. (1973), Com- plete remissions of mycosis fungoides lymphoma induced by topical nitrogen mustard. *Cancer*, **32**, 18.

31 Soft tissue

H.D. Suit, K.H. Proppe
and V.H.C. Bramwell

Under the designation 'sarcoma of soft tissues' are included those malignant neoplasms which arise from the mesenchymal supporting tissues, other than bone, at all anatomic sites. Usually, discussions of this subject do not include sarcomas which arise from parenchymatous organs or hollow viscera. In addition, tumours arising from peripheral nerves are included. The more common sarcomas are named from the tissue of apparent origin, for example, fibrosarcoma, liposarcoma, rhabdomyosarcoma, malignant fibrous histiocytoma, synovial sarcoma, etc. The relative frequencies of these histopathological varieties are given in Table 31.1; these were derived from a study of 1215 sarcomas of soft tissue by the Task Force for Sarcoma of Soft Tissue of the American Joint Commission (Russell et al., 1977). These tumours are not common: the annual incidence in the United States is approximately 4500 newly diagnosed lesions, forming 0.7% of all cancers (Cancer Statistics, 1979). The rarity of this tumour can be further emphasized by noting that there are, among the total numbers of adenocarcinomas diagnosed per year, approximately 102 000 adeno-

Table 31.1 Histopathological varieties of sarcoma of soft tissue (from Russell et al., 1977).

Histopathological variety	Proportion of total cases (1215)
Rhabdomyosarcoma	19.2%
Fibrosarcoma	19.0%
Liposarcoma	18.2%
Malignant fibrohistiocytoma	10.5%
Sarcoma of soft tissue, type unspecified	10.0%
Synovial sarcoma	6.9%
Leiomyosarcoma	6.5%
Malignant Schwannoma	4.9%
Angiosarcoma	2.7%
Other types	1.9%

carcinomas of the colorectal tissues, 91 000 adenocarcinomas of the breast etc. Thus knowledge of the natural history and efficacy of different therapeutic approaches is less well developed for soft tissue sarcomas than for adenocarcinomas and squamous cell carcinomas.

The aetiology of this group of tumours remains unknown. Significant antecedent trauma at the site of the lesion is not a common feature in the history of patients with soft tissue sarcoma. Clearly, genetic factors are involved in a small proportion of patients (Strong, 1977). An example is the high frequency of desmoid tumours among patients with familial polyposis (McAdam and Galigher, 1970). Sarcomas of soft tissue and bone have been observed in patients with bilateral retinoblastoma, a tumour in which strong hereditary factors operate (Jensen and Miller, 1971). Another example is that of von Recklinhausen's disease whose major clinical feature is multiple neurofibromatosis. An important proportion of these patients ultimately exhibit malignant change in one of the neurofibromas (Fraumeni, 1973). Another factor which may play a role in the genesis of sarcoma of bone and soft tissue is virus infection, although this is by no means proven. It is, however, supported by the apparent common antigenicity of cells of human sarcoma of soft tissue and bone (Harris and Sinkovics, 1976). Unfortunately, a small number of patients develop soft tissue sarcomas at the site of prior therapeutic irradiation (Kim et al., 1978). Although the data are limited, this change occurs in less than 1% of patients who were adults at the time of treatment and who have been followed for 5–25 years (Hatfield and Schulz, 1970).

For the series of 1215 tumours, evaluated by the Soft Tissue Sarcoma Task Force (Russell et al., 1977), the male: female ratio was 1.12:1. These lesions are commonest in the extremities with 40% of all tumours being located in the lower limb. In fact, 383 of the 1215 (32%) were in the thigh. These tumours are commoner in older people, especially above the age of 55 years

(35% of all soft tissue sarcomas). The majority of soft tissue sarcomas occurring below the age of 15 years are rhabdomyosarcomas (D'Angio and Evans, 1975), which differ considerably from adult tumours in natural history and response to therapy.

Although these lesions are uncommon, there has been a considerable increase in general medical interest over recent years in the problems of management presented by these patients. This is due to changing management strategies and improved clinical results. In particular, solid evidence has accumulated that in addition to surgery, there are important roles for radiation therapy and chemotherapy in the management of some groups of patients. Until the early 1960s, the consensus of medical opinion was that the only serious prospect for cure of patients with soft tissue sarcomas was radical surgery. Radical surgery, particularly amputation, produced impressive results, but at the cost of major functional loss or cosmetic disfigurement. Clinical studies over the last two decades have suggested that more conservative surgical approaches, when combined with radiation therapy, and in some situations, chemotherapy, may be as effective as the more classical radical surgical procedures. Furthermore, there is considerable optimism that aggressive chemotherapy given to patients who are free of clinically evident metastatic tumour will produce a higher cure rate. This has been achieved for rhabdomyosarcoma of childhood (see Chapter 37).

The excellent results currently being obtained by more conservative treatment strategies are through a multidisciplinary approach to the overall management of these patients (diagnostic evaluation, biopsy, treatment, rehabilitation and follow-up). The multidisciplinary team includes not only the surgeon but also the radiation therapist, chemotherapist and pathologist. The pathologist is an extremely valuable member of the team because the staging system which is now employed for these lesions (other than childhood rhabdomyosarcoma) utilizes histopathological grade as the principal determinant of clinical stage. This chapter will discuss the role of radiation therapy and chemotherapy combined with surgery or given alone, in the management of soft tissue sarcoma in the adult patient. Rhabdomyosarcoma of the paediatric age group is discussed in Chapter 37.

Clinical evaluation

Clinical examination

The most frequent initial complaint is of a painless lump of a few weeks to several months' duration. Occasionally, pain or tenderness precedes the detection of a lump. With progressive growth of tumour,

symptoms appear which are secondary to infiltration or pressure on adjacent structures (e.g. tendons, muscles, nerves) or organs. There are usually no other symptoms except for those occasionally seen which are secondary to metabolic effects of the tumour, e.g. malignant fibrohistiocytoma (Weiss and Enzinger, 1978). We have seen two examples of this: in the first patient fever, anaemia, weight loss and severe weakness disappeared with regression of the lesion during and following radiation therapy; the second patient had marked episodic reactions which were histamine-like and these disappeared completely when the tumour was resected (at the referring hospital).

During physical examination of the site of the primary lesion and regional node areas, precise anatomic location is essential with assessment of involvement of muscle groups, nerves or tendons, vessels, and of evidence of pressure effects on other adjacent structures. The regional lymph nodes need to be examined with care in all patients. They are unlikely to be involved except in high grade lesions, e.g. rhabdomyosarcomas, Grade III synovial sarcomas, and Grade III unclassified sarcomas. We have not seen lymph node involvement from a Grade I sarcoma. Laboratory investigations should include a complete blood count and biochemical assessment of renal and liver function.

Radiographic evaluation

In screening for pulmonary deposits, whole lung tomograms are more valuable than standard chest films (Neifeld *et al.*, 1977) and there is evidence that computerized body tomography (CT) will reveal metastatic lesions missed on conventional tomography (Schanner *et al.*, 1978). This procedure may be justified in the high risk patients, e.g. IIB and higher stage. For the primary site, the following procedures should be performed: soft tissue films, xerograms and where available CT scans. Depending upon the pattern of presentation and the nature of any planned surgery, an arteriogram may be of value. For rhabdomyosarcoma, high grade synovial and unclassified sarcomas, lymphangiograms are usually obtained. Bone scan need not be performed unless specifically indicated.

Biopsy

It is important that an adequate biopsy should be obtained by an experienced surgeon who is part of the multidisciplinary group which will be responsible for the definitive treatment of the patient. Careful thought should be given to the site of the surgical incision, so that the scar is removed at the time of subsequent surgery or encompassed in the post-operative radiation field. In the latter case, the biopsy should be sited so that the scar is exposed to minimal external trauma; necrosis after high-dose radiation therapy almost invariably starts in the surgical scar. Technique of biopsy depends upon the size of the tumour and the clinical presentation. For example, a small lesion (e.g. ⩽ 3 cm) is usually removed by simple excision on the presumption that it is benign. Where the malignant nature of the tumour is suspected, biopsy should be incisional. Formal treatment plans may then be made after the diagnosis has been established. An important detail is that meticulous care should be taken to achieve haemostasis since the patient who presents with extensive ecchymosis at the site of incisional biopsy is a special problem. During the incisional biopsy, the tumour capsule is violated and consequently tumour cells may have travelled along the same tissue planes as the red blood cells. This obviously complicates planning of surgery or radiation therapy.

Needle biopsy does not yield sufficient material for determination of histopathological type and grade, and frozen section diagnosis is also inadequate. The delay in diagnosis caused by waiting for the permanent sections is justified because of the value of a carefully considered diagnosis based on well prepared histological material. However, a frozen section is of value in selecting the best area for biopsy in poorly differentiated or necrotic tumours.

Histopathological diagnosis

Soft tissue tumours offer some of the greatest diagnostic challenges; because of their rarity, the opinions of pathologists with a special interest in these tumours should be sought to increase the accuracy of diagnosis and grading. Since these tumours often exhibit varying histopathological patterns and the neoplastic cells frequently differ from their presumed tissue of origin, wherever feasible a number of sections from different areas of the lesion should be examined microscopically, seeking diagnostic features. Special histochemical stains may be of value. A further aid to diagnosis in selected cases is electron microscopy and we recommended that at the time of biopsy, a small piece of tissue should be placed in glutaraldehyde fixative for later processing, if indicated.

Classification

Although the diagnosis and classification of soft tissue sarcomas is often difficult, accurate typing and an accepted terminology are essential in order to provide the clinician with a sound diagnostic base for planning management of the individual patient. This is also required to assess the relative frequency of the various histological subtypes and the results of the different treatment. It is inevitable that with advancing knowledge new entities may be recognized and a shift in the relative frequency of some histological types may occur. Rhabdomyosarcoma was formerly one of the more commonly encountered neoplasms in the adult but the recent recognition of fibrohistiocytic tumours as a distinct clinical and pathological entity has made inroads into the ranks of rhabdomyosarcoma. Malignant fibrous histiocytic tumours, fibrosarcoma and liposarcoma are in our experience, the most commonly encountered malignant neoplasms and occuring with equal frequency, accounted for 63 of the 112 cases in a recent review of soft tissue sarcomas treated at the Massachusetts General Hospital. In the same material, about 10% were unclassified and designated either as undifferentiated sarcoma or undifferentiated sarcoma, spindle cell type.

In addition to a classification based on the main histological type, many lesions have sub-varieties which are distinctive in their microscopical appearance and clinical behaviour. For example, rhabdomyosarcoma may be of embryonal, alveolar or pleomorphic type, and liposarcoma may be well differentiated, myxoid, round cell type or pleomorphic. Another tumour showing differences in behaviour related to its subtype is synovial sarcoma which may be predominantly biphasic (spindle cell and epithelioid pattern) or monophasic (spindle cell *or* epithelioid) (Moberger *et al.*, 1968). Therefore, these important subdivisions should be part of the histopathological diagnosis.

Grading

In assessing the degree of malignancy of a given neoplasm, it is our practice to evaluate the most aggressive areas of the tumour. Three grades, 1, 2, and 3, are used corresponding to the well established and familiar grading of well, moderately and poorly differentiated tumours. In broadest terms, the assessment of grade is made according to how closely the neoplasm resembles its presumed tissue of origin. Definition of the criteria used for grading every type of tumour is not feasible in this chapter. Microscopic features that are most closely evaluated in grading include degree of cellularity, degree of cytological differentiation and pleomorphism, nuclear pleomorphism and hyperchromatism, frequency of mitoses, loss of polarity and the formation of extracellular substance. The grade of malignancy assigned to a given neoplasm is the result of an evaluation of the above parameters as well as specific histological features. Furthermore, the accuracy of grading is directly related to the quality of the material examined and the experience of the pathologist.

Several studies have shown the importance of grad-

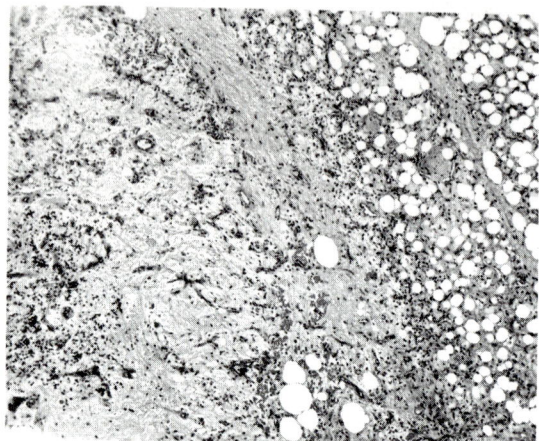

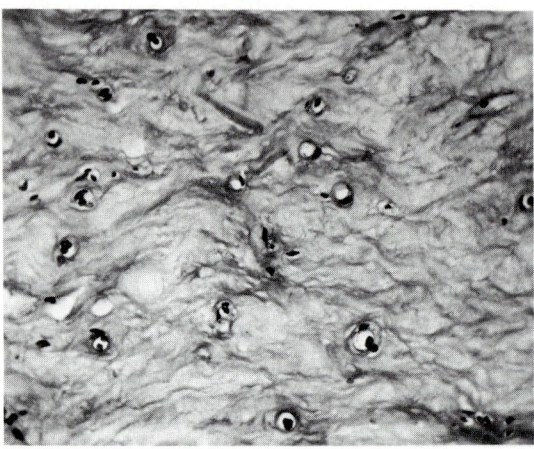

Fig. 31.1 (a, b)   These photomicrographs demonstrate the histopathological patterns in a low-grade liposarcoma (I/III) before and after radiation therapy. This lesion was located in the medial and posterior thigh (distal one-third) and was 12 cm long.

Fig. 31.1 (a)   Liposarcoma, mixed pattern, Grade I/III. The left half of the photograph shows a myxoid liposarcoma; on the right side the tumour appears as a differentiated liposarcoma (hematoxylin and eosin × 100)

Fig. 31.1 (c)   A higher magnification of this tumour post-irradiation which shows finely fibrillar hyalinized connective tissue. In a few areas, such as above, occasional degenerating neoplastic cells were found in the stroma (hematoxylin and eosin × 400).

indicate a good overall correlation between grade and survival regardless of histological type, grade alone should not be used as the exclusive determinant of stage, if the latter is used to select therapy and predict the outcome. Management of each patient must be individualized and based on all parameters known to predict biological behaviour. For example, angiosarcoma of the breast may appear so well differentiated as to be virtually indistinguishable from a benign angioma. Nevertheless, it is a highly malignant and usually fatal neoplasm. Accordingly, histological classification may also be critical in assessing prognosis and in planning patient management.

An attempt should be made to grade all sarcomas of soft tissue as part of a continuous effort to identify subtypes and variants which will allow better prediction of behaviour and selection of treatment. Fig 31.1 (a), (b) shows a typical example of a liposarcoma, before and after treatment.

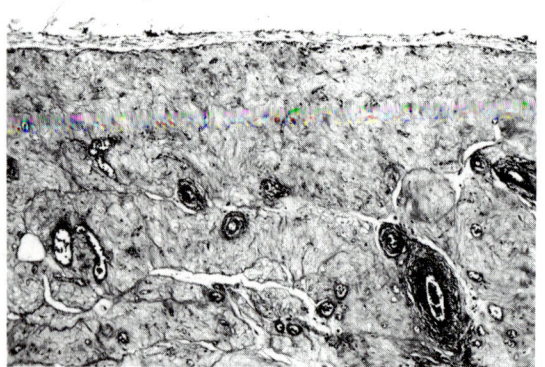

Fig. 31.1 (b)   Representative section of the tumour at 29 days after completion of pre-operative radiation therapy (5400 rad given in 27 fractions over 37 days). The tumour has been transformed into a gelatinous and almost an acellular mass. The blood vessels are thickened and sclerotic due to radiation (hematoxylin and eosin × 100).

ing and its correlation with survival (Castro *et al.*, 1973; Pritchard *et al.*, 1974; Stout, 1948; van der Werf-Messing and Unnik, 1965; Reszell *et al.*, 1966).

Although the available data (Russell *et al.*, 1977)

Staging

The Task Force on Soft Tissue Sarcomas of the American Joint Commission for Cancer Staging and End Result Reporting has established a staging system for soft tissue sarcomas which is an extension of the TNM system to include G for histological grade. Of these parameters, grade of tumour was considered the most important determinant of stage. The staging system is outlined in Table 31.2. Retrospective restaging of 702 cases according to this system showed good correlation

Table 31.2 Staging system for sarcoma of soft tissue (from Russell *et al.*, 1977).

	Stage	GTNM Parameters
Key	Stage IA	$G_1 T_1 N_0 M_0$
G: histopathological grade	IB	$G_1 T_2 N_0 M_0$
(1, 2 or 3)	Stage IIA	$G_2 T_1 N_0 M_0$
T: tumour size		
T_1, tumour < 5 cm in diameter	IIB	$G_2 T_2 N_0 M_0$
T_2, tumour > 5 cm in diameter	Stage IIIA	$G_3 T_1 N_0 M_0$
T_3, invasion of major vessels,	IIIB	$G_3 T_2 N_0 M_0$
nerves or bones	IIIC	$G_{1-3} T_{1-2} N_1 M_0$
N_1: biopsy proven metastases to		
regional lymph node(s)	Stage IVA	$G_{1-3} T_3 N_{0-1} M_0$
M_1: clinically evident distant	IVB	$G_{1-3} T_{1-3} N_{0-1} M_1$
metastases		

between stage and survival. It is essential that the meaning of tumour grade and stage be understood; furthermore, the close and effective collaboration between pathologists and clinicians experienced in soft tissue sarcomas should improve our knowledge of the natural history and response to the various treatment modalities.

Approaches to management of the primary lesion

Our goal in devising a management strategy for the patient with soft tissue sarcoma is the eradication of the primary lesion and any involved regional lymph nodes with a minimum cost in cosmetic and functional loss to the patient together with effective well tolerated treatment for occult metastatic tumour.

Surgery alone

Until some ten years ago, the only therapeutic modality which was accepted as offering a serious likelihood of cure of the patient with soft tissue sarcoma was surgery. The surgical technique commonly employed in the 1930s was simple excision. This was not, however, effective as shown by local recurrence rates of 70–95%. Techniques of radical resection were therefore developed and with these the local recurrence rate was drastically reduced i.e. to 20–30% (Cantin *et al.*, 1968; Martin *et al.*, 1965). During simple excision, the lesion is handled and visualized by the surgeon and all gross disease is removed. The technique of radical resection requires that the biopsy site be included in the surgical specimen and that there be wide margins of normal tissue in three dimensons around the tumour. The tumour should not be visualized during the proce-

dure. When this procedure has been performed and the surgical margins are proven by gross and histopathologic studies to be generous, i.e. > 2 cm, then very low rates of local recurrence may be expected, in the order of 15–20%. There are no published data relating local failure rate to histological grade for soft tissue sarcoma in surgically treated patients. The improvement in results by radical surgery documented above is impressive.

Rationale for combining radiation therapy and conservative surgery

However, radical resection may mean considerable functional loss or disfigurement, particularly if amputation is necessary. The rationale for combining radiation therapy with conservative surgery is that radiation in less than radical doses will eradicate the small number of tumour cells remaining after simple excision; i.e. those which would have been removed by a more radical surgical procedure. That is, radiation

Table 31.3 Radiation dose level (TDF) and local control of soft tissue carcinoma when treated by radiation alone.

Dose (TDF)	Tumour size	< 5	5–9	10–14	> 15
≥ 105		2/2	4/9	2/2	2/3
95–104					0/1
80–94			1/3	0/1	0/3
< 80			1/3	0/1	0/1

could be expected to provide at least the gain over simple surgery that radical surgery has been shown to have. Thus, a combined modality approach would employ surgery to remove the grossly evident tumour mass. This can be accomplished by simple excision in most situations. Moderately high radiation doses should then inactivate the small number of cells in the tissues adjacent to the obvious tumour, although generous fields would be needed to cover microscopic extension along tissue planes. An advantage of radiation therapy is the relative ease with which the treatment volume can be designed to include tissues suspected of involvement without concern for the position of nerve, vessels and tendons. Results from several clinical studies demonstrate that this approach is clinically practical, that survival results appear the equal of those obtained by radical surgery and superior cosmetic and functional results may be obtained. The sequel is devoted to a detailed consideration of how surgery and radiation therapy may be most effectively combined. However, there are patients in whom a lesion in an extremity has caused such extensive tissue destruction that a reasonable functional result cannot be expected; in such instances, prompt amputation is the most effective and practical approach.

Radiation therapy alone

Prior to the discussion of combined radiation therapy and surgery, it is useful to document that radiation therapy alone can be effective in achieving permanent cures of patients with soft tissue sarcomas. Our preference is to combine limited surgery with radiation, rather than using radiation alone. There are, however, patients who, for reasons of anatomic location, medical inoperability, or refusal of any surgery, are not candidates even for a conservative surgical procedure. Leucutia (1935) described one patient who had been treated by deep X-ray therapy for a recurrent fibrosarcoma of the scapula region and who was alive without tumour at ten years after therapy. In 1950, Sir Stanford Cade in his Presidential Address to the Royal Society of Medicine, described 22 patients who for a variety of reasons were treated by radiation therapy alone. Six survived for 5–26 years. A review of results of treatment of soft tissue sarcoma by radiation therapy alone was presented in 1963 by del Regato. Windeyer *et al.* (1966) described results of radiation treatment alone in fibrosarcomas; of 8 patients available for 5-year follow up, 4 were free of local disease, although 1 had required surgery for a recurrence. McNeer *et al.* reported in 1968 their analysis of the results of treatment of 653 patients with sarcomas of soft tissue treated at Memorial Hospital; 25 of the 653 patients had been treated by radiation therapy alone; 14 of the 25

were surviving at 5 years, and 8 of 20 were surviving at 10 years. Local control was achieved in 14 of the 25 patients. Analysis in August 1975 showed that of 18 patients treated at the M.D. Anderson Hospital, with radiation doses in excess of 6300 rad, local control had been achieved in 14 (Suit and Russell, 1977, 1979); the 4 local failures included 1 marginal failure. Of 11 patients who were Stage 1 and 2, 5 are known to have survived 65–168 months with control of the primary tumour.

At the Massachusetts General Hospital, radiation therapy alone has been employed in 21 primary sarcomas and 12 post-surgical recurrent sarcomas since 1970. Data for local control at 1–7 years after therapy are given in Table 31.3, and illustrate the dependence of local control on radiation dose. Local success was infrequent at TDF values of < 105 or approximately the equivalent of 6500 rad delivered as daily treatments of 200 rad, 5 treatments per week. In this group of patients, there was no convincing relationship between control rate and tumour size. However, the largest tumours in this series were treated with truly massive doses i.e. doses of 7000–8000 rad. The late tissue damage was considerable after such doses to large tumours. This approach is not recommended but may be used if surgery is out of the question. Nonetheless, an occasional patient may be salvaged. These data from several centres are convincing evidence that radiation therapy can be effective in the treatment of soft tissue sarcomas (see Fig 31.1 (*a*) for example). Despite this, we are of the opinion that the functional results are clearly superior when more moderate doses of radiation are given in combination with conservative surgery.

Sequence of radiation therapy and surgery

Although not proven by clinical trial, we suggest that radiation therapy is more effective if it precedes surgery. The relative advantages of pre-operative or post-operative radiation are listed below:

Pre-operative radiation therapy
1. Treatment volumes for radiation therapy administered prior to surgery are planned solely on the basis of known and likely extent of disease. In contrast, post-operative irradiation fields should include not only the site of the tumour, but also all tissues handled during the surgical procedure including the stab wound. Therefore, the treatment volume for post-operative radiation therapy will usually be larger than for pre-operative irradiation. This means that acute and late radiation reactions may be expected to be less severe in patients who receive radiation therapy pre-operatively because of the smaller treatment volume.

2. Radiation given pre-operatively reduces the number of viable tumour cells to such small absolute levels that the likelihood of viable cells being spilled into the wound or forced into the blood vascular space is drastically reduced. This should reduce the frequency of wound recurrence and of distant metastasis.

3. Initiation of radiation therapy is not delayed. Where radiation therapy is given post-operatively, delays of 10–14 days or even longer may occur before the treatment is started. This means that residual tumour has an opportunity to grow. Where wound healing delays treatment further, recurrent tumour may be grossly evident at the time of initiation of irradiation (especially where surgery was grossly incomplete and the lesion was of the high grade).

4. At the time of surgery, the tumour is observed to be smaller and usually is surrounded by a relatively dense pseudocapsule. This means that a more conservative approach is feasible. In addition, a lesion previously considered inoperable may regress to such an extent that it becomes operable.

5. If the surgical procedure is conservative, there is seldom a problem in wound healing following the usual radiation dose levels of 5600 rad in 5.5 weeks given at approximately 200 rad per fraction and 5 fractions per week.

6. Histological examination of the surgical specimen usually reveals only a few foci of tumour cells or, not infrequently, intact tumour cells cannot be identified.

Post-operative irradiation

1. The histopathological diagnosis and grade of tumour can be judged on the basis of examination of tissue samples taken from several regions of the tumour rather than on the smaller incisional biopsy specimen.

2. Surgery is immediate.

3. There is no delay in wound healing caused by prior radiation therapy.

4. Post-operative radiation therapy is the only feasible sequence for those lesions which are small and are readily removed by excisional biopsy. This is a relatively common situation as small sarcomas are frequently judged to be benign and are removed by simple excision by the local physician.

Radiation therapy treatment planning

The principal goal in treatment planning is the definition of the target volume and then the determination of the portal arrangements, portal weighting, and beam characteristics which yield the treatment volume most closely approaching the target volume. The target volume is that volume of tissue which is 1. known to contain tumour, and 2. which is judged to have a significant probability of involvement by tumour. Specification of these two volumes will be based upon analysis of the details of the clinical history, the findings on physical examination, histopathologic characteristics and grade of the tumour, the nature of prior surgery, and interpretation of the various radiographic procedures (standard X-rays, xerograms, arteriograms, lymphangiograms, and CT-scan studies). The radiation therapist is usually better informed if he examines the histopathologic material with the pathologist. Similarly, if there has been prior surgery, treatment planning may be facilitated by discussing the operative findings with the surgeon. In order to appreciate the target volume three dimensionally, contours at appropriate levels through the affected region are prepared and the anatomic structures are drawn on each contour. Alternatively, CT scans may be used.

After study of the defined target volume, the radiation therapist, working in conjunction with the radiation biophysicist, assesses which of the various treatment modalities either used alone or in combination will produce the most attractive treatment volume. The possibility of using more than one treatment modality should be considered, e.g. external beam photons or electron beam, interstitial therapy, intraoperative electron beam with surgery, etc. A valuable point to keep in mind in planning treatment is that there may indeed be a failure (recurrence or necrosis) which would require subsequent radical or amputative surgery. The treatment plan should, if feasible, allow for this with careful consideration of the sites of flaps and incision. The treatment plans should feature a uniform distribution of radiation dose throughout the treatment volume with a range in dose which does not exceed ± 5.0% of the central tumour dose. Every possible technical effort should be made to minimize the treatment volume. Where appropriate, the treatment plan should include the use of wedge filters, compensating filters, patient immobilization devices, side lights, tattoo marks, secondary collimation (cerrobend cut-outs), etc. The tattoo marks are placed, whenever possible, on skin that is relatively fixed, e.g. over the anterior iliac crest, over the greater trochanter etc. An example of a patient immobilization device is shown in Fig. 31.2. Here, the leg is rigidly locked into position so that there is virtually no motion during the course of an individual treatment and there is great precision in repositioning of the patient extremity from treatment session to treatment session. To increase the reproducibility of the set up, the position of the patient's head, arms and legs should be comfortable and the position stipulated either by diagrams or photographs. In general terms, for patients in a supine

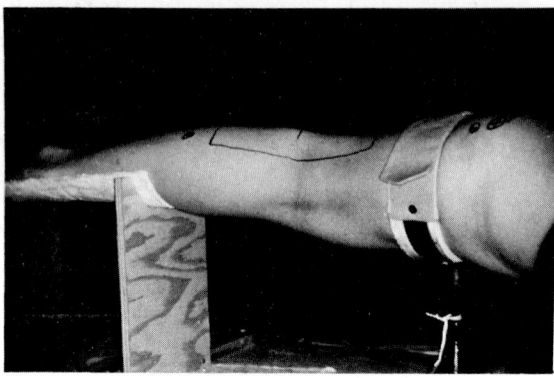

Fig. 31.2 This photograph shows an example of an immobilization system employed in radiation therapy of a lesion in the lateral knee region. Here, an extremely tight immobilization was achieved. Treatment was administered by a pair of anterior and posterior oblique wedge fields.

position, the head should be straight, arms by the side, heels together, toes falling apart; patient position is checked to make sure that the midline of the patient is parallel to the long axis of the couch. Because of the emphasis on obtaining minimum treatment volume, the portal will often be irregular in contour. This is greatly facilitated by using cerrobend cut-outs.

After the patient's position has been secured, attention should be paid to the presence of skin folds in the entry area, e.g. the inguinal area, natal cleft, etc. Masking tape may be applied and then the skin folds pulled back (the tape should not be applied over skin to be irradiated). In determining the treatment plan a simulator is of great practical value. Where a simulator is not available, the actual treatment plan used must be confirmed by study of portal films taken in position on the treatment machine. The points being made are intended to encourage a technical effort comparable with that made in treatment of head and neck tumours, Hodgkin's disease etc. Treatment planning for soft tissue sarcomas has not generally received a high technical effort. Such efforts are handsomely rewarded by improved functional results.

Radiation dose level

This must be substantial if there is to be a high frequency of permanent eradication of disease. In our own experience, low doses are generally ineffective, even for achieving partial regressions. Our general approach has been to irradiate in 5 fractions per week giving 180–200 rad per fraction, using all fields on each treatment day for the first 5000 rad. During this component of the treatment, a bolus is applied over the biopsy or surgical scar (the bolus is usually 1–2 cm wide and thick enough to achieve approximately a 90% dose level on the skin). The treatment volume for this portion of the treatment includes all tissues known to be involved by tumour plus any surrounding tissue that may possibly be infiltrated. At the 5000 rad point the treatment volume is reduced so as to cover areas of known involvement. Where radiation therapy alone is used, the dose is then carried to approximately 7500 rad, usually with one additional field reduction at the 6500 rad level. For patients treated post-operatively, the dose should be approximately equal to 6600 rad if the resection was grossly complete, and approximately equal to 7000 rad, if there was macroscopic residual disease. The treatment, of course, should not be started until the scar is well healed. For patients treated pre-operatively, the radiation dose should be 5600 rad followed by supplemental radiation, given either at the time of surgery (interstitial technique or intraoperative electron beam therapy) or by subsequent external beam technique, with the total dose being 6500–7000 rad. Where interstitial therapy is employed, a convenient approach is to insert thin plastic tubes (e.g. angiocaths) into the tumour bed under direct vision. The radioactive material (e.g. iridium-192) need not be inserted until some 3–4 days later when wound healing is well under way.

Efficacy of radiation therapy in the treatment of patients with soft tissue sarcoma

Pre-operative radiation therapy

We consider that the most efficacious combination of radiation therapy and surgery is pre-operative radiotherapy (approximately equal to 5600 rad/5–6 weeks) followed in approximately 3 weeks by conservative resection (removing minimal or no normal tissue around the partially regressed mass) and then followed by a supplemental dose to the tumour bed. To date we have treated 17 patients by this strategy, all more than 12 months ago. Results in terms of local control and continuous disease free survival are given in Table 31.4. In most of these patients, the primary lesion regressed partially and at surgery was surrounded by a connective tissue shell in nearly all instances. The resection was essentially straightforward in 15 patients (complete removal of the gross disease). For these, local control has been achieved in all instances. However, distant metastases have developed in 3 patients with stage IIIB disease. There were 2 patients in whom resection was grossly incomplete and local control was achieved in only one of these patients; both have developed distant metas-

Table 31.4 Sarcoma of soft tissue treated by radiation therapy followed by conservative resection.

Resection of residual mass		
Stage	Local control	Disease-free survival
IB	3/3	3/3
IIB	4/4	4/4
IIIA	1/1	1/1
IIIB	7/7	4/7
Resection attempted but not completed		
IIIB	1/2	0/2

Table 31.5 Local control and disease-free survival in 100 patients with sarcoma of soft tissue (M.D. Anderson Hospital).

Stage	Local control* (for > 24–130 months)	Disease-free survival at > 40 months
IA	12/12	11/12
IB	8/9	7/11
IIA	20/26	16/27
IIB	14/19	7/26
IIIA	5/5	3/8
IIIB	4/8	2/16
Total	63/79 (80%)	46/100

* Patients dying at less than 24 months with local control are excluded from the analysis of local control.

tases. Technical problems accounting for incomplete removal in these 2 patients were: 1. an extraosseous osteosarcoma in the anticubital space; the median nerve was completely encased in tumour; 2. a malignant fibrohistiocytoma of the buttock which was found to extend through the sciatic notch into the pelvis. An additional 3 patients have been treated pre-amputation (1 patient each IB, IIB and IIIB). Local control was achieved in all 3; unfortunately, all have died of metastatic tumour at 8, 17 and 33 months.

Atkinson *et al.* reported in 1963 on 15 patients with operable sarcoma of soft tissue who were treated by pre-operative radiation therapy (4500 rad in 4–5 weeks) followed 4–6 weeks later by block resection. The tumours were 4–20 cm in size; 10 were recurrent lesions. There has been 1 local failure and no distant metastases in these patients. Median follow up was 3 years, 5 months. In the same clinic block resections were performed on 54 patients with 'comparable lesions', there have been 40 local recurrences. Seven patients developed distant metastases (some with local recurrence). These groups were not strictly comparable. Martin *et al.* (1977) have reported on 10 patients treated at M.D. Anderson Hospital by pre-operative irradiation and resection. There have been no local recurrences (though two have developed distant metastasis). In summary, although limited, experience with pre-operative radiation therapy appears highly promising in treatment of larger lesions.

Post-operative radiation therapy

There is considerable experience in the treatment of patients post-operatively for both primary and recurrent soft tissue sarcomas. The local control and disease-free survival for 100 patients at >40 months after treatment at M.D. Anderson Hospital are presented in Table 31.5 (Suit and Russell, 1977). As

shown by these data, local control was regularly achieved for the Grade I sarcomas (20/21) and in a high frequency for the small lesions (37/43 or 86%). Achievement of local control was less common in the larger and higher grade sarcomas: 18/27 (66%) for IIB and IIIB. Disease-free survival decreased rapidly with stage: 92% for IA to 12% for IIIB. For the higher grade lesions there is a clear need for development of effective treatment for occult metastatic disease.

We present an illustrative case of a patient who has done well following local excision for a small sarcoma and post-operative radiation therapy. Mr. A.R. is a 49-year old white male who was seen in 1967 following excisional biopsy of a 3-cm sub-cutaneous mass overlying the left lateral malleolus. Histopathologically, the tumour was interpreted as being a synovial sarcoma (biphasic pattern), Grade 1. The stage was therefore IA. He declined the recommended amputation and requested a radiation therapy consultation. The appearance of the ankle at 11 years after radical dose radiation therapy is presented in Fig. 31.3. He is free of pain and oedema and has a normal gait. During the past 11 years he has experienced three episodes of painful swelling secondary to insect bites; these were treated conservatively with antibiotics (but avoidance of hot soaks etc.). Radiographically there are changes of minimal radiation osteitis. This is a fair example of the result which may be expected in the treatment of small lesions.

A major problem remains; what is an effective treatment of a patient who is referred after simple excision of a large high grade (2 or 3) lesion? In a number of instances we have recommended further resection followed by radiation therapy. Functional status is decreased modestly by the additional surgery but the impression is that local control rates are higher.

Table 31.6 Complete and partial response rates following various chemotherapy regimes in patients with locally advanced and/or metastatic sarcoma of soft tissue.

Regime			No. evaluable patients	Responses CR + PR (%)	References
CYVADIC			118	59	Gottlieb et al. (1975)
Cyclophosphamide	500 mg/m²		193	52	
Vincristine	1.4 mg/m²	} day 1	60	37	Pinedo et al. (1979a)
Adriamycin	50 mg/m²		15*	'74'	Rodriguez (1977)
DTIC	250 mg/m²	day 1–5	12	'59'	
repeat every 3–4 weeks			20	15	Giuliano et al. (1978)
CYVADACT					
as above except replace DTIC with					
actinomycin D	0.3 mg/m²	days 3–5	199	40	
ACM					
Adriamycin	60 mg/m²				
Cyclophosphamide	600 mg/m²	} day 1	100	36	Lowenbraun et al. (1977)
Methotrexate	25 mg/m²				
repeat every 3 weeks					
STS-1					
Adriamycin	60 mg/m²	day 1			
DTIC	250 mg/m²	days 1 and 2	22	41	
Methotrexate +	50 mg/m²	IV infusion			Subramanian and
folinic acid rescue	over 12–24 hours	days 1			Wiltshaw (1978)
repeat every 3 weeks					
AMe					
Adriamycin	60 mg/m²	day 1 – 45 mg/m² day 22			
MeCCNU	150 mg/m² orally		53	39	Rivkin et al. (1978)
repeat every 6 weeks					

* protected environment, prophylactic antibiotics, escalating doses of adriamycin and cyclophosphamide.

obtained (Benjamin et al., 1974). Methotrexate (Subramanian and Wiltshaw, 1978) and DTIC (Gottlieb et al., 1976) have activity as single agents giving response rates of 36% (15/41 patients) and 16% (10/61) patients respectively. Cyclophosphamide, actinomycin D and vincristine, although active in childhood sarcomas, have not been adequately tested in adults. However, as single agent chemotherapy did not produce any significant prolongation in survival, various multiagent chemotherapy protocols have been investigated.

The most extensively studied drug combination in the treatment of soft tissue sarcoma is CYVADIC (see Table 31.6). This was first described by the South West Oncology Group (Gottlieb et al., 1975) and CYVADIC I produced 18 complete remissions (15%) and 52 (44%) partial remissions in 118 patients. Median survival was 13 months; this was better than the six month median survival time for adriamycin alone. Experience with a later protocol, CYVADIC II has been less good, yielding overall response rates of 52% (SWOG), 37% (60 patients; EORTC; Pinedo et al., 1979b), and 15% (20 patients; Guillano et al., 1978). Another South West Oncology Group protocol

substituted DTIC by actinomycin D (CYVADACT) and achieved an overall 40% response rate.

Other useful combinations are adriamycin, cyclophosphamide and methotrexate (Lowenbraun et al., 1977); methyl CCNU and adriamycin (Rivkin et al., 1978); adriamycin, DTIC and methotrexate (Subramanian and Wiltshaw, 1978); results of which are summarized in Table 31.6. Vincristine, actinomycin D and cyclophosphamide (VAC) although highly effective in childhood rhabdomyosarcoma, show little activity against adult sarcomas (Rosenbaum and Schoenfeld, 1977; Creagan et al., 1976).

In most instances, patients with widespread metastatic disease will be treated by chemotherapy, using radiotherapy and/or surgery to palliate painful or rapidly enlarging local lesions. However, a single metastatic lesion may be amenable to radical resection or radiation therapy.

Pulmonary surgery

Evidence is now available that resection of pulmonary metastases may be worthwhile in selected patients. In one study, resection of all visible tumour was possible in 86 of 102 patients with pulmonary metastases from sarcomas, and overall 5-year survival was 26% (Martini *et al.*, 1974). In another series of 40 patients, pulmonary lesions were completely resectable in 34 and 5-year survival was 33.8% (Feldman and Kyriakos, 1972). Factors such as disease-free interval (time elapsing between resection of the primary tumour and appearance of pulmonary metastases) and tumour doubling time (calculated from measurements of the diameter of pulmonary nodules seen on serial chest X-rays) seem to influence prognosis and certain criteria for selection of patients for surgery have been suggested (Joseph, 1974); 1. control of the primary tumour has been achieved; 2. there is no evidence of extrapulmonary metastases; 3. pulmonary lesions should be resectable; multiple lesions are not a contraindication but if extensive multiple resections are necessary, the failure rate rises; 4. the patient should be fit for surgery as regards general condition and respiratory status; 5. tumour doubling time should be > 40 days.

Desmoid tumours

Desmoid tumours are locally aggressive lesions which do not metastasize. If uncontrolled, they infiltrate adjacent tissues and structures in a relentless and progressive manner; ultimately, such growth involves a critical structure(s) and causes death. Therefore, these tumours must be treated with great respect and effective treatment implemented early. Histopathologic features of these lesions are: an almost purely fibroblastic appearance (comprised almost entirely of collagen and normal appearing fibroblasts); a low incidence of mitotic figures; infiltration of adjacent tissues (there is no pseudocapsule). Metastases from desmoid tumours are presently unknown. There are, however, instances where a lesion has been diagnosed as a desmoid tumour but later in the evolution of the disease during multiple recurrences, the histological character alters to that of a true fibrosarcoma. Aetiology of desmoid tumours is not established. Trauma often precedes clinical manifestations of these lesions. Desmoid tumours were first reported occurring in the anterior abdominal wall of females in the post-partum period. Subsequently, however, they have been shown to occur at virtually all anatomic sites in both sexes and at any age. They may develop in operative wounds (as did two in our series). Fortunately, most of the desmoid tumours arise where a radical resection can be performed. This is the preferred treatment and should be implemented if at all possible. A proportion of the lesions, however, arise at sites where radical resection is not feasible or if attempted, would be associated with major morbidity or mutilation. In such patients, radiation therapy may be effective given alone or in combination with localized surgery.

Several groups have demonstrated that radiation therapy may yield long-term local control in a high proportion of cases (Wara, 1977; Benninghoff and Robbins, 1964; Suit and Russell, 1975). The clinician needs to appreciate that desmoid tumours regress quite slowly even after successful radiation therapy. Thus, although the tumour will ultimately regress completely and permanently, this may require one or two years. Such a slow regression is not surprising in view of the very small cellular content, i.e. the tumour is almost entirely stromal. Accordingly, both the clinician and the patient need to exercise patience. This is not a problem provided the nature of the lesion and its response to radiation therapy has been explained to the patient. Clearly, the goal is permanent control and the pattern of local response is not of great import as long as it is understood.

At the Massachussets General Hospital, ten patients with desmoid tumours have now been treated by radiation therapy and have been followed for more than one year. Seven of these were irradiated for extensive gross disease and three were treated following incomplete surgical resection, i.e. surgical margins were positive or there was gross tumour left in the operative wound, although the tumour was not palpable at the initiation of treatment. The radiation dose level has been 5500 rad to 7000 rad in 6–8 weeks. Tumour regression occurred in all seven of the patients with palpable disease at the time of treatment and six of these remain free of evident local disease or complications. There has been one local failure, this occurred at 1.5 years after treatment to 5500 rad of a 9-year old boy who presented with extensive recurrent disease (after multiple surgical procedures). There were multiple discrete nodules in the neck extending to the submental region to the suprasternal notch. Because of the age of the patient, the radiation dose was kept at a modest level.

We would like to present the case of a relatively typical response in one of the six patients who have been treated successfully for gross disease. This patient is a 27-year old female who presented with a very large tumour in the anterior abdominal wall in the postpartum period. The CT-scan presented in Fig. 31.4 demonstrates that the lesion was quite extensive. It measured 17 cm from superior to inferior; and, as shown, the mass extended far posteriorly into the pelvis. This was considered to be non-resectable. The patient was treated with a full course of radiation therapy: 6100 rad delivered in 34 fractions over 74 days. The extent of regression at 15 months is shown by comparing the CT-scans shown in Fig. 4 (*a* and *b*). At present the patient is 30 months post-treatment and

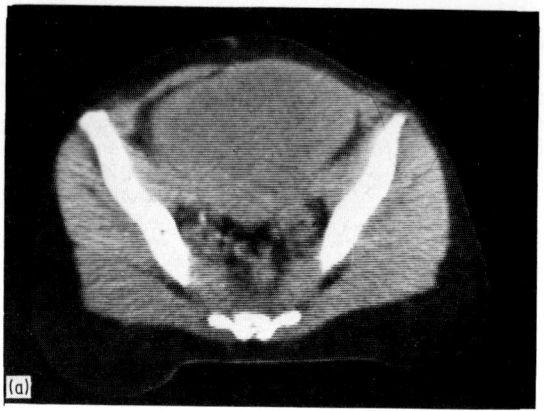

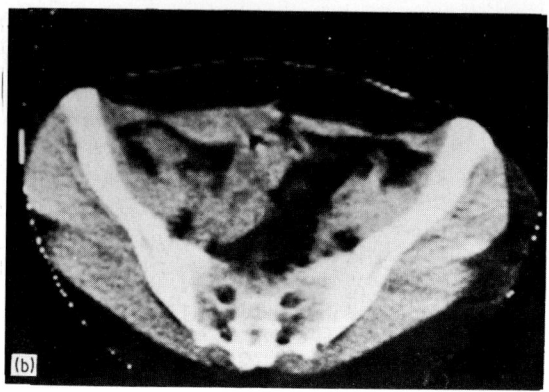

Fig. 31.4 (*a,b*) These CT-scans demonstrate the extent of a massive desmoid tumor of the anterior abdominal wall in a 27-year old female (post-partum) and the degree of regression at 15 months following radiation therapy (6100 rad, 34 fractions over a total time of 74 days). At 30 months there is no clinical evidence of residual disease and the patient is free of abdominal wall or pelvic symptoms.

there is no clinically evident residual tumour. She is free of symptoms and is leading a normal life.

Of the three patients who were treated for incompletely resected tumour, all three are alive without evidence of disease and without complications. These results support fully the experience at the M.D. Anderson Hospital (Suit and Russell, 1975). Wara *et al.* of the University of California, San Francisco, reported in 1977 on a series of 16 patients treated by radiation therapy; 13 of 16 were free of evidence of disease at the time of report. This is further supported by the 1964 paper of Benninghoff and Robbins describing results from Philadelphia.

In summary, the available data clearly warrants the acceptance of high dose precision radiation therapy as an effective modality in the treatment of desmoid tumours and one that can be employed in those situations where radical surgery is not feasible or acceptable. We are not, however, recommending that radiation therapy replace surgery if surgery is possible.

Further reading

Cade, S. (1951), Soft tissue tumours: their natural history and treatment. Section of surgery: president's address. *Proc. Roy. Soc. Med.*, **44**, 19–36.

Enzinger, F.M., Lattes, R., Torloni, H. (1969), International Histological Classification of Tumours. No.3: Histological Typing of Soft Tissue Tumours. World Health Organisation.

References

Atkinson, L., Garvan, J.M. and Newton, N.C. (1963), Behavior and management of soft connective tissue sarcomas. *Cancer*, **16**, 1552–62.

Benjamin, R.S., Wiernick, P.H. and Bachur, N.R. (1974), Adriamycin chemotherapy – efficacy, safety and pharmacologic basis of an intermittent single high-dosage schedule. *Cancer*, **33**, 19–27.

Benjamin, R.S. *et al.* (1976), Cyvadic vs. Cyvadact: a randomised trial of Cyclophosphamide, Vincristine and Adriamycin + DTIC or Actinomycin D in metastatic sarcomas. *Proc. Am. Ass. Cancer Res.*, **17**, 256.

Benninghoff, D. and Robbins, R. (1964), The nature and treatment of desmoid tumors. *Am. J. Roentg.*, **91**, 132–7.

Blum, R.H. (1975), An overview of studies with Adriamycin (NSC-123127) in the United States. *Cancer Chemother. Rep.*, **6**, 247–51.

Cancer Statistics (1979), *Ca-A Cancer Journal for Clinicians*, **29**(1), 6–7.

Cantin, J. *et al.* (1968), The problem of local recurrence after treatment of soft tissue sarcoma. *Ann. Surg.*, **168**, 47–53.

Castro, E.G., Hajdu, S.I. and Fortner, J.G. (1973), Surgical therapy of fibrosarcoma of extremities. *Archs Surg.*, **107**, 284–6.

Creagan, E.T. *et al.* (1976), A comparative clinical trial evaluating the combination of Adriamycin, DTIC and Vincristine, the combination of Actinomycin D, Cyclophosphamide and Vincristine, and a single agent, Methyl-CCNU, in advanced sarcomas. *Cancer Treat. Rep.*, **60**, 1385–7.

D'Angio, G.J. and Evans, A. (1975), Soft tissue sarcomas. In: *Cancer in Children*, (eds H.J.G. Bloom *et al.*) Springer-Verlag, Berlin, Heidelberg and New York, pp.217–41.

Del Regato, J. (1963), Radiotherapy of soft tissue sarcomas. *J. Am. Med. Assoc.*, **185**, 216–8.

Feldman, P.S. and Kyriakos, M. (1972), Pulmonary resection for metastatic sarcoma. *J. Thorac. Cardiovasc. Surg.*, **64**, 784–99.

Fraumeni, J.F. (1973), Genetic factors in the etiology of cancer. In: *Cancer Medicine*. (eds J.F. Holland and E.M. Frei), Lea & Febiger, Philadelphia, Pennsylvania, pp. 7–15.

Guillano, A.E. *et al.* (1978), Failure of combination chemotherapy (CYVADIC) in metastatic soft tissue sarcomas: implications for adjuvant studies. *Proc. Am. Soc. Clin. Onc.*, **19**, 359.

Gottlieb, J.A. *et al.* (1975), Adriamycin (NSC-123127) used alone and in combination for soft tissue and bone sarcomas. *Cancer Chemother. Rep.*, **6**, Pt. 3, 271–82.

Gottleib, J.A. *et al.* (1976), Role of DTIC (NSC-45388) in the chemotherapy of sarcomas. *Cancer Treat. Rep.*, **60**, 199–203.

Harris, J.E. and Sinkovics, J.G. (1976), Immunology and immunotherapy of human tumors. In: *The Immunology of Malignant Disease*, C.V. Mosby Co., St. Louis, Missouri, pp.411–29.

Hatfield, P.M. and Schulz, M.D. (1970), Post irradiation sarcoma: including 5 cases after x-ray therapy for breast carcinoma. *Radiology*, **96**, 593–602.

Jensen, R.D. and Miller, R.W. (1971), Retinoblastoma: epidemiologic characteristics. *New. Engl. J. Med.*, **285**, 307.

Joseph, W.L. (1974), Criteria for resection of sarcoma metastatic to the lung. *Cancer Chemother. Rep.*, **58**, 285–90.

Kim, J.H. *et al.* (1978), Radiation induced soft tissue sarcoma and bone sarcoma. *Radiology*, **129**, 501–8.

Krementz, E.T. *et al.* (1977), Chemotherapy of sarcomas of the limbs by regional perfusion. *Ann. Surg.*, **185**, 555–64.

Leucutia, T. (1935), Radiotherapy of sarcoma of the soft parts. *Radiology*, **25**, 403–15.

Lindberg, R.D. *et al.* (1977), Adjuvant chemotherapy in the treatment of primary soft tissue sarcomas: a preliminary report. In: *Management of Primary Bone and Soft Tissue Tumors*. Year Book Medical Publishers Inc., Chicago, Illinois, pp.343–52.

Lowenbraun, S. *et al.* (1977), Combination chemotherapy with Adriamycin, Cyclophosphamide and Methotrexate (ACM) in metastatic sarcomas. *Proc. Am. Soc. Clin. Onc.*, **18**, 286.

Martin, R.G., Butler, J.J. and Albores-Saavedra, J. (1965), Soft tissue tumors – surgical treatment and results. In: *Tumors of Bone and Soft Tissue*. Year Book Medical Publishers Inc., Chicago, Illinois, pp.333–48.

Martin, R.G., Lindberg, R.D. and Russell, W.O. (1977), Preoperative radiotherapy and surgery in the management of soft tissue sarcoma. In: *Management of Primary Bone and Soft Tissue Tumors*. Year Book Medical Publishers Inc., Chicago, Illinois. pp.299–307.

Martini, N. *et al.* (1974), Surgical treatment of metastatic sarcoma to the lung. *Surg. Clinics. N. Amer.*, **54**, 841–8.

McAdam, W.A.F. and Goligher, J.C. (1970), The occurrence of desmoids in patients with familial polyposis coli. *Br. J. Surg.*, **57**, 618–31.

McNeer, G.P. *et al.* (1968), Effectiveness of radiation therapy in management of sarcoma of soft somatic tissues. *Cancer*, **22**, 391–7.

Moberger, G., Nilsonn, U. and Friberg, S. (1968), Synovial sarcoma. Histological features and prognosis. *Acta Orthop. Scand.*, Suppl. No. 111.

Neifeld, J.P., Michaelis, L.L. and Doppman, J.L. (1977), Suspected pulmonary metastasis: correlation of chest x-ray, whole lung tomograms and operative findings. *Cancer*, **39**, 383–7.

Pinedo, H.M. *et al.* (1979a), Re-evaluation of the CYVADIC regimen for metastatic soft tissue sarcoma. *Proc. Am. Soc. Clin. Onc.*, **20**, 346.

Pinedo, H.M. *et al.* (1979b), Evaluation of adjuvant therapy in soft tissue sarcoma: a collaborative multi-disciplinary approach (EORTC protocol 62771). *Eur. J. Cancer*, **15**, 811–20.

Pritchard, R.J. *et al.* (1974), Fibrosarcoma – clinical and statistical study of 199 tumors of soft tissue of the extremities and trunk. *Cancer*, **33**, 888–97. *Proc. Am. Soc. Clin. Oncol.*, **18**, 320.

Reszell, P.A., Soule, E.H. and Coventry, M.B. (1966), Liposarcoma of the extremities and limb-girdles. A study of 222 cases. *J. Bone Jt. Surg.*, **48**, 229–44.

Rivkin, S. *et al.* (1978), Methyl CCNU-Adriamycin in metastatic sarcomas. *Proc. Am. Soc. Clin. Onc.*, **19**, 331.

Rodriguez, V., Bodey, G.P. and Freireich, E.J. (1977), Increased remission rate and prolongation of survival in patients with soft tissue sarcomas treated with intensive chemotherapy on a protected environment – prophylactic antibiotic programme (PEPA).

Rosenbaum, C. and Schoenfeld, D. (1977), Treatment of advanced soft tissue sarcoma. *Proc. Am. Soc. Clin. Onc.*, **18**, 287.

Rosenberg, S.A. *et al.* (1978), Prospective randomised evaluation of the role of limb sparing surgery, radiation therapy and adjuvant chemotherapy in the treatment of adult soft tissue sarcomas. *Surgery*, **84**, 62.

Russell, W.O. *et al.* (1977), A clinical and pathological staging system for soft tissue sarcomas. *Cancer*, **40**, 1562–70.

Schanner, E.G. *et al.* (1978), Comparison of computed

and conventional whole lung tomography in detecting pulmonary nodules: a prospective radiologic-pathologic study. *Am. J. Roentg.*, **131**, 51–4.

Simon, M.A. and Enneking, W.F. (1976), The management of soft tissue sarcomas of the extremities. *J. Bone Jt. Surg.*, **58A**, 317–27.

Sordillo, P. *et al.* (1978), Adjuvant chemotherapy of adult soft part sarcomas with 'ALOMAD'. *Proc. Am. Soc. Clin. Onc.*, **19**, 353.

Stout, A.P. (1948), Fibrosarcoma. *Cancer*, **1**, 30–63.

Strong, L.C. (1977), Genetic considerations in pediatric oncology. In: *Clinical Pediatric Oncology.* (eds W.W. Sutow *et al.*) C.V. Mosby Co., St. Louis, Missouri, pp.16–32.

Subramanian, S. and Wiltshaw, E. (1978), Chemotherapy of sarcoma. *Lancet*, **i**, 683–6.

Suit, H.D. and Proppe, K.H. (1979), Radiation therapy of soft tissue tumors. Presented at International Cancer Congress, Buenos Aires, Argentina.

Suit, H.D. and Russell, W.O. (1975), Radiation therapy of soft tissue sarcomas. *Cancer*, **36**, 759–64.

Suit, H.D. and Russell, W.O. (1977), Soft part tumors. *Cancer,* **39**, 830–6.

Suit, H.D. and Russell, W.O. (1979), Unpublished data.

Suit, H.D., Russell, W.O. and Martin, R.G. (1975), Sarcoma of soft tissue: clinical and histopathologic parameters and response to treatment. *Cancer*, **35**, 1478–83.

Townsend, C.M., Eilber, F.R. and Morton, D.L. (1976), Skeletal and soft tissue sarcomas: results of surgical adjuvant chemotherapy. *Proc. Am. Ass. Cancer Res.*, **17**, 265.

Van der Werf-Messing, B. and Unnik, J.A.M. (1965), Fibrosarcoma of the soft tissues. A clinicopathologic study. *Cancer*, **18**, 1113–23.

Weiss, S.W. and Enzinger, F.M. (1978), Malignant fibrous histiocytoma. *Cancer*, **41**, 2250–66.

Windeyer, B., Dische, S. and Mansfield, C.M. (1966), The place of radiotherapy in the management of fibrosarcoma of the soft tissues. *Clin. Radiol.*, **17**, 32–40.

32 Bone, cartilage and synovium

C.S.B. Galasko,
Haydn Bush and M.L. Sutton

Although the skeleton is one of the commonest sites of metastatic disease, primary bone tumours are rare and account for approximately 1–1.5% of all deaths from malignant disease.

The aetiology of these tumours is not well understood. Certain oncogenic animal viruses have been implicated (Reilly *et al.*, 1972; Miller *et al.*, 1976) but there is little data demonstrating a causal relationship with human primary malignant bone tumours. There are a number of well recognized predisposing causes: fibrous dysplasia, Paget's disease, osteochondroma and irradiation.

The site of the tumour is important as it affects the prognosis and this will be discussed under the different tumours.

The majority of patients with primary malignant bone tumours die from pulmonary metastases and it has always been said that the primary spread is via the blood stream; but lymphatic spread does occur. For example, at the Christie Hospital, England, 10% of patients with osteosarcoma of the lower limbs have inguinal lymph node involvement. There are no data as to whether the initial spread is via the lymphatics or the blood stream.

The classification of bone tumours is confusing. There has been failure to agree upon a generally acceptable terminology and classification, although recently the World Health Organization has established a Tumour Panel which has produced a workable classification (Schajowicz *et al.*, 1972) which is under continuous revision. The main difficulty is that localized overgrowths of bone, cartilage or fibrous tissue may develop in response to injury, infection or as a result of maldevelopment or hormonal disturbance. Because these lesions present as swellings, they have been described as tumours although they are not neoplasms in the true meaning of the word. They are prob-ably best considered as tumorous conditions of bone and, as such, will not be described in this chapter.

Even when the classification has been agreed upon, it is often difficult to diagnose or classify a particular tumour and this has led to the establishment of Bone Tumour Registries. Unfortunately, the majority of these Registries tend to classify the tumours retrospectively. What is needed are National and Regional Bone Tumour Panels consisting of expert bone tumour pathologists, radiologists, oncologists and orthopaedic surgeons who will be prepared to give a working diagnosis and advice about treatment for an individual patient and at short notice. The definitive diagnosis depends on a combination of the clinical, radiological and histological findings. In comparing different therapeutic regimens, the results obtained in different units or the results obtained at different periods in the same unit, it is essential to compare like with like, i.e. the tissue diagnosis and the staging must be the same and the techniques used standardized.

Gilchrist and his colleagues (1978) and Taylor *et al.*, (1978) have shown that in their unit the survival rates for osteosarcoma improved in succeeding periods without changing the treatment. It is for this reason that the results obtained in studies which rely on comparing a new method of treatment with an historical, retrospective group should be viewed with great caution. Only properly controlled trials can give totally reliable results. This is one of the reasons why the management of bone tumours, particularly the rare tumours, should be centralized in special units which then will deal with larger numbers. It is only in this way that we can hope to improve our knowledge of these tumours and their treatment and prognosis.

Bone consists not only of cells concerned with the formation and maintenance of bone but of many other elements as well: haemopoietic tissue, fat, nerves,

Table 32.1 Classification of bone tumours.

		Benign	Malignant
1.	Bone-forming tumours	Osteoma Osteoid osteoma Osteoblastoma	Osteosarcoma Parosteal (juxtacortical) osteosarcoma

2.	Cartilage-forming tumours	Enchondroma
		Ecchondroma
		Osteochondroma
		  (cartilage capped
		  exostosis)
		Chondroblastoma
		Chondromyxoid fibroma
			Chondrosarcoma
			Juxtacortical
			  chondrosarcoma
			Mesenchymal
			  chondrosarcoma

3.	Giant cell tumour (osteoclastoma)	Giant cell tumour*	Giant cell tumour*
4.	Connective tissue tumours	Desmoplastic fibroma Lipoma	Fibrosarcoma Liposarcoma Mesenchymoma Undifferentiated sarcoma

5.	Marrow tumours		Ewing's sarcoma
			Reticulum cell sarcoma
			  (reticulosarcoma of
			  bone)
			Lymphosarcoma of bone
			Myeloma

6.	Vascular tumours	Haemangioma Lymphangioma Haemangioendothelioma* Haemangiopericytoma*	Angiosarcoma Haemangioendothelioma* Haemangiopericytoma*
7.	Histiocytic reticuloendothelioses†	Eosinophilic granuloma Hand-Schuller Christian	Letterer-Siwe
8.	Tumours of synovium	Synovioma (benign synovioma)	Synovial sarcoma
9.	Miscellaneous tumours	Neurilemmoma Neurofibroma	Chordoma Adamantinoma of long bones

10.	Tumour-like lesions	Solitary bone cysts
		Aneurysmal bone cyst
		Non-ossifying fibroma
		  (metaphyseal fibrous
		  defect)
		Fibrous dysplasia	

* These tumours should probably be classified as intermediate or indeterminate as they tend to be locally
  aggressive and recur but usually do not metastasize until late
† Discussed under Children's Tumours

blood vessels, etc.; tumours can develop from these structures as well as from the bone forming elements and, therefore, all these tumours should be included in a working classification (Table 32.1).

Table 32.2 shows the relative incidence of the malignant bone tumours. It is not possible to give the ratio between the numbers of malignant and benign tumours. Malignant tumours are often referred to special centres whereas benign tumours are treated loc-

ally. However, the majority of bone tumours are benign.

There are three important aspects to the diagnosis of a primary bone tumour:

1. The diagnosis of the tumour and particularly whether it is benign or malignant. Occasionally this may be extremely difficult. Osteochondroma provides a good example when there is some proliferative activity in the cartilage cap. Histologically, the cartilage

Table 32.2 The relative incidence of malignant bone tumours (from Dahlin, 1957).

Tumour	Number	Percentage
Osteosarcoma	469	39
Parosteal sarcoma	21	2
Chondrosarcoma	218	18
Fibrosarcoma	58	5
Giant cell tumour	120	10
Ewing's sarcoma	141	12
Reticulum cell sarcoma	70	6
Chordoma	80	7
Miscellaneous	8	1
Total	1185	100
Myeloma	536	

may look benign whereas clinically it may behave in a more aggressive manner. A correct diagnosis is vitally important as it may mean the difference between major ablative surgery and a minor excision biopsy.

2. The determination of the local extent of the tumour. This is important for therapeutic as well as prognostic reasons. If an osteosarcoma is confined to the distal femur and there is no evidence of involvement of the rest of the bone, a through femur amputation or possibly a wide local resection may be adequate. However, if there is more proximal femoral involvement, this may be followed by stump or local recurrence.

The most useful investigations to delineate the extent of the tumour are arteriography, computerized tomographic (CT) scanning, tomography and skeletal scintigraphy. Arteriography and/or CT-scanning is essential to delineate the size of the lesion and particularly the extent of involvement of the surrounding soft tissues. This is most important if wide local excision of the tumour is under consideration. Tomography may help define the intraosseous spread of the tumour. Skeletal scintigraphy is most useful in diagnosing 'skip' lesions, which may determine the level of amputation.

There is good evidence to suggest that patients with osteosarcomata less than 5 cm in diameter have a better prognosis than those with larger tumours.

3. Determination of the general extent of disease. The majority of patients who die from osteosarcoma develop pulmonary metastases within six to nine months of diagnosis. Cade (1955) therefore advised that the primary tumour should be treated by high doses of irradiation and if the patient had not developed evidence of pulmonary metastases within six

months the limb should be amputated. This technique never gained favour in North America as it was felt that the primary tumour could not be sterilized by radiotherapy alone. There is no doubt that Cade's technique saved many children with occult pulmonary metastases an unnecessary amputation at a time when they were dying from disseminated osteosarcoma. With the recent advances in chemotherapy and the possibility of resection of pulmonary metastases the therapeutic approach has altered. Every attempt should be made to determine the extent of the disease before embarking upon treatment. CT-scanning of the lungs is probably the most useful investigation to detect pulmonary metastases. Skeletal scintigraphy can be of great value in osteosarcoma. Soft tissue deposits may produce sufficient bone to concentrate the bone-seeking isotope so that pulmonary and other soft tissue metastases may be demonstrated on the scintigram. Other techniques of diagnosing metastases such as lung tomography, pulmonary scintigraphy and hepatic scintigraphy are less valuable as the detection rate of occult metastases is low.

Benign tumours of bone

These will not be discussed in detail. However, it is important to be certain of the diagnosis. They may be treated in several ways.

1. Observation, e.g. non-ossifying fibroma, osteochondroma that is not producing symptoms, is not enlarging and which has been found accidentally
2. Curettage, e.g. enchondroma
3. Curettage and bone grafting, e.g. a large enchondroma, bone cyst
4. Excision, e.g. osteochondroma that is producing symptoms or enlarging, ecchondroma

Osteosarcoma

Osteosarcoma refers to those malignant tumours which arise from the primitive bone-forming cell. Usually, osteoid formation is the predominant feature of the neoplasm. Occasionally, bone absorption is prominent as a result of the vascularity of the neoplasm – the telangiectatic or osteolytic osteosarcoma.

Although rare, it probably is the commonest primary malignant tumour of bone (excluding multiple myeloma). It can develop at any age, but particularly occurs during the childhood or adolescent growth spurt or as a complication of Paget's disease. The peak incidence is in the second decade. The tumour arises from the metaphysis, the commonest site being the lower end of the femur (26%), the upper end of the tibia

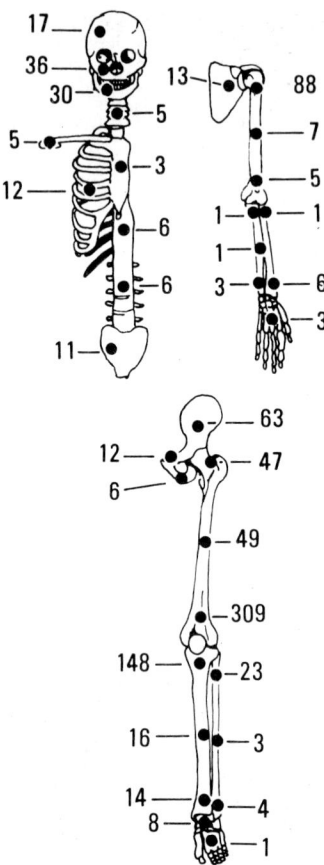

Fig. 32.1 The sites of occurrence of osteosarcoma indicating the numbers of patients in one series.

(18%) and the upper end of the humerus (9%). However, it can arise from virtually any bone, and it may be multiple (Fig. 32.1).

Clinical features

As with most tumours of bone, pain is usually the first symptom. Pain at the end of a long bone in a young person and not otherwise explained requires an X-ray to exclude an osteosarcoma. After some time the patient notices a mass. This interval may be very short in rapidly growing sarcomata. Frequently the symptoms are brought to light by trauma. The tumour is not secondary to the trauma but it is the latter that has brought the patient's attention to the mass. There may be an associated limp.

Clinical examination reveals a diffuse firm mass at the metaphyseal area. The mass may be extremely

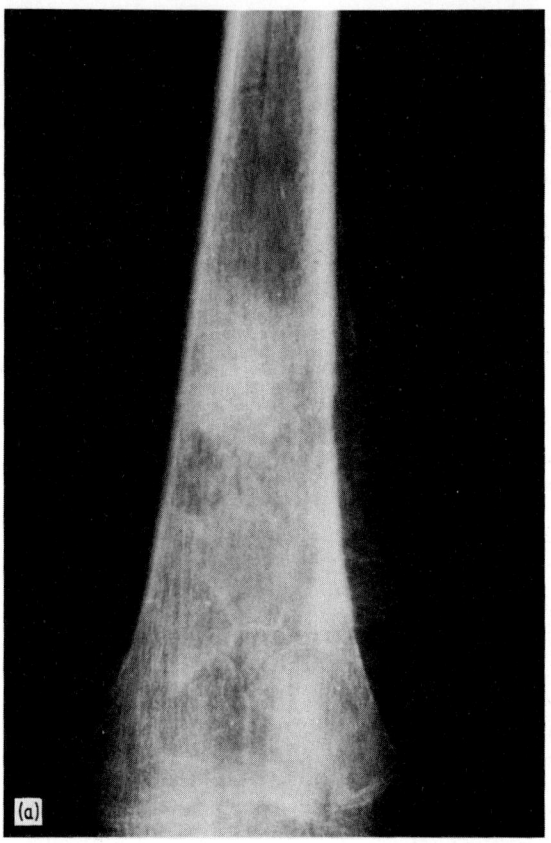

Fig. 32.2 Radiographic appearance of osteosarcoma. (*a*) Classical appearance. Irregular metaphyseal bone destruction, sub-periosteal 'sunray' spiculation with Codman's triangles at the proximal extent of the periosteal elevation. (*b*) More usual appearance of irregular metaphyseal bone destruction and new bone formation within the sub-periosteal extension of the tumour. (*c*) A purely lytic osteosarcoma.

large and tender. The overlying skin is warmer than normal, very vascular tumours may pulsate and a thin periosteal capsule may be associated with a crackling sensation. Very large, rapidly growing tumours may be associated with a leucocytosis, anaemia or pyrexia. The patient's general condition is usually good until the tumour is advanced or widespread.

The diagnosis is confirmed by X-ray and biopsy. Angiography, CT-scanning and skeletal scintigraphy are useful in delineating the extent of the tumour. Chest X-ray, CT-scanning and skeletal scintigraphy are important investigations in determining the degree of dissemination.

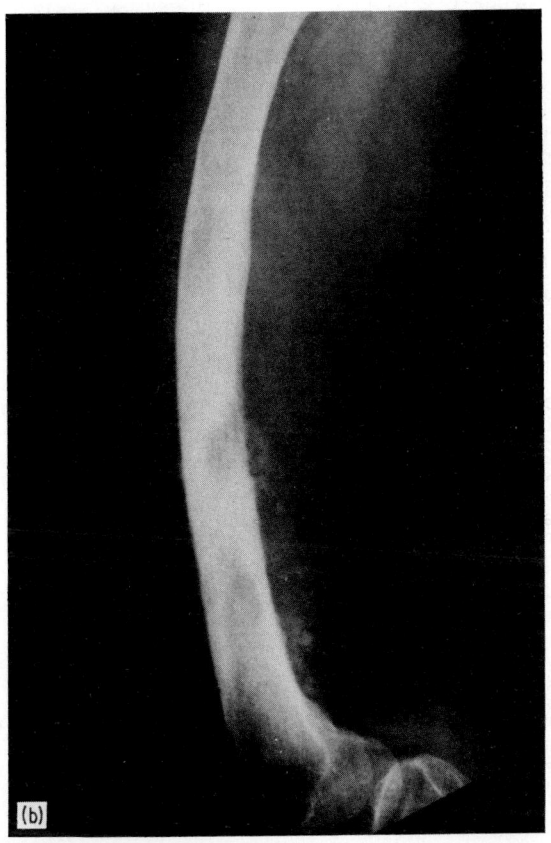

(b)

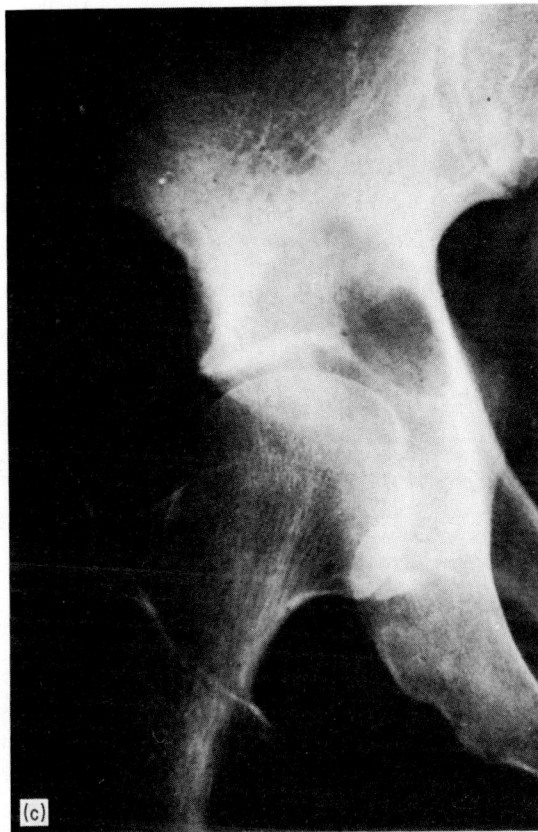

(c)

Radiographic features

The X-rays show an irregular destruction of bone in the region of the metaphysis. With increasing growth, the cortex is breached but vestiges of the original cortex usually remain. The combination of sub-periosteal extension of the tumour and new bone formation within the lesion suggests the diagnosis in half the cases (Lichtenstein, 1977) (Fig. 32.2*a* and *b*).

Pathology

The tumour arises in the metaphysis and extends in two directions – along the medulla or sub-periosteally. In the medulla, the trabeculae are destroyed and the tumour may extend for considerable distances but tends not to transgress the growth plate. Skip lesions are rare (Lewis and Lotz, 1974). The periosteum initially offers an impenetrable barrier, the tumour extending widely beneath it. The periosteal separation stops short at the periosteal attachment to the epiphyseal cartilage. At the edges of the tumour, where the periosteum is raised and still intact, there may be some sub-periosteal new bone formation producing the classical Codman's triangle. The sub-periosteal ossification within the tumour is often perpendicular to the main axis of the bone and gives the typical 'sunray' spiculation.

The macroscopic appearance varies from a soft, fleshy and vascular tumour with areas of haemorrhage and necrosis to a more solid, greyish white neoplasm containing cartilage or bone. The new bone may be scattered throughout the tumour giving it a gritty sensation on cutting. Much of the new bone is reactive rather than neoplastic. Pathological fractures may occur but are not common as the pain and swelling often immobilize the patient.

The histological pattern is extremely variable but in general consists of a frankly sarcomatous stroma and the direct formation of tumour osteoid and bone by this malignant stroma. There is a great variation in cellular morphology. The commonest cell is small and spindle shaped with a hyperchromatic nucleus. The cells may be polyhedral, round, cuboidal or columnar. They vary considerably in size and arrangement. The more anaplastic the neoplasm, the greater the degree of pleomorphism. Giant multinucleated bizarre shaped cells occur and mitotic figures are frequent. The intercellular matrix may be scanty or considerable and may be myxomatous, cartilaginous, osteoid or osseous. Destruction of bone may be associated with osteoclasts. The lesions tend to be vascular with numerous thin walled blood vessels. Different areas in the same tumour may show different histological appearances. There may be minimal osteoid formation and the tumour may appear to be purely lytic (Fig. 32.2c).

Spread

The tumour metastasizes early via the blood stream, particularly to the lungs but it may spread to other tissues including the skeleton. The tumour may also spread via the lymphatics to the draining lymph nodes. McKenna and his colleagues (1966) found such spread in 30% of cases at autopsy.

Prognosis

Prior to the 1970s 5-year survival varied from 5–20% (Cade, 1955; Jaffe, 1958; Lindbom *et al.*, 1961; Price, 1961; Weinfeld and Dudley, 1962; Gilmer *et al.*, 1963; Dahlin and Coventry, 1967). However, in a most significant paper Gilchrist and his colleagues (1978), have demonstrated that at the Mayo Clinic the prognosis improved in succeeding decades, with surgery alone. Their latest group reached a 2-year survival of 40%. As indicated in the introduction to this chapter the authors believe that these results indicate that there may be a change in the natural history of these tumours and that new methods of treatment must be shown to be significantly better than concurrent control groups in which standard treatment is used. This is particularly so when the newer treatments are associated with significant morbidity or even mortality. Prognosis can be correlated with alkaline phosphatase levels (Levine and Rosenberg, 1979).

Treatment

Until recently the standard method of treatment was either amputation or irradiation followed by amputation three to six months later provided no pulmonary metastases had appeared. It had been generally accepted that the majority of patients with osteosarcoma already had pulmonary seeding by the time they presented for treatment, even though the radiographs of the lungs appeared normal. The majority of these pulmonary metastases manifested themselves within six months and led to the patient's death within nine to twelve months of presentation. It, therefore, was felt that an amputation was unnecessary in patients who were likely to develop pulmonary metastases and die from their tumour within months. However the limb was amputated three to six months later in those patients who did not develop metastases partly because irradiation alone did not sterilize the tumour (Lichtenstein, 1977), viable tumour cells being found in virtually all specimens examined and partly because the doses of radiation used (up to 10 000 rad) produced irradiation necrosis. Many surgeons, particularly in North America, did not accept this treatment regimen which was directed at the primary tumour while attempting to spare the limb if the patient developed overt metastases, as they felt that the tumour could continue to metastasize following irradiation and suggested immediate amputation. Sweetnam and his colleagues (1971) showed that there was no difference in the 5-year survival between those patients treated by primary amputation and those patients treated by ablative radiotherapy and subsequent amputation. Irradiation alone produced much poorer 5-year survival rates.

With the development of effective chemotherapeutic agents for metastatic osteosarcoma in the early 1970s important new developments have occurred in the systemic treatment of patients with apparently localized disease in an attempt to prevent or delay the appearance of overt recurrences.

The evaluation of effective single cytotoxic agents subsequently led to the development of more effective chemotherapeutic combinations in metastatic disease and the relevant effectiveness of many of these agents is shown in Table 32.3.

High dose methotrexate (Djerassi *et al.*, 1972) was probably one of the first chemotherapeutic agents shown to produce a response in metastatic osteosarcoma. Table 32.4 shows the response rate for high dose methotrexate alone and in combination. However, many of the studies that attempt to evaluate the responsiveness of osteosarcoma to both single agents and combinations have employed very small numbers of patients with metastatic disease and the interpretation of the overall responsiveness of this tumour should be made with some caution.

It has been demonstrated, in many solid tumours, that combination chemotherapy is more effective in inducing responses than single agents alone (Henderson and Samaha, 1969; De Vita *et al.*, 1975).

Table 32.5 shows the response of metastatic osteosarcoma to a number of combination regimens which have formed the basis of the use of systemic combination chemotherapy in the adjuvant situation.

Table 32.3 Effective single agents in metastatic osteosarcoma.

Chemotherapeutic agent	No. patients	No. responses	% response rate
Cyclophosphamide	28	4	14
Melphalan	33	5	15
Vincristine	11	0	0
Adriamycin	109	28	26
Methotrexate (with citrovorum)	4	0	0
Cis-platinum	8	4	50
Mitomycin-C	17	4	23
Total	210	45	21

Table 32.4 Use of high dose methotrexate (MTX) and citrovorum factor rescue alone and in combination in osteosarcoma (from *Cancer Treat. Rep.*, **62**, Feb. 1978).

Drug regimen	No. patients	No. response	% response rate
MTX + citrovorum	4	0	0
Vincristine + MTX + citrovorum (1st schedule)	14	4	29
Vincristine + MTX + citrovorum (2nd schedule)	8	7	88
Total	26	11	42

Table 32.5 Combination chemotherapy in metastatic osteosarcoma of bone (From *Cancer Treat. Rep.*, **62**, Feb. 1978).

Drug combination	No. patients	No. responses	% response rate
VCR + MTX + Citrovorum	14	4	29
VCR + MTX + Citrovorum	8	7	87
ADM + MTX + Citrovorum	13	7	54
ADM + DTIC	18	8	44
VADIC	46	16	35
CYVADIC	29	7	24
CYVADACT	20	5	25
Total	148	54	36

VCR = vincristine; MTX = methotrexate; ADM = adriamycin; DTIC = imidazole carboxamide; VADIC = vincristine, adriamycin and DTIC; CYVADIC = cyclophosphamide and VADIC; CYVADACT = CYVADIC and actinomycin-D

With the introduction of moderately effective chemotherapy for metastatic osteosarcoma many researchers turned their attention in the early 1970s to the use of such treatment in patients with apparently localized osteosarcoma in an attempt to prevent the development of early pulmonary metastases.

In 1974, Jaffe and his colleagues (1974*a*) reported the use of adjuvant vincristine and high dose methotrexate in a group of 20 patients, comparing their survival with those of historical controls; 78% of the historical controls had pulmonary metastases at twelve months compared with 10% of the group treated with adjuvant chemotherapy and in this group the disease-free rate at two years was 52%.

In a second study Cortes and his colleagues (1974) reported the use of adriamycin. They also used Marcove's (1971) data to produce an historical control group, and reported a disease-free survival rate at two years of 50%. Both Jaffe and Cortes have recently updated their figures (Jaffe *et al.*, 1978; Cortes *et al.*, 1978). In Jaffe's original 20 patients treated with vincristine and high dose methotrexate with citrovorum factor rescue the follow-up is now from 39 to 58 months. Seven of the 20 patients have developed pulmonary metastases and life-table analysis suggests a metastasis-free rate in this group of 32%. In their more recent studies adriamycin has been added to the chemotherapeutic regimen. Twenty-two patients have been treated and 54% remain free of pulmonary metastases at 18 to 36 months. Cortes has now treated 88 patients and the life-table analysis indicates that 39% of these patients will be disease-free at five years. These studies can be criticized because neither treatment nor protocol was always rigidly followed but in those patients in whom there was no violation of either the surgical or chemotherapeutic protocol the '*predicted' disease-free survival* at five years is of the order of 50%.

Unfortunately, both groups of workers relied on an historical control and their results are very little different from the recent figures published by the Mayo Clinic (Gilchrist *et al.*, 1978; Taylor *et al.*, 1978), who reported a survival rate of 40% at two years in patients treated by surgery alone. It is vital in this disease that adequately controlled trials are performed to evaluate fully the use of adjuvant chemotherapy.

Sutow of the South Western Oncology Group has reported an important series of studies. In the first study, which was started in 1963, he used melphalan in 14 patients, only two of whom achieved long-term survival. In 1968 a new programme was introduced with vincristine, actinomycin D and cyclophosphamide used as a three-day pulsed regimen. Eleven children were treated and three (27%) are long-term survivors. In 1971 Sutow introduced a four-drug adjuvant regimen (CONPADRI I) consisting of cyclophosphamide, vincristine, melphalan and adriamycin. At the present time 56 patients have been registered, of whom 44 can be evaluated. Twenty-four patients are alive without evidence of disease with a median follow-up of 37 months. The 1- and 2-year disease-free survival rates are 59% and 55% respectively. In the CONPADRI II regimen high dose methotrexate with citrovorum rescue was included. In the initial study with this programme there were drug related deaths and the period of methotrexate infusion was decreased from 24 hours to 6 hours. The methotrexate blood level has been monitored and subsequently there have been no toxicity problems. The median follow-up is 21.5 months and the 1- and 2-year disease-free survival rates are 62% and 51% respectively.

In the CONPADRI III regimen the doses of methotrexate and adriamycin were increased. The median follow-up is only 14.5 months, and the 1- and 2-year disease-free survival rates are currently 66 and 42% respectively. As a result of these studies, particularly the early ones Sutow (1976) has concluded that most patiets must be considered to be at risk for the development of late metastases for at least three years. In their latest regimen (CONPADRI IV) the dose and frequency of methotrexate has been further increased. It is interesting that the best survival figures available have been obtained with the CONPADRI I regimen. Sutow has demonstrated a pattern of late relapse for which adjustments in adjuvant chemotherapy scheduling dosage and overall time period have been made in the evolution of these programmes.

A recently updated study by Etcubanas and Wilbur (1978) from the Children's Hospital, Stanford, has not confirmed the positive benefit of adjuvant chemotherapy in osteosarcoma reported by the other three groups. Twenty-nine patients were admitted to the study and received combination chemotherapy with high dose methotrexate and citrovorum factor rescue in addition to vincristine, adriamycin and cyclophosphamide. Fourteen (48%) of the 29 patients are currently disease-free at 8 to 48 months follow-up. The present median disease-free survival is 21 months and the projected 4-year disease-free survival is only 13%.

The results of these studies suggest that although chemotherapy may be of importance in the management of localized osteosarcoma, its place is not yet established. The authors of this chapter feel that it is regrettable that these studies have not used properly matched controls. What is needed is an adequately adjuvant chemotherapy, possibly combined controlled, randomized clinical study to evaluate scientifically effective with adjuvant lung irradiation (see below).

These studies have shown that the treatment of the primary tumour is important. Chemotherapy cannot be used to replace ablation of the primary tumour, nor can it be used to compensate for poor surgical technique.

It is now generally accepted that there is little place for pre-operative irradiation. However, there is some debate as to the optimum technique of surgical ablation. In some centres local radical resection with customized prosthetic replacement is being used in an attempt to save the limb. Pre-operative angiograms and CT-scans are essential to delineate the extent of the tumour and ensure that there is at least one plane of normal tissue between the tumour and the neurovascular bundle. There are a number of individuals alive today with an intact limb having had a radical local resection for osteosarcoma. At the present time there are no series with sufficiently large numbers or sufficiently long follow-up to give any significant 5-year survival figures. It should be remembered that osteosarcoma is usually a fatal tumour and that no benefit will be gained in attempting to save the limb if, as a result, the patients die from their malignancy. The authors feel that the techniques of local resection may have much to offer, in defined instances. However, this form of therapy is at an experimental stage and should only be carried out in large centres where there are adequate facilities and where large numbers of patients may be studied prospectively. In this situation local radical resection might be compared with the more conventional amputation, both groups of patients receiving the same adjuvant therapy. Before local radical resection becomes accepted as a reasonable alternative to ablation for localized tumours, it must be shown that the survival is as good.

The level of amputation is also a contentious issue. Most surgeons will agree that when osteosarcoma affects the proximal tibia the limb should be amputated through the femur. However, there is disagreement concerning the level of amputation for sarcomata limited to the distal femur. Through femur amputations are associated with a definite stump recurrence, the incidence varying from 4% (Campanacci and Cervellati, 1975) to 28% (Sweetnam et al., 1971). It is possible that angiography, skeletal scintigraphy and CT-scans may be useful in determining the level of amputation, by defining the intra- and extraosseous extent of the neoplasm. Sweetnam (1975) has indicated that in the pre-chemotherapy era a hip disarticulation was probably necessary and has asked whether through femur amputation will be adequate in the chemotherapy era. This question is still unanswered and also needs prospective evaluation.

The question of prophylactic pulmonary irradiation is also unresolved. With modern techniques disabling pulmonary fibrosis can be avoided. There is some evidence that it may be associated with an improved prognosis, but this needs to be confirmed. An EORTC

trial (Breur et al., 1978) has indeed shown that a dose of 2000 rad in 2 weeks can lead to results comparable to those from chemotherapy, and further trials with both chemotherapy and lung irradiation are in progress.

Recurrent and metastatic disease

It is generally accepted that chemotherapy is of some value in advanced disease although varying response rates have been reported (Tables 32.3 and 32.5). It is also generally agreed that solitary pulmonary metastases should be excised. Most centres would agree that it is often worthwhile excising several lesions but the use of multiple resections for pulmonary metastases is debatable. There have been isolated case reports from several centres where patients have been subjected to 15 to 20 thoracotomies and even if this has been associated with a 4- or 5- year survival one must question the quality of that survival. The possibility that such aggressive treatment of pulmonary metastases is associated with a much prolonged survival needs to be confirmed by other centres. Once again the numbers of patients so treated are too small for any meaningful survival figures.

The developments that have occurred in the past few years in the treatment of osteosarcoma are exciting; nevertheless, caution should be urged in the interpretation of the results for the reasons cited above and future studies must embody a concurrent control group before new methods are introduced into the general management of these patients who die early from metastatic disease.

Parosteal sarcoma

Clinical features

This occurs in a slightly older age group and presents as a painful mass particularly in the region of the knee joint.

Radiographic appearance

The tumour is juxtacortical and densely ossified. Periosteal reaction and sunray spiculation do not occur. The tumours grow slowly, gradually surrounding the bone but eventually destruction of the cortex with invasion of the medullary cavity occurs.

Pathology

The tumour consists of trabeculae of neoplastic bone and osteoid tissue with a definite malignant connective tissue stroma. There may be a fibrous tissue pseudocapsule.

Prognosis

This is better than the osteosarcoma, with a 5-year survival of 50–70% (Johnson, 1970).

Treatment

The treatment is by primary amputation. Occasionally, smaller tumours can be removed by radical excision and the defect grafted or replaced with a custom-built prosthesis. It is too early to say whether radical excision gives as good a prognosis as primary amputation. If the excision does *not* encompass the entire lesion with a minimum of 1–2 cm of muscle and other soft tissue, local recurrence nearly always occurs (Scaglietti and Calandriello, 1962).

Chondrosarcoma

This usually occurs in the 30–60-year age group although it may occur in younger individuals. It tends to be a primary malignancy in younger patients but in the older age group peripheral lesions are often secondary to a malignant change in the cartilage cap of an osteochondroma, particularly in diaphyseal aclasis (hereditary multiple osteochondromata). Central lesions may arise in enchondromata and particularly enchondromatosis (Ollier's disease). The peripheral lesions tend to have a better prognosis in that they usually are circumscribed and operable. Chondrosarcomata may rarely complicate irradiation and even Paget's disease of bone.

Clinical findings

The clinical presentation is frequently vague. An alteration in the size or symptoms of a known osteochondroma or a recurrence of an excised 'benign' cartilage tumour may be the presenting complaint. The neoplasm occurs most commonly in the pelvis, ribs, scapula and femur. Dahlin and Henderson (1956) stated that the nearer a cartilaginous tumour to the axial skeleton and the larger the tumour, the more likely it is to be malignant.

If an enchondroma of a long bone becomes painful in the adult, it is probably malignant, especially if the X-rays show that it has penetrated through the cortex. It has been suggested for many years that incomplete operative removal of simple chondromata may lead to a malignant change, but the malignant change may well have preceded surgery. However, if a chondroma is being removed it should be removed totally. Physical examination usually reveals a firm or hard, but non-tender mass.

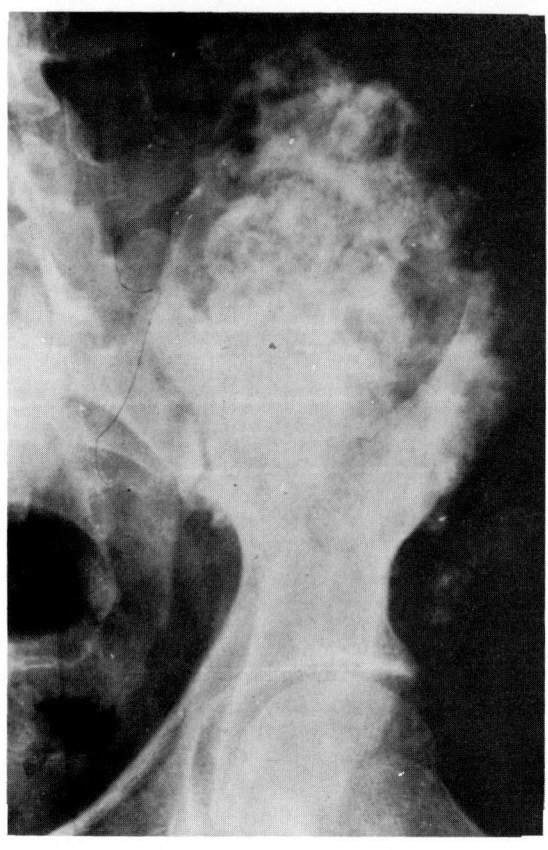

Fig. 32.3 Chondrosarcoma. There is a large tumour arising in the ilium, associated with irregular calcification and bone destruction.

Radiographic features (Fig. 32.3)

The central chondrosarcoma frequently presents as an expanding lesion with irregular calcification and bone destruction. Periosteal new bone formation may be evident. A peripheral tumour often presents as a malignant degeneration of an osteochondroma. Under these circumstances, there is frequently a large soft tissue mass containing large flecks of irregular calcification over the head of the osteochondroma. The appearance of irregular calcification in the cap of an osteochondroma warrants immediate excision biopsy. A benign osteochondroma has a well-defined outline, uniform texture and no abnormal soft tissue shadows.

Pathology

The macroscopic appearance is of a greyish, translucent, fairly vascular tumour which may be lobulated and may contain areas undergoing cystic degeneration and liquefaction.

The diagnosis is often difficult to make, particularly in the low-grade tumours. The tissue must be generously sampled and the worst-looking areas examined. The presence of small fields of (a) many cells with plump nuclei; (b) more than a few cells with two such nuclei and particularly (c) giant cartilage cells, indicate that the neoplasm is malignant (Lichtenstein, 1977).

Histologically, the tumour can be classified in three grades:

Low grade
This is a well differentiated neoplasm. The cells are cartilaginous in type although increased in number and the matrix is well formed. There is local infiltration of the surrounding tissues at the periphery. Almost three quarters of the patients are alive at ten years.

Medium grade
There is a reduction in the amount of matrix, an increase in the cellularity, the cells vary in shape and size and show nuclear irregularities. Less than half the patients are alive at five years and one third at ten years.

High grade
This has a poorly differentiated cartilaginous pattern. Anaplastic cells, frequent mitoses and occasional islands of cartilage are seen. Only 10% patients survive three years.

Mankin (1978) has shown that there are biochemical differences between normal cartilage, low-grade and high-grade chondrosarcomata.

Spread

The tumour often remains localized for years, particularly the peripheral type, despite local recurrence. Spread is via the blood stream to the lungs. Pulmonary metastases tend to occur earlier with central lesions. Metastases are uncommon at other sites, although lymph node involvement does occur.

Prognosis

The overall 5-year survival is approximately 35% but this depends on the grade of the tumour.

Treatment

The treatment of choice is adequate resection. It may be possible to remove many of the peripheral chondrosarcomata by adequate local resection. In doing the operation it is important to maintain normal tissue between the tumour and the scalpel at all times and remove the osteochondroma at its base. If the neoplasm cannot be removed with an adequate covering of normal tissue then amputation is necessary. Central chondrosarcomata which are confined to bone and where there is no extraosseous extension of the tumour can be excised by local resection of either part or the entire bone followed by prosthetic replacement or bone grafting. However, if there is any extraosseous extension of the tumour amputation is indicated.

The tumour tends to recur locally before it metastasizes. Local recurrences can also be treated by radical excision but the risk of dissemination increases with each recurrence. Once a tumour has recurred twice then amputation is indicated and it may be rational to amputate following the first recurrence.

Irradiation, even in large doses has only a limited effect and should be reserved for the palliation of inoperable tumours. Occasionally, tumours arising from the pelvis and the spine may reach enormous sizes. Technically it may not be possible to excise these tumours *en bloc* and they may have to be removed piecemeal, although chondrosarcomata arising in a vertebral body have been excised successfully. Postoperatively the area should be irradiated, although it is doubtful whether the patient will gain much benefit.

A number of authors have reported on the use of combined treatment with radiation therapy and cytotoxic drugs for the local control of chondrosarcomata. Although no prospective studies have been carried out to test irradiation alone versus irradiation plus chemotherapy a number of preliminary reports suggest that local control may be improved by the combination of irradiation with razoxane (ICRF 159). Rhomberg (1978) has suggested that the improved response to this combination may result in local control. Ryall *et al.* (1979) have treated eight patients with 11 chondrosarcomata. Of the 11, five have regressed completely, two partially, in three there was no change and in one there was active progression.

Chemotherapy alone is associated with a poor response rate (Table 32.6).

The initial resection must be adequate and the tumour must be widely excised, even if a hemipelvectomy is needed, to offer the patient the best chances of survival.

Giant cell tumour

This is generally classed as an intermediate or indeterminate tumour as it tends to recur after local removal and occasionally behaves as a frankly malignant tumour metastasizing through the blood stream, particularly once the tumour has recurred. The neoplasm

Table 32.6 Chemotherapy in chondrosarcoma of bone.

Cytotoxic agent	No. patients	No. partial response
Adriamycin	17	1
DTIC (imidazole carboxamide)	1	0
Adriamycin + DTIC	9	0
Adriamycin, DTIC + vincristine	3	0
CYVADIC (cyclophosphamide, vincristine, adriamycin + DTIC)	6	2
Methyl CCNU	2	1
Methyl CCNU + actinomycin-D	10	0
Total	48	4 (8.3%)

occurs most commonly in the third and fourth decades after the epiphyses have closed. The commonest sites are the distal femur, proximal tibia, distal radius and proximal humerus. The tumour arises in the metaphyseal region and extends across the site of the fused growth plate into the epiphysis almost reaching the joint surface. It is usually eccentric.

Clinical findings

The giant cell tumour usually presents with pain and a gradually developing swelling. The onset may be acute following a pathological fracture. The eccentric enlargement at the end of a long bone may be palpable and if the overlying cortex is extremely thinned 'eggshell crackling' may be felt.

Radiographic findings

The radiographic appearance is usually of a lobulated, lytic eccentric tumour involving the metaphysis and epiphysis. The cortex is thinned, expanded and frequently breached. Bone destruction is often incomplete, the residual trabeculae within the tumour giving it the lobulated appearance. There is a sharp line of demarcation between the tumour and the unaffected shaft in contra-distinction to sarcomata. Because the neoplasm is eccentric, the enlargement of the bone end is also eccentric. The tumour very rarely enters the joint, but pathological fractures may occur.

Pathology

The tumour consists of two elements:
1. A vascular and cellular stroma made up of oval shaped cells containing a small elongated, darkly staining nucleus with little eosinophilic cytoplasm. The stromal cells show a varying degree of mitotic activity, pleomorphism and hyperchromatism. The cellular stroma is the critical feature.
2. Giant cells – these are large cells with pink staining cytoplasm filled with numerous and centrally placed nuclei. It has been suggested that they arise from fusion of the stromal cells. The giant cells may become anaplastic.

Macroscopically, the tumour presents as a reddish or grey lesion, with areas of necrosis and haemorrhage.

Histologically, the tumour can be graded depending on its appearance. Approximately half the cases of any large series fall into Grade I. In this group the cytological features indicate the lowest degree of aggressiveness. There is no appreciable atypism of the stromal cells and hyperchromatic nuclei are rare.

Grade 2 neoplasms range from those in which the stromal cells show slight, though definite atypism to those which are markedly atypical but not frankly malignant.

Grade 3 tumours show frank malignant changes, with a sarcomatous type of stroma. Virtually all the nuclei exhibit atypism and are unusually large and irregular.

It is uncommon to see frankly sarcomatous tissue when the neoplasm is first biopsied. These changes are seen usually in a lesion which was initially Grade I or 2 but which has become more aggressive following each recurrence. There is some correlation between the histological grading and the behaviour of the tumour (Hutter *et al.*, 1962; Mnaymneh *et al.*, 1964).

Spread

When malignant, the commonest site of metastatic involvement is the lungs, the tumour metastasizing via the blood stream.

Prognosis

Approximately 35% (Goldenberg *et al.*, 1970) to 62% recur (Hutter *et al.*, 1962) and 10–30% become frankly malignant and metastasize (Hutter *et al.*, 1962). The 5-year survival rate is approximately 66.0% (Thomson and Turner-Warwick, 1955).

Treatment

The treatment depends on the site of the tumour. If the affected bone is one that easily can be removed, for example, the fibula, excision of part or the whole of that bone is recommended. If wide excision of the neoplasm will result in severe disability, e.g. the distal femur, more conservative measures are frequently indicated in the first instance. The treatment of choice probably is thorough curettage and bone grafting. The incidence of recurrence is lower following curettage and grafting than curettage alone. Cryosurgery has been advocated (Marcove *et al.*, 1975), but this technique requires further evaluation.

Although there are many reports of irradiation successfully controlling giant cell tumours there are no well controlled sizeable series with adequate follow-up. The general consensus of opinion is that irradiation is followed by a higher recurrence rate than surgery and an increased risk of sarcomatous change. Goldenberg *et al.* (1970) reported a 7% incidence whereas Dahlin (1957) noted a 19% incidence.

Recurrent lesions should be treated by wide local excision followed by prosthetic replacement or bone grafting. Amputation is indicated for the frankly malignant tumours.

There is little data indicating the responsiveness of these tumours to chemotherapy. Benjamin *et al.* (1974) reported one partial response in two patients treated with adriamycin and Chang *et al.* (1976) reported one partial response in two patients treated with intravenous methyl CCNU.

Fibrosarcoma of bone

These may be primary, follow irradiation (with a long latent interval) or may develop in Paget's disease, in a giant cell tumour of bone, and rarely in fibrous dysplasia, or at the site of an old bone infarct.

Clinical findings

The tumour may arise at any age but commonly occurs in the late third and early fourth decades. The patients usually present with pain and swelling and the femur and tibia are the commonest sites.

Radiographic findings

The tumour arises within the medulla, but eventually penetrates the cortex and extends into the surrounding soft tissues. These present as lytic lesions with little surrounding reaction and must be distinguished from parosteal fibrosarcomata which appear as a faintly outlined, soft tissue shadow; the bone looking normal except for a shallow concavity of the cortex opposite the tumour.

Pathology

The tumour is usually firm, fibrous, glistening and greyish white although occasionally it is more cellular, soft and cystic. The degree of vascularity varies. The parosteal fibrosarcoma may have a pseudocapsule consisting of condensed surrounding tissue.

Histologically, the tumour is a spindle cell fibrosarcoma with a variable degree of collagen formation, although, in the intramedullary varieties there may be virtually no intercellular substance. There is a wide variation in their behaviour, which is often related to their cytological characteristics. The more anaplastic neoplasms tend to metastasize earlier (Gilmer and MacEwan, 1958; Jaffe, 1958; Huvos and Higinbotham, 1975).

Spread

The tumours remain localized for a considerable time, particularly the parosteal fibrosarcomata but ultimately metastasize via the blood stream to the lungs.

Prognosis

The 5-year survival varies from 25 to 40%.

Treatment

Radical excision of the tumour is the operation of choice. In the parosteal variety, this can frequently be accomplished by a wide local excision. Under these circumstances, the prognosis is particularly favourable if the tumour has a pseudocapsule. It is possible that intramedullary fibrosarcomata may be adequately treated by radical excision followed by prosthetic replacement provided the lesion is still confined within the cortex. Once it has broken through amputation is indicated. If the tumour recurs, amputation is indicated providing that the patient has not developed pulmonary metastases. Irradiation or neutron therapy may be useful for treating metastases and for palliation of inoperable local recurrences. There are no separate reports regarding the chemotherapeutic response of fibrosarcomata of bone; these tumours have been included in overall response rates of soft tissue fibrosarcomata and the numbers involved are too small for separate analysis.

Ewing's sarcoma

This usually occurs in the 5–20-year age group and affects males more commonly than females. It arises in the diaphysis of long bones, particularly the tibia, followed by the tibula, humerus and femur. The lesions may be multiple. Although the cell of origin is not clearly defined there is good evidence that it arises in the mesenchymal connective tissue framework of bone marrow (Friedman and Gold, 1968; Kadin and Bensch, 1971).

Clinical findings

There is frequently a history of trauma. The patients complain of pain, usually of some months duration, and the development of a slowly growing tumour. The pain is intermittent and during each attack the tumour may enlarge visibly and there may be a febrile illness and leucocytosis. The tumour is often large and usually tender. The presence of a fever, anaemia and raised erythrocyte sedimentation rate is often associated with a fulminating course (Lichtenstein, 1977).

Radiographic findings

There is diffuse rarefaction of the diaphysis extending over a considerable area. The cortex is involved and at a later stage, periosteal new bone formation, which may be layered (onion peel appearance), is seen. Chronic osteomyelitis may produce a similar radiological appearance (Fig. 32.4). This is followed by gross tumour formation with marked bone destruction.

Pathology

The tumour begins in the marrow of the diaphysis. It is greyish white with areas of necrosis, haemorrhage and cyst formation. The tumour extends in the Haversian canals to the surface, raising the periosteum. Subperiosteal layers of new bone are deposited only to be destroyed. These layers give the 'onion peel' appearance, although this classical radiographic feature is seen infrequently.

The tumour is very cellular and consists of small, round or polyhedral cells arranged in solid cords or sheets. The cells are clearly delineated with boundaries and pseudorosette formation commonly occurs. The nuclei are prominent, round or ovoid and have finely divided or powdery chromatin and usually one or more nucleoli. Reticulin fibres are irregularly distributed and frequently sparse.

The differential diagnosis includes metastases from neuroblastoma, reticulum cell sarcoma, metastatic carcinoma (particularly small cell bronchial carcinoma), Hodgkin's disease and lymphosarcoma of bone. The diagnosis may be difficult and special stains for reticulin fibres and glycogen content may be necessary.

Schajowicz (1959) found that the cells of Ewing's sarcoma contained glycogen, whereas this was not the case with reticulum cell sarcoma. Lichtenstein (1977) did not find this particularly helpful and relied on the cytological characteristics to differentiate the two lesions. Neuroblastoma cells are small and round, with a dense hyperchromatic nucleus, little cytoplasm and are arranged in rosettes. The presence of neurofibrils gives the diagnosis, but may be difficult to demonstrate.

Prognosis

The prognosis for Ewing's sarcoma is particularly poor. Prior to the advent of adjuvant chemotherapy the 5-year survival was probably less than 5%. Historically, survival rates of 10–15% have been reported but many pathologists believe that other round cell tumours were included in these groups. It has even been suggested that the diagnosis was incorrect in the survivors.

The advent of effective chemotherapy has produced important improvements in the early survival of patients with this highly malignant tumour, although it is still too soon fully to evaluate its effect.

Treatment

Prior to the advent of effective chemotherapy, radiotherapy was the treatment of choice. It was often associated with marked amelioration of symptoms and good local control in many patients. However, virtually all patients died within two–three years from generalized skeletal, pulmonary and other visceral metastases. Adjuvant chemotherapy following radiotherapy has improved the survival. Single agent response rates in metastatic Ewing's sarcoma are higher than in many other solid tumours (Table 32.7'. Jaffe *et al.* (1974*b*) demonstrated that the response rate to combinations of cytotoxic drugs could produce even higher response rates. They used a combination of vincristine, actinomycin D and cyclophosphamide (VAC). Soon after this several centres used combination chemotherapy regimens in the adjuvant situation and the accumulted results of these series are shown in Table 32.8. The use of single agent adjuvant chemotherapy in combination

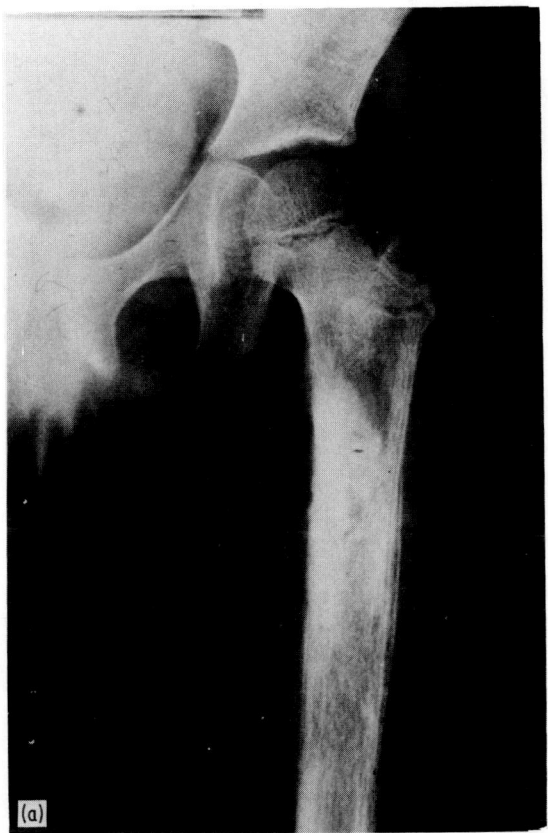

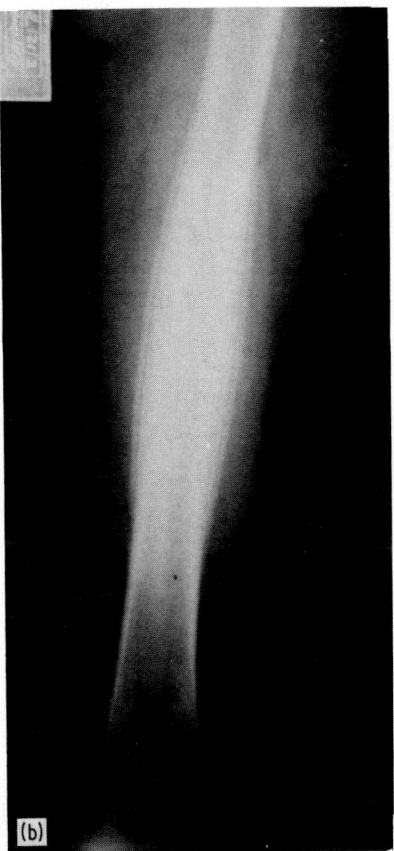

Fig. 32.4 'Onion-peel' appearance. This is due to layered sub-periosteal new bone formation. (*a*) Ewing's sarcoma. There is rarefaction of bone in addition to the new bone formation.
(*b*) Chronic osteomyelitis.

with radiation therapy has been shown to improve both the disease-free interval and survival times (Johnson and Humphreys, 1969; Freeman *et al.*, 1972). Even more favourable results have been obtained using combination chemotherapy (Johnson and Pomeroy, 1972; Rosen *et al.*, 1974; Bacci *et al.*, 1978). It is now known that Ewing's sarcoma may exhibit a late relapse pattern and in this context the data from Johnson and Pomeroy (1975) are of interest. Using a variety of chemotherapeutic protocols, 66 patients who presented with local disease were admitted to their studies. They considered that 43 patients were evaluable. The 5-year survival was 52%. No patient who presented with advanced disease survived five years.

It should be appreciated that although these data represent an important advance in the management of Ewing's sarcoma relapse beyond five years is not uncommon.

The design of adjuvant chemotherapeutic programmes in relation to the behaviour of this particular tumour is of considerable importance if the improved survival rate is to be maintained beyond five years.

Prior to the development of adjuvant chemotherapy there was little indication for surgery in these patients. With the increase in the length of disease-free intervals it needs to be established whether radiotherapy is still the treatment of choice for the local lesion or whether surgical ablation is indicated. Bacci and his colleagues (1978) studied 37 patients. In 10 patients the primary tumour was treated surgically, with post-operative irradiation. The primary tumour was treated by radiotherapy alone in 27 patients. All 37 patients were also given combination chemotherapy. The follow-up of both groups of patients ranged from 12 to 62 months. Only one of the surgically treated group had developed distant metastases and there have been no local recurrences whereas eight of the patients who had radiotherapy alone developed metastases and nine patients developed a local recurrence (including six

Table 32.7   Single agent response rates in Ewing's sarcoma.

Chemotherapeutic agent	No. patients	No. responses	% Response rate	Author
Cyclophosphamide	29	17	59	Haggard (1967) Samuels and Howe (1967) Sutow and Sullivan (1962)
Actinomycin D	5	3	60	Senyszyn *et al.* (1970)
Vincristine	5	1	20	Sutow (1968)
Mithramycin	5	2	40	Kofman *et al.* (1973)
Adriamycin	44	22	50	Gottlieb *et al.* (1972) O'Bryan *et al.* (1973) Oldham and Pomeroy (1972) Tan *et al.* (1972)
BCNU	12	5	41	Palma *et al.* (1972)
Total	100	50	50	

Table 32.8   Adjuvant chemotherapy after radiation therapy for localized Ewing's sarcoma.

Regimen	No. patients	No. disease free	Duration (months)	Author
Cyclophosphamide	3	2	44–52	Johnson and Humphreys (1969)
Various agents	9	4	12–146	Freeman *et al.* (1972)
Cyclophosphamide Vincristine }	15	10	4–91	Hustu *et al.* (1972)
Various agents	43	22	(52% 5-year survival life-table analysis)	Johnson and Pomeroy (1975)
Actinomycin D Adriamycin Vincristine Cyclophosphamide }	12	12	10–37	Jaffe *et al.* (1974b)
Vincristine Cyclophosphamide }	19	6	12–46	Fernandez *et al.* (1974)
Total	101	56 (56%)		

who developed both metastases and a local recurrence).

The cytotoxic effect of the chemotherapeutic agents may be different on the primary tumour and on micrometastasis (Schabel, 1975; Burchenal, 1976). The central core of the tumour may not be destroyed by irradiation, even with doses in excess of 7000 rad. This central area is poorly vascularized, and the cells are hypoxic and resistant to irradiation and cytotoxic drugs. The increase in the disease-free interval may give these viable cells sufficient time to metastasize or develop into a local recurrence. The rationale for amputation or excision is the removal of these cells.

Primary reticulum cell sarcoma of bone

Bone involvement occurs in the leukaemias, lymphomata and Hodgkin's disease. Solid deposits may be seen but these are part of a more generalized disease. However, there is no doubt that localized skeletal involvement as the sole, or at least initial, manifestation of a reticulum cell sarcoma occurs (Parker and Jackson, 1939).

Clinical findings

The tumour occurs most commonly in the second to

fourth decades and primarily affects the femur, tibia and humerus. Pain is usually the first complaint.

Radiographic findings

The initial finding is an osteolytic lesion at the end of a long bone which gradually extends throughout its length. Fragmentation of the cortex is seen and pathological fractures tend to develop. There is little periosteal reaction.

Pathology

The tumour consists of pinkish grey granulation tissue. The cells are identical to those of reticulum cell sarcoma arising in a lymph node. The nuclei are round, oval, indented or lobulated and there is considerable cytoplasm. Mitotic figures are common. Dense reticulin fibres pass between the cells. The lesion must be differentiated from Ewing's sarcoma (*vide supra*).

Prognosis

The 5-year survival varies from 35–50% plus (Parker and Jackson, 1939; Hatcher, 1948; Coley *et al.*, 1950; Boston *et al.*, 1974).

Treatment

Parker and Jackson (1939) studied 17 patients, seven of whom were alive and apparently free of tumour 10 years later. They advocated prompt radical surgery followed by prophylactic irradiation of the regional lymph nodes. However, since then several centres have achieved similar results with primary irradiation. Hatcher (1948) showed that there was no viable residual tumour following irradiation. Lichtenstein (1977) reported a similar case the patient receiving a total tumour dose of approximately 2000 rad. Coley and his colleagues (1950) estimated the 5-year survival rate at 73% and the 10-year rate as high as 55% in those patients with localized lesions treated by irradiation. They advocated a total tumour dose of 3000–4000 rad whereas Wang and Fleischli (1968) and Newall and Friedman (1970) recommended higher doses of 4500–5000 rad. Amputation should be reserved for recurrent tumours or tumours which are not controlled by adequate irradiation.

Chemotherapy has been shown to be of use in the disseminated lymphomata and is being investigated in the treatment of disseminated reticulum cell sarcoma. Unfortunately there is not enough information available to evaluate its efficacy.

Synovial sarcoma

This usually arises from the synovium of joint or tendon sheath, but may arise in sub-cutaneous tissue or muscle.

Clinical findings

The neoplasm usually develops in the third and fourth decades and affects the upper limb more frequently than the lower limb. It usually presents as a painless swelling.

Radiographic features

An extra-articular shadow with or without calcification may be seen.

Pathology

It is a soft, fleshy, tumour with a false capsule. It contains areas of haemorrhage and foci of calcification. There is very cellular stroma made up of spindle cells. Gland-like structures with cuboidal or columnar pseudoepithelial cells are seen.

Spread

The main spread is to lungs via the blood stream. Skeletal metastases occur and there is a 20% incidence of lymph node involvement.

Prognosis

The 5-year survival varies from 10 to 40%.

Treatment

Radical local excision is the treatment of choice. Block dissection or radiotherapy to the lymph nodes may be indicated. There is no separate information available in relation to chemotherapy, these neoplasms being included with soft tissue sarcomata. The EORTC are currently conducting a number of trials in soft tissue sarcomata, which include synovial sarcomata but the results are not yet available.

Skeletal metastases

The skeleton is one of the commonest sites of metastatic disease, metastases accounting for more than half the cases of malignant bone tumours. Abrams and his colleagues (1950) reported on 1000 consecutive autopsies on patients with carcinoma. Overall, skeletal metastases were found in 27%. They were found in

Mankin, H. (1978), Personal communication.

Marcove, R.C. *et al.* (1971), Osteogenic sarcoma in childhood. *N.Y. St. J. Med.*, **71**, 855–9.

Marcove, R.C. *et al.* (1975), Giant cell tumors treated by cryosurgery. A report of 25 cases. *J. Bone Jt Surg.*, **55A**, 1633–44.

Milch, R.A. and Changus, G.W. (1956), Response of bone to tumor invasion *Cancer*, **9**, 340–51.

Miller, C.W., De Blasi, B.R. and Fisher, M.S. (1976), Immunologic studies in murine osteosarcoma. Immunogenicity, growth kinetics and immunotherapy. *J. Bone Jt Surg.*, **58A**, 312–17.

Milner, T.H., Maynard, C.D. and Cowan, R.J. (1971), Evaluation of ^{85}Sr bone scans and roentgenograms in 100 patients. *Archs Surg.*, **103**, 371–2.

Mnaymneh, W.A., Dudley, H.R. and Mnaymeneh, L.G. (1964), Giant-cell tumour of bone. An analysis and follow-up study of the 41 cases observed at the Massachusetts General Hospital between 1925 and 1961. *J. Bone Jt Surg.*, **46A**, 63–75.

Newall, J. and Friedman, M. (1970), Reticulum cell sarcoma. Part II: Radiation dosage for each type. *Radiology*, **94**, 643–7.

O'Bryan, R.M. *et al.* (1973), Phase II evaluation of adriamycin in human neoplasia. *Cancer*, **32**, 1–8.

Oldham, R.K. and Pomeroy, T.C. (1972), Treatment of Ewing's sarcoma with adriamycin (NSC–123127). *Cancer Chemother. Rep.*, **56**, 635–9.

Palma, J. *et al.* (1972), Treatment of metastatic Ewing's sarcoma with BCNU. *Cancer*, **30**, 909–13.

Parker, F. Jr. and Jackson, H. Jr. (1939), Primary reticulum cell sarcoma of bone. *Surgery, Gynec. Obstet.*, **68**, 45–53.

Price, C.H.G. (1961), Osteogenic sarcoma. An analysis of survival and its relationship to histological grading and structure. *J. Bone Jt Surg.*, **43B**, 300–13.

Reilly, C.A. Jr. *et al.* (1972), Immunological evidence suggesting a viral etiology of human osteosarcoma. *Cancer*, **30**, 603–9.

Rhomberg, W.U. (1978), Radiotherapy combined with ICRF 159 (NSC 129943) *Int. J. Radiat. Oncol. Biol. Phys.*, **4**, 121–6.

Roberts, J.G. *et al.* (1976), Evaluation of radiography and isotopic scintigraphy for detecting skeletal metastases in breast cancer. *Lancet*, **1**, 237–9.

Robinson, M.R. and Constable, A.R. (1973), Strontium-87m and the gamma camera in the study of bone metastases from carcinoma of the prostate. *Br. J. Urol.*, **45**, 173–8.

Rosen, G. *et al.* (1974), High dose methotrexate with citrovorum factor rescue and adriamycin in childhood osteogenic sarcoma. *Cancer*, **33**, 1151–63.

Ryall, R.D. *et al.* (1978), Combination of radiotherapy and razoxane (ICRF 159) for chondrosarcoma. *Cancer*, **44**, 891–5.

Samuels, M.L. and Howe, C.D. (1967), Cyclophosphamide in the management of Ewing's sarcoma. *Cancer*, **20**, 961–6.

Scaglietti, O. and Calandriello, B. (1962), Ossifying parosteal sarcoma. Parosteal osteoma or juxtacortical osteogenic sarcoma. *J. Bone Jt Surg.*, **44A**, 635–47.

Schabel, F.M. Jr. (1975), Concepts for systemic treatment of micrometastases *Cancer*, **35**, 15–24.

Schajowicz, F. (1959), Ewing's sarcoma and reticulum cell sarcoma of bone, with special reference to the histochemical demonstration of glycogen as an aid to differential diagnosis. *J. Bone Jt Surg.*, **41A**, 349–56.

Schajowicz, F. *et al.* (1972), *Histological Typing of Bone Tumours*, World Health Organisation, Geneva.

Senyszyn, J.J. Johnson, R.E. and Curran, R.E. (1970), Treatment of metastatic Ewing's sarcoma with actinomycin D (NSC 3053). *Cancer Chemother. Rep.*, **54**, 103–7.

Shearer, R.J. *et al.* (1974), Radio-isotope bone scintigraphy with the gamma camera in the investigation of prostatic cancer. *Br. Med. J.*, **2**, 362–5.

Sutow, W.W. (1968), Vincristine (NSC 67574) therapy for malignant solid tumors in children (except Wilm's tumor). *Cancer Chemother. Rep.*, **52**, 485–7.

Sutow, W.W. and Sullivan, M.P. (1962), Cyclophosphamide therapy in children with Ewing's sarcoma. *Cancer Chemother. Rep.*, **23**, 55–60.

Sutow, W.W., Wilbur, J.R. and Vietti, T.J. (1971), Evaluation of dosage schedules of mitomycin C (NSC 26980) in children. *Cancer Chemother. Rep.*, **55**, 285–9.

Sutow, W.W., Gehan, E.A. and Dyment, P.G. (1978), Multi-drug adjuvant chemotherapy for osteosarcoma; interim report of the South West Oncology Group studies. *Cancer Treat. Rep.*, **62**, 265–9.

Sutow, W.W. *et al.* (1975), Adjuvant chemotherapy in primary treatment of osteogenic sarcoma. *Cancer*, **36**, 1598–1602.

Sutow, W.W. *et al.* (1976), Multi-drug chemotherapy in primary treatment of osteosarcoma. *J. Bone Jt Surg.*, **58A**, 629–33.

Sweetnam, R. (1975), The surgical management of primary osteosarcoma. *Clin. Orthopaed. Rel. Res.*, **111**, 57–64.

Sweetnam, R., Knowelden, J. and Seddon, H. (1971), Bone sarcoma: treatment by irradiation, amputation and combination of the two. *Br. Med. J.*, **2**, 363–6.

Tan, C. *et al.* (1972), Adriamycin in children with acute

leukaemia and other neoplastic diseases. In: *International Symposium on Adriamycin* (eds S.K. Carter *et al.*) Springer-Verlag, Berlin, p. 204–12.

Taylor, W.F. *et al.* (1978), Trends and Variability in survival from osteosarcoma. *Mayo Clinic Proc.*, **53**, 695–700.

Taylor, W.F., Ivins, J.C., Dahlin, D.C. and Pritchard, D.J. (1978), Osteogenic sarcoma experienced at the Mayo Clinic, 1963–1974. In: *Immunotherapy of Cancer. Present Status of Trials in Man* (eds W.D. Terry and D. Windhorst). Raven Press, New York.

Thomson, A.D. and Turner-Warwick, R.T. (1955), Skeletal sarcomata and giant-cell tumours. *J. Bone Jt Surg.*, **37B**, 266–303.

Wang, C.C. and Fleischli, D.J. (1968), Primary reticulum cell sarcoma of bone, with emphasis on radiation therapy. *Cancer*, **22**, 994–8.

Weinfield, M.S. and Dudley, H.R. Jr. (1962), Osteogenic sarcoma. A follow-up of the 94 cases observed at the Massachusetts General Hospital from 1920 to 1960. *J. Bone Jt Surg.*, **44A**, 269–76.

33 Leukaemia – myeloproliferative disorders and supportive care

J.M.A. Whitehouse and J.M. Ford

Unlike many neoplasms, those discussed in this chapter are frequently overtly disseminated at diagnosis. The diffuse distribution of the organ concerned means that accurate assessment of disease extent is relatively crude and that in some instances an accurate diagnosis may be difficult to make in the face of the wide array of alternative cell types. Inevitably, treatment has to be designed for a systemic disorder.

Neoplasms of bone marrow origin include those thought to arise directly or indirectly from haemopoietic stem cells and those arising from other cells populating the marrow. The former include the acute myelogenous leukaemias (AML) and chronic myeloid leukaemia (CML). Acute leukaemias which cannot readily be identified as AML are best classified as acute non-myelogenous leukaemias (ANML); among these are the acute lymphoblastic leukaemias (ALL) and the acute undifferentiated leukaemias (AUL).

Other conditions such as polycythaemia rubra vera (PRV) and myelofibrosis (MF) were included by Damashek in his classification of the myeloproliferative disorders, and although not neoplasms by classical interpretation, they may progress to a terminal state having the characteristics of AML or CML. Other malignancies of bone marrow include chronic lymphocytic leukaemia (CLL) (see p.674), prolymphocytic leukaemia (PLL), myeloma (MM) and hairy cell leukaemia (HCL) (see Chapters 34 and 36).

The subjects discussed in this chapter will therefore be confined to conditions which are believed to arise as a result of dysgenesis of marrow stem cells, namely the acute leukaemias, CML, PRV and MF. Acute leukaemia is further discussed with special relevance to children in Chapter 37.

Incidence

The annual incidence per 100 000 population by sex is summarized for each condition in Table 33.1. It can be seen from this table that these conditions affect both sexes equally apart from ALL and PRV where the male:female incidence is approximately 2:1. Although rare, AML, CML, PRV and MF all appear to have a shallow peak incidence between 50 and 70 years. This is most marked in AML. ALL does show a slightly increased incidence in these decades but by far the highest incidence occurs between 0 and 4 years.

Investigation

Specific investigations indicated for a particular malignancy are dealt with in the appropriate section. In all patients clinical examination should be comprehensive and include examination of the fundi for evidence of haemorrhage or exudates, and of the mouth for gum or nasopharyngeal infiltration and haemorrhagic or infective lesions. The size and extent of lymphadenopathy, the presence of splenomegaly and hepatomegaly should be carefully documented. Both the latter may be measured from identical points at the costal margin to enable continuous comparison. The skin should be examined for evidence of infiltration, infection or haemorrhagic manifestations and since infection is a potentially lethal hazard in neutropenic patients, no external area should be spared scrutiny.

Table 33.1 Leukaemias and myeloproliferative diseases 1973–1974 (from the West Midlands Cancer Registry, by courtesy of Dr. J.A.H. Waterhouse).

Diagnosis	*Annual incidence** *per* 100 000	
	Males	*Females*
Leukaemia:		
acute myeloblastic	2.61	2.38
acute lymphoblastic	1.46	0.76
acute monocytic	0.12	0.21
acute, type unspecified	0.24	0.19
chronic myeloid	0.77	0.85
erythroleukaemia	0.10	0.14
Polycythaemia rubra vera	1.05	0.50
Myelofibrosis	0.22	0.27

* Average annual incidence, using the 1971 census population

Mandatory tests for all patients with suspected haematological malignancy include the following:

1. Full blood count, including differential white count, platelet count and examination of film.
2. ESR.
3. Blood urea and electrolytes.
4. Serum calcium.
5. Serum immunoglobulin and serum protein electrophoresis.
6. Liver function tests.
7. Serum B_{12} and B_{12} binding protein.
8. Serum folate and red cell folate.
9. Serum urate.
10. Chest X-ray, both PA and lateral (to show anterior mediastinum).
11. Bone marrow aspirate and/or trephine (including iron stains).
12. Blood group.

Specific investigations which may be indicated include tests for haemolysis, cytogenetic studies, leukocyte alkaline phosphatase, lymph node biopsy with imprints, histological examination of biopsy material, surface marker studies of cell population, arterial pO_2, blood volume, liver, bone or spleen scans and red cell survival studies.

General management principles

All patients with haematological malignancies must have their progress carefully monitored. Various types of flow chart are now available permitting graphic display of peripheral blood and other selected characteristics. These facilitate treatment supervision, allow an immediate appreciation of impending toxicity and are particularly valuable in the follow-up of patients receiving intensive chemotherapy.

The early management of the chronic leukaemias, PRV and MF, is relatively straightforward. The management of the acute leukaemias is becoming increasingly specialized and where possible should be carried out at a special centre. Within the special centre, supportive care facilities must be available to deal with the problems of severe bone marrow suppression, which result both from the disease and its treatment. Infection should be controlled prior to treatment for the granulocyte response to infection results in an increased risk of selectively ablating the normal granulocytic series, should chemotherapy be administered at that time. Urgent investigation of pyrexia in the neutropenic patient should be followed by therapy with antibiotics – active particularly against gram negative organisms. A detailed appraisal of supportive care follows later in this chapter.

Polycythaemia rubra vera (PRV)

Three categories of disorder associated with an increased haematocrit can be recognized (Table 33.2).

1. Polycythaemia rubra vera or primary polycythaemia for which the cause is unknown.
2. Secondary polycythaemia for which many causes can be recognized.
3. Relative polycythaemia in which the red cell mass is of normal volume but the plasma volume is reduced.

Table 33.2 Polycythaemias.

Primary
    Polycythaemia rubra vera

Secondary
  Hypoxic
    Abnormal haemoglobin (i.e. methaemoglobin)
    Chronic pulmonary disease
    Congenital heart disease (left to right shunt)
    Gross obesity
    High altitude
  Tumours and others
    Bronchogenic carcinoma
    Cerebellar haemogioblastoma
    Hepatoma
    Renal tumours, cysts and hydronephrosis
    Uterine myomas

Relative
    Dehydration
    Stress

Both primary and secondary polycythaemia have an absolute increase in red cell mass. Exclusion of secondary polycythaemia is essential before a diagnosis of PRV is made. Only PRV will be discussed here.

PRV is uncommon and the incidence has been estimated at between 0.6 and 1.8/100 000. The incidence is greatest in men between the ages of 40 and 70 years, and the median survival is about 13 years. Patients with this disorder may present with a wide variety of symptoms, some of which are the result of a rise in blood viscosity resulting from the increase in red cell mass, others with a haemorrhagic tendency. Common presenting features include complaints of headache or a feeling of fullness in the head, dyspnoea, easy fatigability, dyspepsia and flatulence. Haemorrhagic features include epistaxis, gastrointestinal haemorrhage and disturbances of vision. The latter may result from a thrombotic tendency. Peripheral vascular problems also occur. Pruritus is common and may be particularly severe after a hot bath. The cause for this is unknown, although histamine release, anoxia of pain terminals and blood stasis in small vessels have all been proposed to explain this phenomenon. Gout may result from the increased cell turnover and subsequent cellular destruction, and bone pain from an extension of erythropoetic marrow.

Moderate splenomegaly is present in about 60% of cases at presentation, and helps to differentiate the condition from the secondary polycythaemias in which splenomegaly is not a feature. Few other physical signs are helpful diagnostically, although some patients have a marked plethoric facies, conjunctival injection and engorgement of fundal veins which suggest a diagnosis of either primary or secondary polycythaemia. Characteristically, examination of the peripheral blood in PRV reveals a raised haemoglobin, an increased haematocrit and frequently both a leucocytosis and an increase in platelets, but early in the disease only marginal elevation of one of the indices may be apparent. Patients should be fully investigated to exclude causes of secondary polycythaemia (Table 33.2). Measurement of total red cell and plasma volumes will help to distinguish an absolute polycythaemia from a relative polycythaemia. A blood arterial oxygen saturation below 92% indicates a secondary polycythaemia of the kind associated with a reduced blood oxygen saturation. An intravenous pyelogram (IVP) can be helpful in identifying a renal cause for polycythaemia. In specialist laboratories, erythropoietin levels may be measured. These are low or even absent in PRV.

The leucocyte alkaline phosphatase B_{12} and B_{12} binding proteins are usually raised in PRV but normal in secondary polycythaemia. In the patient who has not suffered a recent haemorrhage there is usually little problem in distinguishing PRV from CML, MF or essential thrombocythaemia on the basis of peripheral counts.

Bone marrow examination may not be particularly helpful but an increase in marrow cellularity, in the number and size of megakaryocytes, in the number of eosinophils, in the amount of reticulin or degree of myelofibrosis and depletion of marrow iron stores have all been reported.

A significantly increased incidence of aneuploidy has been demonstrated in PRV, and it has been postulated that in these patients disease is advancing to the accelerated phase.

Progression to MF occurs in many patients and this is manifest by increasing splenomegaly with or without an associated progressive fall in haemoglobin which may then remain stable at a lower level. The peripheral white blood count may show a shift to the left, and although the platelet count may be raised initially, this also falls as the degree of fibrosis increases. A bone marrow trephine examination at this time shows increased fibrosis and new bone formation. Other patients progress to a clinical and haematological state which may be difficult to distinguish from CML.

Treatment

In the early chronic phase of this disease, the major feature is the increased red cell mass and consequent features of hyperviscosity, vascular distension and tissue anoxia. Venesection can control these problems satisfactorily and is particularly useful in those patients with low-grade disease; 500 ml of blood, or less in the elderly, should be removed at 24-hour intervals until the haematocrit lies between 42 and 47%. Current studies indicate that, intermittent venesection should be carried out, at intervals, in order to maintain the haematocrit within the normal range. This may only be required at intervals of several months to maintain the patient symptom-free. Spleen size is unhelpful in monitoring the condition. Occasionally venesection alone may result in an increase in the platelet count. This should be monitored carefully, but the incidence of thrombotic complications is not greater after venesection, and merely reflects the overall myeloproliferation.

The disadvantage of venesection is the lack of influence on the raised platelet count and the continued depletion of iron stores which may result in glossitis and dysphagia, where the iron loss is not restored. In those patients with markedly raised platelet counts, or in whom venesection produces only poor control, treatment with radioactive phosphorus is indicated. Females of child-bearing age should not be treated in this manner and young males should probably also be excluded since azoospermia may result. ^{32}P in a dose of

3 mCi or 5 mCi, administered intravenously, is rapidly taken up by mitotically active cells of the bone marrow and later incorporated in the calcium phosphate of the bone. The irradiation of the marrow usually produces a normal peripheral blood picture in one to two months. If control is still not adequate at three months, a further 3 mCi may be given. The reduction in platelet count also means that subsequent control by venesection is facilitated and further ^{32}P may not be required for a number of years. The incidence of acute leukaemia developing in radiation-treated patients is higher than that of the normal population, so that a limit of 30 mCi ^{32}P has been suggested. However, there is now evidence that the incidence of acute leukaemia is also significantly raised in patients with PRV treated with alkylating agents alone, emphasizing the need for meticulous care in the planning of treatment. Minimal treatment by both ^{32}P and chemotherapy is desirable since leukaemogenesis and other complications will be dose-related.

Busulphan has been used for disease control, but it is less effective and more difficult to control than ^{32}P therapy. It may prove useful in the short term control of thrombocytosis when administered in the same dose regimen as for CML.

Allopurinol should be prescribed for all patients with PRV to avoid the complications of hyperuricaemia. Once the level of nucleoprotein release is reduced and the disease is stable, this may be discontinued.

Pruritus is frequently reduced by venesection, and its return may prompt the patient to request further treatment. In those in whom symptomatic relief is poor, antihistamines have been tried with little benefit. Cholestyramine has, however, produced relief in some patients and merits trial in those who are severely affected and who are unrelieved by other therapy. Recent preliminary studies of cimetidine, a histamine antagonist, have been encouraging.

Surgical procedures are better delayed until good haematological control is achieved. Anticoagulants are only rarely administered to the patient with PRV, and should be monitored with extreme caution. Splenic infarction is best treated conservatively. Late progression of the disease and the development of MF is associated with a fall in haemoglobin and ultimately of thrombocytopenia. Once this situation has developed, little therapy is of value and the clinical course is one of progressive marrow failure.

Myelofibrosis (MF)

This condition may develop *de novo* or as a sequel to other conditions (primary or secondary MF) (Table 33.3). Rarely it may follow exposure to certain chemicals. Frequently patients have only minimal symptoms

Table 33.3   Myelofibrosis.

Primary
    Acute
    Chronic

Secondary
    Benzene
    Chronic infection
    Fluorosis
    Hodgkin's disease
    Irradiation
    Malignant infiltration of marrow
    Marble bone disease
    Mastocytosis with generalized osteosclerosis,
        hepatosplenomegaly and urticaria pigmentosa
    Renal osteodystrophy with osteosclerosis
    Secondary to other chronic myeloproliferative
        disorders
    Syphilis
    Toxic
    Tuberculosis

at presentation, and these may be referrable to the spleen or result from the mild anaemia. Vague non-specific constitutional symptoms may be elicited on close questioning. Gout and renal colic may occur. The physical findings at the time of diagnosis are primarily those of hepatosplenomegaly. Splenic enlargement is usually pronounced and may be gross. Examination of the blood commonly reveals anisocytosis and poikilocytosis, a reticulocytosis (up to 5%), a moderately raised leucocyte count $(15-30\times10^9/1)$ and often a small number of blast cells. The platelet count is often raised initially, trending downwards as the disease progresses. Impaired liver function tests are often found. Hyperuricaemia is common, although overt gout is less so.

The leucocyte alkaline phosphatase score is not particularly valuable as it may be normal, raised or low. Elevated blood and urine histamine levels may be found in many patients and some correlation has been proposed between high levels and the incidence of clinical symptoms.

Bone marrow examination reveals an increase in reticulin, extensive fibroblastic proliferation and new bone formation. Radiological evidence of MF is apparent in about 30% of patients as sclerotic change in bones. This tends to be symmetrical and involves the pelvis, the vertebrae, clavicles and ribs. Islands of increased bone density may be seen in the ends of long bones. Myeloid metaplasia is a feature of this condition, occurring predominantly in the liver and spleen, but extramedullary haemopoiesis may occur at other sites. These are frequently intra-abdominal, but rarely spinal cord compression may occur from an extradural deposit. The median survival of this condition is about four years, death resulting from the consequences of bone marrow failure or of leukaemic transformation.

Treatment

Folate deficiency should be excluded and if present treated appropriately. In the patient with moderate to massive splenomegaly, significant pooling may occur in the spleen leading to the features of hypersplenism. ^{51}Cr labelled RBC survival studies with scanning of the spleen may assist in recognizing such patients and some benefit may be obtained from splenectomy. This operation may also be of value in providing symptomatic relief for the patient with a huge painful spleen. Certainly, the indication for splenectomy is rarely well defined, and each patient has to be carefully assessed individually. ^{51}Cr red cell survival studies and ^{59}Fe utilization studies do not help in any major way the decision to undertake splenectomy. This is usually undertaken on the clinical grounds of discomfort or pain associated with splenomegaly or splenic infarction. Some anxiety exists as to whether splenectomy accelerates myeloid expansion elsewhere, for example in the liver, but the evidence for this is unsubstantiated.

Chemotherapy has little place in the management of MF. Regression of spleen size can certainly be achieved in some patients by the use of alkylating agents, but usually at the cost of peripheral pancytopenia.

Oxymethalone and other androgens have been used in an attempt to raise haemoglobin levels. Therapy needs to be continued for two months before failure to achieve benefit is acknowledged. These hormones are markedly virilizing but may produce an increase in haematocrit in some patients.

Steroid therapy may produce a temporary improvement in the peripheral blood count and an improvement in well being. There may also be some relief of generalized bone discomfort which occurs in some patients.

Allopurinol 200 mg twice daily is advisable where hyperuricaemia is diagnosed.

Palliative therapy is the most important aspect of long-term management and frequently involves the control of infection and of haemorrhagic complications.

Chronic myeloid leukaemia (CML)

Disease characteristics

The symptoms and signs of CML result from the consequences of an accumulation of cells of the granulocytic series in the bone marrow and spleen. The onset of symptoms such as sweats and itching due to a hypercatabolic state, may be insidious. The combined effects of a compromised red cell series and the expansion of the granulocytic compartment within the bone marrow may give rise to a normochromic normocytic anaemia, producing increasing lethargy, easy fatiguability and shortness of breath on exertion. The anaemia is only mild in many patients, while in others its onset may be so slow as to pass almost unnoticed. Examination of the peripheral blood may reveal a raised white cell count which can range as high as 1000×10^9/l, containing 20–50% myelocytes and other precursor cells. An eosinophilia and basophilia may also be noted. Thrombocytopenia is not usually an early feature of the condition. Platelets may be large and atypical and the count may actually be raised initially. The large platelets may be functionally deficient which accounts for the haemorrhagic features sometimes seen in the presence of a raised platelet count. With disease progression (or indeed over-treatment), purpura and other haemorrhagic manifestations develop with increased severity.

Bone marrow examination at the time of presentation reveals a grossly hypercellular marrow, devoid of fat spaces. A reticulin positive myelosclerosis may occur at any stage in the disease. A diagnostic feature is the presence of a marker 22 chromosome, the Philadelphia or Ph^1 chromosome. This anomaly is associated with chromosome G22, the lost portion of a long arm of G22 frequently translocated onto t9, but in about 8% the deleted segment of 22q is translocated onto other chromosomes. Other chromosome abnormalities in addition to the Philadelphia chromosome, appear to represent new clones with aneuploid constitution. The Ph^1 chromosome has been found in myeloid and erythroid tissue and megakaryocytes and its presence implies a clonal origin for the affected cells. The majority of CML patients (80%) demonstrate the Ph^1 chromosome. The remainder may be truly Ph^1-negative or may represent the inability of available techniques to demonstrate all chromosomal abnormalities. There is some evidence, that there may be a correlation between chromsomal changes and the clinical course of the disease, and patients exhibiting a double Ph^1 chromosome have a more aggressive variant of the disease associated with shortened survival. Extension of haemopoiesis into long bones and infiltration of expanding marrow may cause bone pain suggesting an arthropathy. Hepatomegaly is usually only slight, but splenic involvement is frequently manifest by splenomegaly which may be gross. Mechanical problems which result from this include a dragging sensation in the left hypochondrium, a feeling of fullness after small meals, often causing loss of appetite and consequent weight loss. Abdominal pain may result from splenic engorgement and splenic infarction. The latter may mimic signs of pleuritic origin. Recurrent small infarctions may even suggest recurrent pulmonary emboli as a diagnosis, but the discovery of a large spleen and, in some instances, the demonstration of a rub over the infarcted area, will suggest the true diagnosis. Other constitutional features include fever of unexplained origin, general debility and lassitude, even recurring in the presence of a normal haemoglobin.

Rare features of the disease are lymphadenopathy, skin infiltration and priapism. Recently, bizarre neurological symptoms, including visual disturbances have been attributed to hyperviscosity syndromes in patients with high peripheral white counts. Gout is uncommon, although the serum uric acid is often raised.

A low leucocyte alkaline phosphatase is characteristic in this condition and the serum B_{12} and B_{12} binding protein, transcobalamin I may be raised.

The clinical course of CML is frequently one of a benign process, responding rapidly to corrective therapy with intermittent periods of stability. Throughout this time, the patient is well and often little troubled by the condition. Eighty per cent or more of patients with CML have disease which transforms in character from a relatively benign state which is readily responsive to treatment with a single agent alone, to an outright leukaemia. Were it not for this fact there would be a debate over its acceptance as a true neoplasm. Nothing is known of the factors which initiate blast cell transformation. Occasionally, the condition follows a fulminant course (acute blast crisis) but in the majority of patients, this transformation occurs slowly over a period of months as a progressive acceleration of the disease state – the so called 'accelerated phase' of the disease. In some, progression may be much less rapid with patients surviving for several years.

The onset of 'blast crisis' can be suspected in a patient whose slowly rising white count becomes increasingly refractory to standard treatment. The total blast count increases and although absolute definition is irrelevant, more than 50% blasts in the bone marrow confirms the existence of a blast crisis. Often the patient develops prominent symptoms attributable to increasing bone marrow infiltration – pallor, weakness, bone pain, plus fever and splenic discomfort. Haemorrhagic features may become prominent. Rarely extensive bone destruction may result in hypercalcaemia.

Even more rarely, a patient may present in blast crisis with regional lymphadenopathy or a myeloblastic tumour of bone or skin. The clinical features and lymph node or tissue biopsy may suggest an atypical lymphoma, but close examination of the biopsy material will indicate infiltration with myeloid tissue. Frank haematological blast crisis of CML usually follows rapidly and identification of the Ph^1 chromosome establishes the diagnosis. The morphological characteristics of the blast cells are myeloid in 80% of patients, but the remaining 20% have cytological features of a lymphoblastic nature. This distinction has some therapeutic relevance. Newer techniques have facilitated the recognition of the latter population of cells. Antisera raised to cells from patients with established ALL, react with the lymphoblastoid cells of CML blast crisis (CML BC). Furthermore, terminal deoxynucleotidyl transferase which is only found in high concentrations in normal thymus and in ALL cells, is also found to be raised in cells from CML BC of lymphoblastoid character. It is thought that the blastic transformation in these cases arises as a result of transformation in coexisting Ph^1-positive lymphoid cell lines which are undetected in the chronic phase. An alternative suggestion is that they arise from myeloid stem cells but undergo dedifferentiation during the blastic transformation.

Treatment

It is remarkable that this condition, which is sensitive to various treatment modalities, has a marker chromosome and can readily be monitored by following the peripheral blood count and the degree of marrow change, and has a median survival which has been unaffected by recent advances in cancer medicine. The reasons for this are not entirely clear. The proliferating granulocyte population may be reduced by chemotherapy or irradiation but neither method is exclusively selective and bone marrow suppression may be a consequence of either therapy.

Irradiation
Extracorporeal irradiation is no longer practised since the resultant pancytopenia may be severe and there is no selective toxicity for the granulocyte population. A reduction in granulocyte count can be achieved by direct irradiation of the spleen but comparisons with busulphan therapy have shown no advantage for splenic irradiation in relieving the pain of infarction of presplenitis. Both treatments are equally effective at reducing the size of the spleen. However, oral single agent chemotherapy is easier to manage and the overall survival of patients receiving drugs alone is greater than those receiving intermittent irradiation. Splenic irradiation has occasionally been used to achieve temporary palliation of symptoms in patients refractory to chemotherapy, but the risk of bone marrow suppression and thrombocytopenia limits this approach. It may now however be worthwhile having a fresh

approach to the use of irradiation in judicious combination with chemotherapy.

Chemotherapy

Several agents, such as busulphan, dibromomannitol and hydroxyurea, have been shown to be useful in controlling the chronic phase of CML. The majority of patients respond to the alkylating agent busulphan. Comparison of this drug with other alkylating agents and 6-mercaptopurine demonstrated the superiority of busulphan. The earlier comparisons with splenic irradiation revealed that busulphan-treated patients had higher maintained haemoglobins than the irradiated group of patients. Busulphan remains the drug of choice at the present time. Treatment may be commenced using 4 mg daily and continued until the total white count has fallen to between $10-15 \times 10^9$/l. It has been customary to continue on a maintenance dose of between 0.5 mg and 2.0 mg daily of busulphan. However, in patients who receive no maintenance chemotherapy, the delay before counts once again rise is very variable and it is often preferred, once the white count has reached a reasonable level, to discontinue the busulphan and to delay retreatment until there is an obvious upward trend in the total white count, and until levels have reached $25-30 \times 10^9$/l. Thrombocytopenia may indicate busulphan overdosage but can occasionally be an early sign of impending blast crisis. Overdosage may produce a continued fall in the peripheral counts, even when the drug is stopped and in rare instances marrow aplasia may result from which recovery can be incomplete. Other rare side-effects of busulphan include an Addisonian-like syndrome with pigmentation, hyponatraemia and weakness, pulmonary fibrosis, gynaecomastia and testicular atrophy, or amenorrhoea.

All patients receiving treatment with this drug should receive regular follow-up examinations and the peripheral counts should be carefully monitored using flow charts where fluctuations will be readily apparent. It may take between two and four months before the white count reaches satisfactory levels. The response to chemotherapy is associated with a reduction in spleen size and a rise in haemoglobin. The serum B_{12} and B_{12} binding protein levels, the leucocyte alkaline phosphatase score (LAP) return to normal during periods of effective disease control. The bone marrow examination at this time may show a persistence of granulocytic hyperplasia.

Attempts to eliminate the Ph^1-positive clone have been generally unsuccessful, despite varying combinations of splenic irradiation, splenectomy and intensive chemotherapy. Significant reduction of Ph^1-positive cells in the bone marrow has only been achieved in the minority and neither this nor a restoration of bone marrow to apparent normality appeared to confer any obvious benefit in terms of delaying the onset of blast crisis.

Disease progression may be marked by an increasing refractoriness to busulphan therapy so that increased doses are required for control. There may be no obvious evidence of blast crisis throughout this period, although the disease 'acceleration' is often marked by a more rapid rise in the white cell count and platelet counts and evidence of an enlarging spleen. This state may last for weeks or months before frank 'blast crisis' is manifest. Hydroxyurea in a dose of between 0.5 g and 2.0 g daily may be used where escape from busulphan has occurred. It is administered orally and does not have the prolonged marrow suppressive effect of busulphan so that on cessation of therapy, a rapid rise of the white count is often seen. Apart from bone marrow suppression, the side-effects are minimal so that the dose required may be titrated against the total white count. Once escape from this drug follows resistance to busulphan, the implication is that the disease is rapidly progressing to blastic transformation and alternative therapy is indicated.

Splenectomy

Early elective splenectomy has been proposed as a therapeutic manoeuvre since the splenic complications developing in blastic crisis cause significant morbidity. The value of this procedure remains to be evaluated. It does not appear to delay the onset of blast crisis, nor to improve tolerance to chemotherapy and may be an extremely hazardous procedure in those patients with persistent thrombocytopenia, massive splenomegaly or severe splenic symptoms. Death may occur from haemorrhage despite adequate cover with platelet transfusions and the operation, advocated by some where platelet consumption is presumed, cannot yet be justified as routine.

Leucapheresis

Continuous flow centrifuge leucapheresis is readily available as a procedure in most special centres, but has little value in the therapy of this condition except as a means of treating patients with high white counts and obvious hyperviscosity symptoms. It has principally been used to obtain granulocytes from CML donors for use as therapeutic granulocyte transfusions.

Immunotherapy

As in the immunotherapy of other human malignancies, this remains an experimental procedure with little to recommend it therapeutically at the present time.

Treatment of blast crisis

A florid acute leukaemia develops in more than three quarters of the patients with Ph[1]-positive CML. Occasionally, patients may present in blast crisis as an acute leukaemia in which Ph[1] chromosome is later demonstrated. Regional lymphadenopathy or tumours resulting from tissue deposition of myeloid material may precede the acute leukaemic manifestations of blast crisis.

Once diagnosed, these patients should be managed as for acute leukaemia. Local infiltration of skin or lymph nodes may be treated with radiotherapy. The leukaemia frequently responds to the agents used in acute myelogenous leukaemia, but the response is often only partial and the overall survival shorter. Various combinations have been proposed and these are summarized in Table 33.4. An unexpected finding is the response of some patients to vincristine and prednisolone alone, since neither agent has significant activity in AML. However, the majority of responding patients have been found to have blast cells with lymphoblastoid characteristics. One cytogenetic study has suggested that the existence of aneuploidy favours complete remission and that those patients whose blast cells are predominantly hypodiploid are particularly responsive. Hyperdiploid patients rarely responded to vincristine and prednisolone alone. Thus cytogenetic studies and the identification by morphological, biochemical and cytochemical studies of the lymphoblastoid cell population may have some therapeutic value.

No satisfactory chemotherapy maintenance has yet been identified for this condition. Both high dose intermittent chemotherapy and continuous regimens have been tried, but the median duration of survival remains 8–10 months after onset of blast crisis, indicating the need for improved maintenance therapy.

A consequence of the improved survival in some patients is the increase in incidence of meningeal leukaemia which is manifest as in other acute leukaemias, either symptomatically with signs of raised intracranial pressure, or asymptomatically with cytological evidence of disease in the cerebrospinal fluid alone. Intrathecal therapy with methotrexate 12.5 mg twice weekly to a total of ten injections or five injections of methotrexate followed by five injections of cytosine arabinoside may be effective in the eradication of infiltration.

Various experimental procedures are under evaluation for the control of CML BC. One which has theoretical appeal is the attempt to destroy the blast cell population with intensive chemotherapy and radiotherapy followed by bone marrow reconstitution using leucapheresed cells (containing colony-forming cells) or bone marrow cells collected and stored at the time of diagnosis, to restore chronic phase CML. Unfortunately, just as the disease has transformed during its normal course, so it may be expected to do so again from the stored cells repopulating the bone marrow.

Table 33.4　Chemotherapy of blastic transformation of chronic myeloid leukaemia (CML-BC).

Reference	Agents used	No. of patients	Complete remission
Marmont and Damasio (1973)	Vincristine and prednisolone	24	9
Spiers *et al.* (1974)	Thioguanine Daunorubicin Cytosine arabinoside Methotrexate Prednisolone Cyclophosphamide Vincristine L-asparaginase	9	4
Hayes *et al.* (1974)	Cytosine arabinoside BCNU Vincristine Prednisolone	86	4
Shaw *et al.* (1975)	Vincristine and prednisolone	4	1
Canellos *et al.* (1976)	Cytosine arabinoside 6-Thioguanine	13	1

The acute leukaemias (see also Chapter 37 for acute leukaemia in children)

Leukaemic process

The aetiology of most of the acute leukaemias in man remains obscure, although in some animals viruses capable of inducing leukaemia have been identified. Exposure to irradiation or chemicals such as benzene are known to increase the risk of acute leukaemia in man. For instance, the population of Hiroshima and Nagasaki who survived the nuclear explosions of 1945, have developed acute leukaemia at a frequency which is four times greater than that of unexposed Japanese.

The hazards of combining irradiation and chemotherapy in the treatment of malignant disease are now being appreciated in those conditions where long-term survival results from such treatment. In a recent study from Stanford University, patients with Hodgkin's disease who received combined therapy with irradiation and chemotherapy had an incidence of AML which approached 4% at six years. Continuous administration of alkylating agents has also been incriminated, particularly in patients with ovarian carcinoma and myeloma.

For the most part however, the causative factors of both AML and the ANML including ALL are unknown. Nonetheless, there is an increasing understanding of the leukaemic process which may eventually assist in planning therapy. The original concept of actively proliferating leukaemic cells having unusually rapid rates of DNA replication and mitosis has now been discounted. It is now clear that leukaemic cells may synthesize DNA and divide at a rate comparable to, or even less than that of normal blast cells, but that a failure of maturation exists so that the ratio of blast cells to cells committed to differentiation is greater than one. The result is a steadily expanding pool of blast cells, the progressive accumulation of which eventually leads to both marrow failure and the development of clinical features suggesting acute leukaemia.

Discussion has focused around whether AML represents the outcome of a primary maturation abnormality affecting some of the granulocytic precursor cells, which nonetheless retain their capacity for normal maturation progression in the appropriate environment, or whether the leukaemic cells represent a totally separate neoplastic population. The whole population of cells of bone marrow origin would be likely to be affected by the former process, while in the latter, malignant transformation of a solitary stem cell could produce a clone of leukaemic blast cells.

The evidence for and against both interpretations is well reviewed by Clarkson (1972). It seems likely that the leukaemic cell population proliferates alongside the normal one and that the essential dominance of the former confirms its neoplastic role.

The leukaemic cells probably achieve their dominance in part by direct competition with the normal marrow. A degree of differentiation suggests a longer cell turnover time than that of the more primitive cell population. Whether normal controlling mechanisms operate to decelerate normal haemopoiesis as the leukaemic population expands is not clear. Certainly, this would facilitate the rapid establishment of leukaemic cells throughout the marrow stroma and would only require the normal cells to be capable of cell–cell recognition for inhibition of growth. The widespread infiltration of the marrow by leukaemic cells demonstrating identical degrees of maturation can be quoted as evidence both for a clonal origin and for maturation arrest.

The suggestion that external factors may be of relevance in the development of acute leukaemia gains support from reports of leukaemic transformation occurring in normal male cells transplanted into heavily irradiated female siblings with ALL. However, there are no reports yet of this occurring in AML and collective evidence favours the existence of a separate neoplastic population of leukaemic cells in this condition. The existence of a population of tumour cells with distinctive characteristics would lend encouragement to the prospect of cure.

Clinical features

The diagnosis of an acute leukaemia is rarely difficult to make. The history is usually short – four to six weeks or less, often dating back to what is described as an influenza-like illness, the particular features being fever and generalized aching. This is followed by poor recovery and the subsequent development of the symptoms and signs of anaemia, thrombocytopenia or both. Infective complications are less common at the time of presentation, despite the fact that in the myelogenous leukaemias, granulocytic precursor cells are involved in the neoplastic process. Specific physical signs apart from those of anaemia or haemorrhage are uncommon in AML, apart from tissue infiltration of the skin and gums which may occur in monocytic and myelomonocytic variants. In ALL lymphadenopathy, splenomegaly and anaemia are frequently apparent at the time of presentation, but haemorrhagic features are less common than in AML. Although raised peripheral white blood counts frequently imply an underlying leukaemic process, the diagnosis must be confirmed by bone marrow examination. ALL, hypoplastic AML, monoblastic leukaemia and acute promyelocytic leukaemia (APML) may be recognized with some accuracy using morphological characteristics alone. With the exception of APML where daunorubicin has been suggested to be of particular therapeutic value, survival or responsiveness to treatment does not appear to correlate with the degree of cytological differentiation. In recent years, a number of objective laboratory tests combined with standard morphological criteria have led to some advances in the classification of the different sub-types of acute leukaemia (Table 33.5). Cytochemical studies may facilitate typing of leukaemias; sudan black or peroxidase stains are essential to make a firm diagnosis of AML. The periodic acid Schiff stain is useful in identifying ALL where coarsely granular or block positivity on a negative cytoplasmic background is seen. Similar positivity may be seen in CML in blast crisis. Difficulties of interpretation may arise, however, since about 30% of ANML are PAS-negative.

The surface characteristics of the leukaemic cell may well prove to be a useful means of characterizing the cell type. This is particularly true of the lymphoid leukaemias where the identification of surface immunoglobulin or the ability to rosette sheep red cells has permitted the broad differentiation into those lymphoid leukaemias which are presumed to be of T-cell origin, those of B-cell origin and those which have neither marker (the 'null'-cell leukaemias). Attempts have been made to raise anti-sera to leukaemic cells of the different sub-types and in ALL there has been a suggestion that leukaemia-associated antigens may well exist. This is not yet true for AML. The principle value of such anti-sera lies in their application to the study of the leukaemic process and its evolution. Indeed, as previously mentioned, an antigenic similarity has been demonstrated between the leukaemic cell with lymphoid morphology in CML (blast crisis) and ALL cells. Certain biochemical markers can be used to differentiate cerain cell types, for example, serum and urine lysozyme levels are frequently raised in patients

with acute myelomonocytic or monocytic leukaemia, and terminal deoxynucleotidyl transferase which is found in high concentrations in normal thymus is also found in the many leukaemic cells of patients with ALL and in some in blast crisis of CML, particularly those with a lymphoid morphology.

It has been recognized for many years that granulocytic leukaemias can occur with a longer than usual natural history in which the diagnosis of acute leukaemia is certain. These have a low percentage of blast cells in the marrow. This condition has been described under a number of different names: smouldering leukaemia; refractory anaemia with excessive myeloblasts; sub-acute granulocytic leukaemia; preleukaemia; hypoplastic acute leukaemia and oligoblastic leukaemia. It is likely that such patients have been diagnosed as AML and included in trial analysis.

The variability of criteria for the diagnosis of AML and the inclusion of cases of hypoplastic AML which may have a relatively good prognosis, emphasizes the difficulties of analysing data from different centres which are only superficially comparable. The clinical features associated with the different sub-categories of acute leukaemias are reviewed in Table 33.6. At least three of the varieties of acute leukaemia, namely acute monoblastic, acute promyelocytic and hypoplastic leukaemia are sufficiently distinct to warrant separation from the myeloblastic and acute myelomonoblastic groups which form the bulk of AML. The study of patients with acute monoblastic leukaemia and myelomonocytic leukaemia has shown that hypokalaemia, skin infiltration and gum hypertrophy are more common in these groups although these factors have little relevance in predicting the outcome of therapy. Of more importance is the recognition of acute promyelocytic leukaemia, since disseminated intravascular coagulation is an almost invariable complication of this disorder. High blast counts and low platelet counts at presentation appear to have some

Table 33.5 Classification of the acute leukaemias.

Acute myelogenous leukaemias (AML)	Myeloblastic Myelomonocytic Monoblastic Promyelocytic Erythroleukaemia Hypoplastic	
Chronic myeloid leukaemia – blast crisis (CML-BC)	Lymphoblastoid Other	
Acute non-myelogenous leukaemia (ANML)	Lymphoblastic (ALL) –	'T' 'B' NULL
	Undifferentiated (AUL)	

Table 33.6 Clinical features of the acute leukaemias.

	Lymphadenopathy	Splenomegaly	Skin/gum infiltration	DIC
AML				
Myeloblastic	0	0 → +	0	0 → +
Myelomonocytic	0 → +	0	0 → +	0 → +
Monoblastic	0 → ++	0 → +	0 → ++	0 → +
Promyelocytic	0	0	0	++
Erythroleukaemia	0	0	0	0
Hypoplastic	0	0	0	0
CML BC	0 → ++	++	0	0
ANML				
ALL	+ (++ mediastinum – 'T' cell)	+	0	0
AUL	+	+	0	0

0   usually absent
+   usually discrete
++ usually marked

prognostic significance in childhood ALL and AML, observations which are less valid in adults.

Treatment

The management of the patient with acute leukaemia may be regarded as having two stages, the first is a period of intensive chemotherapy (remission induction) during which rapid reduction in disease volume is attempted; this, if successful, results in an apparent disease-free state (complete remission). Throughout this period, specialist supervision is required since expertise in the provision of supportive care may profoundly affect the patient's ability to tolerate the chemotherapy. The second phase involves the maintenance of the disease-free state over a prolonged period of time (remission maintenance). This is particularly important since disease-free survival reflects the ability to eradicate or control the disease process and the way in which this is effected is of considerable importance to the patient's quality of life.

There is a widespread tendency to regard the patient with acute leukaemia as in urgent need of specific anti-leukaemic therapy. Some justification for this can be obtained from the survival of untreated patients with ALL or AML or of those receiving sub-optimal treatment. However, despite this, since an inevitable consequence of giving anti-leukaemic therapy is to produce hypoplasia of normal marrow, there are considerable advantages in ensuring that the patient who is to receive treatment has his clinical state restored to as close to normality as possible prior to therapy. The correction of anaemia, the treatment of infection and prevention of further haemorrhage are a vital prelude to treatment. Since rapid cellular catabolism is a consequence of successful treatment, allopurinol should be commenced prior to treatment and normal renal function ensured. Abnormal hepatic or renal function may affect drug metabolism and excretion and consequently its mode of action and toxicity.

Various principles of chemotherapy administration have evolved from observation of the response to therapy. In the absence of major selective kill of the leukaemic cell population, which may occur in ALL of childhood, the rapidity of achievement of bone marrow aplasia is likely to be of importance so that rapid repopulation by normal tissue may occur. Continued intensive chemotherapy may inhibit such recovery if given at the time of synchronous recovery of the normal stem cell population, and thus permit re-establishment of the leukaemia. These factors encourage caution in the interpretation of the figures for single drug activity; nonetheless, they provided a guide to potentially effective agents.

At the time of presentation, the disease burden probably amounts to some 1×10^{12} cells, representing about 30 doublings of tumour cell mass. It is probable that in acute leukaemia, as in other tumours, the growth rate is Gompertzian in fashion, i.e. the rate of growth of the tumour is high at the outset, but it slows down as the tumour volume increases. What is difficult to comprehend is why following therapy the normal marrow regrowth should be favoured when a degree of aplasia exists and yet the leukaemic population be favoured at the outset when the normal marrow is in dominance.

deaths from MM in the Registrar General's Report for 1976. The death rate per million was five in 1950, had risen to 15 in 1960 and the figure for 1976 was 27. This apparent increase is probably due to improved diagnostic facilities, rather than a true increase. In all the death rates since 1950, there have been an equal number of deaths in both men and women, although individual hospital series have shown up to a 2 : 1 ratio of men to women. The peak number of deaths were in the sixth and seventh decades with less than 1% before the age of 40 years.

Clinical features

Patients are usually symptomatic of their disease by the time they seek medical help, although there are a few patients who are detected on routine screening. When patients present, they usually complain of severe back or rib pain. This presentation is what one would expect in a condition which is primarily a disease of the bone marrow with secondary osteolysis. It is relatively rare, however, to have pain in the skull, despite widespread destruction. The pain is usually precipitated by movement and is often sudden in onset and may be very severe. Persistent localized pain or tenderness often indicates a pathological fracture which may occur with only minimal trauma such as rolling over in bed in extreme cases. The patient may complain of loss of height because of vertebral collapse and subsequent kyphosis of the thoracic spine.

Weakness and lethargy are common symptoms often associated with anaemia. Anaemia may be due to bone marrow replacement but there are also many other factors involved. An increased plasma volume may cause a relative drop in haemoglobin and chronic renal failure is commonly associated with anaemia. There may be blood loss in patients who are thrombocytopenic or have associated coagulation defects. The presence of the tumour or its avidity for folate are other causes of anaemia. The anaemia due to malignancy is normochromic in type, and that due to folate deficiency is megaloblastic and macrocytic. Serum Vitamin B_{12} levels may be low in myeloma but this is due to the low circulating transcobalamin levels.

Renal failure is a frequent and usually ominous manifestation of MM. It occurs in up to half of the patients at some time during their illness. Approximately 20–30% of patients present with significant renal failure and its accompanying symptoms. The renal function is usually chronically affected, although some patients present with acute symptoms. The causes of chronic renal failure include hypercalcaemia and associated dehydration, hyperuricaemia, serum hyperviscosity, urinary tract obstruction and infection, and infiltration of the kidney with plasma cells or amyloidosis. However, these mechanisms were only found to be the cause of renal failure in three out of 16 patients in a recent study by De Fronzo *et al.* (1978). He found, as others have, a strong correlation between the presence and the quantity of Bence Jones proteinuria. Although not statistically significant, λ Bence Jones protein tended to be associated with a higher risk of renal failure. Abnormalities in renal tubule acidifying and concentrating ability were observed only in Bence Jones-producing patients and occurred in the absence of significant reduction in glomerular filtration rate. Severely deranged renal histology was seen only in patients with Bence Jones proteinuria and consisted primarily of tubular atrophy and degeneration. The glomerulus is usually spared. These findings suggest that the Bence Jones protein exerts a direct nephrotoxic effect at the tubular level, the glomerular filtration rate remaining relatively well preserved despite the significant abnormality of the tubules. Although obstructing tubular casts were observed only in patients with severe damage, many patients with similarly impaired renal function had no evidence of such casts. In contrast, Kyle (1975) reported no correlation of renal failure with Bence Jones proteinuria.

Neurological complications are relatively common. In one series (Silverstein and Doniger, 1963), 20% of patients had nerve root compression with radicular, motor and sensory symptoms, and 10% had cord compression. Five per cent of patients with myeloma present with cord compression, commonly in the thoracic spine, leading to paraparesis or paraplegia. This is due to direct extension from, or collapse of a vertebra, or rarely from a solitary extradural deposit.

Cranial nerve lesions are rare and are usually the result of tumour compression around foramina at the base of the skull. Deposits in the orbit may produce exophthalmus as well as cranial nerve palsies. Direct invasion of the central nervous system is rare but odd cases have been reported, as have cases of meningeal involvement.

Peripheral neuropathy is a rare but well documented complication. Amyloidosis may cause a neuropathy by infiltration of the flexor retinaculum with resulting entrapment of the median nerve (carpal tunnel syndrome), by direct infiltration of nerve fibres or due to deposits of amyloid in the perineural blood vessels. In some patients, however, no cause is ever found for the polyneuropathy. Multifocal leukoencephalophy is a rare complication. Organic cerebral disorders are usually secondary to uraemia, hypercalcaemia, hyperviscosity or steroid toxicity.

Hyperviscosity in MM is found in under 5% of cases, in comparison with up to 50% of patients with macroglobulinaemia. The syndrome may present with loss of vision, bleeding (particularly epistaxis), headache, vertigo, congestive cardiac failure, renal failure, somnolence and coma. The hyperviscosity is caused by increased quantity, abnormal aggregates, or polymerization of the paraprotein.

Hypercalcaemia is a common and important reversible complication of myeloma. It is found in one third of patients at presentation and patients may also develop it later in their disease. Hypercalcaemia should be suspected in any patient with anorexia, nausea, vomiting, polydipsia, polyuria and constipation before it leads to renal failure, confusion and coma. Immobile patients with extensive bone disease and poor renal failure are particularly at risk. Prompt treatment is necessary to relieve these distressing symptoms and, most important, the renal failure may be reversible.

The liver may be palpable in up to 20% of cases, although only 5% are palpable more than 5 cm below the costal margin. Likewise, the spleen may be palpable in up to 5%, but in less than 1% of Kyle's (1975) series did it extend more than 5 cm below the costal margin. Lymph nodes also are rarely enlarged.

Kyle (1975) reports histologically proven amyloidosis in 7% of his series, but this is probably an underestimate since not all patients suspected of having amyloidosis were biopsied. In 61 patients with amyloidosis associated with myeloma (Kyle and Bayrd, 1975) a palpable liver, macroglossia, congestive cardiac failure or the carpal tunnel syndrome were the commonest manifestations. Although less common manifestations such as purpura, particularly of the upper eyelids, skin fragility, peripheral neuropathy, malabsorption, nephrotic syndrome and orthostatic hypotension should alert the physician to the diagnosis. The prognosis after documentation of amyloidosis associated with myeloma is very poor, in the region of only four months, although some cases have been reported to have responded to chemotherapy.

Diagnostic criteria

To make the diagnosis of multiple myeloma, two of the three major criteria must be fulfilled (Table 34.1). The presence of certain non-specific disease features such as anaemia, hypercalcaemia, renal failure, demineralization, compression fractures, and hypoalbuminaemia will frequently support the diagnosis.

The diagnosis is usually easy in the advanced cases but great care is required at the earlier stages of the disease, since not all cases will fulfil all three diagnostic criteria and there is a large differential diagnosis for each criterion.

Examination of the bone marrow is required in all cases. The distribution of myeloma cells is often patchy so that the percentage of myeloma cells in the sample will vary greatly from site to site. Even at the same site, a bone marrow aspirate may be negative and the trephine positive, or vice versa. To increase the chance of a positive sample an area should be chosen which is tender or has been shown to be involved by X-ray. The most comfortable site for bone marrow aspiration and trephine is the posterior iliac crest. A negative aspirate and trephine does not exclude the diagnosis, and another sample should be obtained if there is any doubt.

The myeloma cells are moderately large (20–30μm in diameter) with abundant basophilic cytoplasm, eccentric nuclei with a perinuclear halo, and prominent nucleoli. Multinucleated cells are frequently seen. Various intranuclear and cytoplasmic inclusions may also be present.

The diagnosis of MM must be based on the cytological abnormalities of the plasma cells since bone marrow plasmacytosis may be seen in many disorders including chronic infections, rheumatoid arthritis, systemic lupus erythematosis, sarcoidosis, cirrhosis of the liver, agranulocytosis, drug hypersensitivities and metastatic carcinoma. Immunofluorescence or immunoperoxidase methods may be helpful in showing that the cells present are monoclonal.

Table 34.1 Diagnostic criteria.

1. Demonstration of focal or generalized increase in abnormal plasma cells in bone marrow or other tissue
2. Presence of serum or urinary myeloma protein
3. Typical X-ray changes

Two of the three criteria are required for diagnosis

Protein electrophoresis and immunoelectrophoresis are required to detect and characterize the monoclonal protein in the serum. Table 34.2 shows typical results of immunoelectrophoresis in a large group of patients. IgE myeloma not present in this series is extremely rare. The light chains can be detected in the urine of 70–80% of patients, but may be difficult to demonstrate unless the urine is concentrated. The presence of the monoclonal protein in the serum or urine is usually accompanied by suppression of the normal immunoglobulins. Quantitation of the immunoglobulins is routinely performed by radial-immunodiffusion, though for follow-up many centres prefer to quantitate the 'M' protein by densitometry of the electrophoretic strip.

Care must be taken not to equate the presence of a monoclonal peak with myeloma since there are other causes (Table 34.3), the commonest of which is the

Table 34.2   Results of immunoelectrophoresis of serum (from Kyle and Bayrd, 1975).

Immunoglobulin	Number	%
IgG	316	59
IgA	126	23
IgD	6	1
Negative heavy chain	89	17
Total	537	100
Light chain		
κ	320*	60
λ	158*	30
Negative	55	10
Total	533	100

* Includes Bence Jones proteinaemia

Table 34.3   Monoclonal gammopathies (from Alexanian, 1975).

Disorder	%
Multiple myeloma – symptomatic	65
Multiple myeloma – indolent	2
Localized plasmacytoma	5
Macroglobulinaemia of Waldenström	8
Heavy chain disease	< 1
Primary amyloidosis (without myeloma)	< 1
Idiopathic peak	20

idiopathic peak of benign monoclonal gammopathy. An idiopathic peak has been found in the serum of 0.5% of normal individuals over the age of 30 years (Alexanian, 1975). These peaks are usually of less than 30 g/l of IgG. The normal immunoglobulins are not depressed and lytic bone lesions and Bence Jones protein are absent. Patients with idiopathic peaks very rarely develop MM. Idiopathic peaks of IgM are rare and are usually associated with lymphoma or chronic lymphatic leukaemia.

The X-ray changes may be different in both type and extent but with very few exceptions, they are essentially osteolytic (Fig. 34.2). The degree of bone destruction may vary from a diffuse osteoporosis, through small and almost insignificant areas of translucency, to rounded or oval defects with sharply defined margins. The majority of patients show a combination of osteoporosis, lytic lesions and fractures. The verteb-

rae, skull, thoracic cage, pelvis and proximal portions of humeri and femora are the most common sites of involvement. Vertebral collapse is common but erosion of the vertebral pedicles which is frequently seen in metastatic carcinoma is rare. The lesions frequently extend into the soft tissues.

Not all patients will fulfil all three criteria. In a large series (Kyle, 1975) found 21% of patients with negative X-ray studies, 6% with negative bone marrow aspirate, and 9% with no monoclonal protein in the serum, but only three out of 500 patients with no detectable monoclonal protein in the serum or urine. The diagnosis is difficult and I have had referred recently, with a diagnosis of myeloma, patients with a tuberculoma of the rib, chronic osteomyelitis, cytomegalovirus infection, and the most common of all, metastatic carcinoma.

Differential diagnoses

The major differential diagnoses have been discussed under the criteria for diagnosis. MM, however, needs to be distinguished from two rare forms of plasma cell malignancies, the solitary myeloma of bone and extramedullary plasmacytomas. Wiltshaw (1976) concludes that solitary myeloma of bone constitutes a rather unusual presentation of MM but it is essentially the same disease. The majority of patients eventually develop lesions of the same type and distribution characteristic of MM within a few months or years.

Extramedullary plasmacytomas show several differences from MM and solitary myeloma of the bone. They are common in the upper air passages, have a high incidence of metastatic spread to soft tissues, and although spread to bone frequently occurs, there is no preference for bone containing active marrow and wide-spread bone marrow involvement is rare. Prolonged survival may be achieved with therapy for localized disease, and vigorous treatment for disseminated disease may result in longer remissions than those seen in MM.

Staging

In MM, Salmon and co-workers have shown that the absolute number of plasma cells in patients may be derived from the relationship between the *in vitro* production rate of 'M' protein per cell and the *in vivo* 'M' protein production rate (Sullivan and Salmon, 1972) They found that the clinical range of the tumour mass was from approximately 2×10^{11} to 5×10^{12} myeloma cells and that there was a relationship between the number of tumour cells present with the severity of the symptoms of the disease, and survival. This research method of assessing tumour mass is obviously not appl-

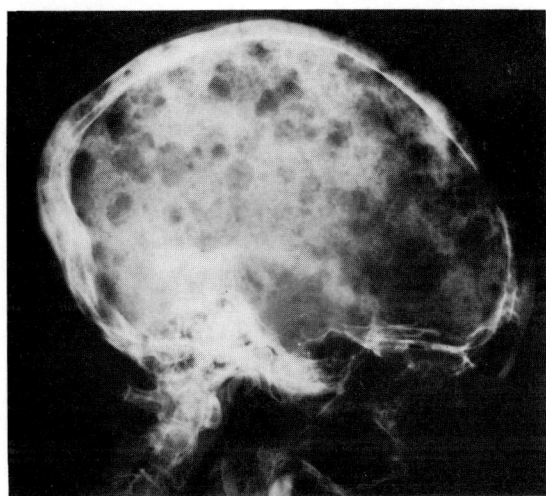

Fig. 34.2 Typical skull X-ray appearance of multiple myeloma.

icable to routine management of patients, but by correlating their tumour mass results with clinical data a staging system has been put forward by Durie and Salmon (1975) (Table 34.4). Woodruff *et al.* (1978) have applied this staging technique to a retrospective series of patients (Fig. 34.3). The staging technique clearly separates the patients into prognostic groups. Unfortunately, however, the majority of patients fall into Stage II and III. It should be noted that the major prognostic factor of renal function has to be taken into account and is denoted by the A and B categories of this staging system.

Tumour kinetics

MM is a 'model tumour' because not only can the tumour mass at any one time be readily estimated but the tumour is easily biopsied and serial studies of cytokinetics performed. Clarification of the growth kinetics may provide a more rational line for future improvement in treatment.

In many animal tumours, including rodent myeloma, tumour growth rates decrease with increasing tumour size, in accord with Gompertzian kinetics. Salmon (1975) has suggested that in myeloma both tumour growth and regression can be described with Gompertzian kinetics. He estimates that the evolutionary period is between two and five years, far shorter than the exponential extrapolation of twenty years proposed by Hobbs. In Salmon's model, as the tumour size decreased with therapy, an increased growth fraction developed which balanced the effects of treatment so that tumour mass remained constant for prolonged periods (plateau phase). In addition, he argues that cycle-specific drugs should be active in the plateau phase. Durie *et al.* (1977) found that the thymidine labelling index (TLI) was significantly higher in patients with low as compared with high tumour cell mass, and that there was a rise in the TLI immediately after chemotherapy, which then fell to a low level. A persistently elevated TLI following each course was associated with an incomplete response or early relapse.

Drewinko and Alexanian (1977) found that although some responding patients had a high thymidine labelling index, the median was similar to that for untreated patients and only during the initial months of treatment did myeloma patients demonstrate a significant increment in the proportion of 'S' phase cells. By using continuous infusions of tritiated thymidine, Drewinko and Alexanian (1978) have made estimates of the growth fraction (GF). All untreated and unresponsive patients had a GF of less than 1%. In four responsive patients, the GF remained the same in two, and in the two further patients increased to 4% and 8% respectively. Relapsing patients, however, with a rapid doubling time had growth fractions ranging from 20% to 47%. The plasma cell generation time was estimated as 8 days and the intrinsic cell loss from 47–83%. Cycle-specific drugs therefore may be of value in the early months of treatment and also at relapse.

Treatment

Although there is a very small group of patients in whom the myeloma is indolent, the majority of patients when they seek medical advice have symptomatic disease with deteriorating laboratory tests and clearly require treatment. Patients who are asymptomatic and whose disease is thought to be indolent should be carefully followed and treatment instigated when there is evidence of progression. Patients treated with palliative radiotherapy and steroids have a median survival of only nine months which is similar to untreated series of patients. There is a continuous fall in the survival curve with approximately 20% of patients alive at two years and less than 5% at five years (Scarffe, 1978). Although radiotherapy and steroids may give good palliation, to prolong survival systemic chemotherapy is required. The treatment of MM can be considered under two headings: (a) supportive (relief of symptoms and the prevention and treatment of complications); and (b) anti-neoplastic (radiotherapy and chemotherapy).

Table 34.4   Myeloma staging (from Durie and Salmon, 1975).

Stage	Criteria	Measured myeloma cell mass (cells × 10^{12}/m²)

I	*All* of the following:
	1. Haemoglobin value > 10 g/100 ml
	2. Serum calcium value normal (≤ 12 mg/100 ml)
	3. On roentgenogram, normal bone structure (scale 0) or solitary bone plasmacytoma only
	4. Low M-component production rates
	  a. IgG value < 5 g/100 ml
	  b. IgA value < 3 g/100 ml
	  c. Urine light chain M-component on electrophoresis < 4 g/24 hours
		< 0.6
		(low)

II	Fitting neither Stage I nor Stage III	0.6–1.20 (intermediate)

III	*One or more* of the following:
	1. Haemoglobin value < 8.5 g/100 ml
	2. Serum calcium value > 12 mg/100 ml
	3. Advanced lytic bone lesions (scale 3)
	4. High M-component production rates
	  a. IgG value > 7 g/100 ml
	  b. IgA value > 5 g/100 ml
	  c. Urine light chain M-component on electrophoresis > 12 g/24 hours
		> 1.20
		(high)

Subclassification:
A = Relatively normal renal function (serum creatinine value < 2.0 mg/100 ml)
B = Abnormal renal function (serum creatinine value ≥ 2.0 mg/100 ml)

Scale: Normal bones (0)
Osteoporosis (1)
Lytic bone lesions (2)
Extensive skeletal destruction and major fractures (3)

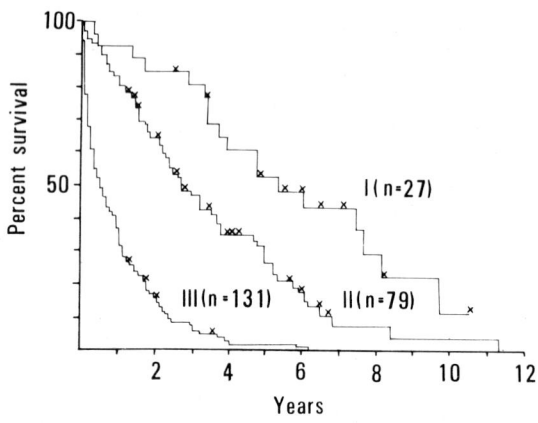

Fig. 34.3   Clinical staging of multiple myeloma (from Woodruff *et al.*, 1979).

x = patient still alive.

Supportive care

The patients, when they present, are often elderly, in severe pain, frightened and depressed. The physician must gain their confidence and give reassurance that although the myeloma cannot be cured, it can be controlled in most patients and their symptoms relieved. Depressive illnesses may easily be missed and the patient's progress retarded. Simple open discussion of the problems with the patient may be helpful, or in some cases, anti-depressive drugs are indicated.

Mobility must be maintained to prevent a negative calcium balance and all the problems of keeping the elderly in bed. Pathological fractures should be internally fixed followed by irradiation to maintain mobility. Adequate regular analgesics should be given and irradiation to localized painful areas. Corsets and back supports are often poorly tolerated but some patients do benefit. As the patient responds to treatment, they should be encouraged to take as much exercise as they can tolerate (often much more than one would expect from their X-rays), but to avoid hazardous procedures such as lifting heavy weights.

Hypercalcaemia should be treated as an emergency since it often leads to renal failure which is reversible in the early stages. Mild hypercalcaemia may be treated with oral prednisolone, 60 mg daily and adequate hydration, until the calcium returns to normal, usually within a few days. Severe hypercalcaemia accompanied by dehydration may require 4–6 l of intravenous normal saline over the first 24 hours along with the prednisolone. The addition of frusemide (Lasix) 40 mg every 4 hours may be beneficial. Specific chemotherapy should be instigated as soon as possible to treat the underlying disease and the patient mobilized. These simple measures control hypercalcaemia in most cases. In resistant cases, intravenous mithramycin, 25 μg/kg of body weight may be effective. Mithramycin inhibits osteoclastic activity and it has been suggested that it may have a specific effect on bone dissolution. Calcitonin, oral phosphate and indomethacin may also be used.

The role of treatment of demineralization of the bones with fluoride, calcium and vitamin D is not clear. Sodium fluoride alone has failed to show any benefit. Kyle and Bayrd (1975) however, showed some benefit with 50 mg sodium fluoride, twice daily with calcium carbonate, 1 g four times daily. Other workers have suggested the use of vitamin D and androgens. These studies require further clarification before this treatment can be generally recommended.

Hyperuricaemia should be prevented during the first few courses of treatment with adequate hydration and the use of the xanthine oxidase inhibitor, allopurinol, 300–600 mg orally daily. Allopurinol should also be used in those patients found to have significant hyperuricaemia or excessive excretion in the urine to prevent the development of uric acid stones or nephropathy. Alkalinization of the urine with sodium bicarbonate and acetazolamide (Diamox) may also be useful.

Renal failure is an important complication of MM. Adequate hydration is required at all times to help excrete light chains, calcium, uric acid and other metabolites. Dehydration should not be allowed prior to procedures such as intravenous pyelography since this may precipitate acute renal failure. Hypercalcaemia, hyperuricaemia, urinary tract infections and hyperviscosity states should be treated promptly to prevent renal damage. The light chain production should be reduced as quickly as possible with chemotherapy. A full dose of alkylating agent should be used with no reduction in dose because of renal failure, providing there is an adequate urine output. Peritoneal dialysis may be useful during an episode of acute renal failure and haemodialysis has been used both for acute failure and for long term maintenance in patients who have achieved a good response.

Russell *et al*. (1977) describe falls in blood ureas of greater than 5 mmol/l in eight out of 16 patients treated with multiple plasma exchanges. The mechanism of the improvement is not known. He postulates that in patients with renal failure, there is decreased catabolism and excretion of light chains by the kidney, and they accumulate in the serum. Removal of the light chains by plasma exchange helps prevent further damage. In one of their patients a single plasma exchange removed 50 times the quantity of light chains being excreted in the urine. Correction of hyperviscosity is another possible method of improving renal function by plasma exchange. I have seen dramatic improvement after plasma exchange of renal function, but it is difficult to be certain whether the improvement is due to the plasma exchange, and not to other supportive measures such as forced alkaline diuresis, and correction of hypercalcaemia. The median survival of Russell's group of patients presenting with renal failure was only 20 weeks. Confirmation of the efficacy of this treatment is required before it is recommended.

Hyperviscosity is readily treated by plasma exchange, using one of the commercially available blood cell separators: 2–3 l can be safely exchanged in 1.5–2 hours. Symptoms rapidly improve, patients previously stuporosed may come round whilst still being exchanged and hold rational conversations. The procedure is only temporary and the paraproteins reaccumulate so chemotherapy should be instituted immediately. Patients who respond poorly to chemotherapy may be maintained symptom-free by long-term plasma exchange.

The haemoglobin in most patients who respond to treatment rises to about 10 g/dl. There are, however, a minority who have an anaemia not associated with iron, B12 or folate deficiencies, excessive chemotherapy, or bone marrow infiltration in whom androgens may be effective therapy. Fluoxymesterone, 15–30 mg daily by mouth may be of value.

Bacterial infections are common and should be treated urgently. The patient should have the appropriate cultures and X-rays as indicated after a careful history and examination, and started on broad spectrum antibiotics until sensitivities are known. Nephrotoxic antibiotics such as gentamycin should be carefully monitored. Prophylactic gamma globulin is not effective in the prevention of infection. Prophylactic antibiotics have been used but I have never found them indicated. Explanation to the patient that he is at risk to infections and should report promptly for treatment is very important.

The carpal tunnel syndrome may be treated by division of the flexor retinaculum and give lasting symptomatic relief. The most important neurological complication is cord compression. Benson *et al.* (1978) have pointed out that the survival in patients who present with cord compression may be long and should be treated aggressively. Surgical decompression followed by radiotherapy gave good results in 11 out of 30 patients with complete paraplegia, and nine out of 22 patients with paraparesis who had symptoms for periods ranging from three weeks to three months. Despite delay in presentation, patients must be treated radically. Dexamethasone, 6–8 mg daily should be used as an adjunct to the other treatment modalities.

Chemotherapy

Before comparing the results of chemotherapy, the reader must consider carefully a number of points. Complete remission in the true sense of the word is never obtained. The majority of authors refer to a response rate to a given regimen, however, different criteria for response are used. An objective response to treatment defined by the Committee of the Chronic Leukaemia and Myeloma Task Force (1973) is as follows:

(a) Reduction of plasmacytomas by palpation or on X-ray by 50% or more in the product of the two largest diameters.
(b) A fall of the M protein to 50% or less of the pre-study value.
(c) If urinary M protein greater than 1 g/24 hours, a fall to 50% of this value; if urinary M protein 0.5 – 1 g a fall to less than 0.1 g/24 hours.
(d) Definite radiographic evidence of skeletal healing.

The South Western Oncology Group (Alexanian, 1977) who have reported some of the largest clinical trials of chemotherapy require both of the following criteria:

(a) A decrease in the production rate of serum myeloma protein to less than 25% of the pre-treatment value.
(b) Disappearance of Bence Jones protein excretion.

Calculation of the serum myeloma production rate takes into consideration the M protein concentration, change in plasma volume, and the change of catabolic rate of IgG protein with changing serum concentrations. The fractional catabolic rate of IgG myeloma protein for the subclasses 1, 2 and 4 decline markedly with a progressive decline in concentration below 30 g/l. Thus changes in tumour mass will be underestimated when calculations are based only on measured decline of the IgG peak.

Salmon and collaborators have taken this a stage further and now report their results in change in tumour cell mass which can be calculated using programmable pocket calculators (Salmon and Wampler, 1977). Bone marrow plasmacytosis is of little value in assessing response because of the patchy nature of the infiltration. Unless there is renal failure, the haemoglobin usually rises to above 10 g/dl and some patients also develop recalcification of bone lesions or recovery of depressed normal immunoglobulins. The objective response is parallelled by a subjective improvement in performance status and many are able to return to an almost normal life.

The next major criterion used for assessment is survival and these results can easily be biased by inclusion of early stage disease with good renal function (see Fig. 34.3). There has also been an improvement in the supportive management of patients and direct comparison with historical controls may not be applicable.

Single agents

Urethane, introduced in 1947 was used for many years until Holland *et al.* (1966) showed that although there may be symptomatic improvement, the survival for a urethane-treated group was worse than those who received placebo alone. Melphalan (L-phenylalanine mustard) was synthesized in 1953 and was first reported useful in myeloma by Russian investigators in 1958. These reports were confirmed and melphalan has become the single most used agent in myeloma, although others (Table 34.5) notably cyclophosphamide and BCNU show similar activity.

Both melphalan and cyclophosphamide have been used either as low dose continuous or high dose intermittent regimens. There is a response rate of between 30 and 50% and prolongation of survival is probably similar for both drugs and both regimens. A Medical Research Council trial of continuous melphalan and cyclophosphamide found that the median survival of both arms was similar (Medical Research Council, 1971). There has been no direct comparison between high dose intermittent melphalan and cyclophosphamide. Although melphalan and cyclophosphamide are both alkylating agents, Bergsagel *et al.* (1972) have used intermittent high dose cyclophosphamide with good results in patients resistant to melphalan. This result was not confirmed by Kyle and Elveback (1976); however, they used a lower dose and less frequent regimen. Steroids have been shown to decrease serum and urinary M protein, but not improve survival. They must therefore have minimal anti-neoplastic effect, the decrease in M protein usually results from increased catabolism. Prednisolone, however, when used in combinations may have a synergistic effect.

Table 34.5 Single agents (from Clarysse, *et al.*, 1976).

	No. studied	% Response
Melphalan	499	42
Cyclophosphamide	413	29
Procarbazine	33	13
BCNU	31	39
Chlorambucil	15	33
Adriamycin	23	13
Prednisolone	39	49

Table 34.6 Response rates from SWOG studies (from Alexanian *et al.*, 1977).

Combination	No. studied	Response rate % evaluable
Daily M	23	14
Intermittent M	54	31
Intermittent M + P	132	59
Intermittent M + P + Pr	226	53
Intermittent M + C + P	84	47
Intermittent M + A + P	76	46
Intermittent C + A + P	64	39
Intermittent M + P + Pr + V	124	59
Intermittent V + M + C + P	86	62
Intermittent V + C + A + P	77	57
Intermittent M + C + B + P	75	49

M = Melphalan   A = Adriamycin
P = Prednisone   V = Vincristine
Pr = Procarbazine   B = BCNU
C = Cyclophosphamide

Combination chemotherapy

The addition of prednisolone to melphalan in the South West Oncology Group studies increased the response rate and median survival (Table 34.6). Costa *et al.* (1973) reported similar findings in a study where the addition of prednisolone increased the response rate from 23% to 55%. The median survival for good risk patients who responded was 53 months, versus 30 months for melphalan alone.

Table 34.6 shows the response rates of trials carried out by the SWOG and assessed by the 75% decrease in the protein production rate described previously. It should be noted that although there are no significant differences between the various combinations and intermittent melphalan and prednisolone, the addition of vincristine to a combination increased the response

rate although the differences were not statistically significant. In part, the improved response of VMCP over MCP alone may be that the MCP was given every three weeks instead of four.

Fig. 34.4 shows the survival curve for the various regimens. The survival curves for MP, MPP, MAP and CAP were all similar but superior to intermittent melphalan alone. The survival for the 305 patients receiving vincristine combinations (VMCP, VCAP and MPPV) was significantly longer than that for the 727 patients receiving six different alkylating agents and prednisolone combinations, without vincristine (p < 0.01). The other four agent regime, MCBP has a similar survival curve to the vincristine combination. The median survival for MPPV was 30 months and the projected median survival for VMCP and VCAP is 34 months, about nine months longer than that for patients treated with MP, MPP, MAP, MCP and CAP.

Alberts *et al.* (1977) have shown that vincristine, when used alone in patients who have already obtained a response with alkylating agents, induced in seven out of eight patients a 24–60% further decrease in total body myeloma cell number. Vincristine has been

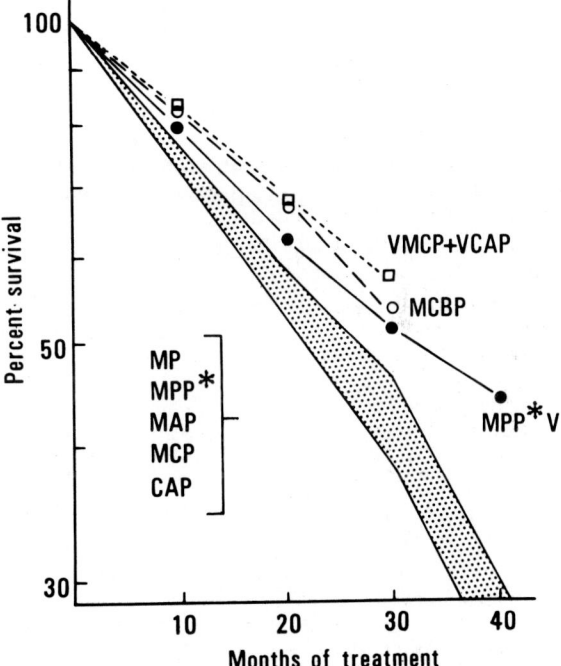

Fig. 34.4 Survival from initial treatment for various drug combinations used by SWOG (A = adriamycin; B = BCNU; C = cyclophosphamide; M = melphalan; P = prednisone; P* = procarbazine) Alexanian *et al.*, 1977).

shown to increase the penetration and accumulation of methotrexate within cells, and some of its action increasing response and survival may be because of a similar action with the drugs used in the combinations, or because of the increased percentage of cells in the S phase of the cell cycle in the early part of the treatment regimen.

In summary, the SWOG studies show that no alkylating agent combination has a better response rate than intermittent melphalan and prednisolone, but the four-drug combinations, give longer median survivals.

A five-drug regimen of melphalan, prednisolone, cyclophosphamide, vincristine and BCNU (the M-2 protocol) (see Table 34.7) has been shown to give excellent results (Case *et al.*, 1977) Of 46 previously untreated patients, 34 were clinical Stage 3, 10 Stage 2 and 2 Stage 1. Forty (86%) of the 46 showed a 50% reduction in M protein. The criteria for response is difficult to equate with the SWOG studies but Case does report that the average maximum tumour cell regression was 76% for responders. The median time in remission is greater than 20 months with 27 of the 40 responders still in remission. This data suggests that the median duration of survival will be at least 12 months longer than the 22 months obtained with melphalan and prednisolone in a previous study at the Memorial Hospital. Thirteen (50%) of 26 patients previously treated with single alkylating agents responded to the five-drug regime. The median time in remission is greater than 22 months with eight patients still in remission. These results in previously treated patients are very impressive since the outlook for patients resistant to melphalan and cyclophosphamide is usually poor.

It is of interest that in the first report of the M-2 protocol (Lee *et al.*, 1974), the vincristine was given on day 21 of their regimen and it was stated that this was perhaps one of the reasons for the protocol's success, but in the last report, it was given on day 1 of the protocol.

The group of patients reported, although many are Stage 3, was a relatively young group for myeloma with an average age of approximately 55 years with a performance status of 70–80% which must make them a reasonably favourable group.

Remission maintenance

The evidence for maintenance treatment is somewhat confusing. In the experience of the SWOG, the survival of patients maintained after response with melphalan and prednisone or BCNU and prednisone was no better than an unmaintained group, retreated with melphalan and prednisone at relapse. Eighty per cent of the unmaintained group achieved second remissions. Following resumption of treatment, the magnitude of tumour reduction was usually less and the remission duration shorter. There was no improvement in a later study when MCBP was compared with azothiaprine and prednisone and periodic courses of MCBP. Case *et al.* (1977) recommend however, that the M-2 protocol should be continued since in their hands, terminating treatment in responding patients was followed by premature and aggressive relapse in six patients, and death within four months in four of them. Alexanian *et al.* (1978) shed some light on the discrepancies of advice. They found that patients with low tumour mass (clinical Stage 1) and those with a complete disappearance of serum M protein had the longest unmaintained remissions (median, 19 months), and that 10 out of 12 evaluable patients responded a second time to chemotherapy with melphalan and prednisone. Patients presenting with intermediate or high tumour cell mass (Stage 2 and 3) or with persistent serum myeloma proteins after 12 months of therapy had short unmaintained remissions. The tumour growth rate is also likely to be important, patients with longer doubling times are likely to have longer survival than those with more rapid tumour growth.

Patients with low tumour mass and with disappearance of M protein are only a small number of cases in most physicians' experience and so maintenance chemotherapy appears necessary in the majority of patients with myeloma, although new approaches are required to lower the number of tumour cells during the plateau phase.

Recommended management

The progress in the management of myeloma described has been achieved by careful study of the disease, both *in vitro* and *in vivo* by special centres. We are now in a position to monitor both the tumour cell number and cell kinetics of a small growth fraction disease and so, hopefully, improve not only our management of this disease but also of the more common solid tumours with small growth fractions in which

Table 34.7   M-2 protocol (from Case *et al.*, 1977).

Vincristine	0.03 mg/kg	i.v. day 1
BCNU	0.5 mg/kg	i.v. day 1
Cyclophosphamide	10 mg/kg	i.v. day 1
Melphalan	0.25 mg/kg	oral days 1–4 inclusive
Prednisone	1 mg/kg	oral days 1–7 tail off over 21 days

Repeat every 35 days

dard dose-time relationships were observed.

A further at-risk group in Stage II as noted above are those patients with more than three nodal areas involved at presentation. The definition of these 'at risk' categories is essential to the further improvement of the results in early stage disease.

Table 35.17 summarizes the conclusions of several studies directed at the assessment of the role of combined radiotherapy and chemotherapy.

The most comprehensive trials have been those carried out at Stanford University and reported recently by Rosenberg *et al.* (1978). In these studies on PS patients, radiation therapy was given first and patients randomized to receive nothing or MOPP chemotherapy. No significant differences in survival have been seen, although (with the exception of PS IB and IIB) the continuously disease-free survival figures for RT + CT are significantly better than those obtained with RT alone. One conclusion of these studies is that chemotherapy deferred until relapse occurs may be no less effective than chemotherapy given electively as part of the first planned treatment. The potential advantage of deferring therapy is to avoid normal tissue sequelae, particularly male sterility and the potential hazard of carcinogenesis (Arseneau *et al.*, 1972).

So far as the latter aspect is concerned, in the Stanford series of 244 patients followed from three to nine years, five developed second malignancies. There was no evidence that second malignancies other than AML were increased in patients receiving irradiation and MOPP. Coleman *et al.* (1977) reported eight patients developing AML of a total group of 680 Hodgkin's disease patients. The actuarial probability of developing AML at seven years was 2% for the entire group and 3.9% for the combined chemotherapy-radiotherapy group.

Involved field versus extended field radiotherapy for Hodgkin's disease

Early observations documenting the frequency with which untreated node areas adjacent to nodes involved by Hodgkin's disease subsequently became the sites of disease led to their elective treatment with radiotherapy. The extended field culminated in the development of the mantle technique first used in Stanford in 1956. An assessment of the merits of the extended field approach has been complicated by the introduction of laparotomy and splenectomy for pathological staging which meant that experience gained in CS patients could not be extrapolated to treatment results obtained in PS patients. The early trial of involved field radiotherapy against extended field techniques carried out on CS patients in Stanford,

Table 35.17 Hodgkin's disease: summary of outcome of combined chemo-radiotherapy vs radiotherapy trials.

		Significant difference in disease-free interval
EORTC (1977)	CS I + II A & B RT ± vinblastine	RT + CT > RT
Rosenberg *et al.* (1978)	RT ± MOPP	
	PS I & IIA	RT + CT > RT
	PS I + IIB	NS
	PS IIIA	RT + CT > RT
	PS IIIB	RT + CT > RT

showed no differences for patients without systemic symptoms but both survival and disease-free survival advantages were demonstrated for 'B' patients treated with the extended field approach (Kaplan and Rosenberg, 1966). The results of a multicentre study (Collaborative Study, 1976) carried out on CS and PS I and II patients treated between 1967 and 1973 in the United States, showed no significant difference between involved field and extended field radiation therapy in terms of survival, although for disease-free survival there was an advantage for the extended field approach.

Rosenberg and Kaplan (1970) have reported the results comparing total nodal irradiation with involved field treatment in CS and PS IA and IIA patients. The former treatment was superior to involved field irradiation in terms of disease-free survival but not survival.

It can be concluded from these studies that an advantage in terms of disease-free survival has been demonstrated using the extended field approach to treat early stage Hodgkin's disease.

Histology and patient survival

The histopathological classification introduced by Lukes and Butler (1966) had clear prognostic significance when tested in older case material before the introduction of radical radiotherapy based on pathological staging procedures and the development of effective chemotherapy. Several recent series have reported little difference between the various subtypes. Thus Fuller *et al.* (1977) in an analysis of 90 patients with Stage I and II disease found no significant difference between MC, NS and LP in terms of disease-free survival (there was only one LD patient in the series).

Figs 35.17 and 18 shows survival and continuously disease-free survival rates by histopathological subtype for PS I–III patients treated at The Royal Marsden Hospital between 1970 and 1976. No significant differences are seen between the different categories.

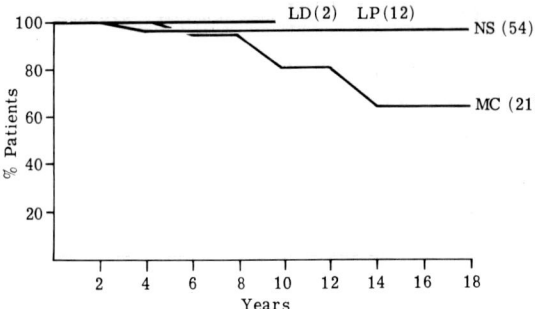

Fig. 35.17 Hodgkin's disease: PS I & IIA survival according to histology (Royal Marsden Hospital 1970 – 1976).

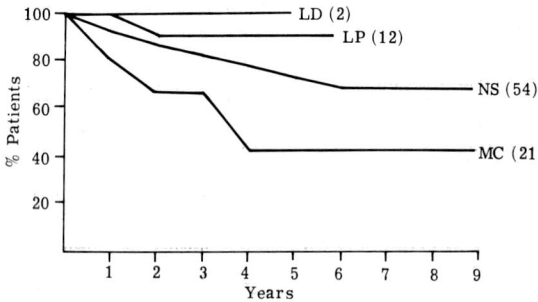

Fig. 35.18 Hodgkin's disease: PS I & IIA continuously disease-free survival according to histology (Royal Marsden Hospital 1970 – 1976).

Within the Stage I–IIIA patients the following significant differences emerged: LP vs MC: disease-free survival (P < 0.002); MC vs NS: survival (P < 0.04); and LP vs NS: disease-free survival (P < 0.006). No significant differences were seen in Stages I–IIIB between the different histopathological sub-types.

Pattern of relapse after chemotherapy: implications for combined chemo-radiotherapy

The documentation of relapse pattern in patients developing further evidence of disease after achieving complete remission with chemotherapy has obvious implications for combined chemotherapy-radiotherapy. In a recent analysis of 52 patients relapsing after achieving complete remission with MOPP, Young *et al.* (1978) have reported that in 92% of cases disease reappeared in previously involved sites. In 71% of relapses, the recurrence was confined to initially involved sites and in the majority of instances disease reappeared in lymph nodes, particularly the mediastinum, para-aortic and left supraclavicular nodes. Nodular sclerosis accounted for 43% of relapses. Systemic symptoms were a highly significant prognostic factor

and appeared to transcend stage. Thus, of 24 complete remitters with Stage II–IVA disease, only two (8%) relapsed, compared with 50/137 (36%) Stage II–IVB patients.

Careful restaging of patients in apparent complete remission following chemotherapy will demonstrate occult residual Hodgkin's disease in a proportion depending upon the restaging procedures employed. Herman and Jones (1977) have recently reported on 82 complete remission patients in 12% of whom occult disease was detected. In all but one patient, as expected, disease was identified in an initially involved site and bulky lymph nodes were particularly at risk.

There are few reports of splenectomy after chemotherapy. Herman and Jones reported five repeat laparotomies in complete remission patients, but all had previously apparently undergone splenectomy before chemotherapy. The spleen-positive rate after chemotherapy is relevant to the use of staging laparotomy in patients treated with combined therapy in whom chemotherapy may eliminate splenic foci and render pathological staging irrelevant.

Childhood Hodgkin's disease

The mode of presentation and natural history of Hodgkin's disease in children does not differ greatly from that in adults, but staging and treatment procedures need to be modified to minimize possible hazards without reducing the chance of cure.

Hodgkin's disease is uncommon in children and rare under the age of five, the incidence increasing with increasing age. It is commoner in boys with a 5:1 ratio in under 10 year olds and about 3:1 at 14 years (Smith *et al.*, 1977). In older children the normal adult distribution is seen. In the United States there is a similar incidence in blacks and whites. Prior tonsillectomy and appendicectomy have been considered as risk factors (Vianna, 1976), and epidemiological studies have suggested that 'clustering' of cases (Vianna *et al.*, 1972) and a higher than average mortality from Hodgkin's disease among teachers (Milham, 1974) and families of children with Hodgkin's disease (Grufferman *et al.*, 1977; Razis *et al.*, 1959) point to an infectious aetiology. However, these findings have not been substantiated and have been criticized on statistical grounds (Smith *et al.*, 1977).

Fig. 35.19 shows the histological distribution in children compared with a group of adults treated in the same period. Nodular sclerosis is even commoner in the first decade as shown here, occurring in up to 63% of cases (Strum and Rappaport, 1970). Fig. 35.20 shows the relationship of histology to age and sex. Lymphocyte predominance is more frequently seen in boys.

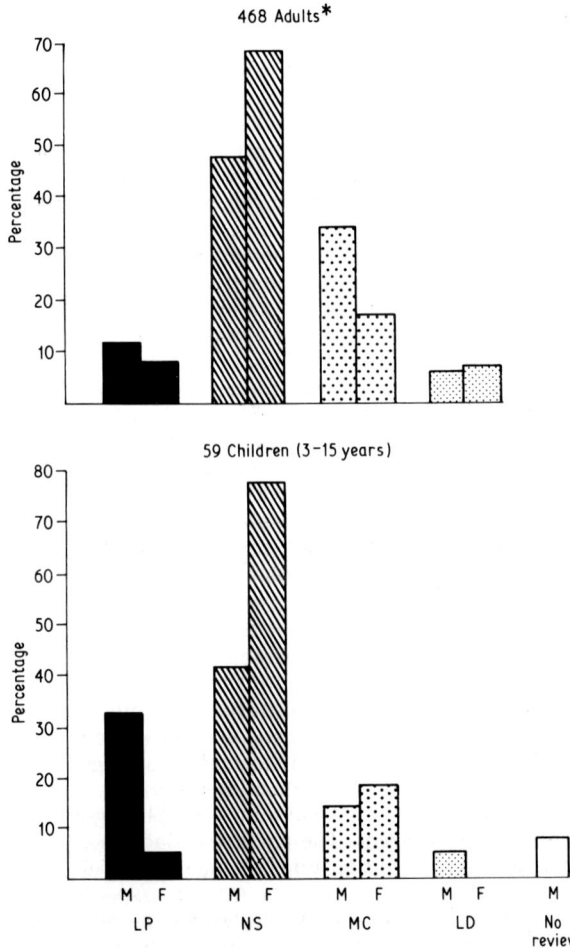

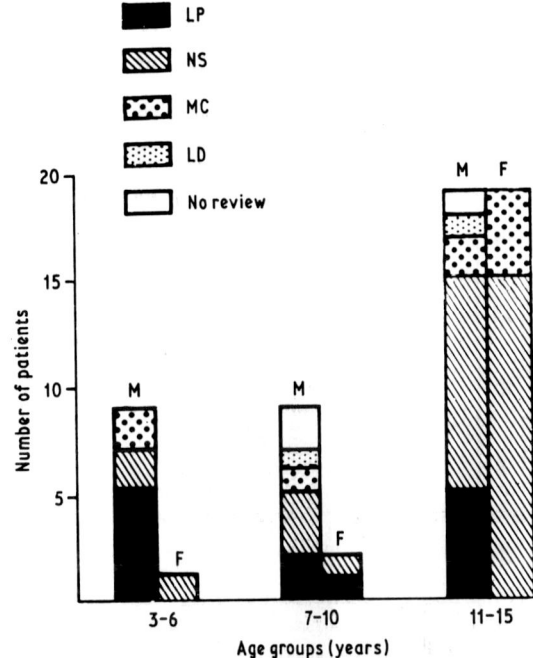

Fig. 35.20 The relationship of histology to age and sex in childhood Hodgkin's disease (M: male; F: female).

Fig. 35.19 A comparison of histological presentations in adults and children with Hodgkin's disease (Royal Marsden Hospital. Consecutive adults with Hodgkin's disease seen at R.M.H. 1968–75).

The most common presenting feature is cervical lymphadenopathy. The nodes may fluctuate in size and children are often treated with antibiotics for presumed infection before the diagnosis is established. A histological pattern of reactive hyperplasia may be seen at first biopsy and is usually due to poor node selection. Systemic symptoms are present in 30% of children. Children should be staged as fully as possible but modifications are necessary compared with the investigations advocated in the adult.

Lymphangiography is performed unless contraindicated by the presence of bulky mediastinal nodes or evidence of Stage IV disease. Although technically more difficult than in adults, the procedure is possible in most children. Sedation is necessary and at The Royal Marsden Hospital all lymphangiograms are performed under general anaesthesia in young children. Mobilization of the dye from the nodes is more rapid than in adults and contrast may disappear as soon as three to six months after lymphangiography.

Laparotomy with splenectomy as a staging procedure in childhood Hodgkin's disease presents a difficult problem. Accurate diagnosis of splenic involvement is not possible except by splenectomy but severe infections and death have been recorded in children after the procedure (Hays *et al.*, 1972). Chilcote *et al.* (1976) have documented episodes of septicaemia and-/or meningitis in 200 children following diagnostic laparotomy and splenectomy. Eleven of these children died. The commonest organisms were penicillin-sensitive pneumococci and streptococci, but *Haemophilus influenzae*, *Listeria*, *Pseudomonas* and *Meningococcus* were also found. Approximately 80% of infections occur within two years of splenectomy and recurrent episodes are not uncommon. A 5% incidence of post-operative bowel obstruction has also been reported (Rosenstock *et al.*, 1974). Thus, although it is desirable in children with clinically localized disease to exclude the presence of intra-abdominal disease and so limit treatment to reduce the

Table 36.4 Microscopical characteristics of the commoner round cell tumours of bone (from Arthur *et al.*, 1970).

	Ewing's tumour	Neuroblastoma	Bone lymphoma
Fibrous septa	Usually present	May be present	Usually absent
Diffuse reticulin	Absent	Absent	Always present
Perivascular cuff	Usually present	May be present	Usually absent
Rosettes	Absent	May be present	Absent
Glycogen	Usually absent	Sometimes present	Usually absent

intravenous pyelography, CAT-scanning (when available), isotope bone scan, serum electrophoresis, bone marrow examination and catecholamine examination of the urine. Obviously these tests must be preceded by a careful clinical examination.

The majority of patients can be categorized in this way. A small number of tumours have some of the characteristics of both Ewing's tumour and of lymphoma of bone. Usually these tumours behave as unpredictably as true Ewing's tumour and can be treated as such.

Management

(a) *Primary lymphoma of bone.* When full investigation reveals no other involvement, radical radiotherapy offers results as good as with surgical ablation. It is essential to irradiate the whole of the affected bone. The omission of a small portion of a bone may be followed by relapse at that untreated site. The 5-year survival rate after radical radiotherapy is about 50% (Wang and Fleischli, 1968; Boston *et al.*, 1974). As most reported series occurred before the availability of modern investigations, it is likely that many patients already had more extensive disease when first seen, and a better survival rate can be hoped for in the future.

The whole of the affected bone is irradiated to a tumour dose of 4000–4500 rad in 4–5 weeks, using a megavoltage machine. The site of many tumours makes it necessary to include major joints in the irradiated volume, with subsequent limitation of movement. Some radiotherapists prefer to treat the whole bone to this dose level, then reduce the treatment volume to the original main tumour and add 1500 rad in 2 weeks. This may reduce the possibility of local relapse. Especially when irradiating to high doses of this order, it is preferable to leave a corridor of unirradiated normal tissue down the length of the limb. Through and through irradiation of an entire limb may be followed

by a complete circle of fibrosis, ensheathing and gradually compressing the limb with eventual impairment of its peripheral blood supply. Intermittent claudication and finally gangrene requiring amputation may follow. Amputation is a hazardous operation after treatment of this type.

Following irradiation, bone recalcification occurs rapidly, being usually visible by the end of treatment. Curative treatment is usually followed by very dense calcification in the tumour bearing area, and these changes may remain permanently. The rapidity and the denseness of the recalcification are characteristic features of this tumour.

(b) *Secondary lymphoma of bone.* When investigation of an apparent primary lymphoma of bone demonstrates distant lymphomatous spread, the treatment becomes that of Stage III–IV lymphoma, and either combination chemotherapy or total body irradiation will be indicated (see below). Local irradiation to the 'primary' bone lesion may be necessary for rapid pain relief, but obviously this may not affect the long-term survival. Using combination chemotherapy, it is customary to treat for at least six courses and to continue with three course of consolidation treatment after complete remission (CR) has been recorded. CR of bony involvement by lymphoma is very difficult to assess. Adequate treatment may be followed by dense recalcification regardless of the quality of remission, and tumour shrinkage may occur only after many months. Repeated bone biopsies are not usually acceptable to the patient and the results may not be indicative of the condition of the whole bone. CR in bone can be assessed only by a combination of careful evaluation of associated findings, and inspired guesswork.

'Small round cell' tumours of bone showing a diffuse infiltration with poorly or undifferentiated lymphocytic cells are rarely caused by other lymphomas. In the author's experience, two patients with bone biopsies showing a 'small round cell' tumour had node biopsies showing Hodgkin's disease. One node was removed at the original bone operation, by an observant orthopaedic surgeon, and the second patient developed positive nodes within four months of the original operation. Both have done extremely well with local radiotherapy and chemotherapy, surviving free of disease for 10 and 17 years respectively. Two other patients with 'primary' bone lymphoma had node biopsies within a few months which showed follicular lymphoma. Both patients died within two years. The prognosis of these four patients differed very greatly in spite of the similarity of the original bone biopsies. If the correct diagnosis is to be established, any enlarged nodes should be removed at the time of the original operation and at any subsequent relapse.

Testicle

The majority of published series have included only a small number of patients. Gowing (1976) reviewed 140 patients from whom the pathology was reviewed by the Testicular Tumour Panel and Registry, amongst a total of 2106 cases at that time referred to the Panel. Five had a plasma cell tumour and in seven the testicular involvement was a necropsy finding only. Of the remaining 128 patients only eight had had other manifestations of lymphoma previously. The following were prominent clinical features of these cases. The peak age incidence was between 60 and 80 years. The testicular swelling was typical of testicular tumours in general. There was a particular tendency for both testicles to be affected, sometimes simultaneously but more often in succession. In the Panel cases, 28 (20%) were known to have bilateral disease. It is very difficult to know how many of these patients had disseminated disease when first seen because of their inadequate investigation by modern standards. Gowing refers to eight patients with known tumour elsewhere before the testicular tumour occurred and 13 who were found to have disease elsewhere at the time of orchidectomy.

Almost all NHL of the testicle are diffuse poorly differentiated or undifferentiated lymphomas. Diffuse well differentiated or follicular lymphomas are unknown, as is primary testicular Hodgkin's disease. The prognosis is as would be expected with this type of tumour although a few may survive for many years, suggesting that some lymphomas are, in fact, limited to the testicle. The management of these tumours depends upon the extent of the disease process after full investigation. Localized disease is usually treated as a seminoma. The likelihood that the opposite testicle will become involved and the probable age of the patient indicate that post-operative irradiation should not spare the opposite testicle, which would be better included within the treatment volume. A tumour dose of 3000–4000 rad in 5 weeks is adequate in most cases. Chemotherapy is indicated in widespread disease. The response of the tumour may be good initially, but long-term results remain poor with cases of this type, sometimes in spite of very vigorous treatment.

Thyroid gland

NHL may present in the thyroid gland, with any of the commoner histological appearances. From the management point of view, it is extremely important to remember that a 'small celled carcinoma' of the thyroid may be very difficult to differentiate from a diffuse well differentiated or poorly differentiated lymphoma. The characteristic features of the 'small celled carcinoma' of the thyroid in the past were its extreme radiosensitivity, followed, almost inevitably, by dissemination within 3–18 months and death. Retrospectively the similarity between these types of tumours is probably best explained by the fact that 'small-celled carcinoma' was often unrecognized NHL. Investigation of a patient with a 'round celled' or 'undifferentiated' thyroid cancer using modern imaging techniques frequently demonstrates the widespread changes of a malignant lymphoma which provides a rational explanation for the extremely rapid 'spread' of the tumour. Excellent reviews of the subject have been published (e.g. Smithers, 1970). Unfortunately these are now mainly of historical interest only, because of modern advances in histological interpretation and imaging techniques.

From the practical point of view any patient with a NHL or an 'undifferentiated' carcinoma of the thyroid must be investigated fully as is usual with NHL. If the disease is finally considered to be localized to the neck, radical irradiation should be given as if the patient had a primary carcinoma of the thyroid. Local irradiation is also indicated as a palliative measure for thyroid enlargement with or without local pressure effects. Should the disease prove to be generalized, the appropriate treatment should be advised as for Stage III–IV disease.

There is a close relationship between NHL of the thyroid and Hashimoto's disease (autoimmune thyroiditis). The differential diagnosis may be very difficult. Hashimoto's disease may show an extreme degree of lymphocytic infiltration often with a marked admixture plasma cells. These appearances are very similar to that found with NHL. The position is further confused because of the occasional finding of a high level of thyroid antibodies in thyroid carcinoma (Doniach *et al.*, 1968).

Treatment

Surgery

The part of the surgeon in the treatment of the NHL is limited in extent. However, when surgery is required, it is often in situations which require very considerable intellectual and technical ability, and where unsuccessful surgery may be disastrous. The very important place of the surgeon in establishing the correct diagnosis and, in some cases, determining the extent of the NHL, has been referred to already under the section on Investigations.

There are three situations where surgery may be the only worthwhile method of treatment.

Gastrointestinal NHL (see Section on special sites)
Most patients with lymphoma arising in the GI tract present to the gastroenterologist or surgeon, often as an emergency in the middle of the night, frequently with intestinal obstruction or perforation. The importance of taking at least an adequate biopsy in an apparently absolutely untreatable, advanced gut 'cancer' cannot be overemphasized: remissions of long duration may be possible if the tumour proves to be a NHL. The importance of removing all operable tumour in even relatively advanced gastrointestinal NHL cannot be overemphasized both from the point of view of attempting to cure the patient and in order to prevent the risks of subsequent perforation after effective radiotherapy or chemotherapy. The surgeon carries a heavy responsibility in many of these cases and it is unfortunate that so often an operation proves to be necessary as an emergency during the night, when highly experienced staff may be unavailable.

Splenectomy

Splenectomy as a therapeutic measure may prove necessary under several circumstances during the management of a patient with NHL.

(a) *Primary splenic lymphoma.* A very small number of patients have been reported where the lymphoma has been limited to the spleen and where splenectomy alone has been followed by very long survival and possibly cure. The patient is found to have a moderately or grossly enlarged spleen, which may or may not be producing symptoms. The blood count may show a low grade lymphocytosis; indeed, most patients are considered initially to have very low grade chronic lymphatic leukaemia, but careful examination of the circulating lymphocytes may reveal the typical appearance of the cleaved follicle centre cell. The cells can be regarded as a spill-over into the blood stream and not a manifestation of established leukaemia. Similarly, bone marrow examination may reveal scattered 'islands' of small darkly staining lymphocytes, which must not be taken as indicating leukaemic infiltration. Splenectomy may be followed by the disappearance of the peripheral lymphocytosis, and the marrow changes. The removed spleen shows changes of follicular lymphoma with or without diffuse areas of replacement with small lymphocytes. The differential diagnosis from very low grade chronic lymphatic leukaemia is clearly difficult: in cases of doubt it is probably safer to remove the spleen and observe the patient over a long period of time. The syndrome is rare. The author's experience includes five patients, three of whom subsequently developed generalization, two with Grade I NHL and one with chronic lymphatic leukaemia, over a period of up to eight years.

(b) *Pain and pressure effects.* Enlargement of the spleen in NHL may itself be painful, particularly when there has been rapid general enlargement with stretching of the splenic capsule or infarction or the enlarged organ may produce painful pressure effects. These include the production of a hiatus hernia with all that this may entail, and, in extreme cases gross painful abdominal distension, and limitation of physical activities. The need for surgical intervention requires careful judgement on the part of the clinician-in-charge. The splenic enlargement may be one manifestation of generalized disease and may respond well to chemotherapy, corticosteroids or splenic irradiation. However, sometimes the splenic enlargement with its accompanying symptoms persists in spite of treatment. Surgical removal then offers the only hope of relief for the patient and should be considered without further delay

(c) *Haemolytic anaemia.* Anaemia in NHL is common and may be due to many factors all of which require careful evaluation. Haemolytic anaemia is characterized by a persistently low haemoglobulin level, and raised reticulocyte count, in the absence of any evidence of chronic blood loss, for example from the gastrointestinal tract. Splenic enlargement may be minimal and there may be fluctuations in the degree of haemolysis making prolonged observations necessary. The diagnosis may be confirmed by a red cell survival study, which should show diminished reduction of the normal half life. It should be emphasized that in NHL, even a severe degree of haemolysis is rarely associated with jaundice or measurably raised bilirubin levels, unless there is associated severe hepatic dysfunction. Whether or not to undertake splenectomy depends upon the clinical situation. With low grade haemolysis, the condition may resolve following treatment for the underlying lymphoma or with corticosteroids. If corticosteroids are necessary, the decision as to whether or not they are to be used for prolonged treatment depends upon the dose necessary for adequate control. The complications of prolonged high dose corticosteroid therapy are well known. It is suggested that if a dose of prednisone 30 mg daily (or its equivalent) is necessary for a period of over three months in order to control the haemolysis, splenectomy should be considered as a preferable alternative (Jelliffe and Nabarro, 1961).

(d) *Hypersplenism*. Many of the manifestations of this syndrome may be due to sequestration of blood elements in a massive spleen. However, the clinical picture of hypersplenism may be seen without a palpably enlarged spleen and it is therefore difficult to explain the syndrome only as one of sequestration. The patient has the typical clinical manifestations of low haemoglobin, a low polymorph count and a low platelet count. All three elements may be low or the depression may be limited to one or two elements. The spleen is usually palpable and may be huge. Bone marrow examination often provides an answer to the problem. In contrast to the low peripheral blood levels, the marrow is normal or hyperactive. For example, if there is a thrombocytopaenia, it is common to see an increase in the number of megakaryocytes. Treatment of the underlying disease particularly with steroids may be of temporary benefit but splenic irradiation is rarely helpful, usually increasing thrombocytopaenia rather than shrinking the spleen. Splenectomy usually provides the only satisfactory solution. The lower the platelet count, the more urgent the need for operation. Platelet infusions should be reserved for the actual operation as their prolonged use may lead to antibody production. Following splenectomy the improvement in the depression of the peripheral blood elements is frequently dramatic (Fig. 36.8).

Central nervous system involvement

Extradural deposits of NHL are common, sometimes as a presenting feature, but more usually in the course of the disease. Extradural deposits of tumour with pressure on the spinal cord represent one of the few surgical emergencies in clinical oncology. Although the extreme radiosensitivity of NHL makes it possible to consider radiotherapy without previous surgical decompression, there are certain advantages in considering surgery. Firstly, the extradural deposit may be due to some other cause. The coexistence of NHL with other tumours is not uncommon. Secondly, a carefully performed surgical decompression of the cord is the quickest way of removing the ever-present risk of pressure from an extradural deposit blocking one of the penetrating spinal arteries. These arteries are end-arteries, and such a block is followed by an irreversible

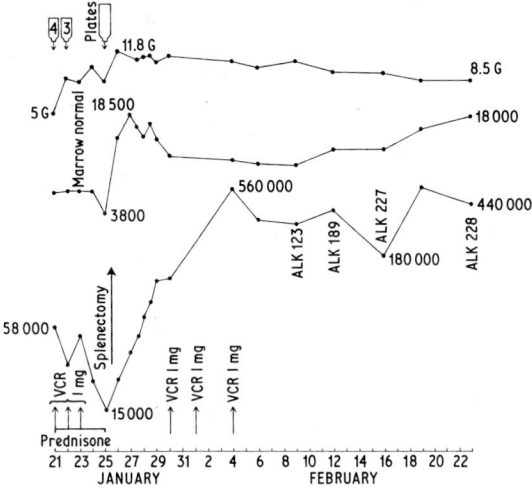

Fig. 36.8 Female aged 54 with Stage IV diffuse undifferentiated NHL. There was a progressively falling white cell and platelet count (nadir, 15 000) which was not affected by steroids and vincristine. Marrow biopsy normal. Splenectomy followed by extremely rapid return to normal blood lines of white cells and platelets.

complete paraplegia progressing rapidly over a few hours. This tragedy must be prevented whenever possible by the removal of the extradural mass with its accompanying pressure on the cord.

The neurosurgeon is also sometimes involved in the management of patients with tumour spread to the CSF and also when there is opportunistic infection of the CSF space, for example with *Cryptococcus neoformans*.

Radiotherapy

The value of radiotherapy in the control of NHL has been recognized for many years. For example, radiotherapists have appreciated that patients with giant follicular lymphoma or Brill Symmer's disease could be controlled, sometimes for many years, by the judicious use of irradiation in relatively small doses to gland masses that were troubling the patient (Levitt, 1952). As with Hodgkin's disease, spontaneous remissions and fluctuations in the progress of this group of disease occurs. This made the long-term evaluation of treatment difficult to assess at a time when cure was regarded as impossible and when there was no detailed classification and accurate staging was impossible.

Using modern pathological classification and staging procedures, it is now possible to approach patients with NHL in a reasonably logical way. Radiotherapy may be used when the disease is apparently localized, when the disease is apparently limited to the main lymph node regions (TNI) and also when the disease is widespread (TBI).

Localized radiotherapy

Although less than 20% of NHL remain as localized Stage I or II disease after full investigation, the value of radiotherapy in this small group is very great as it offers an excellent chance of cure. In an analysis of 233 patients with NHL of primary nodal origin, published in 1969, the patients presenting with localized disease could be controlled for many years with localized radiotherapy even when the histology suggested a poor prognosis (Millett *et al.*, 1969). Of eight patients with localized lymphoblastic lymphosarcoma, five did not survive five years, but all three survivors remained alive and well for periods of 11–17 years and these patients have remained disease-free a further nine years later. This result is particularly satisfactory when it is remembered that all patients had been investigated by what would nowadays be considered totally inadequate means. It is very likely that the five patients failing to survive five years had already developed widespread disease, which had not been demonstrated. Hellman *et al.* (1977) describe the results of irradiation of 65 patients with localized NHL of all histological types and refer to a 5-year survival rate of 80%. In this series, all patients with nodular Stage I disease survived five years, whereas only 50% of patients with diffuse histology, survived for a similar period of time. Long-term survival rates with localized NHL have been reported also by other workers (Lipton and Lee, 1971; Prosnitz *et al.*, 1969; Robinson *et al.*, 1971; Van der Werf-Messing, 1968).

With all available modern methods of tumour localization the possibilities of treating truly localized disease becomes increasingly likely and there is no doubt that in almost all cases of localized NHL, radical localized radiotherapy is essential treatment. The only exception to this rule is in childhood and possibly in the young adult. Although the 'local' lymphoma will often respond very well to radiotherapy, generalization usually occurs rapidly and there should be the least possible delay in inaugurating general treatment, and possibly CNS prophylaxis. The need for adjuvant chemotherapy in the older patient with apparently local lymphoma is not established. Comparative prospective trials are, at present, being undertaken by the British National Lymphoma Investigation.

Because there is less evidence in NHL than in Hodgkin's disease that the disease progresses in an orderly manner, affecting adjacent before distant lymph node groups, it is not logical to treat widely to cover all the adjacent lymph node regions. For example, with Stage I disease limited to one side of the neck, it is not logical to treat a full mantle. Wide local irradiation probably provides adequate treatment. As regards dosage, many patients with Grade I NHL have disease which is extremely radiosensitive and will be cured locally with 3500 rad in 3–4 weeks. With Grade II NHL the response is much more variable. Some cases will respond rapidly requiring not more than 4000 rad in 4 weeks, but others prove to be relatively radioresistant and it may be necessary to increase the dose to up to the limits of local tissue tolerance achieving doses of up to 6000 rad.

Extranodal NHL arising from sites such as Waldeyer's ring and the testicle are usually treated to include those lymph nodes which are normally regarded as draining the extranodal site. Thus a tonsillar lymphoma will be treated with fields which include the cervical lymph nodes as well as the tonsillar bed itself.

Total nodal irradiation (TNI)

Patients with Stage III Hodgkin's disease may be treated logically with TNI combining the mantle with the Y fields because lymph node involvement is usually limited to central axis lymph nodes. This is not always so with NHL. Diagnostic laparotomy and other investigations have shown that there is frequently involvement of mesenteric nodes, of the bowel itself and of other structures removed from those regions normally included in routine TNI as used for Hodgkin's disease. Because of this it may be more logical to include the whole of the abdomen in patients receiving TNI and it is possible that Waldeyer's ring and the epitrochlear nodes should also be treated routinely.

'Routine' TNI

This technique has been studied in depth by the Stanford group (Glatstein *et al.*, 1976). Of 68 patients with clinical or pathological Stage III NHL, 51 had follicular disease. TNI was followed by 5- and 10-year survival rates of 75% and 65%. Of the 28 patients who relapsed, 18 had relapse confined to lymph nodes and six involved previously unirradiated epitrochlear nodes. Over 90% of the relapses were seen in the first five years. The Stanford group conclude that there may be a place for high dose TNI in the attempted cure of Stage III NHL especially with the follicular type, but that this treatment should routinely include the epitrochlear and mesenteric nodes and Waldeyer's ring.

Whole abdomen irradiation

If it is accepted that the bowel is often involved and that microscopical involvement of the liver may be difficult to demonstrate, even after a diagnostic laparotomy, then it might seem more reasonable to

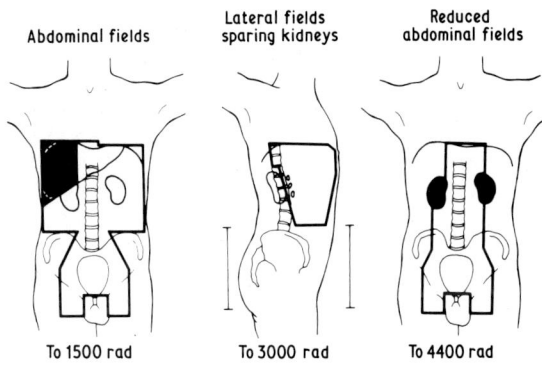

Abdominal fields **Lateral fields sparing kidneys** **Reduced abdominal fields**

To 1500 rad   To 3000 rad   To 4400 rad

Fig. 36.9 Three-way technique of whole abdomen irradiation used at Stanford since 1973. Lead blocks 5-cm thick protect the right lobe of the liver for the first 1500 rad and are also placed over both kidneys and the right lobe of the liver during the final treatment phase. This arrangement gives a dose of up to 4400 rad to the para-aortic and mesenteric nodes and bowel, and up to 2000 rad to the right lobe of the liver and to the kidneys (from Goffinet *et al.*, 1976).

include the whole abdomen in the radiation fields, whether the abdominal lymph nodes are being treated 'locally' or as a part of TNI. Various techniques of accomplishing this type of treatment have been considered in the past. An extremely elegant, safe and apparently effective technique has been evolved at Stanford (Goffinet *et al.*, 1976). This technique combines shrinking anteroposterior irradiation ports with cross-table lateral fields (Fig. 36.9). Effective shielding of the liver and kidneys can be achieved while delivering a total dose of 4400 rad to the main-midline lymph node mass. Blood count depression is no more marked than that with inverted Y irradiation to the abdominal and pelvic lymph nodes.

Total body irradiation (TBI)
Initially used by Heublein (1932) and later reported as being beneficial in the management of some lymphomas (Medinger and Craver, 1942) this technique fell out of favour as increasingly effective cytotoxic drugs were introduced into clinical oncology. Large volume irradiation, usually referred to as X-ray baths, remained in vogue until the late 1950s (Levitt, 1952) but these too became unfashionable.

In 1966, Johnson published results which suggested that total body irradiation could be useful in the management of patients with generalized NHL and there was renewed interest in the subject. Johnson and colleagues (Johnson *et al.*, 1970; Johnson, 1975) have since published several papers on the subject and other authors have confirmed the efficacy of this technique (Hellman *et al.*, 1977; Chaffey *et al.*, 1975).

Techniques vary from a daily dose of 10 rad or 15 rad twice weekly for a total of about 150 rad total body, to a 'half body' technique whereby one half of the body is treated with 50 rad daily for 10 treatments, the patient rests for up to four weeks to allow the platelet count to recover and then the second half is treated similarly, to a total dose of 500 rad. Whether the whole body is treated simultaneously, or in two 'half body' treatments, all normal structures are included in the treatment fields and no attempt is made to shield any particular structures. From the patient's point of view this is relatively undemanding treatment. Whole body doses of 10–15 rad or half body doses of 50 rad, produce little or no side-effects and are well tolerated as an outpatient. Treatment can be given with either telecobalt or a linear accelerator. Obviously many possible treatment positions are possible. A convenient one is that recommended originally by Johnson. The patient is treated with lateral fields, alternating the exposures from the left and the right sides daily. The whole volume of the body can be brought within the width of a conventional supervoltage beam by the adoption of the semi-foetal position on a chair (Fig. 36.10). The doses referred to above are calculated as absorbed doses at the midline of maximum thickness of the trunk. Johnson (1975) reports a median survival of four years in a group of 57 patients treated mainly by this technique with or without additional comprehensive node irradiation. In the same journal there is an initial report of a randomized clinical trial comparing intensive widefield radiotherapy with combination chemotherapy (Canellos *et al.*, 1975) in the treatment of widespread (Stage III, IV) lymphocytic lymphoma. These workers analysed a total of 65 patients, entered and randomized

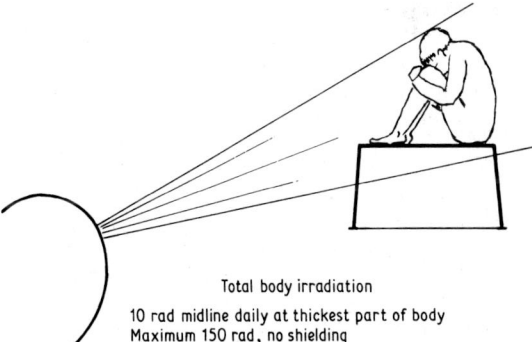

Total body irradiation
10 rad midline daily at thickest part of body
Maximum 150 rad, no shielding

Fig. 36.10 Total body irradiation. Patient is seated on a stool, crouched in the foetal position, thus reducing the height to a size that can be encompassed by a cobalt or X-ray beam. Treatment is from the left and right on alternate days; no normal tissues are shielded. The intended dose is the absorbed dose at the centre of the body at its maximum thickness.

according to stage. At the time of this report, there was no difference between the patients treated initially by chemotherapy or by radiotherapy. In both groups, 80% achieved a response and 55% were grouped as complete responders.

Reference has already been made to the need to examine published reports very carefully before comparing them with reports from other centres because of the complexities of the NHL. For example, Johnson's excellent results refer to only 'lymphocytic' NHL using Rappaport's classification and specifically exclude 'histiocytic' NHL. Thirty-nine of the 57 patients reported by him in 1975 had a nodular or a well-differentiated diffuse pattern, which of course places these patients in the Grade I or favourable category. It is, therefore, not possible to compare Johnson's results with those of the British National Lymphoma Investigation where this technique is under investigation only for the histological Grade II or unfavourable categories. With this group of patients, results are very different with a 2-year survival rate of only 25%. However, it would appear that a small number of patients who achieve complete remission maintain it for a long period of time. (Table 36.5). This small group of patients presumably is comparable with those patients reported by De Vita and colleagues in 1975 with apparently curable diffuse 'histiocytic' lymphoma (see below).

Table 36.5   Follow-up of Grade 2 Stage III, IV NHL. TBI = total body irradiation as recommended by Johnson (1975). CHOP – *see* Table 36.10. Of the small number of patients achieving complete remission, a reasonable percentage remain free of disease (British National Lymphoma Investigation).

Treatment of advanced non-Hodgkin's lymphoma
Survival after CR in Stage III, IV Grade 2 disease

BNLI, 1978

Treatment	Patients achieving CR	Still alive*
TBI	8	6 (75%)
CHOP	13	11 (85%)

* as of May 1978

Chemotherapy

When a lymphoma is generalized, chemotherapy is the most favoured treatment method. The only reasonable contender for Stage IV disease would nowadays be total body irradiation.

Since the introduction of nitrogen mustard by Goodman and colleagues in 1946, it has become apparent that many patients with NHL will respond to a variable degree and for a variable time to almost any of the alkylating agents. By the 1960s it had become accepted that vinblastine and, in particular, vincristine, were effective with this group of disease (Carbone and Spurr, 1968). The efficacy of corticosteroids, most commonly prednisone or prednisolone, in producing objective remissions in the NHL as opposed to Hodgkin's disease, had been recognized for a long time (Jelliffe and Nabarro, 1961; Ezdinli et al., 1969).

With the evolution of combination chemotherapy, it was natural that these three drugs should be combined together in various ways and reports of groups of patients treated with COP or CVP have become frequent (Hoogstraten et al., 1969; Bagley et al., 1972; Schein et al., 1974; Skarin et al., 1974). Response rates of 60–80% were claimed, with high complete remission rates. However, although the initial results were cheering, the relapse rate was high and few patients remained disease-free after three years of follow-up, requiring further courses of treatment. This applied to patients with Grade I (favourable) as well as Grade II (unfavourable) histology.

Stage III, IV Grade I (favourable) histology

The collaborators in the British National Lymphoma Investigation were unimpressed with the initial reports strongly favouring combination chemotherapy in the management of generalized Grade I NHL. In pilot studies carried out during the early 1970s, the BNLI found no obvious therapeutic advantage in using either chlorambucil, COP (with or without additional procarbazine), or total body irradiation. The only prospective trial in the literature comparing single agent with combination chemotherapy was that of Hoogstraten et al. (1969) in which the single agent (cyclophosphamide) had been used for too short a time for it to be effective. From the early work with single agent chemotherapy of the NHL, it was clear that response to low dose continuous treatment with alkylating agents such as chlorambucil and cyclophosphamide could be slow, requiring sometimes up to three months' treatment before a measurable improvement became apparent. Because total body irradiation was being investigated widely at that time, the BNLI decided that there was need for a direct comparison of COP (Table 36.6) with chlorambucil (Table 36.7). From the patients' point of view there were obvious advantages in treatment with a single agent, taken by mouth as an outpatient, with no unpleasant side-effects which interfered with normal life.

A prospective randomized trial comparing COP with chlorambucil was started in 1973. By 1977 certain facts had emerged. The survival rate of those patients treated initially with COP was significantly better than in the group treated with chlorambucil (Fig. 36.11).

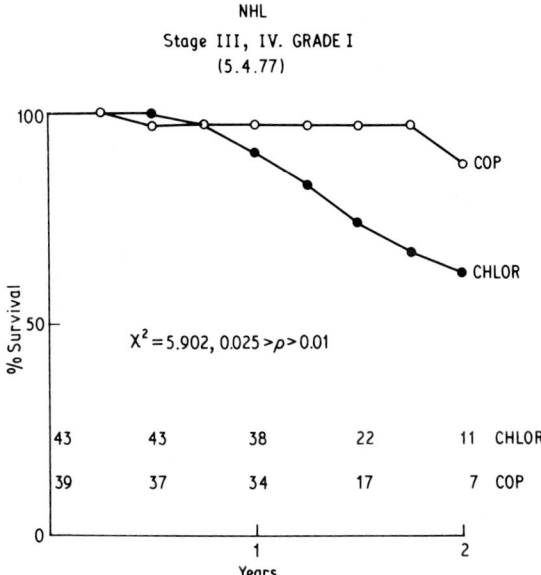

NHL
Stage III, IV. GRADE I
(5.4.77)

$x^2 = 5.902, 0.025 > p > 0.01$

| 43 | 43 | 38 | 22 | 11 CHLOR |
| 39 | 37 | 34 | 17 | 7 COP |

Fig. 36.11 Comparison of crude survival rates in patients with Stage III, IV Grade I NHL treated initially either by COP (*see* Table 36.6) or by chlorambucil (CHLOR, *see* Table 36.7). There is a statistically significant difference between the survival rates, favouring COP (British National Lymphoma Investigation).

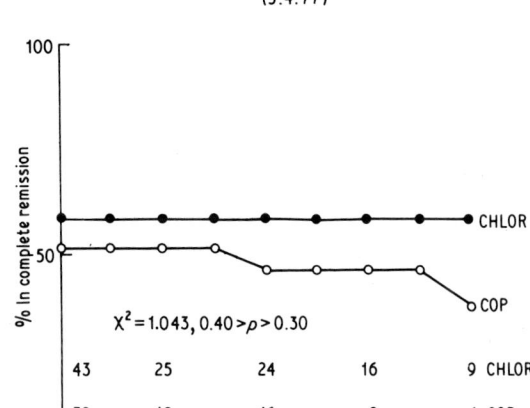

NHL
Stage III, IV. GRADE I
(5.4.77)

$x^2 = 1.043, 0.40 > p > 0.30$

| 43 | 25 | 24 | 16 | 9 CHLOR |
| 39 | 19 | 16 | 8 | 4 COP |

Fig. 36.12 Comparison of relapse-free survival rates in patients with Stage III, IV Grade I NHL treated initially either by COP or by chlorambucil. There is no statistically significant difference between the relapse-free survival rates (British National Lymphoma Investigation).

However, the relapse-free survival rate of the two groups was identical, about one half of the patients in each group continuing free of disease at two years (Fig. 36.12). Detailed examination of patients dying in the two groups demonstrated a marked difference. Amongst the chlorambucil-treated deaths were two due to other cancers and six patients who had been kept on chlorambucil for periods of 6–21 months without evidence of disease control, or treatment with the alternative, COP (Table 36.8). There was clearly a reluctance on the part of the clinicians in charge to change from a treatment which produced no symptoms to combination chemotherapy with all its well recognized complications, in a group of patients who often had no symptoms referable to their illness. The study was completed. It had shown that patients must not be kept on ineffective treatment, that relapse-free survival rates with combination or single therapy were similar and, finally, that the high relapse rate after stopping either treatment suggested that cure might prove impossible or at the very least require a prolonged period of maintenance therapy. A new prospective trial was started with the object of testing these ideas. This study had three phases. Induction therapy over a minimum period of three months uses either COP

Table 36.6 COP.

Cyclophosphamide	600 mg/m²	day 1 + 8 (max. 1 g)
Oncovin (vincristine)	1.4 mg/m²	day 1 + 8 (max.2 mg)
Prednisone	25 mg/m²	Day 1 – 8
Repeat every 2–4 weeks		
Minimum of 6 courses		
Give at least 3 courses after complete remission		

Table 36.7 Chlorambucil.

Initial dose:	0.2 mg/kg daily until complete remission
Maintenance:	0.2 mg/kg daily for 4–8 weeks, then 0.1 mg/kg
Overall treatment:	2 years

(Table 36.9) or chlorambucil. At the end of three months of chlorambucil, or three complete courses of COP, the patient is carefully reassessed and if no progressive improvement is detectable then the patient is changed to the other arm of the trial.

Table 36.8   NHL Stage III, IV Grade I.

Chlorambucil deaths	
Other causes (coronary, cancer of the stomach)	2
Post-splenectomy	1
Possible drug complication	1
Failure also on other combinations	4
Failure on chlorambucil alone	6
Total	14

Patients failing to respond to chlorambucil alone received treatment for 6–17 months

Table 36.9   COP.

Cyclophosphamide	600 mg/m²	day 1 + day 8
Oncovin (vincristine)	1.4 mg/m²	day 1 + day 8
Prednisone	25 mg/m²	day 1 – day 8

Repeat every 3 weeks
Dose reduction according to blood count
Reassess at 3 months
If progressive improvement is occurring, continue for minimum period of 6 months, and for at least 3 months consolidation therapy after complete remission has been recorded

If progressive improvement is recorded, therapy is continued until complete remission (defined as a reversal of all previously abnormal findings) has been obtained. Consolidation is then maintained with the same treatment for three months. At this point patients are carefully watched without further treatment, unless relapse occurs, or they are maintained on chlorambucil for a period of two years (Fig. 36.13). This study will provide useful data comparing chlorambucil with COP for induction therapy, the possible value of the alternative treatment method in patients resistant to the initial treatment method, and the possible value of long-term maintenance therapy, using a single agent.

The original view of the BNLI that combination chemotherapy had not been shown to give better results than single agent therapy in generalized NHL of Grade I (favourable) histology has been confirmed recently. In 1976, Portlock and colleagues published a paper comparing a single agent cyclophosphamide, with combination chemotherapy (CVP) in low or high dosage, in which they show that there is no advantage in combination chemotherapy. More recently Lister *et al.* (1978) have published a paper expressing similar views.

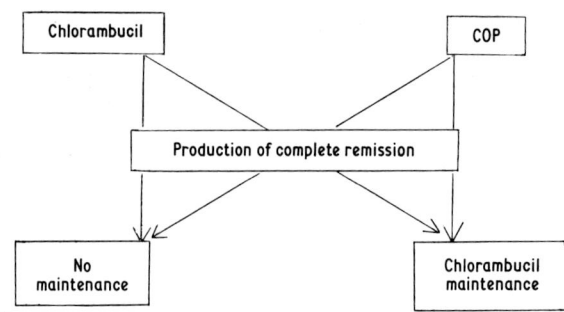

Fig. 36.13   Present trial comparing chlorambucil and COP in the initial management of Grade I Stage III-IV NHL. Following the achievement of Complete Remission, and the administration of Consolidation Therapy, patients are either watched or are given maintenance therapy using chlorambucil (British National Lymphoma Investigation).

Stage III, Grade II (unfavourable) histology
Whereas there seems little doubt that a reasonable number of patients with Grade I generalized disease will respond well to single agent therapy, it is generally accepted that such treatment is not helpful for patients with aggressive treatment with combination chemotherapy and TBI. The BNLI is comparing CHOP (Table 36.10) now somewhat modified from the combination originally published by McKelvey *et al.* (1975) with TBI. The results are poor with either method. The general trend over the world has been to use combination chemotherapy of gradually increasing toxicity in attempts to combat this group of aggressive and depressing diseases. Originally with the success of MOPP in Hodgkin's disease, MOPP was tried for the NHL followed by C. MOPP or (COPP) substituting mustard with cyclophosphamide; during the same period COP or CVP were tried out. The long-term results were disappointing, varying from 20–50% with considerable differences in patient selection. Other drugs have been added including adriamycin and bleomycin to try to improve the results. One interesting approach was that used in BACOP (Skarin *et al.*, 1974; Schein *et al.*, 1975). These programmes were designed particularly to control those lymphomas whose aggressive nature was demonstrated by their tendency to recur rapidly between courses of drugs while the blood count was still low, precluding the further use of myelosuppressive drugs. Basically, the two BACOP regimens adopt the principle of giving bleomycin and steroids in between combinations of more active myelosuppressive drugs. This approach is interesting but no dramatic improvement has occurred following its use. Another new approach has been the use of high dose methotrexate with citrovorum factor

Table 36.10   CHOP (Modified).

Cyclophosphamide	750 mg/m²	i.v. day 1 + day 8
Hydroxydaunorubicin (adriamycin)	25 mg/m²	i.v. day 1 + day 8
Oncovin (vincristine)	1.4 mg/m²	i.v. day 1 + day 8
Prednisone	50 mg/m²	p.o. day 1 – day 8

Repeat every 4–6 weeks
Minimum total 6 courses: 3 courses after CR
Maximum accumulated dose of adriamycin 550 mg/m²

rescue (Pitman *et al.* 1975; Djerassi and Kim, 1976). High remission rates are achieved. Djerassi and Kim reported a total of 22 children of whom all had complete or partial remission. Six patients were free of disease from 2.5–5.5 years after discontinuing treatment. The author's own experience with high dose methotrexate followed by folic acid rescue is limited to 12 adults with generalized Grade II NHL, of whom only two achieved a complete remission for a short time and all of whom died of their disease. It is possible that the responses in children are better than in adults, many of whom are generally unfit or over 60 years.

Generalized Grade II (unfavourable) histology NHL remains an unsatisfactory group of diseases to treat. Occasionally dramatic remission occurs and is followed by long term disease-free survival. The excellent responses of a group of patients with advanced disease reported originally by Lowenbraum *et al.* (1970) and their very encouraging long-term follow-up (De Vita *et al.*, 1975) suggests that in any group of patients of this type there may be a small nucleus of patients who are potentially curable. The second report in 1975 refers to a total of 27 patients with a complete remission rate of 41%. Of the 11 patients achieving a complete remission, 10 were alive and free of disease about ten years later. It should be noted that this group of patients was collected over a 7-year period between 1965 and 1972 and cannot therefore be considered typical of most series. Nevertheless it is very cheering to see that some patients with diffuse undifferentiated (histiocytic) lymphoma are potentially curable.

Non-Hodgkin's lymphoma in childhood and adolescence

The prognosis and management of Hodgkin's disease in children is identical with that in adults, except for the need to consider the effects of irradiation on the epiphysis and other growing tissues, and the possible effects of splenectomy in the very young. These two points must obviously be considered also in the management of NHL, but there are also other features which make the prognosis and management of this group of diseases in the pre-adult phase very different from that in the adult. These differences will be considered in detail.

Histological types

Diffuse well differentiated lymphomas are seen but on the whole they behave in a more aggressive way than in adult life. By far the commonest lymphomas in childhood are diffuse poorly differentiated or diffuse undifferentiated (histiocytic). Included in the poorly differentiated group are the chicken-foot tumour of Lukes' and Burkitt's lymphoma. It is rare to discover that a lymphoma in childhood shows either a follicular pattern or well marked fibrosis, both of which carry a better prognosis.

Primary extranodal involvement

Children are found to have extranodal disease on presentation even more commonly than in adults. The disease effects extranodal sites in 55–60% of children.

Involvement of the mediastinum

Uncommon in the adult, the mediastinum is the primary tumour site in about 20% of children. This tumour is commonly the chicken-foot lymphoma of Lukes, usually considered to be a T-cell lymphoma, characterized by an extremely rapid response of the mediastinal mass to irradiation, and followed by an equally rapid relapse, frequently with meningeal involvement, unless treated initially as a potentially widespread disease (see below). It is common for these children to present with the Mediastinal syndrome (D'Angio *et al.*, 1965).

Later involvement of extranodal tissues

Early involvement of the bone marrow and the central nervous system is common. The development of overt leukaemia is seen in up to 30% of children with mediastinal, nodal and generalized involvement whereas it is less common when the lymphoma appears to originate in the abdomen or head and neck (Jenkins, 1974). Central nervous system (CNS) involvement is seen in a quarter to a third of all children with NHL (Bunn *et al.*, 1976). Obviously a higher rate of involvement will be found by clinicians who are acutely aware of this complication and do not misinterpret the clinical signs produced. In the past a large number of neurological complications including isolated cranial nerve palsies in this group of diseases and in acute leukaemia have been attributed to the use of vincristine whereas the majority of children with symptoms such as this are much more likely to have direct nervous system involvement.

The clinical manifestation of CNS involvement includes personality change, headache and vomiting, all of which may be intermittent, cranial nerve weaknesses or paralyses and concussions. Papilloedema may be found and there may be obvious weakness of cranial nerves. However, there may be few clinical signs and early diagnosis depends upon a good clinical judgement by the clinician-in-charge followed by a lumbar puncture.

When CNS involvement is discovered clinically and confirmed by cerebrospinal fluid (CSF) examination, or by other investigations, treatment will obviously depend upon the extent of the involvement. When there is meningeal involvement confirmed by lumbar puncture and CSF examination, the whole CSF space should be treated with intrathecal methotrexate and/or cytosine arabinoside, and whole cranial irradiation, as in leukaemia. Focal CNS involvement, often associated with macroscopic disease which may be confirmed by myelogram or by bone destruction, e.g. as is seen sometimes in the base of the skull, is an indication for local irradiation.

However, the demonstration of established CNS involvement is usually a confession of failure. Established CNS invasion is very rarely cured. In view of the high probability of bone marrow and CNS involvement it is more profitable to consider the advisability of CNS prophylaxis (see below).

Treatment of childhood non-Hodgkin's lymphoma

From the above account it is clear that NHL in the child is in general a much more agressive disease than in the adult. The rare exceptions to this rule are children with Stage I nodal disease, and those where histological examination shows a follicular pattern or extensive fibrosis.

Excluding these rare presentations, the child with the disease should be treated radically. The treatment is unpleasant, prolonged and may be followed many years later with a higher than expected number of patients with malignant disease. Before starting treatment it is therefore essential to have a very adequate surgical biopsy, which has been well fixed and perfectly prepared by the pathology department. It is important to have more than one opinion on the interpretation of the slides and if, finally, there is any doubt in the pathologist's mind, a second, very adequate biopsy should be obtained. The benefits of this approach cannot be overemphasized. An 'unnecessary' biopsy carries an infinitely smaller morbidity rate than unnecessary treatment. Particular care should be taken in the interpretation of a node biopsy when generalized nodes are very small or when there is only a single large node, particularly from the groin. A careful history is essential with a particular note of any family history of allergies, contacts with infectious diseases or with sources of infectious diseases (e.g. mice, cats, etc.) and drug intake.

Assuming that there is no doubt in the pathologist's minds as to the true nature of the disease and the lymphoma is not one of the rarities suggested above, the following routine will cover most situations.

Local treatment
When the lymphoma arises in a special site such as the abdomen, this will be surgical. Occasionally, as with the anterior mediastinal T-cell lymphoma, local irradiation is indicated to produce relief of obstructive symptoms. However, the dramatic response which can be expected with this treatment must not lead to a postponement of the systemic treatment which provides the only hope of long term cure (Fig. 36.14).

Induction/consolidation chemotherapy
A satisfactory initial response occurs frequently with chemotherapy using cyclophosphamide, vincristine and prednisone. Some workers add other agents but there is no evidence that they help in the production of complete remission. It is usual for the patient to need at least four courses of treatment in order to produce complete remission.

Central nervous system prophylaxis
As with acute leukaemia it has become customary to treat the CNS prophylactically, as a sanctuary site. The whole brain is irradiated to a dose of 2400 rad and the CSF space is treated with intrathecal methotrexate and/or cytosine arabinoside (Chapters 10 and 30). It is normal to avoid a lumbar puncture until the patient has received a reasonable number of induction/consolidation chemotherapy courses in order to prevent the accidental contamination of normal CSF with lymphoma cells carried in by the needle.

Maintenance chemotherapy
On completion of the previous treatment it is necessary to continue with maintenance therapy for up to two years if a complete remission is to have a reasonable chance of continuing. The routines in common use for this purpose are those used satisfactorily in acute leukaemia (see Chapter 33).

The long term results of vigorous treatment of this type are as yet unknown. However it is reasonable to assume that the results cannot be worse than with earlier treatment methods which have resulted in almost total failure in the long-term control of lymphomas in childhood.

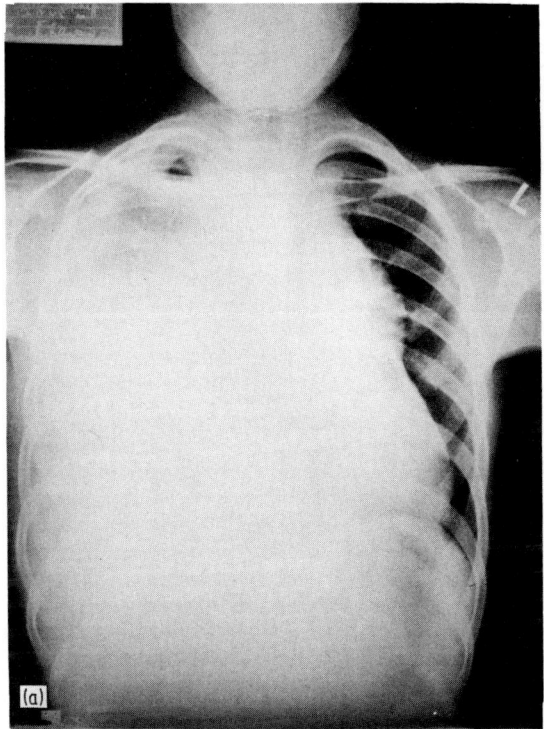

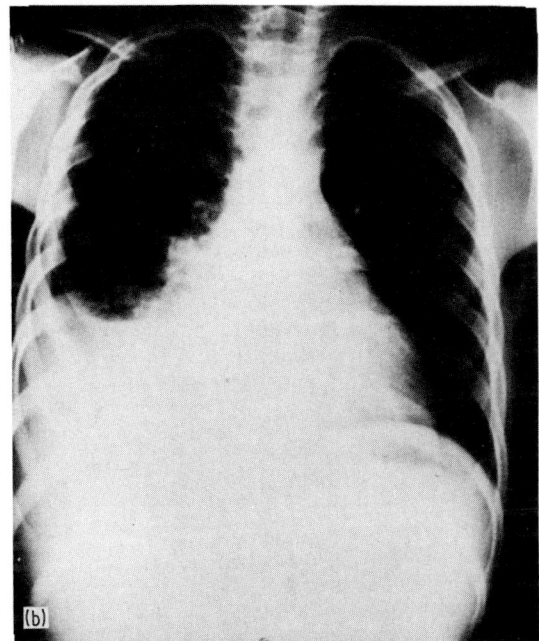

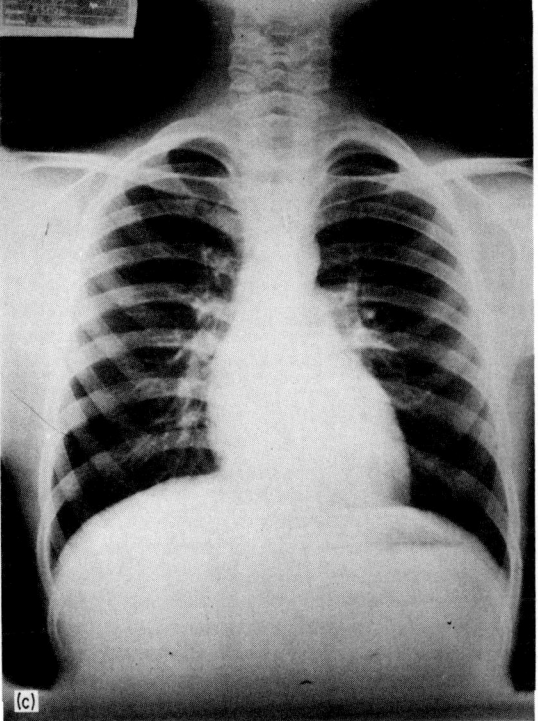

Fig. 36.14 (*a*) Chest X-ray of boy aged 11 admitted with mediastinal syndrome and probably also pericardial infiltration with diffuse poorly differentiated NHL. Irradiation of tumour commenced on day of admission.
(*b*) Chest X-ray after 5 days' irradiation, having received 1500 rad midline.
(*c*) Irradiation completed at tumour dose of 3000 rad in 2 weeks; 20 days after commencing treatment chest X-ray appears normal. Full investigation (excluding laparotomy) showed no evidence of disease elsewhere. Generalization of disease occurred 2 months later, control was not obtained and patient died 5 months after initial presentation.

Follow-up

Complete remission may be defined as the return to normal of all pre-treatment abnormalities, clinical and investigational, provided that it is ethical to repeat the investigation. For accuracy in follow-up it is essential to record several 'markers' which can be repeatedly examined as treatment progresses. Superficial nodes and deep nodes demonstrated by lymphography or CAT-scanning are particularly easy to measure. Liver and spleen enlargements are less easy and abnormalities such as a positive needle biopsy of liver or bone marrow may be very difficult to follow with confidence. The difficulties when following a patient with lymphoma of bone have been referred to already. Lastly, the ESR is not often raised, weight loss is uncommon and systemic manifestations are unusual, unless the disease is progressing very rapidly, so these may be used as progress indicators only with a few patients. Markers, as progress indicators, are of special interest when the patient has received treatment with cytotoxic drugs. Relapse occurs most commonly in those sites previously affected.

After stopping treatment the patient should be seen at regular intervals and it is usual to relate the interval between visits to the tempo of the disease. This may be misleading. For example, it is not unknown for a follicular lymphoma in complete remission to relapse surprisingly soon after stopping chlorambucil, in spite of the low grade histological appearances. It is advisable to follow all patients at intervals of not more than four weeks after stopping chemotherapy, for at least three months, or until it is felt that the tempo of the disease has been accurately assessed. Examinations are made not only to detect early relapse at previously treated sites but also to detect relapse at other sites, the probability of which will depend upon the individual lymphoma. It is obviously particularly important to detect relapse early at sites where further treatment may benefit the patient, in particular extradural extension.

Further reading

Robb-Smith, A.H.T. and Taylor, C.R. (1981), *Lymph Node Biopsy*. Miller Heyden, London.

References

Arthur, J.F. *et al.* (1970), Small round cell tumours of bone, In: *Symposium Ossium* (eds A.M. Jelliffe and B. Strickland) Livingstone, Edinburgh and London, pp. 136–90.

Bagley, C.M. *et al.* (1972), Advanced lymphosarcoma: intensive cyclical chemotherapy with cyclophosphamide, vincristine and prednisone. *Anns Intern. Med.*, **76**, 227–34.

Bagley, C.M. *et al.* (1973), Diagnosis of liver involvement by lymphoma: results in 96 consecutive peritoneoscopies. *Cancer*, **31**, 840–7.

Bennett, M.H. (1975), Sclerosis in non-Hodgkin's lymphomata. *Br. J. Cancer*, **31**, Supplement II, 44–52.

Bennett, M.H. and Millett, Y.L. (1969), Nodular sclerotic lymphosarcoma. A possible new clinicopathological entity. *Clin. Radiol.*, **20**, 339–43.

Bennett, M.H., Farrer-Brown, G. and Henry, K. (1973), A classification of non-Hodgkin's lymphomas. Presented at the Workshop on *Classifications of Non-Hodgkins's Lymphomas*, University of Chicago.

Bennett, M.H. *et al.* (1974), Classification of non-Hodgkin's lymphomas. *Lancet*, **ii**, 405–6.

Bonadonna, G. *et al.* (1975), Staging laparotomy in non-Hodgkin's lymphomata. *Br. J. Cancer*, **31**, Supplement II, 252–60.

Boston, H.C. *et al.* (1974), Malignant lymphoma (so called reticulum cell sarcoma) of bone. *Cancer*, **34**, 1131–7.

Bunn, P.A. *et al.* (1976), Central nervous system complications in patients with diffuse hystiocytic and undifferentiated lymphoma: leukaemia revisited. *Blood*, **47**, 3–10

Canellos, G.P. *et al.* (1975), Therapy of advanced lymphocytic lymphoma. A preliminary report of a randomised trial between combination chemotherapy (CVP) and intensive radiotherapy. *Br. J. Cancer*, **31**, Supplement II, 474–80.

Carbone, P.P. and Spurr, C. (1968), Management of patients with malignant lymphomas: a comparative study with cyclophosphamide and vinca alkaloids. *Cancer Res.*, **28**, 811–22.

Carr, I. *et al.* (1977), *Lymphoreticular Disease*. Backwell Scientific Publications, Oxford and London, pp. 93–100.

Chabner, B.A. *et al.* (1975), Percutaneous liver biopsy, peritoneoscopy, and laparotomy: an assessment of relative merits in the lymphomata. *Br. J. Cancer*, **31**, Supplement II, 242–7.

Chaffey, J.F. *et al.* (1975), Advanced lymphosarcoma treated by total body irradiation. *Br. J. Cancer.*, **31**, Supplement II, 441–9.

Crowther, D.A. and Blackledge, G. (1978), Gastrointestinal lymphomas. *Br. J. Radiol.*, **51**, 75.

D'Angio, G.T., Mitus, A. and Evans, A.W. (1965), The superior mediastinal syndrome in children with cancer. *Am. J. Roentg.*, **93**, 537–44.

De Vita, V.T. *et al.* (1975), Advanced histiocytic lymphoma – a potentially curable disease. *Lancet*, **i**, 248–50.

Djerassi, I. and Kim, J.S. (1976), Methotrexate and citrovorum factor rescue in the management of childhood lymphosarcoma and reticulum-cell sarcoma (non-Hodgkin's lymphomas); prolonged unmaintained remissions. *Cancer*, **38**, 1043–51.

Doniach, D., Roitt, I.M. and Hudson, R.V. (1968), Autoantibodies in thyroid carcinoma. *Lancet*, **ii**, 265–6.

Ezdinli, E.Z. *et al.* (1969), Corticosteroid therapy for lymphomas and chronic lymphocytic leukemia. *Cancer*, **23**, 900–9.

Farrer-Brown, G. *et al.* (1975), Follicular lymphoma. Communication to the *131st Mtg. Path. Soc. G.B. and Ireland.*

Gatti, R.A. and Good, R.A. (1971), Occurence of malignancy in immunodeficiency disease – a literature review. *Cancer*, **28**, 89–98.

Glatstein, E. *et al.* (1976), Non-Hodgkin's lymphomas of Stage III extent: is total lymphoid irradiation appropriate treatment? *Cancer*, **37**, 2806–12.

Goffinet, D.R. *et al.* (1976), Abdominal irradiation in non-Hodgkin's lymphomas. *Cancer*, **37**, 2797–805.

Goodman, L.S. *et al.* (1976), Nitrogen mustard therapy. Use of methyl-bis (β-chloroethyl) amine hydrochloride and tris- (β-chloroethyl) amine hydrochloride for Hodgkin's disease, lymphosarcoma, leukaemia and certain allied and miscellaneous disorders. *J. Am. Med. Assoc.*, **132**, 126–36.

Gowing, N.F.C. (1976), Malignant lymphoma of the testicle. In: *Pathology of the Testis.* (ed. R.C.B. Pugh) Blackwell, Oxford, London, and Edinburgh. pp. 334–55.

Hellman, S. *et al.* (1977), The place of radiation therapy in the treatment of non-Hodgkin's lymphomas. *Cancer*, **39**, 843–51.

Henry, K. (1975), Electron microscopy in the non-Hodgkin's lymphomas. *Br. J. Cancer*, **31**, Supplement II, 73–93.

Henry, K., Bennett, M.H. and Farrer-Brown, G. (1978), Classification of the non-Hodgkin's lymphomas, In: *Recent Advances in Histopathology.* (eds P.P. Anthony and N. Woolf) Churchill Livingstone, Edinburgh, London and New York, pp. 275–302.

Henry, K., Howarth, C. and Farrer-Brown, G. (1976), Primary gastrointestinal lymphomas. Communication to the *132nd Mtg. Path. Soc. G. B. and Ireland.*

Heublein, A.C. (1932), Preliminary report on continuous irradiation of entire body. *Radiology*, **18**, 1051.

Hoogstraten, B. *et al.* (1969), Combination chemotherapy in lymphosarcoma and reticulum cell sarcoma. *Blood*, **33**, 370–7.

Jelliffe, A.M. (1975), Diagnostic laparotomy in non-Hodgkin's lymphoma. *Br. J. Cancer*, **31**, Supplement II, 248–51.

Jelliffe, A.M. and Nabarro, J.D.N. (1961), Corticosteroids in the treatment of the reticuloses. *Br. J. Radiol.*, **34**, 577–80.

Jenkins, R.D.T. (1974), The management of malignant lymphomas, In: *Malignant Diseases in Children.* (ed. T.J. Deeley), Butterworth, London, pp. 319–59.

Johnson, R.E. (1966), Evaluation of fractionated total body irradiation in patients with leukemia and disseminated lymphomas. *Radiology*, **86**, 1085–9

Johnson, R.E. (1975), Management of generalised malignant lymphomata with 'systematic' radiotherapy. *Br. J. Cancer*, **31**, Supplement II, 450–5.

Johnson, R.E., O'Connor, G.T. and Levin, D. (1970), Primary management of advanced lymphosarcoma with radiotherapy. *Cancer*, **25**, 787–91.

Johnson, R.E. *et al.* (1975), Patterns of involvement with malignant lymphoma and implications for treatment decision making. *Br. J. Cancer*, **31**, Supplement II, 237–41.

Jones, S.E., Rosenberg, S.A. and Kaplan, H.S. (1972), Non-Hodgkin's lymphomas. I. Bone marrow involvement. *Cancer*, **29**, 954–60.

Levitt, W.M. (1952), *Handbook of Radiotherapy.* Harvey and Blythe, London.

Lipton, A. and Lee, B.J. (1971), Prognosis of Stage I lymphosarcoma and reticulum-cell sarcoma. *New Engl. J. Med.*, **284**, 230–3.

Lister, T.A. *et al.* (1978), Comparison of combined and single agent chemotherapy in non-Hodgkin's lymphoma of favourable histological type. *Br. Med. J.*, **i**, 533–6.

Lowenbraum, S., De Vita, V.T. and Serpick, A.A. (1970), Combination chemotherapy with nitrogen mustard, vincristine, procarbazine and prednisone in lymphosarcoma and reticulum-cell sarcoma. *Cancer*, **25**, 1018–25.

Lukes, R.J. and Collins, R.D. (1975), A functional classification of malignant lymphomas. In: *The Reticuloendothelial System.* (eds J.W. Rebuck, C.W. Berard and M.R. Abell), Williams and Wilkins, Baltimore.

Medinger, F.G. and Craver, L.F. (1942), Total body irradiation. *Am. J. Roentg.*, **48**, 651.

McKelvey, E.M. *et al.* (1975), Hydroxydaunomycin (adriamycin) combination chemotherapy in non-Hodgkin's lymphoma. *Proc. Am. Assoc. Cancer Res.*, Am. Soc. Clin. Oncol., **16**, 233.

Millett, Y.L. *et al.* (1969), Nodular sclerotic lymphosarcoma. A further review. *Br. J. Radiol.*, **23**, 683–92.

Molassez, M. (1877), Lymphadenoma due Testicle. Bulletins et Memoires de la Societe Anatomique de Paris 52, 176–8.

Moran, E.M. *et al.* (1975), Staging laparotomy in non-Hodgkin's lymphoma. *Br. J. Cancer*, **31**, Supplement II, 228–36.

Nelson, D. F. *et al.* (1977), The role of radiation therapy in localised resectable intestinal non-Hodgkin's lymphoma in children. *Cancer*, **39**, 89–97.

Pitman, S., Tattersall, M.H.N. and Frei, E., III (1975), A phase I–II study of high dose methotrexate with citrovorum factor rescue. *Proc. Am. Assoc. Cancer Res.*, Am. Soc. Clin. Oncol., **16**, 263.

Portlock, C.S. *et al.* (1976), Treatment of advanced

non-Hodgkin's lymphomas with favorable histologies; preliminary results of a prospective trial. *Blood*, **47**, 747–56.

Prosnitz, L.R. *et al.* (1969), The clinical course of Hodgkin's disease and other malignant lymphomas treated with radical radiotherapy. *Am. J. Roentg.*, **105**, 618–28.

Rappaport, H. (1966), *Tumours of the Haemopoetic System*. Armed Forces Institute of Pathology, Washington.

Rappaport, H., Winter W. and Hicks, H.B. (1956), Follicular lymphoma. A re-evaluation of its position in the scheme of malignant lymphomas based on a survey of 253 cases. *Cancer*, **9**, 792–821.

Robb-Smith, A.H.T. (1938), Reticulosis and reticulosarcoma: a histological classification. *J. Path. Bact.*, 457–80.

Robb-Smith, A.H.T. (1964), *The classification and natural history of the lymphadenopathies. (Treatment of Cancer, and Allied diseases)*. 2nd edn, **9**. (eds G.T. Pack and I.M. Ariel), Hoeberg, New York.

Robinson, T., Fischer, J.J. and Vera, R. (1971), Reticulum cell sarcoma treated by radiotherapy. *Radiology*, **99**, 669–75.

Rosas-Uribe, A. and Rappaport, H. (1972), Malignant lymphoma, histocytic type with sclerosis (sclerosing reticulum cell sarcoma). *Cancer*, **29**, 946–53.

Rosenberg, S.A. (1975), Bone marrow involvement in the non-Hodgkin's lymphomata. *Br. J. Cancer*, **31**, Supplement II, 261–4.

Rostom, A.Y. and Peckham, M.J. (1977), Total body irradiation in advanced non-Hodgkin's lymphoma. *Eur. J. Cancer*, **13**, 1241–9.

Schein, P.S. *et al.* (1974), Potential for prolonged disease-free survival following combination chemotherapy of non-Hodgkin's lymphoma. *Blood*, **43**, 181–9.

Schein, P. *et al.* (1975), A new combination chemotherapy programme for diffuse histiocytic (DHL) and mixed (DML) non-Hodgkin's lymphoma. *Am. Soc. Clin. Oncol.*, **16**, 248.

Schein, P.S. *et al.* (1976), Bleomycin, adriamycin, cyclophosphamide vincristine and prednisone (BACOP) combination chemotherapy in the treatment of advanced diffuse histiocytic lymphoma. *Anns Intern. Med.*, **85**, 417–22.

Skarin, A.T. *et al.* (1974), Combination chemotherapy of advanced lymphocytic lymphoma. *Cancer*, **34**, 1023–9.

Smithers, D.H. Sir (1970), *Malignant Lymphomas of the Thyroid Gland in Tumours of the Thyroid Gland*. (ed. Sir David Smithers), Livingstone, Edinburgh and London, pp. 141–54.

Stein, R.S. *et al.* (1976), Bone marrow involvement in non-Hodgkin's lymphoma. Implications for staging and therapy. *Cancer*, **37**, 629–36.

Taylor, C.R. (1977a), *Hodgkin's Disease and the Lymphomas*. Eden Press, Montreal and Lunsdale House, Lancaster, England, p. 11.

Taylor, C.R. (1977b), *Hodgkin's Disease and the Lymphomas*. Eden Press, Montreal and Lunsdale House, Lancaster, England, pp. 26–7.

Van der Werf-Messing, B. (1968), Reticulum cell sarcoma and lymphosarcoma. *Eur. J. Cancer*, **4**, 542–57.

Wang, C.C. and Fleischli, D.J. (1968), Primary reticulum-cell sarcoma of bone with emphasis on radiation therapy. *Cancer*, **22**, 994–8.

37 Paediatric cancer

Jill A. Bullimore and
Martin G. Mott

The treatment of children with cancer carries with it the responsibility of giving the best chance of cure and at the same time causing the least physical and mental damage, so that the child may grow into as normal an adult as possible, able to contribute to the society in which he lives.

The management of children with malignant disease differs in many respects from that appropriate for adults. Carcinomas are the principal neoplasms of adult life, but are uncommon in childhood, where embryonal tumours predominate. Tumours which are common to both age groups, for example, lymphomas and leukaemia, differ in their behaviour and prognosis in the two groups and require differing management. In infancy, many of the embryonal tumours have a tendency to spontaneous maturation and regression which is critically important in deciding appropriate treatment. It is vital that diagnosis is made as early as possible in tumours such as sacrococcygeal teratoma, congenital mesoblastic nephroma, and neuroblastoma, which appear to develop a malignant potential early in infancy. Many of these tumours can, if diagnosed early, be treated with surgery alone. Childhood malignancies have a different natural history to adult tumours, and a period of two years following treatment with no evidence of disease is probably equivalent to cure in many cases. This means that the whole life-span is effectively at risk for late effects of treatment, compared to the relatively short period usually involved for adults. Complications of concern are the anatomical defects following amputation or major surgery, and long-term radiation and chemotherapy effects on developing tissues. There is approximately a 12% cumulative probability of a radiation-induced second neoplasm in the first twenty years of survival (Li *et al.*, 1975) and the risk is possibly increased by concurrent chemotherapy. The genetic sequelae for those who survive to adult life, and the prospects of their bearing normal children or children predisposed to neoplasia, are being studied.

The psychological effects of a serious illness and unpleasant treatment in childhood makes sensitive management of the child and his family essential; this will vary a great deal with the child's age, and should match his understanding and concerns about his illness. In infancy the relationship is predominantly through the parents. Young children must be protected from unnecessary hospitalization and separation from their parents, and every effort must be made to minimize these factors, something which is difficult to achieve outside a paediatric setting. Children commonly interpret unpleasant treatment as a punishment for some supposed misdeed; awareness of their psychological insight and fantasies, by those caring for them, is needed to help them to cope with their illness. Rehabilitation towards as normal a life as possible and strong emotional support should commence on the first day of contact. It is most important that the maximum continuity of care is achieved so that they learn to relate to specific individuals and are not overwhelmed by too many strangers, although it is inevitable that many people will be involved in their care. The child's concepts of death undergo continual evolution and this also needs to be understood if they are to be helped to cope with their fears. Adolescents are a particularly difficult group to manage, because of the paramount importance of their growing independence, which is so threatened by a serious illness. Their reaction to any form of mutilation can be extreme, because of the vital importance of the body image at this stage. The almost universal alopecia from chemotherapy has a far more dramatic impact at this age than it does on younger children. As they mature, concerns about sterilization and potency can become a major issue. Because of the great differences in management with age, it is desirable if possible, to have separate facilities for both adolescents and infants. It is particularly important where facilities such as radiotherapy are shared with adults to provide a separate waiting area or playroom for the children. In our experience adult cancer patients are more upset by seeing children undergoing treatment than *vice versa*.

Incidence

The annual incidence of childhood malignancy recorded in the Manchester Children's Tumour Registry is 100 cases per million children, while that recorded in the third National Cancer Survey in the United States from 1969 to 1971 was 125 cases per million children. Despite its low incidence, malignancy is the leading disease causing death in the age group from 1–14 years, the percentage of deaths rising steadily to 15% in the ninth year and then declining in adolescence to about 6%, as other causes begin to take precedence. The death rate per 100 000 recorded in England and Wales in 1974 shows that the rate from malignancy is at its lowest in the age group 10–14 years, being 5.11 for boys and 4.24 for girls. The rate for boys is consistently higher than that for girls throughout the age range 1–19 years. The majority of tumours occur in infancy, 45% – 50% appearing before five years of age. Leukaemia represents about 30% of childhood cancer, tumours of the central nervous system about 20%, tumours of bone and soft tissue 14% and lymphomas 10%, neuroblastoma 7%, Wilms' 7% and the rarer tumours the remainder. Particular tumours are associated with different age groups; 80% of Wilms' tumours and 80% of neuroblastomas occur in children under five years, whilst about 70% of bone tumours of childhood occur in the age group 10–14 years. Soft tissue sarcomas are spread throughout childhood, but there is a slightly greater number in younger children. Leukaemia is twice as common before five years of age than between 10–14 years, whilst lymphoma shows the reverse pattern.

There are differences in the incidence of particular tumours according to geographical, racial and socioeconomic factors, and the records of cancer incidence and survival vary in reliability from country to country. Nevertheless, apart from the notable exception of Burkitt's lymphoma dominating the cancer incidence in children in Africa, the pattern of leukaemia being most common, with CNS tumours next in frequency is reflected in most national statistics.

Aetiology

The aetiology of the majority of childhood tumours remains unknown. There are however a number of factors which are known to be associated with an increased incidence of childhood malignancy, many of which act in foetal life or early infancy.

Among the environmental causes the best known example is ionizing radiation as demonstrated following the nuclear explosion at Hiroshima. This indicated that relatively low-dose exposure carried a significant risk, and this has been confirmed by studies of children exposed *in utero*, unintentionally, to therapeutic radiation, indicating that there is no safe threshold dose below which there is no carcinogenic effect. The fact that carcinogens can cross the placenta has been demonstrated by the occurrence of a very rare tumour, clear cell adenocarcinoma of the vagina in young women whose mothers were treated with high doses of oestrogens in early pregnancy.

The fascinating association of some tumours of infancy with specific malformations suggests a close link between teratogenesis and oncogenesis which is not well understood (Bolande, 1976). Thus Wilms' tumour is known to be associated with growth abnormalities such as hemihypertrophy, or the full Beckwith-Wiedemann syndrome, as well as being associated with aniridia and genitourinary tract abnormalities. Beckwith's syndrome is also associated with carcinoma of the adrenal cortex and with hepatoblastoma. Common viral infections in pregnancy, such as influenza, have been suggested as possible causative agents of tumours as well as congenital abnormalities. The strongest link so far established between a viral infection and neoplasm is the association between EB virus and Burkitt's lymphoma, which constitutes about half the malignancies occurring in African children from some regions. It occurs primarily in areas with an annual rainfall that exceeds 20 inches and where the mean temperature of the coolest month remains above 60°, locations in which *Anopheles* and *Mansonia* mosquitoes are endemic. The well-nigh universal combined infection with malaria and EB virus in young children living in these areas is almost certainly causally related to the occurrence of Burkitt's lymphoma. The evidence linking Burkitt's lymphoma and EB virus is probably as convincing as it is possible to achieve in a human setting, where experimental infection cannot be considered, and it is perhaps the one example of a childhood tumour where immunization against a putative causal agent is worth considering for the population known to be at high risk.

There are several tumours which are known to have a hereditary basis, although they form only a small proportion of the whole. Genetic associations should nevertheless always be looked for. The thorough documentation of the familial incidence of retinoblastoma is due to successful treatment that has allowed many survivors to reach the age of procreation. There are now many survivors of Wilms' tumour and it is becoming clear that their children may be predisposed to develop the same tumour; as cure rates of tumours increase we may well find that this is a general phenomenon; certainly, isolated reports of similar tumours in siblings, twins, cousins and parent and child, suggest that this is the case. Other well known genetically determined cancers include familial polyposis of the colon and intestinal polyposis (Gardner's syndrome). It is most important to recognize these genetically determined tumours so that adequate genetic counselling concerning the risks to future children can be given.

Survival rates

The American 'End Results Programme' has demonstrated that the 3- and 5-year survival figures for the quinquennia 1955–59, 1960–64 and 1965–69 show a steady improvement, the 3-year survival rising from 32% to 41% (Myers *et al.*, 1975). These figures provide a good index of the likely long-term survival rate, though there may be occasional late relapses. It is premature to extrapolate too much from these data, but it can be said that there has been no improvement since 1969 in the treatment for neuroblastoma and myeloid leukaemia, whereas there has been considerable improvement in the treatment of rhabdomyosarcoma, osteosarcoma and acute lymphoblastic leukaemia. The most effective way to improve survival rates is to ensure that all children receive optimum treatment. Improvements are due to a number of factors such as better staging, better histological classification, effective combined modality treatment and improved supportive care. There is a substantial difference in all of these factors at specialist centres, where there are multidisciplinary teams expert in the treatment of childhood cancer, compared with what can be offered in general hospitals that only rarely see such children. The services required to enable optimum treatment to be given for such a rare disease can only be provided on a regional basis, each region serving a population of two to three million people. The specialist services should be centralized in one hospital complex. Arrangements for maintenance chemotherapy will depend on whether the population is derived from a rural or urban environment. In regions where the population is widely dispersed, diagnostic investigations, staging, and initial surgery, radiation and chemotherapy should take place in the regional centre, but maintenance chemotherapy and follow-up may well be carried out by regional paediatricians who maintain telephone contact with the centre and do joint clinics with one of the central team at intervals. Prompt help must be available for general practitioners to enable them to deal with problems arising in the course of the disease. Centres undertaking this form of treatment should make available facilities for parents to obtain advice at any time.

Paediatric radiotherapy

The aim of radiotherapy is to eradicate tumour within the treated region; a dose and volume capable of achieving this must be used. The dose needed to treat tumours in children does not differ markedly from that needed to ablate adult tumours; however, the developing tissues of children are more susceptible to radiation damage, its severity being related to the amount of radiation given and inversely related to age at the time of treatment.

Some authorities give half of the normal radical dose to children under the age of 18 months and two-thirds between 18 months and three years. It is doubtful if these lower doses are effective if anything other than minimal tumour is present. It may be possible to reduce both field and dose by surgical removal of tumour bulk and by adding chemotherapy. Concurrent chemotherapy with radiation ensures that the systemic micrometastases present outside of the radiation field in most tumours of childhood are not allowed time to progress during the weeks of often protracted local treatment. Caution is necessary when cytotoxic drugs are given concurrently with radiotherapy as radiation effects may be enhanced, particularly by actinomycin D and doxorubicin. Tumour cell kill is greater if chemotherapy and radiation are used concurrently, but the effect on normal tissues is also greater with increased morbidity. Although numerically less rads may be needed to achieve local tumour ablation, the biological effect of combined therapy on malignant and normal tissues is probably as damaging locally as radiation in the higher dose given alone. In practice, it has been found satisfactory to start chemotherapy a few days before radiation and to restrict, where possible, the use of actinomycin D and doxorubicin during radiotherapy. The use of split courses of radiotherapy enables systemic chemotherapy to be continued in the interval.

Many cytotoxic agents may give rise to recall radiation reactions after radiation. These effects can be prevented or alleviated by the concomitant use of steroids.

Immobilization

This is essential if treatment is to be delivered accurately. Every effort is made to treat the child in a comfortable position. If care has been taken to gain the child's confidence, simple sandbags to give support is often all that is needed. Plaster of Paris or plastic moulds, made to measure for each child help to immobilize and aid accuracy of beam direction. Most children over three years of age need no sedation; many under this age can also be persuaded to accept restraint with firm elastic bandages placed across the limbs or trunk, fixing the child to a suitably shaped padded board, which can be accurately located on the treatment bed. Short-lasting anaesthesia with ketamine hydrochloride has proved of great value when daily sedation is required. Rapid recovery from each dose permits the maintenance of normal nutrition in spite of prolonged courses of treatment.

Sequelae of radiation therapy

The long-term effects of treatment of children with cancer have become a major source of concern in recent years. That there are sufficient numbers of children surviving in whom to evaluate these effects reflects the success of treatment.

Effects on normal growth and development, and on the function of vital organs such as the brain, heart, lungs, liver and kidneys, must be considered. The increased risks of a second induced neoplasm in the patient and the possibility of a greater incidence of tumours or abnormalities in his offspring must also be borne in mind.

Megavoltage radiation should almost always be used, to take advantage of the sharp definition of the beam, good depth-doses and skin-sparing effects. Orthovoltage radiation should be avoided, in particular where bony structures will be included in the field. Electrons of low energy are useful for treating superficial lesions, their sharp cut-off at the end of their range minimizing irradiation of deeper structures. Absorbing blocks of lead or other suitable material can be placed in the path of radiation beams to tailor the fields to the required shape, and to protect vulnerable sites such as epiphyses or the eye.

When referring to doses of radiation tolerated by specific tissues and organs and therapy doses given, it is assumed that supervoltage radiation is used, giving 1000 rad per week in 5 fractions, unless otherwise stated, the doses quoted being modal doses. This convention is used throughout the chapter. The doses are those used to treat children over three years of age; a reduction of 50% is used in infants, and intermediate doses between 18 months and three years.

Failure of normal growth may occur resulting in generalized stunting or impairment of growth within an irradiated region.

Generalized stunting

This may be the result of radiation to the pituitary and hypothalamus, to the gonads or to the thyroid. Generalized stunting consequent on cranial irradiation has been reported following treatment of gliomas and CNS prophylaxis in acute lymphatic leukaemia. Doses as low as 2400 rad have been found to impair secretion of growth hormone in a small number of children.

Small doses of radiation in the region of 500 rad to the gonads may result in sub-fertility, but higher doses lead to impaired sexual development and failure of the pubertal growth spurt.

The thyroid in the child is especially sensitive to radiation and some degree of thyroid dysfunction occurs in a high proportion of children who have received 'mantle' irradiation for Hodgkin's disease.

Localized stunting

The damaging effects of radiation on the growing skeleton have been recognized for many years. Arrest or slowing of growth follows epiphyseal irradiation, resulting in shortened limbs and abnormal spinal curvature. Spinal deformity can be minimized by ensuring that whole vertebrae are irradiated and that the dose from side-to-side and front-to-back is equal, so that growth impairment is symmetrical.

Severe radiation damage to soft tissues results in scarring and fibrosis but relatively low doses (in the order of 3000 rad) may lead to diminished muscle bulk and lack of subcutaneous fat. Adults who were treated as children for Hodgkin's disease, with a 'mantle' field, often have noticeably thin necks.

Irradiation of the breast buds results in failure of normal breast development, which unlike that caused by ovarian hypofunction, does not respond to hormone stimulation.

Effects on function

Changes in the gonads caused by irradiation are directly related to the dose received. Girls approaching menarche seem to be particularly susceptible to ovarian damage, and delayed menarche, early menopause, failure of menstruation and infertility, together with impaired growth and breast development, may follow ovarian irradiation.

Testicular radiation even in doses as low as 300 rad results in oligospermia or aspermia in adult life, and higher doses in childhood give rise to failure of pubertal maturation and impairment of the growth spurt, and later sterility.

When it is necessary to include the lungs, liver or kidneys in a radiation field, a dose of 1800 rad, 2400 rad or 1500 rad respectively should not be exceeded if the whole organ is treated, and this may need reduction if concurrent chemotherapy is given. Higher doses may be given if only part of the organ is treated, accepting the loss of function in that part in later life.

Irradiation of the whole of both lungs to 1800 rad may result in some impairment of growth of the thorax and lungs, but lung function, although measurably diminished is not usually clinically significantly impaired.

Acute gastrointestinal damage may be limited to mild vomiting and diarrhoea, but more severe degrees may lead to mucosal ulceration, malabsorption and malnutrition. Later, the small gut may develop varying degrees of villous atrophy, accompanied by malabsorption. Local damage occasionally leads to ulceration, stricture formation or perforation. Whole abdominal radiation should not exceed 3000 rad, though localized areas of gut will tolerate 4500 rad. The tolerance of up to one quarter brain irradiation is 6000 rad, but the spinal cord and brain stem have a lower level of tolerance. If long segments of spinal cord are treated the dose should not exceed 4000 rad.

Recent work on intellectual and psychological changes in children who had received CNS prophylaxis for acute lymphoblastic leukemia (ALL) with 2400 rad plus intrathecal methotrexate has shown subtle defects in memory and increased distractability, though major defects are rare.

The eye is vulnerable to radiation and doses of 600 rad lead to cataract formation. If it is not possible to shield the eye adequately, the risk of a cataract formation is accepted and plans are made to remove it surgically, if necessary.

Following the high doses of radiation needed to treat orbital tumours such as a rhabdomyosarcoma, epilation of the lids and atrophy of the lacrimal glands occur, and the resulting dry eye is prone to repeated infections, conjunctivitis and corneal ulceration. The orbit will fail to grow normally due to the effects on bone and soft tissues and there is likelihood of cataract formation.

Constant care from an ophthalmologist is necessary if the damage is to be minimized, and useful vision retained. Prompt enucleation of a useless eye if it becomes painful, or if the remaining eye is threatened by sympathetic ophthalmia, is essential.

Sequelae of radiation plus chemotherapy

The long-term effects of cytotoxic therapy are as yet even less well catalogued. Many agents used concurrently with radiation increase the severity of radiation sequelae.

Neurotoxicity may result from the use of some cytotoxics, for example, cranial irradiation combined with intravenous methotrexate in doses above 50 mg/m² carries a moderate risk of leucoencephalopathy, and peripheral neuropathy may result from the aggressive use of vincristine. Long-term damage to kidneys and bone has been reported following the use of prolonged methotrexate, and doxorubicin may give rise to cumulative cardiotoxicity.

A high proportion of boys treated with cyclophosphamide are sterile when adult, whereas fertility may be reduced in girls, but sterility is less common.

Both radiation and chemotherapy predispose to the development of a second neoplasm. The risk may be greater when the two modalities are used together than when either is used alone. Many of the second neoplasms reported in children treated for malignancy are not related to the treatment itself but are due to a genetic predisposition to cancer in certain individuals. A number of syndromes which include such a predisposition are well known, while others await recognition.

Leukaemia: acute lymphoblastic leukaemia

Acute lymphoblastic leukaemia (ALL) accounts for more than three quarters of all cases of leukaemia in childhood, and it will therefore be described in this section. Acute myeloblastic leukaemia also occurs but has been fully covered elsewhere (see Chapter 33); children have a better prognosis than adults but in other respects it is the same disease. Chronic myeloid leukaemia also occurs in childhood but is rare. There are two types, the adult type being indistinguishable from the form seen in adults, with the characteristic Philadelphia chromosome. The juvenile type is often associated with a raised haemoglobin F level, and variable clinical features.

Although the incidence of ALL varies from country to country there is no evidence that it has changed during the time that accurate statistical records have been kept. The peak age is at four years with 40% of cases occurring in the 3–5 year group, and is more common in males. Apparent racial differences in incidence are probably related to socioeconomic factors and depend on the sophistication of the medical facilities available for diagnosis and patterns of referral rather than any intrinsic change in disease pattern.

Clustering of leukaemia has been recorded on numerous occasions, but there is no evidence that the incidence of clustering is more than would be expected by chance. Reliance on mortality data can no longer give an accurate picture of the disease as there is a widening difference between incidence and mortality as treatment improves.

There are some defined circumstances in which there is a statistically increased risk of leukaemia (see Table 37.1).

Numerous attempts have been made to subdivide ALL according to cytological differences, such as cell size, nuclear/cytoplasmic ratio, number of nucleoli and cytochemical reactions. A French/American/British (FAB) classification into three types of ALL has recently been proposed (Bennett *et al.*, 1976). Although many cytological features seem to be of some prognostic significance in particular series, none

Table 37.1   Risk of leukaemia (from Miller, 1967).

Group	Approximate risk
Identical twin with leukaemia	1 in 5
Radiation-treated polycythaemia vera	1 in 6
Bloom's syndrome	1 in 8
Hiroshima survivors	1 in 60
Down's syndrome	1 in 95
Radiation-treated ankylosing spondylitis	1 in 270
Sibling with leukaemia	1 in 720
Children under 15	1 in 3000

have been outstanding. The most important prognostic variables are age at diagnosis and initial white count. Prognosis is best for those cases diagnosed between the ages of 2 and 8 years and with an initial white count below 20 000/mm³

Recently it has proved possible to define a most important sub-group of cases of ALL namely those with T-cell leukaemia, which are identified primarily by the existence of cell surface markers which indicate their T-cell lineage. This disease occurs primarily in older boys who present with a mediastinal mass and a high initial blast count. It represents the disseminated stage of T-cell lymphoma (see below) and has a much worse prognosis than ALL of the common type (Chessells *et al.*, 1977).

Clinical features

The presentation and symptomatology of ALL are mainly due to diffuse infiltration of the reticuloendothelial system with immature blasts. The most prominent features are of bone marrow failure, i.e. anaemia, infection and bleeding. Patients frequently present with pallor, fever, purpura and ecchymoses, sometimes accompanied by external bleeding from mucous membranes such as epistaxis or haematemesis and melaena. There may in addition be a degree of generalized lymphadenopathy and hepatosplenomegaly. Non-specific symptoms include anorexia and fatigue, and not infrequently bone and joint pain which may be mistaken for rheumatoid arthritis or osteomyelitis. Half the patients present with a total peripheral white count of less than 10 000/mm³ and a quarter with a platelet count of above 100 000/mm³. A bone marrow aspirate is required for diagnosis, which should not be attempted on peripheral blood findings alone, since a number of viral infections may result in the accumulation of bizarre juvenile white cells in the blood. Although bleeding is usually related to thrombocytopaenia, disseminated intravascular coagulation with abnor-

malities of clotting is not rare in ALL though much less common than in acute promyelocytic leukaemia. Patients may present with evidence of extramedullary disease the most significant of which is meningeal infiltration.

Treatment

The first phase of treatment is to induce a remission of the disease and restore the ill child to good health. This involves reducing the leukaemic cell population from 10^{12} cells at diagnosis to around 10^9 cells, i.e. a three-log kill. At this stage there will be less than 5% of leukaemic blasts in the bone marrow which will have repopulated with normal cells, so reducing the hazards of anaemia, infection and bleeding. Remission induction requires supportive treatment to protect the patient until the disease is controlled; thus slow transfusion with blood until the haemoglobin level is above 10 g% is required with platelet transfusions to control bleeding manifestations, and treatment with intravenous antibiotics, in combination, for infection, since without adequate circulating granulocytes all infections should be presumed to be systemic. Supportive treatment includes care to maintain biochemical balance. Uric acid is frequently raised at diagnosis and rises to much higher levels as specific treatment begins to take effect, so that urate nephropathy is not a rare complication unless preventive measures are taken. We recommend the routine use of allopurinol 300 mg/m²/day in the first few days of treatment, together with a liberal fluid intake and alkalinization of the urine with sodium bicarbonate 3 g/m²/day.

The combination of prednisolone 40 mg/m²/day by mouth and vincristine 1.5 mg/m²/week i.v. results in induction of remission in 90% of patients. The addition of a third drug such as asparaginase or doxorubicin during the induction period may be of benefit in maintaining remission though it will not do much to improve the remission rate.

Complications of induction treatment include hypertension and glycosuria from the prednisolone and alopecia, constipation and neuropathy from the vincristine. Hypersensitivity reactions to asparaginase are nearly always due to a repeat course of therapy, and cardiotoxicity from doxorubicin is a cumulative phenomenon, so they are rarely problems in induction treatment.

CNS Treatment

The blood-brain barrier provides a sanctuary for leukaemic cells in the meninges. Without further treatment, the initial site of relapse will be in the meninges in over half of patients given otherwise effective systemic chemotherapy. The frequency of CNS relapse can be reduced to less than 10% by treatment for occult meningeal leukaemia early in remission. The standard method of treatment used in most centres is cranial radiation with simultaneous intrathecal methotrexate. The cranial radiation is usually given with megavoltage equipment to a dose of 1800 rad in 2 weeks; it is important to treat the whole brain and cranial meninges including the retro-orbital extensions. This is achieved with two lateral opposed fields to cover the cranium, the inferior borders extending from the infra-orbital ridges through the second cervical vertebra. Small lead blocks are placed in the radiation beams to shield the eyes. Intrathecal methotrexate is given at a dose of 10 mg/m² weekly for 5 weeks.

The incidence of CNS leukaemia has been reduced to a similar level in a programme which uses intrathecal methotrexate periodically throughout a three year course of chemotherapy with an intensive multidrug schedule, but without radiation (Haghbin, 1976). The use of higher doses of methotrexate given systemically in order to penetrate the meninges in therapeutic concentrations may make radiation unnecessary. This type of treatment with higher doses of methotrexate cannot be given safely after cranial radiation has interfered with the blood-brain barrier, because of the danger of encephalopathy.

Continuation treatment

Patients who enter remission after one month of prednisolone and vincristine may still have up to 10⁹ leukaemic cells scattered throughout the body, although these cannot be detected by present techniques. If left untreated they will relapse within a few weeks or months. The goal of treatment for childhood ALL is cure, and a period of continuation chemotherapy is therefore required. If given for less than two years, the rate of subsequent relapse tends to increase, whereas after three years the incidence of serious infections with attendant morbidity and mortality becomes the larger problem, so most people favour a period of continuation treatment of about 2.5 years. A large number of different combinations and schedules have been tried but currently the most effective regimen is with oral mercaptopurine at a dose of 75 mg/m²/ day and oral methotrexate at a dose of 20 mg/m²/week, the doses being adjusted to maintain a total white count between 2500 and 3500/mm³ with at least 500 granulocytes and 500 lymphocytes/mm³. There is at present no good evidence that patients in poor prognostic categories such as older age or high white count at diagnosis fare better if given more intensive treatment or a larger number of agents, although there are many trials currently in progress and this situation may change in the future.

After completion of 2.5 years chemotherapy, patients stop all treatment but continue to be watched closely in the clinic. The risk of relapse in the first year off treatment is approximately 10% for girls and 20% for boys, but thereafter the incidence is very low. Patients who relapse off treatment will usually attain a good second remission for a period of several months, whereas the prognosis for patients who relapse while on effective treatment is poor.

With modern treatment it appears that the prognosis for boys may be worse than that for girls. One cause is undoubtedly that T-cell leukaemia, which is commoner in boys and has a much worse prognosis, has in the past usually been categorized as ALL. A further factor may be the incidence of relapse in the testis which may be a sanctuary site like the meninges. It seems more likely however that testicular relapse represents an initial manifestation of systemic disease that is no longer under control. Patients who develop testicular disease should have bilateral radiation to the testes and spermatic cord to the subcutaneous inguinal ring to at least 1200 rad in 8 days, together with aggressive systemic combination chemotherapy.

Complications of treatment

Now that effective treatment with platelet transfusions and correction of clotting disorders has reduced the mortality from bleeding, early deaths, before the disease is controlled, are primarily due to overwhelming sepsis. Deaths during remission are usually related to immunosuppression, the most serious problems being disseminated varicella and *Pneumocystis carinii* pneumonia. Children must not receive live virus vaccines during treatment, and any inadvertent exposure to varicella or zoster should be treated within 72 hours by an infusion of zoster immunoglobulin. *Pneumocystis* pneumonia usually responds readily to high-dose intravenous trimethoprim and sulphamethoxazole, and, if this fails, to pentamidine. The doses required are trimethoprim 20 mg/kg and sulphamethoxazole 100 mg/kg/day, divided into 6-hourly schedule, while the dose of pentamidine is 4 mg/kg/day, intramuscularly, for 14 days.

Concern has recently been expressed about the possible long-term complications of 'prophylactic' CNS treatment with radiation and intrathecal drugs, particularly in terms of intellectual performance and hypothalamic/pituitary endocrine function. The evidence to date is conflicting and it is not yet clear what agents or combinations cause damage or how often it occurs.

Results

About 50% of children with ALL receiving modern treatment can be expected to survive five years free of disease (Mauer and Simone, 1976). As already pointed out, there are a number of known adverse factors that worsen this prognosis, including, age less than 2 or more than 8 years, high initial white count and T-cell disease. Boys do not do as well as girls, and frequently have other high risk factors in addition to their sex with which to contend. The converse is that patients with no poor prognostic features can be expected to do substantially better than the 50% overall survival quoted above.

Future trends

The treatment for good risk ALL is now sufficiently established that most attention is being paid to late effects, with attempts to further simplify treatment without reducing its effectiveness. As we learn more about poor prognostic features, efforts are concentrated on developing better treatment for groups at high risk, e.g. those with T-cell leukaemia. New modes of treatment such as immunotherapy have been tried without any convincing success to date. Bone marrow transplantation is still an experimental procedure and at present offers little to more than a very small proportion of patients with ALL. It may offer a real alternative to patients with poor risk disease on conventional treatment if present problems are overcome and it becomes feasible to transplant other than fully compatible siblings.

Hodgkin's disease

Hodgkin's disease in children resembles that seen in young adults, except that the prognosis appears to be better in the younger age group. This section will, therefore, be restricted to pointing out differences from the full description of the disease given elsewhere (Chapter 35).

Ten per cent of childhood malignancies are lymphomas, of which half are Hodgkin's disease. It is rarely seen below the age of five years, but 50% of the cases in childhood are less than 10 years old. There is a majority of males in the young group with a steadily increasing proportion of girls as age increases. Histologically there is a preponderance of good prognostic categories, i.e. lymphocyte predominant and nodular sclerosis. One third are of mixed cellularity but lymphocyte depletion is rare.

Clinically the usual presentation is with painless adenopathy, principally in the cervical region, and in half of these cases there is involvement of the medias-

tinum. Liver and/or spleen are enlarged in about a third of cases, usually indicating advanced disease, but extranodal primary sites are rare in childhood. Clinical symptoms and signs and investigations are otherwise similar to those in adults. Staging procedures are likewise the same, although this needs to be kept constantly under review. Young children have an increased risk of overwhelming, frequently fatal sepsis after splenectomy, particularly in a disease which is characterized by immunosuppression, that is often augmented by radiation and chemotherapy. Staging laparotomy and splenectomy can only be justified where the results might affect treatment. They should not be considered for patients who have definite evidence of disseminated disease, and their use should be seriously questioned in treatment programmes which involve wide field radiation and chemotherapy whatever the pathological stage. The finding of microscopic disease in individual organs will make no difference to the prognosis if they are going to be encompassed by treatment in any case, so the hazards to the patient have to be weighed against the value of accurate staging, in retrospective evaluation of the effects of different treatment regimens on different stages of the disease. The differential diagnosis in children is predominantly from causes of infectious adenitis (e.g. infectious mononucleosis, tuberculosis, catscratch disease, toxoplasmosis), and other neoplasms.

Treatment

The principles of treatment are the same as in adults except that greater consideration must be given to the late effects of treatment, particularly to those of radiation on growth and development, and the long-term risks of secondary neoplasia in the substantial majority of patients who will be cured of their disease. Patients with (pathological) Stage I disease in favourable sites and with favourable histology, e.g. high cervical, should probably be treated by involved node region (involved field) radiation alone.

Stage II disease that involves the mediastinum can be treated by a mantle field plus coverage of the para-aortic nodes (anchor field). All other Stage I and II patients and those with more disseminated disease should probably be treated by a combination of radiation and chemotherapy. In young children it is worthwhile considering attempting to delay radiation until further growth has occurred; in this situation it is reasonable to consider chemotherapy first in the hope of at least delaying the need for high-dose radiation. The complications of radiation are dose-dependent, and a dose of 3000 rad alone will provide local control in 80% of cases of Hodgkin's disease (Kaplan, 1966). When used together with chemotherapy it is reasonable to consider such a lower dose, with boosts of 500–1500 rad to areas of bulk disease. Chemotherapy has tended to be with the same combinations as are used in adult Hodgkin's disease. The alarming incidence of leukaemia as a second malignancy in patients treated with radiation and MOPP chemotherapy (Cadman *et al.*, 1977) suggests that alternative combinations should be urgently explored, so that highly carcinogenic agents such as procarbazine need not be given to young patients.

Results

The 5-year actuarial survival for all 79 previously untreated paediatric patients seen at Stanford from 1962–1972 was 89%, and no relapses were seen following the combination of radiation and MOPP chemotherapy. Twenty-seven children with previously untreated Hodgkin's disease treated in Toronto from 1972 to 1976 with three cycles of MOPP followed by low dose extended field radiation followed by three further cycles of MOPP resulted in 91% actuarial 3- and 5-year survival and relapse-free survival rates, 25 of the 27 children remaining free of disease from 15 to 64+ months (Jenkin *et al.*, 1979). Paediatric Hodgkin's disease should thus be regarded as a curable disease in almost all patients, who are therefore entitled to the careful and meticulous planning of the finest details of treatment which can only be offered in centres experienced in treating children with this disease.

Non-Hodgkin's lymphoma

In sharp contrast to Hodgkin's disease, childhood non-Hodgkin's lymphoma (NHL) is a distinctly different group of disorders to those seen in adults, although there is some overlap. A major difference is that in childhood it is a disseminated disease at diagnosis in the great majority of cases, with a marked propensity to spread to bone marrow and central nervous system. Although the Rappaport classification is often used, its relevance is strictly limited since there are only three well-defined pathological types of NHL in childhood, and 97% are of the diffuse variety. The types seen are diffuse undifferentiated (DUL; Burkitt's or non-Burkitt's), diffuse lymphocytic poorly differentiated (DLPD; convoluted or T-cell) and diffuse histiocytic (DHL). Leukaemic transformation is almost universal in the DLPD variety, whereas it only occurs in 10% of those with DH histology.

DUL

Burkitt's lymphoma occurring in African children is well known because of its association with the Epstein-Barr virus, and because it accounts for more than half the neoplasms in children in certain geographic areas. Space precludes a detailed description of this tumour which is rarely seen outside Africa. It occurs much more commonly in boys, with a peak age incidence of 5–9 years. It presents most frequently (50%) in the jaw, commencing in the marrow and causing loosening of the teeth. The maxilla is involved three times more frequently than the mandible, usually with intraoral tumour rather than exophthalmos. One third have an abdominal presentation, with massive symmetrical ovarian tumours or ill-defined retroperitoneal masses, often with renal involvement. Paraplegia from spinal extradural lesions is not uncommon.

The disorder (with a similar histology) seen in Europe and America has some common features with the African type, but differs in many respects, one of the most significant perhaps being the frequent presence of systemic symptoms such as fever, chills, anorexia and weight loss which are rarely seen in the African variety. African Burkitt's lymphoma tends to show limited invasion, with regional lymph nodes frequently not involved; leukaemic transformation which occurs in less than 10% is always associated with diffuse liver involvement, in contrast to the 50%–60% frequency in the non-African form; 60% of African Burkitt's lymphoma patients undergoing treatment will develop CNS disease, but only 25% of the non-African type.

DUL shows a high proliferation rate and concomitant high cell death rate. The disease may be multifocal and it is very uncommon to find localized or regional disease. Studies of G6-PD and Ig phenotypes show the disorder to be monoclonal at presentation (Fialkow *et al.*, 1973), though late relapse may be discordant, suggesting the development of new clones.

Effective treatment is not yet established. The only surgery indicated is a biopsy to make the diagnosis. Radiotherapy is of dubious value, though fractionated techniques which take into account the high proliferation rate might prove effective. The drugs more demonstrably effective are high-dose cyclophosphamide and methotrexate. The multiagent combination chemotherapy regimen LSA-L2, otherwise very effective for childhood NHL, is not of great value for this disorder. The combination of cyclophosphamide, vincristine and methotrexate (COM) with radiation reported from the NCI is perhaps the most effective regimen so far described (Ziegler, 1977). Long-term follow-up of the Ugandan patients indicates that Burkitt's lymphoma is probably curable in at least 50% of patients (Ziegler *et al.*, 1979).

DLPD

This disease is typified by presentation with a mediastinal mass in adolescent boys, by rapid evolution to leukaemic transformation, by a high complete response rate to either steroids or local radiotherapy but a median survival of only eight months. Clinical presentation in those with a mediastinal primary is with dyspnoea, cough, pleuritic and sub-sternal pain and generalized features such as fatigue, anorexia, weight loss and fever. Obstruction of the superior vena cava is frequent. Leukaemic transformation is almost universal, and half of those who develop bone marrow disease will also develop disease in the central nervous system. The diagnosis can be made by demonstrating T-cell surface markers on a needle aspirate, on pleural fluid, on bone marrow or CSF blasts. Peripheral blood findings are usually normal unless the disease has already undergone leukaemic transformation and presents as a T-cell leukaemia. Chest X-ray shows a mass in the anterior superior mediastinum that is often huge, may extend up into the root of the neck, and may be associated with a pleural effusion. Uric acid is frequently raised. The usual staging procedures for lymphomas are irrelevant and contra-indicated, since urgent treatment is required. This should consist of liberal hydration, alkalinization of the urine and allopurinol followed by intensive combination chemotherapy, with regimens such as the LSA-L2 protocol (Wollner *et al*., 1976*a*). CNS prophylaxis is warranted because of the known natural history of the disease, though its effectiveness is not yet demonstrated. There is at present no evidence that radiation to the primary site adds to the benefit of chemotherapy, though it increases the risk of immunosuppression and pneumocystis carinii pneumonia. Emergency low-dose radiation of a few hundred rad is however frequently life-saving for complications such as respiratory obstruction from the mediastinal mass or acute renal failure from ureteric obstruction or massive infiltration, which are not uncommon at presentation.

DHL

Relapse in bone marrow and central nervous system is less common than in DLPD disease, and occurs more frequently as a local recurrence or extension. The cure rate has substantially improved since the introduction of intensive combination chemotherapy programmes in addition to radiation.

For NHL presenting in the abdomen, a 70% cure rate can be achieved in those who have complete surgical resection of localized intestinal disease followed by whole abdominal irradiation to a dose of 3500 rad in 3–4 weeks, shielding the kidneys at 1500 rad and liver of 2500 rad. The prognosis remains poor for those with unresectable disease, though intensive combination chemotherapy may alter this situation.

Histiocytosis X

This is a disorder of protean manifestations exemplified by one of its other names, the Hand-Kay-Schüller-Christian syndrome. The classical Kay's triad consists of exophthalmos, membranous bone defects and diabetes insipidus. Histiocytosis X spans a spectrum from benign to highly malignant so that the precise incidence is difficult to assess. Its aetiology is unknown and it is still questionable whether many cases listed as having histiocytosis X truly have a neoplasm. There are a number of rare familial disorders that are very similar both clinically and histologically, and others that are clearly related to immunodeficiency syndromes, that are usually excluded from the group labelled histiocytosis X. Although there are three fairly well defined clinical syndromes, (eosinophilic granuloma, Hand-Schüller-Christian disease, Letterer-Siwe disease) it is clear that many patients merge between these entities. They all share a common histological pattern of diffuse proliferation of histiocytes with or without granuloma formation, together with accumulation of eosinophils, lymphocytes, plasma cells and large histiocytes. It may be possible to split cases into two histological types, of which one is relatively benign and one is malignant.

Solitary eosinophilic granuloma of bone shows a predilection for the skull and long bones and presents with painless swelling associated on X-ray with a lytic lesion with a well defined border, through which pathological fractures may occur. Eosinophilic granuloma of soft tissues may present in the skin, in the CNS, or in the sub-mucosa of the upper gastrointestinal and respiratory tracts. Histiocytosis not uncommonly presents in childhood with chronically draining infected ears with or without destruction of the mastoid and associated cholesteatoma, or with what is misdiagnosed as seborrhoeic dermatitis. Lesions in the vicinity of the pituitary characteristically cause polyuria and polydipsia as diabetes insipidus develops. Clinical features of patients with disseminated disease depend on the organs involved. Common findings include cervical lymphadenopathy, characteristic rash with or without purpuric manifestations, pneumonic infiltration, hepatosplenomegaly, pyrexia of unknown origin and gum infiltration. Diagnosis depends on the characteristic X-ray findings and biopsy to demonstrate the histology.

Treatment

Single eosinophilic granuloma lesions may undergo spontaneous healing, but are frequently treated by biopsy and curettage or low-dose radiation of the order of 500–1500 rad. Patients with multiple lesions may often undergo dissemination and develop visceral lesions, and are therefore usually treated with chemotherapy. Almost all the common cancer chemotherapy agents have been shown to have some effect: thus steroid hormones, vinca alkaloids, alkylating agents, anti-metabolites and antibiotics may all be effective. The drugs most commonly used are prednisone, vincristine, cyclophosphamide and methotrexate. The natural history of the disease makes treatment efficacy difficult to establish, since response to treatment may be slow, with exacerbations and development of new lesions despite a good response. In general, treatment is conservative, provided the disease does not become systemic or undergo rapid evolution. If chemotherapy is indicated it is usually continued for one year after the patient is without evidence of disease.

The most frequent complication is the development of diabetes insipidus which nowadays is relatively easy to treat with the nasal installation of DDAVP; radiation to 1500 rad in 1.5 to 2 weeks to the base of the skull in the region of the pituitary is usually given.

Prognosis

The outlook for isolated eosinophilic granuloma lesions is excellent whatever the treatment given. The outlook for multiple lesions is likewise quite good, but when visceral disease is demonstrated the prognosis must be guarded and will depend on the extent of the disease. Prognosis is known to depend on the age at diagnosis and the degree of organ involvement or organ dysfunction.

Tumours of the CNS

Tumours of the CNS are the commonest form of solid tumour in childhood and are second only to leukaemias in frequency, accounting for between 15% and 20% of the total of childhood malignancies. Over two-thirds are gliomas, most of these consisting of low grade astrocytomas and medulloblastomas. More than half of the childhood intracranial tumours occur in the posterior fossa, about one third being cerebellar astrocytomas and one third medulloblastomas. 25% arise in the cerebral hemispheres, most of these being astrocytomas and ependymomas. Ependymomas form 10% of the total, about the same proportion as brain stem gliomas. Gliomas of the optic nerve and chiasm represent a further 5%, the remainder consists of rarer lesions such as pineal tumours, teratomas, choroid plexus tumours and craniopharyngioma.

Presentation

The presenting clinical features may be produced by raised intracranial pressure due to expansion of tumour or to the obstruction of the CSF pathway, to structural displacement within the intracranial cavity and to direct focal involvement of brain and cranial nerves. A remarkable degree of adaptation and compensation may occur allowing extensive tumour growth before the disease becomes apparent. The typical story is of headaches which are worse in the morning and are often accompanied by sudden vomiting not preceded by nausea. Younger children may fail to thrive and older children may present with personality change or deteriorating performance at school with loss of motor skills, and falling intellectual capability.

Infants may develop enlargement of the head with separation of the cranial sutures resulting in a crackpot sound on percussion of the cranium. The development of a squint, or impaired vision due to papilloedema may be an early sign. Trunkal ataxia may progress to the development of generalized hypertonia, extensor rigidity, neck stiffness and opisthotonus. The focal neurological signs and cranial nerve palsies are common in brain stem gliomas, which often present with facial palsies, disturbances of vision and squint, or difficulty in speech and swallowing sometimes associated with dribbling. Convulsions occur in a minority of cases. Lesions in the vicinity of the hypothalamus may cause diabetes insipidus, growth retardation and precocious puberty.

Investigation

Skull X-ray may show signs of raised intracranial pressure such as sutural separation, erosion of the clinoid processes and occasionally a characteristic 'beaten copper' appearance. Intracranial calcification may occur in teratomas, craniopharyngiomas and some pineal tumours. Arteriography and air encephalography have largely been superseded by computerized tomography as the investigation of choice for locating site and size of intracranial tumours, but they may nevertheless prove very valuable in individual cases, particularly in brain stem lesions. Isotope scans may also be useful in selected cases.

Treatment

Surgery

Raised intracranial pressure should be relieved as quickly as possible if present. Diagnostic lumbar puncture should not be performed except in a Neurosurgical Centre where craniotomy can be immediately performed if tonsillar herniation occurs. The insertion of a shunt from a lateral ventricle to the cisterna magna, thus relieving intracranial pressure, will often allow a more safe definitive surgical procedure two or three days later. Shunting to the right atrium, peritoneal or pleural cavities, may allow seeding of tumour cells into the systemic body compartment and is not therefore recommended where it is possible to avoid this.

Total surgical removal should be attempted where possible. Unfortunately many tumours are infiltrating or are not accessible to surgical ablation and under these circumstances partial removal or simple biopsy is performed. Total surgical removal may be the only treatment required for cerebellar astrocytomas and low grade supra-tentorial ependymomas, some teratomas and choroid plexus papillomas. In the majority of tumours surgical removal is not possible and in these circumstances recurrence is inevitable, even though it may be decades before there are further symptoms in the case of low grade tumours. Where surgical removal has been incomplete radiotherapy is usually indicated. A tissue diagnosis should however be made whenever possible since the curative dose of radiotherapy varies widely from one tumour type to another and radiation tolerance of the normal growing brain is a major limiting factor in planning curative radiotherapy without unacceptable sequelae.

Radiotherapy
CNS tumours are treated with megavoltage radiation. There are three basic radiotherapy techniques for childhood CNS tumours.

1. Radiation to the entire CNS in those tumours known to disseminate through the CSF, such as posterior fossa medulloblastomas and ependymomas, and supra-tentorial high grade ependymomas, choroid plexus carcinomas and germinomas.
2. Tumours treated with wide margins of apparently normal tissue, e.g. an infiltrating glioma.
3. Tumours treated with limited volumes and small margins of normal tissue, e.g. a craniopharyngioma.

Treatment of the latter groups is similar to that of adult tumours as described in Chapter 10.

Gliomas in children over three years of age receive 5000–5500 rad in 6–7 weeks, the dosage being reduced to 4500 rad under this age. The same doses are used to the primary site for medulloblastomas and high grade ependymomas, the remaining CNS and meninges receiving 3500 rad in 5 weeks. The commonest site of recurrence in medulloblastoma remains the posterior fossa which indicates a failure to give a high enough dose to the tumour. It is recommended that the whole CNS and meninges are irradiated in the cases of germinomas, a dose of 3000–3500 rad in 4 weeks in 20 fractions being given.

Chemotherapy
A variety of drugs are known to induce temporary remissions in tumours that regrow following surgery and radiation. The use of adjuvant chemotherapy given together with radiation as primary management for CNS tumours of childhood is currently being tested in a number of large scale trials but there is as yet no unequivocal evidence of benefit.

In theory, the drugs should be lipid-soluble and of low molecular weight to enable them to traverse the blood-brain barrier, although this does not remain intact following radiation to the CNS. The agents most widely used for treatment of brain tumours in childhood include vincristine, the nitrosoureas, methotrexate (intrathecal and high-dose intravenous), VM26 (a podophylline derivative), DTIC and procarbazine. The use of these agents cannot at present be recommended outside of the context of clinical trials.

Medulloblastoma
About half of the cases present in the first five years of life and the tumour is at least twice as common in boys as in girls. The prognosis is worse in young children, probably because they cannot tolerate the doses of radiation required for cure. Many children are gravely ill at presentation and die before adequate surgery or radiation can be undertaken; because of this 5-year survival rates of less than 10% have been recorded. There is a much better outlook for those children who survive the operative period and receive a radical course of radiation. From The Royal Marsen Hospital a 5-year survival rate of 33% for children treated with surgery and radical radiotherapy has been reported (Bloom and Walsh, 1975). The cure rate has improved as radiotherapy techniques have advanced, but the impact of adjuvant chemotherapy is yet to be established.

Surgical ablation is usually impossible because of the infiltrative nature of the lesion, but a sub-total excision is thought by many authorities to be preferable to simple biopsy. The evidence for this is not definitive. The decompression of the posterior fossa afforded by the surgical removal of part of the occipital bone and the neural arches of C1 and sometimes C2 usually prevents CSF obstruction from occurring, but a shunt is sometimes required.

Radiation method
A method for immobilizing the child in an accurately reproducible position for radiotherapy is essential when treating such a large and irregular volume as the

whole CNS over a protracted period of several weeks. A mould of plaster of Paris or other suitable material is therefore constructed which can be located on the treatment couch in the same position every day and in which the child can lie prone, during treatment, in comfort. The mould is made with the child lying supine, with the hips bent at right angles to the back and the knees at right angles to the hips, thus flattening the lumbar curvature so that the spinal cord is at a more uniform distance from the radiation source, facilitating even dosage. The cervical curve is reduced by flexing the head forward as much as the child can tolerate. The mould includes the front of the head, neck, shoulders, upper arms and abdomen down to the iliac crests. The central part of the face (eyes, nose and mouth) are not included but a firm band of plaster crosses the forehead with another crossing the chin. When hardened the mould is inverted and mounted on a base whose height under the thorax and abdomen is the same as the length of the child's thighs so that the child can kneel forward in a comfortable position for treatment. Such a mould is not difficult to make and is well tolerated by children. When treated in a friendly, calm and relaxed atmosphere, it is rare for any form of sedation to be required.

Planning films for accurate location of brain, spinal cord and meninges are taken with the child in the mould in the treatment position. The brain and upper cervical cord are treated by two opposed lateral fields, the caudal ends of these being vertical. Lead shielding is used to tailor the shape of the fields to include only the CNS and meninges. The choice of a lateral field to include not just the head but the upper cervical cord as well enables the inequalities of dose in the neck caused by the cervical curvature to be minimized. A modal dose of 3500 rad is given with these large fields and the volume is then reduced to include the posterior fossa and the region of the third ventricle, pituitary and hypothalamus to which a further 1000 rad is given. An additional 1000 rad is administered in a third reduction in volume extending anteriorly only as far as the posterior clinoid processes giving a maximum dose of 5500 rad to the posterior fossa. The remainder of the spine is treated by direct posterior fields wide enough to cover the cord and meninges and extending to the lower level of S2, to 3500 rad. Two or three spinal fields are used with gaps between the fields calculated according to the geometric and physical properties of the individual machine so that the 50% isodose curves summate at the cord. Two complete plans to include the whole CNS are made with the junctions at different sites to reduce the risk of bands of overdosage occurring at the joins. The two plans are used on alternate days throughout treatment. The spinal and the cranial fields are treated concurrently (Fig. 37.1).

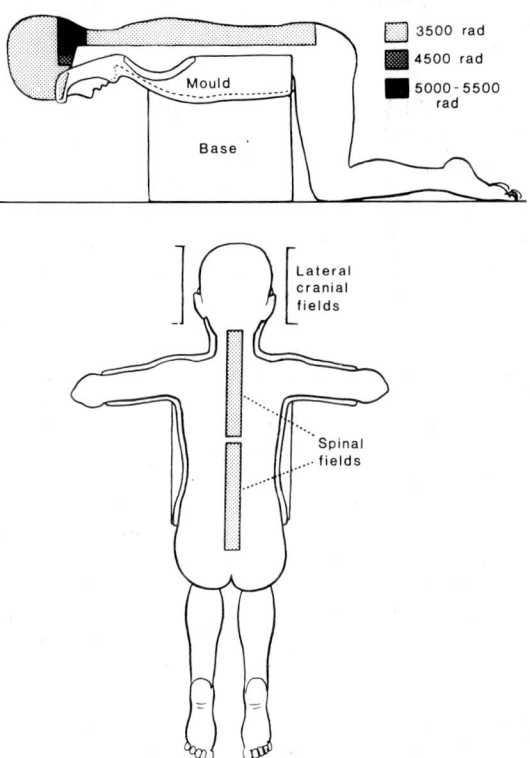

	3500 rad
	4500 rad
	5000 - 5500 rad

Fig. 37.1 Arrangement of fields in the treatment of medulloblastoma.

Prospects for the future

There are at present no obvious surgical refinements which might substantially increase the cure rate for medulloblastoma, though more uniform application of prompt and expert surgical treatment could undoubtedly reduce the number of children who die within a short period of presentation. Radiotherapy techniques are likewise unlikely to result in much further improvement, but the use of radiosensitizers, such as misonidazole, may prove beneficial. Chemotherapy offers the best chance at present.

Wilms' tumour (nephroblastoma)

Wilms' tumour has a stable incidence of one case per 200 000 children per year. It is predominantly a disease of the pre-school child with a peak in the third year, three quarters of all cases occurring in the first five years. In recent large series the sex ratio has been equal.

Aetiology

Wilms' tumour is occasionally familial and is not infrequently associated with a number of congenital abnormalities, particularly aniridia, hemihypertrophy, genitourinary abnormalities and the Beckwith-Wiedemann syndrome. This suggests that genetic factors may interact with an inducing agent that is both oncogenic and teratogenic to the foetus. It is postulated that malignant transformation is a two-step process, a pre-zygotic change accounting for one third of the cases of the hereditary form whereas the other two thirds are induced by two postzygotic changes (Knudson, 1975).

Pathology

The tumour can arise in any part of the kidney, the majority presenting as a single expanding mass surrounded by a pseudocapsule of connective tissue. On section the tumour is fleshy, often with a lobular appearance caused by fibrous septa. There are usually myxomatous areas with patchy haemorrhage and necrosis leading to cystic degeneration. Surrounding kidney tissue is destroyed by compression and invasion, which eventually involves the perinephric tissues. There may be direct extension into the renal pelvis, renal vein and hilar lymph nodes.

Histology may differ from one part of the tumour to another with varying ratios of mesenchymal to epithelial elements. Abortive or embryonic glomerulotubular structures are surrounded by an interstitium consisting of primitive mesenchymal cells, often forming recognizable striated muscle, cartilage, fat and bone.

Recent recognition of a number of histological variants has thrown much new light on the natural history of this tumour. It is important to recognize in infancy, the tumour now usually called congenital mesoblastic nephroma, since surgery alone is usually curative. The association of renal dysplasia with areas of 'nephroblastomatosis', which are often bilateral, in patients with associated malformations or the full Beckwith syndrome, is a distinct entity. At present both of these disorders should be regarded as potential precursors of true Wilms' tumour. The most important advance has been the recognition of sub-groups of Wilms' tumour that have sarcomatous or anaplastic histology. In the recently published American National Wilms' Tumour Study these accounted for 11% of the total cases, but 52% of the deaths from tumour, including seven of the 10 deaths due to tumour in patients diagnosed before 2 years of age. Conversely only 7% of the 378 patients whose tumours did not show these features died of tumour (Beckwith and Palmer, 1978). Precise histopathology must therefore be an integral part of the planning of future treatment for patients with Wilm's tumour. This highlights the necessity for all tumours to be reviewed by a paediatric pathologist with extensive experience of childhood tumours before any radiation or chemotherapy programme is instituted.

Clinical presentation

The most frequent presentation is with an asymptomatic abdominal mass. Abdominal pain from a variety of causes occurs in more than one third of patients and haematuria in more than a quarter. Less common presentations include patients investigated for associated malformations such as hemi-hypertrophy or aniridia, or with metastatic disease in the lung or hypertension. Diagnosis is confirmed by the characteristic finding of splaying and distortion of the calyces on an IVP, the dye being introduced via a foot vein so as to obtain a simultaneous inferior vena-cavagram. A chest X-ray is mandatory to rule out metastases and a skeletal survey to exclude the much more rare bony metastases. Preoperatively, a full blood count is required in case haematuria or bleeding into the tumour substance has produced a degree of anaemia that requires correction before surgery, together with estimation of electrolytes, uric acid and liver function. Urine should undergo microscopy and culture to exclude infection secondary to obstruction before surgery is undertaken. Ultrasound examination and computerized tomography are presently being evaluated. Arteriography has no place as a routine, but may be helpful in more difficult cases. Isotope liver scan may be left until the post-operative period.

Staging

The primary use of a staging system is to aid in planning rational treatment, though it is also helpful in retrospectively evaluating and comparing different treatment regimens. The staging system most commonly employed at present derives from the five groups outlined for the National Wilms' Tumour Study.

Finer details of this staging system are being re-evaluated in the light of the results of present treatment. Details are outside the scope of this limited survey (Table 37.2).

Treatment

The evolution of the present treatment of Wilms' tumour is outlined in the following table (Table 37.3). A compilation of data from the literature by Sutow *et*

Table 37.2 Staging for Wilm's tumour.

Stage I	Tumour localized to kidney and completely resected
Stage II	Tumour extending beyond the kidney but completely resected
Stage III	Residual tumour confined to abdomen, e.g. peritoneal contamination, lymphatic metastases
Stage IV	Haematogenous metastases
Stage V	Bilateral involvement

al. (1978) shows a survival rate of 18% for over 1000 patients treated by surgery alone, and of 31% for almost 2500 patients treated by surgery and radiation. Data from the National Wilms' Tumour Study indicate that over half the patients with Stage II and III disease treated with surgery and radiation remain disease-free at 2 years if given in addition either vincristine alone or actinomycin D alone, and the data for actinomycin D are substantiated by a number of other studies using either single or multiple courses of actinomycin D (D'Angio *et al.*, 1976). This contrasts with an 81% disease-free survival for patients receiving both vincristine and actinomycin D, confirmed by the Medical Research Council trial in which vincristine was given more frequently but with only a single course of actinomycin D (MRC Working Party, 1978). A review of the treatment results for the best regimens in the National Wilms' Tumour Study indicates that it is realistic to state that 90% of patients with Wilms' tumour undergoing modern treatment should be cured.

Surgery

The kidney is always approached through a transverse abdominal incision so that all the abdominal contents

Table 37.3 Nephroblastoma: treatment results.

Treatment	Survival %	Disease-free survival %
S	18	
S + DXT	31	
S + DXT + DAC – single		55
– multiple		62
S + DXT + VCR		55
S + DXT + VCR + DAC single Stages I–III	88	79
S + DXT + VCR + DAC multiple Stages II–III	86	81

S = Surgery   DXT = Radiotherapy   VCR = Vincristine
DAC = Actinomycin D.

can be carefully visualized. The renal pedicle is dissected free and the renal artery and vein ligated with minimal handling of the tumour, taking care to ensure there is not a tumour thrombus growing down the renal vein into the inferior vena cava. The ureter is then identified and tied and the kidney removed *en bloc* with any perinephric extensions of tumour. This should be followed by a dissection of the regional lymph nodes. The extent of the tumour bed is marked with clips to aid the radiotherapist, as is any residual tumour and the limits of the lymph node dissection. Any rupture or spillage of tumour must be detailed. It is important that the opposite kidney is not only visualized but is mobilized for full examination to exclude bilateral tumour.

Radiation

The purpose of post-operative abdominal radiation is the eradication of known residual tumour, and it should be commenced within two weeks of surgery. The dose required to the tumour bed probably does not need to exceed 2000 rad in two weeks, when given in conjunction with chemotherapy and this will limit the long-term morbidity, which is proportional to the dose given.

Simple opposed anterior and posterior fields to cover the tumour bed and adjacent lymph nodes are usually used, care being taken to treat the whole of any vertebra included in this volume.

Radiation of the whole abdomen is not necessary when tumour spill at the time of operation is localized, and should be reserved for those with gross peritoneal contamination (Tefft *et al.*, 1976). When whole abdominal irradiation is undertaken the remaining kidney and, in girls, the contra-lateral ovary, are shielded throughout treatment. Lead blocks are also placed over the femoral heads and acetabula.

Chemotherapy

At present all patients with Wilms' tumour should receive chemotherapy with the combination of vincristine and actinomycin D. The standard dosage schedule consisting of a 5-day course of actinomycin D, 15 μg/kg/day i.v. with vincristine 1.5 mg/m^2 i.v. on days 1 and 5, given at surgery and at 6 weeks, then every 3 months for a period of 15 months. Patients with unfavourable histology should probably receive doxorubicin and cyclophosphamide in addition.

If radiation is indicated, vincristine alone is given weekly throughout the course, and the multidrug regime recommenced two or three weeks from its end. As a result of several large multicentre trials undertaken in the last few years it is now possible to refine the treatment of Wilms' tumour to suit the individual circumstances. Thus, for patients with favourable histology, radiation in Stage I is not necessary and many not be needed in Stage II; chemotherapy should consist of vincristine and actinomycin D and a six-month course may be sufficient.

A more aggressive approach to the treatment of children, who present with metastatic disease, particularly in the lungs, is already giving improved results (Jenkin *et al.*, 1976). The combined approach of excision of the primary with adjuvant chemotherapy and post-operative abdominal irradiation, and whole lung irradiation to 1500 rad in 10 fractions over two weeks, can lead to dramatic regression of disease. Lung metastases which fail to disappear on follow-up whole lung tomography or CT-scan should receive a further booster dose of 500 to 1000 rad in a week to ten days, to very localized fields. Chemotherapy is then continued for at least one year.

Complications of treatment

These are usually acute and reversible. Particular care has to be taken with young infants, whose sensitivity to chemotherapy and radiation makes standard dosages unacceptable. Common problems include almost universal alopecia; vincristine neuropathy which may present as abdominal pain and ileus in the post-operative period; and a syndrome of hepatitis, severe thrombocytopenia and oedema appearing when patients recently undergoing hepatic radiation receive a course of actinomycin D at the full dosage.

Follow-up should be at least monthly for the first year, two monthly in the second year, three monthly in the third year and six monthly thereafter, each examination including a chest X ray. Follow-up IVP should be performed at six months and twelve months. Blood pressure and creatinine clearance should be periodically evaluated.

Future trends

A great deal is now known about the importance of prognostic factors such as tumour histology and weight, the presence or absence of involved regional lymph nodes, and age at diagnosis. It is possible to anticipate excellent chances of cure in good prognostic patients, such that the treatment for these patients will be substantially reduced in the next few years, so reducing the long-term morbidity. For those patients in whom it has come to be recognized that there is a relatively poor prognosis, it should prove possible to devise better treatment combinations to meet their particular needs.

Neuroblastoma

While there have been dramatic advances in the treatment of many childhood tumours in the last decade, this is not true for neuroblastoma. The prognosis for patients with localized disease remains excellent, but two-thirds have disseminated disease at diagnosis and their prognosis remains poor. The annual incidence is approximately eight cases per million children with a slight preponderance of males. It is mainly a disease of pre-school children, 50% of cases occurring before 2 years and 75% before 5 years of age. The incidence of neuroblastoma *in situ*, in autopsies of infants dying from other causes, is as high as 1 in 40, which indicates the frequency with which spontaneous regression occurs. The ability to undergo spontaneous regression is a well documented feature, though how much is due to maturation and how much to immune factors is unknown. Histologically there is a spectrum of maturation from benign ganglion-neuroma through ganglion-neuroblastoma to frank neuroblastoma, and this clearly affects prognosis.

Seasonal and annual variations in incidence have suggested that there may possibly be some environmental agent concerned in aetiology. Unlike Wilms' tumour there is no association with congenital malformations, except possibly skull and brain defects. There is, however, an association with neurofibromatosis and with colonic aganglionosis. Neuroblastoma has occasionally been reported in families.

Pathology

The tumour develops from neural crest tissue and can therefore occur at a primary site anywhere along the craniospinal axis. The primitive sympathogonia cell can differentiate along either a phaeochromocytoma line or a sympathoblastic line. During development, a neuroblastoma is originally firm and encapsulated but later infiltrates and becomes soft and friable with haemorrhage, necrosis, calcification and cyst formation. Histologically it is a densely cellular tumour, the cells containing small round dark nuclei and little cytoplasm. There may be some differentiation with the formation of rosettes and/or neurofibrils. In ganglion-neuroblastoma there is a predominance of undifferentiated neuroblasts with occasional scattered mature ganglion cells. Metastases may show more or less differentiation than the primary tumour. Ganglion-neuromas are firm encapsulated tumours which are benign and do not metastasize. During growth, however, they may envelop nearby structures and extend, for example, through intervertebral foramina to form a characteristic dumb-bell tumour with compression of the spinal cord. Histologically, mature ganglion cells are found scattered throughout a collagenous background laced with neurofibrils in bundles. It is important to recognize that the histological picture in any tumour may vary a great deal from one part to another. Ultrastructural studies reveal membrane bound granules 100μm in size in the cytoplasm, which are similar to the catecholamine granules seen in the adrenal medulla. There may also be larger electron dense granules 500 μm in size, which it is thought may represent storage sites for catecholamines. Attempts to grade neuroblastoma histologically and relate the findings to prognosis have not on the whole been successful.

Clinical features

These will depend on the primary site, which is in the abdomen or pelvis in 60% of patients. A common presenting sign is therefore an abdominal mass which may progress to cause urinary obstruction and infection, or expand through the sacrosciatic notch into the buttock. Thoracic neuroblastoma develops in the posterior mediastinum and will become large before causing respiratory or superior venacaval symptoms. Pain along the neuroaxis may be due to tumour pressure, infiltration of dorsal nerve roots or a dumb-bell projection compressing the spinal cord. Tumours arising in the cervical sympathetic chain may present as a neck mass. Intracranial primaries are rare.

Many patients have symptoms due to metastases, and systemic features, such as irritability, anorexia, weight loss, anaemia, fever and bone pain are common. The tumour shows a predilection for the skeleton, especially the skull, and orbital metastases with proptosis and ecchymoses are a characteristic feature. There may be lymphadenopathy particularly in cervical and supra-clavicular areas, and bluish subcutaneous nodules. Neuroblastoma is a hormonally active tumour producing catecholamines, and catecholamine-related symptoms such as flushing, tachycardia, perspiration, hypertension and headache may occur. Production of a vasoactive intestinal peptide may lead to profuse diarrhoea, hypokalaemia and failure to thrive. There is a rare but fascinating association with acute cerebellar encephalopathy.

Investigations

Due to the disseminated nature of the disease, bone marrow involvement is frequent, resulting in anaemia and thrombocytopenia. Bone marrow aspirate will show infiltration with small round cells that are frequently clumped together around neurofibrillary material to form pseudorosettes. The diagnosis is confirmed by the finding of an excessive excretion of catecholamines, particularly the major metabolites vanillylmandelic acid (VMA) and homovanillic acid (HVA) in a 24-hour urine sample in over 75% of patients. Diagnostic levels may frequently be found in a random urine specimen, and recently attempts have been made to develop screening tests for neuroblastoma e.g. a VMA test strip. Catecholamine excretion is also useful in monitoring the progress of treatment, since levels will fall to normal in 95% of survivors, whereas they will remain elevated or return to high levels in patients whose disease is progressing. Patients with neuroblastoma may also excrete cystathionine in the urine, although this may also occur with other tumours, e.g. hepatoma. Radiology is useful in the investigation of patients suspected of neuroblastoma. For the one third which arise in an adrenal, an IVP done through a foot vein to outline the vena cava will show an extrarenal mass compressing and distorting the kidney, although the intrarenal structure may sometimes also be distorted by invasion. A diffuse speckled calcification can be visualized in 50%. Thoracic lesions may be visualized as a posterior mediastinal mass accompanied by separation of the posterior portions of the ribs, with narrowing and erosion, sometimes associated with widening of the paravertebral shadow. Metastases are primarily lytic and cause bone destruction; they are most frequent in the skull, distal femur and humerus. Aortogram and isotope liver scan may occasionally be useful.

Staging

The staging system most commonly used was proposed by Evans *et al.* (1971), and is based on the site of origin and clinical behaviour (Table 37.4).

Table 37.4 Staging of neuroblastoma.

Stage I	Tumour confined to organ or structure of origin
Stage II	Extension in continuity beyond the organ or structure of origin but not crossing the midline, with or without regional lymph node involvement on the homolateral side
Stage III	Extension in continuity beyond the midline or bilateral lymph node involvement
Stage IV	Remote disease
Stage IVS	Patients, otherwise Stage I or II, but with remote disease confined to liver, skin, and bone marrow (without bony destruction)

Treatment

Treatment for Stage I or II disease consists of total surgical excision which is often curative. Radiation may be used to shrink a tumour and render it operable, and to treat residual post-operative disease, the required dose being 3000 to 4000 rad in 3 to 4 weeks. As a palliative measure radiation is very effective, and good symptomatic relief can be obtained with single fractions of 500 rad. Several chemotherapy agents can be used to obtain temporary control of disease, but no agent or combination has yet been found which eradicates disseminated disease. The agents most frequently used in various schedules and combinations include vincristine, cyclophosphamide and doxorubicin. Other agents which exert some effect include DTIC and VM26. Stage IVS disease is seen in early infancy and is particularly important to recognize since spontaneous regression is common. Treatment should therefore be limited to resection of the primary, and the minimal chemotherapy or radiation required to prevent life-threatening complications, such as respiratory embarassment from extreme hepatomegaly.

Results

Prognosis is related to stage, age, primary site and degree of maturation of tumour. Thus, for example, thoracic or pelvic tumours do better than abdominal tumours. Three quarters of children diagnosed in the first year will be free of disease after two years and potentially cured, compared to 12% of those older than 2 years (Breslow and McCann, 1971). The 2-year disease free survival by stage is 85% for Stage I, 77% for Stage IVS, 63% for Stage II, 37% for Stage III and 6% for Stage IV. It seems clear that for those patients who have an excellent chance of cure, treatment should be by radical surgery alone, aided by radiation or chemotherapy only if necessary. For the many children in whom there is less than a 50% prospect of cure, experimental methods of treatment with new agents possibly combined with radiotherapy are justified. There is great interest in the potential for immunotherapy in this tumour since immune responses to tumour cells in patients and their relatives and spontaneous regression are well documented features. There is, however, no evidence to date that any immunotherapeutic manoeuvres have been of benefit.

Rhabdomyosarcoma

Soft tissue sarcomas account for about 7% of malignant tumours in children, and rhabdomyosarcomas form the largest sub-group, comprising about 50% of the total. They occur throughout childhood, but mainly in the first five years. The estimated annual incidence is 0.27 per 100 000 children under 15 years.

Tumours of the head and neck account for about 35%, common sites including the orbit, nasopharynx, oropharynx, tongue, middle ear and mastoid. Tumours of the genitourinary tract account for a further 20% and may arise from the bladder, uterus, vagina, prostate and paratesticular regions. Lesions of the limbs and trunk comprise the remainder.

Rhabdomyosarcomas are characterized by rapid growth and local infiltration along tissue planes. Many produce blood-borne metastases early in the disease, and bone marrow involvement is present in 20% of patients at presentation. Lymph node spread is seen primarily in genitourinary and limb lesions.

The prognosis is related to the histological type and to the site and extent of the tumour at presentation. Tumours of the orbit have the best prognosis, due partly to their early presentation and relatively late lymphatic and haematogenous spread; tumours of the abdomen and pelvis on the other hand may be late in presentation and have attained a large size at diagnosis. Parameningeal tumours carry a high risk of meningeal involvement, and have a particularly bad outlook.

Pathology

Rhabdomyosarcomas are poorly differentiated, and varied histological appearances may be present in one tumour. There are four main types: embryonal, alveolar, pleomorphic and mixed.

The sarcoma botryoides sub-type of embryonal rhabdomyosarcoma occurs in the bladder, vagina, uterus and nasopharynx, and protrudes in grape-like bunches of nodules; this type has a more favourable prognosis than the alveolar and pleomorphic lesions, the latter being very rare in childhood. Alveolar lesions are commonly found in the limbs and occasionally on the trunk; lymph node involvement is frequently present and early haematogenous spread may result in bony metastases being present at diagnosis.

Presenting features

Rhabdomyosarcomas of the orbit give rise to diplopia, proptosis and chemosis, the condition resembling an acute inflammation of the orbit. Tumours of the retroperitoneum may cause urinary or intestinal obstruction, and haematuria may occur in lesions of the bladder and prostate. A paratesticular lesion usually presents as a lump in the scrotum separate from the testis. A thin blood-stained discharge is a feature of lesions of the vagina and nasopharynx, and lesions of the latter site may present with nasal obstruction, sinusitis, epistaxis, pain and enlarged neck nodes.

Investigations

A biopsy to confirm the histological diagnosis and staging investigations to determine the extent of the disease are essential before treatment.

Chest X-rays and skeletal survey, with isotope bone scans are required in all cases, because of the high incidence of pulmonary and bony metastases. An intravenous pyelogram, micturating cystogram and barium enema may help to define the macroscopic limits of a pelvic or abdominal lesion. Lymphangiography is advisable in tumours of the lower limbs and pelvis. Head and neck tumours frequently require skull tomography to detect bony erosion. Computer assisted tomography (CAT is useful to define the limits of deep-seated tumours and may replace invasive methods of investigation, such as angiography. Early spread to marrow occurs, making trephine and aspiration studies necessary in all cases.

Staging

The treatment plan depends on the stage of the disease at diagnosis, and the staging system used by the American Intergroup Rhabdomyosarcoma Study is a practical one, Table 37.5 being based on this.

Treatment

The aim of treatment is to cure with the minimum morbidity. By using radiotherapy and chemotherapy pre-operatively, it is often possible to reduce substantially the necessity for extensive surgery. In some lesions, notably those of the orbit and nasopharynx, cure can be achieved with radiotherapy and chemotherapy alone. With lesions that arise in the pelvis, it is advisable for at least one course of chemotherapy and radiation to a dose of 2000 rad in 2 weeks to be given pre-operatively. In some instances the tumour may be so reduced as to be rendered macroscopically completely resectable without exenterative procedures.

In Group 1, where the tumour has been completely resected macroscopically, chemotherapy alone is given

Table 37.5   Staging system for rhabdomyosarcoma.

Group 1	Localized disease, totally resected.
Group 2	Regional disease grossly resected.
Group 3	Regional disease with gross residual disease.
Group 4	Distant metastases at diagnosis.

for a period of one to two years. If resection is incomplete as in Groups 2 and 3, radiotherapy is required to the residual tumour and involved lymph nodes. At least one course of chemotherapy is given post-operatively before the start of radiotherapy. If the planned radiation course is protracted, a split course with chemotherapy given in the interval is advisable; in this way systemic treatment of micrometastases is not interrupted.

The treatment of Group 4 disease is palliative in the great majority of cases, but by the judicious use of chemotherapy and radiation, bulky lesions may be reduced in size and pain from bony lesions relieved. Occasionally surgery to relieve symptoms may be required, for example, a colostomy to relieve intestinal obstruction, or internal fixation, combined with radiation to treat a pathological fracture of a limb.

Chemotherapy

Many protocols have made use of combinations of vincristine, actinomycin D and cyclophosphamide (VAC). Doxorubicin and DTIC are also effective against rhabdomyosarcoma and are included in some regimes.

Due to the likelihood of micrometastases being present at diagnosis, chemotherapy should be used in all cases of rhabdomyosarcoma, and should be started as soon as biopsy has confirmed the diagnosis. At least one course is given before surgical resection or radical radiotherapy, and is restarted two weeks from the end of radiation therapy and continued for at least one year. If the radiation course is prolonged, an interval of one to two weeks is made in the course and further cytotoxic drugs given. During radiation, vincristine 1.5 mg/m² may be given once weekly in the absence of neurotoxicity.

The doses of actinomycin D and doxorubicin may be reduced by up to one third immediately after radiation (Table 37.6)

Table 37.6   Treatment protocol for rhabdomyosarcoma Groups 2 and 3.

	1	2	3	Radiation 3000 rad					Radiation 2000–3000 rad					
V	V	.	.	V	V	V	V	V	V	V	V	V	V	V
A	A			Ad					A					Ad
C	C			C					C					C
Weeks	1	2	3	4	5	6	7	8	9	10	11	12	13	14	15

V	= Vincristine 1.5 mg/m²
A	= Actinomycin D 1.5 mg/m²
C	= Cyclophosphamide 1 g/m²
Ad	= Adriamycin 50 mg/m²

Following week 15, VAC and VAdC alternate every three weeks for at least one year.

Radiotherapy

Rhabdomyosarcoma is locally curable by radiation therapy provided that the size of the primary lesion allows the treatment volume to remain small. Cobalt-60 radiation or megavoltage apparatus is usually used but electrons may be more suitable for treating superficially placed lesions. When radiation therapy is to be used as the main form of treatment to the primary disease, for example, when treating rhabdomyosarcoma of the orbit, a dose of 5000–6000 rad given at a rate of 1000 rad per week is required. If the radiation therapy is given in the form of a split course with a gap of two weeks after 2.5–3 weeks of treatment, the higher dose is advisable but if the treatment is given continuously, then the lower dose is appropriate. Chemotherapy is given in the weeks prior to starting radiation therapy and is restarted approximately two weeks from the end of radiation therapy; chemotherapy enhances the effectiveness of radiation against the tumour but will also increase the toxic effects on normal tissues, increasing morbidity.

Surgery

Biopsy of all primary lesions is required for diagnosis and in some lesions, for example paratesticular tumours, the primary lesion may be completely removable surgically. Initial surgical removal of many lesions, particularly those in the head, neck and pelvic regions is not possible without severe mutilation and many lesions are inoperable by virtue of their site. Pre-operative chemotherapy and radiation is frequently given in an attempt to make mutilating surgery unnecessary. Nevertheless, in tumours of the genitourinary tract major surgery involving pelvic exenteration with colostomy and ureterostomy is sometimes needed. At the time of surgery of pelvic lesions biopsy of mesenteric and para-aortic nodes is carried out but routine retroperitoneal node dissection in the case of pelvic and paratesticular tumours is not recommended. If lymph node biopsies have been positive or if there is known residual disease following surgery, radiation and chemotherapy are given.

Treatment of particular sites

Orbit

Radical radiotherapy, combined with chemotherapy, is used in this site. The volume should include the whole of the bony walls of the orbit, and extend posteriorly to the optic chiasm. The dose to the other eye is kept to a minimum; this may be achieved by using wedge pair techniques together with careful choice of beam angles and lead blocks. A dose of 5000–6000 rad in 5–6 weeks is given followed by chemotherapy for at least one year.

Nasopharynx

Following at least one course of chemotherapy, radiation is given to a dose of 5000–6000 rad in 5–6 weeks. The treated volume must include the base of the skull superiorly and extend to the angle of the jaw inferiorly if no nodes are palpable, but may need to extend to the clavicles if lymph node metastases are present.

The anterior limit of the volume is the external nares, and the posterior the mastoid processes. Lead blocks are placed so as to exclude from the radiation fields the eyes, tongue and horizontal portion of the mandibles as far as the anterior faucal pillars.

Pelvic tumours

Radical surgery is the standard treatment in the majority of rhabdomyosarcomas of the bladder, prostate, uterus and vagina. These tumours infiltrate widely and pelvic exenteration may be needed. Colostomy and ureterostomy stomata should be placed on flat abdominal surfaces outside possible radiation fields. However, pre-operative chemotherapy and radiotherapy may enable macroscopically complete removal of the tumour, with less extensive surgery.

Pre-operative radiation to extensive tumours should aim at treating the primary tumour and the whole contents of the pelvis. A simple plan using two opposed anterior and posterior fields is used, with shaped lead shields placed in the path of the anterior and posterior beams to protect the femoral heads from radiation. A dose of 1500–2000 rad is given in 1.5–2 weeks pre-operatively together with chemotherapy.

In treating pelvic tumours the gonads should be spared to allow normal sexual and psychological development to take place subsequently. The testes can be shielded easily with lead blocks, but the ovaries cannot be shielded if pre-operative radiation to the pelvis is given. For this reason, when treating girls, only in the case of very extensive tumours is radiation added to pre-operative chemotherapy. At the surgical removal of the tumour, metal clips are placed to mark its limits and clips are placed on the site of any lymph node biopsies taken. In girls, one or both ovaries are mobilized laterally, and similarly marked with clips, so that they may be avoided when radiation is later given to the pelvis.

In Group 3 tumours, post-operative radiation is given to bring the total to 4500–5000 rad, the fields being tailored to cover the residual pelvic tumour, a suitable arrangement for a bladder or prostate tumour being a direct anterior and two posterior oblique fields, so that radiation to the rectum and femoral heads may be kept to a minimum.

If para-aortic nodes are involved they are treated subsequently to a dose of 4000 rad in 4–5 weeks using anterior and posterior opposed fields to minimize the radiation dose received by the kidneys. Careful planning to avoid overlap or underdosage at the junction of the pelvic and para-aortic fields is necessary. The gap between the lower edge of the para-aortic fields and the upper edge of the pelvic fields is calculated so that the 50% isodose lines meet at the anterior surface of L4.

Radiation treatment as described may become prolonged due to the extent of tumour to be treated, or to side-effects such as enteritis and malaise. In this case, a split course is advisable with a 1–2 week rest from treatment after 2500–3000 rad has been given, during which further chemotherapy is administered, when symptoms have improved.

Testicular and paratesticular tumours
Rhabdomyosarcoma arising in the testes or paratesticular tissues may spread to the lymph nodes in the para-aortic regions. If there is local extension to the scrotum or inguinal tissues, spread to external and internal iliac nodes may also occur.

The primary lesion is removed by inguinal orchidectomy with high ligation of the spermatic cord. Further management depends on the extent of nodal and local involvement. Chemotherapy is given in all cases. Lymphangiography is performed and if no abnormal nodes are demonstrated further surgery and radiotherapy are omitted and chemotherapy alone given. When positive retroperitoneal lymph nodes are demonstrated on lymphangiography, 4000 rad radiotherapy is given to the para-aortic and pelvic nodes using inverted 'Y'-shaped fields extending from the upper border of the body of T10 vertebra to just above the acetabula. If follow-up lymphogram films fail to show resolution of the deposits following radiotherapy and chemotherapy, a laparotomy to remove residual disease in lymph nodes is undertaken. A radical block dissection is usually not possible following extensive radiotherapy, and surgery should be limited to macroscopic removal of these residual masses, relying on chemotherapy to ablate residual microscopic disease.

Trans-scrotal biopsy of a testicular or paratesticular mass is not recommended due to the danger of implantation of tumour in the scrotum; however, should this have been done, the radiation treatment volume must be extended to include the biopsy site. If the tumour has extended to include scrotal tissues, the radiation fields must include the whole of the scrotum and both inguinal regions. When there is need to treat the scrotum it is difficult to avoid irradiating the remaining testis; therefore, this is temporarily transposed to the thigh for the duration of treatment. When treating the inguinal regions, if megavoltage or cobalt radiation is used, considerable dose would be given to the femoral heads; by using low energy electrons, it is possible to

treat the inguinal regions and keep the dose to the femoral heads to a minimum, thereby reducing the risk of arrested growth. Careful matching of the lower margins of the pelvic fields (^{60}Co) and the upper margins of the inguinal fields (electrons) is necessary, to avoid overlap and bands of excessive dose.

Limb and trunk lesions
Wide local excision is performed to include the tumour and the whole muscle in which it has arisen, including the insertions of that muscle and adjacent involved tissues. If the tumour is very extensive, amputation may be necessary, but, with a combination of chemotherapy and pre-operative radiation, this is rarely indicated.

Following incomplete removal of the tumour, postoperative radiation and chemotherapy are given. A strip of normal skin and sub-cutaneous tissue running the length of the treated volume is left untreated in order to preserve some lymphatic drainage and avoid subsequent distal oedema.

A radiation dose of 5000–6000 rad at 1000 rad per week is given to the tumour site; if lymph nodes are involved and have been removed surgically, postoperative radiation to the lymph node site and the adjacent lymph node region is given to a dose of 4000 rad in 4 weeks. If bulk disease has been left postoperatively in the lymph node area, it would be necessary to increase the dose given to 5000–6000 rad in 6 weeks.

Chemotherapy is given both pre-operatively, and for at least one year post-operatively, in all patients.

Results
The three large American children's cancer study groups (CCSG, SWOG and ALGB) joined together to form the Intergroup Rhabdomyosarcoma Study: 423 patients were admitted to this study from 1972 to 1976 and preliminary results have been published (Maurer *et al.*, 1977). Of the first 308 evaluable patients, 16% were Group 1, 28% Group 2, 36% Group 3 and 20% Group 4. A significant incidence of regional lymph node involvement was found only in genitourinary and extremity lesions.

Treatment for Group 1 lesions (by definition completely excised at surgery) consisted of VAC chemotherapy, with a randomization whether or not to receive radiation in addition. No difference in the local relapse rate, disease-free survival or survival in these two groups was found with 80% projected to be disease-free at 60 weeks. Group 2 lesions with microscopic residual disease following surgery all received local radiation, followed by chemotherapy with either VAC or vincristine and actinomycin D without cyclophosphamide for one year; again there was no difference between the two groups, with a projected disease-free survival of 75% at 60 weeks. Groups 3 and 4 received chemotherapy with either VAC or the VAC combination with the addition of doxorubicin, radiation being delayed until the first 6 weeks of chemotherapy have been completed. In these groups combined, there has been as 81% response rate with 30% achieving complete response by 6 weeks, i.e. before radiation; 75% of those who showed a complete response continued without evidence of disease for between 17 and 139 weeks. There was a 16% local recurrence rate, of which half were true recurrences, one quarter involved the development of disease in adjacent sites (meninges), and one quarter were associated with major radiotherapy deviations from protocol. These patients with late disease at diagnosis show a response in more than three quarters, with a complete response achieved in over half, and one quarter achieved complete response before the addition of radiation. It is concluded that a policy of conservative surgery is justified, as is the delay of radiation.

Most of the reports of modern treatment for rhabdomyosarcoma have still only a short follow-up period, so that the long-term prospects for such patients remain uncertain. A recent report, however, gives some reassurance on this point (Sutow *et al.*, 1978). Of 19 patients with head and neck primaries (excluding the orbit) treated at M.D. Anderson Hospital with VAC chemotherapy and radiation, 12 are surviving with no evidence of disease 6.5 to 10 years from diagnosis. It is of considerable significance that 17 of these 19 patients had inoperable disease at diagnosis, though none had distant metastases.

The trends for future management of rhabdomyosarcoma will probably lead to less extensive surgical removal, reduction of radiation dosage when chemotherapy is used concurrently, and the defining of clinical situations where radiation therapy can be omitted. It is clear that chemotherapy is essential in all stages of the disease, but the development of optimal schedules producing maximum survival rates with minimum toxicity has yet to be achieved.

Teratomas

This group of tumours is not confined to childhood but forms a considerable portion of children's neoplasms. The peak incidence is in the third decade, due to the predominance of malignant teratomas of the testes, but there is another peak in childhood in the first five years of life, due to sacrococcygeal and ovarian teratomas, which together comprise 75% of the teratomas of children.

In addition to the gonadal and sacrococcygeal regions, teratomas occur in the mediastinum, and in the retroperitoneal tissues, neck and nasopharynx. Teratomas of the brain are rare but may be found in early infancy, when they are usually poorly differentiated and of considerable size. Germinomas arising in the region of the pineal body or third ventricle should probably be classified as a form of malignant teratoma.

Teratomas are true neoplasms in that their growth is not controlled by normal mechanisms but is continuous and inexorable, though in some the growth rate may be very slow. They are a form of embryonal tumour and approximately 20% are malignant. Malignant teratomas grow more rapidly and have a tendency to recur late, metastases sometimes appearing years after apparently successful surgical removal. They infiltrate locally and commonly disseminate via the blood stream, to give rise to metastases in the lungs and other sites, notably bone; bone marrow involvement occurs in some cases in the absence of discrete bony lesions.

Pathology

Teratomas are characterized by containing tissue from all three germinal layers of the embryo. Neuroectodermal tissue is almost always present; bone, cartilage and fat from the mesodermal layer and epithelia of endodermal origin are usually present and all these tissues may show varying degrees of maturation.

Teratomas which are frankly malignant are usually solid or mixed solid and cystic, and are composed of poorly differentiated tissues. The commonest histological type is embryonal carcinoma, and other malignant tissues include endodermal sinus tumour (yolk sac tumour) and dysgerminoma. Some teratomas contain areas which are composed of relatively benign, well differentiated tissues, alongside embryonal malignant, poorly differentiated tissues. These teratomas must be regarded as malignant and treated along the same lines as the frankly malignant group.

Teratomas of the ovary

Approximately 80% of these are well differentiated. The so-called 'dermoid cyst' of the ovary consists of a teratoma in which there is a large squamous cell component, but other types of epithelia are usually present.

Malignant tumours are usually not mobile and may cause abdominal pain, watery vaginal discharge or occasionally precocious puberty or virilization. They may be composed almost entirely of one type of malignant tissue, but more commonly consist of an admixture of relatively benign and undifferentiated tissues.

Management

Ovarian teratomas are investigated and staged in a similar manner to adult ovarian tumours.

A protein of embryonal origin, α-foeto protein is produced by more than 60% of malignant teratomas and can be detected in minute amounts in the serum by radioimmunassay. It can be used as a marker to measure the response to therapy and to recognize relapse. A positive titre is normal up to the age of six weeks.

Treatment

Surgical removal of macroscopic disease is performed when possible. Hysterectomy and bilateral salpingo-oophorectomy, usually undertaken in adults, is not recommended by many clinicians, but has been advocated by Wollner *et al.* (1976*b*). Chemotherapy is essential in all cases of malignant teratoma, most protocols making use of combinations of vincristine, doxorubicin, cyclophosphamide and actinomycin D.

It has been reported (Cangir *et al.*, 1978) that surgical resection of macroscopic tumour, followed by two years of repeated cycles of vincristine, actinomycin D and cyclophosphamide (VAC) in 21 girls with malignant ovarian tumours, resulted in all patients with Stages I and II disease surviving 18–80 months, 6 out of 7 Stage III patients surviving 25–120 months, and 1 of 5 patients with Stage IV disease surviving 47 months.

Radiotherapy thus has a limited role in the primary management, but is appropriate when the teratoma contains a high proportion of radiosensitive elements, such as dysgerminoma, and possibly where bulk residual disease is present.

Sacrococcygeal teratomas

These tumours form a large percentage of childhood teratomas. They may be found at birth when 90% are composed of well differentiated tissues and have a good prognosis. There is an increasing incidence of malignancy with age, by the age of four months 40% of cases are malignant, and by six months the incidence has increased to over 60%. This makes early diagnosis and treatment of vital importance, as malignant sacrococcygeal teratomas carry a very poor prognosis.

Benign sacrococcygeal teratomas are usually large and obvious at birth as a midline mass between the coccyx and the anus, often ulcerated or causing relative enlargement of one buttock. Interference with bowel function or a bulging anus should lead to pelvic examination which may reveal a teratoma arising from the anterior surface of the sacrum.

Posterior sacrococcygeal teratomas are usually well differentiated and have a good prognosis. Teratomas which lie anterior to the sacrococcygeal region are less common, representing 15–20% of the total and a high proportion are malignant, many being composed predominantly of one tissue, such as endodermal sinus tumour or embryonal carcinoma.

The sacrococcygeal teratomas must be differentiated from meningocele or meningomyelocele, which may also occur in the same children.

Treatment

Benign sacrococcygeal lesions are treated when possible by complete surgical removal. The coccyx is removed completely with the tumour. If the mass extends into the pelvis it may be necessary to perform a laparotomy to free the intra-abdominal portion before the perineal part of the lesion is dissected free.

Malignant sacrococcygeal teratomas are also radically resected whenever possible. Pre-operative radiotherapy and chemotherapy may render resectable locally advanced tumours. A dose of 2000 rad in two weeks to the pelvis, together with VAC chemotherapy is usually used. Even in initially resectable tumours it is now advocated that one or two pre-operative courses of chemotherapy should be given to shrink the tumour and facilitate surgery.

The high incidence of metastatic disease and of local recurrence makes chemotherapy, of the same type as that used in ovarian lesions, essential in all malignant sacrococcygeal teratomas.

When there is residual disease post-operatively, further radiation therapy may be given in addition to chemotherapy. Often it is necessary to include the whole sacrum and coccyx and most of the contents of the pelvis. Fields are arranged to avoid treating the bladder, when this is possible; an arrangement of one posterior and two anterior oblique fields being appropriate. When two opposed pelvic fields are used, care is taken to shield the femoral heads and acetabula.

The sequelae of radiation to the pelvis in infants precludes radical treatment in many cases. If the child is over 5 years, then 4500–5000 rad at 1000 rad per week is given, but in younger children this is reduced to 2500–3000 rad. These lower doses, even when combined with chemotherapy, are unlikely to achieve local cure, but may give good palliation.

Further reading

Bloom, H.J.G. *et al.* (eds) (1975), *Cancer in Children*, UICC Monograph, Springer Verlag.

Jones, P.G. and Campbell, P.E. (eds) (1976), *Tumours of Infancy and Childhood*, Blackwood Scientific Publications, Oxford.

Marsden, H.B. and Steward, J.K. (eds) (1976), *Tumours in Children*, 2nd edn RRCR No. 13, Springer Verlag.

Mauer, A.M., Simone, J.V. and Pratt, C.B. (1977), Current progress in the treatment of the child with cancer. *J. Paediat.*, **91**, 523–39.

Sutow, W.W., Vietti, T. and Fernbach, D.J. (eds) (1977), *Clinical Paediatric Oncology*, 2nd edn C.V. Mosby Co., St. Louis.

References

Beckwith, J.B. and Palmer, N.F. (1978), Histopathology and prognosis of Wilm's tumour. *Cancer*, **41**, 1937–48.

Bennett, J.M. *et al.* (1976), Proposals for the classification of the acute leukaemias. *Br. J. Haematol.*, **33**, 451–8.

Bloom, H.J.G. and Walsh, L.S. (1975), Tumours of the central nervous system. In: *Cancer in Children* (eds H.J.G. Bloom *et al.*) Springer Verlag, pp. 93–119.

Bolande, R.P. (1976), Neoplasia of early life and its relationship to teratogenesis. In: *Perspectives in Paediatric Pathology* 3, Year Book Medical Publishers Inc., Chicago, pp. 145–83.

Breslow, N. and McCann, B. (1971), Statistical estimation of prognosis for children with neuroblastoma. *Cancer Res.*, **31**, 2098–103.

Cadman, E.C., Capizzi, R.L. and Bertino, J.R. (1977), Acute non-lymphocytic leukaemia: a delayed complication of Hodgkin's disease therapy. *Cancer*, **40**, 1280–96.

Cangir, A., Smith, J. and van Eys, J. (1978), Improved prognosis in children with ovarian cancers following modified V.A.C. chemotherapy. *Cancer*, **42**, 1234–8.

Chessells, J.M. *et al.* (1977), ALL in children: classification and prognosis. *Lancet*, **ii**, 1307–9.

D'Angio, G.J. *et al.* (1976), The treatment of Wilms' Tumour: Results of the National Wilms' Tumour Study. *Cancer*, **38**, 633–46.

Evans, A.E., D'Angio, G.J. and Randoph, J. (1971), A proposed staging for children with neuroblastoma. *Cancer*, **27**, 374–8.

Fialkow, P.J. *et al.* (1973), Immunoglobulin and G6PD as markers of cellular origin in Burkitt's lymphoma. *J. Exp. Med.*, **138**, 89–102.

Haghbin, M. (1976), Chemotherapy of ALL in children. *Am. J. Haematol.*, **1**, 201–9.

Jenkin, D. *et al.* (1979), Hodgkin's disease in children: treatment with low dose radiation and MOPP without staging laparotomy. *Cancer*, **44**, 80–6.

Jenkin, R.D.T. *et al.* (1976), Wilms' tumour: adjuvant treatment with actinomycin D and vincristine. *Can. Med. Ass. J.*, **115**, 136–40.

Kaplan, H.S. (1966), Role of intensive radiotherapy in the management of Hodgkin's disease. *Cancer*, **19**, 356–67.

Knudson, A.G. Jnr. (1975), The genetics of childhood cancer. *Cancer*, **35**, 1022–6.

Li, F.P., Cassady, J.R. and Jaffe, N. (1975), Risk of second tumours in survivors of childhood cancer. *Cancer*, **35**, 1230–5.

Mauer, A. and Simone, J. (1976), Current status of treatment of childhood ALL. *Cancer Treat. Rev.*, **3**, 17–41.

Maurer, H.M. *et al.* (1977), The Intergroup Rhabdomyosarcoma Study. A preliminary report. *Cancer*, **40**, 2015–26.

Miller, R.W. (1967), Persons with exceptionally high risk of leukaemia. *Cancer Res.*, **27**, 2420–3.

MRC Working Party on Childhood Embryonal Tumours (1978), Management of nephroblastoma in childhood. *Archs Dis. Child.*, **53**, 112–19.

Myers, M.H. *et al.* (1975), Trends in cancer survival among US white children 1955–1971. *J. Pediat.*, **87**, 815–18.

Sutow, W.W. *et al.* (1978), Long-term evaluation of VAC chemotherapy in childhood rhabdomyosarcoma. *Am. Soc. Clin. Oncol.*, **18**, C98 (abstract).

Tefft, M., D'Angio, G.J. and Grant, W. III (1976), Postoperative radiation therapy for residual Wilms' tumour. *Cancer*, **37**, 2768–72.

Wollner, N. *et al.* (1976*a*), NHL in children: a comparative study of two modalities of therapy. *Cancer*, **37**, 123–34.

Wollner, N. *et al.* (1976*b*), Malignant ovarian tumours in childhood. Prognosis in relation to initial therapy. *Cancer*, **37**, 1953–64.

Ziegler, J.L. (1977), Treatment results of 54 American patients with Burkitt's lymphoma are similar to the African experience. *New Engl. J. Med.*, **297**, 75–80.

Ziegler, J.L. *et al.* (1979), Cure of Burkitt's Lymphoma. *Lancet*, **ii**, 936–8.

Part Three:
Methods and Techniques

38 Medical care

Haydn Bush and M.L. Sutton

The clinical management of patients with malignant disease remains a formidable challenge in oncology. Expertise is required to cover the problems of difficult diagnosis, the early recognition of life threatening emergencies and intercurrent disorders and the evaluation and treatment of secondary complications of malignancy with the attendant consequences of toxic therapies.

This chapter attempts to cover important aspects of day to day clinical oncological practice of increasing concern to medical radiation and surgical oncologists alike. Descriptions are given of common emergencies in oncological practice, selected problems in diagnosis and therapy and some of the serious and often life-threatening consequences of treatment.

Emergencies in oncological practice

In this section several emergency situations are discussed which, although not specific to malignant disease, require special discussion from both the diagnostic and therapeutic standpoints.

Superior vena caval obstruction (SVCO)

This syndrome complex was first described in 1957 by William Hunter. At that time the commonest causes were syphilitic aortic aneurysm and mediastinitis due to tuberculosis (Schecter, 1954). More recently the majority of cases of SVCO are due to malignant disease (Table 38.1). Of all patients with either carcinoma of the bronchus or malignant lymphoma some 3–4% may present with SVCO.

Although SVCO is often associated with a grave prognosis, successful aggressive and early therapy with appropriate supportive treatment may result in a substantial minority (10–20%) of patients surviving for two years (Perez et al., 1978).

The physical findings at presentation include distension of cervical and thoracic veins (67%), facial oedema (56%), and tachypnoea (40%). In more severe cases, oral mucosal engorgement, conjunctival suffusion and papilloedema occur. A histological diagnosis can be made with ease in well over 50% of patients and should be attempted whenever possible. In this situation the positive biopsy rate varies with the diagnostic method used (Table 38.2).

Table 38.1 Causes of superior vena caval obstruction.

Disease	%
Carcinoma of bronchus	85
Malignant lymphoma	10
Benign causes	3
goitre	
constrictive pericarditis	
idiopathic sclerosing mediastinitis	
Other	2
(including: thymoma, teratoma, aortic aneurysm, major vessel thrombotic syndromes, acute lymphoblastic leukaemia (Sternberg sarcoma)	
	100

Table 38.2 Histological diagnosis in SVCO (from Perez et al., 1978).

Method	Positive biopsy rate %
Thoracotomy/biopsy	100
Mediastinoscopy/biopsy	81
Bronchoscopy/biopsy	62
Lymph node biopsy	
(i) scalene	50
(ii) supra-clavicular fossa (palpable nodes)	84
Cytology	
sputum	63
bronchial washings	50
pleural effusion	90–100

The treatment of SVCO includes radiation therapy, chemotherapy and combined approaches together with respiratory supportive care. There is no evidence to support the contention that 'high dose' radiotherapy is more effective than 'low dose' treatment (Perez *et al.*, 1978). Single fractions of radiotherapy may prove as effective as fractionated courses of treatment (Sherrah-Davies, unpublished) but no comparative studies have been performed prospectively.

In SVCO due to bronchogenic carcinoma, cytotoxic drugs including mustine, cyclophosphamide, methotrexate and adriamycin have all been given concurrently with irradiation, but there are few reports of the use of chemotherapy alone. We have seen complete responses in patients with SVCO due to carcinoma of the bronchus using high dose cyclophosphamide (2.5 g/m²) alone.

In general, symptomatic relief with resolution of some of the presenting physical features may be seen in 20% of patients with bronchogenic carcinoma and 75% of patients with lymphoma. No randomized prospective studies have been performed to compare radiation therapy alone, effective chemotherapy alone and combination treatments.

Locally recurrent disease in the mediastinum is very common in patients with bronchogenic carcinoma (>90%) but is less common in malignant lymphoma. Similarly, recurrence of the SVCO syndrome is more common when bronchogenic carcinoma is the cause. In these circumstances one might speculate that survival in SVCO might be improved if the primary treatment was effective chemotherapy, reserving radiation therapy until relapse.

Adjunctive therapy during the early phases have included oxygen, steroids, and diuretics, often given without defined indications. Care must clearly be exercised in the many patients with concomitant chronic airways obstructive disease. It is claimed that both radiation and chemotherapy will induce tissue oedema exacerbating the syndrome. The evidence for this is scanty however, and must be considered carefully in the light of the fact that sudden death in the acute phase is not uncommon, and is presumed to be due to impaired venous return.

Although attempts to make a tissue diagnosis should be swiftly undertaken, SVCO is a life-threatening emergency and effective therapy should be instituted without undue delay.

Spinal cord compression

Acute spinal cord compression due to malignant disease is a medical emergency, often not recognized sufficiently quickly to allow judicious therapy that will prevent permanent neurological disability. Failure to recognize the early symptoms of lower limb weakness, disturbance of gait, paraesthesia and early sphincter disturbance (hesitancy, precipitancy, constipation and spurious diarrhoea) is all too common in oncological practice. Persistent and increasing back pain in the absence of plain radiographic evidence of bone or soft tissue disease may herald spinal cord compression and justify myelography. Indeed it is uncommon for patients with malignant cord compression not to develop back pain, often radicular in nature during the course of their disease. During the development of the syndrome the sequence of events is often pain, motor dysfunction, paraesthesiae and sensory loss. Often, pin-prick and deep pain sensation is retained, if impaired, until much later. Sphincter function too, is often preserved until cord compression is well advanced. Involvement by the malignant process above C^5, although uncommon, may result in neurogenic respiratory failure. Vincristine neuropathy may obscure the development of cord compression. Involvement of the conus medullaris and cauda equina are characterized by saddle anaesthesia, loss of sphincter sensation and urinary incontinence.

Diagnosis includes the neuroanatomic evaluation of the level of spinal cord involvement (bearing in mind that in metastatic disease the cord may be involved at several levels), and the definitive tissue diagnosis. The frequency with which different tumours cause spinal cord compression is shown in Table 38.3.

Table 38.3 Causes of malignant spinal cord compression (from Bruckman and Bloomer, 1978).

Primary tumour	Number	Percentage
Lung	129	16
Breast	94	12
Unknown	91	11
Lymphoma	91	11
Myeloma	68	9
Sarcoma	65	8
Prostate	52	7
Kidney	44	6
GI tract	34	4
Thyroid	24	3
Miscellaneous (each < Thyroid)	116	15
Total	803	100

The anatomical distribution of epidural metastases causing cord compression is similar in many series – cervical 10%, thoracic 70% and lumbosacral 20%. The major aids in diagnosis are clinical neurological evaluation, plain radiology of the spine, lumbar puncture with myelography, computerized tomography, search for a primary tumour and operative biopsy.

Treatment depends on many factors including the duration severity and tempo of the clinical syndrome, the level of spinal cord compression and the histology of the primary tumour.

Opinion varies considerably concerning the right therapeutic approach, but this author considers that the evidence available suggests that laminectomy followed by radiotherapy remains the best single approach, allowing an accurate diagnosis to be made, accurate delineation of the radiation volume for subsequent therapy and often providing the best means of reducing cord compression and producing optimal neurological recovery in the shortest time.

The operative mortality varies from 6–13% in collected series, and some authorities consider that radiation therapy alone may be used in patients with lymphoma, slowly progressive compression with incomplete bock, and epidural metastases to the cauda equina. Patients with rapidly progressing symptoms and signs and complete block should undergo operative decompression. The combined use of laminectomy and post-operative radiotherapy may be of value in those patients in whom the histology is unknown and in those patients with high cervical cord compression at risk from respiratory failure.

Several neurological centres report better results with combined laminectomy and radiation therapy (Wild and Porter, 1963; White *et al.*, 1971), although this is not universally the case (Raichle and Posner, 1970). In malignant lymphoma the use of irradiation alone may produce results that are equivalent or superior to those obtained with combined laminectomy/radiotherapy (Friedman *et al.*, 1976).

Time and dose fractionation considerations are of importance as well as histology in evaluating the results of treatment. Benson has suggested (Benson *et al.*, 1978) that in cord compression due to myeloma doses of radiation close to cord tolerance produce the best results. Similar results have been reported by Khan *et al.* (1976), Murphy and Bilge (1964) and Friedman *et al.* (1976).

Controversy has surrounded the use of initial high dose fractions of radiotherapy. The introduction of concomitant corticosteroid therapy to reduce spinal cord oedema now allows conventional fractionation to be used to maximize early responses.

There are few reports of successful treatment with cytotoxic drugs alone (reviewed by Bruckman and Bloomer, 1978). In general, chemotherapy has a secondary role to play, although full neurological recovery may be achieved in patients with spinal cord compression due to either Hodgkin's disease or non-Hodgkin's lymphoma. A summary of the outcome in relation to tumour type by various treatment modalities is shown in Table 38.4.

In summary, the factors of importance in the successful management of patients with malignant spinal cord compression include a high index of suspicion by the clinician, early neuroanatomical and pathological diagnosis, and the early institution of therapy with surgery radiation therapy and chemotherapy as dictated by each individual case. Notwithstanding these general principles, successful neurological recovery has occurred even when diagnosis and treatment have been delayed for weeks or much more rarely months.

Obstruction of a major viscus

The obstruction of a major viscus by the growth of a

Table 38.4 Treatment results in spinal cord compression in relation to tumour type.

Tumour type	Number of patients	Satisfactory* recovery	Percentage (%)
Lymphoma	147	76	52
Multiple myeloma	40	20	50
Breast	79	26	33
Prostate	35	11	31
Bronchus	101	14	14
Kidney	21	2	10

* Satisfactory implies return of sphincter function and ability to walk independently with simple aids such as walking stick

primary or secondary tumour is not uncommon in oncological practice. Such obstruction often produces a dramatic clinical presentation requiring emergency therapy. Appropriate relief should not be denied any patient because the causative obstructing lesion is incurable. Whilst it is well recognized that adequate palliation may demand aggressive and sometimes radical treatment, the decision to implement major therapy in a terminally ill patient can be extremely difficult.

In patients with known malignant disease, the occurrence of potentially curable intercurrent causes of obstruction is often not considered with the same care as in patients presenting with a primary obstruction of unknown aetiology.

Meticulous attention to diagnostic accuracy and appropriate therapy are as important in oncological practice as in those patients without malignant disease.

Respiratory obstruction
Even advanced tumours of the larynx and hypopharynx seldom present with airways obstruction. Tracheal obstruction is also uncommon. In the latter instance obstruction is usually secondary to extrinsic compression by tumours in the lower neck or upper mediastinum. Most commonly, primary tumours of the thyroid and oesophagus may be responsible, and secondary lymph node masses from a bronchogenic carcinoma, breast, gastrointestinal, bladder or renal carcinoma may obstruct the trachea at the thoracic inlet or in the neck. Rarely malignant lymphomas or thymomas may produce upper airways obstruction.

The symptoms include wheezing stridor dyspnoea and orthopnoea. Cough, usually unproductive, is a common symptom but hoarseness and haemoptysis vary with the site and extent of malignant growth.

Although upper airways obstruction is a gradual process, patients often present as a clinical emergency with cyanosis, tachypnoea, stridor and profound respiratory distress. Soft tissue radiology of the neck and thoracic inlet with tomography where appropriate may help to determine accurately the level of obstruction. Accurate histological diagnosis often helps to determine optimum therapy and biopsy should be undertaken as a routine unless there are specific contraindications. Clearly in a life-threatening situation necessary urgent treatment should not be delayed. Where appropriate endoscopy, tracheostomy, surgical resection, radiation and cytotoxic drugs (with or without steroids) should all be considered. In this respect close liaison from the onset of the medical radiation and surgical oncologist is optimum in order to obtain optimal therapeutic response.

Bronchial obstruction is a common occurrence in patients with bronchogenic carcinoma. This is often a gradual process with one of the major symptoms being increasing effort dyspnoea. Unproductive cough and haemoptysis are not uncommon, and this often signifies an underlying epidermoid carcinoma. Lobar collapse rarely presents with dramatic clinical picture whereas obstruction of a main bronchus with mediastinal shift may rapidly develop into a life-threatening situation, especially in patients with poor pulmonary reserve. Not uncommonly an acute infective exacerbation of underlying chronic obstructive airways disease may precipitate main bronchus obstruction in patients with extrinsic bronchial compression secondary to an underlying carcinoma. The diagnosis is often supported by radiology and may be confirmed judiciously by bronchoscopy and biopsy. Only in a small number of patients with bronchial obstruction due to bronchogenic carcinoma is resection possible (10–25%). With tumours occupying a small volume, radical radiotherapy occasionally produces long-term survivors, but in many, worthwhile palliation of the symptoms due to obstruction may be achieved. Palliative radiotherapy and chemotherapy (especially in small cell tumours) should always be considered in patients with major lower airways obstruction, incapacitated by dyspnoea.

Oesophageal obstruction
Carcinoma of the oesophagus is usually incurable by surgery, radiation therapy and chemotherapy, or even combinations of all three modalities. Although selected series claim 5-year survival rates in excess of 30% (Nakayama, 1959) most patients will require palliative treatment for varying degrees of dysphagia and oesophageal obstruction. With radical radiotherapy alone 5-year survival rates of 30% and 16% have been claimed for tumours of the proximal and distal oesophagus respectively (Rubin *et al.*, 1974). Curative doses of radiation are frequently required to produce any degree of palliation of the obstructive dysphagia. Surgical relief of the obstructed oesophagus includes dilatation, a variety of endo-oesophageal tubes, by-pass surgery and gastrostomy and jejunostomy; the site of the lesion and its extent influencing the choice of procedure (Sise and Crichlow, 1978). Cytotoxic drugs occasionally induce worthwhile palliation of dysphagia and these include bleomycin, methotrexate, actinomycin D and 5-fluorouracil.

Stomach and duodenum
Malignant gastric obstruction is most commonly due to an intrinsic pyloric gastric carcinoma although occasionally a large gastric fundus tumour may produce lower oesophageal, upper gastric obstruction. Duodenal obstruction by contrast is most often due to

extrinsic tumours in pancreas, colon, gall bladder and rarely secondary neoplasms of kidney, adrenal or retroperitoneal structures. Some 20% of patients with gastric cancer may develop the symptoms and signs of obstruction. Diagnosis is made by physical examination, gastric aspiration and lavage (60% may have achlorhydria), contrast radiology, endoscopy and laparotomy. Curative resection can be employed rarely but bypass produces good palliation. Radiation therapy has not yet been demonstrated to be of value in the palliation of gastric obstruction, but combination chemotherapy such as FAM (5-fluorouracil, adriamycin and mitomycin C; Schein *et al.*, 1978 are claimed to produce subjective and objective responses in more than 50% of patients with advanced gastric carcinoma.

Small bowel obstruction

Malignant small bowel obstruction is most commonly due to metastatic intra-abdominal cancer; colorectal, 44.8%, ovary 16.8%, cervix 14.6% and miscellaneous tumours 23.8%. Primary tumours causing obstruction (1–2%) include argentaffin tumours, adenocarcinoma, sarcoma, lymphoma and melanoma.

Symptoms include cramp-like abdominal distension, nausea and vomiting – with the signs of distension, tympany and hyperactive bowel sounds. Plain radiographs of the abdomen (erect, supine and lateral decubitus films) may confirm obstruction, and dilute and double contrast studies may help to identify the site of the lesion. For primary tumours resection with establishment of continuity is important. The prognosis in lymphoma of the small bowel depends on a number of factors including histology, stage and complete resection of all tumour. Some authors stress that abdominal emergency such as obstruction, perforation and peritonitis may adversely affect the outcome of small bowel lymphoma. We have not confirmed this finding (Blackledge *et al.*, 1978). In patients with obstruction due to metastatic or recurrent tumour, guidelines for surgical intervention are more difficult to delineate. Conservative management with nasogastric suction and intravenous fluid and electrolyte replacement may result in improvement in 30% of patients although up to half of these may develop recurrent obstruction (Glass and LeDue, 1973). On relapse surgical intervention is usually necessary. Operative mortality may be as high as 25% (Ketcham *et al.*, 1970), and surgical guidelines have been proposed (Barnett, 1976). Again it should be emphasized that in patients with known carcinoma who subsequently develop small bowel obstruction, it should not be assumed that the obstruction is due to incurable recurrence. Ketcham demonstrated that 25% of such patients had either no recurrence or a second primary tumour and of these some 40% achieved long-term

survival following adequate resection.

Colonic obstruction

Obstruction of the large bowel is less common and is usually due to primary adenocarcinoma, 75% of which are distal to the splenic flexure. Secondary neoplasms causing colorectal obstruction include pelvic tumours such as carcinoma of the cervix and ovary, and intra-abdominal lymphoma.

The symptoms are often insidious and include abdominal pain, constipation (or other change in bowel habit), vomiting, weight loss and rectal bleeding. In the presence of a competent ileocaecal valve, total obstruction results in a closed loop obstruction with increasing abdominal pain and distension. Perforation may occur in 20% of patients particularly if the caecum is involved (Walsh and Donaldson, 1974). Lymphomatous involvement of the caecum, although rare, carries a grave prognosis (Blackledge *et al.*, 1978) and perforation with peritonitis is attended by high operative mortality and a poor overall outlook. Frequently abdominal and rectal examination will reveal a palpable mass and plain abdominal radiographs may confirm the site and extent of obstruction. Barium enema and colonoscopy may confirm the nature of the obstruction. In many series one third of obstructing lesions are within the reach of a sigmoidoscope. Concomitant small bowel obstruction occurs in two fifths of patients and may be the only abnormality in 5%.

Treatment is surgical and delay leading to perforation carries a mortality in excess of 50%. Results from collected series suggest that although 50% of obstructing intrinsic colorectal tumours appear curable by surgery at the time of the primary procedure, 5-year survival rates of 20% only obtain (Glenn and McSherry, 1974). For chronic obstruction due to secondary malignant disease surgical by-pass provides good palliation, allows confirmation of the diagnosis by biopsy and provides details of the anatomic extent of the tumour. The latter may help the radiation therapist to delineate the tumour volume, and the chemotherapist to assess response to therapy.

Renal failure due to malignant disease

Acute renal failure supervenes when there is a rapid reduction in glomerular filtration rate and renal blood flow, resulting in a rise in blood urea and serum creatinine leading to a clinical syndrome of uraemia. Commonly oliguria or anuria accompanies acute renal failure but uraemia may also occur in the absence of a decrease in renal output (Lewinsky, 1966). The causes of renal failure associated with malignant disease are shown in Table 38.5. The secondary replacement of renal parenchyma causing renal failure clini-

Table 38.5   Causes of renal failure in patients with malignant disease.

Directly caused by neoplasm/therapy		Tumour-associated products
Tumour	invasion/metastases	Paraproteinaemia/
	replacement of	hyperviscosity
	renal parenchyma	Uric acid
	obstructive uropathy:	Calcium
	intrinsic	Immune complexes
	extrinsic	FDP's → DIC

Secondarily due to malignant disease		Complications of therapy	
Intravascular fluid loss –		Cytotoxic drugs –	methotrexate
	vomiting		streptozotocin
	diarrhoea		cis-platinum
Diminished intake –nausea			cyclophosphamide
	anorexia	Radiation nephritis	
	cachexia	Anti-microbial agents–	gentamycin
Hypoalbuminaemia			cephaloridine
Hypotension			amphotericin B
Blood loss			
Bacteraemic shock			

cally is uncommon even in lymphoma and acute leukaemia. Autopsy series suggest that renal infiltration in these diseases is more common than is indicated by the incidence of renal malfunction in life. Marked increase in renal size is a common feature of leukaemic and lymphomatous infiltration detected clinically, by plain abdominal radiography and by intravenous pyelography. Death from renal failure due to infiltration by malignant lymphoma is rare. There are few reports of the effects of aggressive chemotherapy on renal failure in this situation (reviewed Garmick and Mayer, 1978). In addition to the clinical and radiological findings other aids in diagnosis include urine microscopy, cytology and biochemistry, ultrasonography, CAT-scanning and renal biopsy.

Treatment is directed toward the remediable causes of renal failure (Table 38.5) and supportive treatment with diet and dialysis as necessary.

Obstructive uropathy is common in oncological practice. Ureteric obstruction, bladder base infiltration and other bladder metastases have been reported in malignant lymphoma and carcinomas of cervix, ovary, colon, bladder, prostate, stomach, pancreas, breast and bronchus. In as many as 70% of patients with carcinoma of cervix, death may be due to obstructive renal failure. In this situation, urinary diversion where possible with ablative surgery, radiotherapy with or without chemotherapy is often the treatment of choice. The decision to institute treatment is often difficult. A uraemic death may be preferable in the situation in which any therapy is either relatively ineffective, toxic, or both.

The renal failure associated with paraproteinaemia,

uric acid, nephropathy, hypercalcaemia and hyperviscosity are dealt with in the chapter on multiple myeloma (Chapter 34).

Cytotoxic drugs causing direct renal tubular cell damage include methotrexate, streptozotocin and cis-diamminedichloroplatinum (cis-platinum). Renal damage may occur with low to medium doses of methotrexate 0.5–3 mg/kg, but more particularly with high dose (grams) regimes. At the latter dose levels a 50% rise in serum creatinine in the first 24 hours may occur in more than half the patients. Prevention includes vigorous parenteral hydration and urinary alkalinization (Pitman and Frei, 1977).

Streptozotocin used in the treatment of pancreatic islet cell tumours produces nephrotoxicity as its major dose-limiting side-effect. Tubular excretion results in the release of an active methylating metabolite causing epithelial cell damage. Renal insufficiency warrants discontinuance of its use until renal function returns to normal.

Cis-platinum, a new effective cytotoxic agent, used in testicular teratoma, ovarian cancer, bladder cancer and head and neck tumours, also induces dose-limiting nephrotoxicity. Dose-related impairment of renal function (diminished creatinine clearance) occurs within 7–14 days, the occurrence of impaired glomerular filtration may herald irrecoverable renal damage. Heavy metal (Pt) deposition is for the most part responsible for the renal damage. Concomitant nephrotoxic antibiotics may exacerbate the renal toxicity due to cis-platinum. Pre-treatment hydration and forced diuresis may decrease the severity of the renal damage.

Pre-existing renal dysfunction may necessitate dose reduction of a number of other cytotoxic drugs that are excreted by the kidney. These include cyclophosphamide, bleomycin, melphalan, 6-mercaptopurine, azathiaprine and rarely anthracyclines such as adriamycin. Mitomycin-C has also been implicated in producing renal damage.

Radiation nephritis may occur following doses of X- or γ-rays exceeding 2300 rad in 4–5 weeks (Luxton, 1961). Acute radiation nephritis increases in the presence of associated hypertension, whilst chronic renal failure may supervene over a period of 10 years.

Some of the common anti-microbial and anti-fungal agents used in the management of severe infections in immunosuppressed and agranulocytopaenic patients with malignant disease, are nephrotoxic (Appel and Neu, 1977). The combination of gentamycin and cephaloridine may cause death from renal failure in a substantial percentage of patients. The decision to use combinations of cephalosporins and aminoglycosides particularly in patients with compromised renal function should be made with caution. Amphotericin-B used in the treatment of systemic mycoses may cause renal damage in as many as 70% of patients treated. The use of an effective non-nephrotoxic anti-mycotic such as miconazole may supplant the use of systemic amphotericin.

As cancer therapy for disseminated malignant disease improves, the importance of secondary renal failure increases. In particular renal failure due to direct infiltration may be recoverable, and its occurrence should not necessarily preclude the institution of optimal therapy with renal support. Renal failure can also be induced and exacerbated by cytotoxic drugs and anti-microbial agents, and in the presence of pre-existing renal dysfunction these agents should be used with care.

Cholestatic jaundice

Malignant cholestatic jaundice frequently presents both diagnostic and therapeutic problems in patients with intrinsic or extrinsic malignant hepatobiliary disease. Intrahepatic metastasis is the commonest cause of malignant jaundice and is due commonly to spread from primary colorectal carcinoma, carcinoma of the breast, bronchus, bladder, malignant melanoma and lymphoma. Primary hepatocellular carcinoma is not considered here. The occurrence of jaundice due to intrahepatic metastases is usually of grave importance, and any degree of hepatic dysfunction requires that cytotoxic drugs undergoing hepatic metabolism for detoxification or activation should be used with caution (e.g anthracyclines, cyclophosphamide, methotrexate etc.). The other causes of malignant

Table 38.6 The causes of malignant jaundice (excluding intrahepatic metastasis) (analysis of 154 cases 1949–1960, after Williams *et al.*, 1960).

Disease	Number of patients	%
Carcinoma of pancreas	94	61
Carcinoma of bile ducts	24	16
Carcinoma of ampulla of vater	16	10
Carcinoma of gall bladder	11	7
Carcinoma of duodenum	4	2.6
Extrahepatic metastases (Grade 2 carcinoma of lymph nodes in portal fissure)	5	3
Total	154	

jaundice are shown in Table 38.6. The symptoms of obstructive jaundice include pain (24–80%, Sise and Crichlow, 1978), weight loss (55–90%), hepatomegaly (36–80%), palpable gall bladder and an abdominal mass. In contrast to metastatic intrahepatic jaundice, malignant jaundice from other causes uncommonly results in markedly elevated hepatocellular enzymes. Total bilirubin levels of 20–30 mmol/l are commonly found with a markedly elevated serum alkaline phosphatase (SAP) level (>500 i.u./l). Following a rise in SAP the γ-glutamyl transpeptidase may rise secondarily. A list of investigations is shown in Table 38.7 and the indications of each are discussed elsewhere (Sherlock, 1975; Sise and Crichlow, 1978).

Where radical operation is not possible (most cases) substantial relief from the symptoms of jaundice may

Table 38.7 Investigation of malignant jaundice.

Stool, urine and serum biochemical characterization of jaundice (including rate of change, periodicity etc.)

Serum alkaline phosphatase, γ-glutamyl transpeptidase

Hepatocellular enzymes, serum cholesterol, lipoproteins etc.

Faecal occult blood

Upper GIT contrast radiology (inc. hypotonic duodenography) (plain films, oral cholecystography, and i.v. cholangiography of less value)

Hepatic scintiscanning ([99]Tc ^{131}I-Rose Bengal)

Coeliacangiography, portal venous angiography

Percutaneous transhepatic cholangiography

Endoscopic duodenoscopy with retrograde cholangiopancreatography

Operative cholangiography and choledochoscopy/ laparotomy/biopsy

Table 38.8 The pathogenesis of malignant hyper-calcaemia.

Exacerbating factors
    Immobilization
    Dehydration   ↓ GFR
    Volume depletion
    Renal failure (tubular)
    Thiazide diuretics
    Hormone therapy (in patients with breast cancer)

Direct tumour invasion and destruction of bone
    (? Grade 2 Osteoclastic responses)
    (? Grade 1 Tumour cell destruction)

Ectopic PTH or PTH-like substance production

Grade 1 Hyperparathyroidism
    Frequency in patients with
            – breast carcinoma
            – chronic lymphatic leukaemia

Osteoclast activating factor
    Breast cancer
    Multiple myeloma

Vitamin D-like substances

Prostaglandin-E

Table 38.9 Malignant hypercalcaemia: manifestations.

Neurological	Cardiovascular
Apathy	ECG changes
Depression	Arrhythmias
Malaise	
Fatigue	*Gastrointestinal*
Weakness	Anorexia
Mental obtundation	Nausea
Pre-coma/coma	Vomiting
	Constipation
Renal	Abdominal cramps
Renal failure (↓GFR and	Paralytic ileus
tubular dysfunction)	(Pancreatitis – rare)
Polyuria	
Nocturia	*Others*
Renal tubular acidosis	Metabolic alkalosis
Glycosuria	Bone pain
Hyperuricaemia	Pruritus
Nephrocalcinosis	Ectopic calcification
Nephrolithiasis	Polydypsia

---

be obtained by a variety of types of drainage procedure. Occasionally palliation may be achieved by irradiation (whole liver, nodes in the portal fissure) or by appropriate chemotherapy depending upon the nature of the causative neoplasm.

Malignant hypercalcaemia

Hypercalcaemia resulting from malignant disease will be considered briefly here (see Chapter 34 on Myeloma). The insidious onset and subtle symptomatology of the clinical syndrome (Tables 38.8 and 38.9) often delays the diagnosis of what may be a treatable condition in which symptomatic relief may be simply achieved. Several surveys indicate that malignant disease may be the commonest cause of hypercalcaemia in populations of hospital patients (reviewed Mazzaferri *et al.*, 1978). As many as 40–50% of patients with metastatic bone disease, metastatic from primary carcinoma of the bronchus, breast, head and neck, kidney and with multiple myeloma may develop hypercalcaemia. Measurement of serum ionized calcium in the presence of protein and paraprotein abnormalities, and disturbances of acid base balance may be difficult, and can be best achieved with a direct measuring calcium ion-sensitive electrode. Therapy however, is often best determined by the patient's clinical condition as is response to a given form of treatment (Table 38.10).

Table 38.10 Treatment of malignant hypercalcaemia.

Rehydration
High fluid, low Ca^{2+} intake
Mobilization
Frusemide   } Ca^{2+}-losing diuretics
Ethacrynic acid
Glucocorticoids
Oral phosphate
Calcitonin
Sodium sulphate
Mithramycin
Indomethacin
Aspirin
Renal dialysis
Specific cytotoxic chemotherapy for causative malignant disease

---

The choice of therapy in patients with malignant hypercalcaemia should be guided by the underlying pathogenesis in any individual (Table 38.8), as well as the severity and course of the clinical syndrome.

In comatose patients or those with marked drowsiness and disorientation, normal saline rehydration-volume expansion with forced diuresis is the treatment of choice. In the absence of bone marrow failure with thrombocytopenia, mithramycin (25 μg/kg) can be given by i.v. push. However, this agent may cause severe thrombocytopenia and may preclude the institution of appropriate cytotoxic therapy for the underlying disease, the latter often providing the best means of controlling malignant hypercalcaemia in the long term. Concomitant glucocorticoid therapy is often of value.

The place of oral phosphate is the subject of some discussion. Whilst undoubtedly effective in both the acute phase and in the long-term maintenance of normocalcaemia, the complications of hypocalcaemia, hypotension, acute renal failure and death cannot be overlooked. These complications of inorganic phosphate administration may be largely avoided if care is taken to monitor dose, dose rate and renal function carefully. In the long term, oral phosphate (1–3 g daily) provides a useful means of controlling hypercalcaemia, but troublesome diarrhoea and ectopic calcification may occur. Mithramycin is thought to exert its effect either by inhibiting osteoblast activity or altering vitamin D metabolism. Major side-effects (occuring more commonly in patients with renal failure) include thrombocytopenia and hepatocellular necrosis. Glucocorticoids are useful in the management of malignant disease but responses to steroids alone are variable and may be slow. Calcitonin is another second line agent that inhibits bone resorption and promotes renal tubular excretion of ionic calcium. Its hypocalcaemic effect is often modest and many patients develop tolerance to calcitonin within a few days of starting therapy. It is however, non-toxic and may be a very useful adjuvant to other forms of hypocalcaemic therapy.

The treatment of malignant hypercalcaemia is often empirical. In general terms the use of rehydration, forced diuresis, steroids and effective chemotherapy will usually control the clinical syndrome both acutely and in the long term.

Respiratory failure

In patients with malignant disease respiratory failure may be consequent upon the underlying neoplasm or less commonly result from therapy. Overwhelming respiratory infection is common in immunosuppressed patients who may also be granulocytopaenic due to their disease or as a result of therapy. Detailed discussion of the causes of respiratory failure and its management will not be given here but some examples of the more difficult diagnostic and therapeutic problems are discussed briefly.

Diffuse metastatic and lymphomatous malignancies may rarely present with such advanced pulmonary parenchymal disease as to precipitate respiratory failure. In Fig. 38.1 a chest radiograph is shown of a patient who developed irreversible respiratory failure due to diffuse alveolar metastatic disease from a

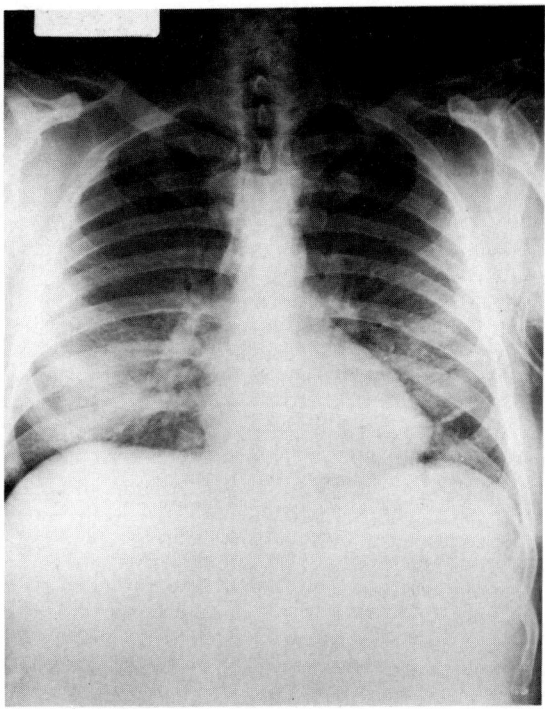

Fig. 38.1 Chest radiograph of a patient with malignant melanoma, who developed diffuse alveoli metastases (confirmed at post mortem) who died of respiratory failure.

malignant melanoma.

Respiratory failure can also be caused by major airways obstruction with lobar or whole lung collapse, opportunistic pneumonic infection, neurogenic respiratory failure, malignant pneumothorax, pleural effusions and as a result of radiation therapy and chemotherapy.

The management of remediable causes of respiratory failure may therefore, involve respiratory support, treatment of the underlying malignancy/infection and therapy for a major airways block (see p. 772). In patients with respiratory failure due to lymphomatous involvement of pulmonary parenchyma, appropriate chemotherapy with steroids may result in rapid amelioration of the respiratory failure.

Opportunist infections causing respiratory failure require a high index of suspicion for diagnosis *ante mortem* and the institution of early therapy. In this context common antimicrobial agents are *Pneumocystis carinii*, *Candida*, *Aspergillus* and Mucormyosis.

Radiation damage after whole lung irradiation may result in an acute alveolitis or result in a chronic fibrosing alveolitis and progressive respiratory failure with doses above 2000 rad. Similarly, several cytotoxic agents used commonly in cancer chemotherapy have been implicated in the induction of pulmonary damage and respiratory failure. The alkylating agents cyclophosphamide and busulphan both produce hyaline membrane changes. Cyclophosphamide is more usually implicated at higher doses than given conventionally (2–5 g) or in association with total body irradiation (e.g. in bone marrow transplantation programmes). Busulphan-induced alveolitis is more commonly seen after long-term administration in patients with chronic myeloid leukaemia, but may occur idiosyncratically.

More recently bleomycin, an antibiotic and antimitotic agent, has been introduced whose major dose-limiting side-effect is interstitial pneumonitis. With doses above 150–250 mg/m² the incidence of pneumonitis increases. However, acute pneumonitis occurring at much lower doses (50 mg) has been reported (Bonadonna *et al.*, 1972). Clinically, the picture is of rapidly developing dyspnoea tachypnoea, cyanosis and respiratory failure. Chest radiographs often reveal diffuse amorphous and reticular shadowing in one or both midzones. Respiratory function tests are consistent with the development of an alveolar-capillary block and treatment can only be symptomatic for the often irreversible and fatal respiratory failure. Sequential respiratory function studies are not helpful in predicting those patients who are at risk of developing an acute alveolitis. Pre-disposing factors include airways obstructive disease, congestive cardiac failure, concomitant lung irradiation, combination chemotherapy and pre-existing pulmonary malignancy or infection.

Infection in patients with malignant disease

Incidence diagnosis and manifestations of infection

Progress in cancer therapy has elevated infection to the position not only of the most serious complication of treatment but also the most frequent cause of death (Ketchel and Rodriguez, 1978). Special factors predisposing to infection include alteration in the integrity of tissues at normal portals of microbial entry, depression of most immune and inflammatory responses, neutropaenia and opportunist infection in patients receiving broad spectrum antibiotic therapy.

In a recent literature review Ketchel and Rodriguez (1978) reported that of 234 patients with acute leukaemia 104 patients with lymphoma, and 380 patients with solid tumours, 74%, 51% and 47% respectively died of acute infection. The majority of bacterial infections in those patients are due to *E.coli*, *Klebsiella* and *Ps. pyocyaneas*; septicaemia and pneumonia (35%,

40%) are the commonest clinical forms of infection. Much less commonly *Staphylococcus aureus*, *Streptocci* and *Listeria monocytogenes* may be responsible for systemic infection. Even more rarely bacterial infections with *Clostridium* bacteroids and *Corynebacterium* species are encountered. Opportunistic infections of the central nervous system have been reviewed recently, and will not be further considered here (Begent, 1977).

It cannot be emphasized too strongly that in as many as 30–50% of all episodes of infection (pyrexia) no organism can be identified. Fungal infections are increasingly recognized as causing serious morbidity due to local infection (mouth, oesophagus, skin, perineum) and mortality because of systemic mycoses. Organisms include *Candida*, *Aspergillus*, *Mucor* and *Cryptococcus*. It is unusual for systemic mycoses to be diagnosed *ante-mortem*, and a high index of suspicion is required.

Virus infections of serious and life-threatening importance include disseminated varicella zoster and cytomegalovirus infections. Parasitic infections with *Pneumocystis carinii* and *Toxoplasma gondii* are also being recognized with increasing frequency. Frequently *Pn. carinii* presents an acute interstitial pneumonitis and is only diagnosed *ante mortem* by special examination of lung bipsy material. Clinical signs of infection are often atypical in cancer patients because of the underlying disease and its therapy. Sites of origin of infection should be carefully identified including the mouth, skin of axillae and inguinal regions, nose, scalp and perianal area. Routine and frequently repeated 'bacteriological sweeps' should include specimens of blood, urine, sputum, faeces and mouth, throat, nasal and skin swabs. Fever is the single most useful index in an otherwise unidentified infection, but patients taking anti-pyretic/glucocortoid medication may require especially careful evaluation.

Excluding fever due to the malignant process, blood products and chemotherapeutic agents (DTIC, bleomycin), 80% of all febrile episodes are likely to be due to infection. Signs of infection are often sparse and unusual. Skin lesions of *Pyoderma gangrenosa* may occur in *Pseudomonas* infection. The lesions of disseminated candidiasis and *Herpes zoster* must be recognized. Bone marrow culture may be of help in the diagnosis of latent mycobacterial and fungal infections and in undiagnosed episodes of septicaemia.

Management of fever/infection

Persistent or recurrent fever above 38°C is suggestive of bacterial infection in immunosuppressed patients with malignant disease. Antibiotic therapy should be instituted promptly after comprehensive bacteriological specimens have been taken. Many different approaches have been suggested (Ketchel and Rodriguez, 1978). We outline our own here.

In *well* patients with an unidentified infection and a pyrexia ≤38°C oral therapy with sulphamethoxazole and trimethaprim (cotrimoxazole) is instituted. If there is no response within 24–48 hours, or if a patient becomes ill with a rising fever before this period has elapsed, parenteral treatment with gentamycin and carbenicillin is started after a further bacteriological sweep. If no response occurs on this regime a cephalosporin is substituted for carbencillin. Gentamycin levels and renal function are monitored daily. In neutropaenic adult patients the positive value of granulocyte transfusions has yet to be objectively established. Our approach is to reserve granulocyte transfusions for patients who have an absolute granulocytopaenia of ≤0.5 × 10⁹/l, and whose fever is unresolved after 48-hours intensive parenteral antibiotic therapy. Care should be exercised in the use of aminoglycoside antibiotics with or without a cephalosporin. Recent reports suggest that they may be responsible for an acute and sometimes fatal pseudomembranous colitis.

The clinical diagnosis of systemic fungal infection is usually difficult. Routine cultures, special cultures and fungal serology should always be performed. In a patient with unresolved fever after the above measures some authors recommend a trial of steroids to indicate such an infection non-specifically. With the advent of less toxic systemic anti-mycotic agents (miconazole) we prefer a therapeutic trial. The clinical development of oral and oesophageal candidiasis (intense burning dysphagia, especially for hot liquids) may precede the development of a fungal septicaemia. Similarly septicaemia may follow a fungal pulmonary infection.

Previously, toxic and relatively ineffective antimycotic therapy has been used in systemic mycoses. Amphotericin B is extremely nephrotoxic producing responses in approximately 70% of patients and 5-fluorouracil produces both fewer responses and hypersensitivity reactions. Newer antimycotic agents (imidazole derivatives) such as clotrimazole and miconazole have been introduced into clinical practice recently. Early experience suggests that their improved effectiveness, and much reduced toxicity may considerably advance the management of systemic fungal disease.

Even newer agents (mycolase) have been reported to be effective in animals with systemic mycotic infections. These drugs comprise selected enzymes known to lyse fungal cell walls, but await clinical evaluation (Davies and Pope, 1978).

Patients with malignant disease who develop systemic viral infections are usually those receiving immunosuppressive chemotherapy and corticosteroids. Inhibitors of viral DNA-synthesis (ARA-A, ARA-C) may in low doses (ARA-C 30–50 mg/m²/day × 5) may be of value in the early phases of the infection. The place of human interferon is presently incompletely evaluated in viral infections in man.

Protozoal infestation with *Pn. carinii* is treated with cotrimazole (trimethaprim/sulpha) or pentamidine (4 mg/kg/day). The latter is nephrotoxic and may be effective in only 50% of infections.

Toxoplasma gondii is another protozoal infection seen in immunosuppressed patients with malignant disease, and may be successfully treated with Daraprim and sulphonamide therapy.

The pathogenesis and management of gram negative bacteraemic shock is summarized in Table 38.11.

Disseminated intravascular coagulation in malignant disease (DIC)

DIC represents a clinico-pathological syndrome complex in which bleeding results from hypercoagulability and the associated increased fibrinolysis. Although several stages may be recognized from a sub-clinical syndrome to catastrophic haemorrhage, classically there is depletion of coagulation factors and platelets with increased fibrinolysis (fibrin dehydration products, FDPs) and the resultant circulating anticoagulants.

Thrombocytopenia due to malignant disease or its therapy may exacerbate the clinical syndrome. The mechanism of the events leading to DIC are reviewed elsewhere (Weick, 1978).

The diagnosis is often made by finding evidence of both fibrinolysis (↑FDPs) and positive tests for soluble fibrin in the serum of affected individuals. In most instances the services of a coagulation laboratory are required to demonstrate the presence of DIC conclusively. A summary of those malignancies with which DIC is known to be associated, is shown in Table 38.12.

There is little agreement about therapy in this group of conditions. No controlled trials have been conducted which support the value or otherwise of agents such as salicylates, epsilon aminocaproic acid or heparin. Indeed, the latter has been implicated in the production of DIC *per se*.

Hypersplenism

Hypersplenism associated with malignant disease (lymphoma, leukaemia and myeloproliferative disorders) may present difficulties in both evaluation and therapy. The resulting pancytopenia makes effective therapy for the underlying disorder difficult or imposs-

Table 38.11 Pathogenesis manifestations and management of gram negative bacteraemic shock.

Pathogenesis
    Ruptured viscus
    Manipulative (endoscopic) procedures
    Vasoconstriction
    Venous pooling
    Hypotension (narrow pulse pressure)
    Disseminated intravascular coagulation (DIC)

Clinical features
    Fever rigors
    Hypothermia
    Prostration
    Tachycardia
    Tachypnoea
    Peripheral cyanosis
    Cold, clammy extremities
    Hypotension
    Oliguric renal failure
    Altered consciousness

Management (includes)
    Central venous pressure monitoring
    Vital signs
    Regulation of peripheral resistance/stroke volume
        (vasoactive drugs, digitalization)
    Maintenance of airway
    Assisted ventilation
    Fluid electrolyte repletion/regulation
    Corticosteroids (large doses)
    DIC – heparinization, aspirin, replacement of clotting
        factors

decision to recommend splenectomy devolves on two clinical problems. The first is symptomatic splenomegaly with abdominal discomfort, repeated splenic infarction with acute or chronic splenic pain. The second is hypersplenism with anaemia increasing transfusion requirement, together with leukopaenia (infection) and thrombocytopenia, making effective chemotherapy difficult often in the face of advancing disease elsewhere. In the first case the indications for splenectomy are largely clinical and referral to a surgeon experienced in both the removal of massive spleens and in the aftercare of such patients is an important consideration.

Table 38.12   Tumours associated with DIC.

Urogenital tumours
    Prostatic cancer/benign prostatic hypertrophy
    Ovarian cancer
    Hydatidiform mole
    Chorion carcinoma

Gastrointestinal tract
    Pancreatic carcinoma
    Gastric carcinoma (microangiopathic haemolytic
        anaemia and DIC)

Other solid tumours
    Bronchogenic carcinoma
    Breast cancer
    Vascular tumours – haemangiomas
                          haemangiosarcomas
    Malignant melanoma

Leukaemia
    Acute progranulocytic leukaemia (88%)
    Acute myeloid/myelomonocytic leukaemia
    Acute lymphocytic leukaemia
    Acute stem cell leukaemia
    Blast transformation of chronic granulocytic leukaemia
    Chronic lymphatic leukaemia

ible, and the indications for splenectomy may be finely balanced in a sick patient with massive splenomegaly. In recent years newer methods of assessing splenic function have been developed and have been reviewed in relation to the indications for splenectomy (Lewis, 1978). Studies of splenic function include estimation of spleen size, measurement of the phagocytic function of the spleen, identification of sites of red cell destruction, measurement of the splenic red cell destruction, measurement of the splenic red cell pool; identification and measurement of splenic extramedullary erythropoiesis, and the evaluation of the contribution of the spleen to lymphocyte recirculation.

With respect to malignant hypersplenism (most commonly seen in non-Hodgkin's lymphomas) the

Although careful estimation of the phagocytic function of the spleen may be predictive of those patients in whom splenectomy is to be of any value, the quantitation and localization of red cell destruction is often the most useful index of hypersplenism in practice.

In the presence of concomitant bone marrow infiltration (e.g. by lymphoma) and possible marrow failure the value of splenectomy for associated hypersplenism may be extremely difficult to assess in an individual patient. We have, however, seen several patients in whom splenectomy has resulted in recovery of pancytopenia despite coexistent marrow infiltration and in whom successful cytotoxic drug therapy was subsequently administered.

Dose-limiting and life-threatening cytotoxic drug toxicity

A comprehensive outline of drug toxicity is given in the chapter on cancer chemotherapy (Chapter 5). This section describes selected important and commonly used drugs whose peculiar unwanted effects may be dose-limiting or life-threatening.

Adriamycin and daunorubicin

The anthracyclines derived from *Streptomyces* species share common dose-limiting toxicities. The most important of these is cardiotoxicity – the production of irreversible congestive cardiac failure due to a degenerative cardiomyopathy. Transient ECG abnormalities occur in one third of patients receiving anthracyclines and are reviewed elsewhere (Cortes *et al.*, 1973). These transient changes are not predictive of those patients who may develop a cardiomyopathy. Reduction of R-wave voltage may occur and is usually irreversible. The transient changes are not associated with morbidity unlike those changes associated with chronic toxicity.

Chronic congestive cardiac failure due to a progressively degenerative and fibrotic cardiomyopathy is related to the total cumulative dose received and to the time period over which that total dose is given. Associated ischaemic or rheumatic heart disease is usually a contra-indication to anthracycline therapy because of the possibility of inducing acute arrhythmias and reproducing the chronic toxicity at much lower doses. In patients with previously normal cardiac status, accumulated doses above 550 mg/m^2 are associated with an increasing incidence of cardiotoxicity that is dose-related. Both transjugular right ventricular endomyocardial biopsy and measurement of the systolic time interval may be useful predictive tests of the development of irreversible cardiotoxicity.

Bleomycin

The pulmonary toxicity of bleomycin is discussed on p. 778. Other major toxicities include skin side-effects including intense pruritus, skin pigmentation, hyperkeratoses and rarely exfoliative dermatis.

Sex hormones

The use of hormone therapy in carcinoma of the breast and prostate is associated with major cerebrovascular morbidity and mortality. In this context the Veterans Administration Study (VACURG; Blackard, 1975) is of major importance. Fluid retention and expansion of the extracellular space may lead to cardiac decompensation.

In many studies oestrogen therapy has been shown to result in a higher incidence of thromboembolic disorders. In the VACURG study, the use of stilboestrol in carcinoma of the prostate results in a higher mortality due to cardiac disorders and cerebrovascular accidents than from the underlying malignancy *per se*.

Vinca alkaloids

The vinca alkaloids, vincristine and vinblastine have been in use for over ten years and their well described neurotoxicity will not be discussed here. Recently a newer semi-synthetic analogue vindesine has been released for clinical use which appears to combine the major toxicities of vincristine (neurotoxic) and vinblastine (myelotoxic). Its importance may lie in its reported lack of cross-resistance to the parent drug. A disturbing additional side-effect recently reported (Vindesine Symposium, London, 1978) is that of an acute painful myalgic syndrome which lasts for several days and may produce profound morbidity.

Gastrointestinal toxicity

The effects of many cytotoxic drugs on the gastrointestinal tract are well known; certain drugs and drug combinations, however, deserve special mention. Their use may result in failure of patient compliance because of profound, unacceptable nausea and vomiting or the production of life-threatening mucositis.

In the former category, the nitrosoureas, mustine, cis-platinum and combinations incorporating imidazole and carboxamide provide good examples.

5-Fluorouracil, methotrexate, adriamycin and bleomycin all produce mucositis as single agents. Their combined use may result in profound gastrointestinal tract epithelial necrosis with the attendant effects of severe pain, diarrhoea, fluid loss and infection. In the presence of hepatic or renal dysfunction the magnitude of these changes may be out of proportion to the doses of drugs used and extreme caution is often required in these circumstances to prevent fatal gastrointestinal tract toxicity.

Cumulative and irreversible bone marrow toxicity

With the use of most cytotoxic drugs the pattern of temporary marrow hypoplasia results in a nadir of peripheral blood counts at 7–10 days with recovery by 14–21 days. Clearly the route, schedule, dose and combinations of drugs may alter this general pattern of recoverable myelotoxitiy.

Certain cytotoxic drugs however, produce cumulative and delayed bone marrow toxicity. Busulphan used over a long period produces peripheral blood leucopaenia with irreversible maturation arrest in the bone marrow. More rarely this kind of toxicity is produced idiosyncratically.

The nitrosoureas are also profoundly myelotoxic causing both a delayed nadir (3–5 weeks) and cumulative marrow hypoplasia. BCNU, CCNU and methyl CCNU all produce this pattern of myelotoxicity, and treatment with these drugs cannot be safely repeated within a six-week period. The newer nitrosoureas, chlorozotocin and streptozotocin are less myelotoxic than the older drugs. Prolonged use of the nitrosoureas often results in cumulative myelotoxicity which is both dose-limiting and often irreversible.

Melphalan, an alkylating agent, commonly used in the treatment of multiple myeloma, also exhibits an interesting pattern of myelosuppression. A biphasic response is seen with a first nadir at 7–14 days, partial recovery and a delayed second nadir at 4–5 weeks. Recovery is usually by six weeks.

Hepatotoxicity

A number of commonly used cytotoxic drugs produce hepatotoxicity. These include methotrexate (reversable enzyme changes, fibrosis, cirrhosis), mithramycin (dose-limiting hepatic necrosis), nitrosoureas (5–25%, reversible enzyme changes and raised serum bilirubin), 5-fluorouracil (reversible enzyme changes leading to hepatic fibrosis especially after hepatic arterial perfusion), imidazole carboxamide, DTIC (reversible changes in hepatic enzymes at 5–14 days, with possible long-term hepatic damage). The combination of irradiation (where the liver is in part or wholly included in the treatment volume) and cytotoxic drugs may precipitate acute hepatic toxicity. This has been seen particularly in young patients with Wilm's tumour where actinomycin D is used concomitantly with abdominal irradiation.

Skin manifestations of malignancy

Descriptions of the various dermatological manifestations of malignant disease are given in standard textbooks of medicine (Beeson and McDermott, 1975) and in a recent review (Staughton, 1978).

A summary of the skin disorders in malignant disease is given in Table 38.13. Many of the accepted markers of visceral malignancy occur very uncommonly, but when present may antedate direct evidence of a malignant process. Non-specific markers often indicate complications of a malignant disease or its therapy, and the proliferation of new cytotoxic drugs has increased the catalogue of disorders of the integument (Table 38.14).

Direct involvement of skin may recur with any metastasizing solid tumour. There are certain sites of predilection. Scalp metastases occur not uncommonly with primary tumours of breast, lung (small cell) and genitourinary tract whilst metastases to skin of the abdominal wall occur secondary to tumours of the stomach, colon, breast and malignant melanoma.

Primary cutaneous infiltrations by lymphoma are not uncommon in the non-Hodgkin group, may present bizarre appearances, and are often associated with a more favourable prognosis. Primary cutaneous Hodgkin's disease has been described but is extremely rare. Skin involvement as part of a generalized lymphoma or leukaemic process is however, not uncommon. In all of these skin infiltrations the differential diagnosis may be difficult. Added to these difficulties are those of the mycosis fungoides group of conditions including all the varieties of pre-mycotic lesions (Samman, 1977).

Of the accepted skin markers for malignant disease, acanthosis nigricans and dermatomyositis are the best known. There are few exceptions to the former occurring in association with malignant disease. The true incidence of malignant disease in patients with dermatomyositis is a matter of some debate with figures ranging from 7% to 50%. However, the occurrence of dermatomyositis in any patient over the age of 50 years should be regarded as a marker of concomitant visceral malignancy.

The care of radiation reactions in skin and mucous membrane

Acute reactions

The degree to which acute tissue reactions in skin and mucous membranes require active management depends on a number of factors arising from the philosophy and practices of the individual radiotherapist. Of these, the most important are:

1. The overall treatment time.
2. The radiation dose per fraction.
3. The concurrent administration of oncolytic drugs.

Long overall treatment times in general reduce the severity of reactions, and may increase the latent period for their development. Some radiotherapists defer X-ray treatments for one or more days in a patient who appears to be developing notable erythema; others regard a planned course of irradiation as virtually sacrosanct, the production of a confluent fibrinous reaction being regarded as an inevitable and even desirable consequence of adequate curative treatment. (Extreme normal tissue reactions are rarely justified in the case of palliative treatments,

Table 38.13 Skin eruptions associated with malignant disease (from Staughton, 1978)

Malignant invasion of skin
 Metastases and infiltration: Stewart-Treves syndrome
         solid tumours   Paget's disease of the breast
         lymphomas
         mycosis fungoides
         leukaemias

Non-specific markers
 Infections: bacterial   Hyperviscosity
        (*Ps.pyocyaneas*)
        viral (*H. zoster*)
        fungal (*Candida*)
 Purpura, petechial ecchymoses
    (marrow replacement, infiltration,
    dysproteinaemias coagulopathies,
    polycythaemia, dysproteinaemia)

Accepted skin markers
 Acanthosis nigricans   Reticulo-hystiocytoma
 Dermatomyositis   Acquired icthyosis
 Pachydermoperiostosis   Exfoliative erythroderma
 Malignant down   (Mycosis fungoides Sézary syndrome)
 Erythema gyratum repens   Scleroderma
 Bowen's disease

Endocrine
 Pigmented striae (ectopic ACTH)   Carcinoid syndrome
 Nelson's syndrome (diffuse post-   Glucagonoma – skin bleeding
    adrenalectomy hyperpigmentation) Acromegaly – skin thickening

Genetic syndromes
 Gorlin's syndrome   Keratoderma pigmentosa
 Gardener's syndrome   Peutz-Jeghers syndrome
 Palmar-plantar keratoderma

Less well established skin markers
 Basex acrokeratosis   Panniculitis
 Follicular muscinosis   Erythema multiforma
 Blistering eruptions

---

especially for instance, in the mouth.)

The following guide to the management of acute reactions is the most applicable to the more marked reactions, but is appropriate in reduced employment to lesser degrees of reaction.

General

Radiation causes depletion of the stem cells component of the basal layers of the epithelium, and this leads to diminished adherence of the superficial layers. These may ultimately separate, with the subsequent leakage of fibrinogen-rich fluid over the denuded area. In the presence of (radiation) killed cells, fibrinogen is converted into fibrin, which forms a pseudomembrane of limited adherence, in which become enmeshed large numbers of polymorphonuclear leucocytes. This membrane constitutes a barrier to further physical, chemical and bacteriological insult, and should not therefore be disturbed. In skin this means that the following must be avoided:

1. Vigorous drying by towels – washed areas must be gently patted dry.
2. Wet-shaving – an electric razor is preferable.
3. The juxtaposition of reacting surfaces where friction can occur, for instance in the infra-mammary region.
4. Pressure during recumbency on treated skin.
5. Constricting or abrasive clothing.
6. The other than very gentle application of bland topical preparations at body or room temperature.

Table 38.14   Cutaneous complications of treatment for malignant disease.

Manifestation	Agent	

Pigmentation – generalized
  punctate
 	
  palmar
	X-irradiation
	Vincristine
	Methotrexate
	Bleomycin
		Bleomycin
		Busulphan
		Hexamethylmelamine

Telangiectasia Atrophy/fragility Sub-cutaneous fibrosis }	Late effects of irradiation	
'Recall' radiation skin reactions (or synergistic)	Actinomycin D Methotrexate Adriamycin Bleomycin	
Local skin and subcutaneous necrosis (due to venous extravasation)	Nitrogen mustard Vinca alkaloids Anthracyclines Actinomycin Imidazole carboxamide	
Erythema Dry desquamation Moist desquamation }	Immediate effects of irradiation	
Alopecia	X-irradiation Anthracyclines Vinca alkaloids Cyclophosphamide	
Keratoses Skin desquamation Erythema Exfoliative dermatitis Pruritus/prurigo }	Bleomycin	

7. Exposure to direct sunlight, or application of hot water bottles.

Any dressing deemed necessary should not be secured by plaster or tape which is adherent to skin likely subsequently to develop a radiation reaction. In general, dressings are best avoided, exposure to the air encouraging the development of a dry adherent crust in the reacting area. This may be further promoted by the local application of 1% gentian violet in water; being a fluid, it can be applied to the skin with the minimum of physical trauma, and it promotes coagulation in the superficial layers of the affected area. It is particularly suitable where larger areas of delicate skin are reacting, for instance in the groins and perineum. Its main disadvantages are that it is unsightly and stains clothing and bedclothes.

A well established skin reaction can be soothed by simple zinc and castor oil ointment, but its use must be limited to the period after the course of irradiation has been completed, otherwise the heavy metal may cause enhanced surface effects.

In circumstances where the integument is reacting but is none the less intact, local cleanliness is best achieved by light dusting with heavy metal-free talc, or starch powder.

Where small skin areas require attention, for instance after treatment of modestly sized skin malignancies, Graneodin ointment or an ointment containing betamethasone plus a topical antibiotic are all that are required. Prolonged use of steroid ointments aggravates the generalized atrophy of irradiated skin, and is therefore to be avoided.

Mucous membranes

Tissue reactions in the mucous membranes generally appear more quickly than in skin, and generally heal more quickly. They are most troublesome in the upper aerodigestive tract, where they may interfere with adequate hydration and nutrition of the patient.

Management is directed to: (a) the avoidance of exacerbating factors, (b) the relief of discomfort and (c) the encouragement of normal tissue recovery.

(a) *The avoidance of exacerbating factors*. These vary from site to site; in the mouth for example, irregular and infected teeth should be removed before the commencement of treatment – where dentures are worn, they should be stored overnight in 1% chlorhexidine to avoid oral sepsis and self-reinfection. Where infection occurs, tetracycline (as syrup) is usually helpful, but it also increases the already higher than normal risk of candidiasis, which in the presence of a fibrinous reaction may be overlooked. Many patients with upper aerodigestive tract malignancies have been long-term abusers of tobacco and alcohol, and these irritants should be withdrawn or minimized. Inveterate spirit drinkers should be instructed to dilute adequately their distillates.

(b) *Relief of discomfort*. Considerable reduction of discomfort is usually possible in the case of reactions in the mouth, pharynx and oesophagus. Paracetamol mucilage taken 10 minutes before meals usually permits the patient to ingest an adequate diet. Mucaine suspension is a useful alternative. The diet itself should be soft, bland and at neither extreme of temperature.

Reactions in the rectal mucosa can be symptomatically minimized by ensuring that the stools are both bulky and soft: this is achieved by daily administration of methyl cellulose granules with liquid paraffin emulsion. It is important that the patient be instructed to continue these measures after discharge from hospital, as in the presence of tenesmus and stool frequency, many patients discontinue their medication on the mistaken impression that they are being given as aperients. The passage of mucus and small amounts of blood per rectum at the height of the reaction are not of great consequence, but occasionally retention enemas containing prednisolone are needed.

Relief of symptoms from bladder mucosal reactions is generally unsatisfactory: treatment of infection (often the result of recent instrumentation of the lower urinary tract) and a moderately high fluid intake is recommended. The use of anticholinergic drugs rarely affords real benefit, and carries some risk of precipitating urinary retention and glaucoma.

When conjunctival reactions are anticipated, sulphacetamide eye-drops should be prescribed routinely.

Persistent crusting may be a problem following treatments which include the nasal cavity, and regular removal of such crusts is of considerable benefit to the patient; this may need to be carried out for many months after the conclusion of treatment.

If reaction is present on the lips, vaseline or grease applied at night will prevent the lips from sticking together during sleep. Dilators prevent adhesions from obliterating the vagina following intracavitary treatments.

(c) *Encouragement of normal tissue recovery*. Many patients are in a poor nutritional state in consequence of age, self-neglect, alcohol abuse and the effects on dietary intake of the neoplasm itself. In particular, deficiencies of vitamin A and C impair healing in mucous membranes, and in the mouth and pharynx, where epithelial cell turn-over is fast, iron deficiency also compromises healing, since rapid cellular proliferation is dependent on adequate availability of iron for the cytochrome oxidase systems. Such deficiencies should be energetically corrected as soon as it becomes clear that therapeutic radiation will be required.

Care of late reactions

Occasionally, in consequence of misjudgement of tissue dose tolerance, trauma, infection, nutritional factors, age or injudicious retreatment of a previously irradiated site, the treated area either fails to heal or subsequently breaks down. Such necroses are usually painful, and healing is characteristically slow and may be incomplete. Secondary infection is common, and may have serious effects on the immediately subjacent devitalized tissues (for instance the laryngeal cartilages or the mandible) requiring major surgical intervention. These grave 'late reaction effects' are commonly a reflection of the extent of destruction caused by the tumour itself, and may more properly be termed 'tumour-related complications of irradiation'; they are discussed by site in the appropriate chapters of this book.

Lesser degrees and smaller areas of breakdown can often be successfully managed conservatively. The general principles of care are as outlined for the acute reactions. On the skin prolonged use of glucocorticoid ointments containing topical antibiotics such as neomycin will often coax a superficial necrosis to heal. Avoidance of cold winds, trauma (from for instance spectacle frames, and undergarment straps) should be avoided. Necroses on the skin of the face and neck not uncommonly follow exposure to strong sunlight, and these necroses nearly all heal with conservative measures. Irradiated skin may be atrophic and deficient in cerumen; whereas steroid ointments are useful for the treatment of acute necroses, their prolonged use increases the atrophy. Irradiated skin at risk of fissuring, with subsequent infection and necrosis, is best protected by regular use of petroleum jelly. Skin necroses greater than 20 cm² often require excision and grafting, preferably by a plastic surgeon experienced in working on irradiated tissue. Where excision of a cosmetically important structure such as the pinna or tip of nose is required, modern materials can be skilfully exploited to produce functionally and socially very acceptable prosthetic replacements.

Late necroses in mucous membranes may heal following the vigorous promotion of local hygiene, and the provision of an adequate diet. Physical factors, such as ill-fitting dentures, need immediate attention. Where conservative or surgical management is impossible or inappropriate, pain can be successfully controlled by repeated use of the cryoprobe, or by diathermy.

Summary

In the past ten years physicians have become increasingly involved in the management of patients with malignant disease. Indeed whatever his specific therapeutic approach any clinical oncologist requires a sound basis in medicine. As therapies are combined and become individually more aggressive multisystem supportive care is required for many patients undergoing treatment of malignant disease. Common emergencies are described here together with the increasingly important complications of both malignant disease and its therapies.

Further reading

Bagshawe, K.D. (ed.) (1975), *Medical Oncology: Medical Aspects of Malignant Disease*. Blackwell Scientific Publications, Oxford.
Holland, J.F. and Frei, E. (eds) (1980), *Cancer Medicine*, 2nd Edn. Lea and Febiger.
Seminars in Oncology (1978), **5**. Emergencies in oncologic practice.

References

Appel, G.B. and Neu, H.C. (1977), The nephrotoxicity of antimicrobial agents. *New Engl. J. Med.*, **296**, 663–70; 722–8; 784–7.
Barnett, W.D. (1976), Problems in abdominal surgery. VI: Intestinal obstruction from peritoneal carcinomatosis. *J. Miss. State Med. Assoc.*, **17**, 325.
Beeson, P.B. and McDermott, W. (eds) (1975) *Textbook of Medicine*. W.B. Saunders Company, Philadelphia, London, and Toronto.
Begent, R. (1977), Opportunistic infections of the central nervous system. *Br. J. Hosp. Med.*, **18**, 402–11.
Benson, W. *et al.* (1979), Spinal cord compression in myeloma, *Br. Med. J.*, **1** (6177): 1541–4.
Blackard, C.E. (1975), Veterans Administration Co-operative Urologic Research Group Studies of carcinoma of the prostate. A review. *Cancer Chemother. Rep.*, **59**, 225–7.
Blackledge, G.B. *et al.* (1979), A study of gastrointestinal lymphoma. *Clin. Oncol.*, **5**, 209–19.
Bonadonna, G. DeLena, M. and Monfardini, S. (1972), Clinical results with bleomycin in lymphomas and solid tumours. *Eur. J. Cancer*, **8**, 205.
Bruckman, J.E. and Bloomer, W.D. (1978), Management of spinal cord compression. *Sem. Oncol.*, **5**, 135–40.
Cortes, E.P. *et al.* (1973), Adriamycin cardiotoxicity in adults with cancer. *Clin. Res.*, **21**, 412.
Davies, D.A.L. and Pope, A.M.S. (1978), Mycolase, a new kind of systemic antimycotic. *Nature*, **273**, 235–6.
Friedman, M., Kim, T.H. and Panahon, A.M. (1976), Spinal cord compression in malignant lymphoma. *Cancer*, **37**, 1485–91.
Garmick, M.B. and Mayer, R.J. (1978), Acute renal failure associated with neoplastic disease and its treatment. *Sem. Oncol.*, **5**, 155–65.
Glass, R.L. and LeDue, R.J. (1973), Small intestinal obstruction from peritoneal carcinomatosis. *Ann. J. Surg.*, **125**, 316.
Glenn, F. and McSherry, C.K. (1974), Obstruction and perforation in colorectal cancer. *Ann. Surg.*, **173**, 983–92.
Ketcham, A.S. *et al.* (1970), Delayed intestinal obstruction following treatment for cancer. *Cancer*, **25**, 406.
Ketchel, J. and Rodriguez, V. (1978), Acute infections in cancer patients. *Sem. Oncol.*, **5**, 167–79.
Khan, F.R. *et al.* (1976), Treatment by radiotherapy of spinal cord compression due to extradural metastases. *Radiology*, **89**, 495–500.
Lewinsky, N.G. (1966), Management of emergencies. V. Acute renal failure. *New. Engl. J. Med.*, **274**, 1016–18.
Lewis, S.M. (1978), Newer methods of assessment for splenectomy. In: *Advanced Medicine*, (ed. D.J. Wetherall) Pitman Medical, Tunbridge Wells, pp. 200–9.
Luxton, R.W. (1961), Radiation nephritis, a long term study of 54 patients. *Lancet*, **ii**, 1221–4.
Mazzaferri, E.L., O'Dorisio, T.M. and LoBuglis, A.F. (1978), Treatment of hypercalcaemia associated with malignancy. *Sem. Oncol.*, **5**, 141–53.
Murphy, W.T. and Bilge, N. (1964), Compression of the spinal cord in patients with malignant lymphoma. *Radiology*, **22**, 495–500.

Nakayama, K. (1959), Statistical review of 5-year survivals after surgery for carcinoma of the oesophagus and cardiac portion of the stomach, *Surgery*, **45**, 883.

Perez, C.A., Preasant, C.A. and Amburg, A.C. Van. (1978), Management of superior vena caval syndrome. *Sem. Oncol.*, **5**, 123–34.

Pitman, S.W. and Frei, E. (1977), Weekly methotrexate – calcium leucovorin regime: effect of alkalinisation on nephrotoxicity. *Cancer Treat. Rep.*, **61**, 695–701.

Raichle, M.E. and Posner, J.B. (1970), The treatment of extradural spinal cord compression. *Neurology*, **20**, 391.

Rubin, P. *et al*. (1974), Cancer of the gastrointestinal tract. II Oesophagus: treatment – localized and advanced. *J. Am. Med. Assoc.*, **227**, 175–85.

Samman, P.D. (1977), Mycosis fungoides. *Bull. Cancer.*, **64**, 177.

Schecter, M.M. (1954), The superior vena caval syndrome. *Ann. J. Med. Sci.*, **227**, 46–56.

Schein, P.S. *et al*. (1978), 5-fluorouracil, mitomycin C and adriamycin (FAM); a new combination chemotherapy program for advanced gastric carcinoma. *Proc. Ass. Clin. Oncol.*, **17**, 264.

Sherlock, S. (1975), *Diseases of the Liver and Hepatobiliary System*. Blackwell Scientific Publications, Oxford.

Sise, J.G. and Crichlow, R.W. (1978, Obstruction due to malignant tumours. *Sem. Oncol.*, **5**, 213–24.

Staughton, R.C.D. (1978), Cutaneous manifestations of malignancy. *Br. J. Hosp.*, **20**, 38–47.

Walsh, J.P. and Donaldson, G.A. (1974), Management of severe obstruction of the large bowel due to malignant disease. *Ann. J. Surg.*, **127**, 492.

Weick, J.K. (1978), Intravascular coagulation in cancer. *Sem. Oncol.*, **5**, 203–11.

White, W.A., Patterson, R.H. and Bergland, R.M. (1971), Role of surgery in the treatment of spinal cord compression by metastatic neoplasm. *Cancer*, **25**, 558–61.

Wild, W.D. and Porter, R.W. (1963), Metastatic epidural tumour of the spine. A study of 45 cases. *Archs Surg.*, **87**, 137–42.

39 The care of advanced disease and psychological factors

Kenneth C. Calman

It is a truism to say that in the management of cancer the clinician must be aware not only of the natural history of the disease and its treatment but of the psychological impact of cancer on the patient. The patient must be treated as a whole. Attention has been focused in the past predominantly on the psychological effects of advanced disease and on patients with terminal illness. Yet this approach neglects the real and clinically important problems which occur early in the disease process. In this chapter psychological effects will therefore be discussed firstly in a general way, then in relation to the management of the patient with advanced disease. In addition the specific problems of terminal illness will be highlighted.

The psychological impact of cancer

While it is pertinent to consider the patient and his or her reaction to cancer, it is also relevant to consider the wider psychological effects of cancer. It is clear, for example, that cancer as a group of diseases engenders more fear in the public at large than any other disease (Aitken-Swan and Easson, 1959). This inbuilt fear not only inhibits discussion of the problem but creates a self-perpetuating cultural view that 'cancer' is a death sentence. What the public know about cancer, its diagnosis and treatment clearly affect the way in which the patients react to their illness. It affects the way we communicate with patients, what we say and how we act. The public expectation of cancer treatment may profoundly affect the attitudes of patients. If over optimistic, then the patient may become disappointed and resentful. If pessimistic, the patient may delay or avoid treatment. As with other aspects of cancer care, the family and friends are part of this communication cycle and their attitudes may also affect the patient.

Just as it is appropriate to consider the natural his-

tory of physical aspects of cancer, so it is important to consider the changes which may take place in the feelings of the patient from the beginning of his or her illness until the end. As the pattern of disease spread unfolds, so the changes in psychological response to the illness also change. The clinician must learn to recognize these changes in response and be ready to offer support accordingly. The greater part of the information on psychological aspects of cancer relates to the dying patient. In addition the effects of specific treatment problems, e.g. mastectomy, colostomy, etc. have also been studied in some detail. There are how-ever enormous gaps in our understanding of the psychological reactions of patients. These are concerned particularly with reactions to the diagnosis, the short-term and long-term effects of treatment and the effects of cancer on the family as a whole. Only tentative, and perhaps personal, conclusions can be drawn in this area.

Cancer also makes a major psychological impression on those caring for patients with cancer. This applies just as much to the care team involved in treating patients with early disease as to those dealing with advanced cancer. Involvement of doctors, nurses and paramedical personnel in the acute problems of the patient may lead to anxiety, depression and disillu-sionment. It is therefore essential that the leader of the cancer care team provides sufficient professional sup-port for the team. He must anticipate problems rather than have to deal with their consequences.

The role of the oncologist in this area of care must not be in doubt. He must make it his responsibility to see that these problems are covered and that sufficient expertise is made available to patients and relatives. Communication is perhaps the major area which links psychological aspects of cancer and terminal care. It should not be forgotten that the fears of the doctor or

nurse may become the fears of the patient. Communication, both verbal and non-verbal, may critically
affect the approach of the patient to his illness.

Psychological aspects of cancer

The psychological consequences of cancer may be
divided into three broad areas. The first of these relates
to physical aspects of cancer which may present as
psychological problems. The most obvious example of
this is brain metastases presenting as an organic
psychosis. The second area deals with the reactions of
the patient to knowledge of the diagnosis and how best
to influence such responses. The third area deals with
the psychological impact of cancer treatment on the
patient. Each of these will now be examined in detail.

Psychological consequences of organic disease

A not uncommon clinical problem is the patient with
cancer who develops confusion or a change in personality. It is not difficult under these circumstances to
ascribe these problems simply to the psychological
effects of the disease. Yet, unless a carefully taken
history and full clinical examination are performed, a
potentially remediable condition may be missed. Even
if the physical problem cannot be eliminated symptomatic improvement may occur.

It is also important to point out that cancer may
present with psychological problems, particularly
depression and non-specific symptoms and these may
often be overlooked or dismissed. This feature may be
related to specific cancers, notably cancer of the pancreas. There is some debate in the literature as to the
relationship between depression and cancer and it
must be assumed therefore that the question remains
open. The mechanism of the depression remains obscure. It may be related to tumour products or to
metabolic effects of the cancer.

Brain metastases may well present with a change in
personality and this may precede the clinical or
radiological picture. Other central nervous system
complications of malignancy such as the carcinomatous neuropathies are in a similar category. The important features are that the patient may not only have
physical signs but there may be loss of cognitive function. This latter possibility should always be checked
before a diagnosis of a psychological disorder is made.

Many of the metabolic complications of cancer may
give rise to symptoms of anxiety, depression and confusion. Cachexia is a common problem and the associated weakness and anorexia may result in depression.
Hypercalcaemia, vitamin deficiencies and the syndromes of inappropriate hormone secretion may result
in overt psychoses or confusion. Many of these compli-

cations can be confirmed by clinical examination and
relatively simple investigations.

In a recent review of patients referred for a
psychiatric opinion, Levine *et al.* (1978) found that
46% were suffering from an organic problem. This
figure illustrates the importance of defining the nature
and mechanism of the psychological problem.

*Psychological problems associated with know-
ledge of the disease*

The general fears which the word cancer arouses are
perhaps natural but the effects of these fears become
apparent when related to individual patients. The
perennial question 'Should the patient be told?' has
been discussed at length. It is clearly a matter on which
the individual oncologist must make up his own mind.
Yet there is surprisingly little evidence in the literature
as to the effects of 'telling' or 'not telling' (McIntosh,
1976). The anxiety begins from the time of diagnosis or
indeed the first symptom experienced by the patient.
This may be the case whether or not the diagnosis is
confirmed by the doctor. The anxiety and depression
experienced is also related to the patient's experience
of cancer in relatives and friends. This may greatly
influence the development of psychological problems.

One thing is clear, however, and that is that clinicians underestimate the psychological morbidity. This
is perhaps because they do not look for it or ask about
it. Anxiety and depression are not the only symptoms
however. Hostility (to the family, friends, the hospital,
the doctor) may be experienced, as may denial (of the
diagnosis, of the symptoms, of the prognosis). Each of
these problems may require a different approach.

In matters of communication it is essential to consider the individual patient; his or her personality, type
of disease, extent of spread, age, prognosis, family, etc.
Thus the approach to the patient with the early breast
cancer is likely to be different than to an elderly patient
with advanced gastric cancer. The oncologist must be
able to adjust his level of communication to the individual patient.

In some cases acute psychological problems may be
experienced and these are often related to diagnostic
or treatment events (Levine *et al.*, 1978). Acute depression or anxiety may require hospitalization and expert
psychiatric attention. With the less acute problems,
once recognized, the clinician must decide on appropriate treatment. In most cases time spent with the
patient will be beneficial – time to talk, to understand
and to define the particular problems. Once these have
been detailed practical help may be given. At the simplest level reassurance alone may be all that is required
or even no more than sympathetic listening. It is likely
however that the patient will need considerable sup-

port over this period of time and this support may be given by any member of the care team. The use of anti-depressants and tranquillizers is essential for a group of patients, though they should not be used in place of spending time with the patient. It is usually obvious when the patient requires expert psychiatric help. Patient referral should be early rather than late. The particular fears and anxieties concerning dying will be considered later.

It is a mistake to assume that all the problems of cancer patients are related to the neoplasm. The psychological problems experienced may also be associated with family matters and work. The use of an experienced social worker may be of great help in this matter. For a group of patients the problems which they have relate to theological questions and in such patients the minister of religion may have a major part to play.

The patient's relatives may also be under considerable strain and may experience psychological problems, anxiety and depression being the most common. This is particularly the case in childhood cancer, where the psychological impact on the parents may be very considerable. Active psychological support is essential in this case. The relatives themselves provide great support for the patient and their willingness to help may be harnessed with mutual benefit.

Treatment related psychological problems

Almost all forms of cancer treatment have side-effects and these effects are not only physical but also psychological. Although each modality will be considered separately, there are obvious overlaps and, as the concept of combined modality therapy gains ground, these interactions will increase (Priestman and Baum, 1976).

Surgical problems

Most surgical procedures carry with them an element of anxiety, though this is usually a temporary problem occurring at the time of the operation. Surgical operations which have attracted most attention from the psychological point of view are mastectomy, colorectal surgery, head and neck procedures and limb amputations.

1. *Mastectomy*. The psychological effects of breast removal are now being increasingly recognized (Morris *et al.*, 1977). In the short term it is thought that 25% of women who have undergone mastectomy will have psychiatric problems and 30% of patients who had an active sexual life before mastectomy will still be having problems 1–2 years later. The long-term problems remain to be defined. Increasingly attention is being

paid before operation to these facts and support programmes are being developed. It is hoped that these will reduce subsequent morbidity.

2. *Colorectal surgery*. There is also very good evidence that the creation of a colostomy may have major effects on the patient from a psychological point of view. Up to 25% of patients may experience clinically detectable problems. Sexual problems related to impotence may not only be related to the operative procedure but also to psychological effects of having a colostomy.

3. *Head and neck operations*. These have particular problems because of the potentially disfiguring effect on the face and neck. Speech problems serve only to accentuate this. Laryngectomy and tracheostomy have similar consequences.

4. *Amputation of limbs*. Particularly in the young this may have a wide ranging effect. The patient's social patterns may have to change. With support and the use of excellent prostheses now available, these problems should be less.

Radiotherapy

One of the unsolved problems of radiobiology is why patients who are having radiotherapy develop weakness and depression (Peck and Boland, 1977). This may occur in the absence of physical signs of side-effects. The depression which occurs is often profound, but resolves spontaneously. Radiotherapy may produce side-effects such as nausea, vomiting and local reactions. These in themselves may induce depression and anxiety.

Chemotherapy

As chemotherapy becomes increasingly used in cancer treatment, it is to be anticipated that the psychological morbidity will increase. It is important therefore that the clinician begins to recognize such problems and anticipate them. Because patients are dependent on regular chemotherapy and because they may have been told that they require treatment to prevent recurrence, they may fail to disclose the extent of their problems to the doctor. The patient is concerned that the doctor's attitudes might change and that the treatment (essential for their survival) might stop. Although drug specific complications may be a problem, it is mainly the non-specific problems of nausea, vomiting and alopecia which cause the major morbidity. Careful explanation before starting treatment may allay these fears but will not necessarily abolish them. Once complications have occurred then it may be more difficult to continue treatment and the patient may refuse therapy. The conflict in the patient's mind at this time should not be underestimated. Chemotherapy requires regular visits to a hospital and this in itself may induce a considerable number of psychological problems. The patient may vomit before coming to the clinic and in the end may refuse to come. An increasingly recognized side-effect of chemotherapy is their alteration of hormonal balance. This may alter mood but more significantly may alter fertility and sexual function. Amenorrhoea is common in pre-menopausal patients having regular chemotherapy. These effects may profoundly influence the relationship between the patient and the family and the psychological consequences of this are just being realized.

The side-effects of chemotherapy may also affect the family in other ways. In particular regular chemotherapy in the childhood malignancies has an enormous effect on the parents and marital problems may occur.

Pain

Although not specifically related to treatment but to the disease itself, pain may have profound effects on the psyche. The continuous unremitting unrelieved pain which can occur may turn a rational patient into a disturbed and changed personality. Adequate pain control may resolve the pain to normal and this will be discussed later. Conversely the use of anti-depressants may alleviate a component of pain.

The oncologist's approach to psychological problems

In this short section some of the psychological problems of the patient have been outlined. How then can the oncologist alter his approach to the patient (Miller, 1977)? He must become aware of the problems and begin to recognize them. He must realize that, if anything, *psychological morbidity is grossly underestimated*.

A prime factor for the patient is time. To allow the patient time to talk and time for the oncologist to understand the problems. When problems arise the patient should be given the advice of the appropriate member of the team and expert psychiatric help sought as soon as possible. Specialists in stoma care and in mastectomy problems should be used where necessary.

The family should be given special consideration and support and should be brought into the decision making process. The staff dealing with patients must also be given psychological help and they should be encouraged to discuss their problems.

Communication is the central theme. Each member of the team should be involved and it is useful to record in the patient's notes what the patient and relatives have been told and their reactions to this. In many hospitals special documents are used for this purpose and are regularly updated by the medical and nursing staff (Soukop and Calman, 1976).

The patient must be considered as an individual. The response to treatment, the prognosis of the tumour and many other factors should be borne in mind.

Terminal care

Terminal care may be defined as the management of patients in whom the advent of death seems certain and not too far off, in whom the diagnosis has been accurately made and in whom care has turned from the curative to the palliative. The crux of the definition is the switch from active anti-tumour therapy to active symptomatic therapy. In the first instance investigations are directed towards identifying tumour spread and treatment towards eliminating the tumour. In terminal care assessment of symptoms, their diagnosis and treatment forms the basis of management. This distinction between care and cure can be difficult. The boundaries are blurred, particularly in children and young adults, where active anti-tumour treatment may be prolonged and many attempts made to control the disease. The decision finally to stop cancer therapy is often extremely difficult, and one which may have to be revised in the light of clinical progress. Symptom control is part of active cancer therapy.

A second implication of the definition is that the diagnosis is established and that the symptoms complained of are related to the cancer. In other words every symptom may not necessarily relate to advancing disease (Byar *et al*., 1973). Before the decision is made to cease anti-tumour therapy it is essential that confirmation of tumour spread is made.

The management of the patient with terminal disease requires clearly defined aims. The first of these aims is to control symptoms and to render the patient comfortable and pain free. The second is to provide the patient with time to talk and allow him or her to discuss particular problems. The third aim is to provide the patient with an environment of caring.

The approach to management

The first essential is to check the diagnosis and confirm that the patient has evidence of advanced cancer. The second is to define the specific symptoms. This requires a careful history, full clinical examination and often simple investigations. The third is to consider whether or not further anti-tumour therapy would be appropriate. The fourth is to consider in detail the social and psychological situation of the patient. When these points have been considered it is then appropriate to deal with the specific symptoms.

The place of death

Most would agree that, where possible, the patient should die in his own home if that is what he wishes. However, this may not be possible for social reasons. The home circumstances may be inadequate. The principal caring relative may be unable to cope either due to infirmity or for psychological reasons. The relative may not be able to leave his employment temporarily. The cost of caring for a sick person at home may be more than the family can afford if the cost of heating the house, preparing special food or regular cleaning of linen is necessary. Lastly, the patient's symptoms may be such that in-patient attention is required. For these reasons alternative accommodation should be considered.

The first of these is the hospital ward where the bulk of the treatment has been carried out. The patient is likely to know the ward staff and may feel at home there. The disadvantage is that the time the nursing and medical staff can spend with the patient may be limited because of other patients with acute problems. Some hospitals have terminal care wards or symptom control units. If properly integrated into the hospital, these are invaluable sources of advice and expertise in terminal care.

As an alternative some hospitals have developed a symptom control team. This is an integrated group of doctors, nurses, social workers and ancillary staff who act as a peripatetic team, visiting patients in other wards and units but having no beds of their own. Advice and special expertise is made available and additional nursing support given as required. This system has the advantage that patients are not removed from the care of the parent unit and still feel they belong.

A further alternative is the hospice. In these units highly motivated medical and nursing staff are able to care for patients with terminal illness. Hospices have become the focus of teaching and development in terminal care and, with the establishment of home care programmes, are now reaching into the community.

The alternatives described above are not mutually exclusive. Indeed it is essential that flexibility of approach is maintained. As the needs of the patient change so the place where he is being nursed may also require changing. The wishes of the patient and relatives must always be borne in mind.

The problem orientated and goal orientated approaches to terminal care

In practical terms it is essential to have a philosophy of management. The two methods to be described need not be seen as opposing each other, rather they represent different approaches.

1. *Problem orientated*. The specific problems of the patient are defined, e.g. a. pain, right hip; b. nausea; c. young family at home. When these problems have been listed, decisions are then made as to the appropriate management, e.g. a. radiotherapy to right hip, start analgesia; b. start anti-emetic; c. contact social worker. Lists such as these simply formalize the clinician's approach and allow him to review at regular intervals the patient's problems. New problems are added and old ones removed.

2. *Goal orientated*. In this approach the patient and the medical team decide on specific goals for the patient to attain. This may be the control of pain, the ability to walk for a short period, the possibility of going home. Each goal must be carefully chosen and be within the limits of possibility. With this approach the patient and the medical team can be seen to be working towards the same aims.

Communication and terminal illness

The problems of communication with the cancer patient have already been discussed. In the patient with terminal illness communication becomes even more important (Hinton, 1974). If the patient has had cancer for some time and has been aware of the diagnosis, then when the period of terminal illness arrives it becomes more natural to discuss this with the patient. It must not be assumed, however, that this is an easy situation to deal with. In the patient who has never had the diagnosis discussed, then the problems may be even greater.

Communication at this stage, however, does not simply involve discussing the diagnosis and the problems of dying. This may be the least important area. Communication at this level implies a coming together and an understanding of the patient's problems. It means allowing the patient time to communicate his or her worries. It involves preserving relationships rather than destroying them (Brewin, 1977).

Communication is not only between the doctor and the patient, but involves the whole team. The relatives should be brought into the decisions to be made and the family brought together to share the experience. This may be extremely difficult to put into practice as it demands time, care and ability to understand the problems involved.

During the period of the terminal illness it has become customary to describe the stages of response through which patients may pass. While recognition of these stages is important, they must not be viewed rigidly. Each stage may require a different approach from the caring team. The first stage is often one of denial and isolation. The patient does not accept the inevitability of death. The second is of aggression and anger. In this stage the patient may ask questions such as 'Why has this happened to me?' or 'Why do I have to suffer?'. To answer these questions each doctor must use his own personal philosophy. There are no easy answers to these questions. The patient may then begin to bargain and clutch at events in the present or in the future which he or she thinks might help. Not surprisingly patients may well become depressed and only time and patience can help the patient at this stage. Where the depression becomes particularly difficult to deal with, anti-depressants may well be of benefit. The aim, of course, is to allow the patient to accept the fact that he is dying but provide him to the end with hope. Hope that symptoms will be controlled and the assurance that someone will be with them at the time of death.

With cancer patients dying of their disease there is often time to help them adjust to their illness. Death does not usually occur suddenly as in other diseases, and there is therefore the opportunity to prepare for the final outcome. The preservation of relationships within and without the family should be the aim during this time (Rees and Lutkins, 1967; Murray Parkes *et al.*, 1969). Each member of the team has a role and, in some patients, the minister or priest has a valuable part to play.

Symptom control

Cancer affects so many organ systems that it is not surprising that the symptoms arising may be very varied indeed. The approach outlined above of assessment and diagnosis of specific symptoms is the only way in which they can be readily and rapidly relieved. Pain is the symptom most commonly associated with cancer, yet it is less often a problem than some of the other distressing problems such as weakness, anorexia, nausea and vomiting.

It is pertinent to mention the prevention of some of these symptoms before discussing them in detail. Nursing care may prevent problems related to the skin and mouth. Thus bedsores, excoriation and dry, painful mouths can, to a large extent, be prevented. The patient should be encouraged to be as mobile as possible, to have daily baths and be out of bed and taking part in the hospital or home routine.

Mouth problems
Regular mouth hygiene may take care of ulceration or soreness. Regular inspection and the use of locally active anti-fungal agents, where appropriate, may relieve symptoms of pain. The use of frequent sips of water, fruit juice or ice will help to relieve a dry mouth.

Anorexia
This is a common symptom in terminal illness. It may

be extremely difficult to control. The use of corticosteroids or anabolic steroids may be of benefit. If the patient so desires, the use of alcoholic beverages before meals may stimulate the appetite.

Nausea and vomiting
If the vomiting is obstructive in origin the use of strong analegesics and anti-emetics may relieve symptoms. The use of a nasogastric tube with suction may be necessary in some instances. Where nausea is the major problem, anti-emetics, often in combination, may be useful. Regular medication is essential and, in severe nausea, this may require to be administered parenterally.

Constipation
This may be related to the tumour, or secondary to the use of analgesics. Regular mild aperients may be all that is required. Where the problem is more severe, locally active suppositories or enemas may be required.

Diarrhoea
This is a particularly distressing symptom and may be related to several things including the tumour, the use of drugs (e.g. antibiotics), impaction or infection. Simple physical examination and bacteriological testing will exclude some of these. Several proprietary preparations may be used to control the diarrhoea. Where previous surgical procedures have been performed, blind-loop syndrome may occur and the use of antibiotics or bile salts may be indicated.

Dysphagia
This is a very troublesome symptom. The patient may have severe pain and, in advanced cases, may not even be able to swallow saliva. Choking and dyspnoea may occur and in this case adequate sedation is essential.

Hiccough
This may be associated with renal failure or diaphragmatic irritation. It can often be controlled with metoclopramide or chlorpromazine.

Ascites
Recurrent ascites can be associated with pain and dyspnoea. Regular paraceutesis may be necessary. The instillation of chemotherapeutic agents may be of benefit but this requires careful consideration in the period of terminal illness.

Cough
This may be caused by the tumour itself or to superimposed infection when several antibiotics may be justified. Control with proprietary cough suppressants or

even diamorphine may be useful, especially if pain is also present.

Dyspnoea

Careful physical examination often with the aid of simple investigations may be necessary to determine the exact cause of breathlessness. It may be related to primary or secondary malignant disease in the chest, pleural effusion, cardiac failure, intra-abdominal pressure or chest infection. The cause should be treated wherever possible. A bronchodilator may help and, where the tumour mass is large, prednisolone may be of benefit. In this symptom, as with many others, anxiety may be a compounding problem and the use of anxiolytic drugs may be indicated. When a distressing rattle is present on breathing, hyoscine may prevent the accumulation of secretions. When dyspnoea occurs suddenly, as with a pulmonary embolism, the use of opiates and hyoscine will rapidly relieve symptoms.

Pruritis

Skin involvement of jaundice may give rise to this symptom. Cholestyramine is indicated where there is obstructive jaundice. Antihistamines or steroids may be necessary when other conditions are present and recently cimetidine has been used.

Insomnia

This frequent complaint is often overlooked. Patients unable to sleep at night may sleep during the day and the whole routine of the home or hospital reversed. It should be remembered that drugs used to treat insomnia may give rise to other symptoms such as confusion.

Confusion

It is essential to exclude a metabolic cause for this and be sure that it is not related to drug overdosage. Treatment for hypercalcaemia (with prednisolone for example) may reduce the confusional state. Where no remedial cause is determined, the use of chlorpromazine or diazepam may be required. Anxiety and depression are common accompaniments of terminal illness and should be treated appropriately.

Local skin problems

Fungating skin lesions may be particularly distressing. Regular dressings may be required and the topical applications of antibiotic creams and solutions may be required.

Pain control

Pain is the symptom most often alleged to be associated with terminal cancer, yet severe pain occurs in only 15–20% of patients. In most instances the pain can be readily controlled, and in only a minority will pain be completely unrelieved. The severe continuous pain which can occur is best described as total pain, an experience which affects the physical, mental, social and spiritual wellbeing of the patient. It completely takes over the patient and pervades all aspects of life.

The fact that pain control can now be more readily achieved is due to the elucidation of certain principles of pain control.

1. The diagnosis of the cause of the pain and the use of specific therapy where indicated.
2. An understanding of the nature of chronic pain and of its ability to wear down the patient.
3. The importance of *regular* therapy. As chronic pain is present all the time, the only method of completely abolishing it is to anticipate the pain and administer analgesia before the pain returns. This may mean increasing dosages and decreasing the time interval between them. The dosages are adjusted to meet the needs of the individual patient.
4. Explanation to the patient. The patient should be involved in the management. He may wish to know why the treatment is being given and what is to be achieved. The patient may be asked to note the response to pain relief and assist in dosage modification.
5. Addiction is not a problem in pain control in terminal illness. Indeed once pain control is achieved, the dosage may even be reduced.

Methods of pain control

There are now many methods available for pain control. Radiotherapy and chemotherapy may be used in some instances specifically to control pain due to cancer spread. In patients with terminal illness due consideration should be given to the ethics of these procedures.

Analgesic therapy is often the simplest way of controlling pain. In general the mildest analgesics are used first and, if given regularly, may be very effective. Recently the use of prostaglandin inhibitors (aspirin and related compounds) have been used specifically to control bone pain related to invasive cancer. If the pain is more severe then the choice of analgesic will have to be reviewed and, in the most severe form of pain, regular diamorphine or morphine therapy may be required. These drugs can be combined with antiemetics or tranquillizers such as chlorpromazine.

There are now many methods of neurosurgical pain relief. These range from the use of local nerve blocks and intrathecal injections to procedures on the spinal cord such as cordotomy.

Because of the wide range of procedures and drugs available there is a case for the development of pain control groups where expertise can be developed and shared.

Terminal care in childhood

The specific problems of terminal care in childhood have already been mentioned. The effects of a dying child involve the family and the whole caring team. Special expertise is required in this area of cancer care. Children have a concept of death which is different to that of adults. They see it not associated with pain or suffering but as a form of separation which may not seem so final as it does in adulthood.

Terminal care – a summary

One of the most frequent comments that a clinician may be tempted to make to the patient or the relatives is 'I'm afraid there is nothing more we can do'. While this may be true of the tumour, it is certainly not true of the patient. To treat patients with advanced cancer and to share in their experience of dying can be one of the most rewarding aspects of cancer care. The relatives must not be forgotten and follow up after bereavement often reveals a host of problems which may require special attention.

Further reading

Cartwright, A. and Anderson, J.L. (1973), *Care of the Dying*, Routledge and Kegan Paul, London.

Hinton, J. (1972), *Dying*, Penguin books, Harmondsworth, Middlesex.

Murray Parkes, C. (1972), *Bereavement: Studies of Grief in Adult Life*, Tavistock Publications, London.

Ross, E.K. (1970), *On Death and Dying*, Tavistock Publications, London.

Saunders, C.M. (ed.) (1978), *The Management of Terminal Disease*, Arnold, London.

References

Aitken-Swan, J. and Easson, E.C. (1959), Reactions of cancer patients on being told their diagnosis. *Br. Med. J.*, **1**, 779–83.

Brewin, T.B. (1977), The cancer patient communication and morale. *Br. Med. J.*, **2**, 1623–7.

Byar, D.P., Mantel, M. and Hankey, B.F. (1973), Predicting survival in terminal cancer. *Br. Med. J.*, **1**, 611–13.

Hinton, J. (1974), Talking with people about to die. *Br. Med. J.*, **3**, 25–7.

Levine, P.M., Silverfarb, P.M. and Lipowski, Z.J. (1978), Mental disorders in cancer patients. *Cancer*, **42**, 1385–91.

McIntosh, J. (1976), Patient's awareness and desire for information about diagnoses but in disclosed malignant disease. *Lancet*, **ii**, 300–3.

Miller, T.R. (1977), Psychiphysiologic aspects of cancer. *Cancer*, **39**, 413–18.

Morris, T., Greer, H.S. and White, P. (1977), Psychological and social adjustment to mastectomy. *Cancer*, **40**, 2301–7.

Murray Parkes, C., Bentamin, B. and Fitzgerald, R.G. (1969), Broken heart: a statistical study of increased mortality among widowers. *Br. Med. J.*, **1**, 740–3.

Peck, A. and Boland, J. (1977), Emotional reactions to radiation treatment. *Cancer*, **40**, 180–4.

Priestman, T.J. and Baum, M. (1976), Evaluation of the quality of life in patients receiving treatment for advanced breast cancer. *Lancet*, **i**, 899–901.

Rees, W.D. and Lutkins, S. (1967), Mortality of bereavement. *Br. Med. J.*, **4**, 13–16.

Soukop, M.S. and Calman, K.C. (1976), Communication and cancer patients. *Practitioner*, **216**, 90–2.

40 Radiotherapy equipment

C.J. Karzmark

Radiotherapy treatment employs both photon and particulate radiations, ranging in energy from about 10 kV to tens of MeV or higher. The treatment units may be conventional X-ray generators or sophisticated particle accelerators. Today, megavoltage photon treatment beams and isocentric mountings predominate, and the electron linear accelerator or linac is rapidly becoming the most widely used treatment unit. Significant improvements in accessories and ancillary equipment have added to their efficacy. Treatment unit designs increasingly incorporate human engineering aspects which improve and simplify treatment.

Equipment for low and medium energy X-rays

Historically, orthovoltage X-rays ranging from 200 to 400 kV in energy were widely used, but the megavoltage beams have largely supplanted them. Where shallow penetration suffices, electron beams often are used in lieu of softer X-rays ranging from 10 to 100 kV. Extensive intracavity therapy frequently employs implants of ^{192} Ir, ^{125} I or other radionuclides. Intraoral and intravaginal X-ray techniques can best be provided by orthovoltage units. Some institutions have found that medium energy X-rays, typically 140 kV and 0.3 mm Cu HVL, provide a useful bridge between superficial and deep therapy, particularly for skin cancers. Such beams are frequently preferable to high energy electrons which do not deposit sufficient dose at and near the skin surface.

Equipment for megavoltage X-rays and electrons

Selection of megavoltage equipment; radiation physics considerations

A number of radiation physics principles determine parameters of substantial clinical significance. A useful general reference is Meredith (1958).

Fig. 40.1 contrasts the central axis depth-dose curves for photon and electron beams of several energies. Near the surface, the photon beams exhibit a significant build up, but electron beams typically have 80% or higher surface dose. The fall-off in dose with depth is particularly rapid for low energy electrons, but as energy increases the electron depth-dose curve increasingly resembles those for megavoltage X-rays. Hence, high energy electron equipment does not appear warranted on this basis. In general, a higher energy unit is likely to be more costly to acquire, house, operate and maintain.

As energy is increased from diagnostic to megavoltage X-ray beam energies, photoelectric absorption is supplanted by Compton interactions as the main mechanism, and physical density rather than atomic number dominates in attenuating the beam. As a consequence, port films show less and less detail as energy is increased, particularly at and above 10 MeV.

Many lesions are treated with parallel opposed X-ray fields. For good dose uniformity to thicknesses of about 15 cm, 4–10 MeV X-ray beams are optimum. However for thick sections, such as the lateral pelvis, these energies entail greater variation in dose with the concomitant problem of sub-cutaneous fibrosis. Here photon energies of 20 MeV or even more provide significant improvements in uniformity. However, the attractive low surface dose of very high energy X-rays is offset by the problem of high exit doses for thinner sections.

X-ray production increases rapidly with energy in the megavoltage region, for example, by a factor of about eight between 4 and 8 MeV. However, the angular distribution is increasingly peaked in the forward direction such that more severe flattening is required. At the higher energies it becomes difficult to achieve and maintain large flat fields.

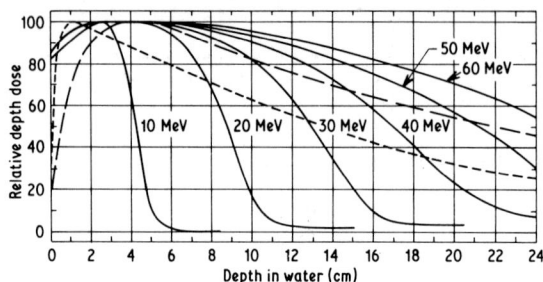

Fig. 40.1   Large field central-axis depth-dose curves for an electron beam at 200 cm SSD. The dotted line is a depth-dose curve for a 5 MeV X-ray beam, 10 × 10 cm field, 100 cm FSD. The broken line is a depth-dose curve for a 22 MeV X-ray beam, 100 cm FSD.

Electron therapy requires less beam current than X-rays for a given dose rate, typically by a factor of 100 to 1000. Hence, for units which provide both modalities, good technical and procedural safety considerations are imperative to ensure radiation safety. Providing a wide variety of flattened electron field sizes is more difficult with electrons. Considerable effort is being expended at this time to improve electron scattering and collimation systems to provide better field uniformity and for simplified, lighter-weight electron collimators.

Electron linear accelerators

Linear particle accelerators evolved at the same time as the better known circular machines, the cyclotron and the betatron. These early physics research machines constitute the historical antecedents of the modern, microwave-powered electron linear accelerator (or linac) now widely used for X-ray and electron radiation therapy.

During and shortly after World War II, high-power, microwave power sources were developed for radar applications. These pulsed diode sources, the magnetron and klystron, are capable of establishing intense electromagnetic fields in suitably designed microwave cavities. The field intensities and frequencies were high enough for linear acceleration of electrons to multimegavolt energies through physically acceptable microwave structures. During the mid-1940s, one group in England and another at Stanford succeeded in building a linear array of coupled cavities capable of both transporting the microwave power and accelerating injected electrons. These programs embraced the wartime hardware and technology in adopting 3000 MHz, a 10-cm free-space wavelength, as the design frequency. Such pulsed linear accelerators can provide high average beam currents and large energy gains in structures

which remain at DC ground potential. These were travelling wave linear accelerators in which the electrons are accelerated by an axial electric field advancing at a suitable velocity down the microwave accelerating structure. Recently developed standing wave microwave electron linacs offer radiotherapy a shorter accelerating structure length for a given energy and microwave power. A general reference for electron linear accelerators for radiation therapy is Karzmark and Pering (1973).

Microwave cavities, power generation and linear accelerator principles

Microwave cavities support specific electric (E) and magnetic (H) field configurations and are ideally suited for use in power generation and in electron acceleration. On the one hand, energetic electrons can generate microwave power by exciting the microwave cavities of klystrons and magnetrons, and, conversely, a linear array of cavities can operate as an electron accelerator by transferring the energy from the cavity fields to an electron beam. Most cavities are cylindrical but other shapes are feasible. The electrical conductors commonly used to transmit power at lower frequencies are inefficient for microwaves. Hollow circular or rectangular pipes, called waveguides, are employed for microwave power transmission. They have field configurations similar to those found in cavities. To improve clarity in microwave structure illustrations, the H field will be omitted since it is of only minor importance for our objectives.

1. *Microwave power generation*. Electromagnetic power at microwave frequencies is generated in appropriately energized cavities. Energy can be abstracted from an electron or electron bunch which has been accelerated by a DC potential and then injected into a cavity at the moment when a decelerating electric field will slow it down. By conservation of energy, the electron kinetic energy is transferred to the oscillating electromagnetic field of the cavity. In broad terms, these phenomena are employed in both klystrons and magnetrons as well as in many other power-generating and power-amplifying microwave devices.

An elementary, two-cavity klystron is shown in Fig. 40.2. An electron beam produced by a cathode and an accelerating DC potential travels axially through the cylindrical cavities and is absorbed by the collector. The first (buncher) cavity bunches the electrons so that they arrive at the second (catcher) cavity as a sequence of electron bunches at microwave frequency. The second cavity is resonant at the arrival frequency of the bunches and a large portion of their kinetic energy is converted into electromagnetic energy in the same manner described above.

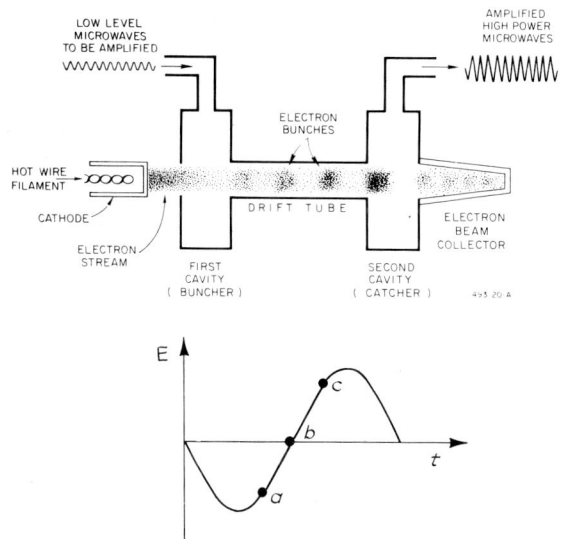

Fig. 40.2 Cross-sectional drawing of an elementary two-cavity klystron tube used as a microwave power amplifier and the phase diagram for the buncher cavity E field. The bunching action of the E field established across the buncher cavity is described in the text.

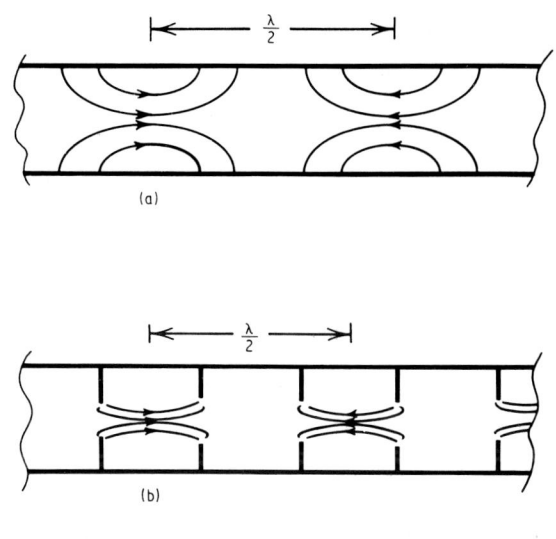

⇌ E field

Fig. 40.3 Spatial travelling wave electric field configuration for: (*a*) smooth cylindrical waveguide and (*b*) disc-loaded cylindrical waveguide. The cross-sections shown contain the cylindrical axis of symmetry.

The bunching operation of the first cavity is called velocity modulation since it alters the velocity but not the number of electrons transversing the tube. In terms of the microwave cycle shown in Fig. 40.2, electrons arriving at the first cavity early in the cycle at time *a* are slowed down by the E field; those arriving midway in time, *b*, are not affected; while those arriving late, *c*, are speeded up. As a result, the electrons arrive at the second cavity in compact bunches.

The magnetron also employs velocity modulation but the geometry is cylindrical in contrast to the linear geometry characterizing the klystron. Typically, magnetrons operating at 10-cm wavelength provide a 2 MW peak power output; klystrons providing 5–10 MW output are used with higher energy linacs.

2. *Travelling wave accelerating structures.* Let us extend our earlier discussion of electron interaction with a cavity for power generation to the converse case where energy is transferred from the cavity to the electron, that is, from the linear accelerator structure. Consider an electromagnetic wave having an axial E field travelling down a cylindrical waveguide into which electrons may be injected. Fig. 40.3a illustrates the E field at one instant of time in such a cylindrical waveguide. A smooth cylindrical waveguide is unsatisfactory for accelerating electrons because the phase velocity v_p of the travelling E field is higher than the

velocity of light, c, the limiting value for particulate velocities. To be accelerated to a prescribed energy and not lost from the beam, electrons must attain the phase velocity of the wave which for megavoltage energies will approach the velocity of light. Many microwave structures exist to reduce the phase velocity to c or less. Fig. 40.3b shows the most common structure in general use, the disc-loaded waveguide which operates as a linear array of coupled cavities. A non-uniform, disc-loaded structure in which phase velocity is gradually increased to $v_p \sim c$ is called a buncher. Electrons, injected at about 80 keV, will be captured and gain energy by travelling with a wave of increasing phase velocity and many will also be bunched, thereby capturing a large portion of the injected electron current on the wave. A buncher section typically constitutes the initial 30 cm of the structure. Thereafter, the structure is uniformly disc-loaded so that $v_p = c$ and the electron velocity v_e asymptotically approaches c as the energy increases.

Travelling wave structures require a terminating load to absorb the residual power at the end of the structure in order to prevent a backward reflected wave and possible electrical breakdown. In general, the microwave input power is divided between the electron beam, the structure and the termination.

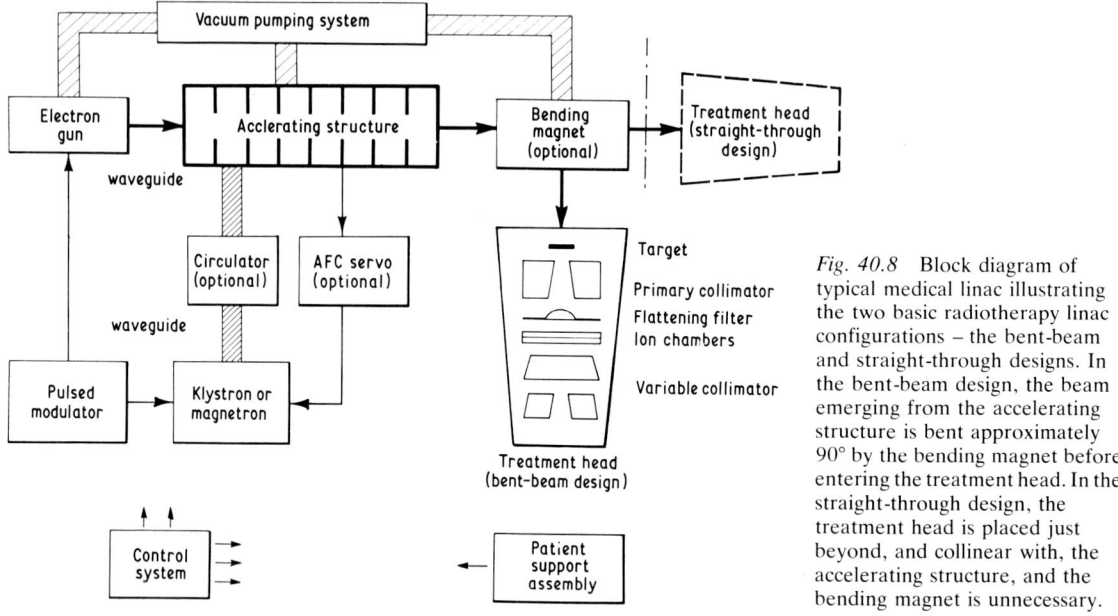

Fig. 40.8   Block diagram of typical medical linac illustrating the two basic radiotherapy linac configurations – the bent-beam and straight-through designs. In the bent-beam design, the beam emerging from the accelerating structure is bent approximately 90° by the bending magnet before entering the treatment head. In the straight-through design, the treatment head is placed just beyond, and collinear with, the accelerating structure, and the bending magnet is unnecessary.

characteristics or the electron energy incident on the vacuum window, the scattering foil or the phantom surface.

Table 40.1 provides a summary of the performance specifications of currently available radiotherapy linacs. All linacs listed operate at S-band frequencies of approximately 3000 MHz corresponding to a free space wave length of about 10 cm. On some units the field size given may be smaller than listed because of rounded corners arising from a conical primary collimator limitation. For many units, large X-ray fields can be provided at increased distances with a corresponding sacrifice in dose rate. Some collimators do not close completely and the minimum field size may, for example, be as large as 3 × 3 cm.

1. *Isocentric mounting*. The isocentric mounting and coordinate motions used in the majority of modern treatment linacs are illustrated in Fig. 40.9. Using this particular combination of couch and accelerator motions, patients can be set-up for treatment rapidly and accurately. For most treatment techniques, the patient lies prone or supine on the treatment couch with the tumour centre located at the isocentre, a point fixed in space and defined by the orthogonal intersection of the horizontal axis of the gantry rotation and the central axis of the X-ray beam. Patient positioning is customarily aided by skin marks and lights which project cross-hair shadows through the isocentre from side and overhead locations. Once the patient is correctly

positioned, the gantry can be rotated rapidly to the treatment angle. A serious geometrical misalignment is unlikely using this coordinate system and set-up procedure.

2. *Ancillary linac features*. The non-mechanical sputter ion vacuum pump developed in the late 1950s has proved eminently satisfactory for radiotherapy linacs. The improved vacuums led to the use of long-lived, low temperature, dispenser oxide and thoriated tungsten cathodes. These new vacuum and cathode technologies encouraged the further development of sealed-off accelerator structures having both long-lived cathodes and ion pumps incorporated in a single assembly, which is easy to replace as a unit.

Improvements in beam transport systems in recent years have resulted in smaller focal spots with decreased penumbra. Typically, linac X-ray focal spot sizes are 1–3 mm in diameter. Beam transport systems for radiotherapy linacs are conveniently divided into collinear (straight-through) and bent-beam designs (Fig. 40.8). In the former, the treatment head is located just beyond, and collinear with, the accelerating structure while in the latter (bent-beam) system, a nominal 90° or 270° magnetic deflection system is incorporated, generally, in an isocentric mounting (Fig. 40.9). Changes of energy, as well as variations of the angle and position of the electron beam on the target, tend to produce detrimental asymmetries in the treatment field. Nominal 270° 'achromatic' magnetic

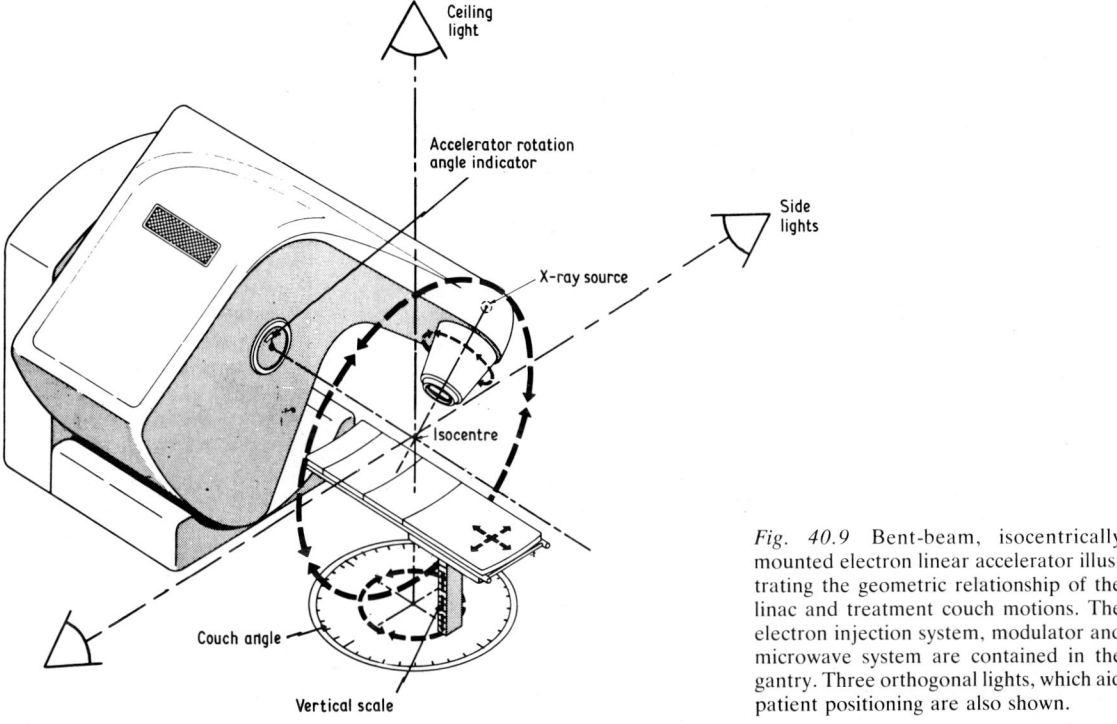

Fig. 40.9 Bent-beam, isocentrically mounted electron linear accelerator illustrating the geometric relationship of the linac and treatment couch motions. The electron injection system, modulator and microwave system are contained in the gantry. Three orthogonal lights, which aid patient positioning are also shown.

deflection systems have been developed which provide improved energy and spatial focusing as compared to nominal 90° systems. The advantage of such systems is that they give a more stable and symmetrical radiation beam.

Linac electronic systems increasingly employ integrated circuit (IC) technology and often have adopted digital, in place of analog, methods. These advances have improved the reliability and decreased the size of electronic systems, often by a factor as large as ten. Maintenance of ICs and discrete components is not routinely required, but, when necessary, is easy because the etched circuit cards, characteristic of the technology, can readily be removed and substitutes tried. The digital systems interface more readily to computers. Small computers or microprocessors can be used to control, monitor and store information pertaining to patient treatment as well as linac operation. They have been used to record a treatment prescription and to verify the daily sequence of treatment. Computers can be used to provide dynamic treatment via programming collimator jaws motion together with movement of the patient with respect to the treatment beam. Dual dosimetry monitors, which provide independent exposure limit backup, are now required. The digital logic of such dosimeter and control systems facilitates rapid programmed self-test regimes of dosimeter and other circuits prior to each treatment exposure. A reference for computer applications in radiology is Sternick (1976).

Microtrons

The microtron is an electron accelerator which combines the principles of both the electron linac and the cyclotron. In it, the electron gains energy from a single microwave cavity and describes orbits of increasing radius in the *H* field. Since megavoltage electrons have an approximately constant velocity, the cyclotron principle by itself cannot be used. Instead, the electrons arrive in the correct phase at the cavity by permitting them to slip an integral number of microwave cycles with each revolution in the magnetic field as they describe orbits of increasing radii. The cavity voltage, frequency and magnetic fields are so adjusted that after each transit through the cavity the electron gains sufficient energy so that its transit time in the magnetic field increases by an integral number of RF cycles. Fig. 40.10*a* illustrates the principle of a conventional microtron.

The principal advantages of the conventional microtron (Fig. 40.10*a*) are: 1. it uses a single cavity for

Table 40.1 Performance specifications of radiotherapy linacs.

Mfr.	Model	Beam energy and modality	SAD (cm)/ isocentre height (cm)	Gantry rotation limits (degree)	Accelerator structure, length and type (TW = Travelling wave SW = Standing wave)
AECL/ CGR-MeV	Therac 6/ Neptune	6 MV X-rays	100/125	365	1.0 on TW
AECL/ CGR-MeV	Therac 20/ Saturne	18 MV X-rays 6–20 MeV electrons*	100/128	365	2.3 m TW
AECL/ CGR-MeV	Therac 40/ Sagittaire	25 MV X-rays 7-32 MeV electrons*	105/114	±105 or 360 w/floor pit	6.0 m TW 2 sections
EMI	EMI Four	4 MV X-rays	100/130	370	0.3 m SW
EMI	EMI Six	6 MV X-rays	100/130	370	0.3 m SW
Philips/ Mel	SL75-5	4–6 MV X-rays	100/118	420	1.25 m TW
Philips/ Mel	SL75-14	8 and 10 MV X-rays 4–14 MeV electrons	100/123	370	2.5 m TW
Philips/ Mel	SL75–20	8 and 16 MV X-rays 5–20 MeV electrons	100/123	370	2.5 m TW
Radiation Dynamics	Dynaray 4	4 MV X-rays	100/122	370	0.75 m TW
Radiation Dynamics	Dynaray 6	6 MV X-rays	100/122	370	1.0 m TW
Radiation Dynamics	Dynaray 10	8 MV X-rays 4–10 MeV electrons	100/122	360	2.25 m TW
Radiation Dynamics	Dynaray 18	6 and 12 MV X-rays 5–18 MeV electrons	100/122	360	2.25 m TW
SIEMENS	Mevatron 6	6 MV X-rays	100/130	390	1.1 m SW
SIEMENS	Mevatron 12/74	10 MV X-rays 5–12 MeV electrons	100/130	360	1.3 m SW
SIEMENS	Mevatron 20	10 or 15 MV X-rays 2.5–18 MeV electrons	100/132	360	1.6 m SW
TOSHIBA	LMR-15	10 MV X-rays 10, 12, 14, 16 MeV electrons	100/124	±210	1.8 m TW
Varian	Clinac 4	4 MV X-rays	80/123	360	0.3 m SW
Varian	Clinac 4/100	4 MV X-rays	100/128	360	0.3 m SW
Varian	Clinac 6X	6 MV X-rays	80/123	360	0.3 m SW
Varian	Clinac 6/100	6 MV X-rays	100/133	360	0.3 m SW
Varian	Clinac 12	8 MV X-rays 6–12 MeV electrons	100/130	±185	1.0 m SW

Microwave power source	Bending magnet (degree)	X-ray field size at SAD cm²	Parameter output for computer interface	Comments or special features
2 MW magnetron	approx 270	40 × 40	yes	No primary collimator cut-off on 40 × 40 cm field. Record and verify as standard. Demountable electron gun.
5 MW klystron	approx 270	40 × 40	yes	No primary collimator cut-off on 40 × 40 cm field. Record and verify as standard. 10 MV X-rays optional; demountable electron gun.
10 MW kylstron	+30, −30 +30, −120	38 × 38	yes	No primary collimator cut-off on 38 × 38 cm field. Record and verify optional; 40 MeV electrons optional; constant gradient structure; 4 magnet achromatic beam transport system. Optional 1000 rad/min/m X-ray beams.
2 MW magnetron	no bend	40 × 40	yes	Computer-based video display; retractable beam stopper; optional record and verify.
2.5 MW magnetron	no bend	40 × 40	yes	Computer-based video display; retractable beam stopper; optional record and verify.
2 MW magnetron	90	40 × 40	yes	Retractable beam shield; demountable electron gun.
2.5 MW magnetron	90	40 × 40	yes	Demountable electron gun.
5 MW magnetron	90	40 × 40	yes	Experimental electron beam. Demountable electron gun; wall mounted gantry.
2 MW magnetron	266	30 × 30	no	5 MV optional.
2 MW magnetron	266	30 × 30	no	6 MV versions of Dynaray 4.
2 MW magnetron	266	35 × 35	no	Electromechanical modality changeover.
5 MW klystron	266	35 × 35	no	Electromechanical modality changeover.
2 MW magnetron	approx 261	35 × 35	no	Retractable beam stopper.
2 MW magnetron	approx 261	35 × 35	yes	Treatment verification system; retractable beam stopper.
7 MW klystron	approx 261	40 × 40	yes	Treatment verification system; retractable beam stopper.
4.8 MW magnetron	105	30 × 30	no	Multileaf collimator; wedge filter interlock.
2 MW magnetron	no bend	32 × 32	no	Original short SW therapy linac.**
2.5 MW magnetron	no bend	40 × 40	yes	100 cm SAD version of Clinac 4; motion interlock.**,†
2 MW magnetron	no bend	32 × 32	no	More efficient guide design, gives higher energy than Clinac 4.**
2.5 MW magnetron	no bend	40 × 40	yes	100 cm SAD version of 6X; motion interlock.**, †
2 MW magnetron	270	35 × 35	no	IC controlled logic; retractable beam stopper.**,†

employed have included neutrons, protons, singly and multiply charged heavier ions as well as negative pi-minus mesons (pions). Heavy ions under study range from carbon to neon. Pion beams being investigated for radiotherapy have been produced by both electron and proton high energy linacs. Such units have first been employed in providing a broad base of dosimetric and radiobiological data as a necessary precursor to clinical use. The performance of a novel pion treatment unit, which employed up to sixty cylindrically convergent beams, has been described by Pistenma *et al.* (1977).

For the charged particle beams, energies of hundreds of MeV may be required to penetrate 20 cm or more of tissue. As a consequence, large laboratory accelerators with fixed beams are often characteristic. An accelerator system intended for routine hospital-based clinical radiotherapy must be cost-effective, reliable and must provide benefits clearly not available from conventional modalities.

Neutron radiotherapy, whose advantage appears tied to the hi-LET component, can be provided with accelerators of 50 MeV or less, and an isocentric neutron therapy unit has been developed commercially. In one version, 42 MeV protons striking a thick beryllium target yield dose rates of about 100 rad/min in air at 125 cm SSD. The depth of 50% dose is about 14 cm. The option of three-dimensional pencil-beam scanning is under investigation. Collimation, dosimetry and treatment planning for heavy particle beams is more complex and crucial than for megavoltage X-rays. A number of clinical trials are currently underway to assess and compare the efficacy of heavy particle therapy (pion, neutron, proton, etc) to more conventional modalities. Two general references are Raju and Phillips (1977) and Rubin (1977). All heavy particle accelerators, including those for neutron therapy, can be used to produce a variety of radionuclides of interest to biology and medicine.

Treatment simulators

The introduction of megavoltage beams, characterized by a small penumbra and a large depth dose, necessitated improved treatment planning. Megavoltage port films provide useful confirmation during therapy but lack the diagnostic quality essential for planning. Conventional diagnostic generators do not adequately duplicate geometric aspects of a treatment unit and beam. This led to the development of simulators which provide this duplication in varying degrees. A general reference on simulators and their use is by the British Institute of Radiology (1976).

The simulator serves two important functions: accurate localization of the tumour volume with respect to surrounding anatomy and verification that the treatment field to be employed covers the tumour as prescribed. Simulation, under proper circumstances, may increase utilization of treatment units. In addition, simulators have been found useful for brachytherapy localization procedures. Most simulators are isocentric with 100 cm SAD. All incorporate radiography and some provide fluoroscopy with image intensification. The simulator should be close to the treatment planning suite; a nearby rapid film processor facilitates the simulation procedure. High output generators are needed for large field, large SSD (e.g. 150 cm) techniques associated with simulation. The more closely a simulator duplicates a specific treatment unit the more readily can the treatment be implemented. However, economics usually dictate that the simulator be used with several different treatment units. Such general purpose simulators are available from a number of manufacturers. Increased versatility adds to simulator cost and mechanical precision is more difficult to achieve and maintain. Where treatment units incorporate confirm-and-record or other computer-assisted features, one may wish to implement some of them on the simulator and to establish a link to the treatment planning computer.

The simulation procedure will benefit from the use of wall or ceiling-mounted light beams which define the entry point on the patient's skin of orthogonal rays directed towards the isocentre. Frequently, simulator fluoroscopy will permit options similar to those of conventional diagnostic fluoroscopy units.

Table 40.2 provides a comparison of some commercial simulator specifications and a recommendation by a BIR working party.

Computerized axial tomographs

The recent introduction of the computerized axial tomograph (CAT) has significant potential for improving tumour localization.

Technological development of CATs is proceeding rapidly and includes improved resolution, both spatial and density, decreased scanning times, synchronization with physiological signals, simplifications in both hardware and software, together with reductions in cost. It has been suggested that CAT-scanning might prove cost-effective for radiation therapy in the United States if only a 3–4% gain were made in the cure of approximately 125 000 patients currently dying of local-regional cancer. The role of CAT-scanning for radiotherapy has been described by Stewart and Simpson (1977).

Accessories

Treatment couches

The movement range and versatility of treatment couches is of paramount importance in the effectiveness of a particular treatment unit. The couch selected should provide comfortable, rapid, accurate and reproducible patient positioning. It should have good rigidity, move smoothly, and incorporate a range of transverse, longitudinal and vertical motions as well as the needed accessories including immobilization devices to accommodate all of the treatment techniques planned for the unit. Simple positive motion locking devices are essential.

If large field treatments, such as the mantle technique, are planned, then the nominal field size together with lowest couch position are of paramount interest. The verticle ram couch provides large SSDs but necessitates a floor pit. Many treatment techniques are facilitated by the presence or absence of a couch centre spine. Hence, couches which provide both options in a single unit are preferable. Openings with or without transparent inserts facilitate many techniques. It is imperative that the patient be adequately safeguarded against mechanical hazard. Where simulators are employed, they should have a couch identical to the treatment unit being simulated. For some treatment techniques, a chair is preferable to a couch and treatment chairs have been incorporated in several treatment units.

Immobilization devices

Ensuring that the tumour remains centred as prescribed is essential in any treatment plan. For many techniques, ancillary immobilization devices are essential. Historically the individual patient's plaster cast has led the way and remains in wide use. More recently fibreglass Light Cast II (Merck, Sharp and Dohme Orthopedic Company, Westpoint, PA, USA.), which 'sets' under an ultraviolet beam, provides a contemporary version. Prior immobilization and positioning of patients for treatment have been recommended as an efficient, cost-effective approach where identical, interchangeable, transportable couches provide an intermediary.

No single device satisfies all of the required criteria for patient immobilization. Hence several techniques must be available to provide for individual patient needs. Whole body casts have been a possibility with modern foam plastics. For head and neck treatments, bite blocks and head holders have been developed. Vacuum moulding devices are especially useful in some situations. Karzmark *et al*. (1975) describe the 'bite-block' and provide a useful bibliography.

Quality assurance

A modern radiotherapy facility is one of the most expensive hospital special care units to construct and operate. High standards of quality assurance (QA), including equipment maintenance and dose calibration, are essential in providing safe, high quality and cost-effective care for the cancer patient. Radiotherapy technologists, with their day-to-day contact with treatment equipment, are in a crucial position to note equipment malfunction and with appropriate direction can implement many of the checks called for. In addition, physicists, engineers and factory service personnel can make important contributions. For optimal patient care, QA must be well organized; maintenance must include scheduled preventive inspections and procedures, and not merely an ill-defined response to unscheduled emergencies.

Equipment performance specifications and assessment procedures for radiotherapy equipment are published by national and international standardizing agencies as well as professional groups. A relevant reference for radiotherapy linacs will soon be completed by the International Electrotechnical Commission (1978) and another is available for Co units from the American National Standards Institute (1974). Complete archival records are essential for QA and each piece of major equipment should have one or more titled, bound notebooks with numbered pages. Every event bearing on a piece of equipment or project should be entered chronologically and signed.

Maintenance scheduling can be organized with the aid of a pegboard to identify and portray the status of various tasks. The equipment with task identifiers are listed vertically on the left alongside each row of holes and a changeable calendar having units of one week is placed across the top. Two colours of pegs are employed corresponding to work finished or yet to be finished. The frequency of attending to various tasks differs and is based on experience with intervals of 1, 2, 4, 8, 13 or 26 weeks being employed. Magnetic boards may also be used and more recently, minicomputers have been programmed to generate a particular week's list of tasks. Such records are signed and may be used to establish maintenance assurance for regulatory agencies.

In general, factory-scheduled maintenance three or four times a year cannot be expected to prevent downtime as effectively as a few hours of preventive maintenance every week with additional effort in the case of identified needs. There is no ready substitute for the acute observation of a concerned user; his sense of sight, hearing and smell will unerringly alert him to almost all problems.

Table 40.2   A comparison of some published simulator specifications.

	Suggested specification	AECL Therasim 750	CASCADE Simulator	EMI Simulator
X-ray head and collimator				
Source axis distance – range	60–100 cm	75–150 cm	90 cm	80–120 cm
Beam limiting diaphragms				
max cm (SSD)	50 × 50 (100)	45 × 45 (100)	40 × 40 (100)	44 × 44 (100)
min cm (SSD)	0 × 0	0 × 0	0 × 0	0 × 0
Field defining wires			fiducial plates	
max cm (SSD)	50 × 50 (100)	45 × 45 (100)	cast 1 cm	43 × 43 (100)
min cm (SSD)	4 × 4	2 × 2	array	2 × 2
Size indication at control desk at SSD	automatic	75, 80, 100 cm automatic digital	none	automatic digital
Collimator rotation – range	± 110°	± 140°	± 180°	± 90°
SSD Indicator – type	optical	optical	optical	optical
– range	60–100 cm	60–200 cm	60–150 cm	60–140 cm
Gantry				
Height of isocentre above floor	<116 cm	120 cm	127 cm	125 cm
Angle of rotation				
⩽100 cm SAD	>360°	±185°	±195°	±185°
>100 cm SAD		±115°		±150°
Speed of gantry rotation	10–360°/min	0–360°/min	*	360°/min
Isocentre tolerance – diameter of sphere	2 mm up to 100 cm	2 mm at 100 cm	3 mm	2 mm at 100 cm
Image intensifier				
Intensifier tube	9 in	choice to 9 in	none	9.5 in
Radical movement of intensifier from isocentre – range	10–60 cm	8–45 cm		15–60 cm
– speed	2.5 cm/s	1.9 cm/s		†
Longitudinal movement – range	±20 cm	±25 cm		±21 cm
– speed	2.5 cm/s	2 cm/s		†
Lateral movement – range	±20 cm	±20 cm		±21 cm
– speed	2.5 cm/s	2 cm/s		†
Intensifier coverage	63 × 63 cm	63 × 73 cm (w/9 in)		63 × 63 cm
Film cassette holder – max	(†)	36 × 43 cm	†	36 × 43 cm
Maximum vertical source to input phosphor distance	190 cm	195 cm		178 cm
Treatment couch				
Vertical movement from isocentre				
– range	+2, −50 cm	39 cm	+3, −72 cm	+7, −58 cm
– speed	0.1–3 cm/s	0–1 cm/s	adjustable †	†
Longitudinal movement – range	130 cm	79 cm	48 cm	100 cm
– speed	2 cm/s	0–5 cm/s	*	†
Lateral movement – range	±20 cm	±20 cm	±15 cm	±20 cm
– speed	2 cm/s	0–5 cm/s	*	†
Couch top rotation – range	>360°	365°	0°	±180°
Couch rotation about isocentre				
– range	±90°	±110°	±90°	±95°

* Not specified;   † Movement motorized but speed not specified;   ‡ Optical projection.

MECASERTO Mo 25 AB	OLDELFT Simulix-Y	PHILIPS Universal Localizer/Simulator	SIEMENS Ximatron IV	TOSHIBA LX-8
X-ray head and collimator				
50–110 cm	50–130 cm	60–130 cm	80–120 cm	80–130 cm
45 × 45 (100)	50 × 50 (100)	35 × 35 (80)	50 × 50 (100)	35 × 35 (80)
0 × 0	0 × 0	0 × 0	0 × 0	0 × 0
45 × 45 (100)	42 × 42 (100)	35 × 35 (80)	50 × 50 (100)	56 × 56 (80)
0 × 0	0 × 0	0 × 0	3 × 3	4 × 4‡
automatic analogue	automatic digital	digital at various SSDs	80, 100, 120 cm	80, 100 cm
360°	±90°	±180°	±100°	−10°, +100°
optical	optical & mechanical	optical	optical	optical
55–120 cm	50–200 cm	60–141 cm	*	65–140 cm
Gantry				
130 cm	126 cm	117 cm	122 cm	117 cm
>360°	±90°	±230° (SAD >100cm) ±120° (SAD <100cm)	±190° (SAD ≤100cm) ±120° (SAD >100cm)	±190° (SSD=130cm, ±90°)
0–360°/min	108–360°/min	3 speeds up to 720°/min	360°/min local 60°/min remote	36–360°/min
2 mm at 100 cm	2 mm up to 130 cm	3 mm at 100 cm	2 mm	2 mm at 100 cm
Image intensifier				
choice	12.5 in DELCALIX	9 or 5 in	Sirecon 2–23 or Sirecon 2–25/17	9 in
0–60 cm	7–55 cm	13–58 cm	40 cm	10–40 cm
1.9 cm/s	1.5 cm/s	3 cm/s	0–1.5 cm/s	†
±15 cm	±19 cm	±17 cm	±19 cm	±20 cm
1.6 cm/s	1.5 cm/s	2 cm/s	0–1.5 cm/s	†
±15 cm	±15 cm	±17 cm	±19 cm	±20 cm
1.6 cm/s	1.5 cm/s	2 cm/s	†	†
53 × 53 cm	62 × 72 cm	57 × 57 cm	63 × 63 cm	35 × 35 cm at 80 cm 44 × 44 cm at 100 cm
36 × 43 cm	43 × 45 cm	35 × 35 cm bigger on request	35 × 35 cm	36 × 43 cm
170 cm	185 cm	188 cm	173 cm	170 cm
Treatment couch				
0, 40 cm	+3, −47 cm	+1, −48 cm	+1, −51 cm	+4, −39 cm
1.6 cm/s	0.8–3.3 cm/s	0–5 cm/s	0–1.8 cm/s	0.17–1.7 cm/s
80 cm	110 cm	80 cm	85 cm	80 cm
1.1 cm/s	0.8–3.3 cm/s	0–5 cm/s	0–1.2 cm/s	†
±25 cm	±25 cm	±20 cm	±20 cm	±15 cm
1.1 cm/s	0.8–3.3 cm/s	0–2.5 cm/s	0–1.2 cm/s	†
>360°	0, 15, 45, 90°	±90°	−150°, +190°	±180°
±100°	±90°	±100°	±100°	±90°

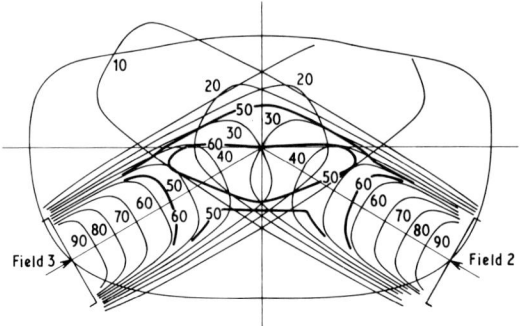

Fig. 41.11   Summation of fields 2 and 3.

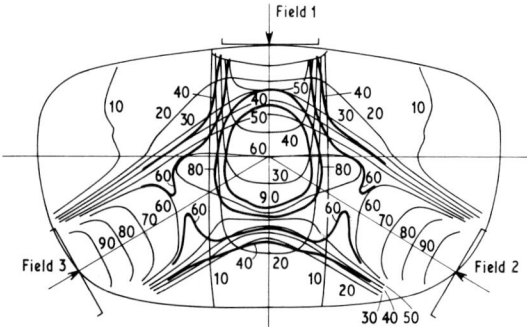

Fig. 41.12   Addition of field 1 to fields 2 and 3.

30% curves of each field intersect, and then to the point where the 20% of field 2 cuts the 40% of field 3, and so on. Where two curves just touch in the way that the 50% and 10% do, the combined 60% isodose curve only just reaches the touching point. After the chart for fields 2 and 3 has been completed it is superimposed on the chart for field 1 as in Fig. 41.12 and the final three-field distribution obtained. Note that the chart for field 1 has to be for a value of 60% at the maximum since this was the weighting chosen for this plan on p. 818 when oblique incidence was not taken into account. If a chart for this weighting is not available, it can be drawn by interpolation from a standard chart having 100% at its maximum. For example the 40% curve on the 60% weighted field will correspond to 40 × 100/60 = 67% on the standard chart and the required curve can be drawn by visual interpolation between the 60 and 70% curves on that chart.

If corrections for obliquity are to be made on any field, a corrected isodose chart has first to be prepared for that field by using the isodose shift technique

described on p. 819. In the same section it was also mentioned that the overall effect of lung tissue on the shape of the final combined isodose chart is small. It is therefore usually satisfactory to draw up the plan ignoring the presence of lung, but finally to adjust the applied doese given on any treatment beam passing through lung by an amount depending on the thickness of lung traversed by the central axis beam. If the weighting used on a 4 MeV X-ray beam for planning purposes was 100% and its central axis passed through 6 cm of lung, then the applied dose that would have been given in the absence of lung must be multiplied by a factor of 100/(100 + 6 × 2.5) = 0.87, since from Table 41.3 the dose beyond lung would be increased by 2.5% per cm of lung traversed.

It is important in Fig. 41.12 to note the size of the high dose zone enclosed in the 90% contour in comparison with the quoted field size. The lateral dimension of this zone is only about 7 cm although 8 × 8-cm fields were used. This difference will be influenced by the convention used for specifying field size on the megavoltage machine being used. A common practice is to specify the field width as the distance between the 50% points on a graph of dose versus distance along a line passing through the build-up maximum perpendicular to the beam axis, when the dose is expressed as a percentage of that at the build-up maximum on the central axis. This convention was used for the field dimensions used in Fig. 41.12, but in some centres the field width is defined as the distance between the 80% points on a cross-plot through the build-up maximum, and the plan of Fig. 41.12 if produced with nominal 8 × 8-cm isodose charts from such centres would give a wider high dose zone. It is important for the radiotherapist to be aware of the field size conventions used on his machines, and of the width of field needed to produce the high dose zone he requires.

Computer methods for isodose charting

Either of the manual methods described in the previous section can be very time-consuming, and is particularly so if repeated attempts have to be made with altered weighting or positions of fields before a satisfactory plan is obtained. It is not surprising therefore that computer systems have been developed to speed up the procedure.

A computer system consists of hardware (the computer itself, a data storage device and suitable peripherals for input of data and output of the plan) and a programme or set of programmes (software) for instructing the computer to carry out the required operations. The hardware that has been used for treatment planning systems can be broadly divided into three types. The first is a general purpose computer system, not necessarily sited in the radiotherapy department or even in the hospital, used in what is called batch mode. Data may be input to the computer in the form of punched cards or punched paper tape, while the treatment planning programme and the necessary field dosage data will normally be held permanently on one of the computer's backing store devices such as a magnetic disc. The minimum requirement for output of a plan is a line printer. Information specifying the type of machine, the field sizes, weights and positions, is punched out as a sequence of numbers in a standard format on cards or paper tape. Details of the patient outline and the contours of any lung or other regions of interest are provided as another string of numbers, the coordinates of points on these outlines so that they are approximately represented by irregular polygons. The cards or paper tape have to be transported to the computer by hand or post or, alternatively the data numbers may be dictated over the telephone to the computer centre and the cards or tape prepared at the centre. The running of the programme with this data may then have to wait for a suitable time slot when the computer has sufficient spare capacity to undertake the job.

If output is restricted to a line printer, the minimum requirement is that the result of the computation should be printed out as a matrix of numbers showing dose values at a grid of points covering the treated area, i.e. an identical output to that obtained by the manual point summation method (Fig. 41.10). Ideally the print-out should be arranged to be life-size so that the numbers are spaced out on the paper at intervals equal to the actual spacing of the points to which they refer. Isodose curves can then be drawn in manually if required. For final presentation of the plan, lines showing the beam axes, field widths and the patient contour have also to be drawn in manually. The line printer output can be arranged to give a visual representation of the isodose contours by printing out the dose values in coded form as shown in Fig. 41.13. If the computer has a graph plotter as one of its devices, isodose contours, field positions and outlines can all be drawn out by the computer.

The main disadvantage of using a remote computer in batch mode for radiotherapy treatment planning is the time that may elapse between preparing the data and receiving the final plan. Obviously this will depend on the local circumstances, but even when communication with the computer centre can be made by a personal messenger service, the turn-round time will often be several hours and may therefore be no shorter than that possible with manual methods. If the plan needs to be revised and run again either due to errors in the input data (which can very easily be undetected at the data preparation stage), or to the dose distribution

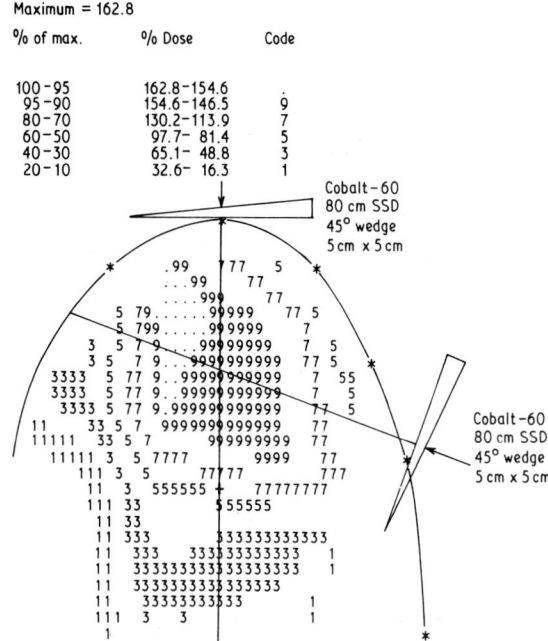

Fig. 41.13 Treatment plan from a computer system having only a line printer for output. Field positions and outline are added by hand.

being unacceptable, then the overall time taken to obtain a satisfactory plan can become considerable. On the credit side, computer planning by any method should provide more consistent accuracy than manual planning, and eliminates the need for trained manual planning staff who may often be very difficult to attract and keep in a job which requires skill and concentration and yet can be very tedious.

The second category of hardware that can speed up the turn-round time considerably is a terminal in the radiotherapy department connected directly by a telephone line to a large computer which supports a multiaccess on-line system. This enables the terminal to be used to input data, set a job running in the main computer and receive output directly the job is completed. In its simplest form the terminal may be no more than a teletype keyboard. The input data for a plan can be typed in as a string of numbers on this keyboard, thus eliminating the need for punched paper tape or cards. Once this step has been completed, a command may be typed which sets the computation running in the main computer. When the computation is completed the output is printed out on the teletype in a form similar to that which has been described above for a line printer. Delays may occur at two stages. The first is at computation and depends on the speed of the main computer, its capability and its workload. The time taken may be several minutes, or more if, for example, the main computer does not have hardware for floating point arithmetic. But with a good multiaccess system the computation time need be only a few seconds. The second delay is caused by the time taken to print out the plan on a teletype. If the printing speed is only 10 characters/s, a plan may take up to 10 minutes to print out, but faster keyboard printers are available and will reduce this time accordingly. A simple on-line terminal system of this kind can therefore reduce the turn-round time so that it is less than that obtainable by manual methods. Its speed and capability can be improved even further by extending the hardware at the terminal end to provide a graphics display and a graph plotter (Crossland *et al.*, 1976). The former can be either a storage or refresh oscilloscope. It enables the data to be checked visually as they are typed in, and provides a rapid means of viewing the final plan. Hard-copy of the plan is available when required from the graph plotter. Such a terminal system may include a small minicomputer and its own to control the display and the plotter and to handle the communication with the main computer.

The third category of hardware is a stand-alone computer system designed primarily for treatment planning and situated in or very close to the radiotherapy department. The computer itself needs to be large enough to run a treatment planning program and will usually have about 32 K bytes of memory. In addition to a teletype keyboard or a visual display unit, a digitizer can be provided which greatly speeds up the input of outlines. Presentation of the data and the plan is on a storage or refresh oscilloscope and a graph plotter provides hard copy. Some form of backing store is required in addition to the computer memory. Magnetic tape was used on the original RAD-8 system (Bentley and Milan, 1971), but it is more usual now to use hard or floppy magnetic discs, or tape cassettes. Compared with an on-line graphics terminal, the cost of stand-alone hardware will be greater, but against this must be set the greater running cost of the terminal system in terms of host computer and telephone charges. Both systems can provide fast interactive radiotherapy treatment planning, and the final choice will depend upon local circumstances.

Several methods of computation are used in computer treatment planning systems. The main differences occur in the quantity and type of beam data that need to be held on the backing store device. Basically the computation process mimics the point summation manual method in that the contribution from each field in turn is added into each point of a dose matrix covering the treatment region. To do this the computer

requires to reproduce a dose distribution for each single field, so that the value of the dose at any point in that field can be determined. One method of making this possible would be to store for each field size of a particular treatment machine, a matrix of dose values corresponding to the dose distribution obtained from that particular field. The dose at any point in the field would then be obtainable by interpolation in this matrix. A rectangular matrix, with say 0.5 or 1.0 cm spacing, would require a large quantity of data to be stored for each field, and it has been shown that sufficient accuracy can be obtained using dose values at a limited number of depths. In the RAD-8 system, dose values for each field size are stored for cross-plots at five depths where they intercept 47 fan lines (see Fig. 41.14), a fan-line being a line radiating from the treatment source. These values have to be obtained and recorded in the backing store before the treatment planning system can be used, and this involves a considerable measurement effort on each treatment machine. Interpolating the values from existing isodose charts is laborious and often of doubtful accuracy.

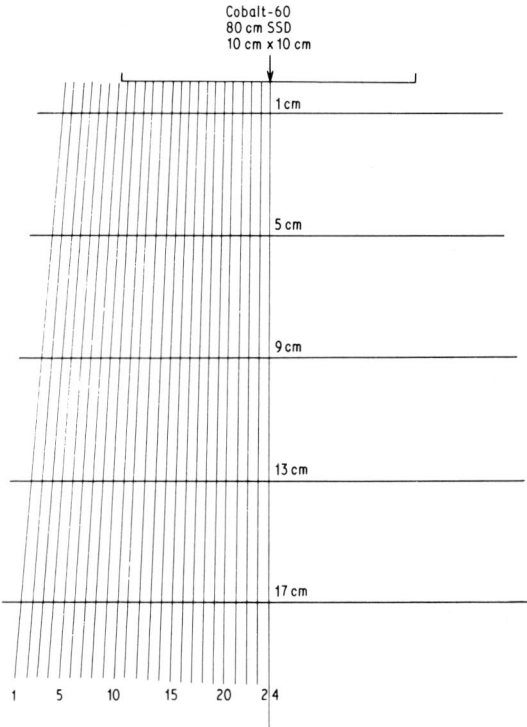

Fig. 41.14 Scheme of fan-lines and cross-lines determining points at which doses are required for specifying a field for the RAD 8 system. (The fan-lines for only half the field are shown).

Remeasurement of the beam data directly in the form required is usually necessary and can be greatly facilitated by the use of an automatic isodose plotter system, several of which are now available commercially. The plotter can be set to drive an ionization chamber or other suitable detector across the beam at a given depth and plot out a graph showing the dose variation along the cross-plot. From this the required dose values for the fan-line intercept points can be read off. The process can be speeded up by controlling the plotter with a small computer (Milan *et al.*, 1976; Redpath *et al.*, 1977) or microprocesser, so that it automatically records the doses at the fan-line intercept points only, and if these records are made on a floppy disc or some other suitable medium, the data can be easily transferred into the radiotherapy planning system computer. This computer may, if conveniently situated, also be the one used to control the plotter.

Because of the considerable amount of data that has to be stored when the above method is used, alternative techniques for deriving the dose at a point from a single field have been used. Cunningham *et al.* (1972), in their programs, use a method based on the concept of separating the primary and scatter dose components and evaluating the scatter by the Clarkson technique of sector summation (Clarkson, 1941). Other methods depend on the property of decrement lines first described by Orchard (1964) and illustrated in Fig. 41.15. He showed that if the dose off the axis is expressed as a percentage of the dose on the central axis *at the same depth*, then points of equal percentage but at different depths lie approximately on straight lines. Thus if the dose profile across the beam is known at two depths, the decrement lines joining points of equal percentage can be drawn and the doses at any other depths deduced. In practice, the profiles at three depths are necessary for the required accuracy but the amount of data requiring storage can thus be reduced. Van de Geijn's programs (Van de Geijn, 1965*b*, 1970, 1972) rely on this projective property of radiotherapy beams. The decrement line position at a given depth also changes regularly with the field size so that interpolation between field sizes is possible and results in a further reduction in the necessary stored data.

An alternative approach is to find empirical mathematical expressions that will fit the measured data and use these for deducing the dose at a point in the field. The only data then requiring storage are the parameters for these expressions. Several expressions for representing central axis depth dose data (Glover, 1966; Sterling *et al.*, 1967; Richter, 1967; Thomas, 1970) and the dose variation across the field (Borger *et al.*, 1972; Thames, 1973; Weinkam *et al.*, 1973; Thomas and Haybittle, 1975; Wilks and Sutcliffe, 1977) have been used satisfactorily. While the use of

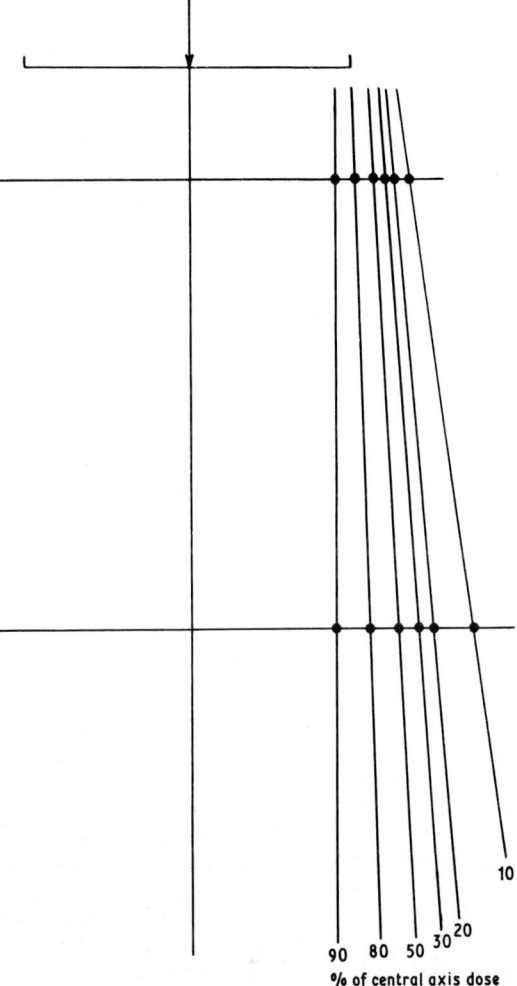

Fig. 41.15 Decrement lines joining points which receive the same dose when expressed as a percentage of the dose on the central axis at the same depth as the point.

these makes the problem of data storage in the computer system trivial, it does not eliminate the necessity for a large number of measurements still to be made on the treatment machines. The parameter values have to be derived from measured data and it is essential that the output of the treatment planning programme for single fields using the parameters is checked against measured isodose curves over a range of field sizes.

Computer methods have made possible the computation of dose distributions in planes other than that containing the axes of the beams or in a situation where the beam axes are not coplanar. A number of programs incorporate this facility. A further development is to achieve fully three-dimensional planning, i.e. a visualization of the body surface, relevant organs and the tumour in three-dimensions and the computation of dose distribution throughout this space. Obviously more patient information is required in the form of outlines and organ shapes in a series of parallel planes, but these can be obtained from transverse axial tomographs or whole body CT-scans. Reinstein *et al.*, (1978) have developed one such system and give an example of its application to the treatment of an oesophageal tumour. Information from five parallel planes was used. Obviously, even without the facilities of such a system being available, the radiotherapist must be concerned about the extent of the tumour in a direction perpendicular to the plane of the beam axes, and be sure that the field dimensions in this direction will produce a high dose zone of adequate size. Fig. 41.16 shows how the area enclosed by the 90% isodose curve in the plan shown in Fig. 41.12 decreases as the distance of the plane of computation from the plane of the beam axes increases. Up to 2 cm from the plane the area remains reasonably constant but at 3 cm it has almost vanished. Thus the maximum dimension of the high dose zone in this dimension is only just over 6 cm as compared with about 7 cm in the plane of the beam axes, even though the field dimension 8 cm is the same in both directions. This illustrates a general point that in order to treat a spherical tumour volume, one should use rectangular fields with dimensions perpendicular to the plane of the beam axes greater than the dimensions parallel to that plane.

Wedge filters

It is often convenient and desirable to treat a lesion by fields directed from one side of a patient only. Fig 41.17 shows such a situation where, since the lesion is in the left hand side of the patient cross-section, it is obviously treated more efficiently by fields from that side where the thicknesses of overlying tissues are less, while normal tissue on the right-hand side will be spared high dosage. If two plain fields are used at right-angles as shown in Fig. 41.17, a high dose area will occur where the fields overlap, but the dose across this area will be far from uniform. In particular the dose at A will be considerably higher than that at B, since A is nearer to the surface for both fields. A more satisfactory dose distribution can be obtained by placing wedge filters in each beam as shown in Fig 41.18. A wedge filter is a wedge shaped piece of metal (usually lead in megavoltage machines) which can be placed in the path of the beam using a special fitting in the treatment head. Its effect on the isodose chart from a single field can be seen in Fig. 41.19*a*, and the resulting two-field distribution is shown in Fig. 41.19*b*. An acceptably uniform distribution over the tumour area has now been obtained.

A variety of wedge filters is usually supplied with a treatment machine. These may each be specified by

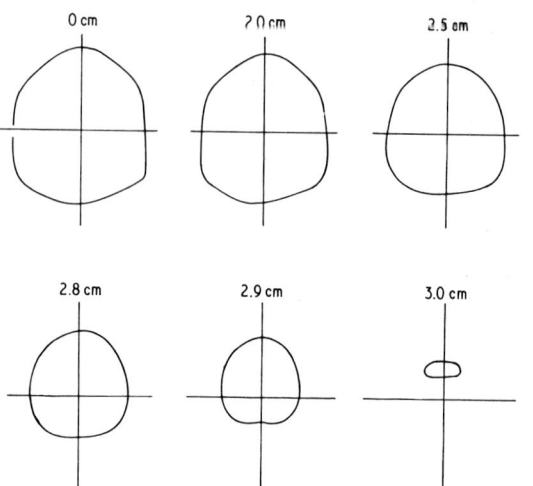

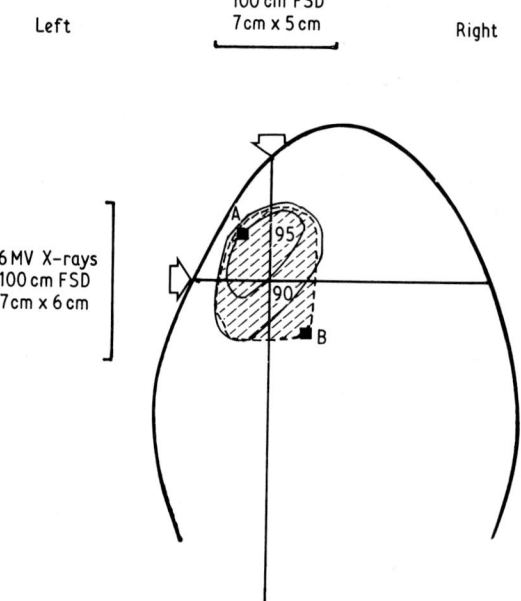

Fig. 41.16   Area included by 90% isodose curve in three-field technique of Fig. 41.6, as distance from the plane containing the beam axes is increased from 0 to 3 cm.

Fig. 41.17   Non-uniform distribution of dose over target volume when two plain fields at right angles are used.

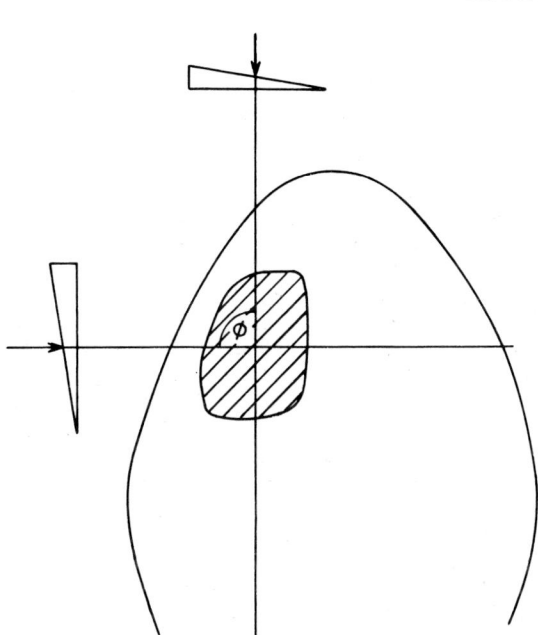

Fig. 41.18 Arrangement of two wedge fields. ϕ = hinge angle.

their 'wedge angle', i.e. the angle θ in Fig. 41.19*a* which the 50% isodose curve makes with the perpendicular to the beam axis. For a two-field wedge treatment the hinge angle is the angle ϕ between the beam axes as shown in Fig. 41.18. If tissue compensators are used, or there is no significant effect of oblique incidence, an arrangement where $\phi = 180° - 2\theta$ will obtain a satisfactorily uniform dose along the bisector of ϕ since the isodose curves from each field will run parallel to each other along this line. A common arrangement is therefore two fields using 45° wedges with beam axes at right-angles to each other. The effect of oblique incidence in a situation such as that shown in Fig. 41.17 would be to counteract to some extent the effect of the wedge. Thus the missing tissue occurs on the same side as the thick end of the wedges and therefore the beam is less reduced in intensity on this side and the isodose chart will be similar to a wedge of smaller wedge angle. Two methods of correcting for this can be used. The first is to increase the hinge angle since from the formula given above, if θ is effectively less, ϕ must be increased. The second method is to use a wedge with a wedge angle larger than 45° to compensate for the effective reduction of the wedge angle by oblique incidence.

Fig. 41.20 shows another common technique using wedge fields. The two parallel opposed fields produce a dose gradient which increases from A to B. The plain

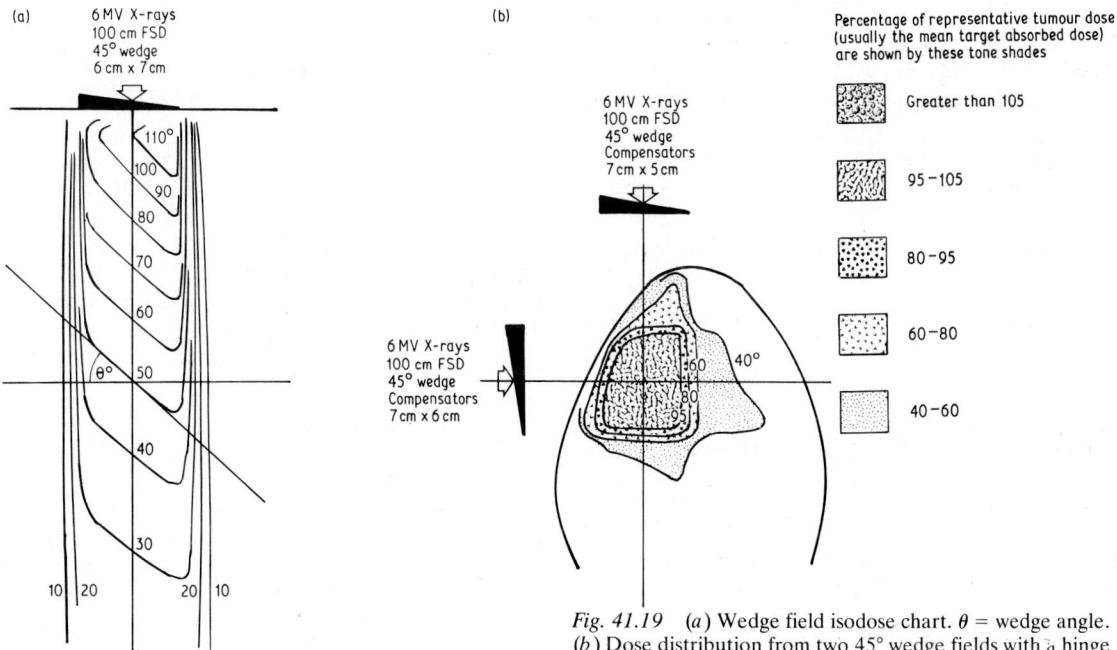

Fig. 41.19 (*a*) Wedge field isodose chart. θ = wedge angle. (*b*) Dose distribution from two 45° wedge fields with a hinge angle of 90° when tissue compensators are used to overcome the effects of oblique incidence.

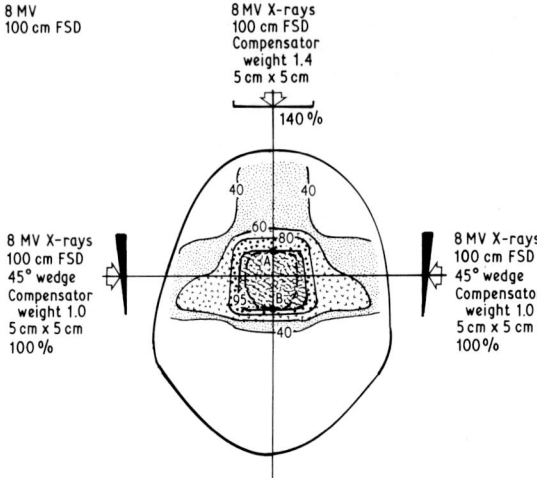

8 MV
100 cm FSD

8 MV X-rays
100 cm FSD
Compensator
weight 1.4
5 cm x 5 cm

140 %

8 MV X-rays
100 cm FSD
45° wedge
Compensator
weight 1.0
5 cm x 5 cm
100 %

8 MV X-rays
100 cm FSD
45° wedge
Compensator
weight 1.0
5 cm x 5 cm
100 %

Fig. 41.20   Combination of two lateral wedge fields and one anterior plain field.

Percentage of representative tumour dose
(usually the mean target absorbed dose)
are shown by these tone shades

Greater than 105

95–105

80–95

60–80

40–60

anterior field produces a dose gradient which increases from B to A. By suitable choice of weighting on the anterior field these two gradients may be made to balance each other so that a uniform high dose area is obtained over the tumour. The calculation for obtaining the weight for the anterior field is identical to that given on p. 819.

When a wedge is inserted in the beam, the applied dose rate is reduced by an amount depending mainly on the primary beam absorption in the thickness of the centre of the wedge. This reduction expressed as a wedge factor (= applied dose with wedge/applied dose without wedge), must be taken into account when the treatment is implemented (see p. 838). It is usual for a wedge to be wide enough for use over a range of field sizes. If its lateral position in the beam remains fixed for all field sizes (Fig. 41.21a) the wedge factor will remain approximately constant (although there will be some small variation with field size due to effects on scattered radiation). This reduces the possibility of calculation error due to reading the wrong wedge factor, but is relatively inefficient in usage of the machine output since on a small field the shaded portion of the wedge in Fig. 41.21a does nothing except reduce the overall output. An alternative method which is sometimes used is shown in Fig. 41.21b where the lateral position of the wedge is changed with field size so that the thin end of the wedge is always aligned with the field edge. This makes more efficient use of the radiation output, but means that the wedge factor will change considerably with field size.

Because of the effect of a wedge filter on both the

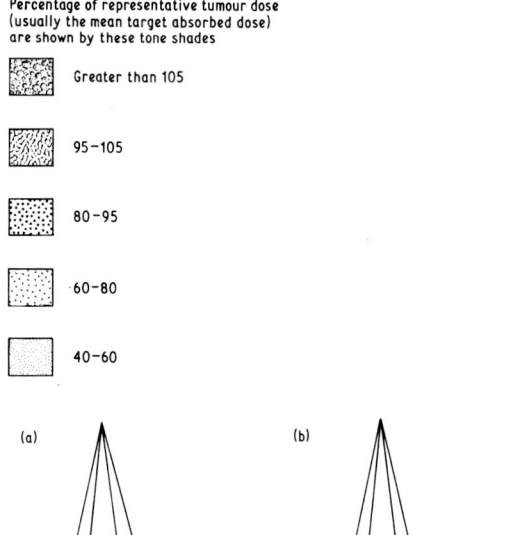

(a)

(b)

Large field
position

Small fiel
position

Small
field

Large
field

Small
field

Large
field

Fig. 41.21   (a) Wedge filter in fixed position in beam for all field sizes. Shaded area shows part of filter which has no wedge effect for small field.
(b) Wedge filter moving with field size so that thin end always coincides with edge of field.

output and the isodose chart, it is most important that the chances of error caused by either omitting a wedge filter or inserting the wrong one should be minimized.

Wedge filter interlock systems are therefore an essential requirement on treatment machines having wedge filters. These ensure that the machine can only be switched on if the wedge filter selected by the operator using a selector switch on the treatment control console coincides with the wedge filter that is inserted in the treatment head. A further major error can occur if the wedge filter is orientated wrongly relative to the patient. Visual indication of the wedge direction can be provided on the treatment head and in the field illumination, and these, combined with markers on treatment shells, can help to guard against such an error. Nevertheless one must still rely heavily on the vigilance of the operator.

Optimization

There are many variables that effect a treatment plan and which ideally should be optimized to provide the 'best' plan for a given set of circumstances. Some, such as field size, are usually determined without much ambiguity from the size of the required treatment volume. But the best values of others, such as field entry point and angulation, weighting, wedge angle are not so immediately obvious, although the experienced treatment planner can often choose initial values which produce an acceptable treatment plan at the first attempt. The calculation of weighting to balance field gradients has already been described on p. 818, and the choice of wedge angle and hinge angle have been discussed on p. 827. Entry point and angle will normally be determined by the planner taking into account the need to deliver the required dose to the tumour as efficiently as possible, i.e. with the minimum irradiation of normal tissue, and the necessity to avoid dosage above a certain level to some sensitive organs.

With the advent of computer methods for treatment planning and their ability to produce different plans very rapidly, it was not surprising that the possibilities of computer optimization were investigated (Hope and Orr, 1965; Bahr et al., 1966). One of the first problems was to quantify the criteria determining the 'goodness' of a treatment plan. Hope *et al.* (1967) attributed to each plan a numerical score based on the dose gradient across the tumour, the dose to the tumour relative to the maximum incident dose, the integral dose, the shape of the high dose area, the doses to vulnerable regions, and the dose in regions of possible direct tumour extension or lymphatic spread. The lower the score value the 'better' the plan. The optimization programme, run on a large multipurpose computer, calculated the score for combinations of field positions, wedge angles and weights in pre-specified ranges, and selected plans with the lowest scores. A very large number of plans needed to be tried and, to reduce computer time, simple dose gradient additions and comparisons were made for optimization purposes and only the finally chosen plan computed fully. More recently Van der Laarse and Strackee (1976) have also described an optimization suite of programs for a large computer, with scores based on very similar criteria to those of Hope *et al.* (1967). On a small dedicated computer the possibilities are more limited, but the treatment planning system described by Redpath *et al.*

(1977) contains an optimization facility which for a given combination of beam directions and sizes finds the optimum weights and wedges for the beams, based on the criterion of uniformity of dose throughout the tumour volume. Hodes (1974) described a program which performs a similar function.

Although it has been demonstrated that computer optimization is a feasible and practical procedure in routine clinical use, it is still not widely used. This is probably because an experienced planner with a non-optimizing computer system can produce acceptable plans very quickly and it is doubtful if in the vast majority of cases the use of computer optimization methods will produce plans that are significantly better clinically.

Isocentric techniques

In any discussion of planning so far it has been assumed that the distance from the source to the skin surface was the standard FSD for which isodose charts were available having their 100% value either at the surface or at the build-up maximum on the central axis. There are many situations in which it is more convenient to position the patient with his tumour centred at the isocentre of an isocentric treatment machine (see p. 836), and maintain this position for all treatment fields. Thus for the three fields in Fig. 41.22, the distance from the source to the tumour centre, O, remains constant, while the FSD for each field is different (F_1, F_2 and F_3). It is not therefore possible to use standard central axis depth dose data and standard isodose charts for treatment planning and calculation in this situation.

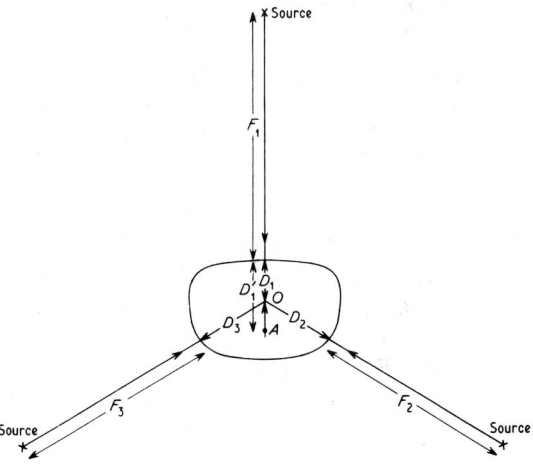

Fig. 41.22   Three-field isocentric treatment.

The usual method of calculation of dose on the beam axis is by means of tables of tissue-air ratios (Gupta and Cunningham, 1965). The tissue-air ratio (TAR) for a depth, D, is the ratio of the dose at the point with D cm of overlying tissue present to the dose at the same point (i.e. the same distance from the source) measured in air with a sufficiently thick cap on the detector to achieve maximum build-up. Since this ratio depends only on the effect of absorption and scatter in the overlying tissue, it will not be affected by the distance of the point from the source. Thus only one table of tissue-air ratios is required for a particular radiation quality showing values of TAR for different field sizes and for different tissue depths, D. Such tables are available in the *British Journal of Radiology*, Supplement 11. It should be noted that the field sizes are measured at the depth, D, *not* at the surface of the patient. Instead of a table of applied dose rates against field sizes for a particular machine, a table of air dose rates at the isocentre is required. Suppose that for the field size being used on field 1 in Fig. 41.22, the TAR is 0.72 for a depth D cm. Then for every 100 rad delivered in air at the isocentre for this field size, the tumour centre will receive $100 \times 0.72 = 72$ rad. It is also possible to calculate the dose at other points on the beam axis of a single field, say A from field 1. First it is necessary to calculate the field size at A by multiplying each field dimension at the isocentre by $(F_1 + D'_1)/(F_1 + D_1)$. The TAR for this field size and depth D'_1 is then found from the table. Supposing it is 0.51. For every 100 rad delivered in air at A, the dose in tissue will be 51 rad. But the dose in air at A will be $(F_1 + D_1)^2/(F_1 + D'_1)^2$ times the dose in air at O. Thus for every 100 rad delivered in air at O the dose at A in tissue will be 51 $(F_1 + D_1)^2/(F_1 + D'_1)^2$.

There are difficulties in measuring directly TAR at energies above 3 MeV, because of the scatter caused by the build-up cap when measuring the dose in air. An alternative approach, valid at higher energies, is to use tissue-maximum ratios (Holt *et al.*, 1970). The tissue-maximum ratio (TMR) for a depth, D, in tissue is the ratio of the dose at the point with D cm of overlying tissue, to the dose at the point when situated at the depth of maximum build-up with full back scatter present. The TMR is in practice the same as the fractional depth dose if the beam were used at infinite FSD, and values of TMR can be obtained from the *British Journal of Radiology*, Supplement 11. Calculations are the same as for TARs but the machine output information now used is a table of applied dose rates for different field sizes when the build-up maximum is situated at the isocentre.

Obtaining a complete isodose chart by manual methods for an isocentric plan of this kind is most easily achieved by the method described by Du Sault (1959). Measurements are made and isodose charts

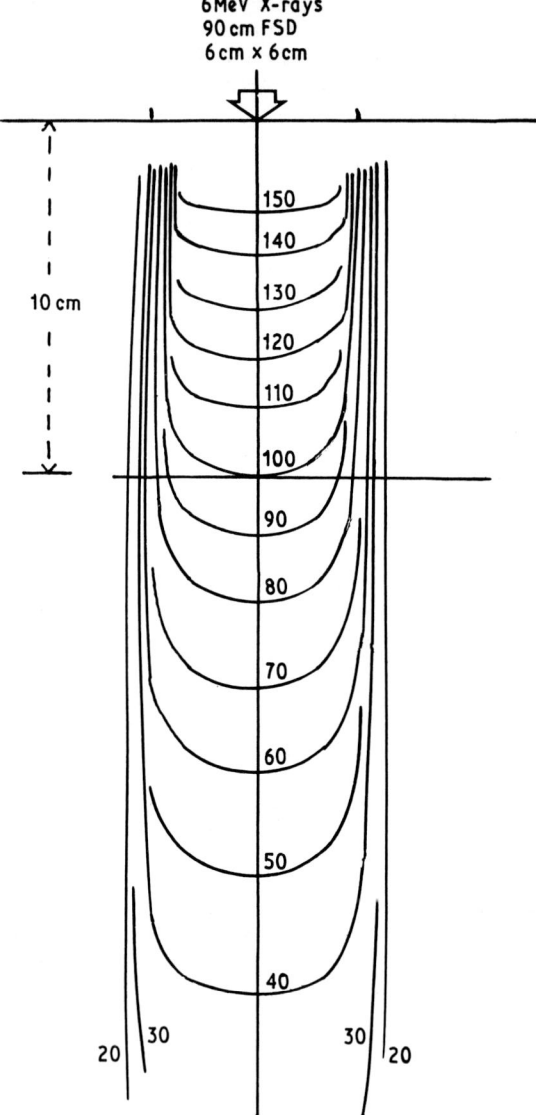

Fig. 41.23   Isodose chart normalized to 100% at 10 cm deep on the central axis.

drawn up with the isocentre at three different depths in the measurement phantom, say 5, 10 and 15 cm. The charts are drawn as shown in Fig. 41.23 with the values normalized to 100% at the isocentre i.e. 10 cm deep in Fig. 41.23. The field size also refers to its dimensions at 10 cm deep. The methods described on pp. 821–22 can now be used, choosing for each field a chart measured at the depth nearest to the depth of the isocentre for that field, i.e. if $D_1 = 8$ cm, a chart for a 10-cm deep isocentre would be used. The final numbers obtained by summation will be relative to 300 rad in tissue at O (if equal weights in tissue at O are given on each field). The TARs for D_1, D_2 and D_3 can then be used to find the air doses required from each field to deliver 100 rad at O. The errors involved in using a 10-cm deep isodose chart for an 8-cm deep situation are very small, as the dose gradient above and below the isocentre varies only to a small extent with its depth.

Computer methods can derive the dose at a point in a field under isocentric conditions from the same data used for non-isocentric treatments. Although extra computation is required, there is no necessity to make extra measurements when initially obtaining the basic dosage data.

Rotation therapy

A natural extension of multiple beam directed techniques is the use of rotation therapy, where the treatment

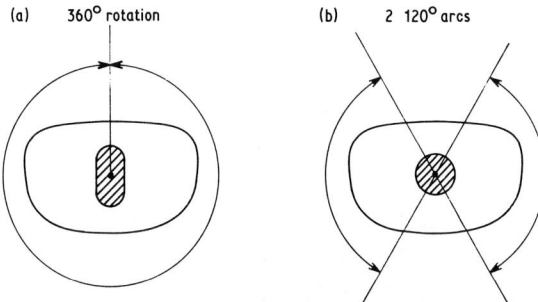

Fig. 41.24 High dose zones from rotation technique using (*a*) full 360° rotation; (*b*) two 120° arcs.

beam remains pointing at the tumour centre (or some other fixed point), but rotates in an arc during the treatment, simulating in effect a fixed field treatment with a very large number of field positions. An isocentric mounting (see p. 836) is essential for this type of treatment, and in modern equipment there is usually a facility for adjusting the speed of rotation so that a pre-selected dose is delivered in one arc.

Although rotation therapy should obtain a higher ratio of tumour dose to normal tissue dose than a three- or four-field technique, it is less easy with rotation to shape and position the high dose volume just as required. A full 360° arc rotation treating a central circular tumour in a circular body cross-section will obtain an ideal central high dose area, but the more common situation is the treatment of a central tumour in an oval-shaped cross-section as shown in Fig. 41.24*a*. In this case a 360° rotation results in a high dose area elongated in the AP direction. A better distribution can be obtained by limiting the rotation to two arcs as shown in Fig. 41.24*b*, but now most of the treatment is given through the regions where there are greater depths of overlying tissue. The expected improvement in tumour/normal tissue dose ratio over that obtained with a three- or four-field technique does not therefore materialize. For this kind of reason, and because of the difficulties of planning such treatments by manual methods, the use of rotation therapy techniques is not widespread. A possibly useful technique was described by Sutherland (1962) and uses two arcs and wedge filters as shown in Fig. 41.25. To see why such a combination produces the resulting isodose chart, it may be compared with the three-field technique shown in Fig. 41.20. When the arcing fields are in their lateral positions they produce a dose distribution similar to that of the two parallel opposed lateral

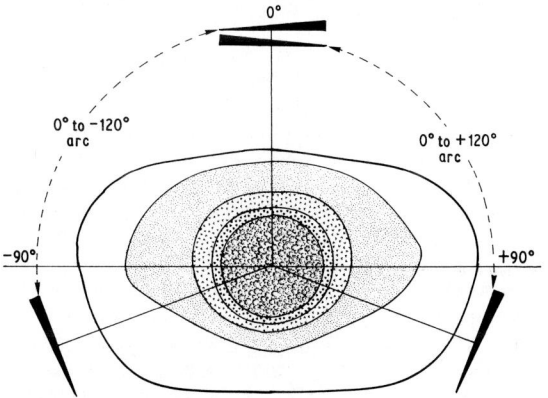

Fig. 41.25 Rotation technique using 9 cm × 9 cm 45° wedge fields; 6 MeV X-rays at 100 cm source-axis distance; two 120° arcs.

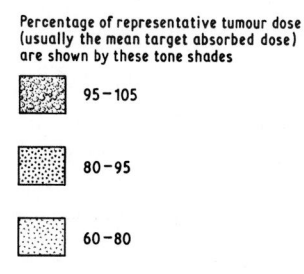

Percentage of representative tumour dose (usually the mean target absorbed dose) are shown by these tone shades

95–105

80–95

60–80

40–60

wedge fields in Fig. 41.20. When the arcing fields are in their anterior position, their wedges cancel each other out and their effect is similar to that of the plain anterior field in Fig. 41.20. This technique has been shown to be very useful in sites such as the bladder where a rapid fall-off of dose posterior to the high dose area is required.

To calculate the dose at the isocentre from a rotation arc it is usual to divide the arc into, say, 10° segments and calculate an average TAR. For each of the distances D_1 to D_n in Fig. 41.26 the TAR for the field size used is found. The average TAR is then calculated from:

$$(TAR)_{AV} = \frac{\frac{1}{2}(TAR)_1 + (TAR)_2 + (TAR)_3 \ldots}{n-1}$$
$$\frac{\ldots + (TAR)_{n-1} + \frac{1}{2}(TAR)_n}{n-1}$$

This average TAR can then be used to find the dose delivered at the isocentre, O, in tissue for every 100 rad in air as on pp. 830–31. A weighting of a half is given to the TARs at the extreme ends of the arc because less time is effectively spent irradiating through these positions.

Large field techniques

The use of large field treatments introduces a number of special problems in treatment planning. In the first place, the required field size may be larger than the maximum obtainable from the treatment machine available at the standard FSD. Supposing a field size of 40×40 cm is required from a unit giving a maximum possible field size of 30×30 cm at 100 cm FSD. To obtain the required 40×40 cm field size, the FSD must be increased in the ratio of the field dimension required to the maximum field dimension available. The FSD to be used will therefore be $100 \times 40/30 = 133$ cm. The applied dose rate will be

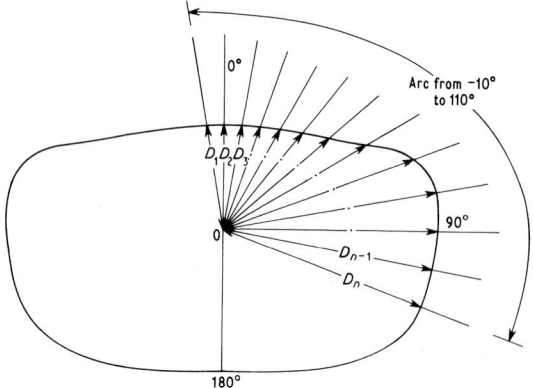

Fig. 41.26   Calculation of axis dose in rotation therapy.

reduced at this new FSD by the ratio $(100/133)^2$. Since the applied dose rate for megavoltage is measured at the build up maximum, a more accurate correction factor for the effect of FSD is $[(100 + D_{max})/(133 + D_{max})]^2$, where D_{max} is the depth of the build-up maximum. This takes into account the effect of the change in FSD but not the effect the increased area will have on the back-scatter contribution. Fortunately for megavoltage treatments this will be a very small change and can in practice be ignored.

Central axis percentage depth doses may also only be available for the standard FSD (F_1) and will need correction for use at the extended FSD (F_2). Let the percentage depth dose for depth D at FSD F_1 be P_1. The percentage depth dose for depth D at FSD F_2 is given by:

$$P_2 = P_1 \times \left[\frac{F_1 + D}{F_1 + D_{max}}\right]^2 \times \left[\frac{F_2 + D_{max}}{F_2 + D}\right]^2$$

P_1 should be read from the depth dose table for the new enlarged area, but this area may well be outside the range of the tables. Fortunately, again, for megavoltage treatments the variation of depth dose with field size is small, and a sufficiently accurate estimate can be obtained by extrapolating a plot of percentage depth dose against side of square field for the depth D.

An alternative method of obtaining large fields is to use two smaller fields adjacent to one another. The problem here is to ensure correct dosage in the area at the join of the two fields. If the field edges are too close there may be overdosage; if too far apart there may be underdosage. To decide the correct separation it is important to know the field-size convention used (see p. 822), as the field illumination is usually set up to correspond with this convention. If the 50% width measure of field size is used, setting up the two fields so that the areas shown by the field illumination exactly adjoin one another will give a reasonably uniform dose at the depth of build-up maximum. However, as shown in Fig. 41.27, the overlap of the fields increases at greater depths due to their divergence, so that the dose is no longer uniform. The actual overlap used must therefore depend on where overdosage or underdosage would be critical. If the field size is specified as the 80% rather than the 50% width and the field illumination set up to correspond, a gap will need to be left between the fields as shown by the illumination. The amount of this gap will depend on the penumbra of the machine, and can be found by reference to the appropriate isodose chart. Even so, if the beam has a narrow penumbra a small error in setting up will quite easily cause a large under- or overdosage. A useful way of overcoming this problem is deliberately to increase the penumbra at the adjacent edges of the fields by intro-

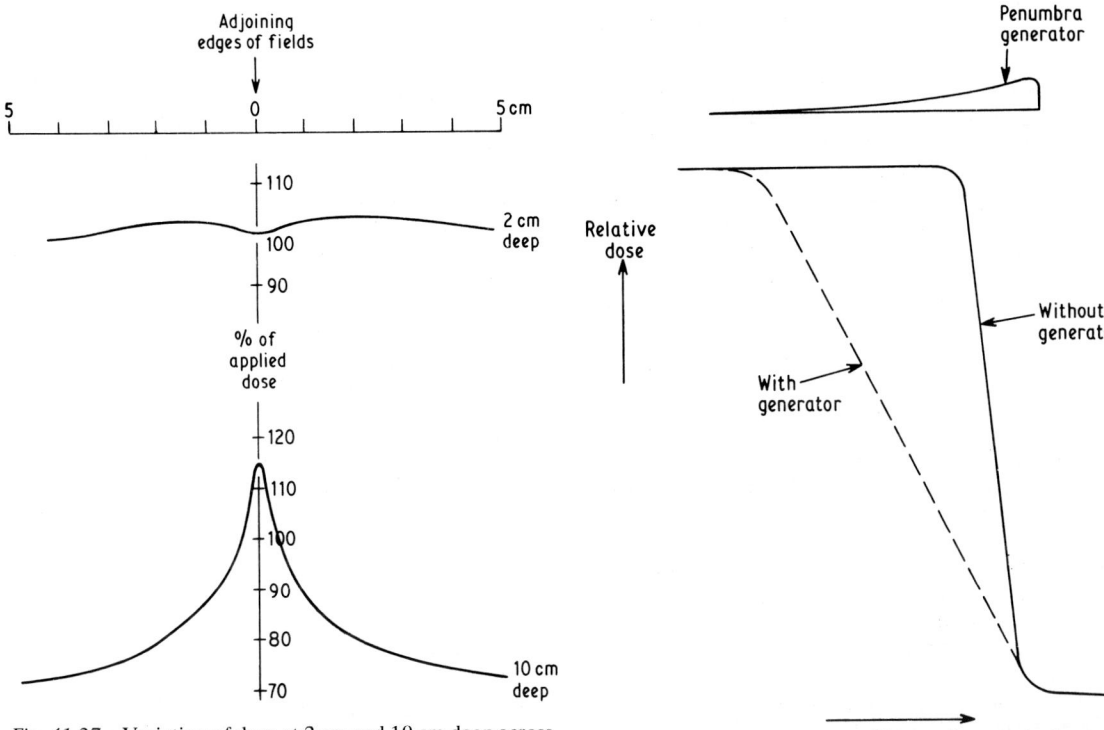

Fig. 41.27 Variation of dose at 2 cm and 10 cm deep across junction of two adjoining 8 MeV linear accelerator fields.

Fig. 41.28 Effect of penumbra generator in broadening penumbra.

ducing a wedge into the beam as shown in Fig. 41.28. Armstrong and Tait, (1973) have described such a wedge for a 6-MeV linear accelerator which increases the penumbral width to about 10 cm at 150 cm from the focus, and have shown that positioning errors of up to ±1 cm can then be tolerated.

An alternative method which is sometimes used for the same purpose is to shift the position of the line where the fields join by about 1 cm each treatment fraction for, say, five fractions and repeat the sequence throughout the treatment course.

Many large field treatments require the fields to be specially shaped to protect sensitive areas. For example, blocks of shielding material may be inserted in the beam to protect the lungs during a mantle treatment for Hodgkin's disease. For megavoltage treatments these blocks have to be quite thick, e.g. 5 cm of lead for ^{60}Co γ-rays, and are usually mounted on a plate attached to the end of the collimator system. They therefore have to be scaled down in lateral dimensions in the same way that is necessary for tissue compensators (see p. 820), and a technique for doing this has been described by Edland and Hansen (1969). Since blocks may have to be made to suit individual patients any method of simplifying the fabrication of the blocks

is an advantage. Edland and Hansen (1969), to avoid casting metal, used lead shot held in a Styrofoam pattern, a 7 cm thickness of shot being equivalent to 5 cm of lead. More recently low melting point alloys have become available and are very easy to handle (Marshall *et al.*, 1975). For example MCP70 made by Mining and Chemical Products Ltd, melts at 70°C and can be cast in expanded polystyrene moulds. The density of MCP70 is 9.4 g/cm³ and about 20% more thickness than lead is therefore required to achieve the same shielding.

Principles of field combination*

To round off this section on radiotherapy field planning it may be helpful to attempt to distil some of the general principles underlying the wide range of practical methods developed for use in particular situations.

In every case in which planning presents any problem the tolerances of some normal tissues are the major factors determining the field arrangements. The

*Contributed by J.S.Orr

dose levels at which damage to normal tissues of various kinds becomes critically important are fairly well defined. For those types of tissue which occur widely in the body, skin and blood vessels for example, there are common dose levels, dependent on the volume of tissue irradiated and the duration of the treatment.

Although no completely fixed procedure can be put forward, because of the measure of uncertainty which always exists in the information available for making decisions on a treatment, and the consequent need for clinical judgement, explicit criteria can be derived. These criteria, listed below, can be used both as signposts in devising field arrangements to achieve the therapeutic intention in some measure, and also as touchstones for judging the methods proposed.

1. The dose within the tumour volume and an appropriate specified margin, including the regions of possible tumour spread, should lie within defined limits. In many cases these limits are so close together that the objective is the achievement of a uniform dose within the volume.

2. The doses to all common tissues outside the tumour volume and specified margin, i.e. the tumour region, and the doses to skin and subcutaneous regions, should be as much below the dose given to the tumour region as possible.

3. The volume of tissue lying outside the tumour region but receiving the same dose as the tumour region should be as small as possible.

4. The doses to certain specific tissues, such as the spinal cord, the kidneys or the eyes, should be minimized and should not exceed the particular tolerance dose appropriate to the region affected.

5. The integral dose should be minimized, usually by delivering as much dose to the tumour region as possible by the shorter paths.

6. The treatment method should be such as to minimize the difficulties of arranging the patient and the treatment unit.

7. Every treatment plan should have a clearly defined basis, and the groups of treatments with a common theme should be sufficiently large to allow statistically significant comparisons to be made.

The requirements of these criteria are normally conflicting and a compromise must be reached. The extent to which each criterion can be satisfied depends on the physical and geometric attributes of the radiation fields and their interaction. The approach to uniformity of dose throughout the tumour region depends on the balance of the vector values of dose gradient from the individual fields. The closeness with which the tumour region can be outlined by the edge of the high dose region depends on the position and size of the individual fields, and on the extension outside of the tumour region of the parallel-sided figure common to

all the fields and formed by the pairs of sides of each of the fields. The doses to general vulnerable tissues, and the integral dose, depend on the steepness of the central axis depth dose curves, the distance each beam has to traverse from the skin to the tumour region, the relative incident dose given to the fields, and the number of fields. The sparing of particular vulnerable tissues depends on the factors mentioned in the previous sentence and also on the relationship between the tissues and the edges of the fields. The ease and speed of implementing a treatment depends on the design of the treatment unit and its suitability for the particular field directions and configurations demanded. The merits of dose distribution are determined by all these factors and their interactions.

If it is accepted that the principles of field combination depend on the features of single fields, the therapeutic intention, and the above criteria, an out-

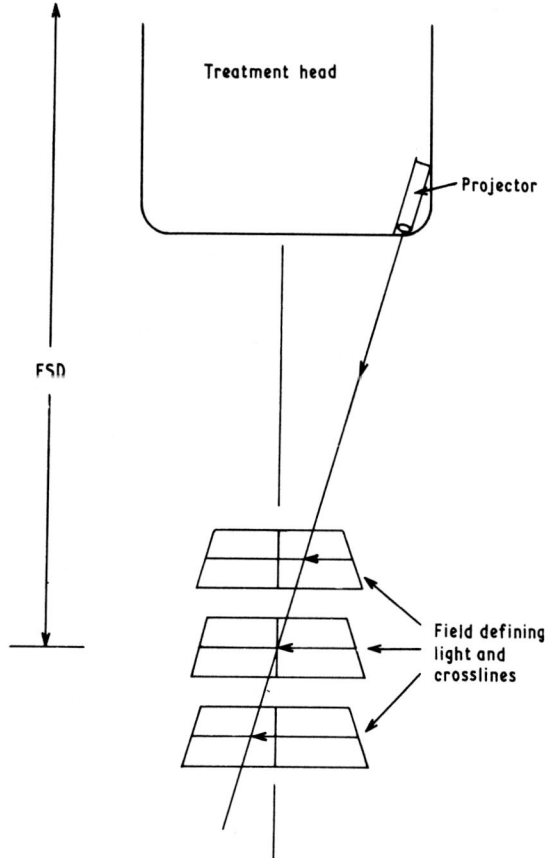

Fig. 41.29   Schematic diagram of optical front pointer and FSD indicator.

line procedure can be set down, as follows:

A. A single field is first considered. The two criteria which may compel the addition of a second field are:

1. The non-uniformity of the dose within the tumour region.
2. The ratio of the subcutaneous dose to the dose to the tumour region.

Only the first of these criteria may be satisfied if the two fields are opposed. Both criteria may be better satisfied if the second field is used to pick out and raise the dose level of only a part of the path of the first field.

B. The positions, weighting and wedging of the two fields should be selected to satisfy the criteria:

3. The geometric matching of the high dose treated volume to the tumour region.
4. The dose to specific vulnerable regions.
5. The integral dose.

C. If criterion 2 cannot be satisfied with two fields, then a third, fourth or fifth field can be added. The choice of number of fields is also influenced by criterion 3.

D. Once the decision to use more than two fields has been made, the position, weighting and wedging of the fields should be selected to satisfy criteria 3, 4 and 5, just as in B.

E. In all cases account should be taken of criteria 6 and 7.

Typical field arrangements fall into a series of patterns of increasing complexity. The selection of a basic pattern is determined first, and then the pattern is modified to achieve the best compromise between the requirements of the criteria.

Beam direction

Equipment aids

In superficial and orthovoltage equipment the treatment beam is usually defined by applicators which extend to the full extent of the FSD and whose cross-section at that end corresponds exactly to the field size. If the centre of the applicator end (marked by cross-wires) is set up in contact with an entry point marked on the patient's skin, then the entry point of the beam, its orientation and the FSD are satisfactorily determined.

Megavoltage beams are defined by collimator systems which have to be some distance from the skin so that the skin-sparing effect can be maintained. The area is illuminated on the skin by means of a light and mirror system in the treatment head that projects a beam of light as if it originated from the radiation source. The accuracy of this projection depends on the

lamp and mirror positions and should be regularly checked. As already described on p. 822, the illuminated area may be set to show the area within the 50% contours, or some other value such as 80%, but it is important that the user should be aware of the convention adopted. Cross-lines are also projected to show the centre of the beam.

The FSD can be determined either by an optical system or a mechanical front pointer. The former is illustrated in Fig. 41.29. An illuminated V or other shape is projected at an angle to the beam so that the point of intersection with the central axis occurs at the standard FSD. If the patient surface is either above or below the correct point, the V and the cross-lines from the field illumination lamp will not coincide. A more sophisticated version projects an illuminated scale instead of a V and the distance to the skin can be set up to any required value by observing the reading on the scale where it is cut by the central cross-line. A mechanical front pointer is also usually fitted with a scale showing the distance from the focus to the tip of the pointer.

A mechanical back pointer attached to the treatment head, as shown in Fig. 41.30, enables accurate beam direction of a treatment field provided that the required entry and exit points (E and X respectively) can be marked on the patient or on a treatment shell (see p. 837) worn by the patient. The back pointer is mounted so that it can rotate about the beam axis, but the pointer QP always coincides with the beam axis, although it can be moved in and out to suit different thicknesses of patient. If the machine is adjusted so that its front pointer set to the required FSD (or its optical system) is aligned with E and the back pointer aligned with X, the beam will accurately pass through the centre O of the treatment volume.

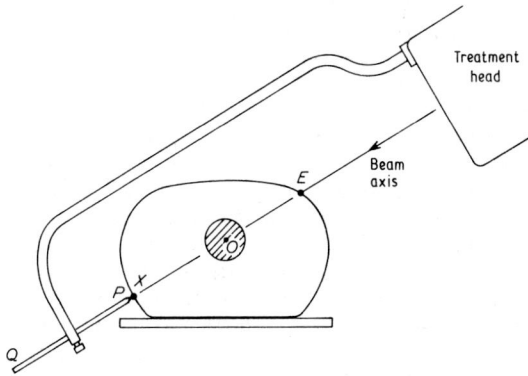

Fig. 41.30 Mechanical back pointer for beam alignment using entrance and exit marks, E and X.

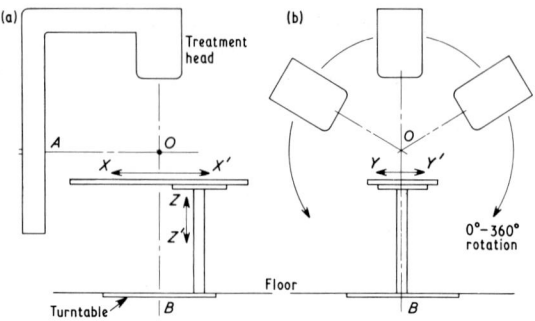

Fig. 41.31 Schematic diagram showing movements of an isocentric treatment machine.

Isocentric mounting

To facilitate setting up treatments and also to provide for rotation therapy, most modern megavoltage units incorporate an isocentric mounting in their design. Fig. 41.31 shows the essential features of such a design. The treatment head is mounted on an L-shaped arm (or an arm projecting from a drum) so that the head can be rotated through a full 360° about the axis AO with the beam axis always passing through O, the isocentre. The couch top has two translational movements, XX' and YY', and is mounted on a ram which can be adjusted to provide a vertical movement ZZ'. So that the treatment head has clear passage under the couch, the ram is usually off-centred from the vertical axis OB passing through the isocentre, but mounted on a turntable in the floor which rotates about the axis OB. The couch top may have removable panels so that treatments may be given below without absorption of the beam in the material of the top or its supports.

An isocentric mounting may be used for setting up treatment in two ways. Fig. 41.32 illustrates the situation when it is required to treat all fields with the same FSD, and this FSD is the distance from the radiation source to the isocentric axis, i.e. the source-axis distance, SAD. The movements of the couch top and the vertical couch movement are first used to adjust the patient so that the entry point of the beam coincides with the isocentre. This may be done with the treatment head at any rotational angle as the isocentre can be located either with the mechanical front pointer or the optical system. The rotation angle can now be adjusted to bring the back pointer to the level of the exit point, X. In general the back pointer will still not coincide with X when viewed from above but a final adjustment to bring them into coincidence can be made by means of the couch rotation. Note that because the angulation and couch rotation movements rotate about the isocentre, the initial setting of the

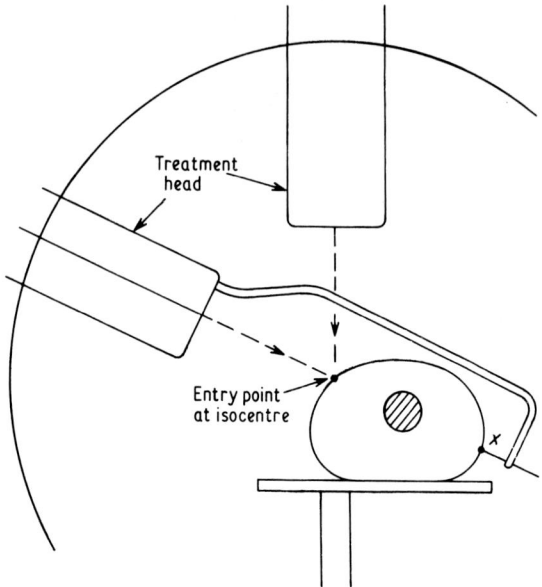

Fig. 41.32 Using a back pointer with an isocentric mounting to set up a treatment field with the entry point at the isocentre.

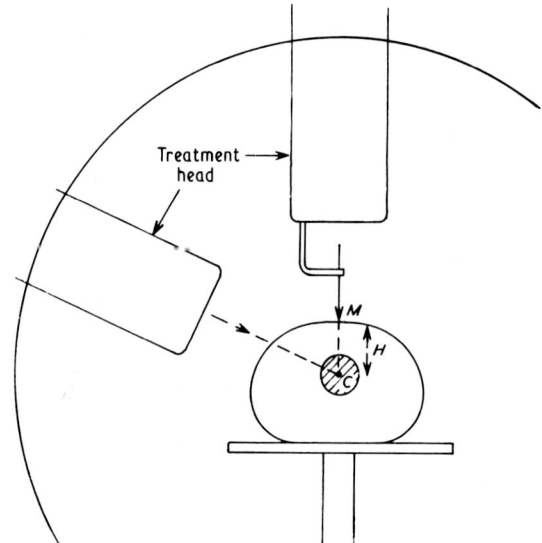

Fig. 41.33 Arrangement of isocentric machine with tumour centre at the isocentre.

entry point will remain unchanged.

The second method of using an isocentric mounting is shown in Fig. 41.33. In this case the distance from the source to the centre of the treatment volume, C, is kept fixed for all fields and this is achieved by locating the

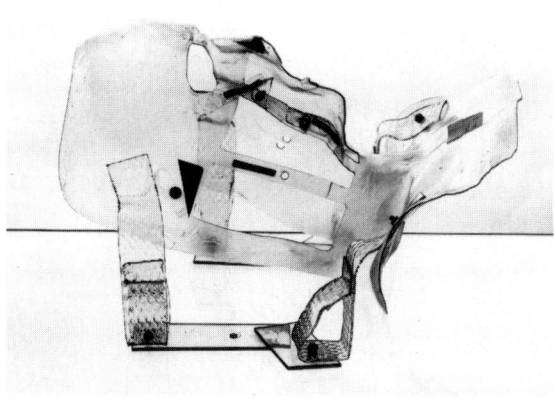

Fig. 41.34 Treatment shell.

centre of the treatment volume at the isocentre. It is necessary to know the distance H of C below a skin mark M placed vertically above C when the patient is lying flat. This distance can be determined from radiographs as described on p. 814. With the tube head pointing vertically downwards and its front pointer set to a distance equal to $SAD - H$, the couch movements are used to bring the front pointer into coincidence with the skin mark M. C is now at the isocentre and the treatment head can be adjusted to any required rotational angle still maintaining the beam axis passing through C. For each field direction the depth of C below the field entry point can be determined by observing the FSD on the front pointer scale.

Treatment shells

The use of skin marks on a patient has certain disadvantages. The marks may get rubbed off between treatments, and the skin itself may move in relation to underlying tissues and thus introduce errors. For these reasons, treatment shells are often used for small field beam directed treatments, particularly in the head and neck region. A treatment shell is worn during the treatment and is made of some material that is easy to mould into a good fit of the part of the patient to be treated. Entry and exit points of treatment fields are marked on the shell rather than on the patient, and other indicators may be fixed to the shell to remind the radiographer of the direction of any wedge that is required or the compensator to be used. In order to preserve skin-sparing with supervoltage treatments the majority of the shell material in the treatment field is cut away just leaving two cross-bars to support the entry point mark as shown in Fig. 41.34.

The treatment shell also plays an important part in the planning stage as has already been described on p. 814. The internal contour of the shell at the level of the plane containing the beam axes can be obtained and used as the outline for the calculation of the treatment plan.

Simulation and check films

A treatment simulator is a machine having all the movements of a treatment machine and its couch, but with a diagnostic tube head fitted instead of a treatment head. In addition to a normal diagnostic-type light beam diaphragm for adjusting the beam size, the machine also has radio-opaque cross-wires which can be adjusted to outline any rectangular shape within the beam.

In use the simulator may be positioned so as to reproduce exactly the set-up of a treatment field on a patient. The cross wires are set to the size of the treatment field to be used and the main diaphragms opened wider so as to include neighbouring organs and structures. In screening mode, the image intensifier picture will enable the radiotherapist to check that the treatment field is centred correctly, includes the whole of the volume required to be treated, and does not include some adjacent sensitive organ. A radiograph can provide a permanent record of the set-up of each field. Ideally the machine parameters for each field (i.e. size, angulation, couch positions, etc.) can be recorded and used to ensure an exact reproduction of the set-up on the treatment machine, but this requires a uniformity of scale conventions on all the treatment machines in a department and on the simulator, and such uniformity unfortunately seldom exists.

Whether or not a simulator is available, it is often useful to check a field position by taking a radiograph with the actual treatment machine when set up on the patient. Although bone does not show up very well on radiographs using high energy radiation, air cavities and changes in tissue density are quite well delineated, so that useful information can be obtained from such a check film. Fig. 41.35 shows a check film taken on a linear accelerator. A comparatively insensitive film is usually used, sandwiched between lead screens to reduce soft scattered radiation, and can often be left in position for the whole of a normal treatment exposure on the field (Wollin *et al.*, 1972).

The prescription and its implementation

Superficial and orthovoltage treatments

The calibration of a superficial or orthovoltage treatment machine will usually provide tables showing applied dose rates for each of the applicators available under given conditions of kV, mA and filtration. Pro-

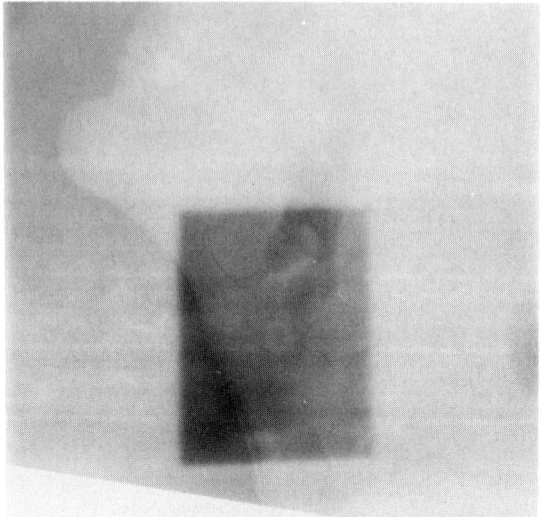

Fig. 41.35   Check film taken on 6 MeV linear accelerator using Kodak Industrex MX5 film. An exposure of 5 rad was given on the treatment field and then a further 5 rad given with the field enlarged so as to show up surrounding structures. (Reproduced by permission of Professor M.J. Peckham, Royal Marsden Hospital.)

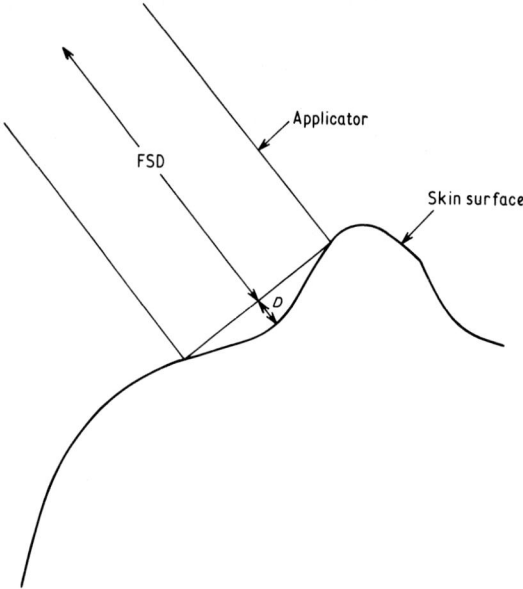

Fig. 41.36   Stand-off of applicator caused by re-entrant surface in treatment area.

vided that the kV and mA readings are maintained at their correct values the radiation output should correspond to the calibration figure, although machines will usually also have a monitor ionization chamber, the output from which is shown on a meter on the control desk and provides a check on the constancy of the machine's performance. The delivery of the required applied dose is then obtained by setting up a time on a treatment timer that controls the termination of the exposure. The time required for a particular field is calculated by dividing the unit applied dose required on that field by the applied dose rate for the applicator used. Thus if 500 rad is required using an applicator for which the applied dose rate is given as 50 rad/min, the treatment time will be 500/50 = 10 min.

Sometimes, as mentioned on p. 816, a lead cut-out may be used to modify the field size. This will alter the dose rate because of the difference in back-scatter, and this must be taken into account in calculating the treatment time. What is called the Back-scatter Factor (BSF) is the ratio of the dose rate at the entry point of the beam with tissue persent to the dose rate at the same point in air, and the tables of BSFs for different field sizes and different radiation qualities are available in the *British Journal of Radiology*, Supplement 11 (1972). When a lead cut-out is used its area must be

found and the corresponding BSFs for that area and for the applicator looked up in the tables. The applied dose rate for use with the cut-out is then calculated from:

$$\text{Applied dose rate with cut-out} = \text{Applied dose rate for applicator} \times \frac{\text{BSF for cut-out}}{\text{BSF for applicator}}$$

A situation may arise as shown in Fig. 41.36 where the end of the applicator cannot be placed directly in contact with the lesion to be treated but is stood off by a distance D cm. This again reduces the effective applied dose because of the inverse square law. The applied dose rate to be used in calculating the treatment time is given by:

$$\text{Applied dose rate with stand-off} = \text{Applied dose rate for applicator} \times (F/F + D)^2$$

where F is the standard FSD for the applicator.

Megavoltage treatments – γ-ray therapy units

Gamma-ray therapy units are similar to superficial and orthovoltage X-ray machines in that the accurate delivery of the required dose is determined by a treatment timer. No monitor ionization chamber is necessary in the beam because of the steady radiation output from the source which is only affected by radioactive decay. For cobalt-60 the half-life is 5.3 years, which means that the output decreases by 1.1% per month.

Tables of applied dose rates for different field sizes therefore need to be corrected every month to take this reduction into account. Treatment times are calculated in a similar way to that described in the previous section, remembering that when a wedge filter is used the applied dose rate for the plain field must be multiplied by the appropriate wedge factor (p. 828).

Megavoltage treatments – linear accelerators and other X-ray units

The radiation output from linear accelerators and other megavoltage X-ray generators is not sufficiently constant to enable dose delivery to be determined by a treatment timer. A monitor ionization chamber in the treatment beam is therefore used to integrate the dose delivered and terminate the treatment when the required level has been reached. The output of the monitor chamber is in arbitrary dose units which do not correspond to applied dose in rad, and for which the factor converting them into rad will vary with field size. The calibration of the machine now provides tables showing the conversion factor C, in rad per monitor unit, for each field size, and the treatment is determined by setting up on the control console the number of monitor units required. These are obtained by dividing the unit applied dose by the conversion factor. Thus if C is 1.10, an applied dose of 500 rad will be delivered by $500/1.10 = 454$ monitor units. The use of a wedge must be allowed for by multiplying C by the appropriate wedge factor.

Electron beams

Linear accelerators and betatrons can provide useful beams of high energy electrons for treatment purposes, if the X-ray target is replaced with a scattering foil. The percentage depth dose curves from such beams are shown in Fig. 41.37, and have the following characteristics:

1. There is only a small skin sparing effect, very much less than that obtained with megavoltage X-ray beams.
2. The dose maximum extends over a broad plateau of length depending on the energy.
3. Beyond this plateau the dose falls rapidly because of the finite range of the electrons.
4. There is a 'tail' of more penetrating radiation which may be about 5% of the maximum.

These characteristics make electron beams particularly suitable for single field treatments of tumours extending from just under the surface to some centimetres deep, where beyond the tumour there are

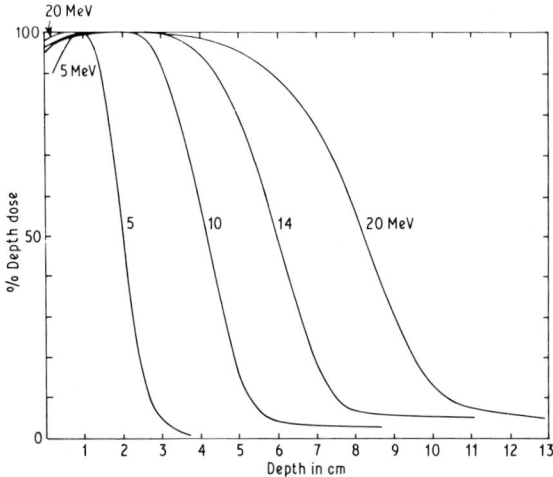

Fig. 41.37 Central axis depth dose curves of electron beams of various energies produced by Philips Medical Systems SL75/20 linear accelerator; 20 cm × 20 cm field at 95 cm FSD.

sensitive organs to which dose must be kept to a minimum. If the effective depth of treatment is taken to be where the dose falls to 90% of the maximum, then it can be seen from Fig. 41.37 that the effective treatment depth in cm is about one-third of the beam energy in MeV. The range of electrons in cm, i.e. to the end of the steeply falling part of the curve, is about half the beam energy in MeV. The 'tail' of the curve is due to high energy X-rays (bremsstrahlung) generated by electrons being stopped in the scattering foil, the collimating system and also in the patient.

The curves of Fig. 41.37 are for beams in unit density soft tissue. The presence of other tissues will affect the depth dose curve mainly because of density differences. Corrections can be made by assuming that the attenuation for broad slabs by a thickness, T, of inhomogeneity is equivalent to the attenuation by a thickness $T \times C_{ET}$ of water, where $C_{ET} = 0.5, 1.1$ and 1.8 for lung, spongy bone and compact bone respectively (ICRU, 1972). The effect of small inhomogeneities is more complex. In particular, small air cavities can produce just beyond the cavity, doses higher than would be expected from consideration solely of the lower density in the cavity. Increases of 60% above the normal tissue maximum have been reported by Starchman and Chao (1972), and are a factor to be taken into account when using electron beams in the region of the mouth, neck and sinus cavities.

Fig. 41.38 shows a typical isodose chart for an electron beam. The beam edges are not so well defined as for an X-ray beam from a linear accelerator, and tend

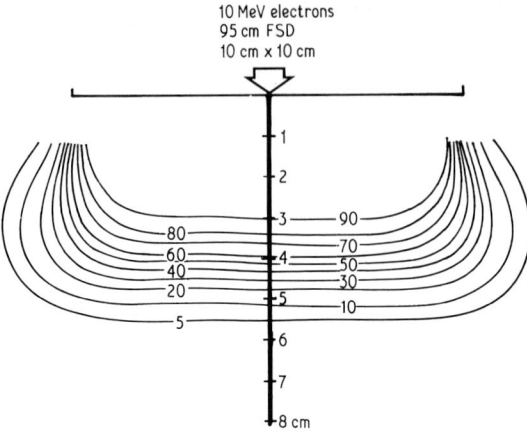

10 MeV electrons
95 cm FSD
10 cm x 10 cm

Fig. 41.38 Isodose chart for a 10 cm × 10 cm 10 MeV electron beam.

to bulge outwards towards the end of the range. Within the beam the 90% isodose curve is not flat over the whole of the nominal field width, so that a wider field may need to be specified to treat the full lateral extent of a tumour adequately.

Mould room facilities

A radiotherapy department requires adequate facilities for making the various treatment aids needed for individual patients such as shells and lead cut-outs. The space for such facilities (designated a Mould Room from the days when a large part of the work was making external radium moulds) should be conveniently placed for patient access, and also be close to the simulator room or diagnostic equipment for taking check films. A small suite of rooms is required since in addition to the main workroom, a separate room with sink should be available for work directly involving the patient such as making plaster casts and fitting treatment shells. One also needs a storeroom for materials and an office for keeping documentation and other paper work. An adjacent mechanical workshop containing a lathe, milling machine, drilling machine and other similar equipment is very convenient, although the main purpose of this mechanical workshop will be for more general work in connection with the radiotherapy machines.

The Mould Room will need to have an adequate set of small tools of its own and also to be equipped with specialist equipment, in particular a vacuum moulding machine for moulding plastic sheet onto the plaster casts, and mixing bowls, etc. used in making these casts. Materials are available which can be cold-moulded directly on to the patient (see Lewinsky and

Walton, 1976) and the use of these would avoid the use of plaster and might obviate the need for a moulding machine. Another item is a device for tracing the contour from the inside of treatment shells. If compensators are used, then the Mould Room will be the place where the compensator blocks and plates are kept, made up and suitably labelled so as to be uniquely identified for a particular field on a particular patient.

Brachytherapy – interstitial, intracavitary and 'mould' treatments*

The use of arrays of sources consisting of sealed containers of radioactive material emitting ionizing photons, commonly called interstitial implants when implanted into tissue, is a very valuable tool for radiotherapy. When such arrays are lying against or very close to tissue surfaces but not actually within tissue they are termed intracavity insertions or external moulds depending on their anatomical location.

The common features of these procedures fall into two categories. The first category includes the nature of the containers and the mode of preparation, handling and use. Many sources are used for all three types of procedure. Nearly all the procedures present problems in controlling the radiation dose to staff. The second category includes the physical principles underlying the geometry of the array of sources and the clinical objectives.

The ideal treatment by these procedures could be one in which all the malignant tissue was uniformly saturated with radioactive sources emitting very short range radiation. Then the tumour could be uniformly irradiated while sparing normal tissue. The details of the practical methods in use are influenced by the deviations from an ideal imposed by a number of constraints.

1. The radiation has considerable penetration with a fall-off from a point source approximating to the inverse square law over at least the dimensions of the tumour. Because of this, uniformity of absorbed dose can only be approached in an interstitial implant by increasing the density at which sources are located around the periphery of the tumour volume. Otherwise, if the sources are uniformly arranged the dose at the centre will be roughly double the dose at the periphery.

2. The anatomy of tumour sites can force the therapist to use only medially placed sources as for treatment of the cervix or uterus or frontally placed sources as for treatment of the tongue, or centrally placed sources as for treatment of the lip, or externally placed sources for mould treatments.

*Contributed by J.S. Orr

3. The limited number of radioactive substances available, and the strength and shapes of the containers which are required to withstand rough handling yet be easily inserted into tissues or narrow tubes, limit the options open to the manufacturers of sources and to the radiotherapist. The geometry and absorption of the containers also affect the dose distribution.

Methods of reducing or overcoming some or all of the radiation hazard problems include remote handling and afterloading methods for the safety of radiotherapists and technical and theatre staff, the use of ^{125}I seeds which can also reduce dose to nursing staff, and a variety of remotely controlled equipments for intracavitary treatments which are safe for all staff (Simon, 1971; Paine, 1972; Pierquin, 1964).

The radioactive materials commonly available are listed in Table 41.4 together with some of their physical properties.

Most of the rules and tables for deciding on the total amount of radioactive substances to be used for a particular patient and the rules for deciding on the arrangements of sources were worked out for radium. The roles of all the substances listed in Table 41.4 are so similar with respect to these rules that it has often proved convenient to measure the strength of each in terms of the equivalent number of milligrams of radium. Then the rules can be used directly with only minor corrections although radioactive decay must be taken into account.

One way to get a simple overall view of the physical basis of the rules used in practice is to start with the concept of a point source and consider the radiation emanating from it. The strengths or effective activities of the sources are defined on the basis of the dose rate on the surface of a sphere of 1 cm radius with the source at the centre of the sphere. If the spherical surface round the source is increased in radius, r, the area of the surface, which is derived from the formula πr^2, increases in proportion to r^2. Then, since dose is usefully regarded as a concentration, it can be seen that the radiation is diluted in space over the larger area. The dilution factor is evidently r^2, and if the dose rate at the surface of the larger sphere is to be the same as that for the standard 1 cm sphere, the strength of the sources at the centre must be increased by this same factor r^2.

In clinical applications the external surface of the volume to be treated normally receives the lowest dose rate, and since this must not fall below the minimum lethal tumour dose, it is roughly true that the same total dose, allowing for overall time, is given to this external surface. As indicated above, the strengths of sources to achieve this must be proportional to the area of the external surface.

If the sources were all at the centre a non-uniform distribution would result, and, where this is not the aim, the sources are normally concentrated near the periphery if practicable. Such a peripheral arrangement requires an increase in strength over the simplest central case. In addition, if the volume is asymmetrical, for example, elongated, a further increase in strength is required since the surface presented to the radiation is relatively increased.

The practical rules developed from thorough theoretical bases embody these simple features, which are also implicit in empirical rules which have evolved purely from clinical experience.

A well known and widely used set of rules suitable for any of the above radioactive substances, but particularly for those whose source strengths are expressed by their equivalence to radium mg, is the Manchester System. This is clearly described by Meredith (1967), and also by Paterson (1963) and Howell (1972).

Two examples using the tables from Meredith (1967) will illustrate the procedures. In each case a total dose of 7000 roentgens (on which unit the tables are based) is to be given in one week.

Table 41.4

	Half-life	*Photon energy*	*Half value layer (lead)*
Cobalt-60	5.3 years	1.17, 1.33 MeV	12 mm
Iodine-125	60 days	27–35 keV	0.025 mm
Caesium-137	30 years	660 keV	6 mm
Tantalum-182	115 days	0.07–1.2 MeV	12 mm
Iridium-192	74 days	0.3–0.6 MeV	4.5 mm
Gold-198	2.7 days	412 keV	4.5 mm
Radon-222	3.8 days	0.24–2.2 MeV	13.0 mm
Radium-226	1600 years	0.18–2.2 MeV	13.0 mm

A   A planar implant is to treat a volume 4 cm × 6.5 cm by 1 cm thick with the radioactive sources placed centrally 0.5 cm from each of the two larger surfaces. The appropriate table gives 442 mg hours per 1000 R for such an implant with sources distributed in a plane over an area of 26 cm². Therefore, since 7000 R is required in 168 hours, the total strength required is

$$\frac{(442 \times 7)}{168} = 18.4 \text{ mg radium equiv.}$$

In the reference, rules are given for the arrangement of the sources to achieve a stated degree of uniformity of dose over the two large surfaces.

B   A volume implant is to treat a cylinder of tissue 2 cm in radius and 3.5 cm high. The volume of tissue is 44 cc and the appropriate table gives 447 mg hours per 1000 R for sources distributed throughout the volume. Thus 18.6 mg radium equivalent would be required.

Note that surfaces of the treated volumes indicated in these examples both have areas of about 70 cm² but that the sources are distributed more peripherally in the second example.

Of all the substances listed in Table 41.4 and used for interstitial implants, iodine-125 has the special attraction of minimizing the radiation to ward nursing staff. This is because of the very low energy, less than 35 kV, of the X-rays. ^{125}I is supplied in the form of titanium seeds 4.5 mm long and 0.8 mm wide containing a radio-opaque gold marker and two spheres of ion exchange resin holding the ^{125}I (Hilaris, 1975).

The half-life of 60 days makes ^{125}I considerably different from other sources used for permanent interstitial implants. The dose rate is low which makes handling and insertion safer and the total dose given is normally above 16 000 rad over a year. The low energy also allows the release of patients earlier than for other substances. One empirical formula for calculating the activity required is based on the average length of the three mutually perpendicular dimensions of the volume to be treated, $(A+B+C)/3$. This is multiplied by a factor which may be approximated by a constant or taken as decreasing as the average dimension increases.

Clinical experience has shown that care and accuracy in all aspects of brachytherapy, including planning and dosimetry, can give improved results whatever sources are used.

Further reading

Johns, H.E. and Cunningham, J.R. (1974), *The Physics of Radiology*. Thomas, Springfield.
Meredith, W.J. and Massey, J.B. (1977), *Fundamental Physics of Radiology*. 3rd edn, Wright, Bristol.

References

Armstrong, D. and Tait, J. (1973), The matching of adjacent fields in radiotherapy. *Radiology*, **108**, 419–22.
Bahr, G.K. *et al*. (1966), The method of linear programming applied to radiation treatment planning. *Radiology*, **91**, 686–93.
Battista, J.J., Rider, W.D. and Van Dyk, J. (1980), Computed tomography for radiotherapy treatment planning. *Int. J. Rad. Oncol. Biol. Physics*, **6**, 99–107.
Bentley, R.E. and Milan, J. (1971), An interactive digital computer system for radiotherapy treatment planning. *Br. J. Radiol*., **44**, 826–33.
Borger, F, Simpson, L. and Ovadia, J. (1972), An analytical model for a 6 MeV X-ray beam. *Phys. Med. Biol*., **17**, 444.
British Journal of Radiology (1972), Central axis depth dose data for use in radiotherapy. Supplement 11.
Clarke, H.C. (1969), A contouring device for use in radiation treatment planning. *Br. J. Radiol*., **42**, 858–60.
Clarkson, J.R. (1941), A note on depth dose in fields of irregular shape. *Br. J. Radiol*., **14**, 265–8.
Clayton, C.B. and Thompson, D.J. (1970), An optical apparatus for reproducing surface outlines of body cross-sections. *Br. J. Radiol*., **43**, 489–92.
Crossland, P., Haybittle, J.L. and Jameson, D.G. (1976), An on-line computer graphics terminal for radiotherapy treatment planning. *Br. J. Radiol*., **49**, 868–74.
Cunningham, J.R., Shrivastava, P.N. and Williamson, J.M. (1972), Program IRREG – calculation of dose from irregularly shaped radiation beams. *Comput. Prog. Biomed*., **2**, 192–9.
Doolittle, A.M. *et al*. (1977), An electronic patient-contouring device. *Br. J. Radiol*., **50**, 135–8.
Du Sault, L.A. (1959), A simplified method of treatment planning. *Radiology*, **73**, 85–94.
Edland, R.W. and Hanson, H. (1969), Irregular field shaping for ^{60}Co teletherapy. *Radiology*, **92**, 1567–9.
Giessan, P.H. (1973), A method of calculating the isodose shift in correcting for oblique incidence in radiotherapy. *Br. J. Radiol*., **46**, 978–82.
Glover, J.R. (1966), A more general form of the power law for tissue/air ratios. *Phys. Med. Biol*., **11**, 607–8.
Greene, D. and Stewart, J.G. (1965), Isodose curves in non-uniform phantoms. *Br. J. Radiol*., **38**, 378–85.
Gupta, S.K. and Cunningham, J.R. (1966), Measurement of tissue-air ratios and scatter functions for large field sizes for cobalt-60 gamma radiation. *Br. J. Radiol*., **39**, 7–11.

Hall, E.J. and Oliver, R. (1961), The use of standard isodose distributions with high energy radiation beams. The accuracy of a compensator technique in correcting for body contours. *Br. J. Radiol.*, **34**, 43–52.

Hilaris, B.S. (ed) (1975), *Handbook of Interstitial Therapy*. Publishing Services Group, Inc., Acton, Mass., USA.

Hobday, P. *et al*. (1979), Computed tomography applied to radiotherapy treatment planning: Techniques and results. *Radiology*, **133**, 477–82.

Hodes, L. (1974), Semi-automatic optimization of external beam radiation treatment planning. *Radiology*, **110**, 191–6.

Holt, J.G., Laughlin, J.S. and Moroney, J.P. (1970), Extension of the concept of tissue-air ratios to high energy X-ray beams. *Radiology*, **96**, 437–46.

Hope, C.S. *et al*. (1967), Optimization of X-ray treatment planning by computer judgement. *Phys. Med. Biol.*, **12**, 531–42.

Hope, C.S. and Orr, J.S. (1965), Computer optimization of 4 MeV treatment planning. *Phys. Med. Biol.*, **10**, 365–73.

Howell, J.B. (1972), *Radium Recipes for Cutaneous Cancer*. Charles C. Thomas, Springfield.

ICRU, (1972), *Radiation Dosimetry: Electrons with Initial Energies between 1 and 50 MeV*. Report 21, ICRU, Washington.

Lanzl, L.H. *et al*. (1970), An automatic patient-contouring measuring apparatus. *Am. J. Roentg.*, **108**, 162–71.

Lewinsky, B.S. and Walton, R. (1976), Lightcast: an aid to planning treatment and immobilization in radiotherapy and research. *Int. J. Radiat. Oncol. Biol. Phys.*, **1**, 1011–5.

Lillicrap, S.C. and Milan, J. (1975), A device for the automatic recording of patient outlines on the treatment simulator. *Phys. Med. Biol.*, **20**, 627–31.

Marshall, T.J., Mott, G.T. and Grieveson, M.H. (1975), A technique for using low melting point alloy for individual patient shielding in radiotherapy. *Br. J. Radiol.*, **48**, 924–6.

Massey, J. (1962), Dose distribution problems in megavoltage therapy. 1. The problem of air spaces. *Br. J. Radiol.*, **35**, 736–8.

Meredith, W.J. (1967), *Radium Dosage, The Manchester Method*. E. and S. Livingstone, Edinburgh and London.

Milan, J. *et al*. (1976), On-line beam data acquisition for a dedicated radiotherapy planning computer. *Br. J. Radiol.*, **49**, 172–5.

Orchard, P. (1964), Decrement lines: a new presentation of data in cobalt 60 beam dosimetry. *Br. J. Radiol.*, **37**, 756–63.

Paine, C.H. (1972), Modern afterloading methods for interstitial radiotherapy. *Clin. Radiol.*, **23**, 263.

Parker, R.P., Hobday, P.A. and Cassell, K.J. (1979), The direct use of CT numbers in radiotherapy dosage calculations for inhomogeneous media. *Phys. Med. Biol.*, **24**, 802–9.

Paterson, R. (1963), *The Treatment of Malignant Disease by Radiotherapy*. Williams and Wilkins, Baltimore.

Pierquin, B. (1964), *Précis de Curiethérapie*, Masson et Cie, Paris.

Redpath, A.T., Vickery, B.L. and Duncan, W. (1977), A comprehensive radiotherapy planning system implemented in Fortran on a small interactive computer. *Br. J. Radiol.*, **50**, 51–7.

Reinstein, L.E. *et al*. (1978), A computer-assisted three dimensional treatment planning system. *Radiology*, **127**, 259–64.

Richter, J. (1967), A new formula for tissue-air ratios in ^{60}Co therapy. *Br. J. Radiol.*, **40**, 479–80.

Simon, N. (ed.) (1971), *Afterloading in Radiotherapy*. US Dept of Health, Education and Welfare.

Starchman, D.E. and Chao, J.H. (1972), Perturbation of isodose distributions adjacent to cavities in tissue-equivalent media during irradiation by 10–35 MeV electrons. *Radiology*, **104**, 177–86.

Sterling, T., Perry, H. and Weinkam, J. (1967), Automation of radiation treatment planning; VI: A general field equation to calculate percent depth dose in the irradiated volume of a cobalt 60 beam. *Br. J. Radiol.*, **40**, 463–8.

Sutherland, W.H. (1962), Arc therapy with wedge-filtered beams of cobalt 60 radiation. *Br. J. Radiol.*, **35**, 478–81.

Thames, H.D. (1973), A new method for computer generation of dose distributions for external X- and gamma-ray sources. *Radiology*, **106**, 199–208.

Thomas, R.L. (1970), A general expression for megavoltage central axis depth doses. *Br. J. Radiol.*, **43**, 554–7.

Thomas, R.L. and Haybittle, J.L. (1975), A widely applicable method for computing dose distributions from external megavoltage beams. *Br. J. Radiol.*, **48**, 749–54.

Van de Geijn, J. (1965a), The construction of individualised intensity modifying filters in cobalt 60 teletherapy. *Br. J. Radiol.*, **38**, 865–70.

Van de Geijn, J. (1965b), The computation of two and three dimensional dose distributions in cobalt 60 teletherapy. *Br. J. Radiol.*, **38**, 369–77.

Van de Geijn, J. (1970), A computer program for 3-D planning in external beam radiation therapy, EXTDOS. *Comput. Prog. Biomed.*, **1**, 47–57.

Van de Geijn, J. (1972), Revised and expanded version of EXTDOS, a program for treatment planning in external beam therapy. *Comput. Prog. Biomed.*, **2**, 169–77.

Van der Laarse, R. and Strackee, J. (1976), Pseudo

optimization of radiotherapy treatment planning. *Br. J. Radiol.*, **49**, 450–7.

Weinkam, J.J., Kolde, R.A. and Sterling, T.D. (1973), Extending the general field equation to fit the dose distributions of a variety of therapy units. *Br. J. Radiol.*, **46**, 983–90.

Wilks, R.J. and Sutcliffe, J.F. (1977), A simple model of ^{60}Co beams for computerized radiotherapy planning. *Phys. Med. Biol.*, **22**, 737–46.

Wilks, R. and Casebow, M.P. (1969), Tissue compensation with lead for ^{60}Co therapy. *Br. J. Radiol.*, **42**, 452–6.

Wollin, M. *et al.* (1972), A photographic method of defining radiotherapeutic portals. *Br. J. Radiol.*, **45**, 73–4.

Worthley, B. (1966), Equivalent square of rectangular fields. *Br. J. Radiol.*, **39**, 558.

42 Radiation hazards and protection

R.E. Ellis

The statutory requirements in the United Kingdom under the Health and Safety at Work Act (1976) and the European Economic Community Directive on Radiation Protection (1976) have made it essential for all employers to reappraise their existing radiation protection arrangements to ensure the safety of their staff and members of the public who may enter their facilities or who live in the neighbourhood of establishments utilizing radiation. Other countries too are having to reconsider their radiation protection arrangements in the light of the International Commission on Radiological Protection (ICRP) Publication 26 (1977) which has considerably changed the general philosophy behind the setting of the maximum permissible dose levels. Emphasis has now been placed on quantifying the probability of deleterious effects occurring in the irradiated person whereas in previous reports maximum permissible dose levels had been set without identifying the order of risk other than that it was small and considered to be acceptable by the worker.

In the context of this book the emphasis in this chapter on radiation protection is to pick out for radiotherapists those aspects which will be of particular concern in their specialty. Therefore some aspects of radiation protection, e.g. attenuation of shielding materials, will be given only passing mention and the reader is referred to one of many texts available, some of which are referred to in the bibliography at the end of the chapter.

The chapter is divided into three main sections. The first gives in some detail the radiobiological evidence of the effects and risks of radiation using particularly data drawn from epidemiological studies of patients who have received radiation treatment. Consideration is given both to the acute effects occurring in a matter of weeks after irradiation and to the long-term effects of irradiation.

The second section summarizes the current ICRP philosophy and gives details of the revised recommendations for dose-equivalent limits for occupational exposure and for members of the public.

The third section summarizes the current legislation in the European Economic Community and their application in the UK with attention drawn to the existence of Codes of Practice, notes for guidance and various texts produced in the USA, which together provide sources of advice for good practice in the various aspects of radiology and radiotherapy.

The biological effects of radiation

Acute effects

Whole body irradiation
The likelihood of an accident involving whole body irradiation occurring in a radiotherapy department is small; nevertheless such accidents have occurred. The cause of such accidents has usually been the mechanical failure of a shutter or source movement or the operation of accelerators under irregular conditions. Studies of the cells in the circulating blood have been correlated with dose for a number of accidents including those in the nuclear power industry where so termed 'criticality accidents' have occurred. These latter accidents occur when a quantity of fissile material, which is normally handled with great care at subcritical concentrations, has accidently come together in critical amounts. The ensuing explosion releases flash doses of up to several thousand rad of penetrating γ-rays. The Institute of Nuclear Studies at Oak Ridge has combined blood cell data from these accidents with data from patients given whole body irradiation of up to about 200 rad of γ-rays for the control of leukaemia. The pooled data are given in Figs. 42.1, 2 and 3 for external whole body doses of 100, 300 and 450 rad respectively.

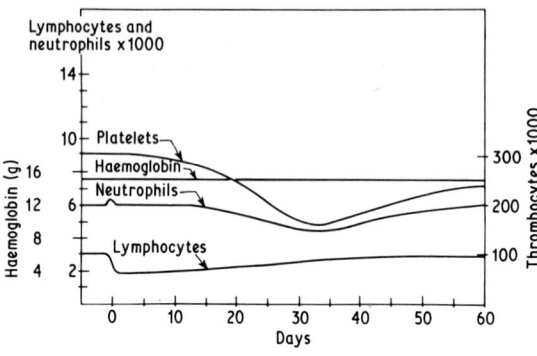

Fig. 42.1　Typical haematologic response to 100 rad.

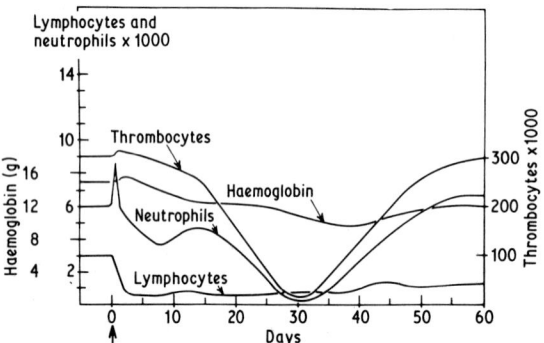

Fig. 42.2　Typical haematologic response to 300 rad.

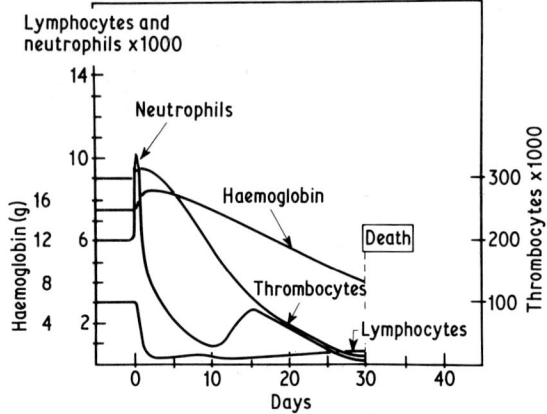

Fig. 42.3　Typical haematologic response to 450 rad

It can be seen from these graphs that the early drop in circulating lymphocytes may be used as a measure of the radiation dose. At doses in excess of about 150 rad the drop in lymphocytes is such as to leave the person susceptible to infection and regimes of isolation of the patient and the use of broad-spectrum antibiotics have been used to help the accident cases survive. The other cell types tend to reach their minimum number at about 30 days post-irradiation and it is at this time that death may occur from the so-termed haematological death. Deaths that occur within a few days of the irradiation are due to the more severe gastrointestinal reactions and disturbances of the fluid and electrolyte imbalance and these effects occur after doses of several hundred rad up to about 800 rad. At doses above this level the central nervous system is affected almost immediately, observations indicate a staggering in gait occurring half a minute after doses of the order of 1000 rad or so.

The 'haematological death' occurring at 30 days (Fig. 42.3) is typical of most mammalian species and is used to compare the mean lethal dose, i.e. that dose which will cause 50% of the irradiated population to die within 30 days. This is often referred to as the LD50 (lethal dose for 50% death) but should be stated as the LD50%/in 30 days. For man this is usually stated as being in the 450–500 rad range but obviously depends on the amount of medical care available to the irradiated person. The newer techniques being practised in a few radiotherapy centres for the treatment of leukaemia involve whole body irradiation of about 800 rad of γ-rays to destroy the immune response and such treatments and subsequent medical and nursing techniques obviously enhance the probability of survival. These facilities and techniques will obviously aid accident cases which may occur in the future.

Partial body irradiation
The radiation doses quoted in the previous section that lead to death or severe changes in the blood cell picture only apply to those instances where absolutely total body irradiation occurs. Should any portion of the bone marrow be shielded from irradiation then that marrow will be available to help prevent the extreme drop in cell types. There are many reports of animal studies that illustrate this effect as well as information indicating a generalized reduction of response as the fraction of the body irradiated is reduced. The results of experiments on mice in which the intestine was irradiated as part of whole body irradiation, or the intestines were shielded but the rest of the mouse irradiated or the intestine alone was irradiated, showed that the mean dose for death from gut damage occurred at 800, 1200 and 2000 rad respectively.

Biological dosimetry using leucocyte chromosome aberrations
The techniques of preparing cultures of peripheral leucocytes and undertaking chromosome karyotyping

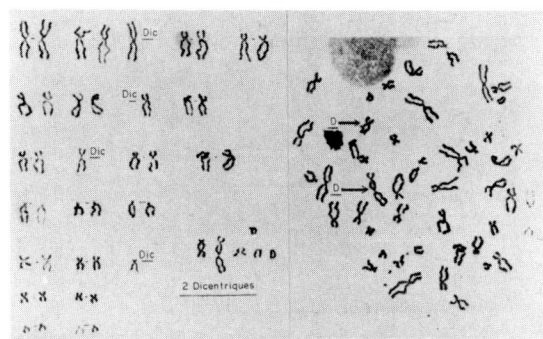

Fig. 42.4 Chromosome abnormalities after irradiation of 600 rad of X-rays.

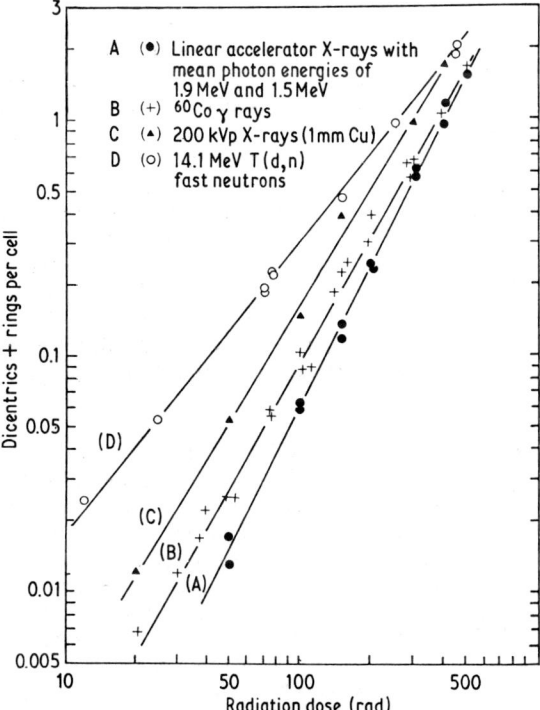

Fig. 42.5 Dose-response relationship for dicentrics plus rings for different qualities of radiation (cells irradiated *prior* to culture and cultured for *fifty* hours).

after 54 hours of culture has enabled the frequency of aberration yield in the chromosomes to be used as a biological dosimeter. The technique is simple in that only 10 ml of peripheral blood is required from the donor and the estimation of the number of dicentrics plus rings per cell can be obtained within three days.

Fig. 42.4 shows a typical karyotyping obtained from an occupational worker in which four chromosomes were shown to be abnormal and the dicentrics and fragments of chromosomes are shown together. Similar studies have been made of patients treated for ankylosing spondylitis as well as low dose whole body irradiation. A comprehensive account of the data obtained by this technique was published by UNSCEAR (1969).

The technique is sufficiently sensitive to determine whole body doses down to 5 rad of γ-rays. The response is dependent on radiation quality being more sensitive at higher LETs (Linear Energy Transfer). The response to 200 kV X-ray and 14 MeV neutrons being twice and seven times as sensitive per rad compared with cobalt-60 γ-rays at a dose of 20 rad (Fig. 42.5).The technique has proved very useful in those accident cases where there is some doubt as to the level of exposure particularly at low doses up to 100 rad where there is little evidence of a change in blood count. The National Radiological Protection Board at Harwell, Oxon, operates a postal service in the UK and the result is available within five days of receipt of the sample.

Other acute effects

Other acute effects may be utilized to identify the level of localized radiation doses. For example, the skin reaction may be used for cases of irradiation by X-rays up to about 400 kV or from β-rays and electrons. The erythema occurs after doses in excess of 400–600 rad of low energy 100 kV radiation. Somewhat higher doses are required at X-ray energies up to about 400 kV. At this energy and above the maximum dose then begins to be just under the surface and less erythema occurs. The erythema threshold is however dependent on the person's skin colouration and pigmentation.

Loss of hair (epilation) occurs some 10–20 days after radiation from a single X-ray dose of 450–600 rad. At higher doses of about 1000 rad permanent loss of hair will occur. A similar effect can be seen from protracted irradiation received by occupational workers, e.g. the loss of hair on the back of the phalanges in people involved with high hand doses. This apparently occurs at somewhat lower dose levels and may be due to an increased fragility of the hair.

Long-term effects

The effects of radiation may be classified as somatic effects which affect the individual who receives the irradiation and the genetic effects which cause deleterious effects in the subsequent offspring of the irradiated person. It is also necessary to distinguish between those effects which occur with a low probability and therefore can be considered to be 'a chance' that the specific deleterious effect will occur and those effects that will occur in all irradiated individuals if a specific tissue or organ receives a given dose.

Somatic effects – summary

The long-term effects of irradiation of an individual are to increase the risk of somatic injury resulting in:

(a) The induction of cancer: leukaemia, thyroid cancer, cancer of the breast, bone cancer, lung cancer, other cancers at other sites.
(b) Development abnormalities in the irradiated foetus or in growing bone or other tissues.
(c) Non-specific reduction in life span.
(d) Opacities of the lens of the eye (cataracts).
(e) Chromosomal abnormalities.
(f) Decreased fertility

Induction of leukaemia

The incidence of leukaemia induction expressed in numbers of excess leukaemia induced per million population irradiated by unit dose has been derived from two main sources. One source is the study of survivors of the atom bomb explosions at Hiroshima and Nagasaki in 1945 and the other the study of 13 352 patients who received X-ray treatments for ankylosing spondylitis in the year 1935–1955. In the earlier study of these patients Court Brown and Doll (1955) identified that some 0.3% of the patients subsequently developed leukaemia. In the latest of the studies of this group Smith and Doll (1978) have shown that for those patients who received only one course of treatment the excess risk of developing leukaemia rose soon after the treatment ended, the mean latent period was about ten years and the excess risk dropped to zero within 20 years (Fig. 42.6). A similar distribution of leukaemia induction was shown by the atom bomb survivors with the excess incidence dropping back to zero by 1970, i.e. after 25 years. The skin doses given to the ankylosing spondylitic patients were in the range 1000–2000 rad given over periods of two or three weeks. The average dose to the whole bone marrow was 350 rad. The fields were sited over the spine from the cervical spine down to the lumbar spine and generally across the sacroiliac joints. The dose received by the atom bomb survivors was in the range of a few rad to several hundred rad of mixed radiation of γ-rays and neutrons.

The risk rate for the induction of leukaemia has been taken in these studies to be in the range 20–40 cases induced per million man rem (20–40 cases per 10^4 man Sv).

A survey of patients who had received X-ray or radium treatments to the pelvis for the treatment of metropathia haemorrhagica were shown by Smith and Doll (1976) to have an increased incidence of

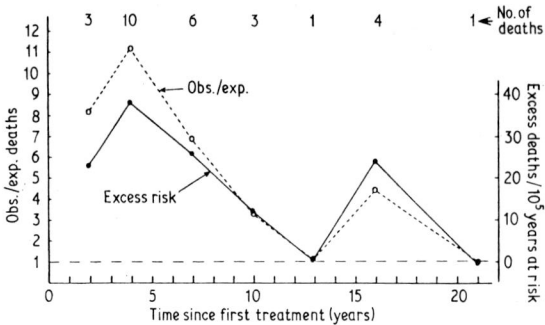

Fig. 42.6 Observed and expected numbers of deaths from leukaemia according to the time since first treatment.

leukaemia of 17 per million man rad. However no surveys have indicated an increase in leukaemia in those patients treated at much higher doses for carcinoma of the cervix. A possible explanation may be that considerably more cell killing is likely to take place in the volumes of bone marrow in the pelvis in these latter treatments and hence less cells are present to undergo a neoplastic change.

Induction of other cancers

The workers with X-rays who suffered damage from ionizing radiation in the early part of this century were

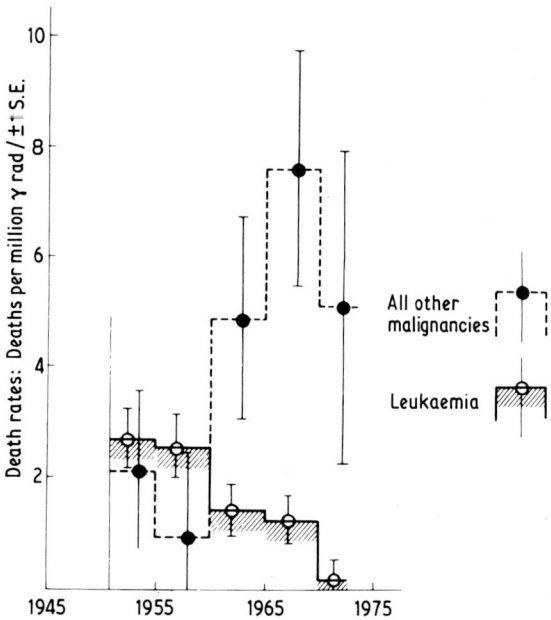

Fig. 42.7 Variation of death rates from leukaemia and from all other malignancies with time since exposure.

aware that radiation could cause neoplastic changes. Many of these workers were to become the early martyrs of radiology. To commemorate their lives there is a memorial in Hamburg with several hundred names inscribed upon it.

However, with the early reports of the increased leukaemia incidence in the atom bomb survivors attention was not focused on the increase in generalized cancers until the early 1960s. The reason for this is the longer latent period for the induction of generalized cancers compared with that of leukaemia. Fig. 42.7 shows the incidence curve of generalized cancers in the atom bomb survivors compared with the leukaemia incidence. The ankylosing spondylitic population referred to previously was also studied to see whether there was an increase in the generalized cancers for those tissues which were heavily irradiated, i.e. in the direct path of the X-ray fields which were applied to the spine from the posterior–anterior direction. Court Brown and Doll (1965) showed that there was a similar increase and in the recent report by Smith and Doll (1978) the incidence of observed cancers compared with those that were expected is higher for a number of sites (Fig. 42.8). The latent period of these cancers, shown in Fig. 42.9, shows that there is a 20–30 year period when cancers may arise. In fact from the data of the atom bomb survivors shown in Fig. 42.7, who obviously were all irradiated in August 1945, it is clear that it will be some years after the 25 years to 1970 before the generalized cancer frequency returns to that of the general Japanese population.

A further interesting feature of the recent ankylosing spondylitic study is that the incidence of the excess induced cancer increases with the age at the first irradi-

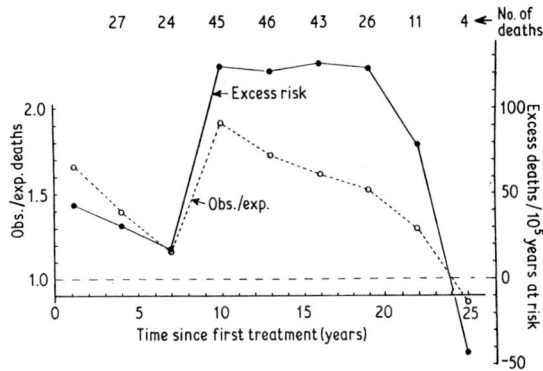

Fig. 42.9 Observed and expected deaths from cancers of heavily irradiated sites according to the time since first treatment.

ation which may be interpreted as indicating that there may be a synergistic effect between radiation and other carcinogenic agents.

An increase in cancers in the pelvic region was reported in 1956 by Palmer and Spratt for patients who had received radiation for the induction of an artificial menopause by placing radium tubes in the uterus. There was a greater than expected incidence of cancers of the fundus uteri, cervix, ovary, rectum, bladder, vagina and vulva: 4% of the patients developed malignancies compared with the 0.7% expected. These patients would have received radiation doses of about 2500 rad close to the sources and average doses of about 700 rad in the pelvis.

Thyroid cancer

There are four sources of information that give information of the induction of thyroid cancer. These are the atom bomb survivors; fishermen from the Marshall Islands in the Pacific who were, for three days, in the fall out from an American nuclear weapon, and two groups of young people who received radiation from medical treatments.

The first of the two medically treated groups is the group of children who were treated in the USA during the period 1927–1957 for enlarged thymus glands. Irradiation was given to anterior and posterior fields with total average doses to the thyroid of 200 rad. Because of the direction of the applied fields the thyroid gland was in the direct beam for the larger field sizes. Surveys by Pifer (1963) and Hempelmann (1975) showed that some 0.6% of the children subsequently developed thyroid cancer.

The second group were children who, in the years up to the late 1950s, were given four- and five-field treatments to the head with doses of 450–550 rad/field to

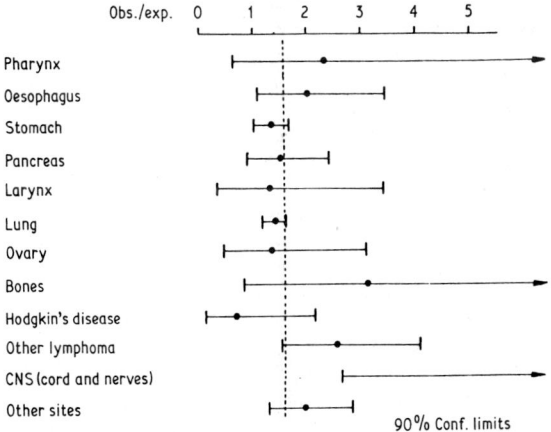

Fig. 42.8 Ratio of observed to expected number of deaths from cancers of heavily irradiated sites three or more years after first treatment.

cause epilation and for subsequent treatment of ring-worm of the scalp. The thyroid gland was subjected to direct radiation of the order of 4–17 rad per total treatment. Since the 1960s drug treatments have been used instead.

The risk of subsequent thyroid cancer is given in Table 42.1 for the four sources. It is interesting to note the similarity of the estimates.

Table 42.1   Thyroid cancer induction.

	Risks per 10^6 rad
Atom bomb survivors	
male	20
female	47
Marshallese Islanders	145
Thymus irradiation	10–180
Ringworm irradiation	140

Breast cancer

Two studies have shown an increased sensitivity of the breasts to the induction by radiation of cancer. The study by Wanebo *et al.* (1968) showed an increased occurrence in female survivors of the A-bomb in Hiroshima and Nagasaki. The mean dose was about 130 rad and the induction rate was 24×10^{-6} per rad. No difference was found in the marital status, parity or length of lactation between the 16 women with breast cancer and the 7819 women in the control group. Studies of mortality rather than occurrence of breast cancer do not give such a definite relationship with excess mortality rates between $\frac{1}{3}$ and $\frac{1}{6}$ of the incidence rates. The incidence rates vary with age and show higher rates in the 10–35 year age groups about twice those for women over 35 years.

The other study relates to women who were in sanatoria in Nova Scotia and were being treated for tuberculosis during the 1930s and 1940s. At this time artificial pneumothorax was used to collapse the affected lung and diagnostic X-rays were used to monitor the progress of the patients' treatment. Myrden and Hiltz (1969) reported 22 cases of breast cancer in 300 patients treated with pneumothorax (7.3%) and four cases in 483 patients (0.8%) who did not have this treatment.

It has been difficult to estimate retrospectively the radiation doses received by these patients during their fluoroscopic X-ray examinations. They mainly were irradiated with their breasts towards the X-ray tube. Elsewhere in the world such patients were usually positioned with their backs to the tube. Assuming that the radiation doses received by the surface of the breasts were in the region 600–3000 rad the incidence rates appear to be in the range $30–140 \times 10^{-6}$ per rad.

It has been important to consider this increased risk of breast cancer in planning mammography screening programmes for well women. Recommendations such as Ellis (1972) indicated that the dose to the breast per examination should be kept below 2 rad per examination to ensure that there should be a low incidence of induction of breast cancer from such screening programmes. With the newer techniques of fast film screen combinations it has been possible to reduce the breast dose to 0.1–0.2 rad per examination. Most screening regimes now recommend X-ray examinations to be used only to supplement every two or three years the more regular inspection by palpation.

Lung cancer

Miners who are occupationally exposed to the α-emitting decay products of radon gas provide the main source of data on the induction of lung cancer. Uranium miners in Colorado and in Czechoslovakia and non-uranium miners in Sweden show an increase of lung cancer with life-time exposure. Studies have also been made of a reported association of an increase in cancer incidence in the miners who smoke as distinct from non-smokers. However, at the moment the reported sizes of the non-smoking groups are too small to make a valid judgement.

The incidences of lung cancer reported are 200–450 cases per million rad delivered to the bronchial epithelium. If a weighting factor of 5–10 is assumed for α-particles then an incidence rate for low LET radiation would be about 50 cases per 10^6 rad.

In comparison with these reports the atom bomb survivors show an incidence rate which varies from 70 cases per 10^6 rad at doses between 10–49 rad falling to 8 per 10^6 rad for exposures over 200 rad.

There is therefore a broad agreement between these sets of data which would indicate that the lung, is, like the female breast, one of the important organs to consider when specifying the tissues at risk from radiation.

Bone tumours

The induction of bone cancers would appear to be caused by a neoplastic change in the epithelial cells lining bone surfaces rather than in the irradiation of the bone matrix itself. There have been a number of studies involving groups of luminizers who painted figures on to watch and dial faces during the first world war and who ingested radium-226 by licking their brushes to get a fine point. During a 20–40 year period a significant proportion of these workers have shown radiological changes in their skeletons and for those with higher body burdens an increase of bone sarcomas.

Table 42.2 Body burdens and radiographic changes in radium luminizers.

Body Burden (μ Ci)	No.	None	Minimal	Mild	Moderate	Advanced	Malignant change
< 0.001	17	14	3	0	0	0	–
0.001–0.01	28	28	0	0	0	0	–
0.01–0.1	90	80	8	1	1	0	–
0.1–1.0	61	25	13	9	9	5	3
> 1.0	40	1	–	2	5	4	28
Total	236						

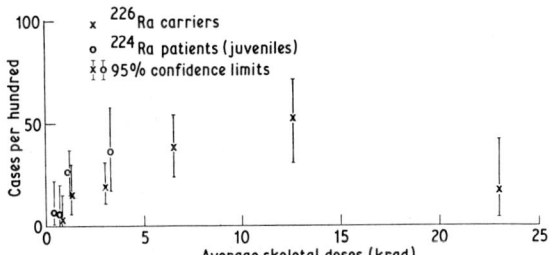

Fig. 42.10 Incidence of bone sarcomas in carriers of ^{226}Ra burdens and in ^{224}Ra-treated patients against average skeletal dose.

During the same period a number of patients were injected with radium-226 solutions as a cure for arthritic conditions and these too have presented with bone sarcomas.

Despite this information, in the late 1940s in Germany a considerable number of patients including young children were injected with radium-224 solutions.

The study of these groups has been very important for yet another reason: it is one of the very few instances where large groups of patients and workers have ingested radioactivity which has subsequently caused a neoplastic change due to internal irradiation of an organ as distinct from external irradiation.

The correlation between the body content many years after the initial contamination and the radiological and pathological findings is illustrated in Table 42.2. The incidence of bone sarcomas is shown in Fig. 42.10 where it is seen that the incidence increases at lower doses and then decreases at the higher doses due, it is considered, to the killing by the radiation of some of the cells potentially at risk. These bell-shaped induction curves have been clearly identified in a number of experimental carcinogenic studies undertaken with rodents.

The incidence rates from these studies show values of 20–25 cases per 10^6 rad for high LET radiation from $_s^{224}$Ra, 9 and 850 per 10^6 rad at the 9 rad and 100 rad level from ^{226}Ra whereas at low LET a value of 3–5 cases per 10^6 rad would appear to be appropriate.

From calculations of the dose from $0.1\,\mu\text{Ci}\ ^{226}$Ra in the skeleton an annual dose of about 30 rem was deduced. As at one time this latter activity was one tenth of the body level observed in any irradiated subject who had developed a bone sarcoma, the 30 rem/year was used as the criterion for any other internally deposited bone seeker. One half of the value, i.e. 15 rem/year, was used as the maximum permissible dose for other internal emitters concentrating in organs other than bone. These criteria were used in fixing maximum permissible values for the period 1959–1977 until the issue of ICRP 26 (see p. 856).

Development abnormalities
Radiation is known to cause damage when delivered during the development of the embryo and the foetus and a very considerable volume of experimental animal information is available. These indicate the lethal effects during the period of major organogenesis, the disturbances of growth and the malformations that may result, for example, microcephaly and malformations of the skeleton and extremities.

The data indicate that the period of major organogenesis is a vital period and in man this is considered to be from day 9 to day 60 after intercourse. By day 60 major organization of heart structures, limbs, eye and eyelids and digits has occurred and the embryo is approaching 3–4 cm long. The foetal period is taken to start at about 60 days and continue to the end of pregnancy. Irradiation during that period does not lead to gross malformations but rather defects of growth, e.g. central nervous system and gonads and at higher doses, about 350 rad and above, to foetal death. The incidence of microcephaly and subsequent mental retardation has been well illustrated by the analysis of the survivors of the atom bomb who were *in utero* at the time the atom bomb was exploded. Fig. 42.11 illustrates the percentage of the newborn children who had head circumferences below 50% of the normal and indicates that there is a 10 in 100 chance at a dose of about 20 rad and 40 in 100 chance at 50–149 rad.

An analysis of mental retardation in 18-year olds who were irradiated *in utero* in Hiroshima and Nagasaki showed (Table 42.3) that there was a 6% chance of being mentally retarded following a dose of 50–99 rad. It has to be noted that in Hiroshima about one fifth of the total dose was from neutrons and the relative biological effectiveness for the production of microcephaly by neutrons may be 10–20.

The other major concern following the irradiation *in utero* is the subsequent carcinogenesis which may occur during the first ten years of life. This effect has been extensively studied by Dr Alice Stewart in the UK and by McMahon in Canada. The studies were made on children who were X-rayed *in utero* for obstetric abdomen and pelvimetry examinations. These examinations are normally undertaken late in pregnancy. The estimates indicate that there is a risk of 0.23 per 1000 of childhood malignancies occurring for every rad received by the foetus. One half of these malignancies are likely to be leukaemia and one quarter of the central nervous system. Some countries, e.g. Denmark, recommend that if for any reason a dose of 10 rad has been received by a foetus then elective surgical abortion should be considered alongside the social implications of allowing the pregnancy to go on. Certainly, in the UK careful consideration has been given to this situation if foetal doses in excess of 20 rad have been received.

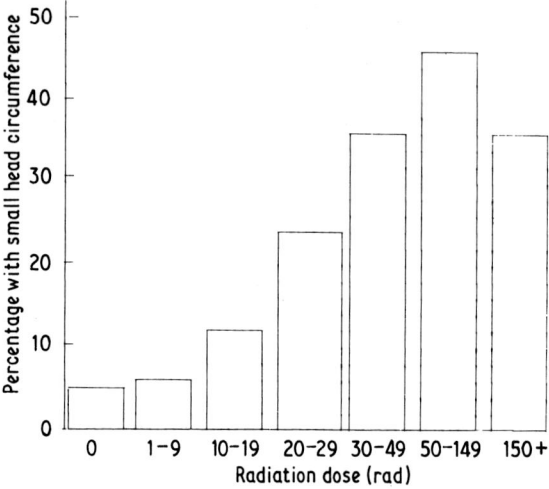

Fig. 42.11   Hiroshima children exposed before 18th week gestation.

Table 42.3   Mental retardation after exposure *in utero* in Hiroshima and Nagasaki.

Dose (rad)	Sample	Cases	Relative risk
Not in city	830	5	1.0
0–9	145	3	3.4
10–49	189	2	1.8
50–99	47	3	10.6
100–199	29	4	22.9
200–299	8	3	62.3
300+	6	2	55.3

Cataract formation
Radiation can cause the permanent induction of cataracts in the lens of the eye. With low LET radiation single doses of 200 rad will cause cataract but with fractionated doses the threshold level of dose is increased to about 1500 rad. The threshold for cataract formation from high LET radiation is much reduced and may be of the order of 50–75 rad. Animal experiments indicate that microscopically observable opacities can be induced from a few rad upwards of both high and low LET.

In radiation protection practice, consideration must be given to the reduction of dose to the eyes from operators handling sealed sources of radiation and to radiologists using overhead screening techniques. For patients having radiotherapy involving beams close to the lens of the eye accurate beam direction is required if it is hoped to ensure that the dose is kept below the cataract threshold levels.

Since the early 1960s, considerable attention has been drawn to the damage that can be caused by radiation to the vascular supply, particularly in the micro circulations found in capillary beds. The retina of the eye is one such site. Radiation doses of 500 rad can cause damage to capillaries, and retinal doses in the range 1000–3000 rad can cause long-term deleterious effects in 20% of cases, particularly where the irradiation is around the macula. Complete loss of vision can be caused where there is damage to the fine vascular supply of the optic nerve or the macula.

It is important to use eye-shields which completely shield the globe in any treatments close to, or involving, beams which potentially can pass through the globe and strike either the lens or the retina.

Life-span reduction
Animal experiments indicate that whole body doses of 100 rad will reduce the life-span of rodents by 1–1.5%.

A study by Court Brown and Doll (1958) into the causes of death of British radiologists prior to 1921 compared with post-1921, in relation to the causes of death of other physicians, indicated no difference in the post-1921 group but showed an excess of cancers in the pre-1921 group. The choice of 1921 as the date in the survey was prompted by the fact that in that year the first British recommendations were published regarding the safety of X-ray operators.

A survey by Seltzer and Sartwell in 1965 in America showed that American radiologists in the 65–79 age group had a higher mortality rate compared with other physicians for the three periods 1935–1944, 1945–1954 and 1955–1958. However, the excess rate was decreasing. For the age group in 1955–1958 there was no difference (see Table 42.4). The improvements in technique and the awareness of the need for radiological protection since the 1940s would be sufficient to reduce the occupationally received doses and hence explain these findings.

Reduction of fertility
Spermatagonia, the first stage of the formation of the sperm, is sensitive to irradiation and hence sperm formation, and therefore fertility is reduced following irradiation. Fertility will fall after pre-existing sperm and those formed from surviving spermatocytes are eliminated from the genital track. Reduction of fertility such that the sperm count drops to zero will be caused by doses of 500–600 rad. However, after a period of up to three to five years sperm count may return through the eventual regeneration of the seminiferous epithelium. A single dose of 25 rad will reduce sperm count by about 30% starting 6 weeks after exposure and recovering in 40 weeks; a single dose of 50 rad may produce a brief temporary sterility.

Several surveys report a degree of successful parenthood in patients treated for neoplastic disease such as Hodgkin's disease and seminoma of the testes, e.g. in a survey in Dresden of 492 patients some 18 had 21 children who were conceived after radiotherapy of one of the parents.

Little information is available on man of the effects of protracted irradiation. In a dog, however, dose rates of 0.6 rad/week showed no detectable change in sperm count whilst sterility occurred within months at a dose rate of 3 rad week.

In women the irradiation of the ovary will cause a cessation of normal menstruation, and the degree of temporary sterility will depend both on the radiation dose to the ovary and the age of the subject. Temporary sterility will be induced by doses of 50–200 rad.

Radiation has been used therapeutically to induce an artificial menopause and such permanent sterility may be produced by ovarian doses of 500–600 rad in women of about 40–50 years. In younger women these doses may only produce temporary sterility. Fractionated regimes for these treatments require radiation doses of 1000–1500 over a few weeks.

Animal data, and a limited amount of human information, indicates that low doses, up to 65 rad to the ovaries, may increase the fertility, particularly in those with a history of infertility. The animal data would indicate that this may be due to an increase in ovulation leading to an increase in litter size.

It is not yet possible to identify what the incidence of increased genetic abnormality would be in offspring conceived after the radiation doses reported in this section. An estimate may be made by reference to the next section.

Genetic effects

Compared with the data on the direct effects of irradiating an individual the information on the hereditary effects is relatively sparse. There is a considerable wealth of knowledge relating to the irradiation of mice and the fruit fly *Drosophila* but this has to be corrected for species difference which is extremely difficult.

The report of UNSCEAR 1977 (see Bibliography) gave a detailed account of the present state of knowledge and Table 42.5 has been derived from these data to simplify the presentation and to indicate the major findings. On the basis that a large population was to receive 1 rad per generation of low LET radiation at

Table 42.4 Unspecific ageing (death rates/1000 person years) (from Seltzer and Sartwell, 1965).

	Age	Radiologist	Physicians	ENT and eye specialists
1935–44	65–79	66.5	52.6	38.9
1945–54	65–79	61.2	47.2	39.0
1955–58	35–49	2.1	2.1	3.2
	65–79	56.1	41.8	39.8

Table 42.5   Effects of 1 rad per generation of low dose LET radiation.

Type of defect	Current incidence per 10^6 live born	Effects per 10^6 fertilized embryos from irradiation of spermatogonia*	No. of effects per 10^6 live born first generation	
			Basis	
			Direct experiment	Doubling dose = 100 *rad*
Dominant and lethal mutations	11 000	64	20	20
Chromosomal disease	4 000	51–261	2–10	38
Congenital constitutional degenerative disease	90 000	Low	Low	5
Totals	105 000	115–325	22–30 plus 11–55 recognized abortions 22–109 early embryonic losses	63
Percentage	100	0.1–0.3	0.02–0.03	0.06

* Note that the effect of irradiation on oocytes is very low

low dose rate, the number of genetic effects that would be observed per million live births in the first generation are shown in the last two columns. Each set of data relate to deductions based on experiment (column 4) or to an assumption of 100 rad being the dose that would double the incidence rate of each type of defect (column 5). It will be seen that, on a percentage basis, 1 rad per generation might increase the rate of live born children having genetic effects by up to 0.06%. It will be observed from column 3 entries, that there will be about five times more effects produced in fertilized embryos but that 80% of these will be lost either at early embryonic stage or as recognized spontaneous abortions.

To extrapolate to a higher rate of radiation dose is difficult as the results of mouse experiments showed that the mutation rate decreased as the dose rate decreased.

The observed rate of mutation of seven easily recognized point loci, such as the colour of eyes etc., showed that if the dose was given at a higher dose rate, the mutation rate for a given dose was three times greater than when given at 0.8 rad/min and that a further reduction in dose rate had no measurable effect. This indicates that there is a repair/recognition facility which can exclude the genetic defect from appearing in a live-born mouse. Nevertheless, at any given dose rate it would appear that a linear dose relationship exists and that the number of effects is approximately proportional to the dose received.

The other important aspect of Table 42.5 is to note that the effects are predominately due to the irradiation of spermatogonia and that the effect of irradiation on oocytes is very small when considering genetic effects. It would appear that there may be a mechanism which is effectively checking the maturing ovum to identify that it is not in some way deficient. It may then be absorbed before appearing as a mature oocyte ready for fertilization.

Considerably more data are required to identify genetic damage from irradiation but the current philosophy would indicate that the relative risk from 1 rad is about three or four times greater for a somatic effect than it is for a genetic effect in a subsequent offspring.

ICRP recommendations

Dose equivalent

The recommendations of the ICRP in terms of the dose

equivalent have to be framed in a manner that takes into account three factors:

(a) The absorbed dose in rad.

(b) The biological effect of the radiation compared with low LET radiation.

(c) The relative risk of irradiating the specified organ compared with the risk of irradiating the whole body.

To define exactly for an occupationally exposed individual the limits of radiation exposure it would be necessary to know for any particular biological effect how it varies with LET. Unfortunately, our present knowledge does not permit us to know the relative biological effectiveness (RBE) for different radiations for all the possible deleterious effects produced by radiation – so called 'end-points', and this is likely to be the position for many years. Therefore, instead of using the RBE related to LET to correct for particular 'end-points' it is necessary in radiation protection to select a representative RBE for a particular radiation type and LET value and to use this representative value for all effects and end-points. This representative RBE value is called the Quality Factor, Q, and the choice of values is such that the value of Q is unlikely to be exceeded by the actual RBEs which might obtain. The effect of this choice is that the value of the dose equivalent will be maximized.

The risks of radiation have been clearly stated in the early part of this chapter and it can be seen that whole body radiation will give rise to a statistical probability of causing a particular deleterious somatic effect. There is therefore a random chance that the effect will occur in any one particular individual; the effect is therefore referred to as a stochastic or random effect, i.e. having a chance of say one in ten thousand of occurring after a certain dose. As the dose increases a proportionate increase occurs in the statistical probability of the effect occurring. On the other hand there are some effects such as the cell depletion in circulating peripheral blood or the skin erythema which will occur in all individuals when particular dose levels are received. These effects are referred to as non-stochastic or certain or unavoidable effects.

The stochastic or random risk of inducing deleterious effects following irradiation of the whole body can be calculated by summation of the various risks of inducing deleterious effects in the various tissues of the body and obviously the total risk to the whole body must be the sum of the individual risks to the parts. From this statement ICRP recommends that if only a part of the body is irradiated then the annual dose equivalent limit for that part of the body will be greater than that for the whole body by the ratio of the risk per unit dose to the whole body following whole body irradiation to the risk per unit dose following the irradiation of the part of the body.

To summarize the statements in this section on dose equivalence in a mathematical form:

The dose equivalent $H = D$, absorbed dose in Gray ($=100$ rad)
multiplied by
Q, the quality factor of the radiation (see Table 42.6)
multiplied by
N, the product of any other modifying factor specified by the Commission
$\therefore$ Dose equivalent $H = D \times Q \times N$
in Sievert (Sv)
($=100$ rem)

Table 42.6 Variation of quality factor with linear energy transfer value of different types of radiation.

$L_\infty - Q$ Relationship		X-rays, γ-rays and electrons	1
L_∞ in water (keV/μm)	Q	Neutrons, protons and singly-charged particles of rest mass greater than one atomic mass of unknown energy	10
3.5 (and less)	1	α-particles and multiply-charged particles (and particles of unknown charge), of unknown energy	20
7	2		
23	5		
53	10		
175	20		

The specification of the weighting factors to the annual dose equivalent limit which apply when only partial body irradiation has occurred is based on the risk data reported earlier in the chapter and is simplified by ICRP 26 into Table 42.7

Mathematically:

$$H_T = H_{WB} \times \frac{1}{W_T}$$

where H_T = annual dose equivalent limit for part of body; H_{WB} = annual dose equivalent limit for whole of body; W_T = weighting factor for part of body. If the part of the body contains several of the organs specified in Table 42.7 then the value of W_T used must be the sum of the appropriate values of W_T.

Table 42.7 Weighting factors for separately irradiated tissues.

Tissue	W_T
Gonads	0.25
Breast	0.15
Red bone marrow	0.12
Lung	0.12
Thyroid	0.03
Bone surfaces	0.03
Remainder	0.30

Annual dose equivalent limits

Occupational exposed workers

(a) For Non-stochastic effects (i.e. effects certain to happen)

| All tissues except lens of | 0.5 Sv | (50 rem) |
| the eye | 0.3 Sv | (30 rem) |

(b) For stochastic effects (random effects)

Whole body	50 mSv	(5 rem)
Gonads ($W_T = 0.25$)	200 mSv	(20 rem)
Breast ($W_T = 0.15$)	330 mSv	(33 rem)
Red bone marrow		
($W_T = 0.12$) and lung	420 mSv	(42 rem)
*Thyroid and bone		
surfaces ($W_T = 0.03$)	1660 mSv	(166 rem)
Remainder ($W_T = 0.3$)	170 mSv	(17 rem)

Occupational exposure of women of reproductive capacity

It is anticipated that if exposure was received at a regular rate an embryo is unlikely to receive more than 5 mSv during the first two months of pregnancy. Strictly, in one sixth of a year the dose equivalent received at the limiting rate would be 50/6 mSv, i.e. 8 mSv. For the remaining period of the pregnancy when the worker would know that she was pregnant she should be employed in a category of work (called Working Condition B) where it is most unlikely that the annual exposure will exceed three tenths of the annual dose equivalent limit, i.e. 15 mSv (1.5 rem/y). Therefore, the foetus is unlikely to receive more than 5 mSv + (7/12 × 15) = 5 + 9 = 14 mSv (1.4 rem).

* As in the above table the dose equivalent limits for stochastic effects in the thyroid and bone surfaces exceed those for non-stochastic effects, it is necessary to lower the annual dose equivalent limits to these individual tissues to 0.5 Sv (50 rem).

Annual dose equivalent limits for individual members of the public

To an individual 5 mSv (0.5 rem)

This individual is considered to be part of a critical group and when the dose is averaged over the whole population the average dose equivalent limit is expected to be one tenth of this individual value. At this public level of 0.5 mSv (50mrem/year) this risk rate would be approximately 50 cases per million man rem.

ICRP recommendations

In the above paragraphs the main data from ICRP Publication 26 has been condensed into easily referable tabulations. There are a considerable number of recommendations and philosophical points made in that publication particularly to the way in which analyses of the risk to the irradiated tissues should be balanced against the cost of the radiation protection facilities. There are also publications (ICRP 22) on such cost benefit analyses and publication ICRP 26 discusses problems involved in developing an index of harm.

Basis for comparison

It is important when considering the effects of radiation to be able to compare the radiation received as part of one's work with that which will be received from naturally occurring radiation sources. The levels of animal dose received by members of the population living in normal western style accommodation is given in Table 42.8 for the gonads, bone marrow and cells lining the bone surfaces. It is seen that the sources are mainly from external radiation from cosmic rays and building materials used in the construction of our homes.

The annual dose of 100 mrad/year, i.e. equivalent to about 0.1 mSv/year gives a guide to what is an acceptable level for populations to receive. The extra man-made radiation doses are predominantly from the medical use of X-rays. The present estimates for the annual genetically significant dose from those sources in the UK is about 10 mrad (0.01 mSv) whereas the mean dose to the bone marrow is about 30–40 mrad/year (0.03–0.04 mSv).

Legislation

In most countries a considerable volume of local legislation controls the use of radiations, the transport of radioactive materials and the disposal of liquid, solid and gaseous radioactive wastes. In the European

Table 42.8   Annual tissue absorbed dose in mrad.

	Gonads	Red bone marrow	Cells lining bone surfaces
1. External radiation			
Cosmic rays	28	28	28
Terrestrial sources	32	32	32
2. Internal radiation			
Potassium-40	15	27	15
Lead-210	0.6	0.9	3.4
Carbon-14	0.5	2.2	2.0
3. Other	1.9	1.9	5.6
Total	78	92	86

Economic Community there is a general EEC directive which came into force in mid-1980, and from this, each member country is having to prepare its own local control legislation. In the UK this will be controlled by the Health and Safety Executive (HSE) who will be issuing three levels of controls:

1. Regulations which are mandatory.
2. Approved codes of practice which will also be mandatory and will apply to specified areas of work.
3. Notes for guidance which will give advice to employers and employees as to their general mode of conduct in specified areas of work.

This legislation will be incorporated in the main through the Health and Safety at Work Act.

It will be necessary for Radiation Protection Advisors, (RPA), usually physicists trained in radiation protection, to undertake the detailed interpretation of these controls in a particular work area.

The particular areas of work described in the codes and notes for guidance will be subdivided into:

1. Diagnostic radiology.
2. Nuclear medicine and unsealed radiopharmaceuticals.
3. Radiotherapy.

   (a) γ-ray teletherapy units.
   (b) X-ray installations including linear accelerators.
   (c) Brachytherapy – the use of small sealed sources at short distances.

Guidance will also be given on aspects of the general organization of protection services, patient protection and the requirements of equipment used in radiotherapy.

A series of booklets prepared by the United States National Council for Radiation Protection on aspects of radiation protection in the medical field are also very useful for factual information and advice on shielding problems of treatment rooms for radiotherapy and on general radiation protection. All these sources of information are essential for the radiation protection adviser and many radiotherapists would find them of value when considering new projects.

Administration of radiopharmaceuticals to a patient

When a clinician wishes to administer radiopharmaceuticals for diagnosis, investigation or treatment, or to use sealed radioactive sources on or in patients he has, in the United Kingdom, to hold a certificate issued under the Medicines Act. A committee called the Administration of Radioactive Substances Advisory Committee advises the Health Minister on the issue of such certificates. The clinician, the scientist responsible for the scientific services and the RPA each have a part to play in this work and details of each aspect have to be completed on the application form.

In these ways it is hoped that all countries will be able to apply the basic ICRP recommendations in a manner which will lead to good practices in all aspects of radiological work.

Further reading

1. International Recommendations and Regulations. ICRP

ICRP (Nov. 1969), *Protection of the Patient in X-ray Diagnosis*. Publication 16, a report prepared by a task group of Committe 3 of the ICRP and adopted by the Commission.

ICRP (Sept. 1969), *Protection of the Patient in*

Radionuclide Investigations. Publication 17, a report prepared for the ICRP and adopted by the Commission.

ICRP (Oct. 1974), *Report of the Task Group on Reference Man*. Publication 23, adopted by the Commission.

ICRP (Nov. 1976), *The Handling, Storage, Use and Disposal of Unsealed Radionuclides in Hospitals and Medical Research Establishments*. Publication 25, a report of Committees 3 and 4 of the IRCP and adopted by the Commission.

ICRP (Jan. 17, 1977), *Recommendations of the ICRP* Publication 26.

2. UK Legislation and Codes of Practice

Official Journal of the European Communities (12 July, 1976; revised May 1978), **19**, L 187. In Joint Consultative Document Ionising Radiations, Health & Safety Commission, National Radiological Protection Board ISBN 0 11 883237 9 HMSO, 1979.

Code of Practice for the Protection of Persons against Ionizing Radiations arising from Medical and Dental Use (1972) DHSS.

3. WHO Technical Reports on Radiation Protection in Hospitals

WHO (1977), *Use of Ionizing Radiation and Radionuclides on Human Beings for Medical Research, Training and Nonmedical purposes*. WHO Expert Committee, Technical Report Series No. 611.

Braestrup, C.B. and Vikterlof, K.J. (1974), *Manual on Radiation Protection in Hospitals and General Practice*. **1**, *Basic Protection Requirements*, WHO.

Frost, D. and Jammet, H. (1975), *Manual on Radiation Protection in Hospitals and General Practice*. **2**, *Unsealed Sources*, WHO.

Keane, B.E. and Tikhonov, K.B. (1975), *Manual on Radiation Protection in Hospitals and General Practice*. **3**, *X-ray Diagnosis*, WHO.

Koren, K. and Wuehrmann, A.H. (1977), *Manual on Radiation Protection in Hospitals and General Practice*. **4**, *Radiation Protection in Dentistry*, WHO.

4. USA National Committee on Radiation Protection (NCRP) Reports on Medical and Allied Aspects

NCRP (Sept. 15, 1976), *Structural Shielding Design and Evaluation for Medical use of X-rays and Gamma-rays of Energies up to 10 MeV*, Report No. 49.

NCRP (March 1, 1977), *Review of NCRP Radiation*

Dose Limit for Embryo and Fetus in Occupationally Exposed Women, Report No. 53.

NCRP (July 15, 1977), *Medical Radiation Exposure of Pregnant and Potentially Pregnant Women*, Report No. 54.

5. United Nations and IAEA General Texts on Effects of Radiation

United Nations Scientific Committee on the Effects of Atomic Radiation (1977), Report. *Sources and Effects of ionizing Radiation*.

IAEA (1976), *Biological and Environmental Effects of Low-Level Radiation*. **1**, IAEA, Vienna.

IAEA (1976), *Biological and Environmental Effects of Low-Level Radiation*. **II**, IAEA, Vienna.

IAEA (1976), *Diagnosis and Treatment of Incorporated Radionuclides*. Proc. Sem., 8–12 December, 1975, IAEA, Vienna.

6. Laboratory Design and Safety

Everett, K. and Hughes, D. (1975), *A Guide to Laboratory Design*. Butterworth.

BOHS (1975), *A Guide to the Design and Installation of Laboratory Fume Cupboards*. Hygiene Technology Guide Series No. 1. British Occupational Hygiene Society, c/o Mr P.J. Hewitt, Bradford University.

References

Court Brown, W.M. and Doll, R. (1957), Leukaemia and aplastic anaemia in patients irradiated for ankylosing spondylitis. Medical Research Council, Special Report Series No. 295 HMSO, London.

Court Brown, W.M. and Doll, R. (1958), The expectation of life and cancer mortality of British radiologists, Second United Nations Conf. *Peaceful Uses of Atomic Energy*, A/CONF15/P/99.

Court Brown, W.M. and Doll, R. (1965), Mortality from cancer and other causes after radiotherapy for ankylosing spondylitis. *Br. Med. J.*, **ii**, 1327–32.

Ellis R.E. (1972), Breast cancer following irradiation (abstract). *Br. J. Radiol.*, **45**, 538, 795–6.

Hempelmann, L.H. *et al.* (1975), Neoplasms in persons treated with X-rays in infancy: fourth survey in 20 years. *J. Nat. Cancer Inst.*, **55**, 519–30,

ICRP, *Implications of Commission Recommendations that Doses Should be Kept as Low as Reasonably Achievable*. ICRP 22, ISBN 0 08 017694 1.

ICRP (1977), *Problems Involved in Developing an Index of Harm*. Anns ICRP 1, 4. ICRP 22.

MacMahon, B. (1962), Prenatal X-ray exposure and childhood cancer. *J. Nat. Cancer Inst.*, **28**, 1173–91.

Myrden, J.A. and Hiltz J.E. (1969), Breast cancer following multiple fluoroscopies during artificial pneumothorax treatment of pulmonary tuberculosis. *Can. Med. Assoc. J.*, **100**, 1032–4.

Palmer, J.P. and Spratt, D.W. (1956), Pelvic carcinoma following irradiation for benign gynaecological diseases. *Am. J. Obstet. Gynecol.*, **72**, 497–505.

Pifer, J.W. *et al.* (1963), Neoplasms in children treated with X-rays for thymic enlargement. I Neoplasms and mortality. *J. Nat. Cancer Inst.*, **31**, 1357–77.

Seltzer, R and Sartwell, P.E. (1965), The influence of occupational exposure to radiation on the mortality of American radiologists and other medical specialists. *Am. J. Epidemiol.*, **81**, 2–22.

Smith, P.E. and Doll, R. (1976), Late effects of X-irradiation in patients treated for metropathia hemorrhagica. *Br. J. Radiol.*, **49**, 224–32.

Smith, P.E. and Doll, R. (1978), Age and time dependent changes in the rates of radiation-induced cancers in patients with ankylosing spondylitis following a single course of X-ray treatment. IAEA Proc. Symp. *Late Biological Effects of Ionizing Radiation*, March, 1978. pp.205–14.

Stewart, A.M. and Kneale, G.W. (1970), Radiation dose effects in relation to obstetric X-rays and childhood cancers. *Lancet*, **ii**, 1185–8.

Wanebo, C.K. *et al.* (1968), Breast cancer after exposure to the atomic bombing of Hiroshima and Nagasaki. *New Engl. J. Med.*, **279**, 667–71.

43 Cancer clinical trial protocols

Richard J. Sylvester, David Machin and Maurice J. Staquet

While there is an ever-growing literature on the design and analysis of clinical trials, the fact remains that little guidance is available when it comes to the important task of actually writing a protocol. Often after the trial has started it becomes apparent that there is an important omission or a lack of clarity in the protocol and that certain modifications are required. In some cases the entire value of the protocol may be jeopardized if the problems are serious enough. In order to aid investigators in the preparation of protocols, some practical guidelines are proposed. While these guidelines were designed for cancer chemotherapy protocols, they are quite general in nature and may also be used for other types of studies.

As there is now a vast literature on the design and analysis of clinical trials, a selected bibliography of some of the most important and recent works arranged by subject matter is also included. In this manner an investigator interested in a particular topic can find at a glance the appropriate references.

The protocol

A clinical trial may be defined as a carefully designed scientific experiment whose purpose is to answer certain specific questions concerning the treatments under investigation. The most important item in any trial is the protocol, a self-contained document which gives a detailed written description of the objectives of the study and describes how the trial is to be carried out. The success or failure of the trial may well depend on how well the protocol is written since a poorly designed, ambiguous or incomplete protocol may result in a trial which will not be able to answer the questions of interest.

A protocol should address itself to an important and interesting question. The question should be important enough to justify the time and expense necessary to carry it out and must have enough interest to attract the required number of investigators and ensure their continued collaboration throughout the course of the study.

Given the available resources, the trial must be designed in such a manner that it will be technically feasible to carry out. The protocol should not be so complicated that only a few of the more experienced investigators can carry it out. In general, a simple straight forward protocol with two arms is to be preferred to a more complicated protocol involving many arms or several randomizations.

The required number of eligible patients must be recruited in a short period of time. If patient intake exceeds two to three years, investigators may lose interest in the trial before the required number of patients have been entered, new more promising therapies may become available in the meantime, and the final results, when available may no longer be of interest.

The following guidelines, which are summarized in Table 43.1, are proposed as an aid to investigators in the preparation of protocols.

Background and introduction

This section should give the background and rationale for undertaking the trial and should convince the reader that there is a real need for doing the study. The natural history of the disease and results of previous studies of related interest should be quoted along with the rationale for choosing the particular treatment regimens under investigation. All appropriate references should appear in a separate section at the end of the protocol. When new drugs are being studied it is especially important to reference all previous clinical and pre-clinical work with the drug.

Table 43.1 Protocol contents.

Objectives of the trial

The objectives of the trial should be clearly spelled out along with the criteria that will be used to evaluate the treatments under study. Depending on the type of study this might include an evaluation of the treatments with respect to the response rate, duration of response, the disease-free interval, disease-free survival, survival, or the quality of life. The use of survival as an end-point may be misleading if the duration of survival following relapse depends on the subsequent treatment received since this is usually left to the discretion of each investigator and may change with time.

Patient selection criteria (eligibility criteria)

The population of patients to be studied should be defined as precisely as possible through the listing of specific objective patient inclusion and exclusion criteria. Such criteria might include:

1. The tumour site, the stage of the disease, the TNM classification, and the histological type.
2. The presence of measurable disease.
3. The patient's age, sex and performance status.
4. The type and amount of previous treatment received.
5. The patient's haematological status and values of specific hepatic and renal function tests.
6. The presence of other diseases, concomitant therapy, a second tumour, or contra-indications for any of the treatments under study.

Subjective criteria should be avoided as much as possible, especially in multicentre studies. If one is to generalize the results of a trial to a given population of interest it is important that the population be well

defined and that all eligible patients presenting themselves in the institution be included in the trial.

Trial design

This section should give a short summary of the trial to include:

1. The time at which patients are to be registered or randomized and what stratifications, if any, are done. While stratification by institution in multicentre trials is generally to be recommended, the need for stratifying patients by prognostic factors is much debated. If stratification is used, the number of additional stratifying variables should be kept to a minimum (one or at most two) as too much stratification can be harmful. Stratification at the time of randomization does not relieve one of the necessity to stratify restrospectively at the time of analysis.
2. Definition of the treatment arms and duration of treatment.
3. In advanced disease specification of the minimum duration of treatment, the time of evaluation and the treatment policy to be followed as a function of the response: should treatment be continued, crossed-over, left to the investigator's discretion, or should the patient be entered in a phase II study?
4. In multimodality trials the maximum delay permitted between surgery, radiotherapy, and the start of chemotherapy or immunotherapy.
5. The frequency of follow-up and duration of study.

In addition, there should be a schema which summarizes at a glance the main details of the study.

Therapeutic regimens and toxicity

The dose, schedule, method of administration, and duration of treatment should be clearly spelled out. Dose adjustments based on weight, body surface area, or age should be indicated along with whether or not dose escalation is permitted. Indicate whether supportive therapy such as steroids or radiotherapy may be given during the course of the study and if so, under what circumstances and in what amounts. Any medication which is strictly contra-indicated should be clearly stated as such. One should also include any special instructions concerning drug supply, storage and availability.

The most frequent toxicities (haematological, renal, hepatic, cardiac, mucous, and skin for example) for each treatment should be listed along with a standardized grading scale to be used for assessing toxicity severity. The schedule for monitoring toxicity should be clearly stated. Based on this grading scale dose modifications should be presented in an easy to read form. Do you reduce the dose by a certain prescribed amount or do you wait until a full course can be given? What is the maximum delay permitted between courses and under what conditions should the patient leave the protocol due to toxicity? For drugs where the total allowable amount received is limited due to toxicity, the limiting dose should be clearly indicated along with what the treatment policy is once the maximum dose has been received.

In adjuvant studies precise details concerning the surgical procedure to be used and/or radiotherapy given should be indicated along with what complications might arise. The primary treatment should be standardized as much as possible in adjuvant studies. Otherwise any differences which appear between the adjuvant treatments may in fact be due to differences in the primary treatment received.

Required clinical evaluations, laboratory tests and follow-up

The required pre-treatment examinations should be listed along with what examinations are required after entry on-study and at what intervals they should be repeated. All patients should be followed up at the same frequency and the same criteria and methods used at each evaluation in order to eliminate possible bias.

The time at which patients with advanced disease are to be evaluated for treatment response should be clearly indicated along with what examinations are required to confirm the response. When evaluating response to treatment it is strongly recommended, whenever practical, that the same clinician evaluates the same patient throughout the course of the study in order to eliminate interobserver variation. Evaluations should, when possible, be blind with respect to the treatment received.

In multicentre trials procedures from one laboratory to another should be standardized as much as possible in order to minimize inter laboratory variation.

Criteria of evaluation

The end-points with respect to which the treatments will be evaluated should be given with all terms clearly defined. In patients with advanced disease precise objective definitions for terms such as complete response, partial response, no change, progression, early death, and toxic death must be given along with the time points at which patients are to be evaluated. For some examples see Moertel and Hanley (1976), Scott *et al.* (1975) and Hayward *et al.* (1977). In addi-

tion, starting and end-points for terms such as duration of survival, disease-free interval and partial or complete response should be defined (see also Chapters 1 and 5).

The protocol should specify how patients who are lost to follow up, receive insufficient treatment or have protocol violations are to be evaluated. Finally, all patient records should be reviewed by an independent extramural review committee to assess both patient eligibility and treatment results.

Registration and randomization of patients

Clear instructions concerning when and who the clinician should contact to register or randomize a patient should be given along with what information the clinician must supply at the time of registration. In multicentre trials a *centralized* randomization by telephone or telex is essential for the following reasons:

1. To insure that the randomization is done correctly since envelope randomization can easily be abused.
2. To know at all times how many patients have been entered on a study.
3. To be able to request overdue forms for all patients entered on-study.

Forms and procedures for collecting data

This section should include copies of the forms to be used and information concerning when and how often each form should be filled out and to whom the forms should be sent. Forms should be kept as simple and as short as possible in order to concentrate on obtaining all of the really important data for each patient entered on-study.

Statistical considerations

Based on the principal end-points of interest and the expected accrual rate, one should calculate the total number of patients required, the expected duration of patient entry, and the expected duration of the study. The exact information required and the techniques used to calculate these quantities can be found in papers included in the selected bibliography which follows. One should specify whether a fixed sample or sequential type of analysis will be performed, if a formal stopping rule will be used in the case of early treatment differences, and how often and to what use interim statistical analyses will be made.

Administrative responsibilities

This paragraph should contain the name, address, and telephone number of the study coordinator or members of the protocol committee, the chairman of each subcommittee (the Central Pathology Review Committee for example) and the data processing and statistical centre. In addition, the principal participating centres should be listed along with the principal investigators in each centre.

References

Only standard formats and accepted abbreviations should be used. Consult the Royal Society of Medicine Guide or the Index Medicus for recommendations and examples.

Appendices

Possible appendices would include the TNM classification or staging system used (AJC, 1977), the performance status classification used (Karnofsky *et al.* (1948) or ECOG/Zubrod (1960) 5-point scale) and a nomogram or table giving the body surface area as a function of height and weight (Gehan and George, 1970) (see also Chapters 1 and 5, and most chapters in Part Two).

References

American Joint Committee for Cancer Staging and End Results Reporting (1977), *Manual for Staging of Cancer 1977*. American Joint Committee, Chicago.

Gehan, E.A. and George, S.L. (1970), Estimation of human body surface area from height and weight. *Cancer Chemother. Rep.*, **54**(1), 225–35.

Hayward, J.L. *et al.* (1977), Assessment of response to therapy in advanced breast cancer. *Cancer*, **39**, 1289–94.

Karnofsky, D.A. *et al.* (1948), The use of the nitrogen mustards in the palliative treatment of carcinoma. *Cancer*, **1**, 634–56.

Moertel, C.G. and Hanley, J.A. (1976), The effect of measuring error on the results of therapeutic trials in advanced cancer. *Cancer*, **38**, 388–94.

Scott, W.W. *et al.* (1975), Comparison of 5-fluorouracil (NSC-19893) and cyclophosphamide (NSC-26271) in patients with advanced carcinoma of the prostate. *Cancer Chemother. Rep.*, **59**(1), 195–201.

Zubrod, C.G. *et al.* (1960), Appraisal of methods for the study of chemotherapy of cancer in man: comparative therapeutic trial of nitrogen mustard and triethylene thiophosphoramide. *J. Chron. Dis.*, **11**, 7–33.

A selected bibliography on the design and analysis of cancer clinical trials

The clinician or statistician who wishes to become acquainted with the statistical concepts involved in the design and analysis of cancer clinical trials has an ever-increasing literature to consult. In this section some of the most important publications dealing with the design and analysis of clinical trials have been grouped together according to the topic discussed. Emphasis has been placed on the most recent ideas and developments. While most of the publications included in this bibliography are suitable reading for non-statisticians, statisticians will find more technical articles referenced in a number of the works listed below. Many of the articles included in this bibliography have themselves quite an extensive list of references, especially the general works section.

Section A deals with Phase I studies, the initial human clinical pharmacological evaluation, and also includes several references concerning preclinical toxicology studies. Phase II trials, the initial efficacy screen in humans, are referenced in section B while section C is concerned with comparative Phase III trials. Section D presents a number of general works which discuss many different aspects of clinical trial design and analysis (including Phase I and Phase II trials) and are recommended reading for all clinicians who wish to learn the general principles of clinical trial design and analysis. Of particular interest are the many references which the articles in this section contain.

A. Phase I Trials

Freireich, E.J. *et al.* (1966), Quantitative comparison of toxicity of anticancer agents in mouse, rat, hamster, dog, monkey, and man. *Cancer Chemother. Rep.*, **50**, 219–44.

Gold, L. (1962), Coordinated phase I studies for cooperative chemotherapy groups. *Cancer Chemother. Rep.*, **16**, 99–105.

Robinson, J.A. (1978), Sequential choice of an optimal dose: a prediction intervals approach. *Biometrika*, **65**, 75–8.

Schein, P.S. (1977), Preclinical toxicology of anticancer agents. *Cancer Res.*, **37**, 1934–7.

Schneiderman, M.A. (1966), Man to mouse: statistical problems in bringing a drug to clinical trial. In: *Proc. 5th Berkeley Symp. Mathematical Statistics and Probability* (eds L. Lecam and J. Neyman), **IV**, University of California Press, Berkeley, pp. 855–66.

Schneiderman, M.A. (1966), Experimental design considerations in multiclinic trials. In: *Clinical Pharmacology, the International Encyclopedia of Pharmacology and Therapeutics* (eds G. Peters and

C. Redouco-Thomas) Pergamon Press, New York, Section 6, Chapter 31, pp.617–36.

B. Phase II Trials

Carter, S.K. (1972), Study design principles for the clinical evaluation of new drugs as developed by the chemotherapy programme of the National Cancer Institute. In: *The Design of Clinical Trials in Cancer Therapy* (ed. M.J. Staquet), Editions Scientifiques Européennes, Brussels, pp. 242–89.

Gehan, E.A. (1961), The determination of the number of patients required in a preliminary and follow-up trial of a new chemotherapeutic agent. *J. Chron. Dis.*, **13**, 346–53.

Muggia, F., McGuire, W. and Rozencweig, M. (1978), Rationale, design and methodology of phase II clinical trials. In: *Methods in Cancer Research* (eds V. De Vita and H. Busch), Academic Press, New York, pp. 199–214.

Muggia, F. *et al.* (1980), Methodology of Phase II clinical trials in cancer. In: *Recent Results in Cancer Research*, **70** (eds S.K. Carter and Y. Sakurai), Springer-Verlag, Berlin, pp. 53–60.

Sylvester, R.J. and Staquet, M.J. (1979), Design of Phase II clinical trials in cancer using decision theory. *Cancer Treat. Rep.*, **64**, 519–24.

C. Phase III Trials

Multicentre trials

George, S.L. (1976), Practical problems in the design, conduct and analysis of cooperative trials. In: *Proc. 9th International Biometric Conference*, **1**, The Biometric Society, Raleigh, pp. 227–44.

Machin, D., Staquet, M.J. and Sylvester, R.J. (1979), Advantages and defects of single center and multi-center clinical trials. In: *Controversies in Cancer: Design of Trials and Treatment*, (eds H.J. Tagnon and M.J. Staquet), Masson Publishing, New York, pp. 7–15.

Staquet, M.J. (1976), The practice of cooperative clinical trials. *Eur. J. Cancer*, **12**, 241–3.

Staquet, M.J. *et al.* (1977), The EORTC data center. *Eur. J. Cancer*, **12**, 14–9.

Randomization, stratification

Bailar, J.C. (1976), Patient assignment algorithms: an overview. In: *Proc. 9th International Biometric Conference*, **1**, The Biometric Society, Raleigh, pp. 189–206.

Block, J.B. *et al.* (1975), Nonevaluable patients in clinical cancer research. *Cancer*, **36**, 1169–73.

Byar, D.P. *et al.* (1976), Randomized clinical trials: perspectives on some recent ideas. *New Engl. J. Med.*, **295**, 74–80.

Byar, D.P. (1979), The necessity and justification of randomized clinical trials. In: *Controversies in Cancer: Design of Trials and Treatment*, (eds H.J. Tagnon and M.J. Staquet) Masson Publishing, New York, pp. 75–82.

Chalmers, T.C., Block, J.B. and Lee, S. (1972), Controlled studies in clinical cancer research. *New Engl. J. Med.*, **287**, 75–8.

Gehan, E.A. (1978), Comparative clinical trials with historical controls: a statistician's view. *Biomedicine,* special issue, **28**, 13–19.

Gehan, E.A. and Freireich, E.J. (1974), Nonrandomized controls in cancer clinical trials. *New Engl. J. Med.*, **290**, 198–203.

Green, S.B. and Byar, D.P. (1978), The effect of stratified randomization on size and power of statistical tests in clinical trials. *J. Chron. Dis.*, **31**, 445–54.

Pocock, S.J. (1977), Randomized clinical trials (letter). *Br. Med. J.*, **1**, (6077), 1661.

Pocock, S.J. (1979), Allocation of patients to treatment in clinical trials. *Biometrics*, **35**, 183–97.

Schneiderman, M.A. (1975), How do you know you've done any better. *Cancer*, **35**, 64–9.

Simon, R. (1979), Heterogeneity and standardization in clinical trials. In: *Controversies in Cancer: Design of Trials and Treatment*, (ed. M.J. Staquet), Masson Publishing, New York, 37–49.

Staquet, M. (1976), The randomized clinical trial: a prerequisite for rational therapy. *Eur. Urol.*, **2**, 265–70.

Staquet, M. (ed.) (1978), *Randomized Trials in Cancer: A Critical Review by Sites.* Raven Press, New York.

Weinstein, M.C. (1974), Allocation of subjects in medical experiments. *New Engl. J. Med.*, **291**, 1278–85.

White, S.J. and Freedman, L.S. (1978), Allocation of patients to treatment groups in a controlled clinical study. *Br. J. Cancer*, **37**, 849–57.

Zelen, M. (1974), The randomization and stratification of patients to clinical trials. *J. Chron. Dis.*, **27**, 365–75.

Sample size determination

Freiman, J.A. *et al.* (1978), The importance of beta, the type II error and sample size in the design and interpretation of the randomized conrol trial. *New Engl. J. Med.*, **299**, 690–4.

Gail, M. (1973), The determination of sample sizes for trials involving several independent 2×2 tables. *J. Chron. Dis.*, **26**, 669–73.

Gail, M.H. and Gart, J.J. (1973), The determination of sample sizes for use with the exact conditional test in 2×2 comparative trials. *Biometrics*, **29**, 441–8.

George, S.L. and Desu, M.M. (1974), Planning the

size and duration of a clinical trial studying the time to some critical event. *J. Chron. Dis.*, **27**, 15–24.

Makuch, R. and Simon, R. (1978), Sample size requirements for evaluating a conservative therapy. *Cancer Treat. Rep.*, **62**, 1037–40.

Analysis, determination of prognostic factors

Armitage, P. (1975), *Sequential medical trials*. 2nd edn, Blackwell Scientific Publications, Oxford.

Armitage, P. and Gehan, E.A. (1974), Statistical methods for the identification and use of prognostic factors. *Int. J. Cancer*, **13**, 16–36.

Breslow, N. (1979), Statistical methods for censored survival data. *Environ. Hlth. Perspect.* (in press).

Dunnett, C.W. and Gent, M. (1977), Significance testing to establish equivalence between treatments, with special reference to data in the form of 2×2 tables. *Biometrics*, **33**, 593–602.

Gehan, E.A. (1978), Adjustment for prognostic factors in the analysis of clinical studies. In: *Methods and Impact of Controlled Therapeutic Trials in Cancer* (eds P. Armitage *et al.*), UICC Technical Report Series 36, Geneva, Part 1, pp.35–73.

Gross, A.J. and Clark, V.A. (1975), *Survival distributions: Reliability Applications in the Biomedical Sciences*. John Wiley and Sons, New York.

Herson, J. (1980), Evaluation of toxicity: Statistical considerations. *Cancer Treat. Rep.*, **64**, 463–8.

Hill, C. and Sancho-Garnier, H. (1979), Interim analysis and early results in clinical trials. In: *Controversies in Cancer: Design of Trials and Treatment* (eds H.J. Tagnon and M.J. Staquet) Masson Publishing, New York, pp. 51–3.

McPherson, K. (1974), Statistics: the problem of examining accumulating data more than once. *New Engl. J. Med.*, **290**, 501–2.

Peto, R. *et al.* (1977), Design and analysis of randomized clinical trials requiring prolonged observation of each patient, II. Analysis and examples. *Br. J. Cancer*, **35**, 1–39.

Pocock, S.J. (1979), Can sequential methods be used for the analysis of cancer clinical trials? In: *Controversies in Cancer: Design of Trials and Treatment* (eds H.J. Tagnon and M.J. Staquet) Masson Publishing, New York, pp. 63–74.

Staquet, M.J. (ed.) (1975), *Cancer Therapy: Prognostic Factors and Criteria of Response*. Raven Press, New York.

Sylvester, R.J., Machin, D. and Staquet, M.J. (1978), A comparison of the alternative methods of calculating survival curves arising from clinical trials. *Biomedicine*, special issue, **28**, 49–53.

Vietta, T. (1980), Evaluation of toxicity: clinical issues. *Cancer Treat. Rep.*, **64**, 457–61.

Ware, J.H. and Byar, D.P. (1979), Methods for the analysis of censored survival data. In: *Perspectives in Biometrics*, (ed. R. Elashoff) **2**, Academic Press, New York, (in press).

D. General Works

Burdette, W.H. and Gehan, E.A. (1970), *Planning and Analysis of Clinical Studies*. Charles C. Thomas, Springfield.

Carter, S.K. (1977), Clinical trials in cancer chemotherapy. *Cancer*, **40**, 544–57.

Carter, S.K. (1978), Clinical trials. *Cancer Immunol. Immunother.*, **3**, 215–18.

Gehan, E.A. and Schneiderman, M.A. (1973), Experimental design of clinical trials. In: *Cancer Medicine* (eds J.F. Holland and E. Frei), Lea and Febinger, Philadelphia, Chapter VIII, pp. 499–519.

Johnson, F.N. and Johnson, S. (eds) (1977), *Clinical Trials*. Blackwell Scientific Publications, Oxford.

Meier, P. (1975), Statistics and medical experimentation. *Biometrics*, **31**, 511–29.

Peto, R. (1978), Clinical trial methodology. *Biomedicine*, special issue, **28**, 24–36.

Peto, R. *et al.* (1976), Design and analysis of randomized clinical trials requiring prolonged observation of each patient, I. Introduction and design. *Br. J. Cancer*, **34**, 585–612.

WHO Handbook for Reporting Results of Cancer Treatment (1979), WHO offset publication no. 48, Geneva.

Williams, C.J. and Carter, S.K. (1978), Management of trials in the development of cancer chemotherapy. *Br. J. Cancer*, **37**, 434–7.

Descriptions of cancer clinical trials in progress

Cancerline, International Cancer Research Data Bank Program, NCI, Silver Springs, Maryland.

Compilation of Clinical Protocol Summaries (1980), 4th edn, Publication No (NIH) 80–1116, US Department of Health, Education and Welfare.

Flamant, R. and Fohanno, C. (eds) (1978), *Controlled Therapeutic Trials in Cancer*, UICC Technical Report Series 32, Geneva.

Staquet, M. (ed.) (1980), *Current Research of the EORTC Cooperative Groups, Project Groups, Clubs, Task Forces and Working Parties*. European Organization for Research on Treatment of Cancer, Brussels.

Acknowledgement

This work was supported by Grant Number 2R10 CA11488–10 awarded by the National Cancer Institute. DHEW.

44 Statistical aspects of cancer trials

Richard Peto

Curiously, the chief statistical difficulties in cancer trials derive not from abstruse aspects of probability theory, but rather from two simple facts which are well-known to every doctor involved in the treatment of cancer.

First, cancer patients differ very markedly from each other for no obvious reason. It is unfortunately a common experience that a woman whose breast cancer seems relatively unaggressive when she first presents may nevertheless run a disastrous clinical course, and be dead within a year or two of mastectomy. Conversely, some breast cancer patients do survive for a decade or more despite having presented with what looked like a really horrible Stage II tumour.

We can recognize some very important measurable prognostic features (such as TNM stage or histological invasiveness for solid tumours, and cell counts or blood biochemistry for others), but despite this there remains great heterogeneity of survival among apparently similar patients, and each doctor who tries to predict to incurable patients how long they are likely to live must be able to recall a fair number of patients who survived very much shorter or longer than expected.

Second, although it may be relatively easy to shrink an unresectable tumour temporarily, it is extremely difficult to cure it. During the first half of this century there was a steady improvement in diagnostic radiology and in the ability to undertake progressively larger and larger operations without killing the patient, and so the proportion of locoregional cancers cured by surgery increased steadily. By the 1950s, however, standards of surgery fairly similar to those of today had been achieved, and for the past quarter of a century the survival probabilities for the major cancers (lung, large intestine, breast, stomach) have been depressingly constant, despite material improvements in the treatment of embryonal and haematopoietic tumours. This suggests that large improvements in the treatment of the ordinary carcinomas (which account for 90% of our

cancer deaths) are more difficult to devise than perusal of the large number per year of apparently positive clinical trial results would suggest. I am not arguing that no *worthwhile* improvements in the treatment of carcinomas are likely in the near future. There are, for example, well over 100 000 'early' breast cancers diagnosed each year in Europe and North America alone, and so if some widely practicable modification of surgical or radiotherapeutic primary treatment or (perhaps more plausibly) some not-too-toxic hormonal or cytotoxic adjuvant treatment can be devised which will reduce the proportion of deaths within 10 years of mastectomy from (say) 0.5 to 0.4, then this would clearly be enormously *worthwhile*. What I am suggesting, however, is that in the near future we are unlikely to devise treatments for any major category of carcinomas which have very *large* effects (such as preventing or substantially delaying as many as half of the deaths now expected). If this is accepted, then, when the survival probabilities associated with two plausible treatments are being compared in a clinical trial, the aim of the trial should be seen as being to distinguish reliably between two medically plausible alternatives: *either* there is no material difference in survival between them, *or* there is a moderate but worthwhile difference in survival.

Corollary: If 1. cancer patients are very heterogeneous, and 2. realistic but moderate improvements in survival need to be assessed, then *large, randomized trials* will be needed.

Suppose the observed difference between the average survival in a group of patients given one treatment and a group given another treatment is to be used to determine whether or not the treatments differ *moderately* in efficacy. Now, unless the groups are quite large, the observed proportions surviving at a given time may not be accurately estimated. Consequently, the difference between these two proportions due to purely random errors may actually exceed in magnitude the difference that would be expected if the two treatments did differ *moderately* in efficacy.

Likewise, misleading differences of this magnitude may arise unless the groups were separated from each other strictly at random, for otherwise the method of deciding which patients to include and which to exclude in each group may have been slightly different, which may in turn appreciably bias the observed difference between the proportions surviving in the two groups. In short, although crude methodology may suffice to pick out gross differences between treatments, reliable and convincing detection of the sort of *moderate* differences which are medically plausible requires that *random* errors be small in comparison with plausible real differences (i.e. that the study be large), and that *systematic* errors be negligible (i.e. that the study be randomized). A further reason for preferring randomization is that it is usually much easier to cheat, either consciously or subconsciously, in a non-randomized study (e.g. by witholding active, toxic treatment from patients so ill that they could not tolerate it and then excluding them from the treated group while leaving such patients in the controls). Because everybody knows it is fairly easy to introduce quite large biases in non-randomized studies, non-randomized trial results are less widely trusted than randomized trial results are. Consequently, even if you do happen to get the answer right with a non-randomized study, people who do not want to believe your results will have quite reasonable methodological grounds for not doing so.*

I shall now briefly review some of the optimal statistical methods for clinical trial analysis. I shall do this chiefly by reference to places in the cancer literature where these methods are already adequately described, because although these optimal methods are certainly worth using, trial organizers are usually fairly willing to accept them without dispute; indeed, once trial organizers have seen any of their real, interesting data analysed by such methods they will probably not want to revert to using anything else in future studies. By contrast, the large majority of the 2000 or so cancer trials currently in progress around the world are almost completely vitiated either by failure to randomize or, even more commonly, by failure to enter enough patients, and the chief intent of this chapter is to argue the need for the wider use of randomization and, especially, for more realistic estimates during the design of cancer trials about the magnitudes of the differences between treatments that can plausibly be anticipated, as a corollary to which the need for much larger trials than are currently commonplace will be obvious.

Standard statistical methods for analysis of time to death or time to recurrence

There have been, for at least a quarter of a century, a variety of texts setting out the statistical considerations that arise in the design of clinical trials and describing the statistical methods needed to analyse such trials. Some of these texts are written in statistics and some are written in English; some of them describe the statistical methods appropriate for acute disease, while others emphasize more the statistical methods appropriate to the interpretation of cancer data, where death may be considerably delayed. The most appropriate, for clinicians undertaking cancer trials, is perhaps the ten-author paper in the *British Journal of Cancer* (Peto *et al.*, 1976; 1977).

It is chiefly written in non-technical language, and it deals not only with principles of trial design but also detailed methods of trial analysis. There have existed for more than ten years now methods of analysis of survival data which are quite clearly optimal, combining maximal statistical sensitivity with a format which is fairly easily understood by the non-statistician (which, after all, includes almost everyone to whom the results of clinical trials are directly relevant). These optimal methods, which are described in detail in the paper, may be summarized as:

Life tables

Plot graphs of the 'Kaplan-Meier' survival curves for various non-overlapping categories of patient (e.g. male/female on one graph, young/middle/old on another graph, and treatment A/treatment B on a third graph). Each graph gives one line per category of patient, indicating the estimated percentages that will be surviving at various times after study entry; as time passes, of course, these percentages decrease from their initial values at time zero of 100%.

Logrank Os and Es

Compare the Observed, O, number of deaths in each category with the logrank Extent of Exposure to risk of death, E, in that category. (E is sometimes called the

---

* Different hospitals with apparently similar catchment areas, referral patterns, patient assessment criteria, and treatment methods may achieve surprisingly different long-term results. Even at one hospital among nominally similar patients, there may be over a period of perhaps a year or two temporary fluctuations in the proportion responding satisfactorily to treatment which are too large to be attributed just to chance, but for which no satisfactory explanation ever emerges.

'logrank expected' number of deaths.) The sum of the Os for any one complete set of categories (e.g. young-/middle/old) necessarily adds up to the total number of deaths in the whole study, as does the sum of all the Es for those categories. If O exceeds E in one category of patient (i.e. if the relative death rate, O/E, in that category exceeds unity), then the patients in that category have fared worse than the average in the whole study. Conversely, if O is less than E in some category then the patients in that one category have a relative death rate, O/E, of *less* than unity and have fared better than average.

Logrank P-values: tests for trend

If the life table graphs for different categories of patients look interestingly different, or if any of the differences between the Os and Es in particular categories look substantial, then formal statistical significance tests (logrank P-values) may be calculated to help judge which such differences can plausibly be ascribed to chance alone. Particularly, the P-value derived for the Os and Es calculated for the different categories of randomized treatment will help us decide whether any material treatment differences really exist.

Retrospective stratification: comparing like with like

Often, the patients entered into a trial can be subdivided into 'strata', such that although it would seem natural to compare members of one stratum on treatment A with other patients in that stratum on treatment B, it is not natural to compare patients on treatment A in one stratum with patients on treatment B in another stratum. (For example, in a multicentre trial we might have one stratum per centre, or we might instead split all the patients in the whole trial into a dozen or so strata on the basis of age and/or sex and/or initial disease condition.) The Os in each treatment category may then be compared with 'retrospectively stratified' Es, to yield an analysis for which O differs only randomly from E unless there exist systematic differences between survival on the alternative treatments even when (comparing like with like) patients are compared only with other patients in the *same* stratum as themselves.

Analysis of time to disease recurrence

This can be done equally easily instead of analysis of time to death using the same statistical methods (Kaplan-Meier curves and logrank Os, Es and P-values). However, the curves now describe the esti-mated percentage who are *alive and free of recurrence* (instead of, as before, the percentages alive), and the Os and Es now both relate to numbers of *recurrences plus deaths without recurrence*. (Counts of recurrences alone which do not also include patients who died without recurrence may be misleading if there is any possibility that some of the deaths without recurrence might have been caused by, or prevented by, one or other treatment.)

Since these statistical methods are all described in full in the *British Journal of Cancer* two-part paper, I do not wish to describe them in detail here; that paper is reasonably readable, and I would urge anyone seriously concerned with cancer trials to try it. A computer program (written in standard FORTRAN for easy transplantability from the Oxford computer to computers elsewhere) exists which implements these cancer trial analysis methods in a way which is quick and convenient to use. Copies of this, together with documentation of how to use it and a worked example of its use, are available on request.

Thus far, all I have written has been fairly standard statistical rhetoric; it all needs to be taken seriously, but you would probably get similar advice from most statisticians. If you ignore it, and particularly if you ignore the need for really large numbers of patients, then your trial will probably be among that large majority of the 2000 or so cancer trials around the world (median size ~ 50) which are of little or no scientific value. Further reasons for needing large numbers of patients are discussed in the previously cited paper, and a list of sixteen suggestions (at least one or two of which may be of some use to you) about practical tricks for getting more patients into trials may be found in Peto (1978). Perhaps the most important of these is that to be really large, trials must be really simple, for, whatever they promise when a trial is being planned, in the long run clinicians will not collaborate as wholeheartedly with a complicated trial as with a simple one. It is *not* necessary in most trials to solicit sufficient documentation to convey a clinical picture of each patient to the trial organizer (Peto, 1980), and often all that is necessary is a yes/no answer from an infrequent, simple examination for disease recurrence, together with a count of deaths via the Registrar General's office, which can provide mortality data on all British patients automatically. Much of the documentation in many trials contributes literally nothing to the main aim of comparing the randomly allocated treatments, and its net effect is simply to waste time and to reduce the eventual trial size unnecessarily. The feeling that each patient must be individually understood, and that large trials somehow deny the special peculiarities of each different patient is the exact opposite of the truth. Statisticians recommend large trials precisely *because* they understand how different each patient may be from another superficially similar patient. It is only when comparing two really large groups of patients with each other that the proportions in each group who would have fared well on standard treatment can be relied on to be approximately the same, as can the proportions who would have fared badly.

I would like to conclude this section by a fairly detailed warning against the common practice of reporting: 'Well, overall there's no significant difference, but if we look into one particular sub-group we do find a striking effect.' I think that such 'effects' found only in particular sub-groups are often illusory, but since this proposition is not as generally accepted by statisticians or by doctors as I would wish, I shall argue it at disproportionate length in comparison with the earlier sections. If you are a doctor and some of the statistical points in what follows are not immediately obvious to you, then pretend that this chapter stops here.

Interpretation of apparent interactions

If you are comparing treatment A with treatment B, and A seems somewhat better (e.g. about two standard errors better, which might be suggestive but not conclusive), then whether or not the effect is real, you are more likely than not to find some sub-group of your patients in which there's quite a striking effect. After all, if the standard error (SE) of the treatment difference (in some arbitrary units) in the whole study is x, then the SE of the treatment difference in half the patients (e.g. those with even birthdays) will be $x\sqrt{2}$, the SE of the treatment difference in the remainder (with odd birthdays) will likewise be $x\sqrt{2}$, and the SE of the *interaction* (i.e. the difference between the treatment difference in the evens and the treatment difference in the odds) will be $2x$. If the actual magnitude of the interaction turns out by chance to exceed $2x$ (which will happen with probability $\frac{1}{3}$) then *either* the people with odd birthdays *or* people with even birthdays will have a treatment difference of more than $3x$ ($P<0.05$), while the other people will have a 'strikingly discrepant' treatment difference of less than x.

When we remember that in any trial there are at least a few (and perhaps several) explanatory variables available initially, it is clear that *whether or not* there is any *real* difference between the two treatments, if the *overall* difference is nearly two standard errors then we will usually be able to find one sub-group in which there is apparently a big effect and another sub-group in which there is apparently no effect. (The situation is even worse when there are a dozen or so explanatory variables, as there is a 1 in 10 chance that the interac-

tion will exceed $3.2x$ by chance alone, yielding a $P<0.01$ treatment effect of $3.6x$ in the even birthdates and $0.4x$ in the odd birthdays, or vice versa.) The safest general rule is to be guided in your judgement as to whether or not the treatments really differ chiefly by the *overall* P-value, and if this is not conclusive (e.g. $0.01 <P<0.1$) then even if, you probably will, you do find one sub-group of patients in whom nearly all the treatment benefit seems to be concentrated, then note and report this fact but do not believe it!

It should be clear from the foregoing that tests for interaction have extremely low power. If, despite this, you perform a formal statistical significance test for an interaction, and you get a highly significant (e.g. $P<0.01$) result, indicating, for example, a greater treatment effect in males than in females, then (unless your overall trial result is *very* highly significant) the apparent treatment effect in females will almost certainly be very small, or even in the opposite direction from that in males. If a treatment effect is seen in males but not in females, and if a test for interaction between sex and treatment is clearly significant, this does not imply *or even suggest* that the treatment does not work at all in females, unless there existed some very strong *prior* reason for expecting this.

Misinterpretation of the implications of tests for interaction is widespread even among statisticians, as is misinterpretation of striking but non-significant interactions, and can be made to sound quite wise by saying things like, 'Of course, nowadays we do not just do clinical trials to find out which treatment is better; what modern clinical trials are for is to find out which patients need which treatments.' Before talking sensibly about interactions, it is necessary to distinguish carefully between qualitative and quantitative interactions. A *qualitative* interaction exists when the true answer to the question 'which is better, A or B?' differs in different sub-groups of patient. (The true answer, of course, can only be 'A' or 'B', or 'Neither'; there are only three possibilities.) A quantitative interaction exists when the true answer to the question 'How much difference is there between A and B?' differs in different sub-groups. (The true answer is in units of whatever measure of response is of interest, e.g. per cent survival, per cent recurrence, turnover, shrinkage, etc.). Let us ignore the common 'null hypothesis' case when there is no material difference between the effects of A and B in any sub-group, and consider only those treatment comparisons which are not more or less equivalent in their effects. Now, my prior hypotheses in interpreting any such data would be as follows.

I am almost certain *a priori* that a *quantitative* interaction will exist between treatment and any categorization of the patients which subdivides them into groups with materially different survival expectancy. Thus, if some measure of age, stage, biochemistry or histology does correlate with survival, I would expect the difference between the effects of treatments A and B to be different in different categories of patient. I would continue to imagine this to be true even if none of the optimal statistical tests for interaction yielded significant results, because they are so insensitive to real interactions. Finally, I would not be greately interested to learn that certain interactions were statistically significant, because I knew there were real interactions anyway and so I am not learning anything new.

If someone tells me good *prior* reasons for expecting a qualitative interaction with a certain variable, then I shall consider this suggestion on its scientific merits largely independently of the trial results. Oestrogens may well prolong the survival of prostatic cancer patients without heart disease, but shorten the survival of patients with heart disease. Oophorectomy or certain other hormonal manoeuvres may well be relevant to pre-menopausal but not to post-menopausal breast cancer patients; local radiotherapy might well be useful in certain tumours if the primary operation was limited but not if it was extensive; myocardial infarction patients may well benefit (in terms of limitation of final infarction size) if fibrinolytic treatment or β-blockade is instituted within a few hours of infarction, but not if it is started a few days after infarction when the tissue is already dead, and so on. In all of these cases there is a reasonable expectation, based on established scientific information, of a *qualitative* interaction.

In cases where the scientific reasons are not obvious, or when they were only constructed *post hoc* to explain away an apparent interaction, I have a strong prior hypothesis that although *quantitative* interactions almost certainly do exist, *qualitative* interactions probably do not. All standard statistical tests for interaction are tests for *quantitative* interaction, and significant results in them do not constitute any kind of evidence for the existence of qualitative interactions, unless in addition there were strong prior scientific reasons for anticipating qualitative interactions. For example,

suppose when testing an anti-platelet agent (aspirin) in stroke prevention, we observed an effect of $4x \pm 1.5x$ in males ($P=0.01$) and an effect in the opposite direction of $-x \pm 2x$ in females (interaction $=5x \pm 2.5x$, $P<0.05$). I would chiefly base my inferences about whether aspiring has any merits on the weighted mean overall effect of $1.86x \pm 0.86x$ ($P<0.05$). Moreover, although I would note that the quantitative benefits in males do seem to exceed those in females, I would not believe this strongly until it was supported by other evidence (which it has now been, incidentally). However, I would be most reluctant to accept, as the United States FDA have already done, that aspirin helps males but is of no value whatsoever for females, since this seems *a priori* so unlikely.

In summary, quantitative interactions are *a priori* very plausible but qualitative interactions are not, and when the overall treatment effects are not overwhelming, trials can be expected to generate a number of apparent qualitative interactions even if no interactions at all exist. Consequently, whether or not there exist interactions which are statistically significant, and whether or not qualitative interactions appear to exist, a statistician who on principle does not infer that A is better than B for one category of patient but not for another (but is instead chiefly guided by the overall results of the whole trial) will in the long run make fewer mistakes than one who is more closely guided by the detailed pattern of the data.

References

Peto, R. *et al*. (1976; 1977), Design and analysis of randomized clinical trials requiring prolonged observation of each patient. Part I: Introduction and Design; Part II: Analysis. *Br. J. Cancer*, **34**, 585–612; **35**, 1–39.

Peto, R. (1978), Clinical trial methodology. *Biomedicine*, special issue, **28**, 24–36.

Peto, R. (1980), Monitoring of cancer patients in clinical trials need not be precise. In: *Cancer: Assessment and Monitoring* (eds T. Symington, A.E. Williams and J.G. McVie) Churchill Livingstone, Edinburgh.

Index

Italic page numbers refer to figures and tables